Anatomy of

Domestic Animals

Systemic & Regional Approach

11th edition

Chris Paquini, DVM, MS
Professor of Anatomy
St. George's University

Tom Spurgeon, PhD
Associate Professor of Anatomy
Colorado State University

Susan Pasquini, DVM
Lecturer
St. George's University

Contributors
Mike Smith, MS, PhD
Newel McArthur, DVM, MS, PhD
Joe Morgan, DVM
Jessica Franchini, MS
Diane Aisenberg
Dave Barbee, DVM
Charles Hutchinson, DVM
Charles Peugh, DVM, PhD
Dr. Rodolfo Bruhl-Day, DVM
Lynn Lankes
Lee Klopp
Lisa Shubitz

Illustrations
Chris Pasquini

Cartoons
Chris Pasquini
John Roberts

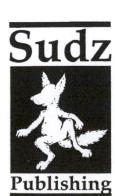

Sudz

Publishing

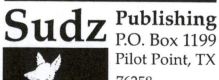

Sudz **Publishing**
P.O. Box 1199
Pilot Point, TX
76258

Phone: (940) 686-9208
Fax: (940) 686-0164
web site: www.sudzpublishing.com
e-mail: sudzpub@mac.com
    sudzpub@hotmail.com

to **Barrett**
my son—who brings
much pride & joy
to my life!

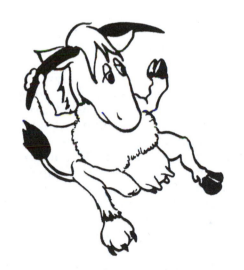

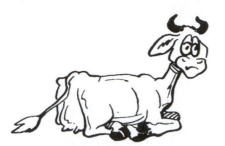

Introduction

Introduction to the 9th & 10th Editions

The 9th edition chiefly corrects some errata discovered by Cathy Schapp, Ph.D., adds a page on quadrants/divisions of the abdomen (page 300) and updates and expands the index.

The 10th edition fine tunes the nerve and arterial pages to make them clear and more complete. Although a few points have been expanded on certain pages, all other pages are the same, keeping page assignments for the 8th, 9th or 10th editions the same.

Our appreciation and gratitude to Dr. Cathy Schapp.

Introduction to First Edition

The Anatomy of the Domestic Animals is to make learning anatomy more pleasant and longer lasting for the student.

The Anatomy of the Domestic Animals is a systems-oriented book, that is a heavily illustrated summary of essential anatomical facts labelled with Arabic numerals, with less important anatomical structures indicated by lower case letters. Capital letters indicate important structures that are emphasized (numbered) on other pages. Such an orientation allows students to fulfill their curiosity without overwhelming them and makes the book helpful to veterinary students as a comparative overview and a good review for surgery classes.

It makes knowledge as easily accessible as possible. Over 700 drawings give ample visual representation to the text; figures are grouped with the supporting text so structural information can be visualized on the same or the facing page.

This book was designed for use in a lab class using prosected dogs, with prosections of the other domestic animals supplementing the dogs. Illustrations of dogs are numerically labeled with the structures named so that important structures are seen without consulting the legend. Following closely are illustrations of the horse and ox, numbered or numbered and named on the drawing. The numbered illustrations allow the students to self test what they have learned from the other species. Illustrations of the other domestic animals (pig, cat, goat, sheep, and llama) are used where species differences are significant.

The accompanying text gives the essentials of each structure in outline form. Expanded introductory paragraphs are used for especially complicated information. Species differences follow in the outline. Clinical applications end each group of structures to put a little "life" into the facts.

Special thanks goes Tom Spurgeon, who edited the book, and whose lectures provided information used in the explanatory paragraphs. Thanks also to Susan Pasquini, who input the information and pasted up the final product. And thanks to Robin Pederson, Michelle Stout, Sheri "llama" Amsel, and Barrett Pasquini for contributing illustrations. I would like to also thank Dr. Jerry Newbrey, Tom McCracken, John Daugherty, Dr. Ray Whalen, Dennis Giddings, Dr. Robert Kainer, Dr. Stephen Roper, Rita Bice, Mike Smith, Bobby Biondini, Joe Waters, Corky Johnston, Dr. Keith Banks, and Dr. Butch "bucks" Kettel for their support and encouragement.

Illustrations were used from *The Atlas of Equine Anatomy* and *The Atlas of Bovine Anatomy*. Supplemental illustrations were done from dissections. *N.A.V.*, 1983 was followed, with an attempt to anglisize the names where it wouldn't add confusion.

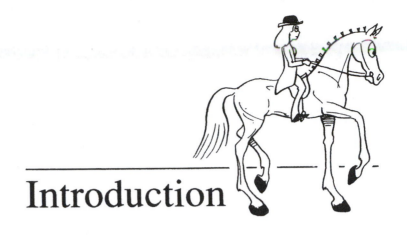

Introduction

Introduction to Fifth Edition

The last two and a half years of teaching Canine Anatomy, Comparative Anatomy, and Applied Anatomy at Ross University have stimulated this fifth edition. *The Anatomy of Domestic Animals* was originally made for an undergraduate veterinary anatomy class. Interest in it by Veterinary students has stimulated additional editions. The goal was to add information for the Veterinary student and still make it manageable for the undergraduate and veterinary technicians. This is still the goal for this edition. This book is still for the undergraduate and the future practising veterinarian, not for future PhDs in anatomy. Added Applied and Clinical Anatomy have been placed in shaded boxes to increase interest in anatomy. The Appendix has been increased with applied anatomy topics that have been difficult for many students here to learn - Nerve Blocks in the horse, Neuroanatomy, and Abdominal Exploration of the ox. These are probably to advanced for the undergraduate, but may stimulate their interest. The radiology section in the appendix should help both the veterinary student and the undergraduate.

Susan Pasquini has since the first edition been responsible for getting this book put together. She has typed, edited and pasted up the pages. While taking Canine and Comparative anatomy at Ross University (soon to be a DVM) she has edited and suggested things for this edition. With out her this and all previous editions would not have been possible.

Mike Smith, from Colorado State University, came down to the Caribbean to take over may class and edited the text while I worked on this edition. Many anatomy discussions were held overlooking the Caribbean sipping a "cold one".

Dr. Charles Hutchison, the Head and other half of the Anatomy Department, through his encyclopedic knowledge and great lectures was a constant stimulus to me and my text. The Neuroanatomy in the appendix evolved from taking notes of his lectures and then editing them from other sources. Dr. Hutchison then edited the final draft.

The radiology section was started by taking notes of Dr. Charles Peugh's lectures when he was here. This was used In DR. Bruhl-Day's radiology class and in Canine Anatomy and modified over the semesters. Dr. Barbee from Washington State edited and changed it to come up with the final product.

Lynn Lankes a second semester student at Ross edited the text as she learned anatomy, and was invaluable.

Dr. Rudolfo Bruhl-Day and Dr. Sandra Mattoni are in the process of translating this book into Spanish.

I would also like to thank all the anatomist who did the work in anatomy and wrote texts on the subject. Their work and my teaching veterinary students have resulted in this text that hhopes to simplify, not define anatomy.

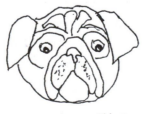

Abbey

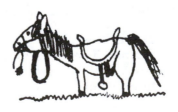

Gina

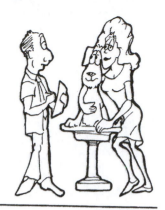

Note to the Student

Illustrations

Illustrations are on the same page as the related text or on the facing page..

Labels

1,2,3 or I,I,II - Arabic numerals or Roman numerals preceding structures in the text refer to numbers in the illustrations on the same or facing pages. These are structures to be learned. Arabic numerals, followed by structure names on the illustrations (usually the dog) allow identification without consulting the text. These are followed closely by illustrations (usually the horse or ox) that have numbers only, allowing you to test yourself.

A,B,C - Capital letter labels of the illustrations are important structures learned on another page (where they usually were Arabic numerals).

a,b,c - Small letter labels in the illustrations are less important structures not needed to be learned by the undergraduate student. In some illustrations, they are important structures (to be learned on another page) that help orient the drawing.

Phonetic (FOH-net-ik) spelling

Phonetic spellings follow commonly mispronounced words.

Etymology

The etymology appears in brackets following some terms. The term's language, root word and its meaning are given. The language is indicated by abreviations (e.g. L. = Latin, G. = Greek, Fr. = French).

Text organization

The text is organized into general information, species differences, and clinical information. The general information comes first and is true for all the species considered. Species differences follow, and then clinical applications to help give "life" to the facts.

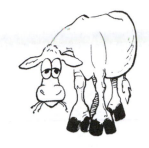

Note to the Student

Regional headings _____

Thoracic limb-88

Thoracic limb-**536**

117-Thoracic limb-143

Regional headings are located in the upper right hand corner of each page, followed by the next page which to turn. In most cases, the next page is the following one, indicated by a normally printed page number (e.g., Thoracic limb-88). When the next page is somewhere else in the text, the page number is bold print (e.g., Thoracic limb-**536**). When a page follows another part of the text, the regional heading is preceded by this page number in bold type (e.g., **117**-Thoracic limb-143).

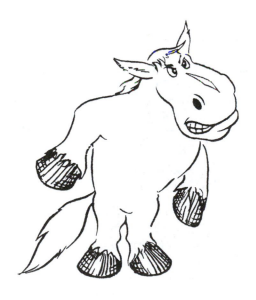

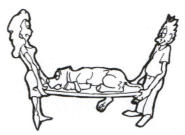

Table of Contents
Systemic

Table of Contents - Systemic

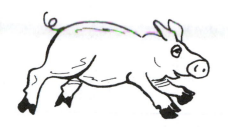

Table of Contents
Regional

Table of Contents - Regional

SELECTED REFERENCES

DeLahunta, A. *Veterinary Neuroanatomy and Clinical Neurology*, 2nd edition, W. B. Saunders Co., Philadelphia, PA, 1983.

Dyce, KM, CJG Wensing. *Essentials of Bovine Anatomy*. Lee & Febiger, Philadelphia, PA, 1971.

Dyce, KM, WO Sack, CJG Wensing. *Textbook of Veterinary Anatomy*. W. B. Saunders Co., Philadelphia, PA, 1996.

Getty, R. *Sisson and Grossman's The Anatomy of the Domestic Animals*. W.B. Saunders Co., Philadelphia, PA, 1975.

Goshal, NG, T Koch, P Papesco. *The Venous drainage of the Domestic Animals*. W.B. Saunders Co., Philadelphia, PA, 1981.

Habel, RE, A de Lahunta. *Applied Veterinary Anatomy*, W.B. Saunders Co., Philadelphia, PA, 1986.

Howard, JL. *Current Veterinary Therapy - Food Animal Practice*. W. B. Saunders Co., Philadelphia, PA, 1981.

Koch, T. *Lehrbuch Der Veterinar-Anatomie*, Band III. Jena, Veb Gustav Fisher Verlag, 1970.

Nickel, R, A Schummer, E Seiferle. *Lehrbuch der Anatomie der Haustiere. Band IV*. Verlag Paul Perry, Berlin, 1975.

Nickel, R, A Schummer, E Seiferle. *The Locomotor System of the Domestic Mammals*. Verlag Paul Perry, Berlin, 1986.

Nickel, R, A Schummer, E Seiferle, WO Sack. *The Viscera of the Domestic Mammals*. Springer Verlag, NY, 1973.

Nickel R, A Schummer, E Seiferle. *The Circultory System, the Skin, and the Cutaneous Organs of the Domestic Mammals*. Verlag Paul Perry, Berlin, 1981

Nomina Anatomica Veterinaria. International Committee on Veterinary Anatomical Nomenclature, Vienna, 1983.

Oliver Jr., JE, ZF Hoerlein, IG Mayhew. *Veterinary Neurology*. W. B. Saunders Co., Philadelphia, PA, 1987.

Pasquini, C, S Pasquini, J Hoover. *Tschauner's Guide to Small Animal Clinics*. Sudz Publishing, Pilot Point, Tx. 1995

Pasquini, C, S Pasquini, J Kirpatrick. *Guide to Bovine Clinics*. Sudz Publishing, Pilot Point, Tx. 1995

Pasquini, C, S Pasquini, P Woods. *Guide to Equine Clinics, Vol. 1*. Sudz Publishing, Pilot Point, Tx. 1995

Pasquini, C, H Jann, S Pasquini. *Guide to Equine Clinics, Vol. 2 - Lameness*. Sudz Publishing, Pilot Point, Tx. 1995

Pasquini, C, S Pasquini, R Barr, H Jann, *Guide to Equine Clinics, Vol. 3 - Lameness Diagnosis*. Sudz Publishing, Pilot Point, Tx. 1995

Popesko, P. *Atlas of the Topographical Anatomy of the Domestic Animals*, W.B. Saunders Co., Philadelphia, PA, 1977.

Sack, WO, RE Habel. *Rooney's Guide to the Dissection of the Horse*. Veterinary Textbooks, Ithaca, NY, 1977.

Schaller, O. *Illustrated Veterinary Anatomical Nomenclature*. Ferdinand Enke Verlag, Stuttgart, 1992.

Schummer, A, H Wilkens, Vollmer, B Haus, KH Habermehl, *Anatomy of Domestic Animals. Vol. 3, The Circulatory System, the Skin, and the Cutaneous Organs of the Domestic Mammals*. Springer Verlag, NY, 1981.

Seiferle, E. *Anatomy of Domestic Animals. The Nervous System, the Endocrine Glands, and the Sensory Organs of the Domestic Mammals*. Verlag Paul Perry, Berlin, 1984.

Shively, MJ. *Veterinary Anatomy*. Texas A&M University Press, College Station, TX, 1984.

Sisson, S, JD Grossman. *The Anatomy of the Domestic Animals*. 4th ed. Philadelphia PA, W.B. Saunders Co., Philadelphia, PA, 1967.

Stashak, TS. *Adam's Lameness in Horses*. Lea & Febiger, Philadelphia, PA, 1987.

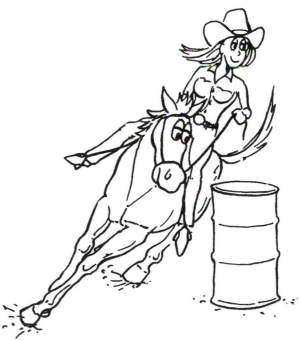

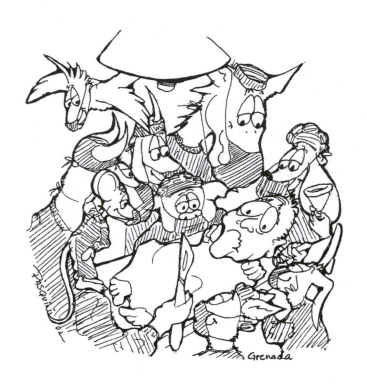

Chapter I
Descriptive Terms

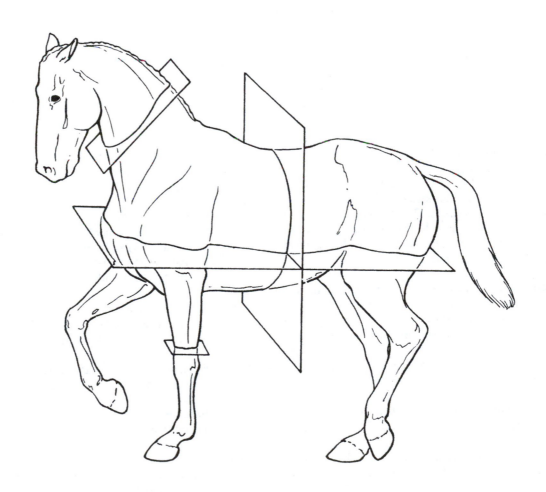

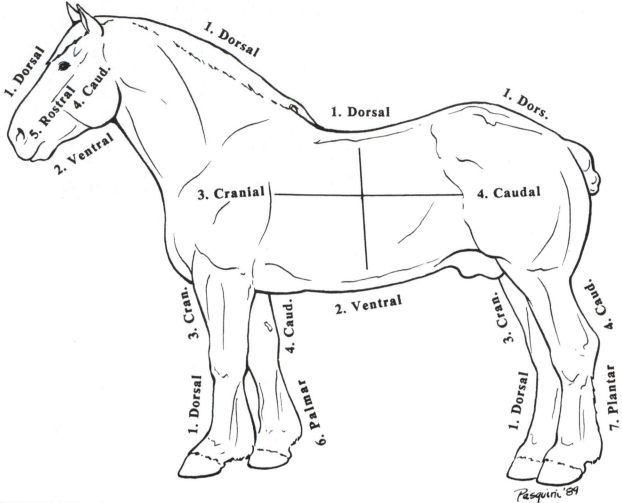

Pasquini '89

DESCRIPTIVE TERMS: precise descriptive terms are used to describe the position of structures and relationships between structures in quadrupeds (four-footed animals). For such terms to have meaning, the quadruped must be in the anatomical position, standing on its four limbs. The anatomical position for humans is standing with the arms at the side and the palms pointing forward. Some human terminology is acceptable for use in certain structures of the animal head.

1. Dorsal (dors.): away from the ground. Also, the surfaces below the proximal (see below) ends of the carpus (wrist in humans) and tarsus (ankle in humans) opposite the palmar and plantar surfaces (see below). (The vertebrae are dorsal to the heart).

2. Ventral (ventr.): toward the ground (The tongue is ventral to the nasal cavity).

3. Cranial (cran.): towards the head. (The neck is cranial to the tail.) Anterior is substituted for cranial in the eye.

4. Caudal (caud.) (L. *cauda*, tail): towards the tail. (The hindlimb is caudal to the forelimb.) Posterior is substituted for caudal in the eye.

5. Rostral (rostr.) (L. *rostrum*, beak): a part on the head closer to

the nose (corresponds to cranial for the rest of the body). (The nose is rostral to the ears). A part behind another part on the head is called **caudal** as in the rest of the body.

6. Palmar (palm.): the surface below the proximal ends of the carpus directed caudally or towards the ground, thus replacing caudal for this part of the limb. (The dew claw of the ox is on the palmar surface of the forelimb). The opposite, cranially facing side is the **dorsal** side.

7. Plantar (plant.): the surface below the proximal end of the tarsus directed caudally or toward the ground. As in the forelimb, the opposite side is the **dorsal** side.

8. Medial (med.): towards the median plane (pg. 18). (The chest is medial to the thoracic limbs).

9. Lateral (lat.): farther from the median plane. (The shoulder is lateral to the ribs).

10. Proximal (prox.) (L. *proximus*, next): nearest the trunk or point of origin of a limb, vessel, nerve or organ. (The elbow is proximal to the digit).

11. Distal (dist.) (L. *distans*, distant): farther from the trunk or

DESCRIPTIVE TERMS

point of origin of a limb, vessel, nerve or organ. (The carpus is distal to the elbow).

12. Superficial (supf.): nearer the surface. (The biceps brachii muscle is superficial to the humerus).

13. Deep: farther from the surface. (The femur is deep to the thigh muscles).

Peripheral (per-IF-er-al): distant from its point of origin; near the surface of the body. (nerves are peripheral to the central nervous system [brain and spinal cord]).

Axial and abaxial: indicate relative position to the longitudinal axis of the limb. These terms are restricted to the digits where the axis is considered to pass between the third and fourth digits.

• **Axial**: closer to the longitudinal axis. (The inside of a digit is the axial side).

• **Abaxial**: further from the longitudinal axis of a limb. (The outside of a digit is the abaxial side)

External (ext.): closer to the outer surface of a structure. (The capsule is external to the kidney).

Internal (int.): closer to the center of a structure. (The medulla is internal to the cortex).

Supra (L. "above"): a prefix signifying above or over (supraspinatus, supraorbital).

Infra (IN-frah)(L. *infra* beneath): a prefix signifying below or beneath (infraspinatus, infratrochlear).

Human terms:

• Anterior: toward the front. This corresponds to ventral and cranial on the limbs of animals, and rostral in head (Anterior chamber, anterior cruciate).
• Posterior: toward the back. Posterior corresponds to dorsal and caudal aspect of the limbs or animals and to caudal in the head (posterior chamber, caudal cruciate).
• Superior: higher. Sometimes replaces dorsal for head structures (levator labii superioris muscle).
• Inferior: lower. Sometimes replaces ventral for structures of the head (inferior palpebra).

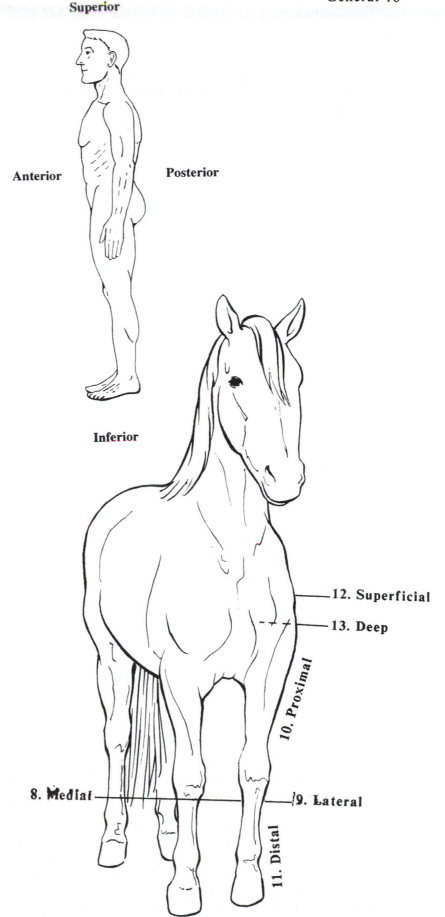

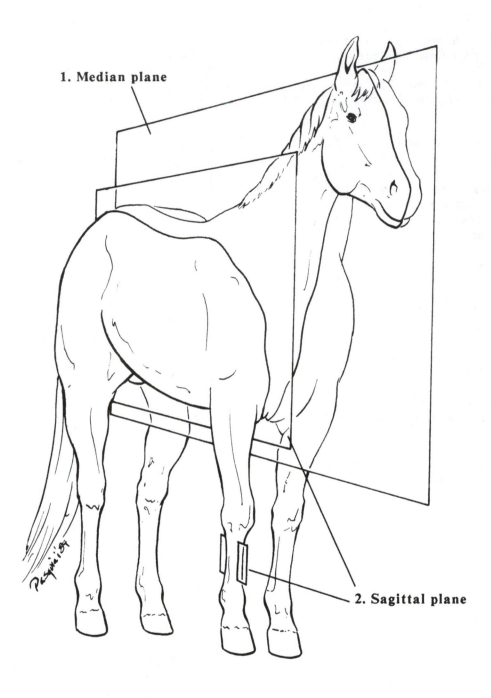

1. Median plane

2. Sagittal plane

PLANES: an imaginary or real surface on which any two points can be connected by a straight line.

1. Median (mid-sagittal) **plane** (on midline): the plane dividing the body into equal right and left portions.

2. Sagittal (paramedian or parasagittal) **plane** (SAJ-i-tal) (off midline): a plane dividing the body into <u>unequal</u> right and left portions. It is parallel to the median plane.

3. Transverse plane: a plane perpendicular to the median plane, dividing the body into cranial and caudal parts. A transverse plane also crosses an organ or limb at a right angle to its long axis.

4. Frontal (dorsal) **plane**: a plane perpendicular to both median and transverse planes, dividing body into dorsal and ventral portions.

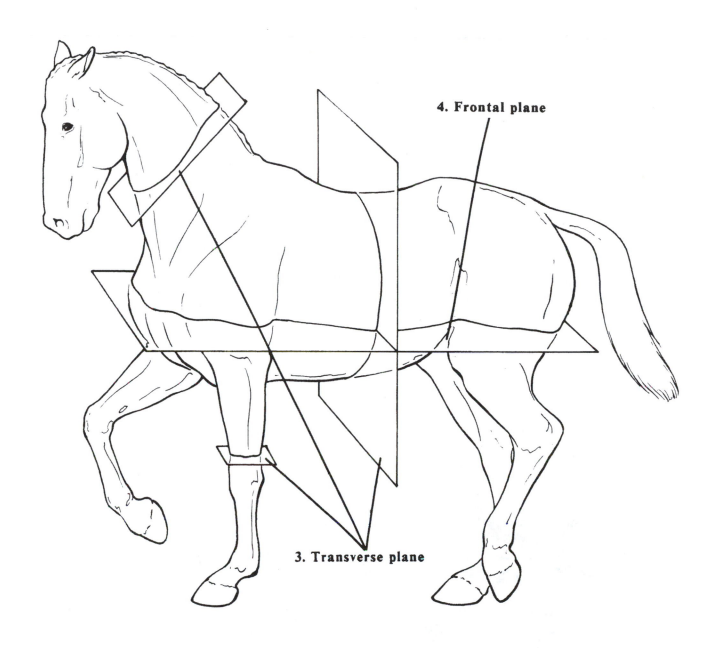

4. Frontal plane

3. Transverse plane

SECTIONS: cuts through various planes of the body to display internal structures. Therefore, sections through these different planes have the same name (e.g., median section is through the median plane).

Longitudinal section (L. *longitudo*, length): a cut parallel to the long axis of an organ or limb. Longitudinal sections may be cut in the median, sagittal or frontal planes.

Transverse section or **cross section**: a cut through the transverse plane of a structure.

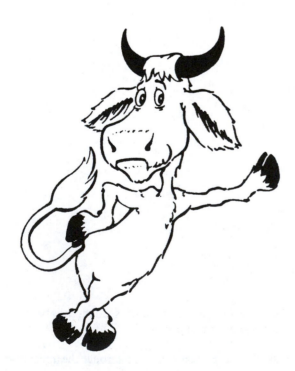

Chapter II
Bones

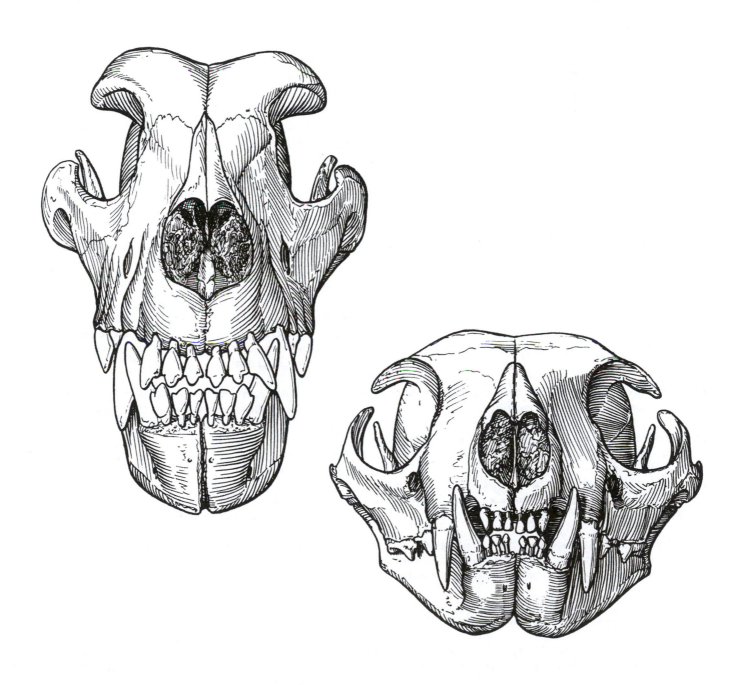

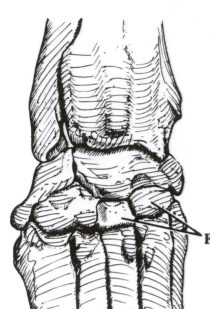

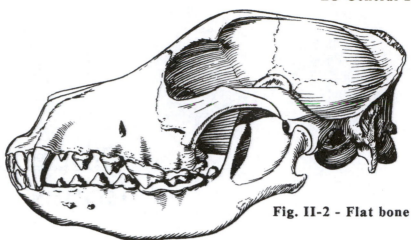

Fig. II-2 - Flat bone

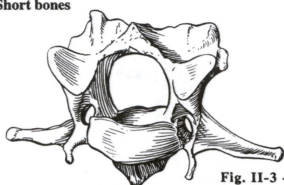

Fig. II-1 - Short bones

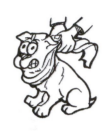

Fig. II-3 - Irregular bone

BONES or **OSSEOUS TISSUE** (G. *osteon* bone): the hard, semi-rigid, calcified connective tissue forming the skeleton. Bones are classified as short, flat, irregular, sesamoid and long bones by their shape.

Osteology (G. *osteon* bone + *logos* study) is the study of bones.

Short bone: a cube-shaped bone (e.g., carpal and small tarsal bones).

Flat bone: two plates of compact bone, separated by cancellous bone (e.g., some bones of skull and ribs).

Irregular bone: a complex and irregularly-shaped bone (e.g., vertebrae and certain facial bones).

Sesamoid (SES-ah-moid) **bone**: a small bone embedded in a tendon; resembling a sesame seed (e.g., patella, proximal and distal sesamoid bones).

Long bone: a bone longer than wide, consisting of a diaphysis (body) and two epiphyses (extremities) with their articular cartilage (e.g., humerus, radius, femur, tibia, metacarpals and metatarsals).

• **1. Diaphysis** (dy-AF-i-sis): the long shaft (body) of a long bone.

• **2. Epiphysis** (e-PIF-i-sis)(pl. = epiphyses [e-PIF-i-seez]): the two enlarged ends (proximal and distal extremities) of a long bone.

• **3. Metaphysis** (me-TAF-i-sis): the joining point of the diaphysis and the epiphysis in a growing bone. This is the part of the epiphyseal cartilage ("physis", growth plate) being replaced by bone.

• **4 Periosteum** (per'ee-OS-tee-um): the fibrous covering around the bone that is not covered by articular cartilage. This layer is necessary for bone growth, repair, nutrition and attachment for ligaments and tendons.

• **5. Articular surface**: the smooth layer of hyaline cartilage covering the epiphysis where one bone forms a joint with another bone.

• **6. Medullary** (MED-yoo-lar'ee) **cavity**: the space in the diaphysis containing the marrow.

• **7. Endosteum** (en-DOS-tee-um): the fibrous and cellular tissue lining the medullary cavity of a bone.

• **8. Apophysis** (Gr. "an offshoot"): any outgrowth of a bone - a process.

• **9. Cortex**: compact bone surrounding the medullary cavity.

• **10. Epiphyseal cartilage, growth plate**: the plate of cartilage between the diaphysis and epiphyses of immature long bones. This is where lengthening of long bones takes place. Synonyms are - epiphyseal plate, physis, metaphyseal plate, growth plate and growth cartilage.

SHAPES OF BONES

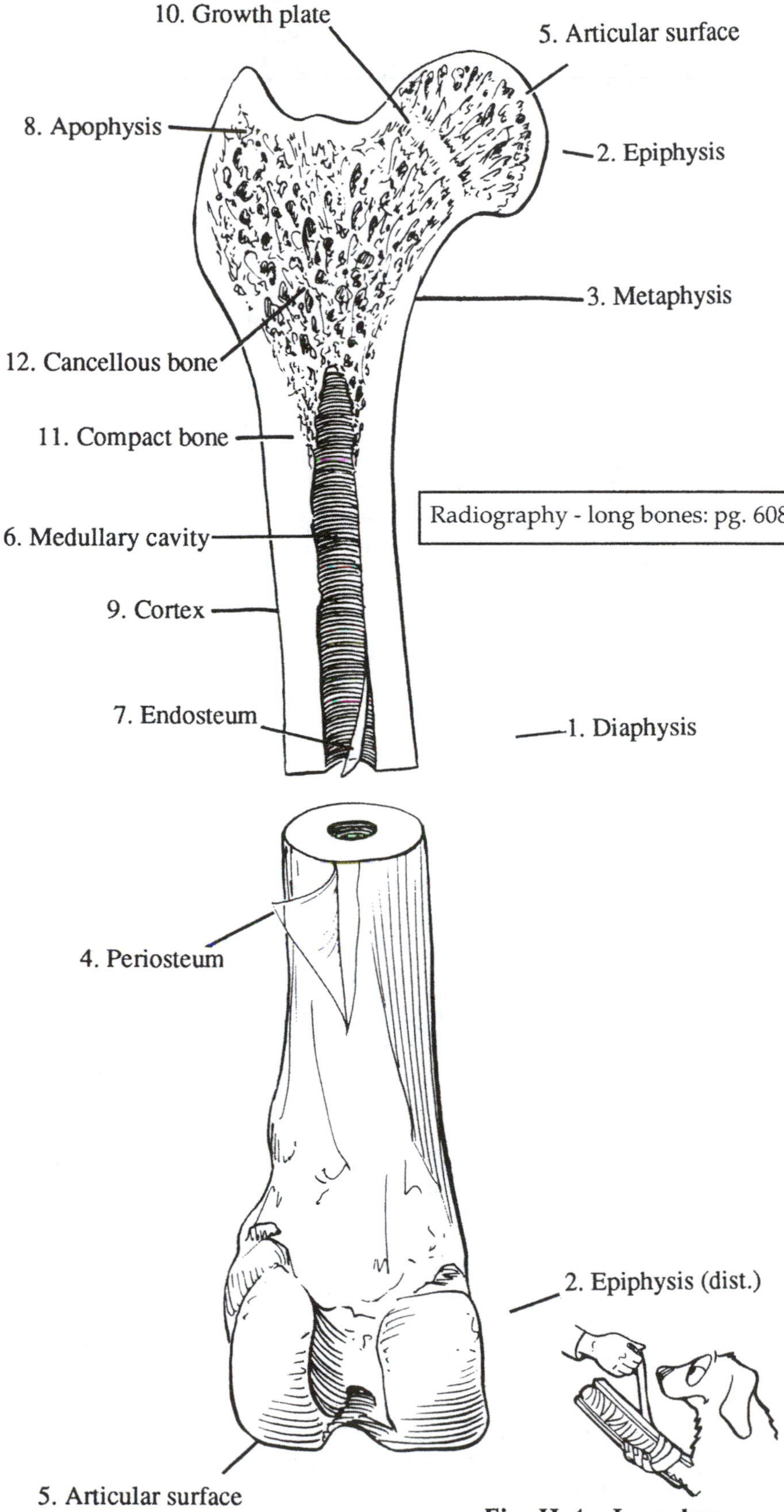

10. Growth plate

5. Articular surface

8. Apophysis

2. Epiphysis

12. Cancellous bone

3. Metaphysis

11. Compact bone

Radiography - long bones: pg. 608

6. Medullary cavity

9. Cortex

7. Endosteum

1. Diaphysis

4. Periosteum

2. Epiphysis (dist.)

5. Articular surface

Fig. II-4 - Long bone

Endochondral ossification: the formation of long bones in the fetus by transforming a cartilaginous model into bone. Bone replacement takes place in three primary ossification centers - the diaphysis and the two epiphyses. This results in a bone capped with articular cartilage and two cartilage discs (growth plates) between the diaphysis and the two epiphyses. Lengthening of bone occurs at the outer side of the growth plate (side next to the epiphysis). Lengthening stops when the growth plates are completely replaced by bone. During growth, radiographically, the epiphyseal cartilage appears as a radiolucent line (dark line) separating the diaphysis from the two epiphyses. The growth in diameter is the result of bone deposited beneath the periosteum (subperiosteal intramembranous ossification).

Intramembranous ossification: forms the flat bones of the head and doesn't use a cartilaginous model.

11. Compact bone: gross term for the part of bone that looks solid.

12. Cancellous bone: gross term for bone with visible spaces in it. It has a trabecular structure of strands of bone separated by spaces and is located at the epiphyseal ends of the marrow cavity.

Woven bone: histological name for immature bone that has been laid down but not organized by secondary remodeling, this can be compact or cancellous bone.

Haversian bone: histological term for adult bone that has been remodeled. This also can be compact or cancellous bone.

CLINICAL

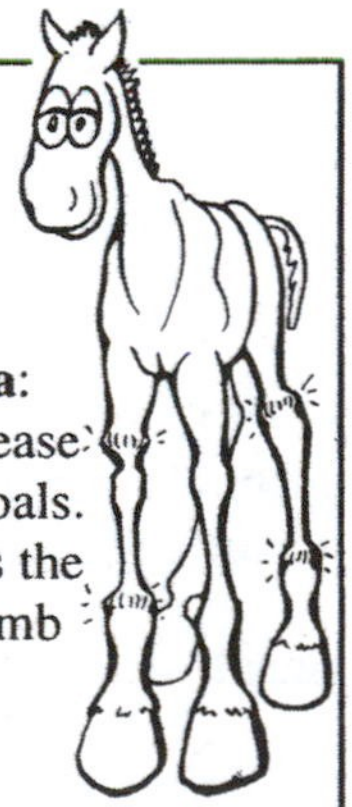

Physis: easily fractured in growing bones.

"Physitis", physeal dysplasia: developmental orthopedic disease common in rapidly growing foals. Swelling of the distal radius is the #1 presenting sign. Angular limb deformities are a sequela to a damaged physis.

Cancellous bone can be harvested surgically and moved to a fracture site to aid in repair. Sources of cancellous bone:
- Tibial tuberosity
- Greater tubercle of the humerus
- Greater trochanter of the femur
- Wing of the ileum

BONE PROCESSES

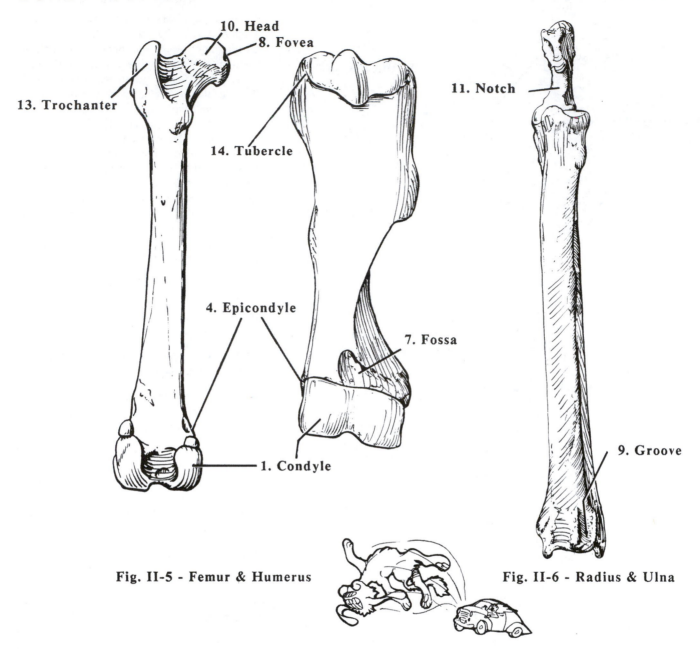

10. Head
8. Fovea
13. Trochanter
14. Tubercle
4. Epicondyle
7. Fossa
1. Condyle
11. Notch
9. Groove

Fig. II-5 - Femur & Humerus

Fig. II-6 - Radius & Ulna

MARKINGS ON BONES: the bumps, holes and depressions on a bone's surface. These markings can be either articular or nonarticular. The following list is in alphabetical order.

Canal: a tunnel through one or more bones (e.g., vertebral canal).

1. Condyle (KON-dyl) (G. knuckle): a large articular prominence (e.g., occipital condyles of the skull and the condyles of the humerus, femur and tibia).

2. Cotyloid (KOT-i-loid) **cavity**: a deep articular depression (e.g., acetabulum of the hip joint).

3. Crest: a prominent border or ridge (e.g., crest of the hipbone).

4. Epicondyle (G. *epi*, upon): a prominence just proximal to a condyle (e.g., lateral epicondyle of the humerus or femur).

5. Facet (F. little faces): a smooth, flat surface (e.g., articular facet of a thoracic vertebra for attachment to a rib). Articular facets are covered with hyaline cartilage.

Fissure (FISH-ur) (Fig. II-33,h): a narrow, cleft-like opening between adjacent bones.

6. Foramen (foh-RAY-men) (L. an aperture): an opening through a bone (e.g., infraorbital foramen, obturator foramen, foramen magnum).

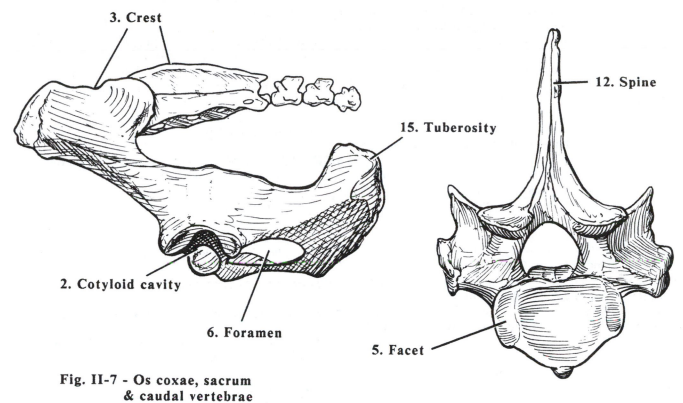

3. Crest

12. Spine

15. Tuberosity

2. Cotyloid cavity

6. Foramen

5. Facet

Fig. II-7 - Os coxae, sacrum
& caudal vertebrae

Fig. II-8 - **Horse** - 7th Cervical vertebra
- caud. view

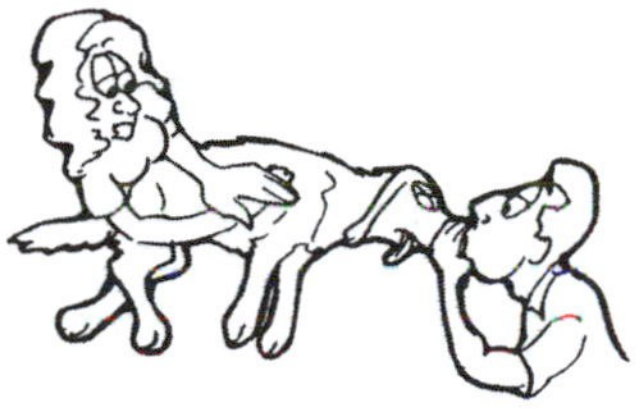

7. Fossa (FOS-a) (L. pit) (pl. fossae): a small hollow (e.g., mandibular fossa, olecranon and radial fossae of the humerus).

8. Fovea (FOH-vee-a) (L. a pit): a shallow, nonarticular depression (e.g., fovea capitis on the head of the femur).

9. Groove (L. *sulcus* furrow): a long, narrow furrow accommodating a vessel, nerve or tendon (e.g., grooves on the distal end of the radius).

10. Head: a rounded articular process (e.g., head of the femur or humerus).

Line (Fig. 11-108,c): a ridge less prominent than a crest.

Meatus (mee-AY-tus) (L. a passage) (pl. meati or meatuses) (Fig. 11-27,7): a tube-like canal through a bone (e.g., external auditory meatus).

11. Notch: a depression at the edge of a bone (e.g., semilunar

notch of the ulna, popliteal notch of the tibia).

15 (1,3,4,5,10,12,13,14). Process: any prominent, roughened projection from a bone (e.g., crest, spine, trochanter, tubercle, tuberosity, etc.).

12. Spine (L. *spina* thorn): a sharp, slender process (e.g., spine of a vertebra, spine of the scapula).

13. Trochanter (troh-KAN-ter): a large, blunt process found only on the femur (e.g., greater trochanter of the femur).

Trochlea (TROHK-lee-a) (pg. 96,#7): a pulley shaped structure (e.g., trochlea of the femur).

14. Tubercle: a small, rounded process (e.g., greater tubercle of the humerus).

15. Tuberosity or **tuber**: a large, usually roughened process (e.g., ischial tuberosity).

THE SKELETON (G. dried): the skeleton is divided into the axial skeleton, the appendicular skeleton and the visceral skeleton. The subdivisions of the axial and appendicular divisions are listed below with the bones that make them up.

AXIAL SKELETON: the bones and cartilages protecting the soft structures of the head, neck and trunk; consisting of the skull, hyoid apparatus, vertebral column and thorax.

1. Skull: the bones of the face and the cranium. These can be furthur subdivided into bones of the cranium and bones of the face.

2. Hyoid apparatus: the bones holding the larynx in place and serving as a major attachment for the tongue.

3, 14. Vertebral column or backbone: the variable number of irregular bones (vertebrae) joined by cartilaginous intervertebral discs. It helps maintain posture and participates in body movements. It houses and protects the spinal cord. The vertebrae are grouped into cervical, thoracic, and lumbar vertebrae, the sacrum (fused sacral vertebrae) (14) and caudal vertebrae. The column forms the central axis of the body and makes up the skeleton of the tail.

4, 5. Thoracic: the **ribs** (4) and **sternum** (5) protecting the thoracic organs.

APPENDICULAR SKELETON: the bones of the limbs and the bones connecting the limbs to the axial skeleton (limb girdles).

6-13. Thoracic limb or **pectoral limb** (PEK-toh-ral)(**"forelimb"**): the scapula, humerus, radius, ulna, carpal bones, metacarpal bones, phalanges and their sesamoid bones.

6. Thoracic girdle or **shoulder girdle**: the two **scapulae** (6) in domestic animals. In man the **clavicle** is included and provides a strut to hold the shoulder laterally. In the domestic animals, which need their limbs under them, it is at best vestigial, with no functional significance. The girdle connects the bones of the arm to the axial skeleton by muscular attachments (syssarcosis), not by a conventional articulation.

7. Arm or **brachium**: the humerus (7).

8, 9. Forearm or **antebrachium**: the **radius** (8) and **ulna** (9).

10-13. Manus: the carpus, metacarpus and digits. In the carnivores, it is also called the forepaw.

10. Carpus: the **carpal bones** (10).

11. Metacarpus: the **metacarpal bones** (11).

12, 13. Digits: the **phalanges** (12) and associated **sesamoid bones** (13).

15-21, 12, 13. Pelvic limb (**"hindlimb"**): the os coxae, femur, patella, tibia, fibula, tarsal bones, metatarsal bones, phalanges and their sesamoid bones.

15. Pelvic girdle: the two hip bones (**ossa coxarum**) (15) attached to each other ventrally and to the **sacrum** (14) dorsally. They connect the pelvic limbs to the axial skeleton. With the sacrum, they form the **bony pelvis** surrounding and protecting the pelvic organs.

16. Thigh: the **femur** (16).

16, 17, 18 & 19. Stifle: the joint between the thigh and crus, along with its menisci and the **patella** (17).

18, 19. Leg or **crus** (L. leg): the **tibia** (18) and **fibula** (19).

20, 21, 12, & 13. Pes (L. foot): the tarsus, metatarsus and digits. It is also called the hindpaw in carnivores.

20. Tarsus or **hock**: the **tarsal bones** (20).

21. Metatarsus: the **metatarsal bones** (21).

12, 13. Digits: the same as the thoracic limb, consisting of the **phalanges** (12) and associated **sesamoid bones** (13).

VISCERAL or **SPLANCHNIC SKELETON**: consists of bones that develop in the viscera or soft structures such as the **os penis** (22) in carnivores and the ossa cordis in the ox and sheep.

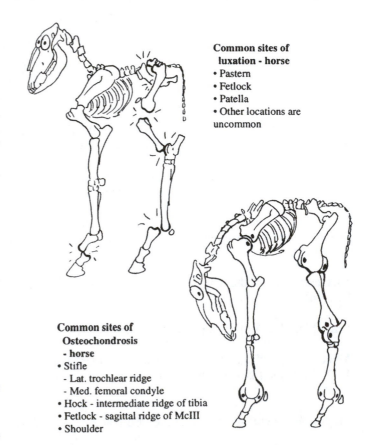

Common sites of
 luxation - horse
• Pastern
• Fetlock
• Patella
• Other locations are
 uncommon

Common sites of
 Osteochondrosis
 - horse
• Stifle
 - Lat. trochlear ridge
 - Med. femoral condyle
• Hock - intermediate ridge of tibia
• Fetlock - sagittal ridge of McIII
• Shoulder

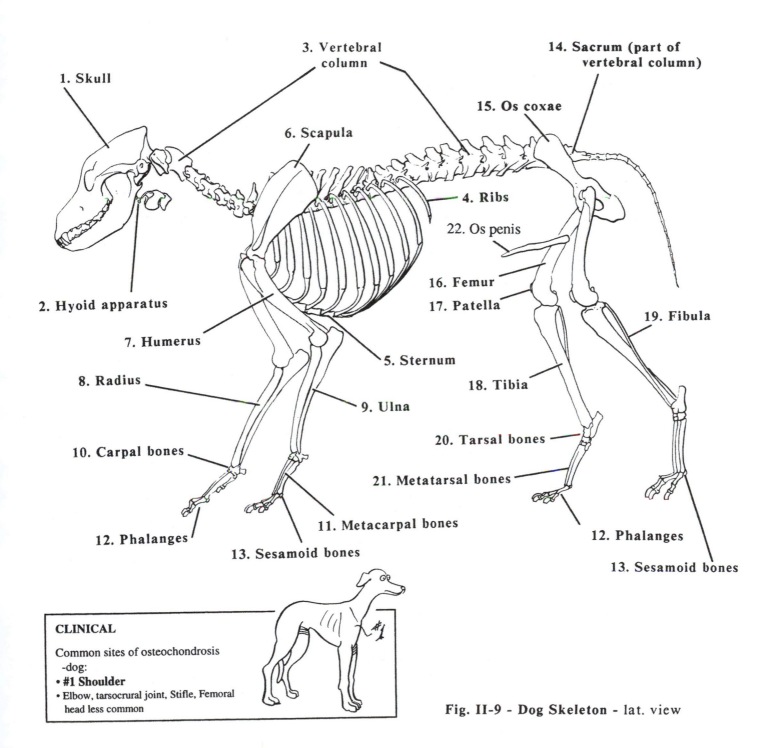

3. Vertebral column

14. Sacrum (part of vertebral column)

1. Skull

15. Os coxae

6. Scapula

4. Ribs

22. Os penis

2. Hyoid apparatus

16. Femur

17. Patella

7. Humerus

19. Fibula

5. Sternum

8. Radius

18. Tibia

9. Ulna

10. Carpal bones

20. Tarsal bones

21. Metatarsal bones

12. Phalanges

11. Metacarpal bones

12. Phalanges

13. Sesamoid bones

13. Sesamoid bones

CLINICAL

Common sites of osteochondrosis
 -dog:
• **#1 Shoulder**
• Elbow, tarsocrural joint, Stifle, Femoral
   head less common

Fig. II-9 - Dog Skeleton - lat. view

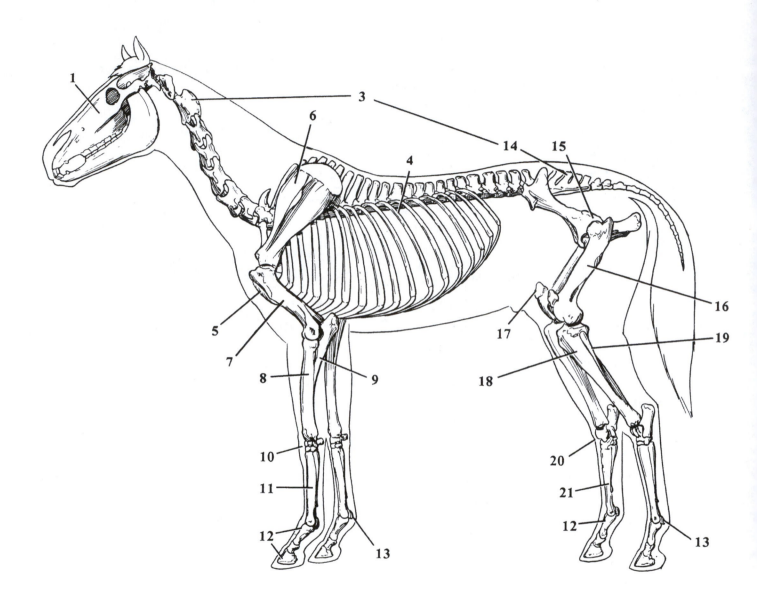

Fig. II-10 - Horse - Skeleton - lat. view

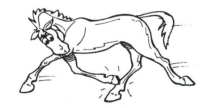

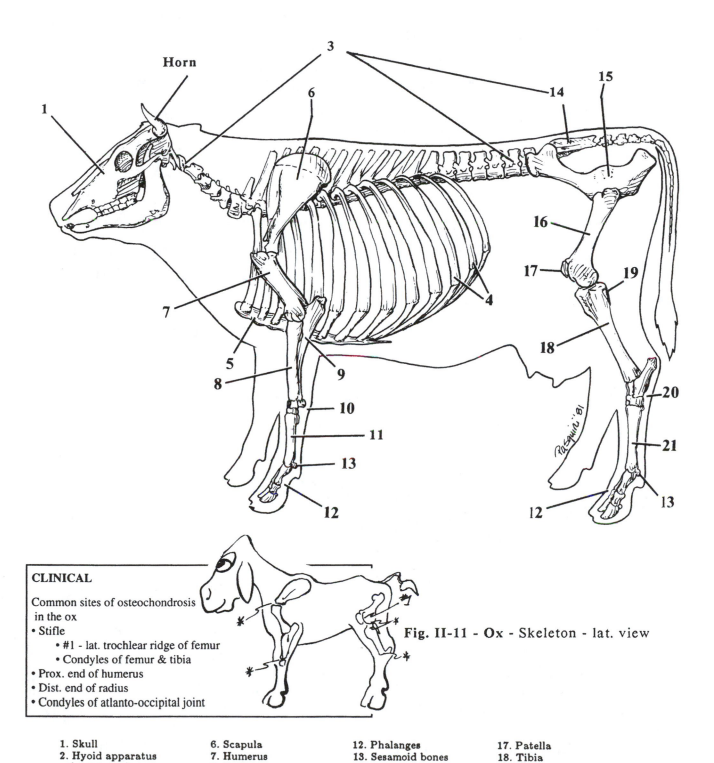

Fig. II-11 - Ox - Skeleton - lat. view

CLINICAL

Common sites of osteochondrosis
  in the ox
• Stifle
  • #1 - lat. trochlear ridge of femur
  • Condyles of femur & tibia
• Prox. end of humerus
• Dist. end of radius
• Condyles of atlanto-occipital joint

1. Skull
2. Hyoid apparatus
   (not shown)
3. Vertebral column
4. Ribs
5. Sternum

6. Scapula
7. Humerus
8. Radius
9. Ulna
10. Carpal bones
11. Metacarpal bones

12. Phalanges
13. Sesamoid bones
14. Sacrum (part of
    vertebral column)
15. Os coxae
16. Femur

17. Patella
18. Tibia
19. Fibula
20. Tarsal bones
21. Metatarsal bones

29

PIG & CAT - SKELETON

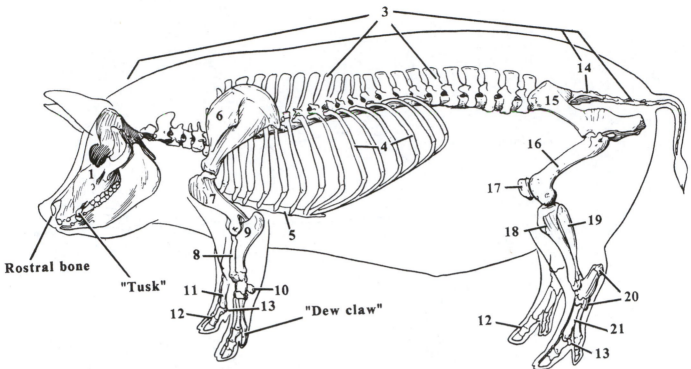

Rostral bone

"Tusk"

"Dew claw"

Fig. II-12 - Pig - Skeleton - lat. view

Fig. II-13 - Cat - Skeleton - lat. view

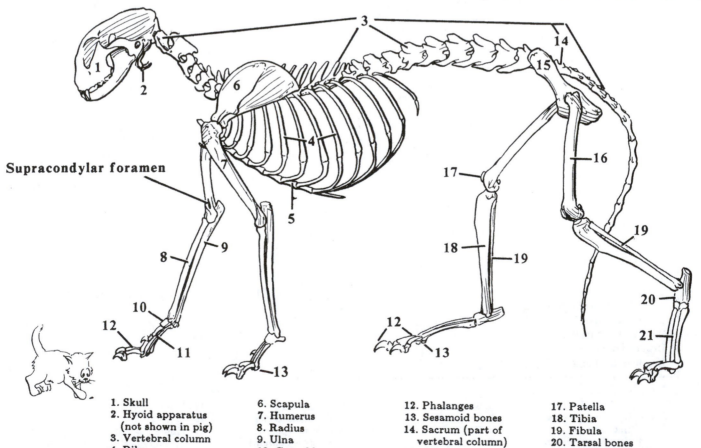

Supracondylar foramen

1. Skull	6. Scapula	12. Phalanges	17. Patella
2. Hyoid apparatus	7. Humerus	13. Sesamoid bones	18. Tibia
(not shown in pig)	8. Radius	14. Sacrum (part of	19. Fibula
3. Vertebral column	9. Ulna	vertebral column)	20. Tarsal bones
4. Ribs	10. Carpal bones	15. Os coxae	21. Metatarsal bones
5. Sternum	11. Metacarpal bones	16. Femur	

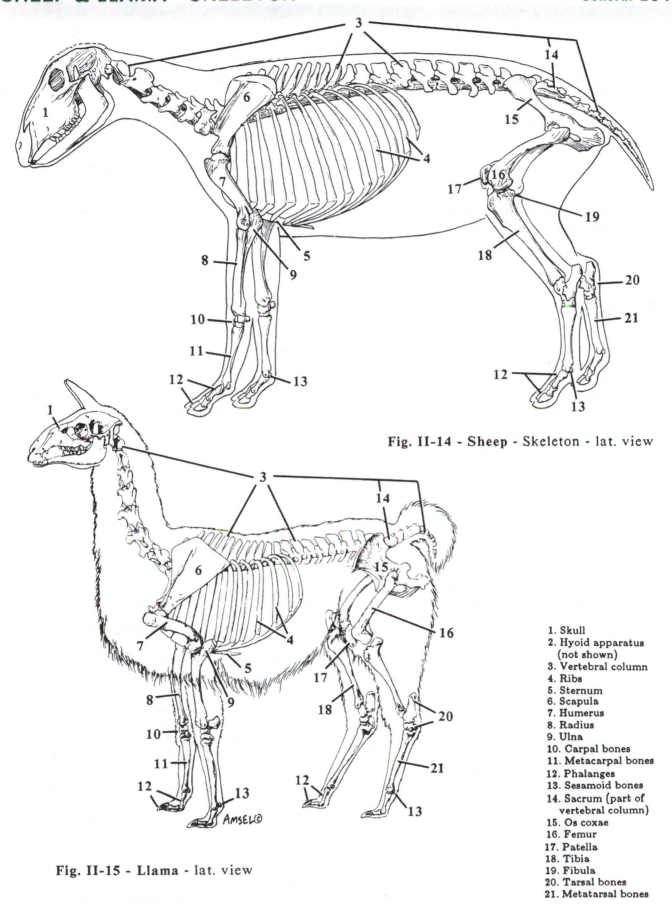

Fig. II-14 - Sheep - Skeleton - lat. view

Fig. II-15 - Llama - lat. view

1. Skull
2. Hyoid apparatus
   (not shown)
3. Vertebral column
4. Ribs
5. Sternum
6. Scapula
7. Humerus
8. Radius
9. Ulna
10. Carpal bones
11. Metacarpal bones
12. Phalanges
13. Sesamoid bones
14. Sacrum (part of
    vertebral column)
15. Os coxae
16. Femur
17. Patella
18. Tibia
19. Fibula
20. Tarsal bones
21. Metatarsal bones

SKULL BONES

CRANIUM (KRAY-nee-um): the bones surrounding the brain, forming the cranial cavity.

Roof of the cranium: the paired **frontal** and **parietal** bones in most domestic species.

Occipital region: the caudal aspect of the skull formed by the **occipital bone**.

Temporal region: the lateral walls of the cranium formed by the **temporal bones**.

The floor of the cranium: the ventral aspect of the cranium formed primarily by the unpaired **sphenoid bone**.

The rostral wall of the cranium: the rostral aspect of the cranium formed by the unpaired ethmoid bone.

1. **Occipital** (ok-sip-i-tal) **bone**: the caudal aspect of both the cranial cavity and the skull as a whole.

2. **Temporal bone**: the caudolateral wall of the cranial cavity.

3. **Parietal** (pa-RY-i-tal) **bone** (L. *paries* wall): together with the frontal bone forms the roof of the cranial cavity in all domestic animals, except the ox and pig.

4. **Frontal bone** (L. *frons* forehead): the rostral part of the roof of the cranial cavity in most domestic species. In the ox and pig, it forms the entire roof.

5. **Ethmoid bone**: the unpaired bone forming the rostral wall of the cranial cavity.

6. **Sphenoid** (SFEE-noyd) **bone** (G. *sphen* wedge): the unpaired bone forming the floor of the cranial cavity.

FACIAL PART OF THE SKULL: the part enclosing the nasal and oral cavities. Among the species, this part can show variations in length (e.g., horse vs. cat). The dog shows great variation within the species whereas, it is fairly uniform in the other domestic species. The facial region is divided into oral, nasal and orbital regions.

Oral region: the **incisive, maxillary**, and **palatine bones** and the **mandible** surrounding the oral cavity.

Nasal region: the **nasal, maxillary, palatine**, and **incisive bones** surrounding the nasal cavity.

Orbital region: the bony socket holding the eye, formed by portions of the **frontal, lacrimal, palatine, sphenoid**, and **zygomatic bones**.

7. **Nasal bones**: along with the cranial part of the frontal bone form the osseous roof of the nasal cavity.

8. **Maxillary bone** (MAK-sil-ler'-ee) or **maxilla**: the lateral part of the face and the part of the hard palate holding the upper cheek teeth.

9. **Incisive bone**: the rostral bone holding the upper incisors (front teeth).

10. **Palatine** (PAL-a-tyn) **bone**: forms the hard palate, along with the maxillary and incisive bones.

11. **Zygomatic bone** or malar bone (L. *mala* cheeks): the cranial part of the zygomatic arch.

12. **Lacrimal** (LAK-ri-mal) **bone** (*lacrima* tear): the medial surface of the orbit.

13. **Ventral nasal concha** (KONG-kah): a scroll of bone located in the nasal cavity.

14. **Pterygoid** (TER-i-goid) **bones**: the small, paired bones in the caudal part of the nasopharynx.

15. **Vomer** (plowshare): the unpaired bone forming part of the osseous nasal septum.

16. **Mandible** (L. *mandere* to masticate): the large bone articulating with the skull that supports all the lower teeth.

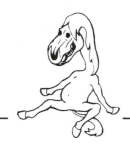

SPECIES DIFFERENCES

Interparietal bone (Fig. II-20,a): the bone found only in the **horse** and **cat**, between the two parietal bones, rostral to the occipital bone. In other species, it is present in the fetus but then fuses with surrounding bones before birth.

Frontal bone: forms the entire roof of the cranium in the ox and pig.

Rostral bone: unique bone found in the nose of the pig.

Dog: there are three types of skulls in dogs relative to the proportions of the facial bones and the cranial vault.

• **Mesaticephalic**: the average conformation (i.e., beagle)

• **Dolichephalic** (dal-i-hoh-se-FAL-ik): has a larger facial component (i.e., collie)

• **Brachiocephalic**: has a shorter facial component (i.e., Boston Terrier).

SKULL BONES - DOG

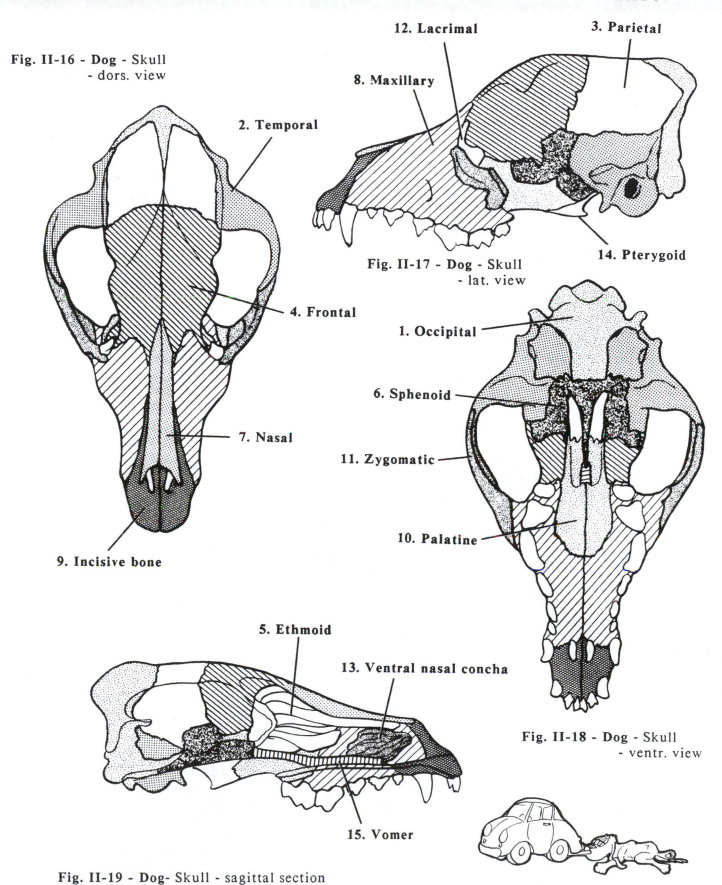

Fig. II-16 - Dog - Skull - dors. view

12. Lacrimal

3. Parietal

8. Maxillary

2. Temporal

Fig. II-17 - Dog - Skull - lat. view

14. Pterygoid

4. Frontal

1. Occipital

6. Sphenoid

7. Nasal

11. Zygomatic

10. Palatine

9. Incisive bone

5. Ethmoid

13. Ventral nasal concha

Fig. II-18 - Dog - Skull - ventr. view

15. Vomer

Fig. II-19 - Dog- Skull - sagittal section

Fig. II-20 - **Horse** - Skull
- dors. view

Fig. II-21 - **Horse** - Skull - ventr. view

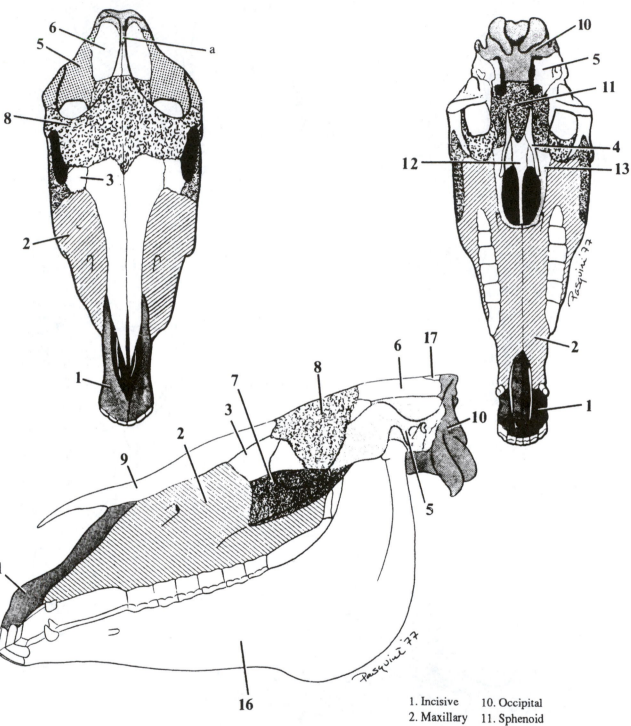

Fig. II-22 - **Horse** - Skull - lat. view

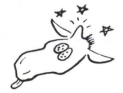

1. Incisive	10. Occipital
2. Maxillary	11. Sphenoid
3. Lacrimal	12. Vomer
4. Pterygoid	13. Palatine
5. Temporal	14. Ethmoid (not shown - horse)
6. Parietal	15. Ventr. nasal concha
7. Zygomatic	16. Mandible
8. Frontal	17. Interparietal (separate only in
9. Nasal	horse & cat)

SKULL BONES - OX

Fig. II-23 - Ox - Skull - lat. view

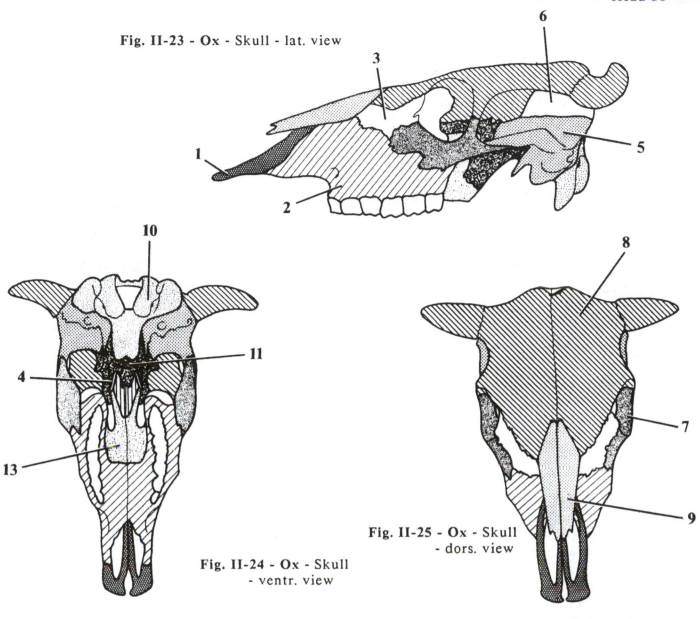

Fig. II-24 - Ox - Skull - ventr. view

Fig. II-25 - Ox - Skull - dors. view

Fig. II-26 - Ox - Skull - sagittal section

SPECIES DIFFERENCES

Frontal bone: forms the entire roof of the cranium in the ox and pig

SKULL - LATERAL VIEW

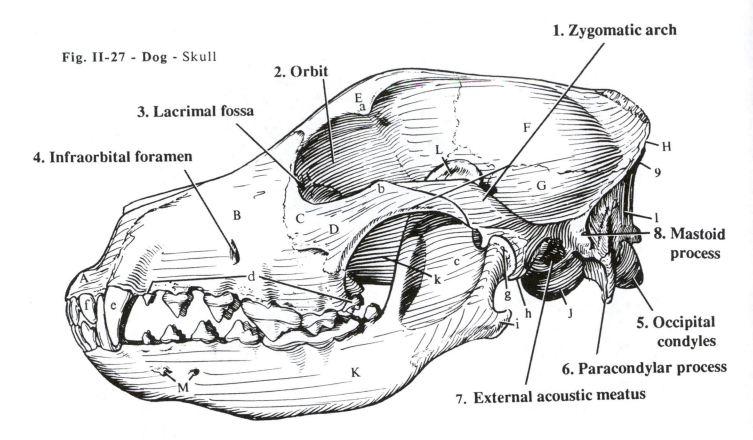

Fig. II-27 - Dog - Skull

1. Zygomatic arch

2. Orbit

3. Lacrimal fossa

4. Infraorbital foramen

8. Mastoid process

5. Occipital condyles

6. Paracondylar process

7. External acoustic meatus

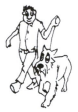

A. Incisive bone	H. Nuchal crest (not shown in ox)	a. Zygomatic process	h. Retroarticular process
B. Maxillary bone	I. Occipital bone	b. Frontal process	i. Angular process (carnivores)
C. Lacrimal bone	J. Tympanic bulla	c. Ramus of mandible	j. Angle of mandible (horse & ox)
D. Zygomatic bone	K. Mandible	d. Cheek teeth	k. Pterygopalatine fossa
E. Frontal bone	L. Coronoid process	e. Canine tooth	
F. Parietal bone	M. Mental foramen	f. Incisor tooth	
G. Temporal bone		g. Articular process	

1. Zygomatic arch: the bony arch forming the lateral wall of the orbit. It consists of the zygomatic bone and the zygomatic processes of the temporal bone.

2. Orbit (F. circle): the bony socket holding the eye.

3. Lacrimal fossa: the depression in the medial margins of the orbit. It collects tears and sends them through the lacrimal canal which opens into the nasal cavity.

4. Infraorbital foramen: the rostral opening of the infraorbital canal, located in the maxillary bone.

5. Occipital condyles: the paired structures lateral to the foramen magnum that articulate with the first cervical vertebra (atlas).

6. Paracondylar (jugular) process: the ventral projection near the occipital condyles.

7. External acoustic meatus: the large opening caudal to the zygomatic arch where the external ear attaches. In life it is covered by the ear drum (tympanic membrane) which separates the external and middle ear.

8. Mastoid process: located caudal to the external acoustic meatus. It is an attachment site for muscles.

9 External occipital protuberance: the caudal process of the occipital bone.

SPECIES DIFFERENCES

Bony orbit: complete in the horse and ruminants, is incomplete in the carnivores but is completed by the orbital ligament.

Facial crest: in horses, the ridge on the lateral surface of the face

Facial tuberosity: in ruminants, the process on the lateral surface of the face.

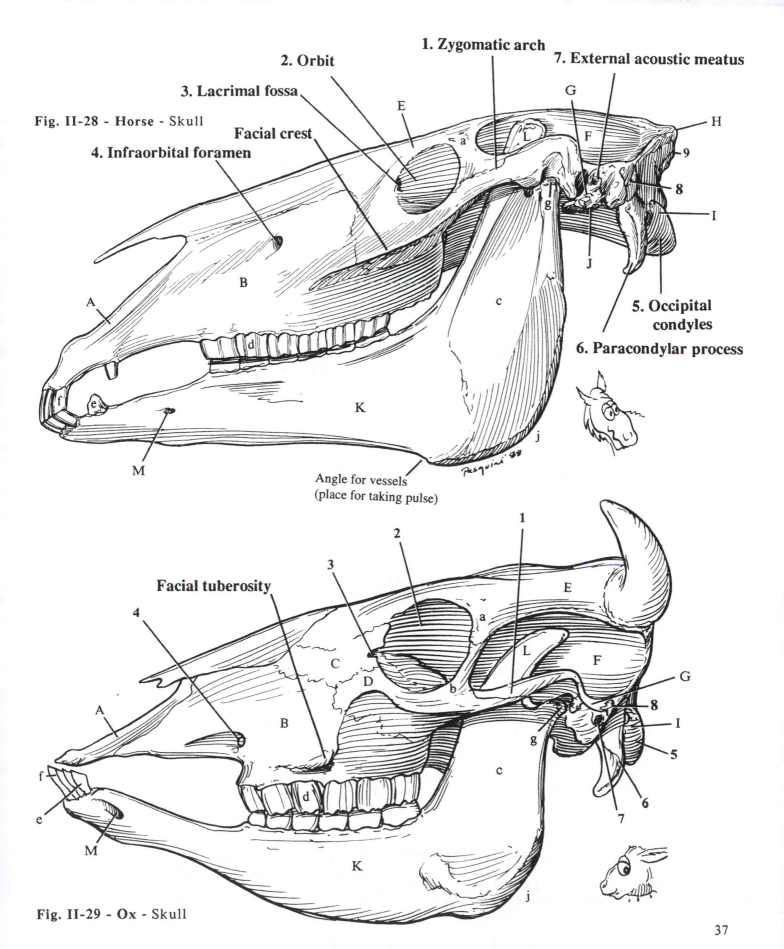

1. Zygomatic arch
2. Orbit
3. Lacrimal fossa
4. Infraorbital foramen

Facial crest

7. External acoustic meatus

Fig. II-28 – Horse - Skull

5. Occipital condyles

6. Paracondylar process

Angle for vessels
(place for taking pulse)

Facial tuberosity

Fig. II-29 – Ox - Skull

1. Nuchal crest

Fig. II-30 - Dog - Skull

b

2. Temporal fossa

B

i

D

a

A

f

C

h

E

g

F

G

3. Nasal aperture

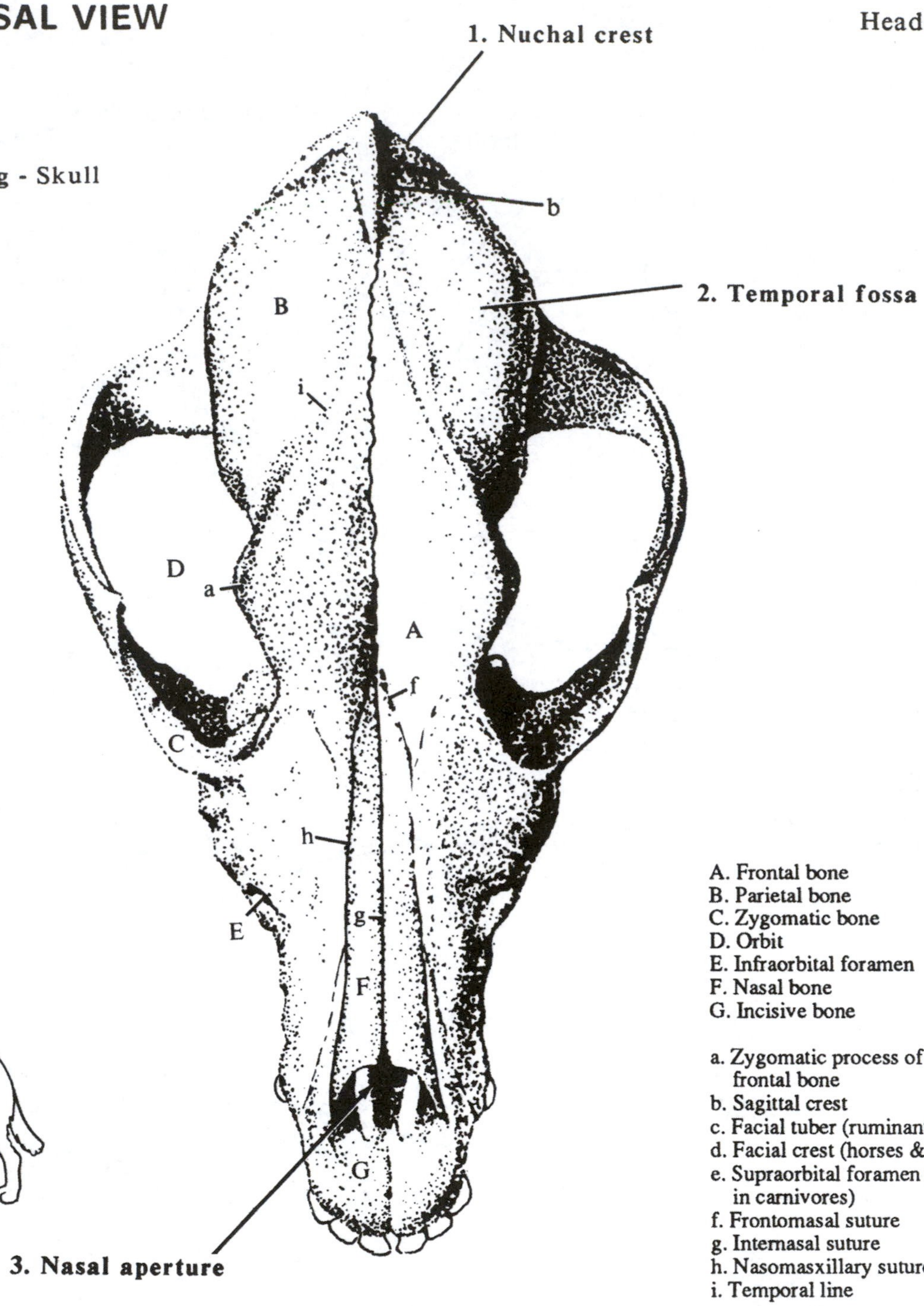

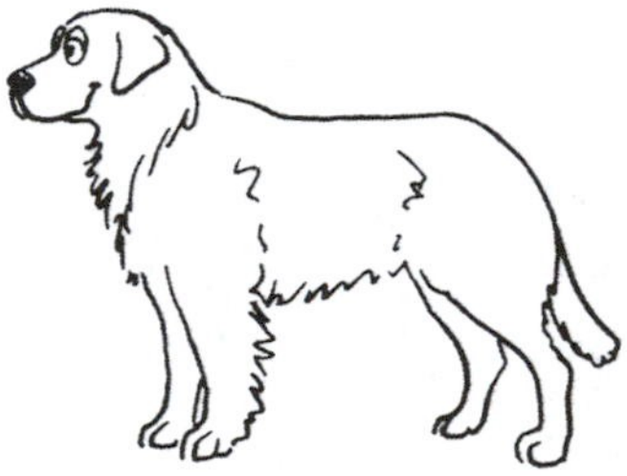

A. Frontal bone
B. Parietal bone
C. Zygomatic bone
D. Orbit
E. Infraorbital foramen
F. Nasal bone
G. Incisive bone

a. Zygomatic process of
   frontal bone
b. Sagittal crest
c. Facial tuber (ruminants)
d. Facial crest (horses & pig)
e. Supraorbital foramen (absent
   in carnivores)
f. Frontomasal suture
g. Internasal suture
h. Nasomasxillary suture
i. Temporal line

Skull radiographs: pg. 606

DORSAL SURFACE OF THE SKULL

1. Nuchal crest (NOO-kal): the transverse ridge at the transition from the dorsal to the caudal (nuchal) surfaces of the skull.

2. Temporal fossa: the depression formed by the temporal and parietal bones.

3. Nasal aperture: the rostral bony opening into the nasal cavity.

4. Median sagittal crest: extends rostrally from the external occipital protuberance on the midline (absent ruminants).

SPECIES DIFFERENCES

6. Cornual process: the process of the frontal bone of horned **ruminants** that is enclosed by the horn.

Temporal fossa (2): in **ruminants** has been pushed to the lateral side of the skull by the frontal bone.

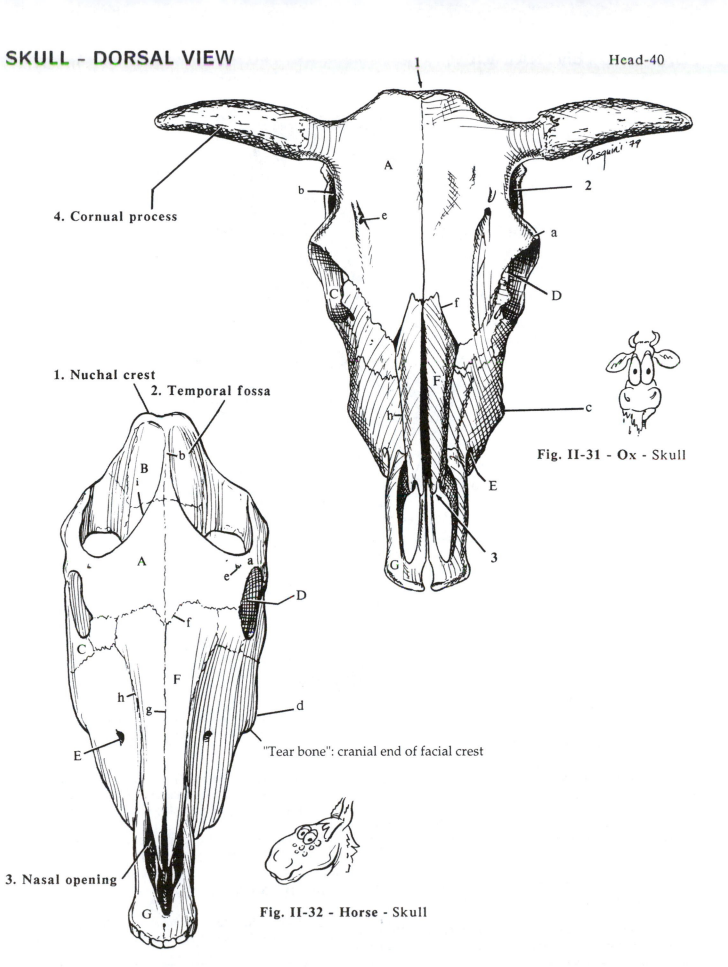

4. Cornual process

1. Nuchal crest

2. Temporal fossa

Fig. II-31 - Ox - Skull

"Tear bone": cranial end of facial crest

3. Nasal opening

Fig. II-32 - Horse - Skull

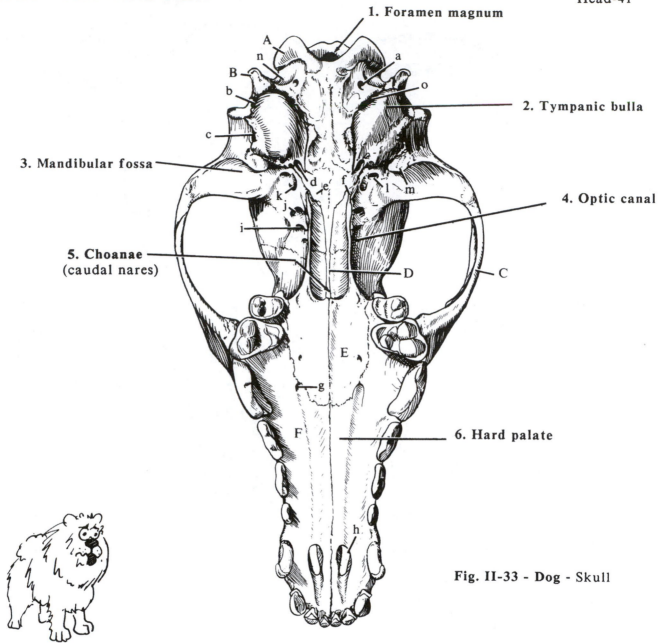

1. Foramen magnum

2. Tympanic bulla

3. Mandibular fossa

4. Optic canal

5. Choanae
(caudal nares)

6. Hard palate

Fig. II-33 - Dog - Skull

Skull radiography: pg. 606

VENTRAL SURFACE OF THE SKULL

1. Foramen magnum: the large opening into the cranial cavity for continuity of the spinal cord and brain.

2. Tympanic bulla (tim-PAN-ik): the smooth bulbous enlargement on the ventral side of the temporal bone housing the middle ear.

3. Mandibular fossa: the area on the zygomatic arch for articulation with the articular process (condyle) of the mandible.

4. Optic canal: the passageway for the optic nerve from the eyeball to the brain. It is rostral to many other foramina that allow passage of other cranial nerves.

5. Choanae (koh-AY-nee) (sin.= choana) or **caudal nares**: the two bony openings, at the caudal end of the hard palate, leading from the nasal cavity into the pharynx.

6. Hard palate: the horizontal parts of the incisive, palatine and maxillary bones, separating the nasal and oral cavities.

SPECIES DIFFERENCES

Foramen orbitorotundum: found in ruminants and pigs, it is the joining of the round and orbital foramina of other species.

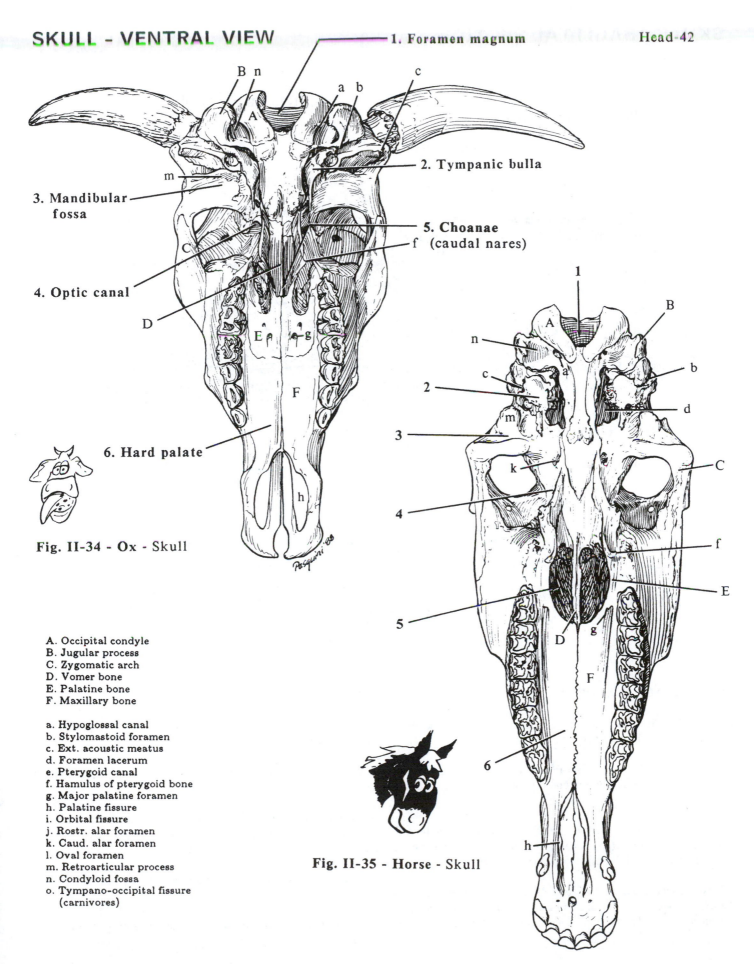

1. Foramen magnum

B n

a b

c

A

2. Tympanic bulla

m

3. Mandibular fossa

5. Choanae
   (caudal nares)

f

C

4. Optic canal

D

E e g

F

6. Hard palate

h

Fig. II-34 - Ox - Skull

Pasquini

1

A

n

B

c

a

b

2

d

m

3

C

k

4

f

5

E

D g

F

6

h

Fig. II-35 - Horse - Skull

A. Occipital condyle
B. Jugular process
C. Zygomatic arch
D. Vomer bone
E. Palatine bone
F. Maxillary bone

a. Hypoglossal canal
b. Stylomastoid foramen
c. Ext. acoustic meatus
d. Foramen lacerum
e. Pterygoid canal
f. Hamulus of pterygoid bone
g. Major palatine foramen
h. Palatine fissure
i. Orbital fissure
j. Rostr. alar foramen
k. Caud. alar foramen
l. Oval foramen
m. Retroarticular process
n. Condyloid fossa
o. Tympano-occipital fissure
   (carnivores)

9. Petrous temporal bone

8. Frontal sinus

Fig. II-36 - Dog - Skull

1. Cranial cavity

7. Ethmoid bone

6. Dorsal nasal concha

5. Ventral nasal concha

4. Nasal cavity

2. Hypophyseal fossa

3. Cribriform plate of ethmoid bone

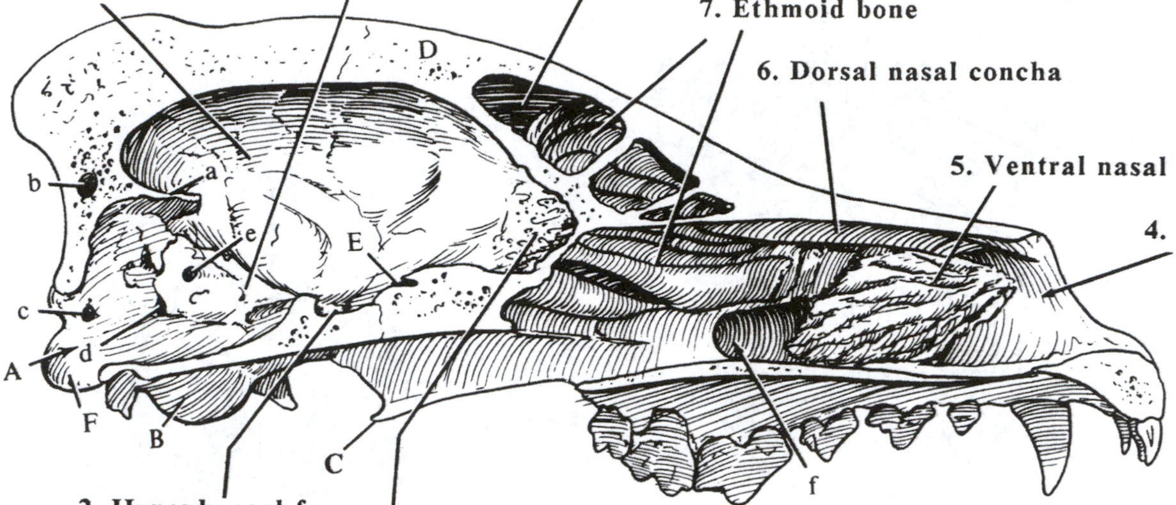

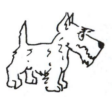

A. Foramen magnum
B. Tympanic bulla
  (not shown in horse)
C. Pterygoid bone
D. Frontal bone
E. Optic canal
F. Occipital bone
G. Vomer (not
  shown in dog)

a. Tentorium osseum
  (absent in ox)
b. Transverse canal
  (absent in ox)
c. Hypoglossal canal
d. Jugular foramen
e. Int. acoustic meatus
f. Entrance to maxillary
  recess (canine)

g. Palatine sinus (ox)
h. Sphenopalatine sinus
  (horse)
i. Mandibular foramen (not
  shown in dog)
j. Sphenoid sinus (ox & carnivores)
  (not shown in dog)

SAGITTAL SECTION OF THE SKULL

1. Cranial cavity: the space in the cranium containing the brain, its meninges and blood vessels.

2. Hypophyseal fossa (hy'poh-FIZ-ee-al): the depression in the floor of the cranial cavity (sphenoid bone) holding the pituitary gland (hypophysis).

3. Cribriform plate (L. *cribum* sieve): the rostral part of the wall of the cranial cavity. Many holes in this part of the ethmoid bone allow the passage of the olfactory nerve (CN I).

4. Nasal cavity: the hollow space behind the nose, surrounded by the facial bones. It is divided in half longitudinally by the nasal septum and is filled by the ventral nasal conchae and ethmoturbinate bones.

5. Ventral nasal concha (KONG-ka): a scroll of bone filling the rostral part of the nasal cavity.

6. Dorsal nasal concha: the largest nasal turbinate of the ethmoid bone.

7. Ethmoid bone: the bone in the caudal nasal cavity. It has many bony scrolls called ethmoturbinates and its cribriform plate forms the rostral wall of the cranial cavity.

8. Frontal sinus: the cavity (paranasal sinus) within the frontal bone.

9. Petrous temporal bone: dense bone containing structures of the inner ear

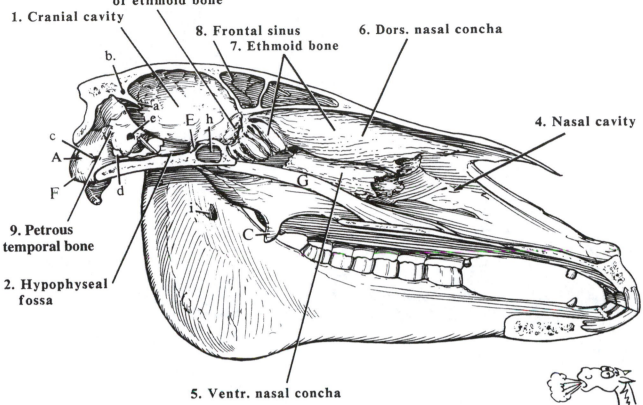

3. Cribriform plate
of ethmoid bone

1. Cranial cavity

8. Frontal sinus

7. Ethmoid bone

6. Dors. nasal concha

b.

a

e

E h

c

A

F

d

i

G

C

4. Nasal cavity

9. Petrous
temporal bone

2. Hypophyseal
fossa

5. Ventr. nasal concha

Fig. II-37 - Horse - Skull

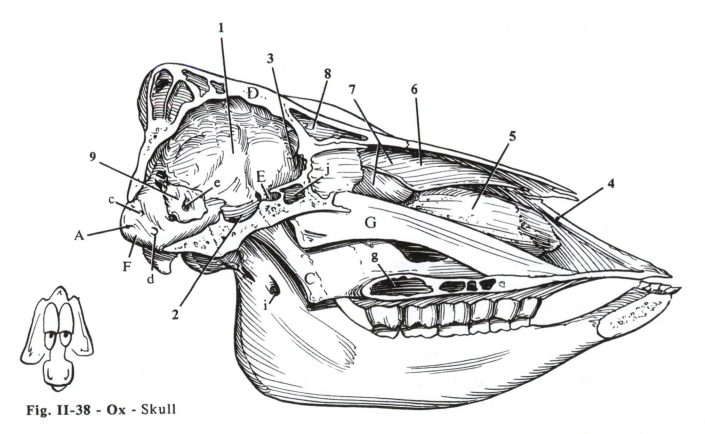

1

3

8

7

6

Đ

9

e

E

j

c

A

F

d

2

i

C

G

g

5

4

Fig. II-38 - Ox - Skull

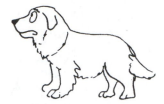

Fig. II-39 - Dog - Mandible - med. view

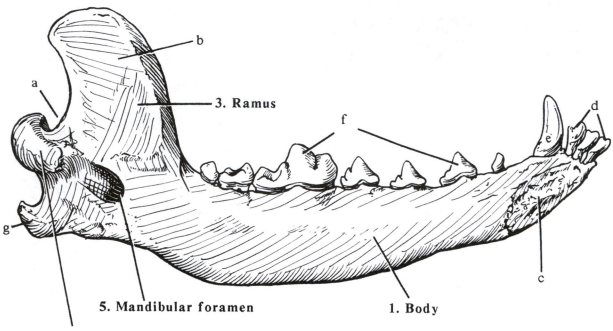

3. Ramus

5. Mandibular foramen

4. Articular (condyloid) process

1. Body

a. Mandibular notch	f. Cheek teeth
b. Coronoid process	g. Angular process (carnivores)
c. Mandibular symphysis	h. Angle of jaw
d. Incisor teeth	i. Masseteric fossa
e. Canine tooth	(not shown-dog)

MANDIBLE (L. *mandere* to masticate) or **lower jaw bone**: the largest and only mobile bone of the mammalian skull. It holds the lower teeth and consists of a right and left half united at the **mandibular symphysis** (c).

1. Body: the horizontal part bearing the lower incisor, canine, premolar and molar teeth.

2. Mental foramen (L. *mentum* chin): the rostral opening of the mandibular canal. (Not visible in the dog illustration)

3. Ramus: the vertical part of the mandible bearing no teeth.

4. Articular (condylar) **process** (KON-di-lar): the smooth proc-

ess which articulates with the mandibular fossa of the temporal bone to form the temporomandibular joint.

5. Mandibular foramen: the opening on the medial side of the ramus leading into the mandibular canal.

Clinical

"Lumpy jaw", Actinomycosis: *Actinomycoses bovis* (bacteria) invades abrasion into bone, resulting in a hard, immovable bony mass of mandible.

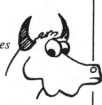

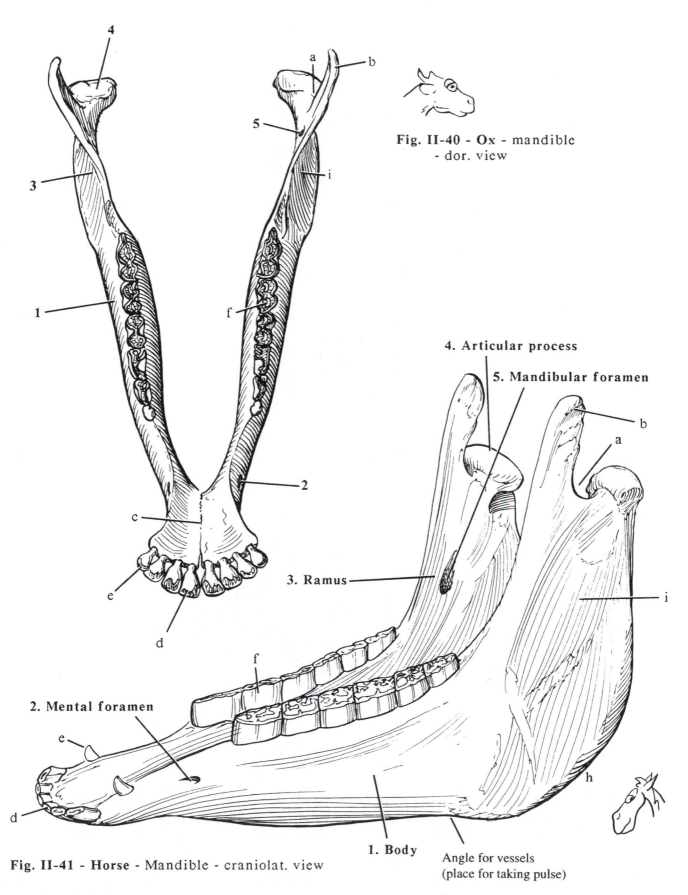

Fig. II-40 - **Ox** - mandible
- dor. view

4. **Articular process**

5. **Mandibular foramen**

3. **Ramus**

2. **Mental foramen**

1. **Body**

Angle for vessels
(place for taking pulse)

Fig. II-41 - **Horse** - Mandible - craniolat. view

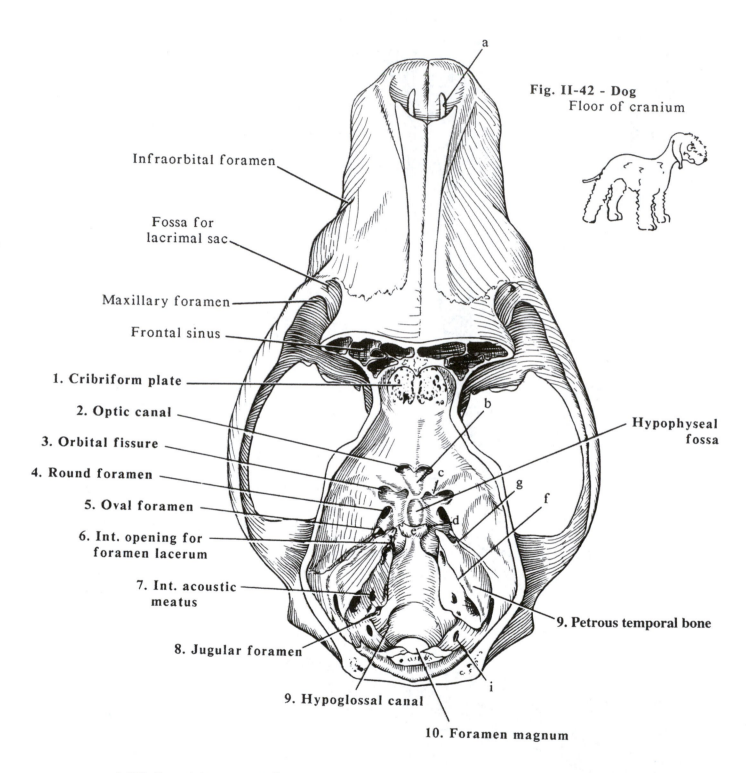

Infraorbital foramen

Fossa for lacrimal sac

Maxillary foramen

Frontal sinus

1. Cribriform plate

2. Optic canal

3. Orbital fissure

4. Round foramen

5. Oval foramen

6. Int. opening for foramen lacerum

7. Int. acoustic meatus

8. Jugular foramen

9. Hypoglossal canal

10. Foramen magnum

Hypophyseal fossa

9. Petrous temporal bone

Fig. II-42 - Dog
Floor of cranium

1. Cribriform plate	6. Formen lacerum	a. Palatine fissure	f. Petrosal crest
2. Optic canal	7. Int. acoustic meatus	b. Sulcus chiasmatis	g. Canal for trigeminal n.
3. Orbital fissure	8. Jugular foramen	c. Rostr. clinoid process	h. Canal for transverse sinus
4. Round foramen	9. Hypoglossal canal	d. Caud. clinoid process	i. Condyloid canal
5. Oval foramen	10. Foramen magnum	e. Dorsum sellae	

Fig. II-43 - Horse
-Floor of cranium

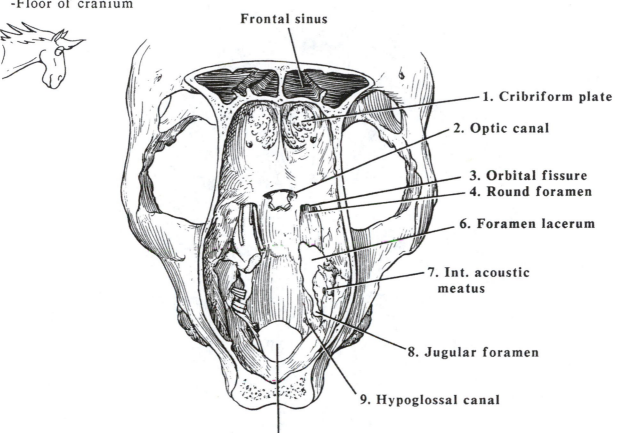

Frontal sinus

1. Cribriform plate

2. Optic canal

3. Orbital fissure
4. Round foramen

6. Foramen lacerum

7. Int. acoustic
   meatus

8. Jugular foramen

9. Hypoglossal canal

10. Foramen magnum

Fig. II-44 - Ox - Floor
of cranium

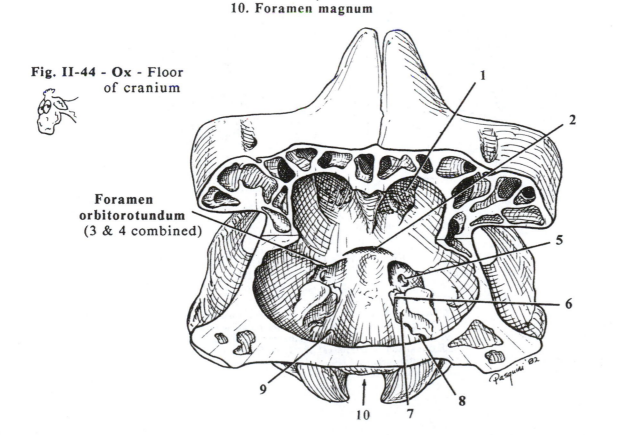

Foramen
orbitorotundum
(3 & 4 combined)

1

2

5

6

9   10   7   8

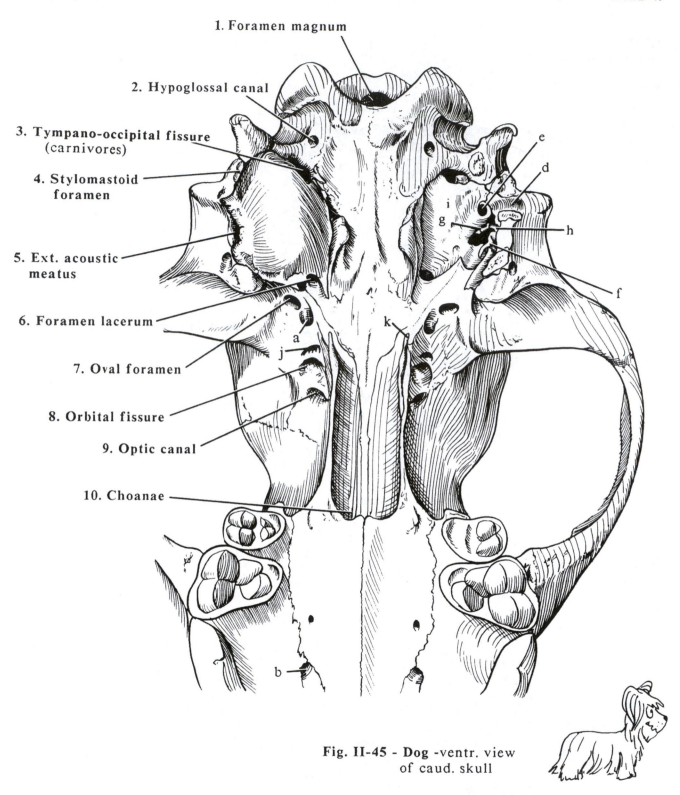

1. Foramen magnum
2. Hypoglossal canal
3. Tympano-occipital fissure (carnivores)
4. Stylomastoid foramen
5. Ext. acoustic meatus
6. Foramen lacerum
7. Oval foramen
8. Orbital fissure
9. Optic canal
10. Choanae

Fig. II-45 - Dog -ventr. view of caud. skull

1. Foramen magnum
2. Hypoglossal canal
3. Tympano-occipital fissure (carnivores)
4. Stylomastoid foramen
5. Ext. acoustic meatus
6. Foramen lacerum

7. Oval foramen
8. Orbital fissure
9. Optic canal
10. Choanae (caudal nares)
11. Jugular foramen (#3 ext. opening in carnivores)

a. Caud. alar foramen
b. Major palatine foramen
c. Supraorbital canal
d. Canal for facial n.
e. Cochlear window

f. Malleus
g. Stapes
h. Incus
i. Promontory
j. Rostr. alar foramen
k. Hamate process of pterygoid bone

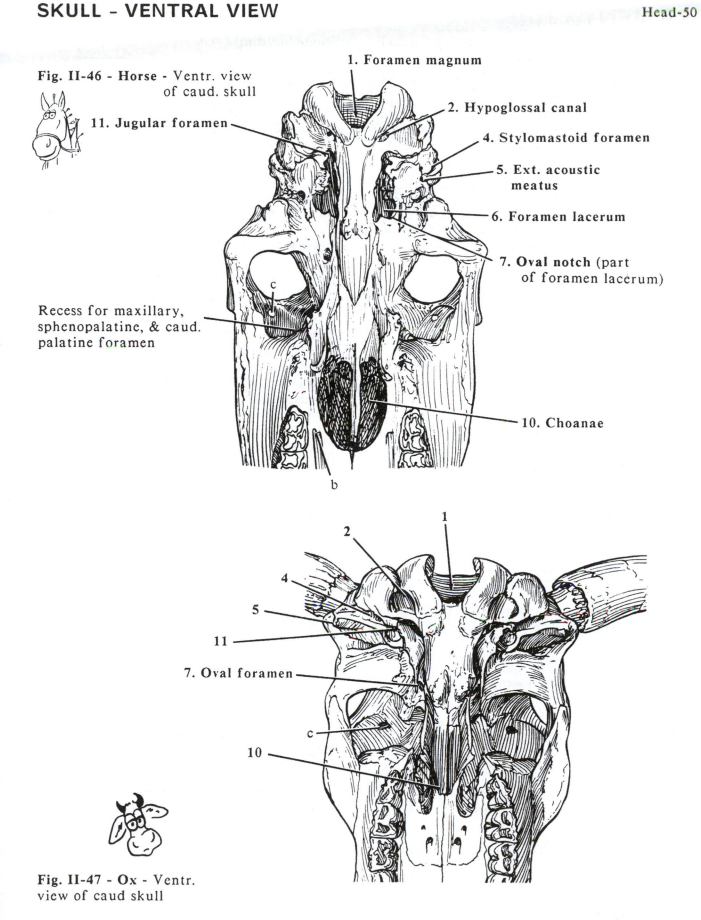

Fig. II-46 - Horse - Ventr. view of caud. skull

11. Jugular foramen

1. Foramen magnum

2. Hypoglossal canal

4. Stylomastoid foramen

5. Ext. acoustic meatus

6. Foramen lacerum

7. **Oval notch** (part of foramen lacerum)

Recess for maxillary, sphenopalatine, & caud. palatine foramen

10. Choanae

b

c

2

1

4

5

11

7. Oval foramen

c

10

Fig. II-47 - Ox - Ventr. view of caud skull

FORAMEN (selective)

Openings	Structures passing through	[Bone location] Facts
Loosely associated with the cranial cavity		
• **Cribriform foramina**	Olfactory n. (I)	[Ethmoid] openings in cribriform plate
• Ethmoid foramen	Ethmoid a., v., n.	
• **Optic canal**	Optic n. (II)	[Sphenoid] into orbit
• **Orbital fissure** (Car, eq)	CrN III, IV, VI, V/1 (ophthalmic)	[Sphenoid] into orbit
• **Round foramen** (Car, eq)	Maxillary n. (V/2)	[Sphenoid] opens into alar canal
• Alar canal (Car, eq):	Maxillary a.	Canal through side of sphenoid bone
- Rostral alar foramen	Maxillary a.., n. (V/2)	[Sphenoid] into pterygopalatine fossa
- Caudal alar foramen	Maxillary a.	[Sphenoid] caudal opening of alar canal
• **Foramen orbitorotundum** (Ru & su)	CrN III, IV, VI, V/1 & V/2 (ophthalmic & maxillary)	Ru & su: combined orbital fissure & round foramen
• **Oval foramen** (Car, Ru)	Mandibular n (V/3)	[Sphenoid] part of foramen lacerum in eq & su
• Carotid foramen	Internal carotid a.	[Sphenoid] also called the foramen lacerum in carnivores. Eq & Su: fuses with oval foramen to form enlarged foramen lacerum
• **Foramen lacerum**	Internal carotid a.,	[Sphenoid, temporal, occipital] in eq & su: large, includes carotid, oval foramina & is continuous with the jugular foramen caudally, although all are separated by tissue in the live animal
• **Internal acoustic meatus**	Vestibulocochlear n. (VIII)	[Temporal]
• **Jugular foramen**	CrN IX, X, XI	[Temporal, occipital] present in all; eq & su: continuous with foramen lacerum
• **Tympanoccipital fissure** (Car, Ru)	CrN IX, X, XI	[Temporal, occipital] external opening of jugular foramen (Car,Ru)
• **Stylomastoid foramen**	Facial n. (VII)	[Temporal] caudal to ear
• **Hypoglossal canal**	Hypoglossal n. (XII)	[Occipital] near occipital condyle
• **Foramen magnum**	Spinal cord	[Occipital]
Rostral pterygopalatine fossa:		3 foramina
• **Maxillary foramen**	Infraorbital a., v., n. (V/2)	[Maxilla] caudal opening of infraorbital canal for maxillary n., most dorsal of 3
• Sphenopalatine foramen	Sphenopalatine a., v., n.	Leads to the nasal cavity
• Caudal palatine foramen	Major palatine a., n.	To major palatine foramen in hard palate, most ventral of 3
Bones of face:		
• **Infraorbital foramen**	Infraorbital a., n. (V/2)	[Maxilla] rostral opening of infraorbital canal
• **Supraorbital foramen**	Ophthalmic division (V/1)	[Frontal] Above orbit
Hard palate:		
• **Major palatine foramen**	Palatine a.	[Palatine, maxilla] through hard palate
• Interincisive canal	Palatolabial a.	[Incisive] caudal to central incisors
• Palatine fissure	Closed in live animal	[Incisive, maxilla] lateral to palatine process of the incisive bone
Mandible:		
• **Mandibular foramen**	Mandibular alveolar n. (V/3)	[Mandible] proximal opening of mandibular canal
• **Mental foramen**	Mental n. (V/3)	[Mandible] distal opening of mandibular canal
Others:		
• **Choanae (caudal nares)**	Air	Opening between nasal cavity & nasopharynx
• **External acoustic meatus**	Sound waves	[Temporal] closed by ear drum from middle ear
• **Lacrimal foramen**	Tears	[Lacrimal] from lacrimal fossa to nasolacrimal canal
• **Nasal aperture**	Air	[Nasal, incisive]

Abbreviations

bo	=	ox	cap	=	goat	eq	=	horse	ov	=	sheep	su	=	pig
ca	=	dog	Car	=	carnivores	fe	=	cat	Ru	=	Ruminant	Un	=	ungulate

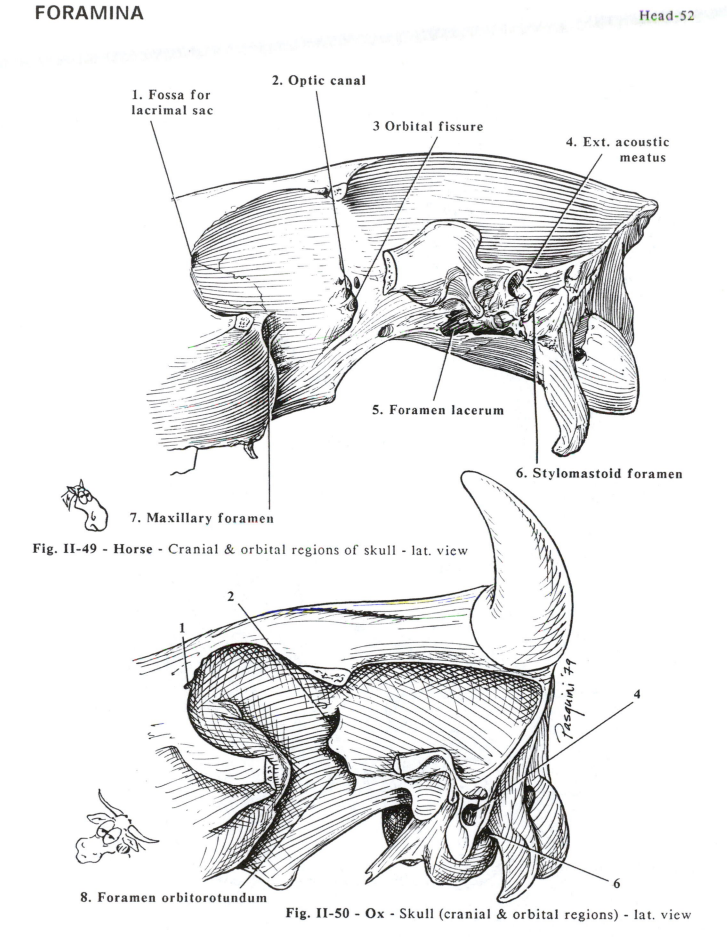

1. Fossa for lacrimal sac

2. Optic canal

3 Orbital fissure

4. Ext. acoustic meatus

5. Foramen lacerum

6. Stylomastoid foramen

7. Maxillary foramen

Fig. II-49 - Horse - Cranial & orbital regions of skull - lat. view

8. Foramen orbitorotundum

Fig. II-50 - Ox - Skull (cranial & orbital regions) - lat. view

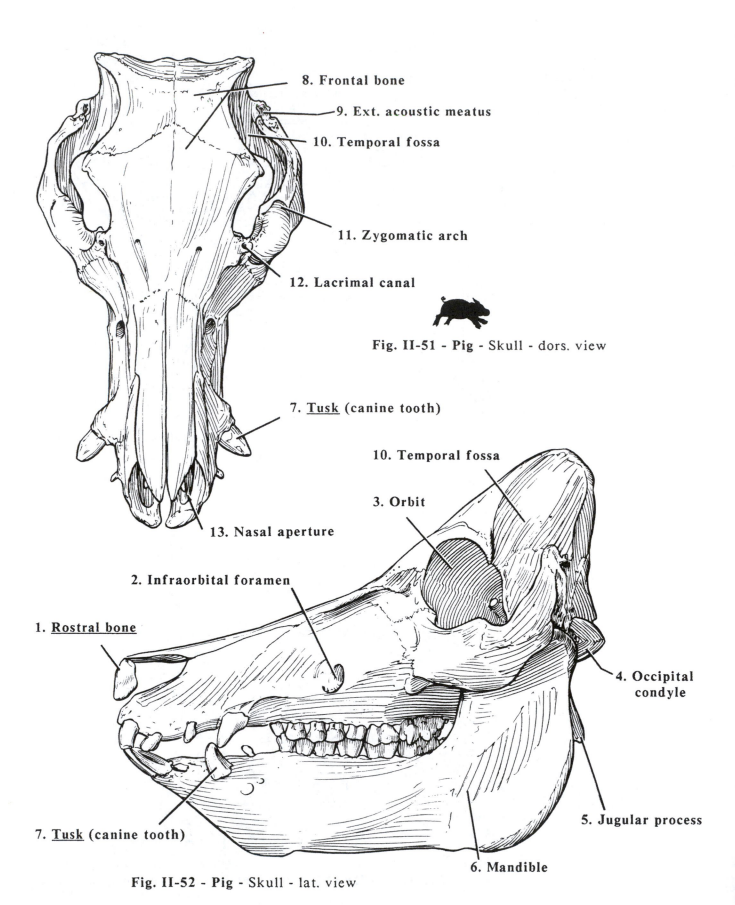

8. Frontal bone

9. Ext. acoustic meatus

10. Temporal fossa

11. Zygomatic arch

12. Lacrimal canal

Fig. II-51 - **Pig** - Skull - dors. view

7. <u>Tusk</u> (canine tooth)

10. Temporal fossa

3. Orbit

2. Infraorbital foramen

1. <u>Rostral bone</u>

4. Occipital condyle

13. Nasal aperture

7. <u>Tusk</u> (canine tooth)

5. Jugular process

6. Mandible

Fig. II-52 - **Pig** - Skull - lat. view

SKULL - CAT

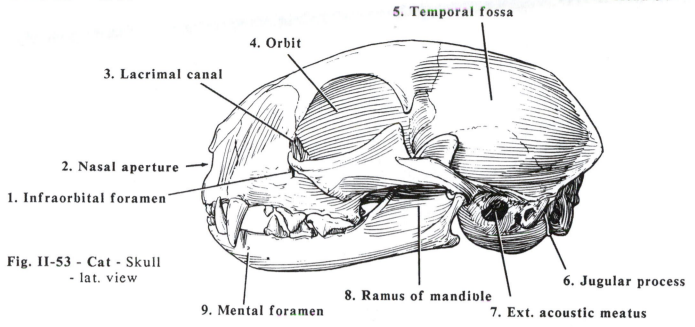

5. Temporal fossa

4. Orbit

3. Lacrimal canal

2. Nasal aperture

1. Infraorbital foramen

Fig. II-53 - Cat - Skull
- lat. view

9. Mental foramen

8. Ramus of mandible

6. Jugular process

7. Ext. acoustic meatus

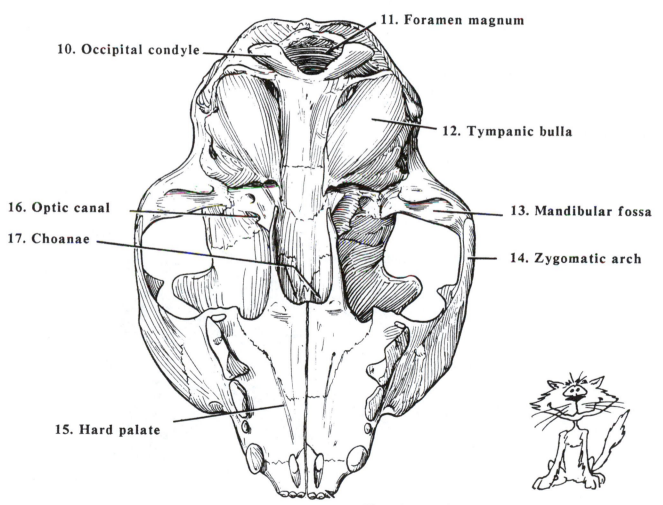

11. Foramen magnum

10. Occipital condyle

12. Tympanic bulla

16. Optic canal

17. Choanae

13. Mandibular fossa

14. Zygomatic arch

15. Hard palate

Fig. II-54 - Cat - Skull - ventr. view

SKULL – GOAT

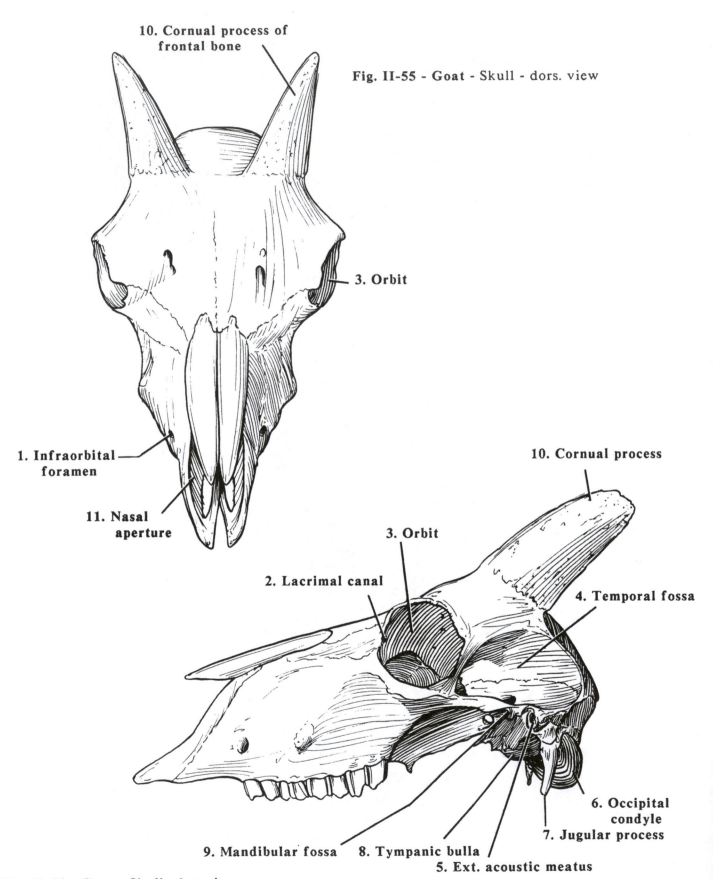

10. Cornual process of frontal bone

Fig. II-55 - Goat - Skull - dors. view

3. Orbit

1. Infraorbital foramen

11. Nasal aperture

10. Cornual process

3. Orbit

2. Lacrimal canal

4. Temporal fossa

6. Occipital condyle

7. Jugular process

9. Mandibular fossa

8. Tympanic bulla

5. Ext. acoustic meatus

Fig. II-56 - Goat - Skull - lat. view

54

SKULL - SHEEP

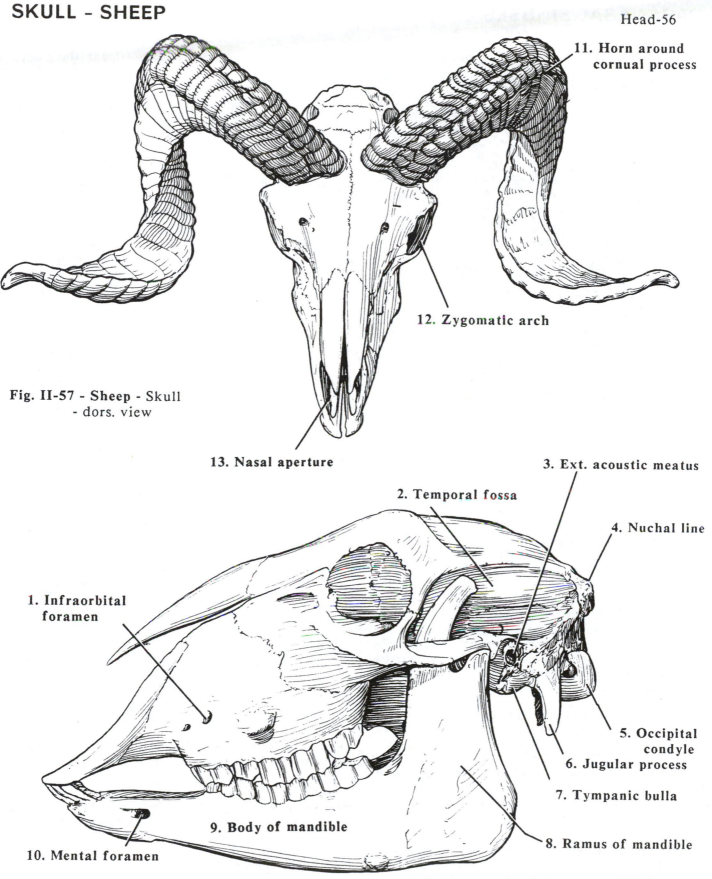

11. Horn around cornual process

12. Zygomatic arch

Fig. II-57 - Sheep - Skull - dors. view

13. Nasal aperture

3. Ext. acoustic meatus

2. Temporal fossa

4. Nuchal line

1. Infraorbital foramen

5. Occipital condyle

6. Jugular process

7. Tympanic bulla

9. Body of mandible

8. Ramus of mandible

10. Mental foramen

Fig. II-58 - Sheep - Skull - lat. view

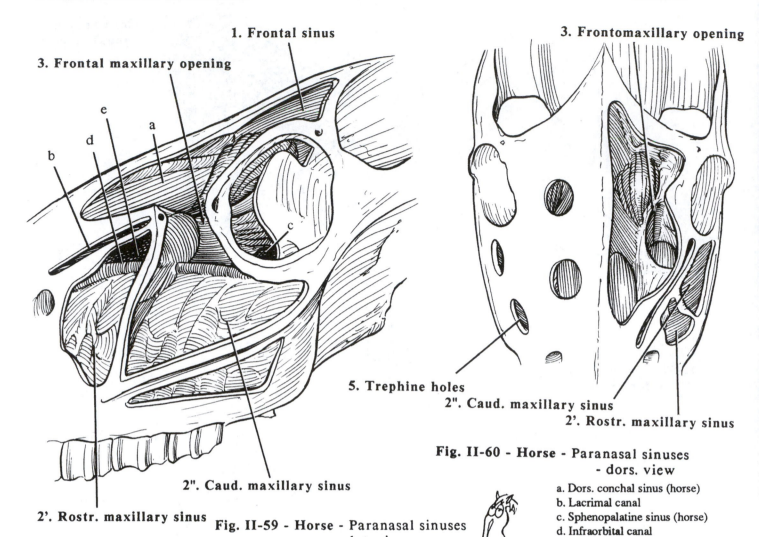

1. Frontal sinus

3. Frontal maxillary opening

3. Frontomaxillary opening

e

a

d

b

c

5. Trephine holes

2". Caud. maxillary sinus

2'. Rostr. maxillary sinus

Fig. II-60 - Horse - Paranasal sinuses
- dors. view

2". Caud. maxillary sinus

2'. Rostr. maxillary sinus   **Fig. II-59 - Horse** - Paranasal sinuses
- lat. view

a. Dors. conchal sinus (horse)
b. Lacrimal canal
c. Sphenopalatine sinus (horse)
d. Infraorbital canal
e. Nasomaxillary opening (horse)
f. Palatine sinus (ruminants)

PARANASAL SINUSES (par'a-NAY-zal SY-nus-seez): the air-filled cavities within some bones of the skull. They are lined by a mucous membrane and communicate with the nasal cavity. The frontal and maxillary sinuses are the best known, but several others may be present, including the sphenoid, palatine, lacrimal and conchal sinuses.

1. FRONTAL SINUS: the paranasal sinus found in the frontal bones of all domestic species.

2. MAXILLARY SINUS: the paranasal sinus in the maxillary bone. It opens into the nasal cavity through the nasomaxillary opening (e).

SPECIES DIFFERENCES

Frontal sinus: in the dorsal part of the skull, between the orbits in the **horse, small ruminants** and **carnivores.** In the **ox** and **pig** the frontal sinus extends to the back of the skull. In the ruminant it has a number of diverticula besides the cornual diverticulum.

Conchofrontal sinus: in horses, the joined frontal and dorsal conchal sinus.

3. Frontomaxillary opening: in the <u>horse</u>, the large opening between the caudal maxillary sinus and the frontal sinus.

4. Cornual diverticulum: the direct continuation of the frontal sinus into the cornual process in horned **ruminants.**

Dog: has a **maxillary "recess"** (Fig II-36,f) between bones in the area of the maxillary bone, not inside the maxillary bone.

Horse: has two maxillary sinuses separated by a bony septum, the **rostral maxillary sinus** (2') and the **caudal maxillary sinus** (2").

Pig and **ruminants:** have a single maxillary sinus.

Lacrimal bulla: paper thin caudal extent of the maxillary sinus in the ruminants.

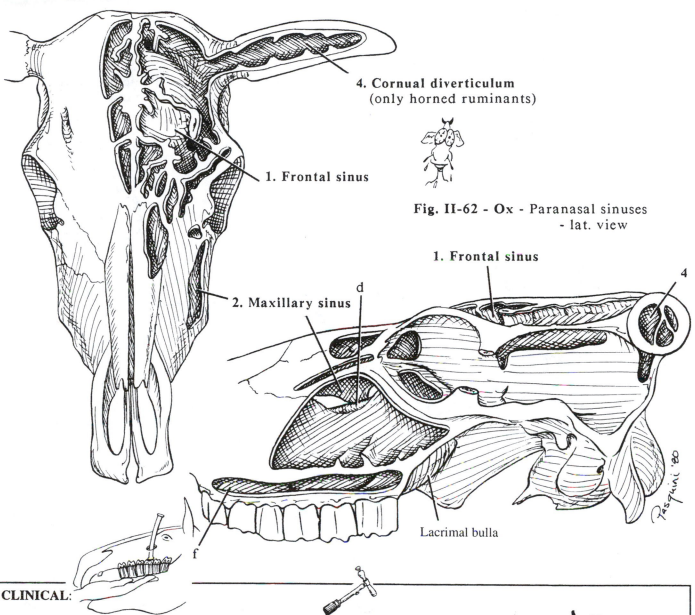

Fig. II-61 - Ox - Paranasal sinuses
- dors. view

4. Cornual diverticulum
(only horned ruminants)

Fig. II-62 - Ox - Paranasal sinuses
- lat. view

1. Frontal sinus

1. Frontal sinus

2. Maxillary sinus

d

4

Lacrimal bulla

f

CLINICAL:

5. Trephination (tree-FYN-ay-shun): the drilling of holes (trephine holes) into the paranasal sinuses.

Horse: "cheek teeth PM3, PM4, M1 & M2 can be removed (repelled) through trephined holes in the maxillary sinuses. The last cheek tooth (M3) is reached by trephining the conchofrontal sinus (1 inch off midline between the medial canthi of the eyes), then using a curved punch through the frontomaxillary opening. Care must be taken to avoid the infraorbital canal (d) and the lacrimal canal (b).

Boundaries for trephination of the maxillary sinus in the **horse**:
• Dorsal - line from medial canthus to infraorbital foramen.
• Ventral - Facial crest.

Cornual diverticulum (4) of the frontal sinuses is often opened in dehorning, and thus a possible entrance for inflammation (sinusitis).

Ox - Trephination of the four compartment frontal sinus:
• Rostral compartment - between the eyes 1 inch from the midline.
• Postorbital diverticulum - 1 - 1 1/2 inches caudal to the lateral canthus of eye.
• Nuchal diverticulum - caudal, halfway between midline and the base of the horn.

Sinusitis: inflammation of the paranasal sinuses. Trephination may be used to drain such infections.

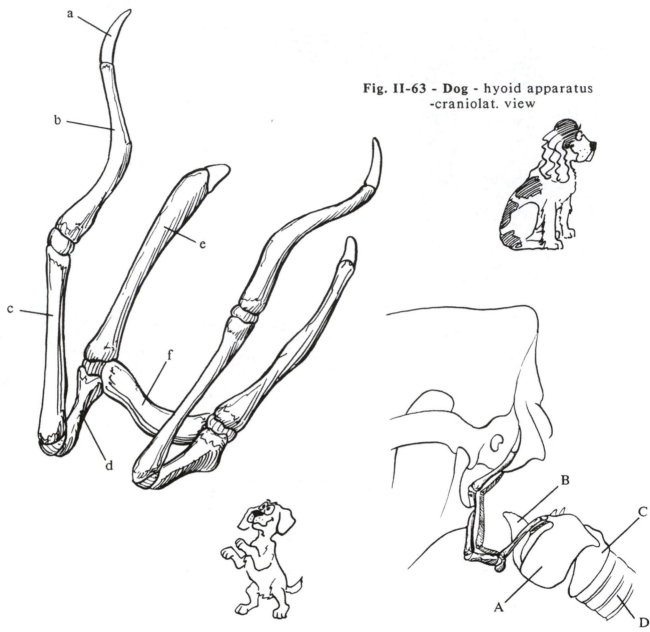

Fig. II-63 - **Dog** - hyoid apparatus
-craniolat. view

Fig. II-64 - **Dog** - Hyoid apparatus
- lat. view

A. Thyroid cartilage
B. Epiglottic cartilage
C. Cricoid cartilage
D. Trachea

a. Tympanohyoid cartilage
b. Stylohyoid bone
c. Epihyoid bone
d. Ceratohyoid bone
e. Thyrohyoid bone
f. Basihyoid bone

HYOID APPARATUS (HY-oid) (G. *hyoedes* u-shaped): a number of connected bones suspending the larynx and tongue from the skull. The hyoid apparatus consists of the basihyoid, thyrohyoid, ceratohyoid, epihyoid, and stylohyoid bones and tympanohyoid cartilage.

Basihyoid bone: unpaired hyoid bone crossing the midline where it can be palpated.

Memory aid: to the order of the hyoid bones in relationship to each other – **S**ick **E**lephants **C**an **B**e **T**reated.

SPECIES DIFFERENCES

1. Lingual process: the rostral projection of the basihyoid bone into the tongue. Carnivores lack such a process, but the horse has a long one and the ox a short one.

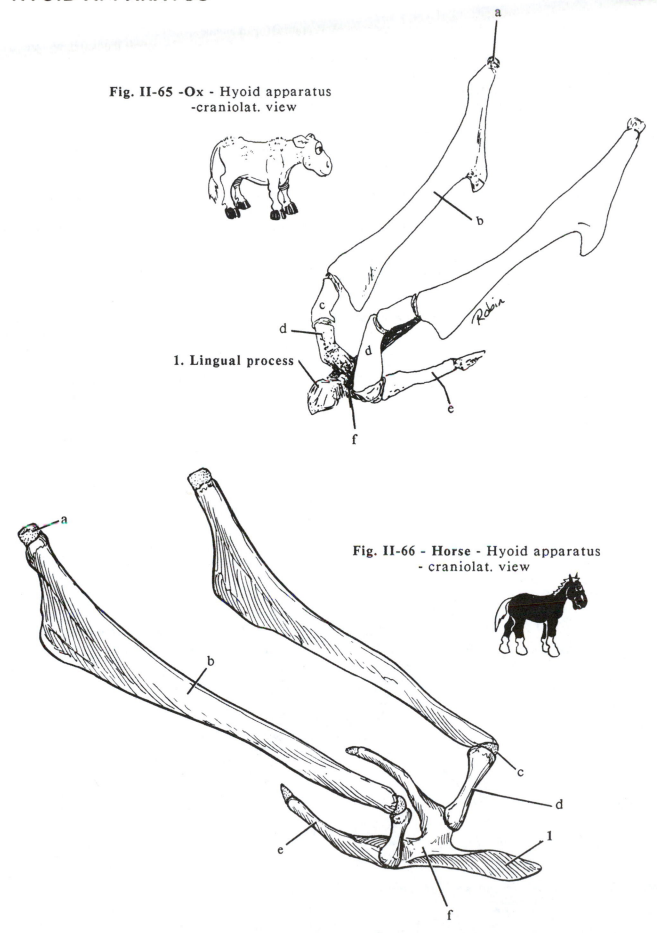

Fig. II-65 -Ox - Hyoid apparatus
-craniolat. view

1. Lingual process

Fig. II-66 - Horse - Hyoid apparatus
- craniolat. view

VERTEBRAE

VERTEBRAL COLUMN, spine or backbone: protects the spinal cord, supports the head and serves as attachment for the muscles effecting body movements. It extends from the skull through the tail and consists of irregular bones - vertebrae. The vertebrae are firmly joined by slightly moveable joints. All the vertebral joints together allow a great amount of movement.

VERTEBRAE (VER-te-bree) (sin. = vertebra): the irregularly-shaped bones making up the spinal column. They are grouped by location into cervical (neck), thoracic (cranial back), lumbar (loin), sacral (croup) and caudal (tail) vertebrae. Each group is represented by its first letter followed by the number representing how many are in each section. C7 T13 L7 S3 Ca *n* is the vertebral formula of the dog. The number of each type of vertebrae is constant except the caudal ones. Twenty can be used as a rough estimate of the caudal vertebrae with some dogs having more and some less. **Common features of a typical vertebra** are the body, vertebral arch, vertebral foramen and processes.

1. Intervertebral foramen: the opening between vertebrae formed by caudal and cranial notches of adjacent vertebrae. These openings allow passage of the spinal nerves.

2. Intervertebral discs: the fibrocartilages connecting the bodies of adjacent vertebrae.

3. Vertebral arch (VER-tee-bral): the dorsal part of a vertebra that arises from the body. It consists of two upright pedicles forming the walls of the vertebral foramen. From the pedicles two lamina project to the midline and form the roof of the vertebral foramen.

4. Vertebral foramen: the space formed by the vertebral arch and the body. The vertebral foramina of all the vertebrae form the vertebral canal, housing the spinal cord.

Vertebral canal: formed in the live animal by all the vertebral foramina.

5. Body: the thick, spool-shaped ventral portion of the vertebra. It is convex cranially and concave caudally to articulate with adjacent vertebrae.

The 7 processes of the vertebral arch: the spine and the two transverse processes provide sites for muscle attachment. The four articular processes form <u>synovial joints</u> with adjacent vertebrae.

6. Spinous process or spine: the dorsal projection of the vertebral arch.

7. Transverse process: the lateral extension of the vertebral arch. They divide the muscles of the back into dorsal (epaxial) and ventral (hypaxial) groups.

8. Articular processes: the four articular processes, two cranial and two caudal (8' and 8"), articulate respectively with the caudal and cranial articular processes of adjacent vertebrae. These form synovial joints.

VERTEBRAL FORMULA:				
Carnivore	C7	T13	L7	S3	Ca20-24
Pig	7	11-15	6-7	4	20-23
Horse	7	18	6	5	15-21
Ox	7	13	6	5	18-20
Sheep	7	13	6-7	4	16-18

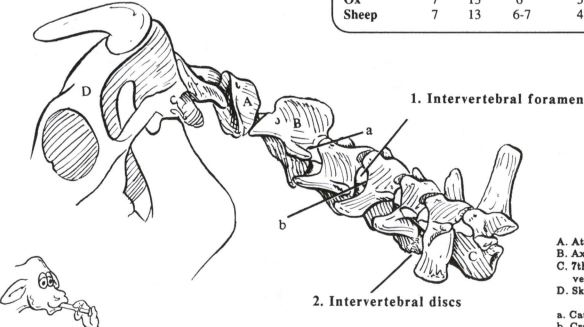

1. Intervertebral foramen

2. Intervertebral discs

A. Atlas
B. Axis
C. 7th cervical vertebra
D. Skull

a. Caud. notch
b. Cran. notch
c. Pedicle
d. Lamina

Fig. II-67 - Ox - Cervical vertebrae - lat. view

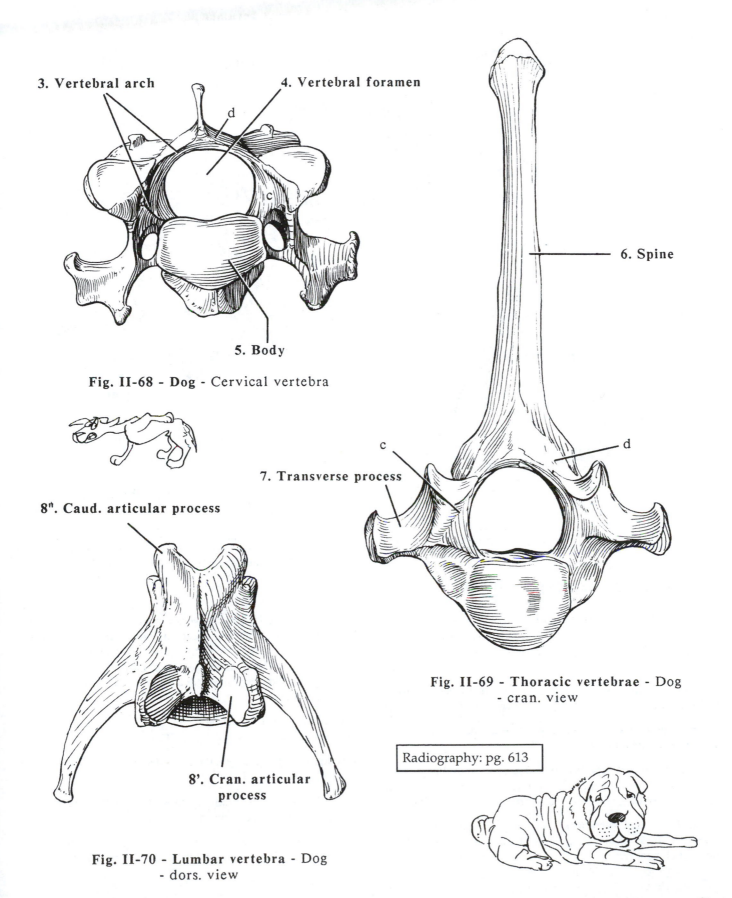

3. Vertebral arch

4. Vertebral foramen

d

c

5. Body

Fig. II-68 - Dog - Cervical vertebra

6. Spine

7. Transverse process

c

d

8ⁿ. Caud. articular process

8'. Cran. articular process

Fig. II-69 - Thoracic vertebrae - Dog - cran. view

Radiography: pg. 613

Fig. II-70 - Lumbar vertebra - Dog - dors. view

CERVICAL VERTEBRAE

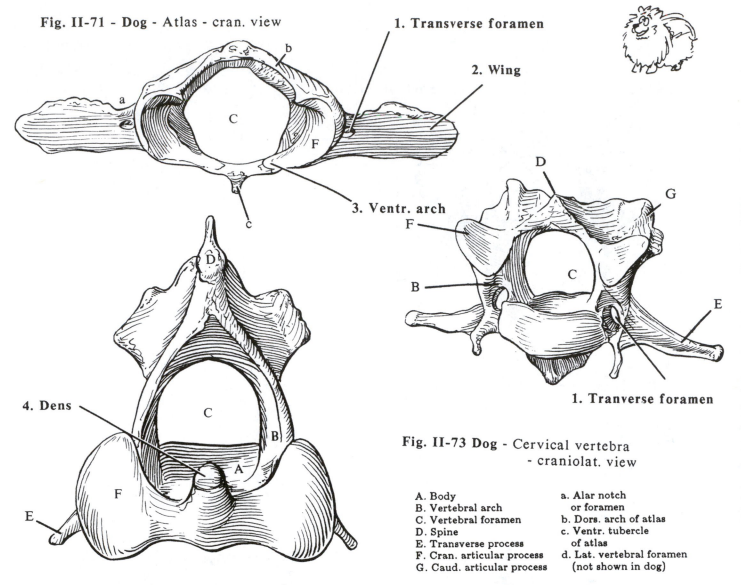

Fig. II-71 - Dog - Atlas - cran. view

1. Transverse foramen

2. Wing

3. Ventr. arch

4. Dens

Fig. II-72 - Dog - Axis - cran. view

1. Tranverse foramen

Fig. II-73 Dog - Cervical vertebra
- craniolat. view

A. Body
B. Vertebral arch
C. Vertebral foramen
D. Spine
E. Transverse process
F. Cran. articular process
G. Caud. articular process

a. Alar notch
or foramen
b. Dors. arch of atlas
c. Ventr. tubercle
of atlas
d. Lat. vertebral foramen
(not shown in dog)

CERVICAL VERTEBRAE (*cervix*, neck): the seven vertebrae of the neck in all mammals, characterized by a transverse foramen (except C7). The 1st (atlas) and 2nd (axis) cervical vertebrae are atypical.

1. Transverse foramen: the hole through the transverse process of C_1-C_6, together forming the **transverse canal.**

Transverse process: of the cervical vertebrae are divided into ventral and dorsal tubercles.

Sixth cervical vertebrae's transverse process: is a large ventral projection. On a radiograph it is used as a landmark and is often called the sled of the sixth cervical vertebrae and looks like a sled.

Seventh cervical vertebrae: has a higher spinous process, no transverse foramen and articular facet on its caudal surface for the head of eh first rib.

ATLAS (C_1): the 1st cervical vertebra, named for its support of the head. It articulates with the occipital condyles to form the atlanto-occipital joint (the "yes" joint). The atlas is atypical because it lacks a body and a spinous process. It articulates with the occipital condyles of the skull allowing flexion and extension ("yes movement").

2. Ventral arch: the portion of the atlas replacing the body of other vertebrae.

3. Wings (alae): the large lateral masses that are modified transverse processes.

AXIS (C2): the long second cervical vertebra. It has a large ridge-like spinous process and the dens.

4. Dens: the peg-like cranial process forming a pivot articulation with the atlas, allowing pivotal motion (the "no" joint).

CERVICAL VERTEBRAE

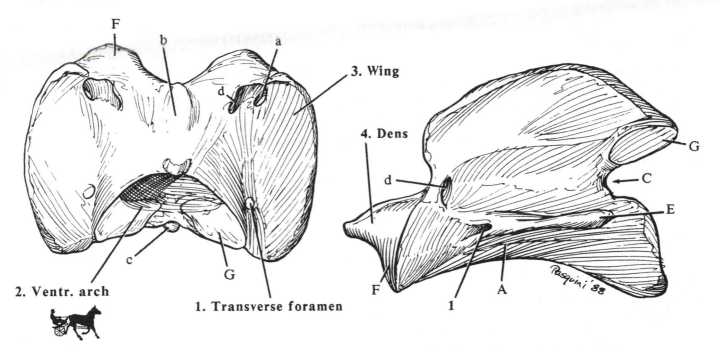

Fig. II-74 - Horse - Atlas
- dors. view

3. Wing

4. Dens

Fig. II-67 - Horse - Axis - lat. view

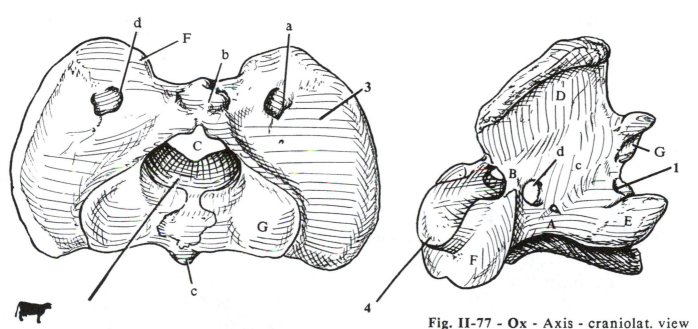

Fig. II-76 - Ox - Atlas - caudodors. view

Fig. II-77 - Ox - Axis - craniolat. view

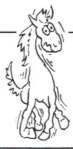

CLINICAL

Wobbler syndrome, equine sensory ataxia: there are two types of stenosis of cervical vertebral canal (static and dynamic). Focal compression of the dorsal spinal cord causes proprioceptive loss (sensory ataxia) with normal motor activity, resulting in a clumsy, tin soldier walk.

Cervical spondylomyelopathy, canine "wobbler": disease of the cervical vertebrae in large breeds causing stenosis of the vertebral canal resulting in ataxia.

THORACIC VERTEBRAE

THORACIC VERTEBRAE: the vertebrae of the thorax, characterized by <u>articular</u> <u>facets</u> for the pair of ribs they bear.

Anticlinal vertebra: the thoracic vertebra with the most vertically oriented spine, usually the eleventh (T11) in the dog. All spines cranial to this vertebra are inclined caudally, all caudal ones incline cranially. This is often used as a landmark in reading radiographs of the thorax or back.

1. Costal fovea: the two facets for articulation with a rib's head, located on the caudal and cranial end of the vertebral bodies of most of the thoracic vertebrae.

2. Transverse costal fovea: the facet on the transverse process that articulates with the tubercle of the same numbered rib.

SPECIES DIFFERENCES		
Species	# of thoracic vertebrae	Anticlinal vertebra
Carnivores	13	11
Horse	18	16
Ox	13	13
Sheep	13	13
Pig	14-15	10
Chicken	7	-

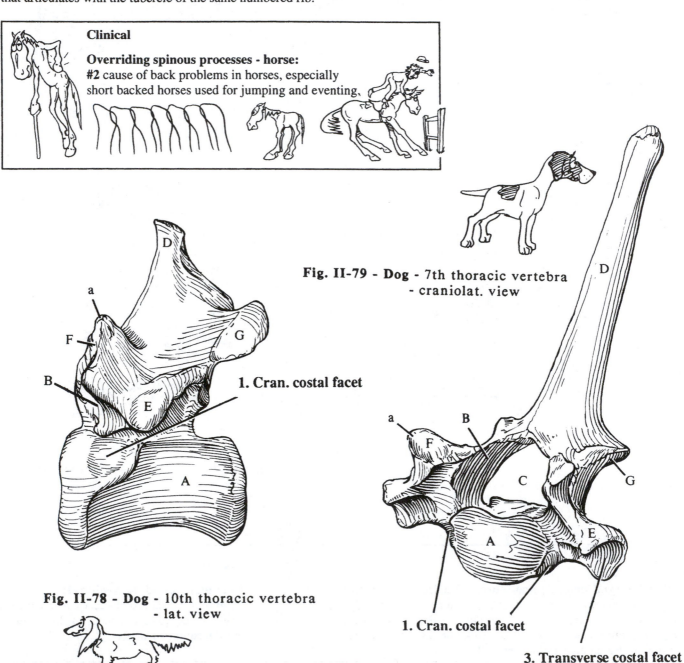

Clinical

Overriding spinous processes - horse:
#2 cause of back problems in horses, especially short backed horses used for jumping and eventing.

Fig. II-79 - Dog - 7th thoracic vertebra - craniolat. view

1. Cran. costal facet

Fig. II-78 - Dog - 10th thoracic vertebra - lat. view

1. Cran. costal facet

3. Transverse costal facet

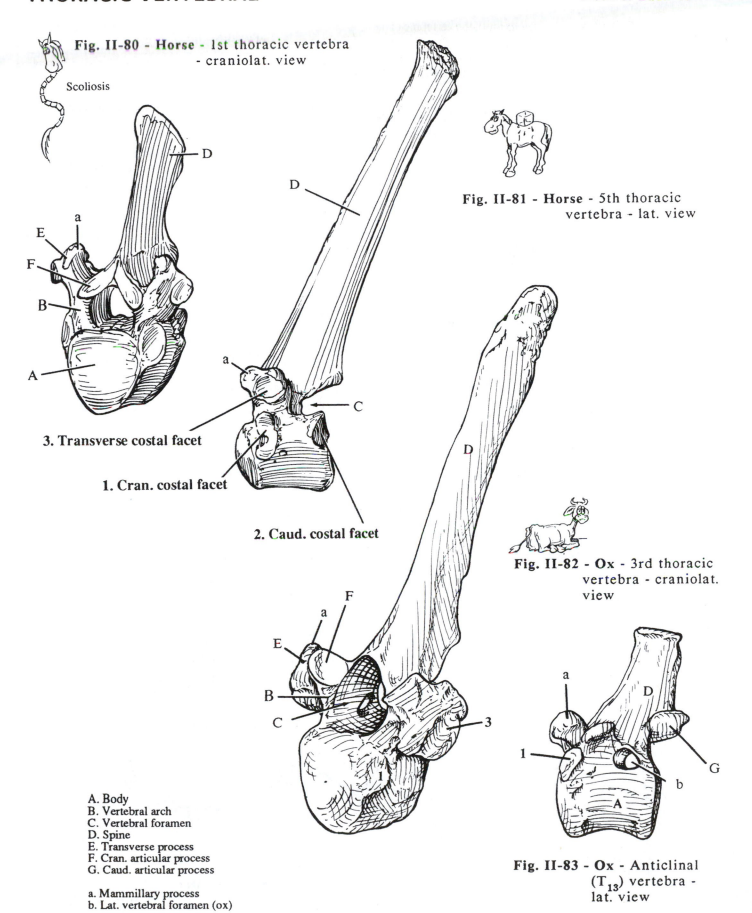

Scoliosis

Fig. II-80 - Horse - 1st thoracic vertebra - craniolat. view

3. Transverse costal facet

1. Cran. costal facet

2. Caud. costal facet

Fig. II-81 - Horse - 5th thoracic vertebra - lat. view

Fig. II-82 - Ox - 3rd thoracic vertebra - craniolat. view

Fig. II-83 - Ox - Anticlinal (T_{13}) vertebra - lat. view

A. Body
B. Vertebral arch
C. Vertebral foramen
D. Spine
E. Transverse process
F. Cran. articular process
G. Caud. articular process

a. Mammillary process
b. Lat. vertebral foramen (ox)

LUMBAR VERTEBRAE

LUMBAR VERTEBRAE (Fr. *lumbus* loin): the vertebrae of the lumbar (lower back, loin) region, characterized by their large size and long plate-like transverse processes (1). They can be distinguished from the last throracic vertebrae by their lack of costal facets.

Accessory processes (d): are found from the midthoracic to the lumbar vertebrae. These can be seen through the intervertebral foramen in radiographs and shouldn't be confused with a ruptured intervertebral disc.

SPECIES DIFFERENCES	
Species	# of lumbar vertebrae
Carnivores	7
Horse	6 (5 in some Arabians)
Ox	6
Sheep	6-7
Pig	6-7
Chicken	14 (lumbrosacral)

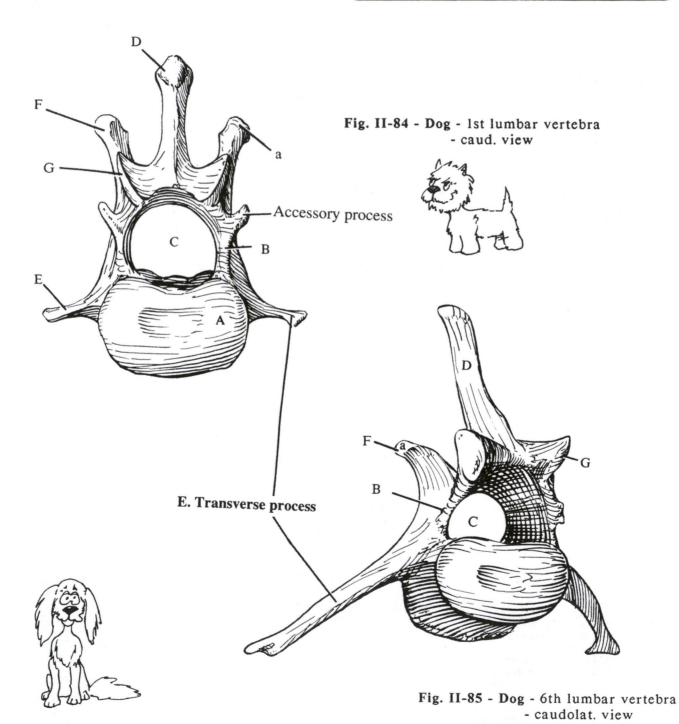

Fig. II-84 - Dog - 1st lumbar vertebra - caud. view

Accessory process

E. Transverse process

Fig. II-85 - Dog - 6th lumbar vertebra - caudolat. view

LUMBAR VERTEBRAE

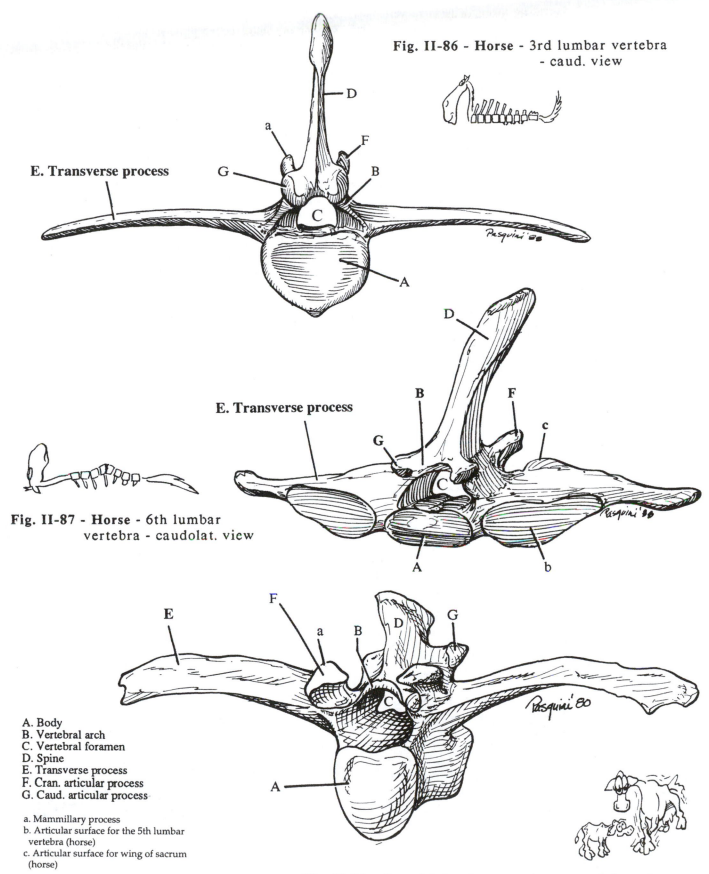

Fig. II-86 - Horse - 3rd lumbar vertebra - caud. view

E. Transverse process

E. Transverse process

Fig. II-87 - Horse - 6th lumbar vertebra - caudolat. view

A. Body
B. Vertebral arch
C. Vertebral foramen
D. Spine
E. Transverse process
F. Cran. articular process
G. Caud. articular process

a. Mammillary process
b. Articular surface for the 5th lumbar vertebra (horse)
c. Articular surface for wing of sacrum (horse)

Fig. II-88 - Ox - 4th lumbar vertebra - craniolat. view

SACRUM

SACRUM: the bone formed by the fusion of the sacral vertebrae. It articulates with the hip bones forming the sacroiliac joint. The portion of the vertebral canal through the sacrum is called the **sacral canal.**

1. Dorsal and **2. ventral sacral foramina:** the openings on the dorsal and ventral surfaces of the bone for passage of spinal nerves.

3. Wings: the lateral parts of the sacrum articulating with the hip bones to form the sacroiliac joint.

SPECIES DIFFERENCES:

4. Spinous processes: the unfused processes in the **horse** and **carnivores.**

5. Median sacral crest: the fused sacral spinal processes in the **ruminants.**

Species Differences	
Species	Fused vertebrae
Carnivores	3
Horse	5
Ox	5
Sheep	4
Pig	4

CAUDAL (coccygeal) VERTEBRAE: the vertebrae of the tail varying in number between the species and within the species. They become progressively smaller distally.

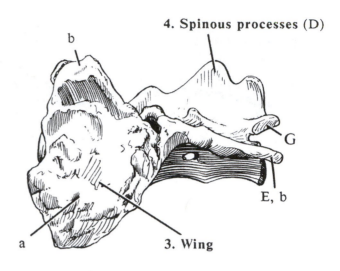

4. Spinous processes (D)

3. Wing

Fig. II-90 - Dog - Sacrum - lat. view

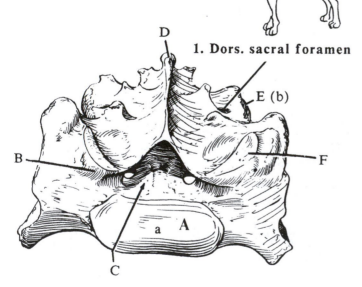

Fig. II-89 - Dog - Sacrum - dorsocran. view

1. Dors. sacral foramen

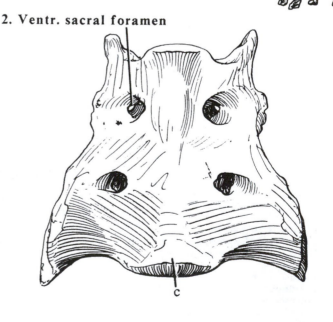

2. Ventr. sacral foramen

Fig. II-91 - Dog - Sacrum - ventr. view

SACRUM

Fig. II-92 - Horse - Sacrum - dorsolat. view

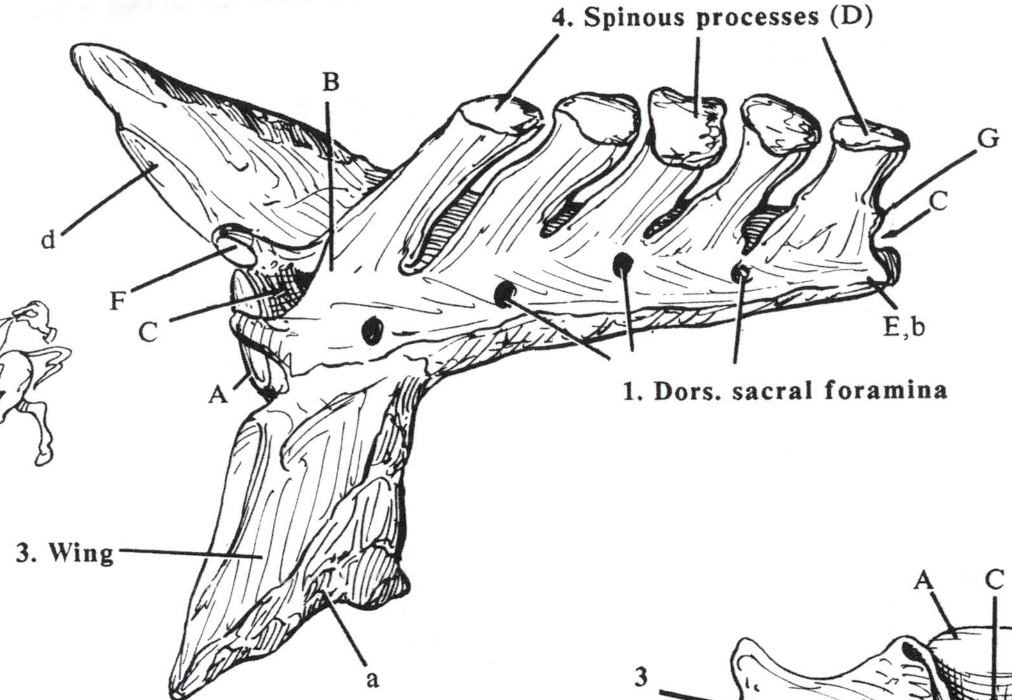
4. Spinous processes (D)
B
G
C
d
F
C
E,b
A
1. Dors. sacral foramina
3. Wing
a

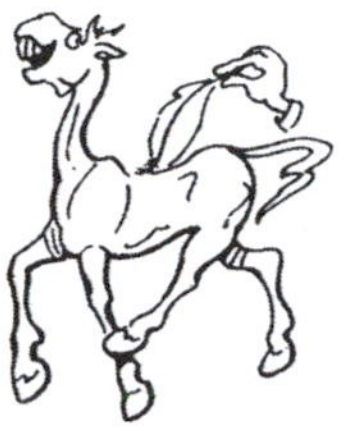

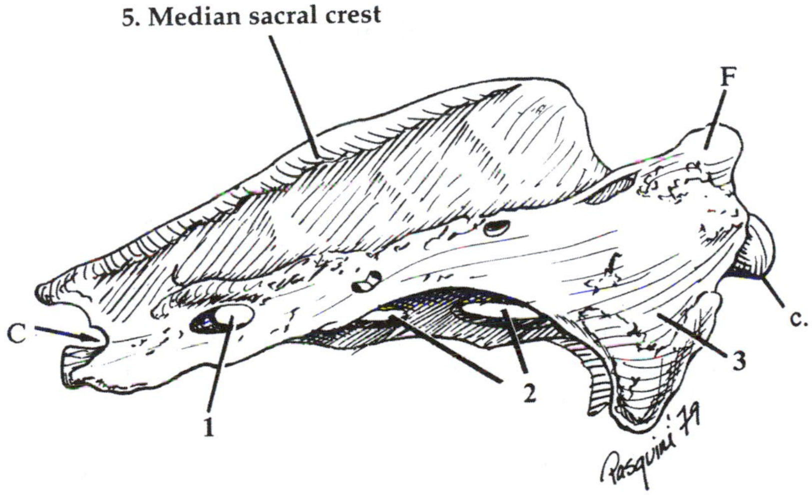
5. Median sacral crest
F
C
c.
3
2
1
Pasquini 79

Fig. II-93 - Ox - Sacrum - lat. view

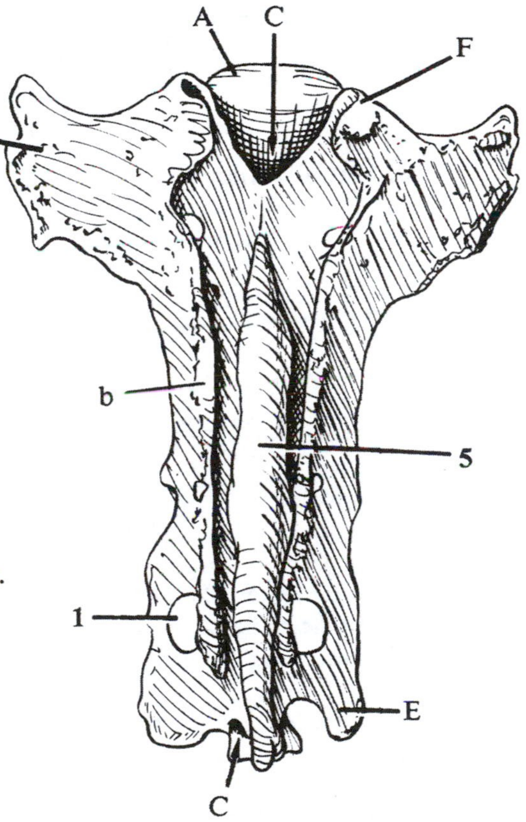
A
C
F
3
b
5
1
E
C

Fig. II-94 - Ox - Sacrum - dors. view

A. Body
B. Vertebral arch
C. Vertebral (sacral) canal
D. Spine
E. Transverse process
F. Cran. articular process
G. Caud. articular process

a. Articular (auricular) surface for ilium
b. Lat. sacral crest
c. Promontory
d. Surface for articulating with transverse process of last lumbar vertebra (horse)

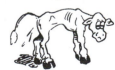

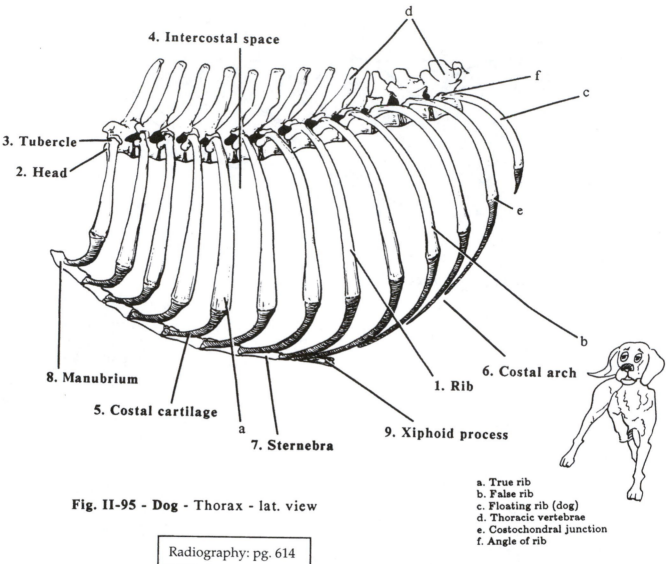

4. Intercostal space

d

f

c

3. Tubercle

2. Head

e

b

8. Manubrium

6. Costal arch

1. Rib

5. Costal cartilage

a

9. Xiphoid process

7. Sternebra

Fig. II-95 - Dog - Thorax - lat. view

a. True rib
b. False rib
c. Floating rib (dog)
d. Thoracic vertebrae
e. Costochondral junction
f. Angle of rib

Radiography: pg. 614

THORAX: the bony cavity formed by the sternum, the ribs, the costal cartilages, and the bodies of the thoracic vertebrae. The thorax encloses and protects the thoracic organs.

1. RIBS (L. *costae*): the long, curved bones forming the lateral wall of the thorax.

• **True ribs** (a) (sternal ribs) articulate directly by their costal cartilage with the sternum.

• **False ribs** (b) (asternal ribs): all ribs that are not true ribs. Their costal cartilages unite to form the costal arch, indirectly joining them to the sternum in all but dog

• **Floating ribs** (c), last false ribs found in the dog & man. They end in costal cartilage that does not join to the sternum or other costal cartilage.

2. Head of the rib: articulates with caudal and cranial costal fovea of adjacent thoracic vertebrae and the intervening intervertebral disc.

3. Tubercle of the rib: articulates with the transverse process of the same numbered vertebra.

4. Intercostal space: the space between two adjacent ribs.

5. COSTAL CARTILAGE (L. *costa*, rib): the bars of hyaline cartilage either connecting the bony rib to the sternum or to the costal arch or ending freely.

6. Costal arch: the curved structure formed by the costal cartilages of the false ribs.

7. STERNUM or **breastbone:** the unpaired bones (sternebrae) forming the floor of the thorax.

70

THORAX

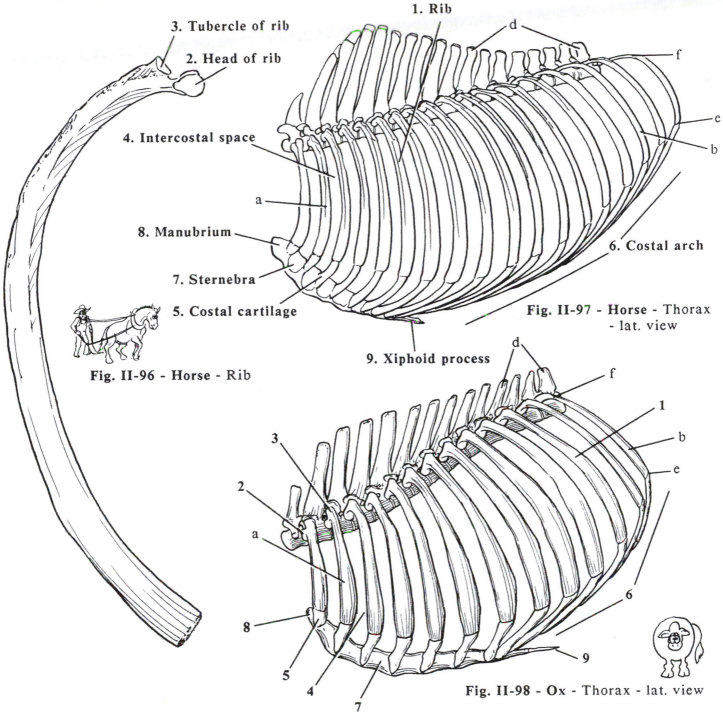

3. Tubercle of rib

2. Head of rib

4. Intercostal space

1. Rib

8. Manubrium

7. Sternebra

5. Costal cartilage

9. Xiphoid process

6. Costal arch

Fig. II-96 - Horse - Rib

Fig. II-97 - Horse - Thorax - lat. view

Fig. II-98 - Ox - Thorax - lat. view

8. Manubrium (ma-NOO-bri-um) (L. handle): the expanded first sternebra.

9. Xiphoid process (ZY-foyd) (G. *xiphos*, sword): the last sternebra which is a thin, horizontal bone capped by the **xiphoid cartilage**.

10. "THORACIC INLET" or **cranial thoracic opening**: formed by the last cervical vertebra, first pair of ribs and the sternum.

11. "THORACIC OUTLET" or caudal thoracic opening: sealed by the diaphragm.

SPECIES DIFFERENCES

Floating ribs: last pair in dogs only.

Number of sternebrae: carnivores - 8, pig, horse and man - 6, ruminants - 7.

DOG - SKELETON - THORACIC LIMB

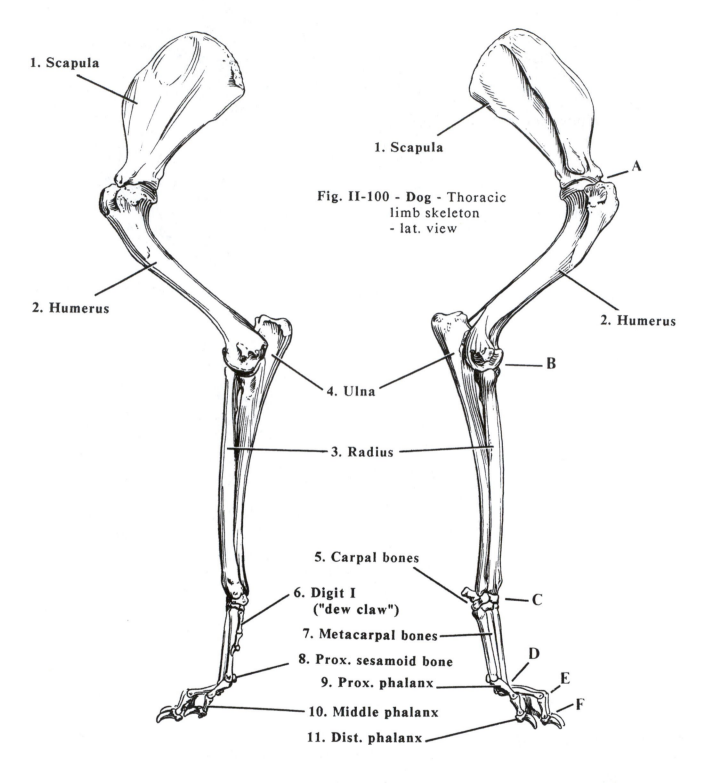

1. Scapula

1. Scapula

Fig. II-100 - Dog - Thoracic limb skeleton - lat. view

A

2. Humerus

2. Humerus

B

4. Ulna

3. Radius

5. Carpal bones

6. Digit I ("dew claw")

C

7. Metacarpal bones

D

8. Prox. sesamoid bone

9. Prox. phalanx

E

10. Middle phalanx

F

11. Dist. phalanx

Fig. II-99 - Dog - Thoracic limb skeleton - med. view

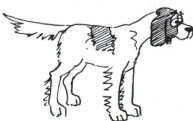

A. Shoulder joint
B. Elbow joint
C. "Carpal" articulations
D. Metacarpophalangeal articulations
E. Prox. interphalangeal articulations
F. Dist. interphalangeal articulations

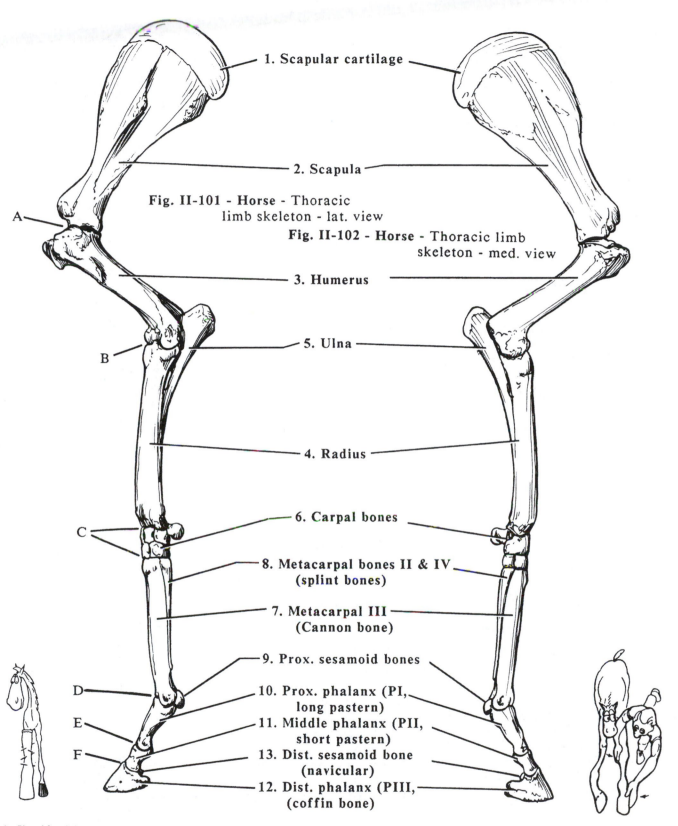

1. Scapular cartilage

2. Scapula

Fig. II-101 - Horse - Thoracic
limb skeleton - lat. view

Fig. II-102 - Horse - Thoracic limb
skeleton - med. view

3. Humerus

5. Ulna

4. Radius

6. Carpal bones

8. Metacarpal bones II & IV
(splint bones)

7. Metacarpal III
(Cannon bone)

9. Prox. sesamoid bones

10. Prox. phalanx (PI,
long pastern)

11. Middle phalanx (PII,
short pastern)

13. Dist. sesamoid bone
(navicular)

12. Dist. phalanx (PIII,
(coffin bone)

A. Shoulder joint
B. Elbow joint
C. "Carpal" articulation
("knee")

D. Metacarpophalangeal
articulation (fetlock joint)

E. Prox. interphalangeal
articulation (pastern joint)
F. Dist. interphalangeal
articulation (coffin joint)

OX - SKELETON - THORACIC LIMB

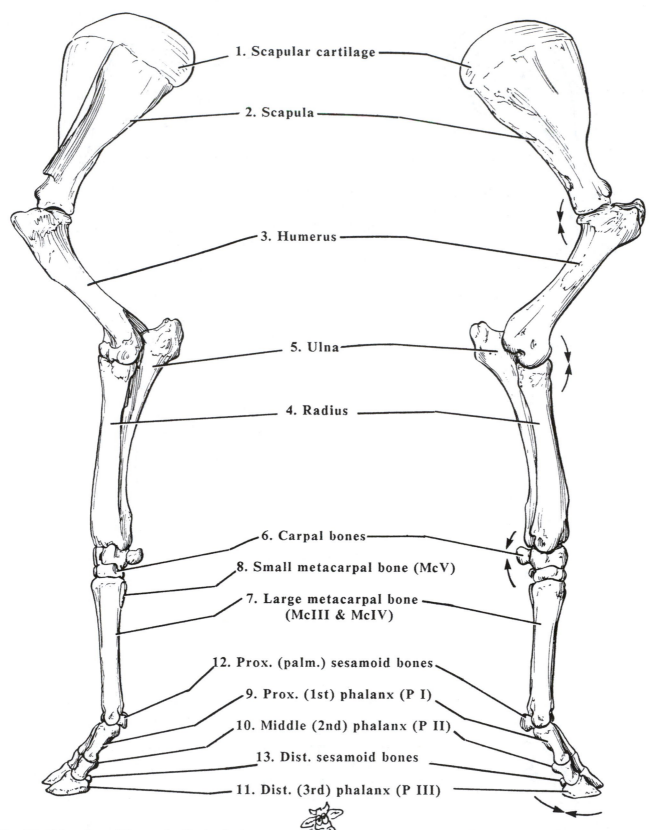

1. Scapular cartilage

2. Scapula

3. Humerus

5. Ulna

4. Radius

6. Carpal bones

8. Small metacarpal bone (McV)

7. Large metacarpal bone (McIII & McIV)

12. Prox. (palm.) sesamoid bones

9. Prox. (1st) phalanx (P I)

10. Middle (2nd) phalanx (P II)

13. Dist. sesamoid bones

11. Dist. (3rd) phalanx (P III)

Fig. II-103 - Ox - Thoracic limb skeleton
- lat. view

Fig. II-104 - Ox - Thoracic limb skeleton
- med. view

PIG – SKELETON – THORACIC LIMB

Fig. II-105 - Pig - Thoracic limb skeleton
- lat. view

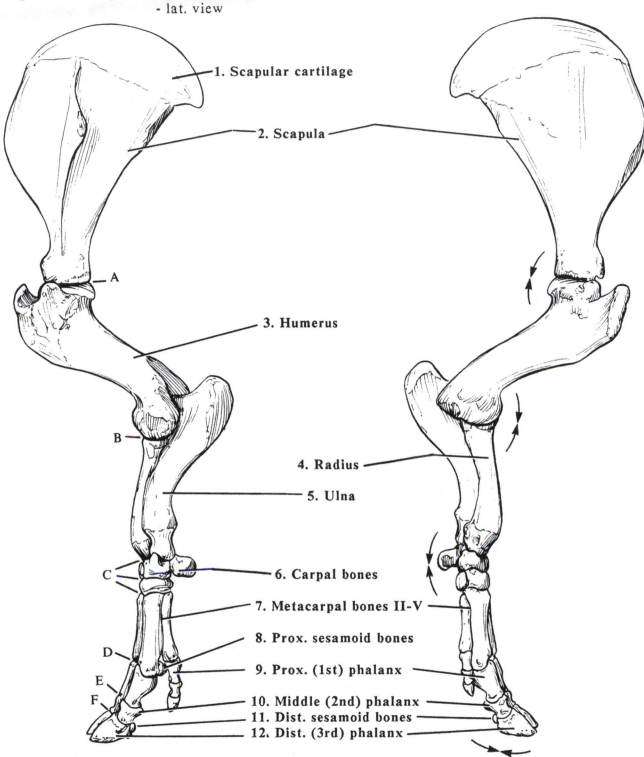

1. Scapular cartilage

2. Scapula

A

3. Humerus

B

4. Radius

5. Ulna

C

6. Carpal bones

7. Metacarpal bones II-V

8. Prox. sesamoid bones

D

9. Prox. (1st) phalanx

E

10. Middle (2nd) phalanx

F

11. Dist. sesamoid bones

12. Dist. (3rd) phalanx

Fig. II-106 - Pig - Thoracic limb
skeleton - med. view

A. Shoulder joint
B. Elbow joint
C. "Carpal" joints

D. Metacarpophalangeal joint
E. Prox. interphalangeal joint
F. Dist. interphalangeal joint

Converging arrows
indicate angle of
flexion of joint

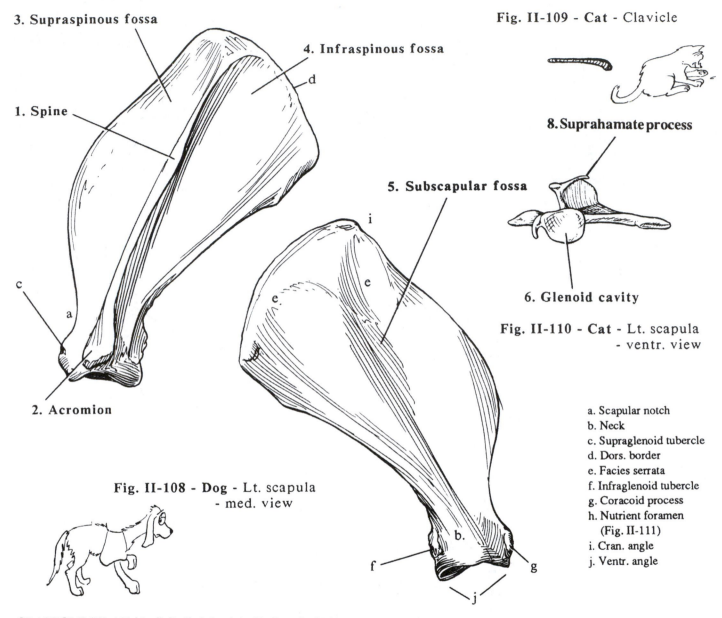

Fig. II-107 - **Dog** - Lt. scapula - lat. view

3. Supraspinous fossa

4. Infraspinous fossa

1. Spine

Fig. II-109 - **Cat** - Clavicle

8. Suprahamate process

5. Subscapular fossa

c

a

2. Acromion

6. Glenoid cavity

Fig. II-110 - **Cat** - Lt. scapula
- ventr. view

Fig. II-108 - **Dog** - Lt. scapula
- med. view

a. Scapular notch
b. Neck
c. Supraglenoid tubercle
d. Dors. border
e. Facies serrata
f. Infraglenoid tubercle
g. Coracoid process
h. Nutrient foramen
   (Fig. II-111)
i. Cran. angle
j. Ventr. angle

CLAVICLE (KLAV-i-kul) (L. little key) (collar bone): the bone articulating with the shoulder and the sternum in man to maintain the shoulder in a lateral position. The domestic animals need their thoracic limb under their bodies, so the clavicle is absent or rudimentary.

SCAPULA (SCAP-yoo-la) ("shoulder blade"): the flat, triangular bone of the shoulder. The two scapulae make up the thoracic girdle.

1. Spine of the scapula: the long projection dividing the scapula's lateral surface and ending as the acromion.

2. Acromion (a-KROH-mee-on): the expanded distal end of the spine of the scapula.

3. Supraspinous fossa (soo'-pra-SPY-nus): the area cranial to the spine providing attachment for the supraspinatus muscle.

4. Infraspinous fossa: the area caudal to the spine providing attachment for the infraspinatus muscle.

5. Subscapular fossa: most of the medial (costal) surface of the scapula providing attachment for the subscapular muscle. The dorsal part of the costal surface is the serrated surface (e) for the attachment of the serratus ventralis muscle.

6. Glenoid cavity: the shallow cavity articulating with the head of the humerus to form the shoulder joint.

7. Scapular cartilage: the cartilaginous structure on the dorsal border of the scapula.

SCALPULA

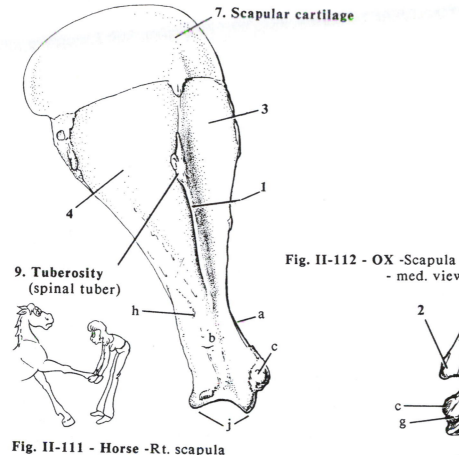

7. Scapular cartilage

3

1

4

9. Tuberosity
(spinal tuber)

h

a

b

c

Fig. II-111 - Horse -Rt. scapula
- lat. view

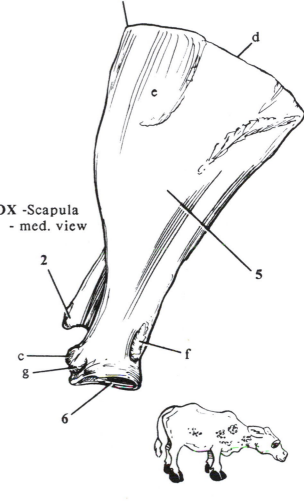

i

d

e

2

5

c

g

f

6

Fig. II-112 - OX -Scapula
- med. view

Radiography: pg. 643

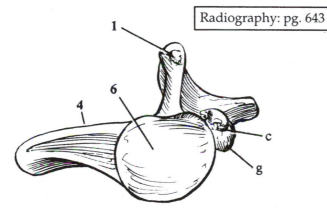

1

4

6

c

g

Fig. II-107 - Ox - Rt. scapula - ventr. view

Supraglenoid tubercle: the process near the cranial aspect of the glenoid cavity, providing attachment for the biceps brachii muscle.

Coracoid process (KOR-ah koid) (Gr. crowlike)(g): the small process on the medial side of the supraglenoid tubercle for the attachment of the coracobrachialis muscle.

8. Suprahamate process: the caudal projection of the acromion found only in the **cat**. The distal end of the spine can be called the acromion or hamate (L. hooked) process.

SPECIES DIFFERENCES:

Clavicle: Cat - a separate, non-articulating bone, seen radiographically. **Dog** - a rudimentary structure attached to the deep surface of the brachiocephalic muscle, rarely seen radiographically. **Horse** and **Ox** - absent.

Acromion (2): absent in the **horse and pig.**

9. Spinal tuber: a bony enlargement of the scapular spine found in the **horse** and **pig** (poorly developed in the cat and ox).

Scapular cartilage (7): a narrow band in the dog, while in the **horse, ruminants** and **pig** it is a broad, thin structure.

CLINICAL

Clavicle: in the cat can be mistaken for a bone in the esophagus on lateral radiographs.

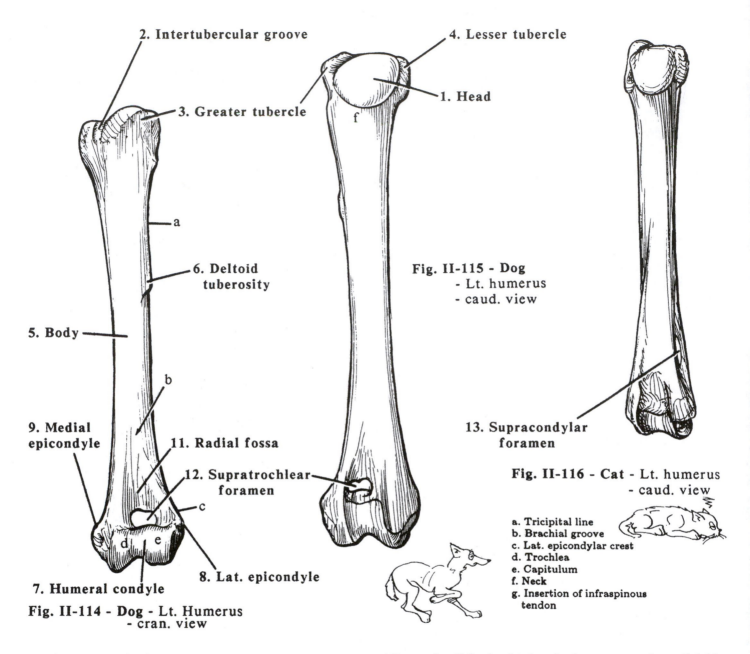

2. Intertubercular groove

4. Lesser tubercle

3. Greater tubercle

1. Head

f

a

6. Deltoid tuberosity

5. Body

Fig. II-115 - Dog
- Lt. humerus
- caud. view

b

9. Medial epicondyle

11. Radial fossa

12. Supratrochlear foramen

c

13. Supracondylar foramen

d e

Fig. II-116 - Cat - Lt. humerus
- caud. view

8. Lat. epicondyle

7. Humeral condyle

Fig. II-114 - Dog - Lt. Humerus
- cran. view

a. Tricipital line
b. Brachial groove
c. Lat. epicondylar crest
d. Trochlea
e. Capitulum
f. Neck
g. Insertion of infraspinous tendon

HUMERUS (HYOO-mer-us) (arm or brachial bone): the largest bone of the thoracic limb. It articulates proximally with the scapula, forming the shoulder joint; and distally with the radius and ulna, forming the elbow joint.

1. Head: the rounded process articulating with the scapula's glenoid cavity to form the shoulder joint.

2. Intertubercular (bicipital) **groove:** the sulcus between the greater and lesser tubercles through which the tendon of the biceps brachii muscle runs.

3. Greater (lateral, major) **tubercle:** the large process cranio-lateral to the head to which many muscles attach. The **point of the shoulder** is a surface feature formed by the greater tubercle.

4. Lesser (medial, minor) **tubercle:** the process on the medial side of the head.

5. Body (shaft, diaphysis): the cylindrical part connecting the two ends (epiphyses) of the bone.

6. Deltoid tuberosity: the large tuberosity on the lateral side of the humerus.

7. Humeral condyle: the entire distal extremity of the humerus, including the two articular areas (humeral capitulum and humeral trochlea), the two fossae (three fossae in the cat) and the lateral and medial epicondyles.

8. Lateral epicondyle: the lateral side of the humeral condyle, giving rise to the extensors of the forearm. Functionally it is

HUMERUS

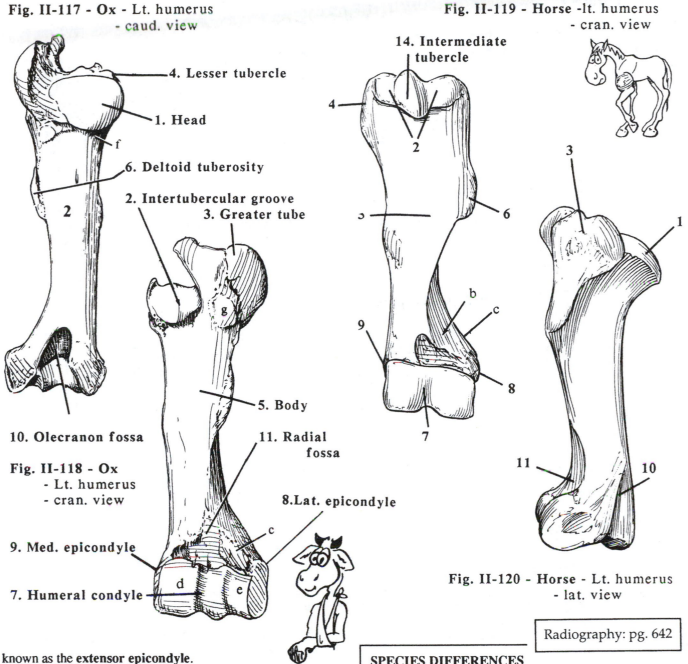

Fig. II-117 - Ox - Lt. humerus - caud. view

4. Lesser tubercle

1. Head

f

6. Deltoid tuberosity

2

2. Intertubercular groove

3. Greater tube

5. Body

10. Olecranon fossa

11. Radial fossa

g

Fig. II-118 - Ox - Lt. humerus - cran. view

9. Med. epicondyle

8. Lat. epicondyle

7. Humeral condyle

c

d   e

Fig. II-119 - Horse -lt. humerus - cran. view

14. Intermediate tubercle

4

2

5

6

9

b

c

8

7

3

1

b

c

11

10

Fig. II-120 - Horse - Lt. humerus - lat. view

Radiography: pg. 642

known as the **extensor epicondyle**.

9. Medial epicondyle: the medial-most point of the humeral condyle, functionally known as the **flexor epicondyle** because it provides attachment for the flexor muscles of the forearm.

10. Olecranon fossa (oh-LEK-ra-non): the caudal excavation receiving the proximal end of the ulna on extension of the elbow.

11. Radial fossa: the excavation opposite the olecranon fossa receiving the proximal end of the radius on flexion of the elbow. The cat has a small coronoid fossa medial to the radial fossa for the medial coronoid process of the ulna on flexion of the elbow.

SPECIES DIFFERENCES

12. Supratrochlear foramen: the hole between the olecranon and the radial fossa found in the dog and sometimes the pig. Nothing passes through it.

13. Supracondylar foramen: the opening in the medial epicondyle present only in the **cat**. To remember which side it is on, the median nerve and brachial vessels pass through it.

14. Intermediate tubercle: a prominence in the **horse's** intertubercular groove.

3. Greater tubercle: is divided into cranial and caudal parts in the **horse** and **ox**.

ULNA & RADIUS

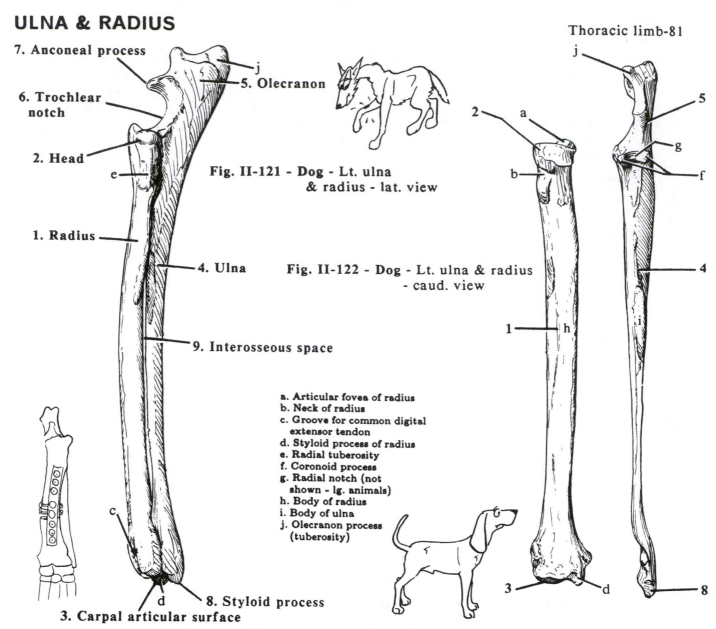

7. Anconeal process

6. Trochlear notch

2. Head

1. Radius

4. Ulna

9. Interosseous space

5. Olecranon

Fig. II-121 - Dog - Lt. ulna & radius - lat. view

Fig. II-122 - Dog - Lt. ulna & radius - caud. view

a. Articular fovea of radius
b. Neck of radius
c. Groove for common digital extensor tendon
d. Styloid process of radius
e. Radial tuberosity
f. Coronoid process
g. Radial notch (not shown - lg. animals)
h. Body of radius
i. Body of ulna
j. Olecranon process (tuberosity)

8. Styloid process

3. Carpal articular surface

1. RADIUS (L. spoke of a wheel): the main weight-bearing bone of the forearm, articulating with the humerus and ulna forming the elbow joint and with the carpal bones and ulna forming the antebrachiocarpal joint. Three distal grooves on its cranial surface accommodate tendons.

2. Head: the proximal part of the radius which articulates (fovea capitis, a) with the humerus (capitulum) and ulna.

3. Carpal articular surface: the articular surface on the distal end of the radius (trochlea) which articulates with the carpal bones.

Styloid process of radius (d): distal end of the radius.

4. ULNA (L. elbow): the long, thin bone serving mainly for muscle attachment and formation of the elbow joint. Proximally it articulates with the humerus and radius, distally with the radius and the carpal bones.

5 . Olecranon (Oh-LEK-ra-non): the proximal part of the ulna

providing a lever arm for the extensor muscles of the elbow. It forms the point of the elbow.

6. Trochlear notch (TROHK-lee-ar) (semilunar notch): the depression for articulation with the humerus and ending in the anconeal process.

7. Anconeal process: the proximal end of the trochlear notch which fits in the olecranon fossa of the humerus when the elbow is extended.

Medial coronoid process (f): the large distal end of the trochlear notch.

8. Styloid process of the ulna: the pointed, distal end of the ulna.

9. Interosseous space: the space between the ulna and radius, readily seen in the carnivores and pig. The horse has a proximal interosseous space and the ox has proximal and distal ones.

ULNA & RADIUS

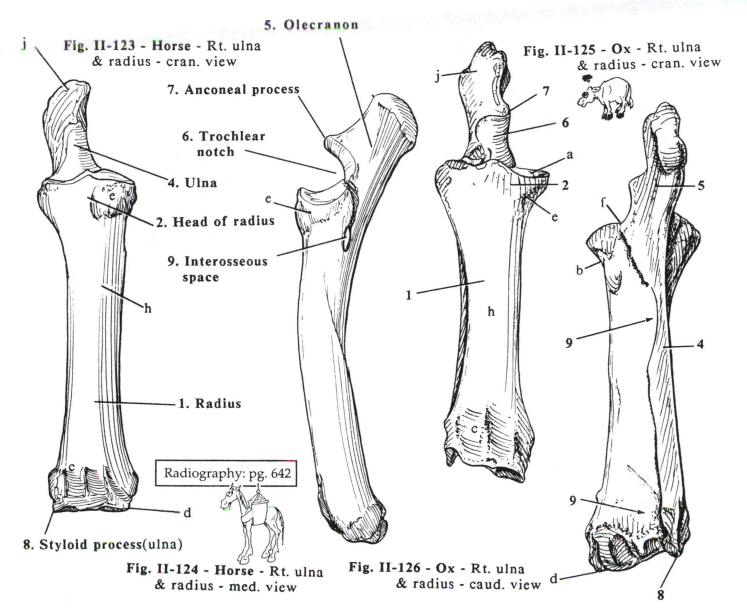

Fig. II-123 - Horse - Rt. ulna & radius - cran. view

5. Olecranon

7. Anconeal process

6. Trochlear notch

4. Ulna

2. Head of radius

9. Interosseous space

1. Radius

Radiography: pg. 642

8. Styloid process(ulna)

Fig. II-124 - Horse - Rt. ulna & radius - med. view

Fig. II-125 - Ox - Rt. ulna & radius - cran. view

Fig. II-126 - Ox - Rt. ulna & radius - caud. view

SPECIES DIFFERENCES

Ulna: fuses with the radius in the **horse** and **ruminant**; therefore, these animals cannot supinate or pronate their forearm. It is not fused in the **carnivores** and **pig,** allowing pronation and supination.

Styloid process of ulna: the distal epiphysis of the **horse's** ulna is fused with the radius, and in essence becomes a part of the radius.

CLINICAL

Ununited anconeal process: failure of the secondary ossification of the anconeal process to unite with the ulna after five months of age.

Fragmented medial coronoid process

(f): can cause degenerative joint disease of the elbow.

Premature closure of the epiphyseal growth plate (epiphyseal cartilage, physis): can occur in the distal radius or ulna. The other bone will continue growing causing deformities of the bones distal to the carpus and joint problems in the elbow.

Angular limb deformities in foals: can be caused by opposite sides of the distal growth plate of the radius growing at different rates. If caught early it may be surgically corrected. A staple may be driven on either side of the physis to slow its growth and allow the other side to catch up. This must be removed when the limb straightens or the limb will deviate the opposite way. Periosteal stripping is the cutting of the periosteum on the side of the physis that is growing slowly. This may speed up its growth to catch up with the other side.

CARPUS

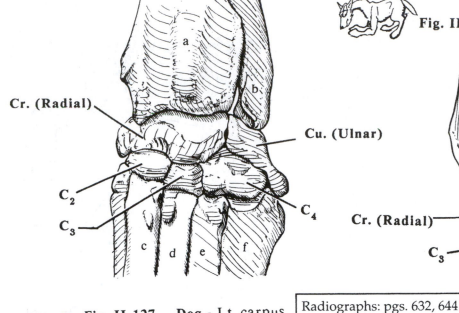

Fig. II-128 - Dog - Lt. carpus - lat. view

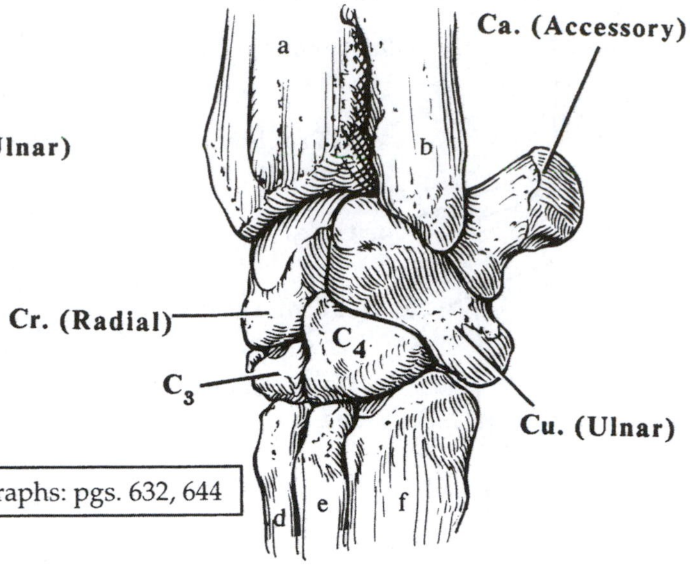

Fig. II-127 - Dog - Lt. carpus - dors. view

Radiographs: pgs. 632, 644

MANUS: the distal part of the thoracic limb, consisting of the carpus, metacarpus, phalanges and their associated sesamoid bones. It is also called the **forepaw** in the carnivores.

CARPUS (KAR-pus) (L. wrist): the carpal bones; also the compound joint formed by these bones, or the region between the forearm and metacarpus.

CARPAL BONES: the two rows of bones forming the carpus. The number of carpal bones varies between species due to fusion between bones or absence of one or more bones. The pig has the generalized pattern of eight bones. The proximal row consists of the radial carpal, intermediate carpal, ulnar carpal and accessory carpal bones. The distal row, from medial to lateral, consists of carpal bones 1-4.

Proximal row:
- **Cr. Radial**: the largest carpal bone, medial
- **Ci. Intermediate**: between the radial and ulnar carpal bones.
- **Cu. Ulnar**: lateral bone in the proximal row.
- **Ca. Accessory**: projects behind (palmar) the carpus, articulating with the ulnar carpal. (only carpal bone to which muscles attach - flexor carpi ulnaris and extensor carpi ulnaris).

Distal row: consists of the 1st, 2nd, 3rd and 4th carpal bones (C_1, C_2, C_3 & C_4) in the generalized pattern.

SPECIES DIFFERENCES

Pig (Fig. II-143-144): has the "generalized" carpus of eight bones.

Horse: conforms to the generalized pattern of eight bones unless the 1st carpal bone is missing, or rarely if a fifth one is present.

Dog and cat: have seven carpal bones due to fusion of the radial and intermediate carpal bones to form the dog's "radial" carpal bone.

Ruminant: has six carpal bones. The 1st carpal bone is missing and the 2nd and 3rd carpal bones are fused.

CLINICAL

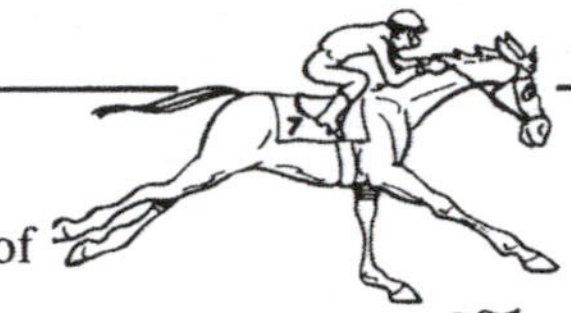

Chip fractures of carpus: #1 fracture of racehorses, caused by overextension at speed. They are usually on the dorsomedial aspect of carpus and thus best viewed with a DMO (dorsomedial oblique) radiograph. The distal radial carpal is the #1 site in Thoroughbreds and the proximal third carpal is the #1 site in Standardbreds.

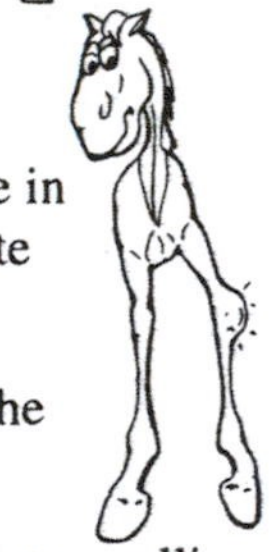

Slab fractures: occur in racehorses most commonly in the third carpal bone followed by the intermediate carpal.

Sesamoid bone of the oblique carpal extensor (abductor pollicus longus) tendon: located on the medial side of the carpus and shouldn't be mistaken for a chip fracture.

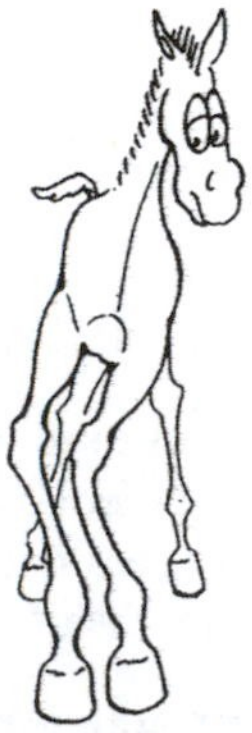

Valgus and varus: terms for deviation of the bones distal to a joint. These can be caused by premature closure of the distal growth plates of the ulna or radius in carnivores or by differential growth rates of the distal physis of the radius in foals.
- **Carpus valgus**: lateral deviation of the bones distal to the carpus. (Memory aid - "L" in vaLgus for lateral deviation.)
- **Carpus varus**: medial deviation of the bones distal to the carpus.

CARPUS

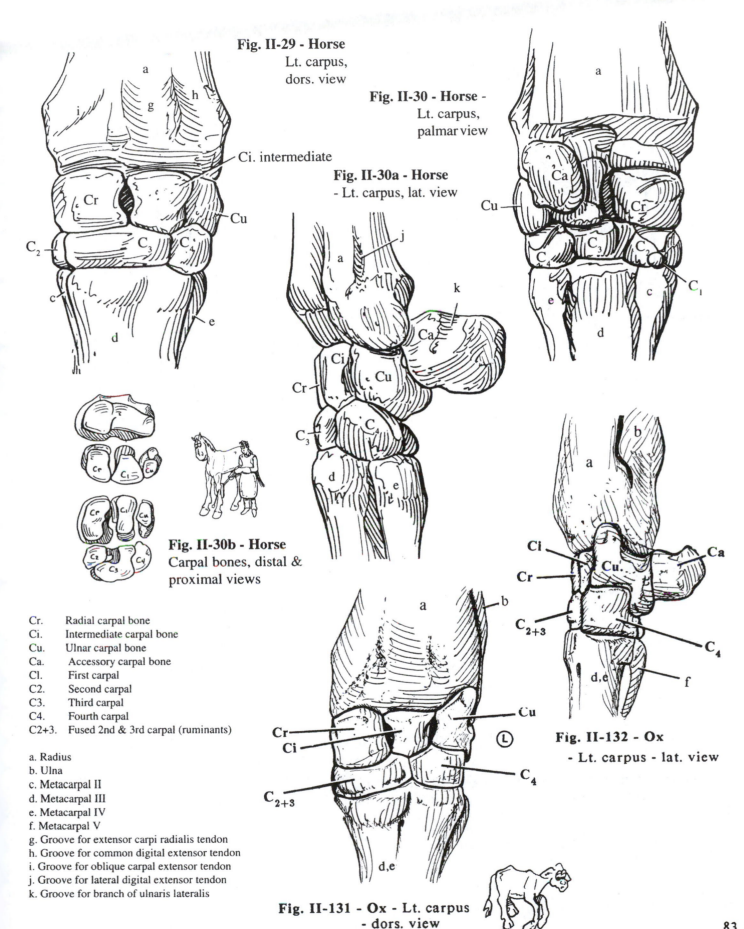

Fig. II-29 - Horse
Lt. carpus, dors. view

Fig. II-30 - Horse -
Lt. carpus, palmar view

Fig. II-30a - Horse
- Lt. carpus, lat. view

Ci. intermediate

Fig. II-30b - Horse
Carpal bones, distal & proximal views

Cr.   Radial carpal bone
Ci.   Intermediate carpal bone
Cu.   Ulnar carpal bone
Ca.   Accessory carpal bone
Cl.   First carpal
C2.   Second carpal
C3.   Third carpal
C4.   Fourth carpal
C2+3. Fused 2nd & 3rd carpal (ruminants)

a. Radius
b. Ulna
c. Metacarpal II
d. Metacarpal III
e. Metacarpal IV
f. Metacarpal V
g. Groove for extensor carpi radialis tendon
h. Groove for common digital extensor tendon
i. Groove for oblique carpal extensor tendon
j. Groove for lateral digital extensor tendon
k. Groove for branch of ulnaris lateralis

Fig. II-132 - Ox
- Lt. carpus - lat. view

Fig. II-131 - Ox - Lt. carpus
- dors. view

83

METACARPAL BONES

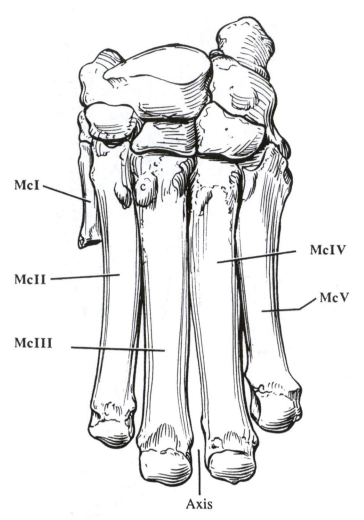

Axis

Fig. II-133 - Dog - Lt. metacarpal
bones - dors. view

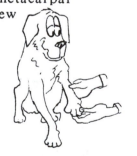

McI
McII
McIII
McIV
McV

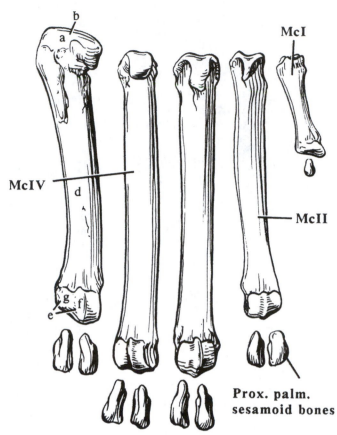

McI

McIV

McII

Prox. palm.
sesamoid bones

Fig. II-134 - Dog - Lt. metacarpal bones
- palm. view

McI Metacarpal I	a. Base
McII Metacarpal II	b. Carpal articular surface
McIII Metacarpal III	c. Metacarpal tuberosity
McIV Metacarpal IV	d. Body
McV Metacarpal V	e. Head
	f. Sagittal ridge
	g. Condyles (med. & lat.)

METACARPUS: the region of the manus located between the carpus and digits.

METACARPAL BONES: the generalized metacarpus has five bones numbered I-V from medial to lateral. The species differ due to absence or fusion of bones. Each bone is composed of a base articulating with the carpus, a head articulating with the proximal phalanx of a digit, and a shaft connecting the two extremities. Two sesamoid bone are associated with each weight bearing metacarpal bone.

CARNIVORE METACARPAL BONES: the generalized pattern of five metacarpal bones. Metacarpal I (McI) is much reduced, bears no weight, has one associated sesamoid bone. It is part of the dew claw.

METACARPAL BONES

PIG METACARPAL BONES (Fig. II-143 & 144): has four metacarpal bones. The 1st metacarpal bone (McI) is missing. Metacarpal bones II and V (McII and McV) are greatly reduced and don't bear weight. The weight is borne by metacarpals III and IV (McIII and McIV).

HORSE METACARPAL BONES: has three metacarpal bones, the 1st and 5th are missing.

Splint bones: the common name for the greatly reduced metacarpals II and IV (McII and McIV). The splints end distally in small swellings called the **"buttons of the splints"**.

Cannon bone: the common name for the large metacarpal III (McIII). It is the only metacarpal to articulate with the digit.

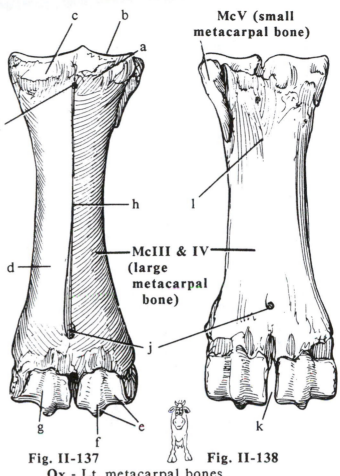

McV (small metacarpal bone)

McII & IV (large metacarpal bone)

Fig. II-137   **Fig. II-138**
Ox - Lt. metacarpal bones
- dors. view   - palm. view

RUMINANT DIFFERENCES
h. Dors. longitudinal groove   k. Intertrochlear incisure
i. Prox. metacarpal canal   l. Palm. longitudinal groove
j. Dist. metacarpal canal

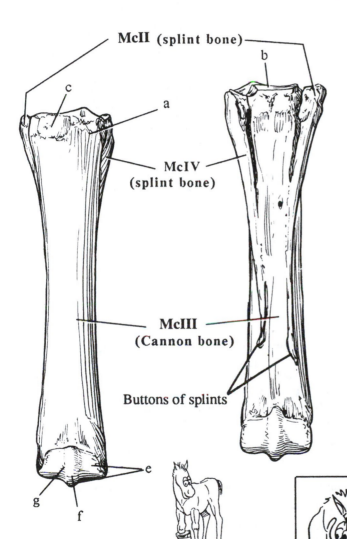

McII (splint bone)

McIV (splint bone)

McIII (Cannon bone)

Buttons of splints

Radiography: pg. 642

Fig. II-135   **Fig. II-136**
Horse - Lt. Metacarpal bone
- dors. view   - palm. view

RUMINANT METACARPAL BONES: two metacarpal bones. The 1st and 2nd (McI and McII) are missing and the 3rd and 4th are fused.

Large metacarpal bone (cannon bone): the common name for <u>fused</u> metacarpals III & IV.

Small metacarpal bone: the common name for the greatly reduced metacarpal V (McV).

CLINICAL - HORSE METACARPUS

"Bucked shins": the inflammation (periostitis) of the dorsal surface of the horse's cannon bone affecting horses mostly under three years of age.

"Splints": an inflammation of the horse's interosseous ligament and build up of bone between the splint bones and the cannon bone (not to be confused with the splint bones).

"Fractured splint": a fracture of a splint bone.

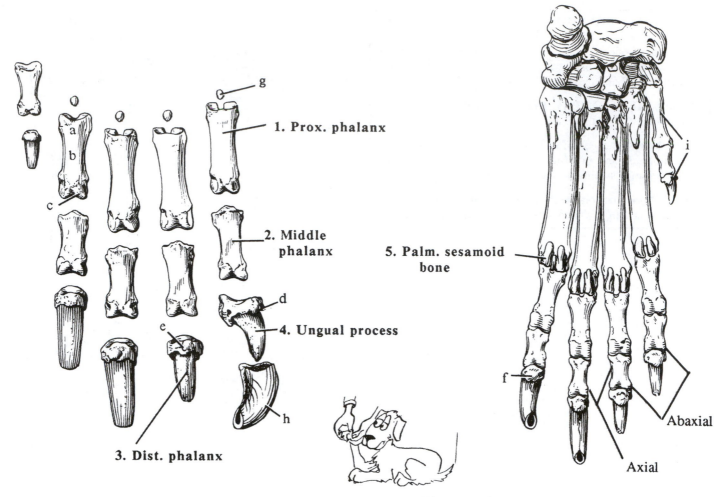

Fig. II-139 - Dog - Lt. digits - dors. view

1. Prox. phalanx
2. Middle phalanx
5. Palm. sesamoid bone
4. Ungual process
3. Dist. phalanx

Abaxial

Axial

Fig. II-140 - Dog - Lt. manus - palm. view

DIGITS: regional subdivision of the manus and pes, correspond to the fingers and toes of man. There are five digits in the generalized digital pattern, numbered from medial to lateral (I-V). Species differences are due to reduction in the number of digits. The digits generally consist of three phalanges, a number of sesamoid bones, tendons, ligaments, vessels, nerves and skin.

Dew claw or paradigit: a digit not bearing weight.

CARNIVORE - DIGITS: four main weight-bearing digits (II-V).

Dew claw (i): the 1st digit and the 1st metacarpal bone. The 1st digit is reduced in size having only two phalanges, the proximal and distal, and one proximal sesamoid bone. Some dog breeds have double dew claws.

1. Proximal phalanx (FAY-lanks): the first phalanx divided into the base, body, and head.

2. Middle phalanx: the second phalanx with the same structure as the proximal phalanx, but shorter. It is not present in the first digit.

3. Distal phalanx: the third phalanx carries the horny claw. The flexor process (f) on the palmar side provides insertion for the deep digital flexor tendon. The **extensor process** (e) located on the dorsal proximal part of the four main digits provides insertion for the tendons of the common digital extensor muscle (long digital extensor muscle in the hindlimb).

4. Ungual process: the tapered, cone-shaped process covered by the horny claw.

Horny claw (h): the fingernail-like structure covering the ungual process.

5. Palmar sesamoid bones: the nine small bones at the metacarpophalangeal joint; two for each of the four main digits and one for the 1st digit.

Distal sesamoid bones: are represented by cartilage in the carnivores and rarely ossify.

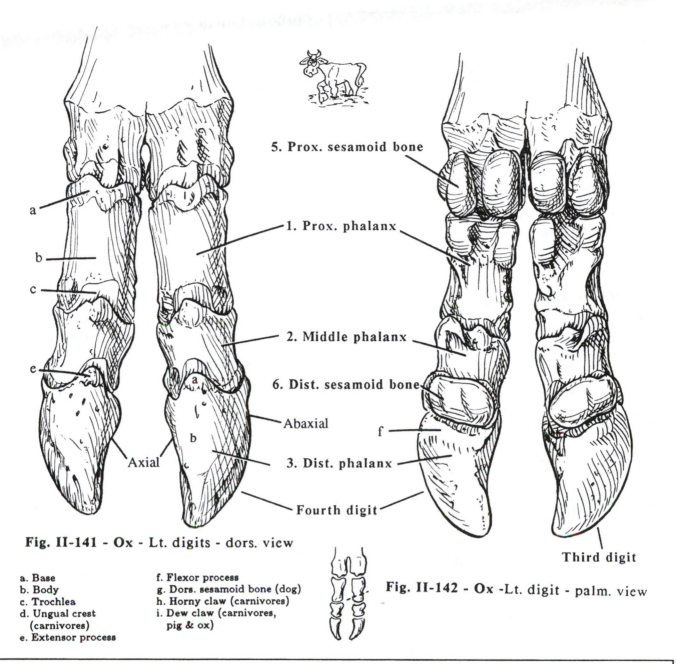

5. Prox. sesamoid bone

1. Prox. phalanx

2. Middle phalanx

6. Dist. sesamoid bone

Abaxial

Axial

3. Dist. phalanx

Fourth digit

a
b
c
e
b
a

Fig. II-141 - Ox - Lt. digits - dors. view

Third digit

Fig. II-142 - Ox -Lt. digit - palm. view

a. Base
b. Body
c. Trochlea
d. Ungual crest
   (carnivores)
e. Extensor process

f. Flexor process
g. Dors. sesamoid bone (dog)
h. Horny claw (carnivores)
i. Dew claw (carnivores,
   pig & ox)

OX - DIGITS: four digits, two weight-bearing and two non-weight-bearing. The 1st digit is missing. The second and fifth digits are vestiges (improbable to find) externally manifested as horny dew claws behind the fetlock.

Third and fourth digits: fully developed weight-bearing digits consisting of three phalanges and three sesamoid bones each. They are numbered medially to laterally.

1. **Proximal phalanx**: the <u>long</u> <u>pastern</u> as in the horse.

2. **Middle phalanx**: the <u>short</u> <u>pastern</u>.

3. **Distal phalanx**: the <u>coffin</u> <u>bone.</u>

Sesamoid bones: two proximal (5) at the metacarpophalangeal joint and one distal (6) at the distal interphalangeal joint for each digit.

CLINICAL

Amputation of digit: possible in cattle because they have another digit. Amputate through the distal end of the proximal phalanx with a Gigli wire.

Wooden block: often attached to one digit to raise the opposite, injured digit off the ground while it heals (ulcerations of sole, subsolar abscess and claw cracks and fractures of distal phalanx).

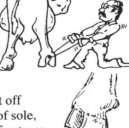

DIGITAL BONES

PIG - DIGITS: four digits, the 1st is missing. The second and fifth are reduced and do not bear weight and are called dew claws. They are fully formed except that they lack a distal sesamoid bone. The main digits (3rd and 4th) consist of three phalanges, two proximal sesamoids and one distal sesamoid.

Fig. II-143 - Pig - Lt. manus - dors. view

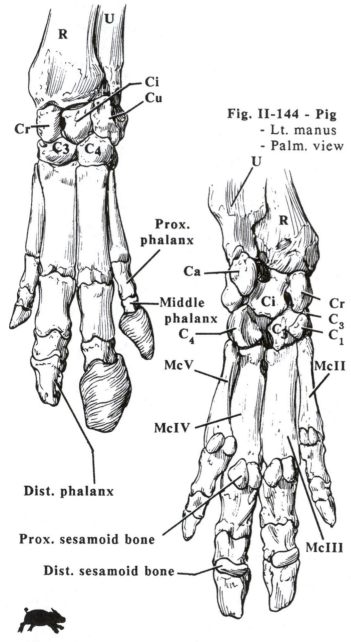

Fig. II-144 - Pig - Lt. manus - Palm. view

Cr — Radial carpal bone
Ci — Intermediate carpal bone
Cu — Ulnar carpal bone
Ca — Accessory carpal bone
C_{1-4} — 1st, 2nd, 3rd & 4th carpal bones

R — Radius
U — Ulna
McII-V — Metacarpal bones

HORSE - DIGITS: one digit per limb supporting Mc III.

1. Proximal phalanx: the **long pastern**.

2. Middle phalanx: the **short pastern**.

3. Distal phalanx, coffin or pedal bone. It fits into the hoof and has an extensor process for the insertion of the digital extensor tendon.
• Parietal surface (a): surface next to the hoof wall.
• Sole surface (b): surface facing the ground.
• Medial and lateral solar foramina (h): entrances to the solar canal for the continuations of the digital arteries.
• Solar canal: the canal between the solar foramina for the terminal arch of the arteries.
• Palmar processes, "angles" or "wings" (c): of the coffin bone.
• Parietal grooves: sulci on the parietal surface.

4. Proximal sesamoid bones or "sesamoids": the two small bones on the palmar side of the metacarpophalangeal (fetlock) joint. The lateral one is taller radiographically than the medial one. This bone is situated between the suspensory ligament and the distal sesamoidean ligaments. Together these make up the suspensory apparatus of the fetlock joint.

5. "Navicular bone" (L. little ship) or distal sesamoid bone: unlike other sesamoid bones it is not embedded in a tendon but is between the deep digital flexor tendon and the middle and distal phalanges. It has articular and flexor surfaces and proximal and distal borders.

CLINICAL - HORSE

Sesamoiditis: common problem of racehorses associated with tearing of suspensory ligament attachments.

Sesamoid fractures: common in racehorses (apical, midbody or basilar locations). This is a suspensory apparatus problem. Breaks to both sesamoids cause disruption of the suspensory apparatus of the fetlock.

Ringbone: periosteal bone deposition on the phalanges, occurring near the pastern joint (proximal interphalangeal joint) is a **high ringbone**; near the coffin joint (distal interphalangeal joint) is a **low ringbone**.

Osselets: ringbone around the metacarpal/metatarsal phalangeal joint (fetlock).

Buttress foot (pyramidal disease): bone deposition at the extensor process of the coffin bone.

"Navicular" disease: a lameness blamed on problems with the distal sesamoid bone and/or the deep digital tendon passing over this bone.

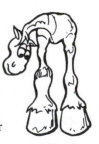

Pedal osteitis: a demineralization of the horse's coffin bone due to inflammation.

Sidebones: ossification of lateral cartilages

DIGITAL BONES

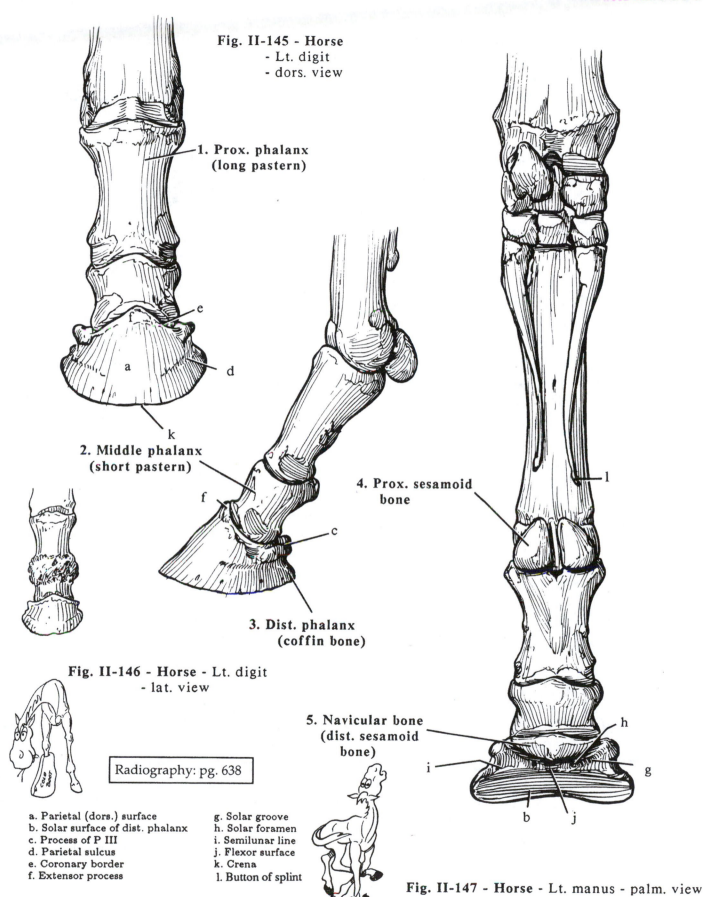

Fig. II-145 - Horse
- Lt. digit
- dors. view

**1. Prox. phalanx
(long pastern)**

**2. Middle phalanx
(short pastern)**

**3. Dist. phalanx
(coffin bone)**

**4. Prox. sesamoid
bone**

**5. Navicular bone
(dist. sesamoid
bone)**

Fig. II-146 - Horse - Lt. digit
- lat. view

Radiography: pg. 638

a. Parietal (dors.) surface
b. Solar surface of dist. phalanx
c. Process of P III
d. Parietal sulcus
e. Coronary border
f. Extensor process

g. Solar groove
h. Solar foramen
i. Semilunar line
j. Flexor surface
k. Crena
l. Button of splint

Fig. II-147 - Horse - Lt. manus - palm. view

89

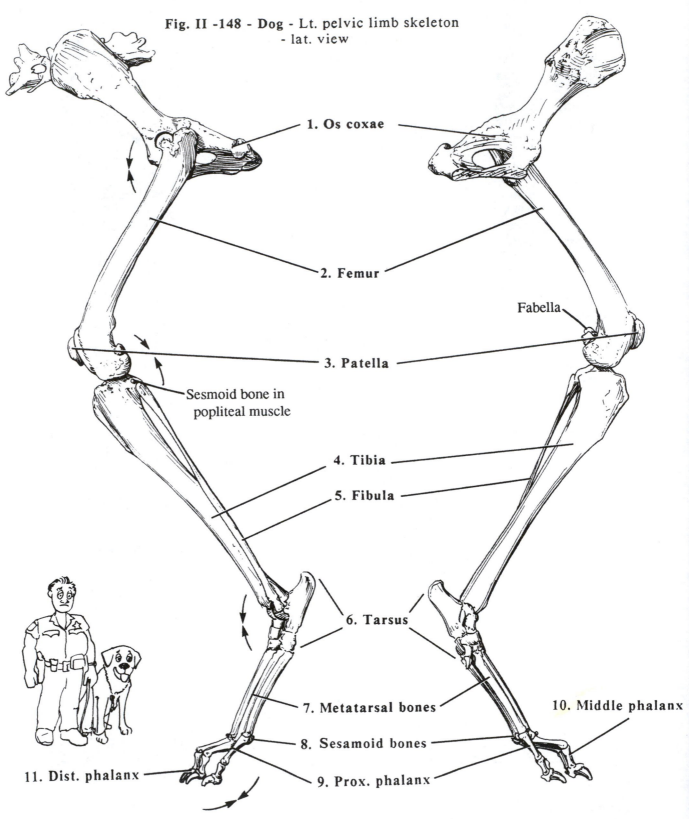

Fig. II -148 - Dog - Lt. pelvic limb skeleton
- lat. view

1. Os coxae

2. Femur

Fabella

3. Patella

Sesmoid bone in
popliteal muscle

4. Tibia

5. Fibula

6. Tarsus

7. Metatarsal bones

10. Middle phalanx

8. Sesamoid bones

11. Dist. phalanx

9. Prox. phalanx

Fig. II-149 - Dog - Lt. pelvic limb skeleton
- med. view

HORSE – SKELETON – PELVIC LIMB

Fig. I-150 - Horse - Lt. pelvic limb skeleton
- lat. view

Fig. II-151 - Horse
Lt. pelvic limb
skeleton - med. view

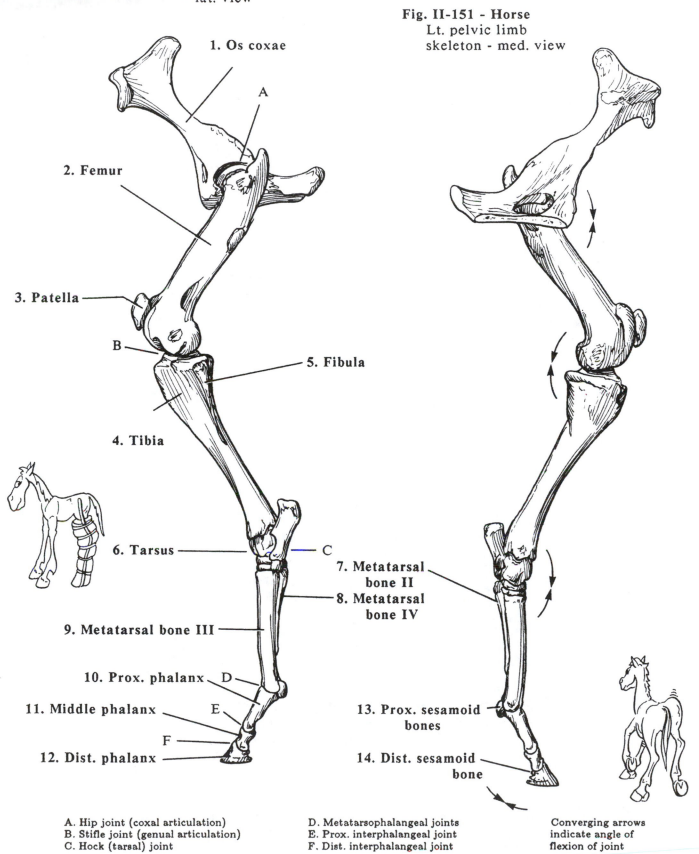

1. Os coxae

A

2. Femur

3. Patella

B

5. Fibula

4. Tibia

6. Tarsus

C

7. Metatarsal
bone II

8. Metatarsal
bone IV

9. Metatarsal bone III

10. Prox. phalanx   D

11. Middle phalanx   E

F

12. Dist. phalanx

13. Prox. sesamoid
bones

14. Dist. sesamoid
bone

Converging arrows
indicate angle of
flexion of joint

A. Hip joint (coxal articulation)
B. Stifle joint (genual articulation)
C. Hock (tarsal) joint

D. Metatarsophalangeal joints
E. Prox. interphalangeal joint
F. Dist. interphalangeal joint

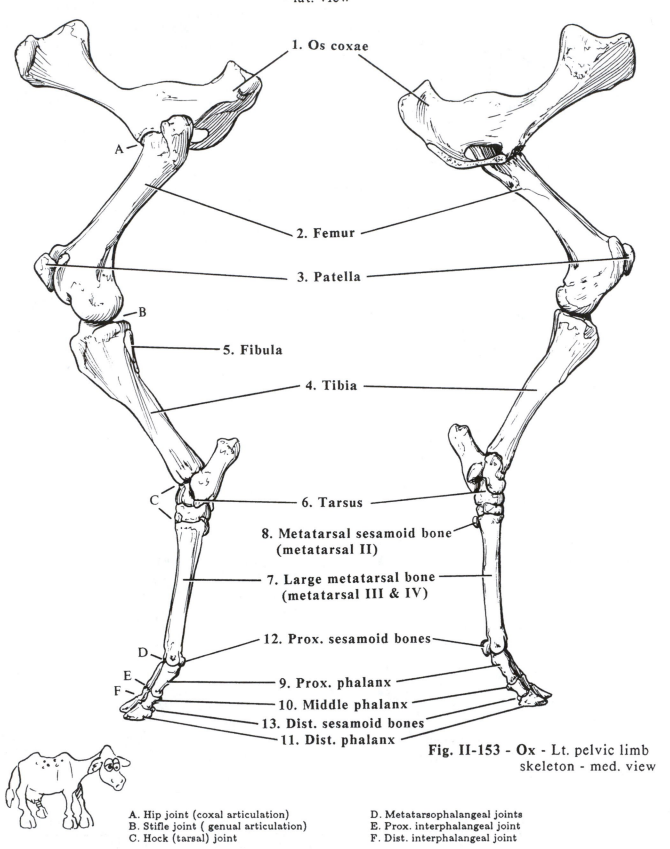

Fig. II-152 - Ox - Lt. pelvic limb skeleton
- lat. view

1. Os coxae

2. Femur

3. Patella

5. Fibula

4. Tibia

6. Tarsus

8. Metatarsal sesamoid bone
(metatarsal II)

7. Large metatarsal bone
(metatarsal III & IV)

12. Prox. sesamoid bones

9. Prox. phalanx

10. Middle phalanx

13. Dist. sesamoid bones

11. Dist. phalanx

Fig. II-153 - Ox - Lt. pelvic limb
skeleton - med. view

A. Hip joint (coxal articulation)
B. Stifle joint (genual articulation)
C. Hock (tarsal) joint

D. Metatarsophalangeal joints
E. Prox. interphalangeal joint
F. Dist. interphalangeal joint

Fig. II-154 - Pig - Lt. pelvic limb skeleton
- lat. view

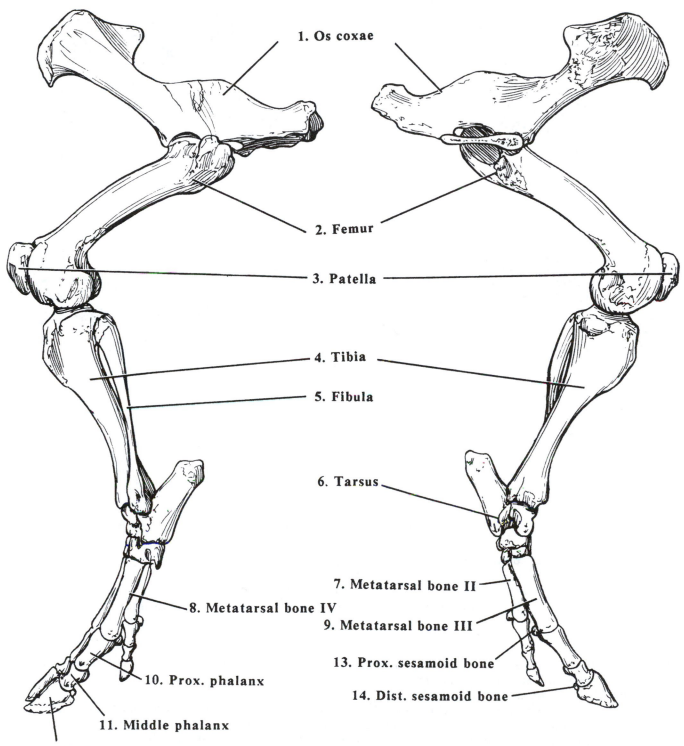

1. Os coxae

2. Femur

3. Patella

4. Tibia

5. Fibula

6. Tarsus

7. Metatarsal bone II

8. Metatarsal bone IV

9. Metatarsal bone III

13. Prox. sesamoid bone

14. Dist. sesamoid bone

10. Prox. phalanx

11. Middle phalanx

12. Dist. phalanx

Fig. II-155 - Pig - Lt. pelvic limb skeleton
- med. view

93

PELVIC GIRDLE

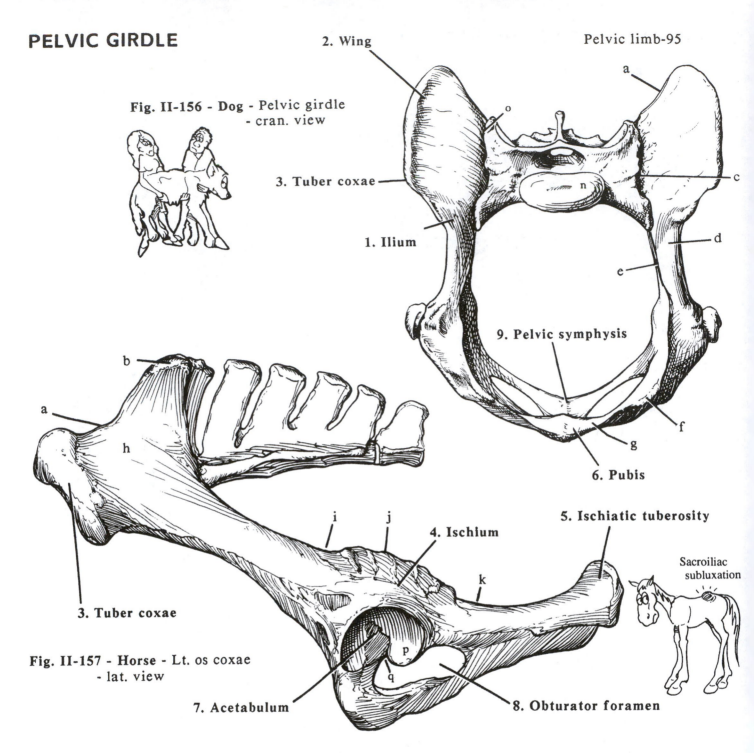

Fig. II-156 - Dog - Pelvic girdle - cran. view

2. Wing

3. Tuber coxae

1. Ilium

9. Pelvic symphysis

6. Pubis

Fig. II-157 - Horse - Lt. os coxae - lat. view

3. Tuber coxae

4. Ischium

5. Ischiatic tuberosity

Sacroiliac subluxation

7. Acetabulum

8. Obturator foramen

PELVIC GIRDLE or **bony pelvis**: consists of the joining of the two hip bones (ossa coxarum), sacrum and first few caudal vertebrae. It encloses the **pelvic cavity**. The **"pelvic inlet"** is the cranial opening into the pelvic cavity. The **"pelvic outlet"** is the caudal opening out of the pelvic cavity. The widest horizontal distance of the pelvic cavity is the transverse diameter. The vertical diameter from the pelvic symphysis to the sacrum (promontory).

HIP BONE or **os coxae**: the fused ilium, ischium, pubic and acetabular bones. The acetabular bone is in the center of the acetabulum and fuses early leaving no visible indication of its presence.

Hip bones or **ossa coxarum**: the two hip bones. They are joined at the pelvic symphysis.

1. ILIUM: the largest and most cranial part of the os coxae. It consists of a wing and a body. It forms the cranial part of the acetabulum and articulates with the sacrum. The ischiatic spine (j) separates the greater (i) and lesser (k) ischiatic notches.

2. Wing: the lateral masses of the ilium that articulate with the sacrum. The gluteal surface (h) is the lateral aspect of the wing where the middle gluteal muscle arises. The auricular surface (c) articulates with the sacrum forming the sacroiliac joint. The iliac crest (a) is the cranial edge of the wing.

PELVIC GIRDLE

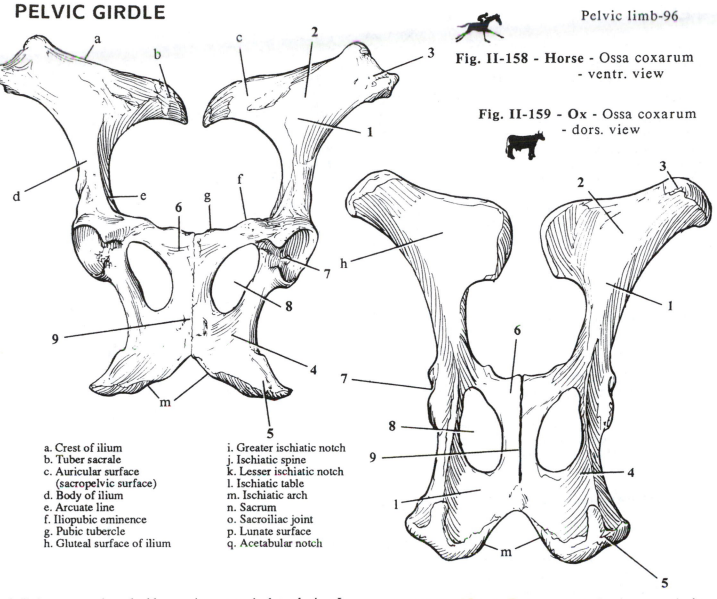

Fig. II-158 - **Horse** - Ossa coxarum - ventr. view

Fig. II-159 - **Ox** - Ossa coxarum - dors. view

a. Crest of ilium
b. Tuber sacrale
c. Auricular surface (sacropelvic surface)
d. Body of ilium
e. Arcuate line
f. Iliopubic eminence
g. Pubic tubercle
h. Gluteal surface of ilium

i. Greater ischiatic notch
j. Ischiatic spine
k. Lesser ischiatic notch
l. Ischiatic table
m. Ischiatic arch
n. Sacrum
o. Sacroiliac joint
p. Lunate surface
q. Acetabular notch

3. Tuber coxae: the palpable prominence on the lateral wing. In the ox it is called the "hook".

Tuber sacrale (b): the medial process of the wing next to the sacrum.

4. ISCHIUM (G. hip): the caudal-most part of the os coxae. The ischiatic table (l) is the horizontal part caudal to the obturator foramen.

5. Ischiatic tuberosity ("pin bone" in the ox): the thick, caudal part of the ischium providing attachment for the caudal thigh muscles.

Ischiatic arch (m): the caudal indentation between the ischiatic tuberosities.

6. PUBIS: the cranioventral part of the os coxae. The pubis consists of a central body and two branches (rami). The cranial ramus forms part of the acetabulum and the caudal ramus is medial to the obturator foramen. The pecten is the cranial border of the two pubic bones (pubes). The pectineus muscle attaches to the iliopubic eminence (f).

7. ACETABULUM (as'e-TAB-yoo-lum) (L. vinegar cup): the concavity articulating with the femoral head. It is formed by the fusion of the ilium, ischium, pubic and acetabular bones. The ligament of the femoral head attaches to the fossa in the acetabulum. The lunate surface (p) articulates with the head of the femur.

8. OBTURATOR FORAMEN (OB-too-ray'ter): large opening in the floor of the os coxae.

9. PELVIC SYMPHYSIS: the junction of the right and left os coxae between the two pubic and two ischial bones.

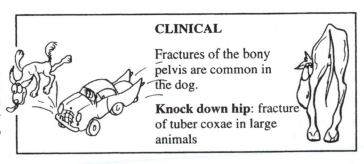

CLINICAL

Fractures of the bony pelvis are common in the dog.

Knock down hip: fracture of tuber coxae in large animals

FEMUR

FEMUR (thigh bone): articulates proximally with the hipbone (forming the hip joint) and distally with the tibia (forming the stifle joint).

1. Head: the smooth process articulating with the acetabulum of the os coxae, forming the hip joint. It has a depression (fovea) (h) for the round ligament of the femur. The <u>neck</u> (a) joins the head to the body of the femur.

2. Greater (major, lateral) **trochanter** (troh-KAN-ter): the large prominence lateral to the head.

3. Lesser (minor, medial) **trochanter:** the prominence distal to the head.

Trochanteric fossa (j): depression on the caudal aspect of the femur between the trochanters.

4. Third trochanter: the prominence on the lateral side, distal to the greater trochanter.

5. Medial and **6. lateral condyles** (G. knuckles): the two large prominences articulating with the tibia and the menisci (fibrocartilage discs between femur and tibia).

Extensor fossa (e): depression on the lateral condyle for the attachment of the long digital extensor muscle.

7. Patellar surface or **femoral trochlea** (L. pulley): the groove articulating with the patella, bounded by two ridges, the medial one being the thicker in all species.

8. PATELLA (pa-TEL-a) (L. little plate) (knee cap): the largest sesamoid bone of the body, articulating with the patellar surface of the femur.

SPECIES DIFFERENCES

9. Trochlear tubercle: the large prominence on the medial ridge of the patellar surface in the horse. The patella locks over this structure when the stay apparatus is in use (pg 198).

4. Third trochanter (4): absent in the **ruminants.**

10. Fabellae (L. bean): the two small sesamoid bones embedded in the heads of the gastrocnemius muscle of the carnivores.

96

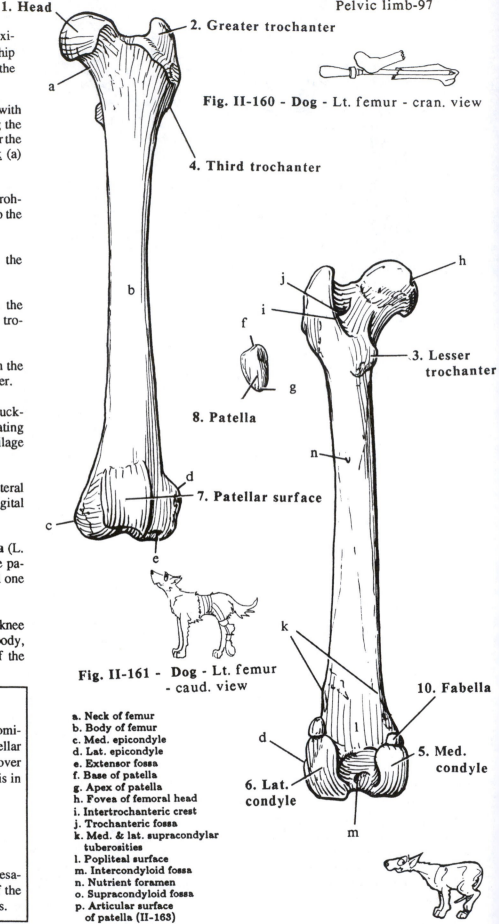

2. Greater trochanter

Fig. II-160 - Dog - Lt. femur - cran. view

4. Third trochanter

3. Lesser trochanter

8. Patella

7. Patellar surface

Fig. II-161 - Dog - Lt. femur - caud. view

10. Fabella

5. Med. condyle

6. Lat. condyle

a. Neck of femur
b. Body of femur
c. Med. epicondyle
d. Lat. epicondyle
e. Extensor fossa
f. Base of patella
g. Apex of patella
h. Fovea of femoral head
i. Intertrochanteric crest
j. Trochanteric fossa
k. Med. & lat. supracondylar tuberosities
l. Popliteal surface
m. Intercondyloid fossa
n. Nutrient foramen
o. Supracondyloid fossa
p. Articular surface of patella (II-163)

FEMUR

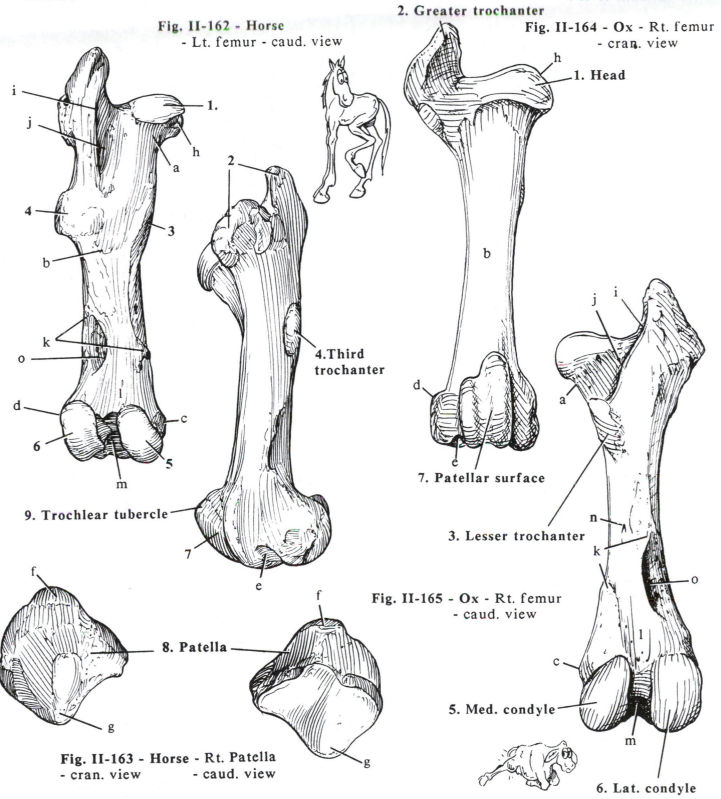

Fig. II-162 - Horse
- Lt. femur - caud. view

1.
i
j
h
a
4
3
b
k
o
d
c
6
5
m

9. Trochlear tubercle

7
e

2. Greater trochanter

Fig. II-164 - Ox - Rt. femur
- cran. view

h
1. Head

b

d
e
7. Patellar surface

2
4. Third trochanter

Fig. II-165 - Ox - Rt. femur
- caud. view

3. Lesser trochanter

5. Med. condyle

j i
a
n
k
o
l
c
m
6. Lat. condyle

f
8. Patella
g

f
g

Fig. II-163 - Horse - Rt. Patella
- cran. view   - caud. view

	CLINICAL
Sesamoid bone of the popliteal tendon in carnivores: shouldn't be mistaken for a chip fracture in radiographs.	**Mid shaft fractures in carnivores**: result in the caudal displacement of the distal fragment due to the pull of the gastrocnemius muscle.
Patellar fibrocartilage: in the horse and ox attaches the medial patellar ligament with the patella.	

TIBIA & FIBULA

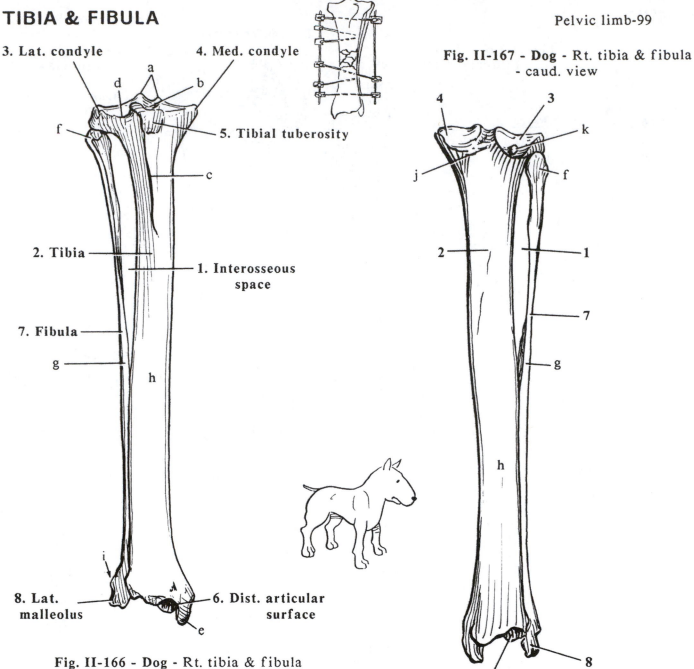

3. Lat. condyle   4. Med. condyle

5. Tibial tuberosity

2. Tibia

1. Interosseous space

7. Fibula

8. Lat. malleolus   6. Dist. articular surface

Fig. II-166 - Dog - Rt. tibia & fibula - cran. view

Fig. II-167 - Dog - Rt. tibia & fibula - caud. view

LEG SKELETON (L. *crus*): the tibia and fibula.

1. INTEROSSEOUS SPACE: separates the tibia and fibula.

2. TIBIA ("shin bone"): the medially located long bone.

3. Lateral and **4. medial condyles** (G. knuckles): the two processes articulating with the corresponding femoral condyles and fibrocartilage discs (menisci).

5. Tibial tuberosity: the large proximal cranial process where muscles and the patellar ligament(s) attach.

6. Distal articular surface or **cochlea**: the two grooves, separated by a ridge, articulating with the trochlea of the tibial tarsal bone.

7. FIBULA (L. pin or skewer) ("calf bone"): the long, thin bone bearing little weight, serving mainly for muscle attachments. It articulates distally with the tibia and the fibular tarsal bone. It is the more lateral of the two bones of the leg

8. Lateral malleolus (mal-LEE-oh-lus): the distal end of the fibula.

TIBIA & FIBULA

Fig. II-168 - Horse - Lt. tibia & fibula
- cran. view

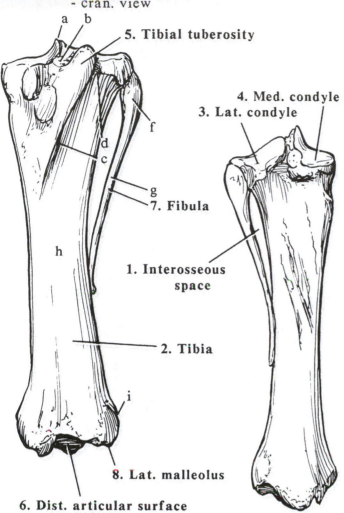

5. Tibial tuberosity

4. Med. condyle
3. Lat. condyle

f

d
c

g
7. Fibula

h

1. Interosseous
space

2. Tibia

i

8. Lat. malleolus

6. Dist. articular surface

Fig. II-169 - Horse - Lt. tibia
& fibula - caud. view

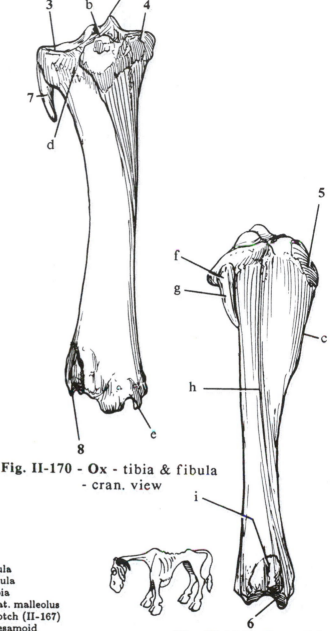

3 a 4
b

7
d

4. Med. condyle
3. Lat. condyle

8
e

Fig. II-170 - Ox - tibia & fibula
- cran. view

5

f
g

c

h

i

6

Fig. II-171 - Ox - tibia
& fibula - lat. view

a. Intercondylar eminence
b. Cran. intercondylar area
c. Cran. border
d. Muscular groove
   (extensor sulcus)
e. Med. malleolus

f. Head of fibula
g. Body of fibula
h. Body of tibia
i. Groove of lat. malleolus
j. Popliteal notch (II-167)
k. Popliteal sesamoid
   bone (carnivores)

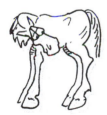

SPECIES DIFFERENCES

Carnivores and pig: the tibia and fibula are not fused.

Ruminants: the head of the fibula fuses to the tibia. Most of the body of the fibula fails to develop, therefore the proximal and distal fibula are not connected and there is no interosseous space. The distal end of the fibula (lateral malleolus) remains separate from the tibia.

Horse: the fibula is a reduced bone that reaches only half way down the tibia. The true distal end of the fibula (lateral malleolus) is fused with the tibia.

CLINICAL

Growth plates in dogs: unite by one year of age. The one for the tibial tuberosity can be mistaken for a fracture in all species.

TARSUS

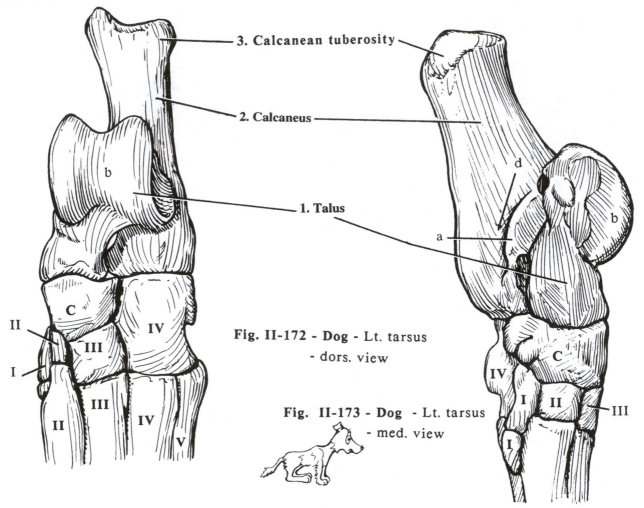

3. Calcanean tuberosity

2. Calcaneus

1. Talus

Fig. II-172 - Dog - Lt. tarsus - dors. view

Fig. II-173 - Dog - Lt. tarsus - med. view

TARSUS (G. *tarsos* flat) or **"hock"**: the two (or two and a half) rows of bones between the crus and the metatarsal region. The proximal row consists of the talus (tibial) and calcaneus (fibular) tarsal bones. In the generalized pattern seen in the carnivores and pig, the distal row consists of central, 1st, 2nd, 3rd, and 4th tarsal bones. The central tarsal bone is actually between the proximal row and the numbered tarsal bones. It doesn't span the whole tarsus because of the "two story" fourth tarsal bone.

1. Talus (L. ankle bone) or **tibial tarsal bone** : the largest bone of the tarsus, located on its dorsomedial side. It articulates by its trochlea (b) with the tibia (the tibia and fibula in the dog).

2. Calcaneus (kal-KAY-nee-us) (L. heel) or **fibular tarsal bone**: the second bone of the proximal row, lateral to the talus.

3. Calcanean tuberosity: the large process of the fibular tarsal bone serving as a lever arm for the common calcanean tendon.

Sustentaculum tali (a): the medial "shelf" of the calcaneus over which the tendon of the lateral head of deep digital flexor crosses.

SPECIES DIFFERENCES

Carnivores and **pigs**: have seven tarsal bones.

Ruminants: have five tarsal bones due to fusion of four bones

to form two bones - centroquartal bone (fused central and fourth) and fused second and third.

Horse: has six tarsal bones due to fusion of two bones - fused 1st and 2nd.

Ruminant and **pig**: have two trochlea to their talus.

CLINICAL

Bone spavin, osteoarthritis of distal tarsal joints: #1 problem of the hock in horses, #1 lameness in Standardbreds, common in western horses and jumpers. Wear and tear disease of the distal intertarsal and tarsometatarsal joints.

Osteochondrosis dissecans (OCD): 2nd most common hock problem. The most common sites in tarsus are the intermediate ridge of the distal tibia followed by the lateral trochlear ridge. Fast growing cartilage grows past its nutritional supply and necrosis. Trauma may cause a dissecting cartilage flap. Clinically there is effusion of the tibiotarsal joint.

Fig. II-174 - Horse - Rt. tarsus - med. view

Fig. II-175 - Horse - Rt. tarsus - plant. view

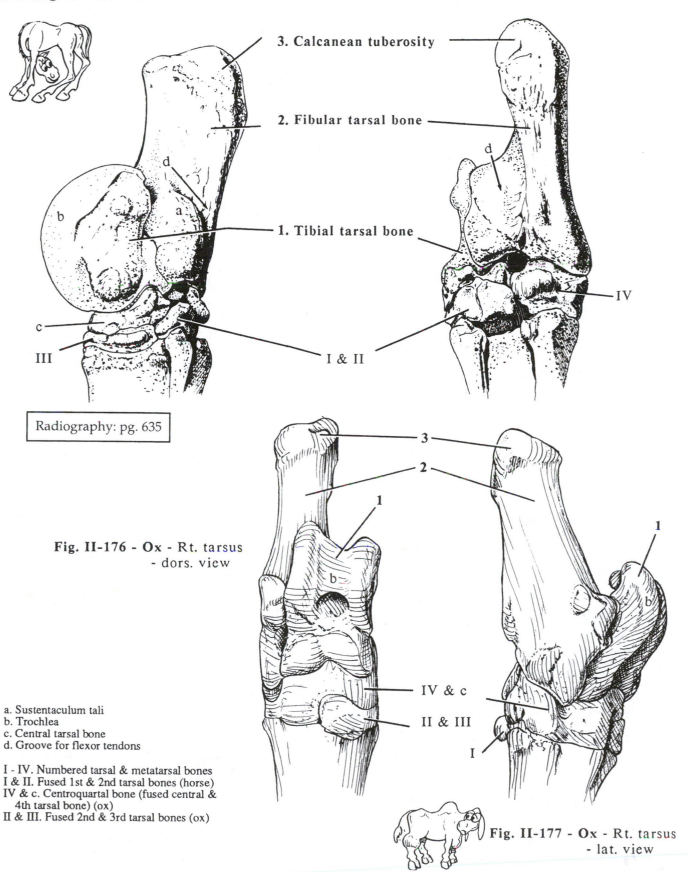

3. Calcanean tuberosity

2. Fibular tarsal bone

1. Tibial tarsal bone

I & II

III

IV

Radiography: pg. 635

Fig. II-176 - Ox - Rt. tarsus
- dors. view

3
2
1

IV & c

II & III

I

a. Sustentaculum tali
b. Trochlea
c. Central tarsal bone
d. Groove for flexor tendons

I - IV. Numbered tarsal & metatarsal bones
I & II. Fused 1st & 2nd tarsal bones (horse)
IV & c. Centroquartal bone (fused central &
    4th tarsal bone) (ox)
II & III. Fused 2nd & 3rd tarsal bones (ox)

Fig. II-177 - Ox - Rt. tarsus
- lat. view

METATARSAL BONES

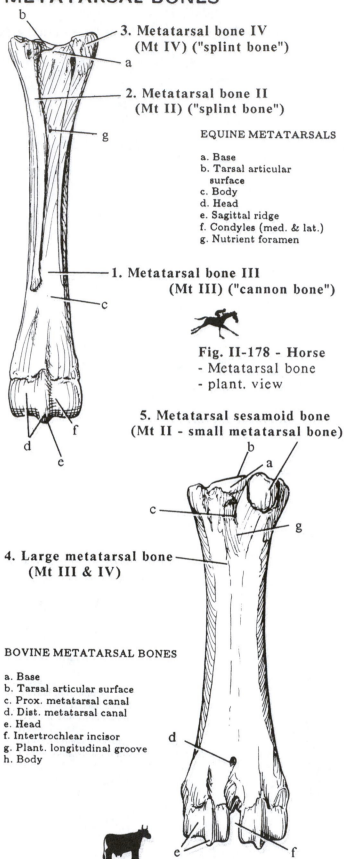

3. Metatarsal bone IV
(Mt IV) ("splint bone")

2. Metatarsal bone II
(Mt II) ("splint bone")

EQUINE METATARSALS

a. Base
b. Tarsal articular
   surface
c. Body
d. Head
e. Sagittal ridge
f. Condyles (med. & lat.)
g. Nutrient foramen

1. Metatarsal bone III
(Mt III) ("cannon bone")

Fig. II-178 - Horse
- Metatarsal bone
- plant. view

5. Metatarsal sesamoid bone
(Mt II - small metatarsal bone)

4. Large metatarsal bone
(Mt III & IV)

BOVINE METATARSAL BONES

a. Base
b. Tarsal articular surface
c. Prox. metatarsal canal
d. Dist. metatarsal canal
e. Head
f. Intertrochlear incisor
g. Plant. longitudinal groove
h. Body

Fig. II-179 - Ox - Metatarsal bone
- plant. view

METATARSAL BONES and DIGITS (met'a-TAR-sul): their pattern is the same as in the thoracic limb of the horse and pig.

SPECIES DIFFERENCES

Carnivores: the first metatarsal bone is even more reduced than in the front limb and the first digit (dew claw) is often absent.

Ruminants: the fifth metatarsal bone is absent. A metatarsal sesamoid bone is present and is often called the "small metatarsal" or metatarsal II.

**Fig. II-180 - Pig - Lt. pes
-dors. view**   **Fig. II-181 - Pig - Lt.
-plant view**

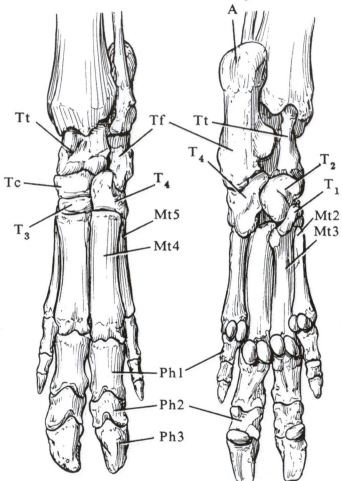

PORCINE METATARSALS

A   Calcanean tuberosity
Tt   Tibial tarsal bone
Tf   Fibular tarsal bone
Tc   Central tarsal bone
T 1-4 Tarsal bones 1-4
Mt 2-5 Metatarsal bones 2-5
Ph 1-3 Prox., middle & dist.
       phalanges

Chapter III
Joints

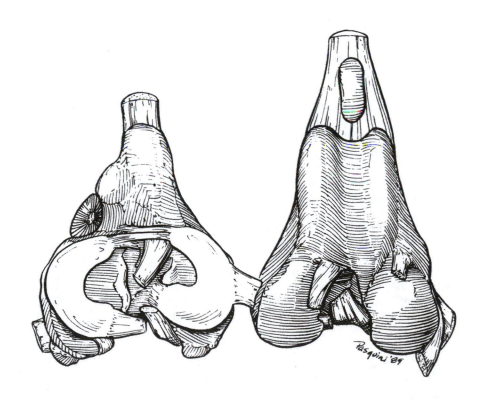

JOINTS

ARTICULATION (ar-tik'-yoo-LAY-shun) or **JOINT**: union or junction between two or more bones of the skeleton.

Arthrology (G. *arthros*, joints + *logos*, study): the study of joints.

JOINT CLASSIFICATION: Joints can be classified by several criteria.

SIMPLE OR COMPOUND JOINTS: classified by the number of bones articulating with each other.

• **Simple joints**: articulations with two articulating bones.

• **Compound joints**: articulations with more than two bones articulating (e.g., stifle).

STRUCTURAL CLASSIFICATION: classified by their uniting medium into fibrous, cartilaginous and synovial joints.

• **Fibrous joint**: articulation united by <u>fibrous tissue</u>, allowing little or no movement, as in a suture or syndesmosis. These are often temporary joints that later ossify (synostosis).

• **Cartilaginous joint**: articulation united by <u>fibrocartilage</u>, <u>hyaline cartilage</u>, or both, as in a synchondrosis or a symphysis. These also can be slightly movable or immovable.

• **Synovial joint**: an articulation united by a <u>synovial joint capsule</u>. These are freely movable.

FUNCTIONAL CLASSIFICATION OF JOINTS: indicates the degree of **motion** possible.

• **Immovable joint** or synarthrosis (sin'-ar-THROH-sis) (pl.= synarthroses) (synarthroidal joint) (*syn*, together; *arthro*, joint): the fixed tight union allowing little or no movement and having great strength (e.g., suture between two facial bones).

  – **Suture** (SOO-chur): a **fibrous** joint between the skull bones. They may ossify with age.

  – **"Hyaline cartilage joint"** or synchondrosis (sin'kon-DROH-sis): an immovable, temporary joint of **hyaline cartilage**, e.g., the cartilaginous epiphyseal plate uniting the diaphyses and epiphyses (pg. 22 of immature bones). The epiphyseal plate allows growth of the bone and then ossifies with age. This process eliminates the joint by forming a synostosis (ossified joint). A few synchondroses persist through life, such as the costochondral junctions (pg. 131).

• **Slightly movable joint** or amphiarthrosis (am-fee-ar-THROH-sis) (amphiarthroidal joint): a joint connected by either connective tissue or fibrocartilage (e. g., between the vertebral bodies). Amphi, as in amphibian, implies both immovable and movable (which it is), allowing only slight motion.

  – **"Ligamentous joint"** or syndesmosis (sin'-dez-MOH-sis)

(G. *syndesmos*, ligament): a **fibrous** joint uniting two bones by a sheet of fibrous connective tissue (e.g., attachments between the costal cartilages in the costal arch [pg. 71] and the interosseous ligament [pg. 111, e] between the radius and ulna in carnivores).

  – **Symphysis** (SIM-fi-sis): the **fibrocartilaginous** (or possibly hyaline cartilaginous) joints that occur on the midline of the body. Although they may or may not ossify with age, they always limit the motion of the joint. Examples are the pelvic symphysis (pg. 118) and joints between sternebrae (pg. 131,1) and vertebral bodies (pg. 130). Fibrocartilage, a strong form of cartilage, is found where bones need to be strongly bound together and still allow some movement.

• **Freely movable joint** or diarthrosis (dy'ar-THROH-sis) (diarthroidal joint): synovial joints. The uniting medium may be considered the joint capsule.

  • **Synovial joint**: discussed on pg. 106.

GOMPHOSIS (gom-FOH-sis): the name for the fibrous implantation of the teeth into the alveoli of the jaw bone. This is not a true joint because the teeth are not part of the skeleton. This peg-and-socket joint is held together by fibrous connective tissue, the **periodontal ligament**, that attaches each tooth in its socket.

Authors note: The proper terms for the different classification of joints (synarthrosis, synchondrosis, syndesmosis, synostosis, amphiarthrosis, etc.) are confusing, easily forgotten, and probably won't make you a better veterinarian.

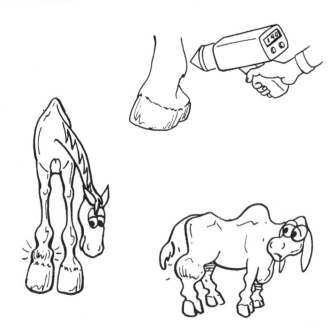

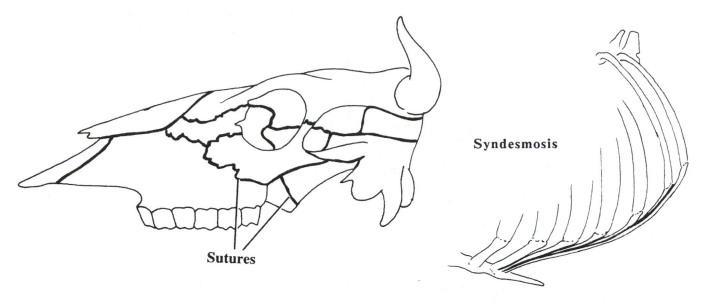

Sutures

Syndesmosis

FIBROUS

CARTILAGINOUS

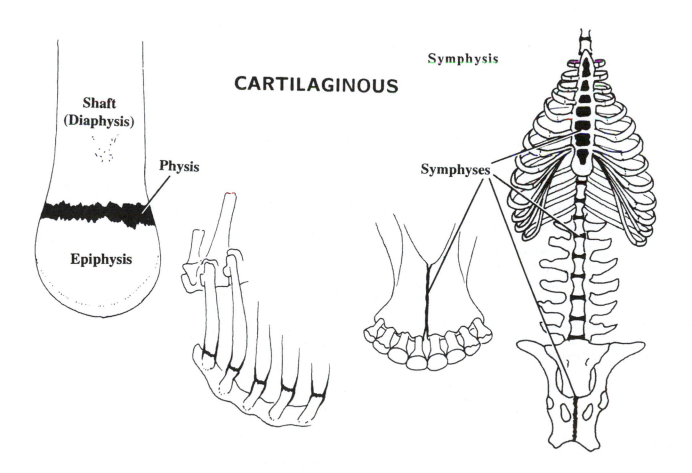

**Shaft
(Diaphysis)**

Physis

Epiphysis

Symphysis

Symphyses

Fig. III-1 - Fibrous & cartilaginous joints

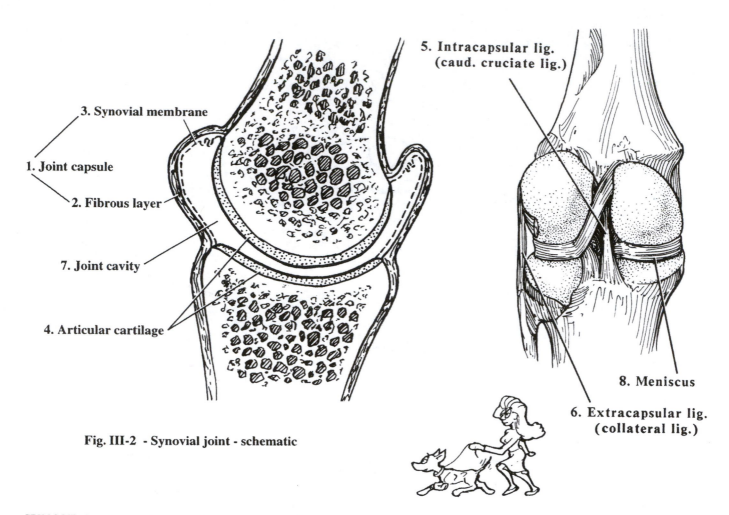

3. Synovial membrane

1. Joint capsule

2. Fibrous layer

7. Joint cavity

4. Articular cartilage

Fig. III-2 - Synovial joint - schematic

5. Intracapsular lig. (caud. cruciate lig.)

8. Meniscus

6. Extracapsular lig. (collateral lig.)

SYNOVIAL (sin-OH-vee-al) (diarthroidal) **JOINT** (movable joint): characterized by its mobility, joint cavity, articular cartilage, synovial membrane and fibrous capsule. This is the most common type of joint. Functionally it is freely movable.

1. Joint capsule: the two-layered structure surrounding the joint, made of an outer fibrous layer and an inner synovial membrane.

2. Fibrous layer (capsular ligament): the white and yellow elastic fibrous part of the joint capsule. It attaches to the periosteum on or near the margin of the articular cartilage. Its thickness varies from joint to joint and within each joint.

3. Synovial membrane: the inner lining of the fibrous layer. It is highly vascular, nerve rich, and produces synovial fluid. The membrane may extend outside the fibrous layer to communicate with a synovial sheath or to form a bursa under a tendon or ligament.

Synovial fluid: the viscous liquid produced by the synovial membrane to lubricate the joint, supply nutrients, and remove waste from the hyaline articular cartilage. It has the consistency of raw egg white.

4. Articular cartilage (ar-TIK-yoo-lar KAR-ti-lij): the translu-cent, bluish-tinged cartilage, usually hyaline, covering the articular ends of bones. It reduces the effects of concussion and friction by its compressibility, elasticity and smoothness. Varying in thickness between and within joints, the cartilage is thickest in areas of highest pressure and friction. Having no vascular or nerve supply, articular cartilage depends on synovial fluid to supply nutrients and remove waste products.

Ligaments (5-6): strong bands of white fibrous connective tissue uniting bones. They function to keep joint surfaces in apposition and still allow movement. They are usually inelastic and may be intracapsular or extracapsular.

5. Intracapsular ligaments: ligaments located within the joint capsule. They are not within the joint space because the synovial membrane reflects over them (e.g., cruciate ligaments of the stifle).

6. Extracapsular ligaments: ligaments developing outside of or as part of the joint capsule (e.g., the collateral ligaments on the sides of all hinge joints).

7. Joint cavity: a unique feature of a synovial joint. It is little more than a potential space containing a trace of synovial fluid.

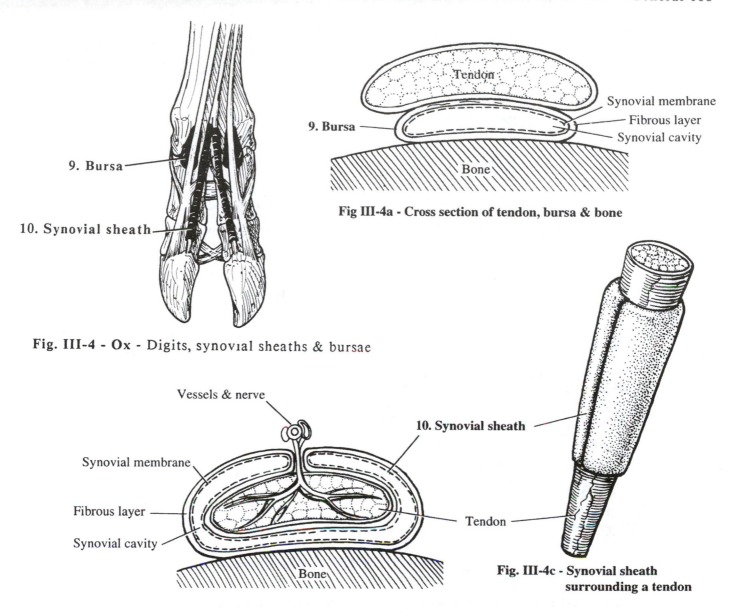

9. Bursa

10. Synovial sheath

Fig. III-4 - Ox - Digits, synovial sheaths & bursae

Tendon

9. Bursa

Synovial membrane
Fibrous layer
Synovial cavity

Bone

Fig III-4a - Cross section of tendon, bursa & bone

Vessels & nerve

Synovial membrane

Fibrous layer

Synovial cavity

Bone

10. Synovial sheath

Tendon

Fig. III-4c - Synovial sheath
surrounding a tendon

Fig. III-4b - cross section of tendon surrounded by a synovial sheath

8. Meniscus or **disc**: a plate of fibrocartilage partially or completely dividing a joint cavity. It functions to allow a greater variety of motion and alleviate concussion. Discs are found only in the stifle (pg. 120) and temporomandibular joints (pg. 127). The intervertebral discs do not divide a joint space.

9. BURSA (BUR-sa) (synovial): a sac-like structure between different tissue that reduces friction between these tissues. Resembling a synovial joint capsule, its walls consist of a fibrous layer lined by a synovial membrane. Bursae are located between skin and bones, tendons and bones, muscles and bones, and ligaments and bones.

10. SYNOVIAL SHEATH: a structure similar to a bursa that wraps completely around a tendon. It reduces friction between the tendon and underlying bones.

CLINICAL

False joints: a joint formed in an unreduced (unhealed) fracture, having all the structures of a synovial joint.

Excess synovial fluid: since synovial fluid in the healthy animal is minimal, the amount of fluid present indicates the state of health of the joint.

Luxations or dislocations: an articular separation, usually due to injury or degenerative changes, but may also have predisposing genetic factors (e.g., patellar dislocation in toy poodles).

Bursitis (bur-SY-tis): inflammation of a bursa.

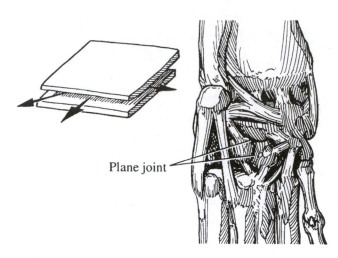

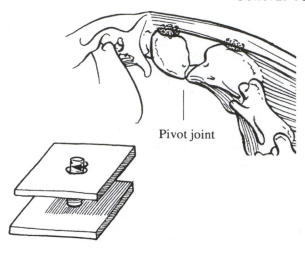

Plane joint - Dog - Intercarpal joints

Pivot joint - Horse - Atlantoaxial joint

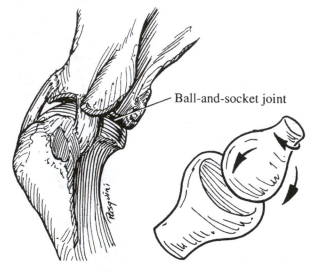

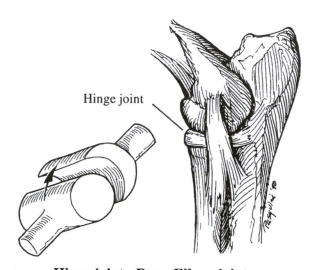

Ball-and -socket joint - Dog - Shoulder joint

Hinge joint - Dog - Elbow joint

CLASSIFICATION of SYNOVIAL JOINTS: Synovial joints are freely movable joints classified in several ways - by the number of articular surfaces, by the shape of the articular surfaces, or by the particular function of the joint.

NUMBER of ARTICULAR SURFACES: a joint is either simple or compound.

• **Simple joint**: two articular surfaces enclosed in a joint capsule (e.g., shoulder joint).

• **Compound joint**: more than two articular surfaces enclosed within the same joint capsule (e.g., stifle).

CLASSIFICATION BY MOVEMENT: the contraction of muscles crossing a joint and the shape of the joint produce its characteristic movements.

• **Plane** (arthrodial) **joint** (ar-THROH-dee-al): multiaxial articulations having flat articular surfaces allowing a simple gliding or sliding motion (e.g., carpal, small tarsal bones, cranial and caudal

articulation between vertebrae).

• **Ball-and-socket** (spheroidal) **joint**: a multiaxial articulation consisting of a spheroidal head fitting into a pit or socket allowing universal movement - flexion-extension, abduction-adduction, medial and lateral rotation, and circumduction (e.g., shoulder and hip joints).

• **Hinge** (ginglymus) **joint** (JIN-gli-mus): a uniaxial joint allowing movement at right angles to the bones involved (flexion and extension) (e.g., elbow joint).

• **Pivot** (trochoid) **joint** (TROH-koyd): a uniaxial joint allowing rotation around a longitudinal axis of a bone (e.g., atlanto-axial joint).

• **Condylar joint**: a uniaxial joint formed by two condyles of one bone fitting into concavities of another bone. Flexion and extension and a little rotation are permitted by such a joint (e.g. femorotibial joint, the temporomandibular joints [both together

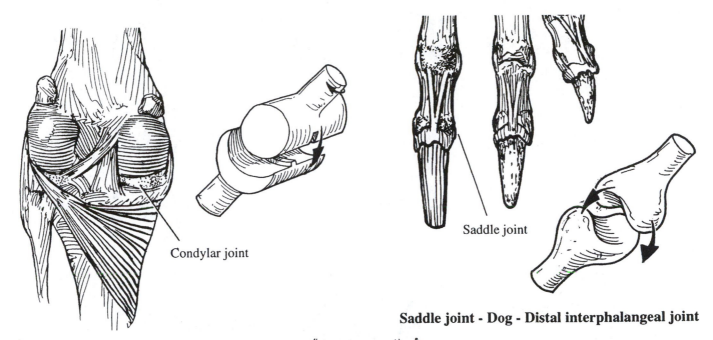

Condylar joint

Condylar joint - Dog - femorotibial joint

Saddle joint

Saddle joint - Dog - Distal interphalangeal joint

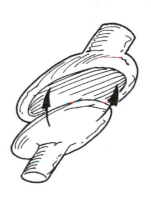

Elipsoidal joint

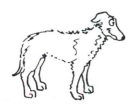

Elipsoidal joint - Dog - Antebrachiocarpal joint

form a condylar joint]).

• **Ellipsoidal joint**: a biaxial joint formed by an ellipsoidal, convex surface fitting into a concavity. Movement in two planes is allowed (flexion-extension; abduction-adduction) with a small amount of rotation (e.g. radiocarpal joint).

• **Saddle joint**: a biaxial joint with the articular surface of the two bones concave in one direction and convex in the other. These surfaces fit together like two saddles, one rotated 90 degrees. A saddle joint allows the same motions as the ellipsoid (flexion-extension; abduction-adduction) and some rotation (e.g., distal interphalangeal joints).

MOVEMENT OF SYNOVIAL JOINTS: Synovial joints may show one or more of the following movements, depending on their shape and where the muscles cross them.

• **Flexion** (FLEK-shun): decreasing the angle between two bones.

• **Extension** (ek-STEN-shun): increasing the angle between two bones.

• **Dorsal** and **ventral flexion**: bending the spinal column dorsally or ventrally.

• **A-B-duction** (ab-DUK-shun): moving a part away from the median plane, or a digit away from the axis of the limb.

• **A-D-duction** (ad-DUK-shun): moving a part toward the median plane or a digit toward the axis of the limb.

• **Circumduction**: movement circumscribing a cone shape, accomplished by combining flexion, abduction, extension and adduction in order.

• **Rotation**: movement around the long axis of a part (e.g., radio-ulnar joints in carnivores).

• **Universal**: all the above movements (e.g., shoulder joint).

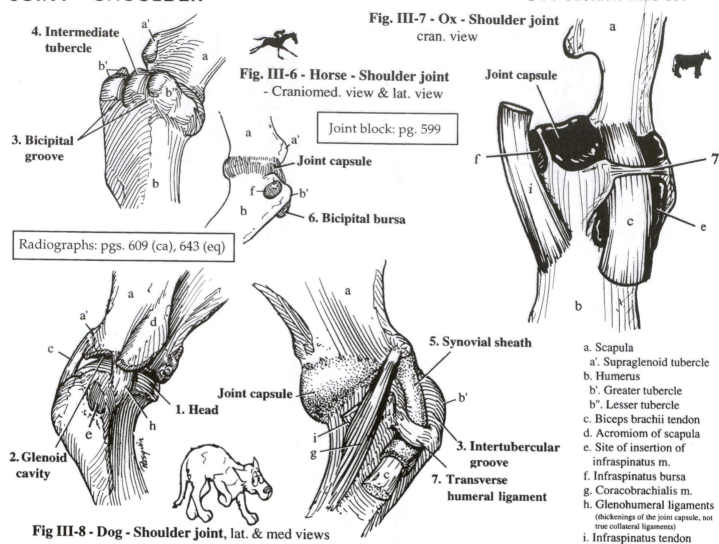

4. Intermediate tubercle

3. Bicipital groove

Fig. III-6 - Horse - Shoulder joint
- Craniomed. view & lat. view

Joint block: pg. 599

Joint capsule

6. Bicipital bursa

Radiographs: pgs. 609 (ca), 643 (eq)

Fig. III-7 - Ox - Shoulder joint
cran. view

Joint capsule

5. Synovial sheath

Joint capsule

1. Head

2. Glenoid cavity

3. Intertubercular groove

7. Transverse humeral ligament

Fig III-8 - Dog - Shoulder joint, lat. & med views

a. Scapula
a'. Supraglenoid tubercle
b. Humerus
b'. Greater tubercle
b". Lesser tubercle
c. Biceps brachii tendon
d. Acromiom of scapula
e. Site of insertion of infraspinatus m.
f. Infraspinatus bursa
g. Coracobrachialis m.
h. Glenohumeral ligaments
(thickenings of the joint capsule, not true collateral ligaments)
i. Infraspinatus tendon

SHOULDER JOINT, glenohumeral or scapulohumeral joint: a ball-and-socket (spheroid) type synovial joint between the glenoid cavity and the humeral head. It has a loose joint capsule with no true collateral ligaments. The muscles crossing this joint provide enough support so shoulder luxation is rare in the dog. It is functionally a freely movable (diarthrodial) joint.

Movement: capable of universal motion, but chiefly flexion and extension in the domestic animals.

1. Head of humerus: fits in glenoid cavity to form shoulder joint

2. Glenoid cavity: forms shoulder joint with humeral head

3. Intertubercular (bicipital) groove: sulcus between grater and lesser tubercle holding the biceps brachii tendon

4. Intermediate tubercle: prominence in the horses intertubercular groove

5. Synovial sheath of biceps brachii tendon: an extension of the joint capsule around the tendon of the biceps brachii muscle as it passes in the bicipital (intertubercular) groove of the humerus in carnivores, pigs and sheep.

6. Intertubercular (bicipital) bursa: located between the bicipital (intertubercular) groove and the bicipital tendon in the horses, ox and goat. Unlike the synovial sheath in dogs, it doesn't communicate with the shoulder joint capsule.

7. Transverse humeral ligament: attaches to the greater and lesser tubercles and holds the biceps tendon in the intertubercular (bicipital) groove.

CLINICAL

Osteochondrosis: a failure of cartilage maturation. Pressure on such a defective cartilage will cause it to crack and may cause a piece ("joint mouse") to be separated and float in the synovial space (osteochondrosis dissecans). This is most common on the head of the humerus in dogs.

Joint blocks: in the horse the bicipital bursa and the shoulder must be blocked separately because they don't communicate.

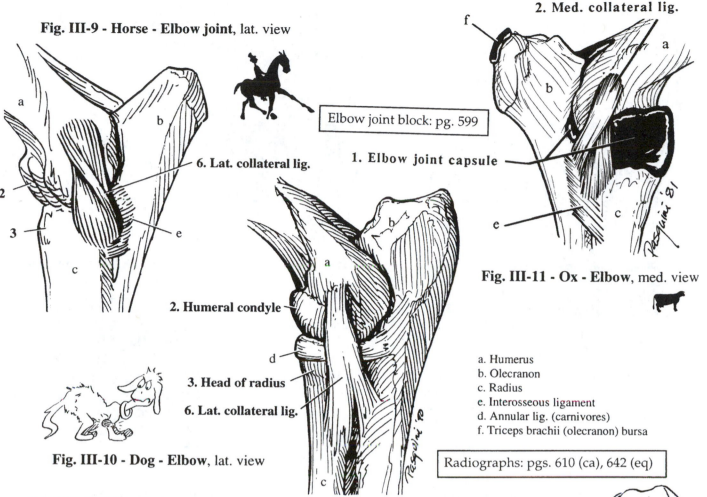

Fig. III-9 - Horse - Elbow joint, lat. view

6. Lat. collateral lig.

2
3
e
a
b
c

Elbow joint block: pg. 599

2. Med. collateral lig.

f
a
b
c
e

1. Elbow joint capsule

Fig. III-11 - Ox - Elbow, med. view

2. Humeral condyle

d

3. Head of radius

6. Lat. collateral lig.

Fig. III-10 - Dog - Elbow, lat. view

a. Humerus
b. Olecranon
c. Radius
e. Interosseous ligament
d. Annular lig. (carnivores)
f. Triceps brachii (olecranon) bursa

Radiographs: pgs. 610 (ca), 642 (eq)

ELBOW JOINT (cubital articulation, humeroradioulnar): a hinge (ginglymus) type of synovial joint allowing flexion and extension. It is also a compound joint formed between the humerus, the radius and the ulna.

1. Joint capsule: the sac enclosing all three articular parts.

2. Humeral condyle: consisting of a capitulum and a trochlea articulates with the head of the radius

3. Head of radius: articulates with the capitulum of the humeral condyle and the ulna

4. Trochlear notch of ulna: articulates with the trochlea of the humeral condyle.

5. Anconeal process of ulna: fits in the olecranon fossa of the humerus.

6. Collateral ligaments (medial and lateral): located on the sides of the joint restricting movement to just flexion and extension.

Proximal radioulnar joint: the joint between the proximal radius and proximal ulna. This joint is fused in the horse and ruminants. In carnivores and the pig, along with the distal radioulnar joint, it allows 90° supination of the manus.

Anular ligament of the radius (d) of the carnivores: a thin band of connective tissue passing transversely around the head of the radius and attaching at both ends to the ulna. With the ulna it forms a ring in which the radius can turn when the forearm is rotated.

CLINICAL   Capped elbow

Olecranon bursitis or **capped elbow**: a false subcutaneous bursa between the skin and the olecranon due to repeated trauma. This is called "shoe boil" in horses due to the repeated contact between the hoof or shoes with the elbow when the animal is laying down.

Elbow luxation: uncommon in the dog due to the anconeal process projecting into the olecranon fossa. It is more common laterally than medially because of the large medial epicondyle. To reduce a lateral luxation the joint should be maximally flexed so the anconeal process can be negotiated back into the olecranon fossa.

Ununited anconeal process, fragmented medial coronoid process and **osteochondrosis of the humeral trochlea**: can all cause lameness of the elbow.

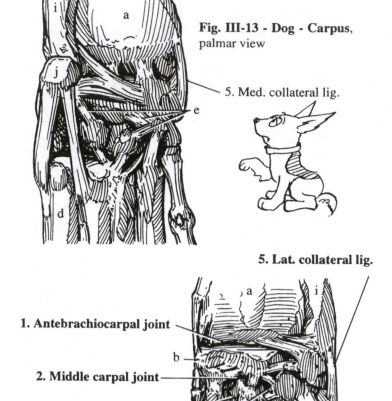

Fig. III-13 - Dog - Carpus, palmar view

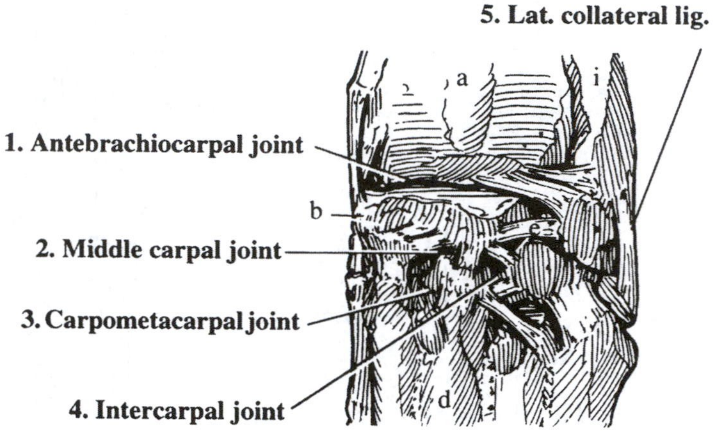

5. Med. collateral lig.

5. Lat. collateral lig.

1. Antebrachiocarpal joint

2. Middle carpal joint

3. Carpometacarpal joint

4. Intercarpal joint

Fig. III-14 - Dog - Carpus, dors. view

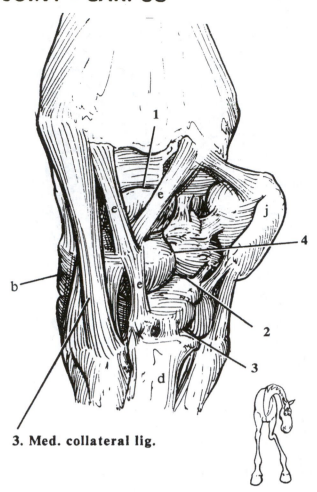

3. Med. collateral lig.

Fig. III-12. Horse - Lt. carpus
- caudomed. view

Radiographs: pgs. 632, 644

DISTAL RADIOULNAR JOINT: between the distal radius and ulna. It is part of the antebrachiocarpal joint with which it shares a joint capsule. With the proximal radioulnar joint it is responsible for the rotation allowed in the forearm of the carnivores and pigs. It is fused in the horse and ruminants.

CARPAL JOINTS: a hinge (ginglymus) type of synovial joint, allowing flexion and extension with some lateral movement. It consists of three main joints - antebrachiocarpal, middle carpal and carpometacarpal.

1. Antebrachiocarpal joint ("radiocarpal" joint): between the distal radius and ulna and the proximal row of carpal bones. There is a lot of movement in this joint.

2. Middle carpal joint: between the two rows of carpal bones. It communicates with the carpometacarpal joint. Although less than the antebrachiocarpal joint, it also has a lot of movement.

3. Carpometacarpal joint: between the distal row of carpal bones and the metacarpal bones. It communicates with the middle carpal joint. There is very little movement in this joint.

4. Intercarpal joints: plane joints between the individual carpal

bones.

INTERMETACARPAL JOINTS: articulations between the proximal ends of the metacarpal bones.

5. Collateral ligaments, medial and lateral: on the side of the hinge joint.

Intercarpal ligaments: between individual carpal bones.

Palmar carpal ligament or **fibrocartilage**: covers the palmar side of the carpus providing a smooth surface to the carpal canal.

6. Flexor retinaculum: thickening of the deep fascia that connects to the medial side of the carpus and the accessory carpal bone. With the carpal bones it forms the carpal canal.

Carpal canal: formed by the accessory carpal bone laterally, the other carpal bones dorsally and the flexor retinaculum on the palmar side.

Structures passing through the carpal canal:
• Tendons and synovial sheaths of the superficial and deep digital flexors
• Ulnar and median nerve
• Arteries and veins.

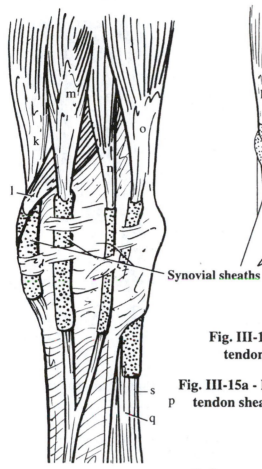

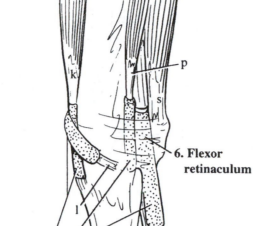

Synovial sheaths

6. Flexor retinaculum

Fig. III-15b - Horse - Tendons & tendon sheaths, caudomed. view

Fig. III-15a - Horse - Tendons & tendon sheaths, craniolat. view

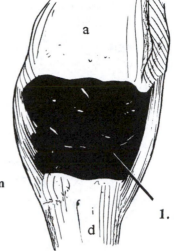

1. Joint capsule

Fig. III-16 - Ox - Synovial membranes, fibrous capsule removed - Craniolateral view

Carpal joint block: pg. 598

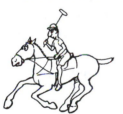

a. Radius
b. Radial carpal bone
c. Ulnar carpal bone
d. Metacarpal bone
e. Intercarpal ligaments
f. Radiocarpal synovial sac
g. Middle carpal - synovial sac

h. Carpometacarpal - synovial sac
i. Ulna
j. Accessory carpal bone
k. Extensor carpi radialis
l. Oblique carpal extensor
m. Common digital extensor
n. Lateral digital extensor

o. Lateral ulnar m.
p. Flexor carpi radialis
q. Deep digital flexor
r. Superficial digital flexor
s. Flexor carpi ulnaris

SPECIES DIFFERENCES

"Knee": a popular term for the horse's carpus.

"Radiocarpal joint": popular, though erroneous, term for the entire antebrachiocarpal joint

CLINICAL

Carpitis or **"popped knees"**: traumatic arthritis of the carpus in horses.

Chip fractures of carpus: common in racing horses. They are usually located on the dorsomedial aspect of the carpus.

Carpal hygroma: subcutaneous bursa on the dorsal surface of the carpus, caused by trauma.

VaLgus: lateral deviation of the bones distal to the joint in question. *Memory aid*: the **L** in valgus indicates lateral deviation distal to the joint.

Varus: medial deviation of the bones distal to the joint in question (No **L**, so medial).

Knocked knees or **carpal valgus**: lateral deviation of the joints distal to the carpus.

Bow legged or **carpal varus**: medial deviation of the bones distal to the carpus.

Carpal joint blocks (see pg 598).

"Splints": inflammation of the horse's metacarpal interosseous ligament between the splint bones and the cannon bone.

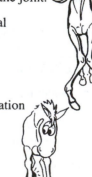

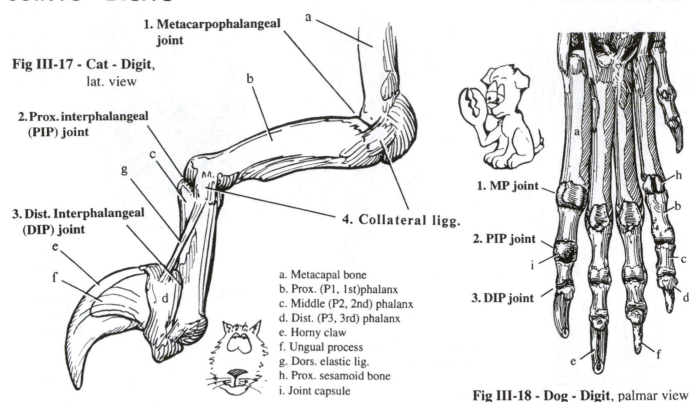

1. Metacarpophalangeal joint

Fig III-17 - Cat - Digit, lat. view

2. Prox. interphalangeal (PIP) joint

3. Dist. Interphalangeal (DIP) joint

4. Collateral ligg.

a. Metacapal bone
b. Prox. (P1, 1st)phalanx
c. Middle (P2, 2nd) phalanx
d. Dist. (P3, 3rd) phalanx
e. Horny claw
f. Ungual process
g. Dors. elastic lig.
h. Prox. sesamoid bone
i. Joint capsule

1. MP joint

2. PIP joint

3. DIP joint

Fig III-18 - Dog - Digit, palmar view

1. METACARPOPHALANGEAL (MP) JOINTS: the articulations between the metacarpal bones and the proximal phalanges, including the palmar sesamoid bones. It is a modified hinge (ginglymus) joint allowing extension and flexion.

PHALANGEAL JOINTS:

2. Proximal interphalangeal (PIP) joints: synovial joint between the proximal and middle phalanges.

3. Distal interphalangeal (DIP) joints: the saddle type of synovial joint between the middle and distal phalanges.

4. LIGAMENTS: medial and lateral collateral ligaments stabilize the sides of all metacarpophalangeal and phalangeal joints. Many ligaments attach to the proximal sesamoid bones. These sesamoidean ligaments are important in the horse's suspensory apparatus & thus stay apparatus (pg. 196).

FLEXOR SYNOVIAL SHEATH: surrounds the deep & superficial digital flexors as the cross the fetlock & digital joints.

SPECIES DIFFERENCES

Dorsal ligaments: paired ligaments found in **carnivores**. They are responsible for keeping the claw retracted in the cat. Flexion of the distal interphalangeal joint by the deep digital flexor is responsible for protrusion of the claw.

Declawing or **onychectomy** (Gr. *onyx* nail): removal of the distal phalanges through the distal interphalangeal joint in cats.

Proximal and **distal interdigital ligaments** in the **ox**: prevent abnormal separation of the two digits. When removing one claw it is wise to leave the proximal interdigital ligament to give support to the remaining digit.

"Fetlock joint" (1): popular term used for the metacarpophalangeal (front limb) and metatarsophalangeal (hindlimb) joints in the horse, and occasionally in ruminants.

"Pastern joint" (2): popular term used for the proximal interphalangeal joint in the horse and often in ruminants.

"Coffin joint" (3): popular name used for the distal interphalangeal joint in the horse and often in ruminants.

Suspensory apparatus: in the horse consists of the suspensory ligament, the proximal sesamoid bones and the "distal sesamoidean ligaments". They act as a unit to support the fetlock joint. Disruption in any one of the three components will result in the fetlock sinking.

"Sesamoidean ligaments", "X, Y, V ligaments" - horse: an unofficial term referring to the straight (Y), oblique (V) and cruciate (X) ligaments that anchor the sesamoid bones distally to proximal & middle phalanges. They are part of the suspensory apparatus, counteracting the pull of the suspensory ligament.

Navicular (podotrochlear) bursa: located between the navicular bone and the deep digital flexor tendon in the **horse**. Its inflammation is associated with navicular disease which is more prevalent in the forelimbs. The pain causing lameness may be eliminated by digital neurectomies (cutting the digital nerves).

JOINTS OF DIGITS

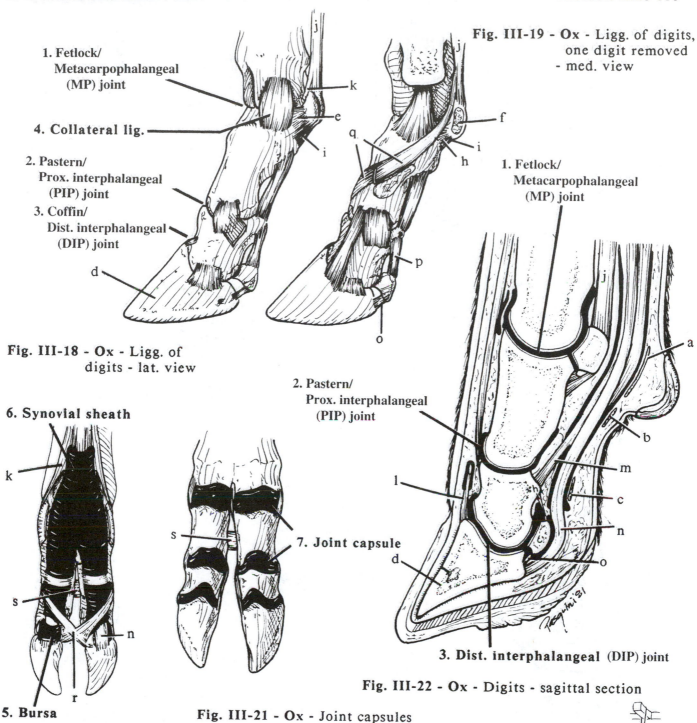

1. Fetlock/
Metacarpophalangeal
(MP) joint

4. Collateral lig.

2. Pastern/
Prox. interphalangeal
(PIP) joint

3. Coffin/
Dist. interphalangeal
(DIP) joint

d

Fig. III-18 - Ox - Ligg. of digits - lat. view

Fig. III-19 - Ox - Ligg. of digits, one digit removed - med. view

6. Synovial sheath

7. Joint capsule

5. Bursa

Fig. III-20 - Ox - Synovial sheaths & bursae - palm. view

Fig. III-21 - Ox - Joint capsules - dors. view

1. Fetlock/
Metacarpophalangeal
(MP) joint

2. Pastern/
Prox. interphalangeal
(PIP) joint

3. Dist. interphalangeal (DIP) joint

Fig. III-22 - Ox - Digits - sagittal section

a. Palm. anular lig.
b. Prox. digital anular lig.
c. Dist. digital anular lig.
d. Dist. phalanx
e. Collateral sesamoidean lig.
f. Intersesamoidean lig.
g. Supf. (straight) dist. sesamoidean lig. (absent in ox)
h. Middle (oblique) dist. sesamoidean lig.

i. Deep (cruciate) dist. sesamoidean lig.
j. Suspensory lig.
k. Extensor br. of suspensory lig.
l. Common digital extensor (tendon)
m. Supf. digital flexor (tendon)
n. Deep digital flexor (tendon)

o. Dist. sesamoidean impar (navicular) lig.
p. Suspensory navicular lig.
q. Middle br. of suspensory lig. (absent in horse)
r. Dist. interdigital cruciate lig.(III-20) (absent in horse)
s. Prox. interdigital cruciate lig.

115

JOINTS - DIGIT

1. MP (fetlock) joint

2. Prox. IP (pastern) joint

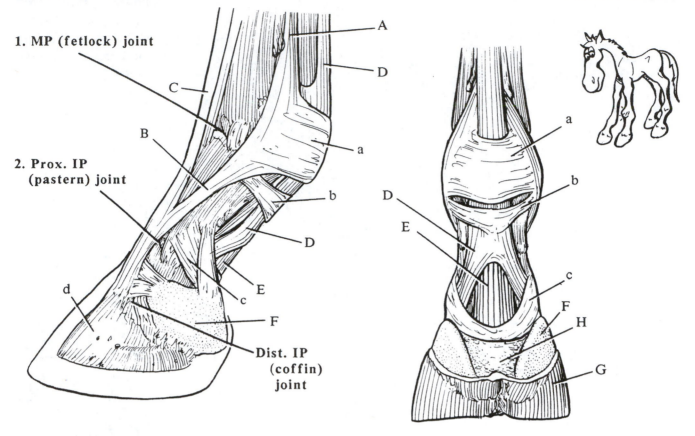

Dist. IP (coffin) joint

Fig. III-23 - Horse - Digit - lat. view

Fig. III-24 - Horse - Digit - palm. view

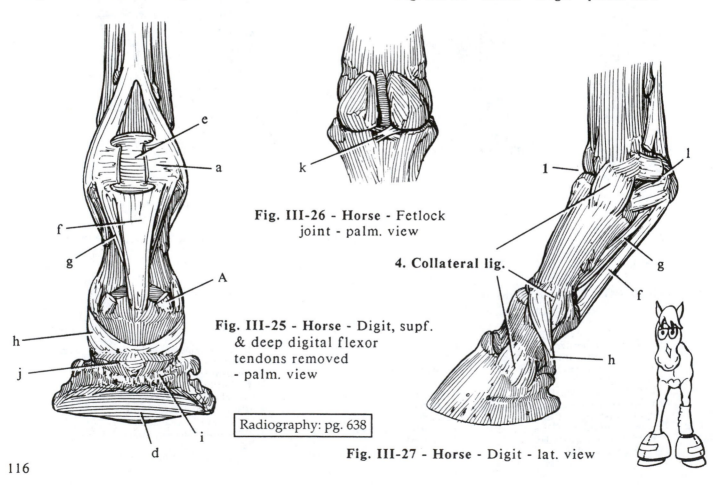

Fig. III-26 - Horse - Fetlock joint - palm. view

4. Collateral lig.

Fig. III-25 - Horse - Digit, supf. & deep digital flexor tendons removed - palm. view

Radiography: pg. 638

Fig. III-27 - Horse - Digit - lat. view

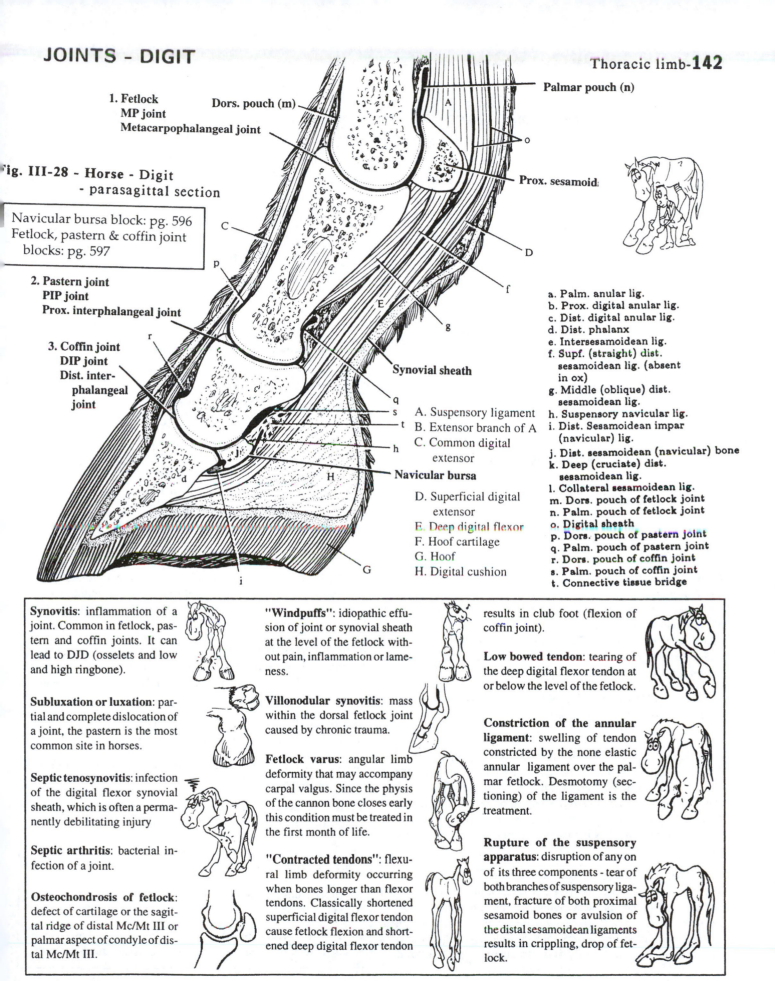

Fig. III-28 - Horse - Digit - parasagittal section

Navicular bursa block: pg. 596
Fetlock, pastern & coffin joint blocks: pg. 597

1. **Fetlock**
   MP joint
   Metacarpophalangeal joint

2. **Pastern joint**
   PIP joint
   Prox. interphalangeal joint

3. **Coffin joint**
   DIP joint
   Dist. interphalangeal joint

Dors. pouch (m)
Palmar pouch (n)
Prox. sesamoid
Synovial sheath
Navicular bursa

A. Suspensory ligament
B. Extensor branch of A
C. Common digital extensor
D. Superficial digital extensor
E. Deep digital flexor
F. Hoof cartilage
G. Hoof
H. Digital cushion

a. Palm. anular lig.
b. Prox. digital anular lig.
c. Dist. digital anular lig.
d. Dist. phalanx
e. Intersesamoidean lig.
f. Supf. (straight) dist. sesamoidean lig. (absent in ox)
g. Middle (oblique) dist. sesamoidean lig.
h. Suspensory navicular lig.
i. Dist. Sesamoidean impar (navicular) lig.
j. Dist. sesamoidean (navicular) bone
k. Deep (cruciate) dist. sesamoidean lig.
l. Collateral sesamoidean lig.
m. Dors. pouch of fetlock joint
n. Palm. pouch of fetlock joint
o. Digital sheath
p. Dors. pouch of pastern joint
q. Palm. pouch of pastern joint
r. Dors. pouch of coffin joint
s. Palm. pouch of coffin joint
t. Connective tissue bridge

Synovitis: inflammation of a joint. Common in fetlock, pastern and coffin joints. It can lead to DJD (osselets and low and high ringbone).

Subluxation or luxation: partial and complete dislocation of a joint, the pastern is the most common site in horses.

Septic tenosynovitis: infection of the digital flexor synovial sheath, which is often a permanently debilitating injury

Septic arthritis: bacterial infection of a joint.

Osteochondrosis of fetlock: defect of cartilage or the sagittal ridge of distal Mc/Mt III or palmar aspect of condyle of distal Mc/Mt III.

"Windpuffs": idiopathic effusion of joint or synovial sheath at the level of the fetlock without pain, inflammation or lameness.

Villonodular synovitis: mass within the dorsal fetlock joint caused by chronic trauma.

Fetlock varus: angular limb deformity that may accompany carpal valgus. Since the physis of the cannon bone closes early this condition must be treated in the first month of life.

"Contracted tendons": flexural limb deformity occurring when bones longer than flexor tendons. Classically shortened superficial digital flexor tendon cause fetlock flexion and shortened deep digital flexor tendon

results in club foot (flexion of coffin joint).

Low bowed tendon: tearing of the deep digital flexor tendon at or below the level of the fetlock.

Constriction of the annular ligament: swelling of tendon constricted by the none elastic annular ligament over the palmar fetlock. Desmotomy (sectioning) of the ligament is the treatment.

Rupture of the suspensory apparatus: disruption of any on of its three components - tear of both branches of suspensory ligament, fracture of both proximal sesamoid bones or avulsion of the distal sesamoidean ligaments results in crippling, drop of fetlock.

JOINTS OF PELVIS

Fig. III-29 - Dog - Ligg. of the pelvic girdle
- lat. view

Fig. III-31 - Horse - Ligg. of the hip joint
- ventr. view

6. Accessory lig.

4. Lig. of the head of the femur

2. Sacrotuberous lig.

3. Pelvic symphysis

Block: pg. 602b

Radiography: pg. 611

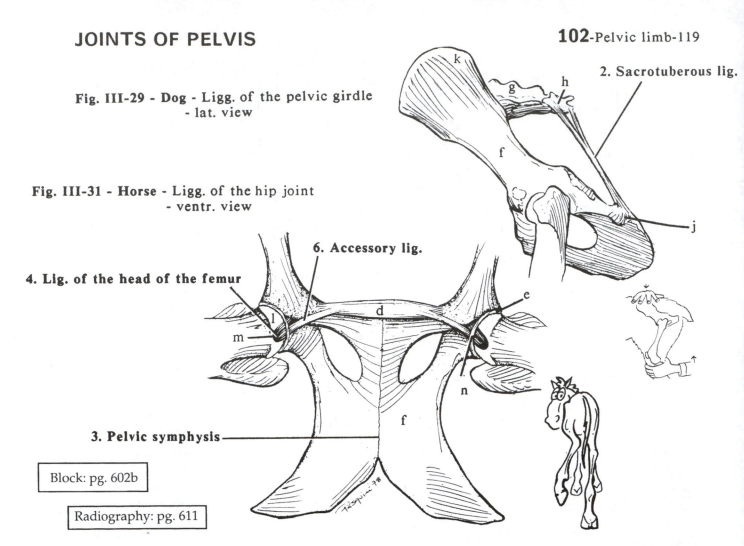

1. SACROILIAC JOINT (Fig. III-33): the relatively immovable articulation between the wings of the sacrum and ilium. This is a combined cartilaginous and synovial joint. Fibrocartilage unites the surfaces of the wings of the sacrum and ilium, forming a sacroiliac synchondrosis. There is a tight joint capsule along the margin of the joint reinforced by dorsal and ventral sacroiliac ligaments.

2. SACROTUBEROUS LIGAMENT: the connective tissue extending from the sacrum and first caudal vertebrae to the ischiatic tuberosity.

3. PELVIC SYMPHYSIS: the symphyseal, slightly movable (fibrocartilaginous) joint between the two hip bones (os coxae). The bones are united by cartilage in the young animal; in the adult, the cartilage is gradually replaced by bone. The front part is formed by the pubic symphysis between the pubic bones. The caudal part is formed by the ischial symphysis between the ischii bones.

HIP JOINT, coxal (KOK-sal) or coxofemoral articulation: the ball-and-socket (spheroidal) type synovial joint between the head of the femur and the acetabulum of the hip bone. It has no collateral ligaments. Its integrity depends on the round ligament of the femur, its strong roomy joint capsule and the muscle mass surrounding it. Functionally, it is a freely movable (diarthrodial)

joint allowing universal movement (flexion-extension, abduction-adduction, medial and lateral rotation and circumduction). As in any joint, what is gained in freedom of movement is offset by loss of stability.

4. Ligament of the head of the femur: formerly the **round ligament of the femur**, it is the short intracapsular ligament extending from the acetabular cavity to the notch on the head of the femur (fovea capitis).

Acetabular lip: the band of fibrocartilage around the rim of the acetabulum increasing the depth of the acetabulum.

Acetabular notch: normal defect in the ventromedial aspect of the acetabulum.

Transverse acetabular ligament (n) crosses the acetabular notch completing the acetabular cavity.

SPECIES DIFFERENCES

Sacrotuberous ligament: Dog – a band of connective tissue (2). Absent in the **cat**.

5. Broad sacrotuberous ligament of the **horse** and **ox**: ("sacrosciatic ligament"): a sheet of connective tissue attaching to the

Fig. III-32 - Ox - Ligg. of the pelvic girdle
- lat. view

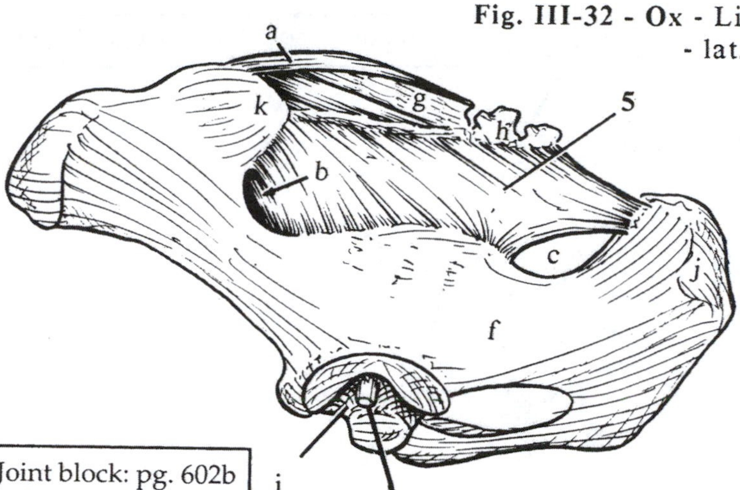

Fig. III-33 - Ox - Ligg. of the pelvic
girdle - cran. view

1. Sacroiliac joint

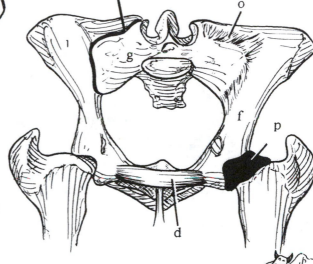

Joint block: pg. 602b

a. Dorsal sacroiliac ligament
b. Greater ischiatic foramen
(absent in carnivores)
c. Lesser ischiatic foramen
(absent in carnivores)
d. Cranial pubic ligament
e. Acetabular margin (lip)
(cotyloid ligament)
f. Os coxae
g. Sacrum

h. 1st caudal. vertebra
i. Acetabulum
j. Ischiatic tuberosity
k. Sacral tuberosity
l. Head of femur
m. Fovea capitis
n. Transverse acetabular ligament
o. Ventral sacroiliac ligament
p. Joint capsule (hip)

ilium, ischiatic spine, and the ischiatic tuberosity, thereby completing the lateral pelvic wall. Between the broad sacrotuberous ligament and the greater and lesser ischiatic notches (Pg. 95, i,k) of the hip bone are two openings: the greater and lesser ischiatic foramina (b,c).

6. Accessory ligament of the head of the femur: the ligament found only in the **horse**. It extends from the prepubic ligament through the acetabular notch under the transverse acetabular ligament. It attaches with the round ligament of the femur to the fovea capitis of the head of the femur. It stabilizes the hip and also makes it harder for a horse to kick to the side (cow kick), but doesn't prevent it.

Trochanteric bursa in the horse: between the insertions of the medial and the superficial gluteal and the greater trochanter

CLINICAL

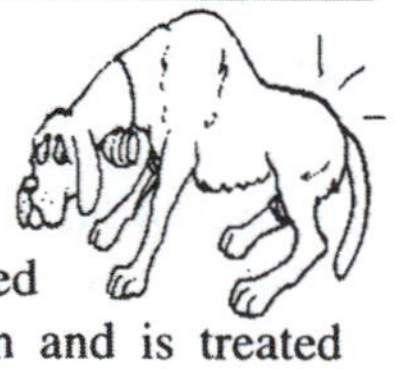

Hip dysplasia: malformed hip joint resulting in a progressive degenerative disease, having a high incidence in some breeds. It is evaluated radiographically. This condition causes pain and is treated many ways; cutting the pectineus muscle (pectineal tenotomy), cutting the neck and head of the femur off (head and neck osteotomy), or remodelling the acetabulum by cutting up the hip bones and repositioning them.

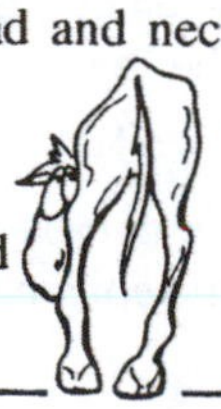

Knocked down hip: incorrect term for a fractured tuber coxae in large animals.

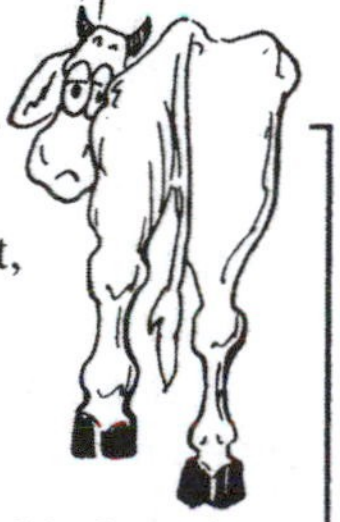

Hip luxation: more common in dogs and cattle than horses. The ox has a weaker round ligament, no accessory ligament, and a more shallow acetabulum.

Craniodorsal hip luxation: the most common direction a hip luxates in all species. To evaluate hip luxation of the dog place your thumb in the space between the greater trochanter and the ischiatic tuberosity. Then rotate the limb outward (laterally). If the hip joint is intact the thumb will be forced out. If the thumb remains, the joint is luxated or the neck of the femur is broken.

Subluxation of sacroiliac joint: uncommon condition in jumping horses which results in "jumper's bump" on healing.

Trochanteric bursitis: rare inflammation of either or both trochanteric bursae causing a **horse** to favor the injured side by cocking the hip towards the good side. This configuration during movement is called **"dog trotting"**.

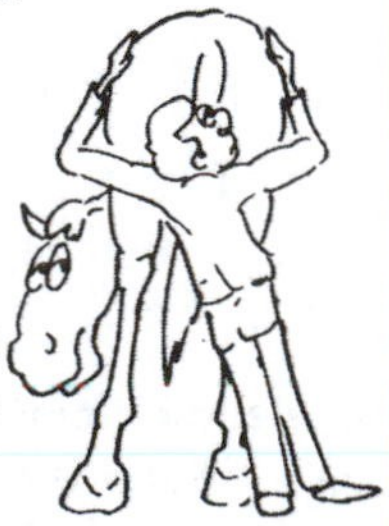

"Jumper's bump"

Compression test - horse: have a kick board in place, stand behind the horse and palpate the greater trochanter on both sides for heat, pain and evidence of swelling associated with bursitis. Press maximally with palms over the greater trochanters.

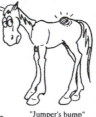

1. Patellar lig.

Radiography: pg. 612 (ca), pg. 643 (eq)

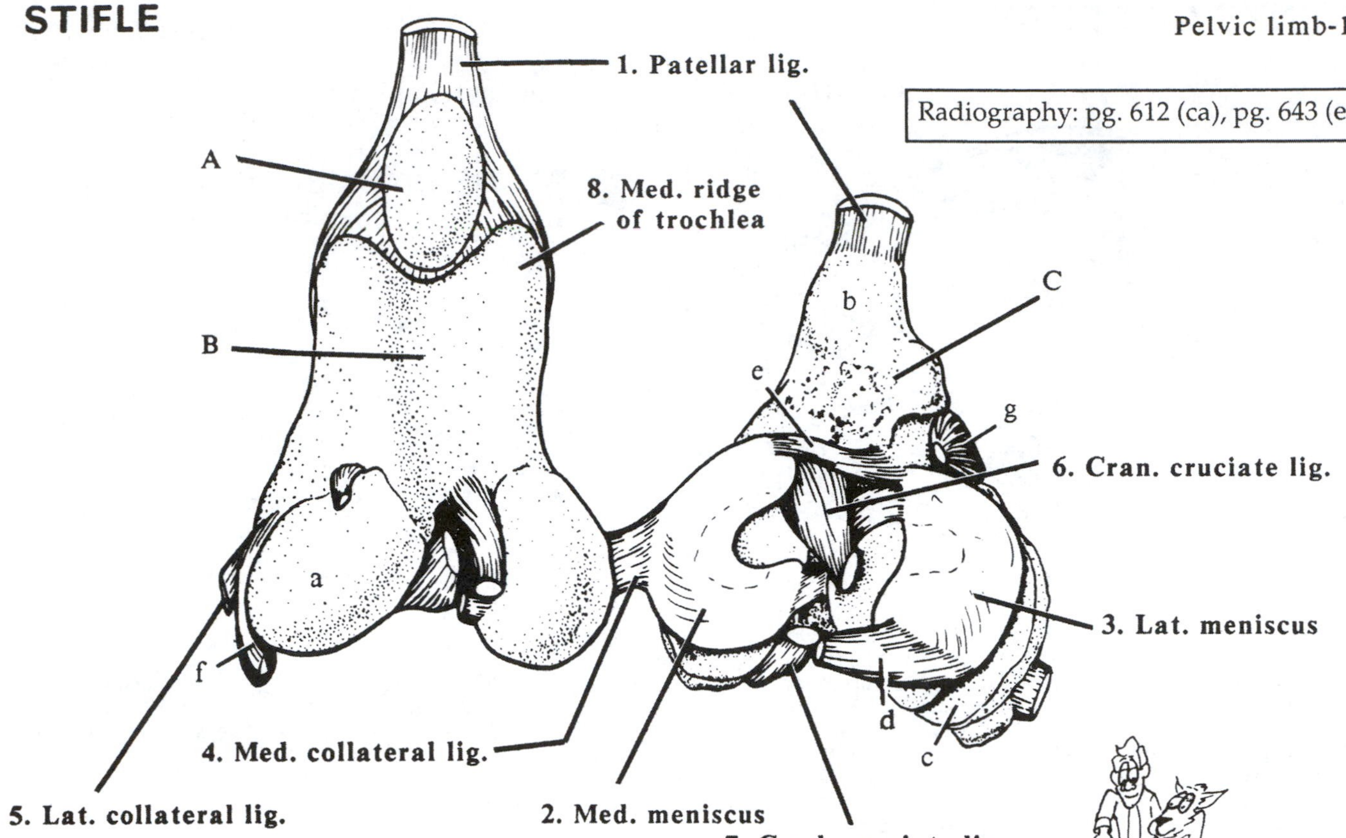

8. Med. ridge of trochlea

A

B

C

6. Cran. cruciate lig.

3. Lat. meniscus

4. Med. collateral lig.

5. Lat. collateral lig.

2. Med. meniscus

7. Caud. cruciate lig.

Fig. III-35 - Dog - Rt. stifle opened, dist. end of femur & prox. end of tibia

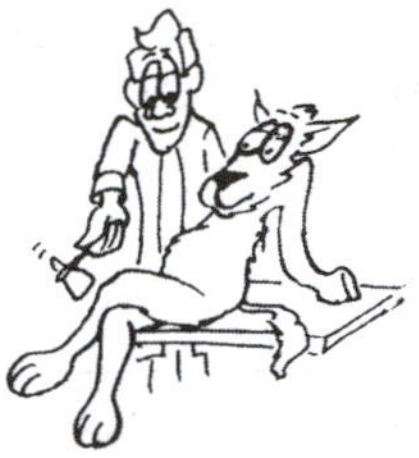

STIFLE JOINT or genual articulation (L. *genu*, knee): the compound joint between the femur and patella and the femur and tibia. It is a condylar joint which acts like a hinge joint with a little rotation.

Femoropatellar joint: the articulation between the patella and trochlea of the femur. It has a spacious joint capsule.

1. Patellar ligament(s): the part of the tendon of insertion of the quadriceps muscle between the patella and the tibial tuberosity. (The patella is a sesamoid bone within the tendon of the quadriceps muscle.)

Femorotibial joint: the articulation between the femoral condyles and tibia (and the interposed menisci).

2,3. Medial and **lateral menisci** (G. crescents; sin. = meniscus) or **semilunar cartilages**: the wedge shaped, crescentric fibrocartilaginous discs between the tibial and femoral articulating condyles. They compensate for incongruence of the articulating bones and absorb some concussive forces. The many ligaments of the menisci help stabilize the joint.

4, 5. Medial (tibial) and **lateral (fibular) collateral ligaments**: strong stabilizing bands on the medial and lateral sides of the stifle.

4. Medial (tibial) collateral ligament: strong stabilizing band on the medial side of the stifle. It fuses with the joint capsule and the

medial meniscus.

5. Lateral (fibular) collateral ligament: the strong band connecting the lateral epicondyle to the head of the fibula. It is separated from the lateral meniscus by the tendon of the popliteus muscle.

6,7. Cranial and **caudal cruciate** (L. resembling a cross) **ligaments**: 2 intra-articular ligaments named for their <u>tibial</u> attachment.

6. Cranial cruciate ligament: inserts <u>cranially</u> on the <u>tibia</u>. It arises from the caudolateral femur. It prevents cranial movement of the tibia in relationship to the femur.

7. Caudal cruciate ligament: inserts <u>caudally</u> on the <u>tibia</u>. It arises from the craniomedial distal femur. It prevents caudal movement of the tibia in relationship to the femur.

LAMP: *memory aid* for which side the cranial (anterior) and caudal (posterior) cruciate ligaments are on - lateral and medial respectively.

Femoral ligament of the lateral meniscus or meniscofemoral ligament (d): connects the caudal part of the lateral meniscus to the femur. It is the only ligament connecting the mensici to the femur.

Femoropatellar ligaments, medial and lateral (m): extend from the epicondyles to the patella.

STIFLE

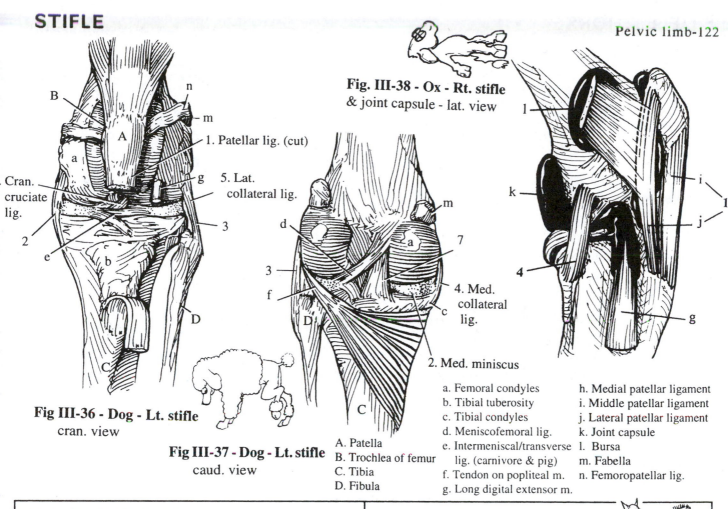

Fig III-36 - Dog - Lt. stifle
cran. view

Fig. III-38 - Ox - Rt. stifle
& joint capsule - lat. view

Fig III-37 - Dog - Lt. stifle
caud. view

1. Patellar lig. (cut)
5. Lat. collateral lig.
. Cran. cruciate lig.
4. Med. collateral lig.
2. Med. miniscus

a. Femoral condyles
b. Tibial tuberosity
c. Tibial condyles
d. Meniscofemoral lig.
e. Intermeniscal/transverse lig. (carnivore & pig)
f. Tendon on popliteal m.
g. Long digital extensor m.
h. Medial patellar ligament
i. Middle patellar ligament
j. Lateral patellar ligament
k. Joint capsule
l. Bursa
m. Fabella
n. Femoropatellar lig.

A. Patella
B. Trochlea of femur
C. Tibia
D. Fibula

SPECIES DIFFERENCES

Carnivores, pigs and **small ruminants**: have one patellar ligament.

Horse and **ox**: have three patellar ligaments - lateral, middle (intermediate) and medial (h-j).

8. Medial ridge (trochlear tubercle) of the femoral trochlea (Fig. III-41): the enlarged process in the **horse** that is consciously forced between the medial and middle patellar ligaments to cause the "patellar lock" of the stay apparatus (pg. 196).

Parapatellar fibrocartilage: the hook of fibrocartilage attached to the medial side of the patella. The medial patellar ligament attaches to it. It hooks over the medial patellar ridge when the stay apparatus is engaged.

CLINICAL

"Upward fixation of the patella": the involuntary (pathological) "catching" of the patella on the medial ridge of the femoral trochlea. Conditioning the horse may resolve problem. Surgical cutting of the medial patellar ligament is a last resort because it may result in degenerative changes in the apex of the patella.

Cranial ("anterior") drawer sign: the pathological movement of the tibia cranial to the femur due to rupture of the cranial cruciate ligament. Common in small animals due to trauma from the lateral side (HBC [hit by car]), which also usually tears the medial collateral ligament, and the medial meniscus since it is attached to the medial collateral ligament.

Horse: the synovial joint cavity of the stifle is divided into three sacs - the medial and lateral femorotibial sacs and the femoropatellar sac. These sacs may or may not communicate. This is clinically important because if one sac is infected, the other two may be also. When anesthetizing these joints in lameness diagnosis all three joints have to be injected individually (see pg. 600).

Patellar luxation: the displacement of the patella medially or laterally out of the femoral patellar surface (trochlea). Medial luxation is more common in small breeds and lateral luxation more common in large breeds of dogs.

Gonitis: inflammation to the stifle. This can be due to soft tissue or bony lesions.

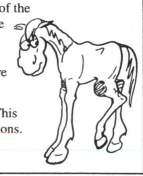

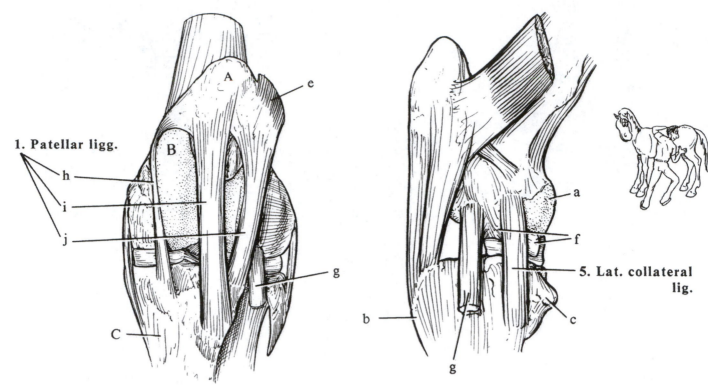

1. Patellar ligg.
 h
 i
 j

Fig. III-39 - Horse - Lt. stifle
   - cran. view

Fig. III-40 - Horse - Lt. stifle - lat. view

5. Lat. collateral
    lig.

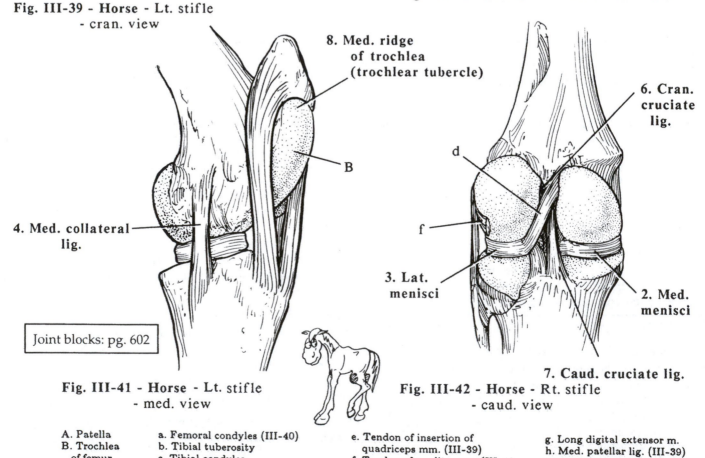

8. Med. ridge
 of trochlea
 (trochlear tubercle)

6. Cran.
 cruciate
 lig.

4. Med. collateral
   lig.

Joint blocks: pg. 602

3. Lat.
 menisci

2. Med.
 menisci

7. Caud. cruciate lig.

Fig. III-41 - Horse - Lt. stifle
    - med. view

Fig. III-42 - Horse - Rt. stifle
    - caud. view

A. Patella	a. Femoral condyles (III-40)	e. Tendon of insertion of quadriceps mm. (III-39)	g. Long digital extensor m.
B. Trochlea of femur	b. Tibial tuberosity	f. Tendon of popliteus m. (III-40, removed in III-39)	h. Med. patellar lig. (III-39)
C. Tibia	c. Tibial condyles		i. Middle patellar lig.
	d. Meniscofemoral lig. (III-42)		j. Lat. patellar lig.

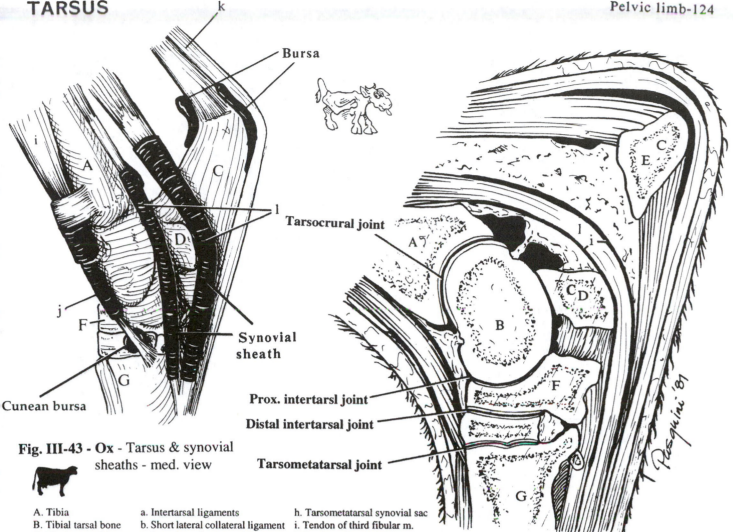

Fig. III-43 - Ox - Tarsus & synovial sheaths - med. view

Fig. III-44 - Ox - Tarsus - sagittal section

A. Tibia	a. Intertarsal ligaments	h. Tarsometatarsal synovial sac
B. Tibial tarsal bone	b. Short lateral collateral ligament	i. Tendon of third fibular m.
C. Fibular tarsal bone	c. Long lateral collateral ligament	j. Tendon of cranial tibial m.
D. Sustentaculum tali	d. Joint capsule	k. Tendon of superficial digital flexor m.
E. Calcanean tuberosity	e. Tibiotarsal synovial sac	l. Tendon of deep digital flexor m.
F. Central tarsal bone	f. Proximal intertarsal synovial sac	m. Tendon of long digital extensor m.
G. Metatarsal bone	g. Distal intertarsal synovial sac	n. Tendon of long fibular m.

TIBIOFIBULAR JOINT: between the lateral condyle of the tibia and the head of the fibula. They differ between the species due to variations in fibular development. Its joint capsule is an extension of the lateral sac of the femorotibial sac of the stifle joint.

TARSUS or "hock" (TAR-sus) (G. *tarsos*, flat): a compound hinge (ginglymus) type of synovial joint. It is a composite, uniaxial joint articulation like the carpal joint, allowing flexion and extension.

Tarsocrural ("tibiotarsal") joint: articulation between the proximal row of tarsal bones (talus and calcaneus) and the tibia and fibula. The trochlear ridges of the talus fit into the cochlea of the tibia. The ridges and grooves are off the sagittal plane so that the hindpaw passes lateral to the forepaw in a gallop. This is the most movable of the tarsal joints. Its synovial sac communicates with the proximal intertarsal sac and the synovial sheath around the tendon of the lateral digital flexor.

• Species differences of tarsocrural joint:
  - Ruminants and pig: formed between the tibia, fibula, talus and calcaneus
  - Horse and carnivores: calcaneus not involved

Proximal intertarsal joint: articulation between the proximal row (talus and calcaneus) and the central and fourth tarsal bones. It communicates with the talocrural sac.

• Distal trochlea of the talus: present in the pig and ruminant giving the proximal intertarsal joint more mobility than the other species.

Distal intertarsal (centrodistal) joint: articulation between the central tarsal and tarsal bones I, II and II. The distal intertarsal joint doesn't cross the whole tarsus because the fourth tarsal bone crosses it on the lateral side.

Tarsometatarsal joint: articulation between the distal row of tarsal bones and the metatarsal bones I to V.

Intertarsal joint: the plane articulations between the individual tarsal bones, as apposed to the proximal and distal intertarsal joints which are between the rows of tarsal bones.

Tarsal joint capsule: as in all synovial joints, consists of fibrous and synovial parts. The **fibrous part** extends from the distal end of the tibia and fibula to the proximal end of the metatarsal bones. Its plantar surface is thickened to smooth the deep wall of the tarsal canal. The **synovial part** encloses the individual tarsal joints and these are called synovial sacs - **talocrural sac, proximal intertarsal sac, distal intertarsal sac** and **tarsometatarsal sac**. The intercommunication between the different joints of the tarsus is important clinically in horses for intra-articular injections in lameness diagnosis (see appendix).

123

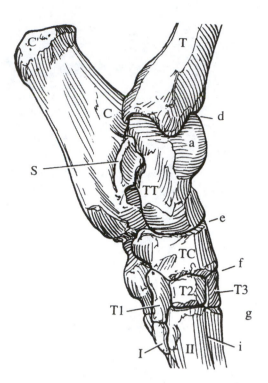

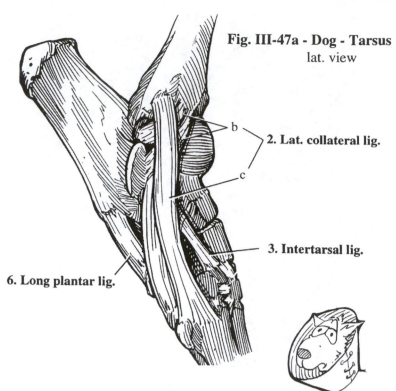

Fig. III-47a - Dog - Tarsus
lat. view

2. Lat. collateral lig.

3. Intertarsal lig.

6. Long plantar lig.

Fig. III-47a - Dog - Tarsus - Ligg.
lat. view

		a. Trochlea of talus
T. Tibia	T1. 1st tarsal bone	b. Short collateral lig.
TT. Tibial tarsal bone	T2. 2nd tarsal bone	c. Long collateral lig.
C. Calcaneus	T3. 3rd tarsal bone	d. Tibiotarsal joint
C'. Calcanean tuberosity	T4. 4th tarsal bone	e. Prox. intertarsal joint
S. Sustentaculum tali	I-V. Metatarsal bone	f. Dist. intertarsal joint
TC. Central tarsal bone		g. Tarsometatarsal joint
		h. Dist. tibiofibular joint
		i. Intermetatarsal joint

1, 2. Medial and **lateral collateral ligaments**: the strong bands on either side of the tarsus. Both have long and short parts.

3. Intertarsal ligaments: numerous connective tissue bands holding the tarsal bones together.

4. Proximal extensor retinaculum: the transverse ligament across the distal end of the tibia holding down the tendons of the long digital extensor and cranial tibial muscles.

5. Distal extensor retinaculum: the transverse loop that holds the tendon of the long digital extensor muscle.

6. Long plantar ligament: the well developed ligament on the plantar side of the fibular tarsal bone (calcaneus) connecting the fibular tarsal bone to the metatarsus.

Flexor retinaculum: thickening of the deep fascia over the plantar aspect of the tarsus

Tarsal canal: passage formed by the tarsal bones and the flexor retinaculum containing:
• Tendon and sheath of long digital extensor
• Plantar branch of saphenous artery and vein
• Medial and lateral plantar nerves

INTERMETATARSAL, METATARSOPHALANGEAL and IN-TERPHALANGEAL JOINTS: resemble the analogous joints of the thoracic limb.

SPECIES DIFFERENCES

Proximal tibiofibular joint:
• **Carnivore, horse** and **pig**: the head of the fibula articulates with the tibia by a plane type of synovial joint.
• **Ruminant**: the head of the fibula is fused to the tibia.

Distal tibiofibular joint:
• **Carnivore, ruminant** and **pig**: the distal fibula (lateral malleolus) forms a synovial joint with the distal tibia. Its joint capsule is a continuation of the talocrural joint.
• **Horse**: the distal fibula (lateral malleolus) fuses with and becomes a part of the tibia.

CLINICAL

"Curb" (desmitis): enlargement of the long plantar ligament in the horse.

Horse's talocrual pouches: the part of the joint capsule not tied down by bones or ligaments allowing access for arthrocentesis (dorsomedial, medioplantar and lateroplantar pouches).

Spavin: the common term for problems of the horse's tarsus.

• **Bone spavin**, true spavin: osteoarthritis and periostitis usually of the distal intertarsal, tarsometatarsal joint of the hock. The disease usually begins on the dorsomedial aspect of these joints under the cunean tendon. Lameness manifests as an asymmetrical gluteal rise ("hiking"). The horse raises the affected limb's hip during motion to minimize flexion of the hock. Resulting periosteal bone formation can bridge and even fuse the joints (ankylosis). Ankylosis will cure the lameness.

• **"Jack spavin"**: an especially large form of bone spavin.

• **"High spavin"**: bone spavin of the proximal tarsus.

TARSUS

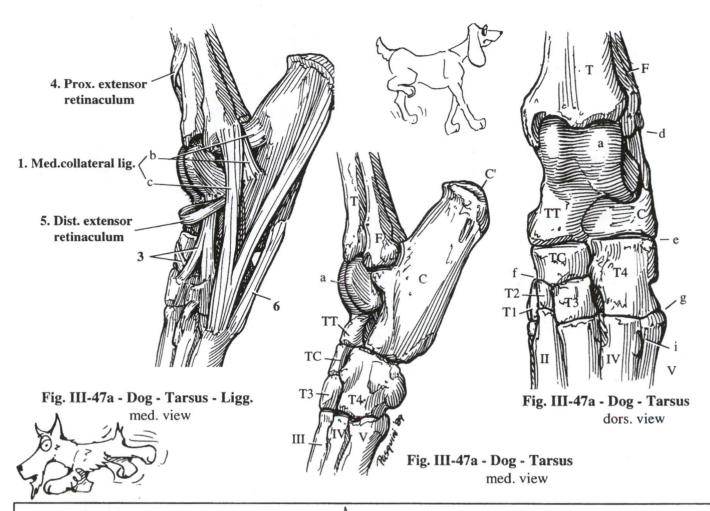

4. Prox. extensor retinaculum

1. Med. collateral lig. { b c

5. Dist. extensor retinaculum

3

6

Fig. III-47a - Dog - Tarsus - Ligg.
med. view

Fig. III-47a - Dog - Tarsus
med. view

Fig. III-47a - Dog - Tarsus
dors. view

• **Blind (occult) spavin**: a lameness of the tarsus with no palpable or radiological changes.

• **Bog spavin**: the distension of the tarsal synovial pouches with excess synovial fluid seen in horses and cattle.

• **Blood spavin**: an enlargement of the medial saphenous vein over the tarsus.

Spavin test: the procedure to test for lameness due to problems in the tarsus. Lift the leg and flex the hock for one minute. Set the leg down and immediately trot the animal. This will exacerbate a spavin for several steps. Mild positive reactions to a spavin test may be due to stifle problems so view with suspicion.

Cunean bursitis - horse: inflammation of the cunean bursa. The bursa is located over the common site of bone spavin, so bursitis must be differentiated from bone spavin.

Cunean tenotomy - horse: cutting the medial branch of the cranial tibial muscle (cunean tendon) to relieve the clinical signs of bone spavin or cunean bursitis. This doesn't cure the animal or prevent further problems if stress is continued.

Capped hock (hygroma): acquired SQ bursa of the point of the hock in horses and cattle.

Tarsal conformation: the correct orientation of the horse's tarsus should be vertical. Deviation from this orientation results in conformational defects.

• **"Sickle-hocked"** or **"curby"**: a conformational defect where the tarsus is angled (flexed) when viewed from the side.

• **"Cow-hocked"**: a conformational defect where the two tarsi deviate medially towards each other. The tarsi should be straight and parallel when viewed from behind.

Thoroughpin: inflammation of the tarsal synovial sheath of the DDF tendon. Pushing on the swelling doesn't distend other tarsocrural pouches as it does with bog spavin.

Septic tarsitis: infection of the hock causing severe lameness and swelling.

Luxation of tarsal joint: frequent in cattle and horses.

Tarsal cellulitis/hygroma: common in cattle due to chronic trauma. Worry about invading joint and causing septic tarsitis.

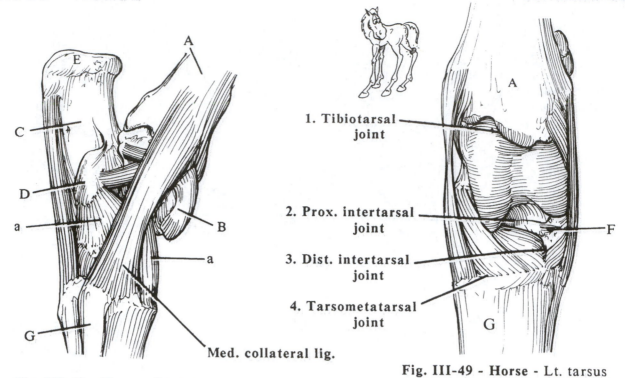

1. Tibiotarsal joint
2. Prox. intertarsal joint
3. Dist. intertarsal joint
4. Tarsometatarsal joint

Med. collateral lig.

Fig. III-48 - Horse - Lt. tarsus - med. view

Fig. III-49 - Horse - Lt. tarsus - cran. view

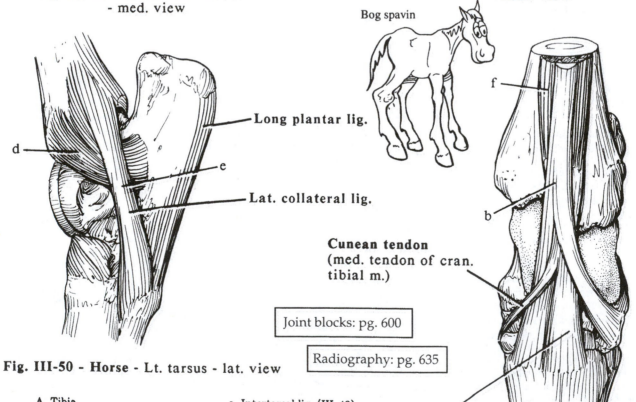

Bog spavin

Long plantar lig.

Lat. collateral lig.

Cunean tendon (med. tendon of cran. tibial m.)

Joint blocks: pg. 600

Radiography: pg. 635

Fig. III-50 - Horse - Lt. tarsus - lat. view

A. Tibia
B. Tibial tarsal bone (talus)
C. Fibular tarsal bone (calcaneus)
D. Sustentaculum tali
E. Calcanean tuberosity
F. Central tarsal bone (III-49)
G. Metatarsal bone

a. Intertarsal lig. (III-48)
b. Tendon of third fibular (peroneus tertius) m. (III-51)
c. Lat. tendon of cran. tibial m.
d. Short lat. collateral lig. (III-50)
e. Long lat. collateral lig.
f. Cranial tibial m. (III-51)

Fig. III-51 - Horse - Tendons - dorsal view

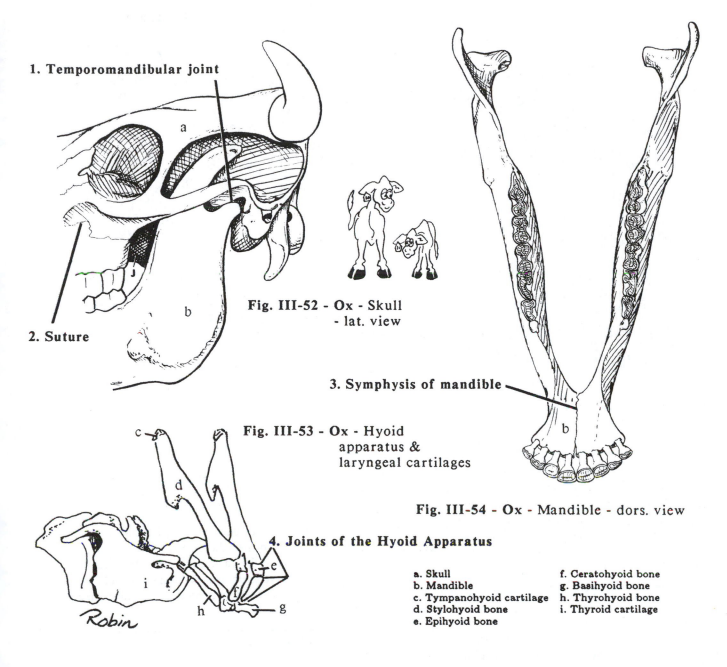

1. Temporomandibular joint

2. Suture

Fig. III-52 - Ox - Skull - lat. view

3. Symphysis of mandible

Fig. III-53 - Ox - Hyoid apparatus & laryngeal cartilages

Fig. III-54 - Ox - Mandible - dors. view

4. Joints of the Hyoid Apparatus

Robin

a. Skull
b. Mandible
c. Tympanohyoid cartilage
d. Stylohyoid bone
e. Epihyoid bone
f. Ceratohyoid bone
g. Basihyoid bone
h. Thyrohyoid bone
i. Thyroid cartilage

1. TEMPOROMANDIBULAR JOINT: a condylar joint between the condyles of the mandible and the mandibular fossae of the temporal bones. It has a loose joint capsule whose lateral side is strengthened to form a lateral ligament.

Articular disc: a thin meniscus lying between the two articular surfaces of the joint.

2. SUTURES OF THE SKULL: the immovable, fibrous joints between the skull bones.

3. SYMPHYSIS OF THE MANDIBLE: the cartilaginous joint joining the right and left mandibular bodies.

JOINTS OF THE AUDITORY OSSICLES: the ear bones articulate with each other via synovial joints. The stapes articulates with the vestibular window by a fibrous joint (syndesmosis). The auditory ossicles are held in place by a number of ligaments (See Ch. VIII).

4. JOINTS OF THE HYOID APPARATUS: the synovial articulations between the bones of the hyoid apparatus and between the thyrohyoid bone and the cranial cornu of the thyroid cartilage. The tympanohyoid cartilage forms a fibrous (syndesmosis) articulation with the skull.

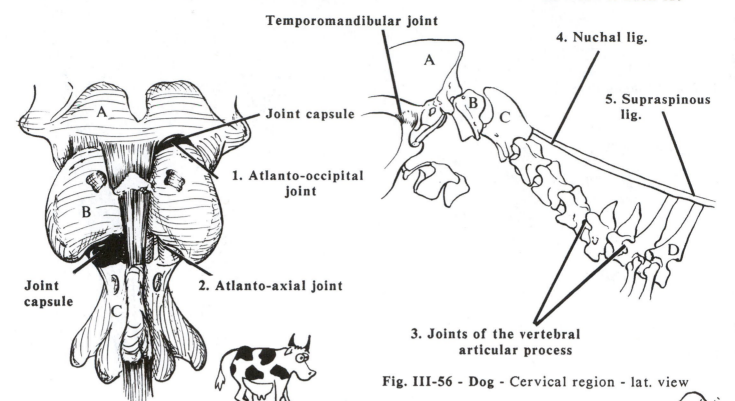

Temporomandibular joint

Joint capsule

1. Atlanto-occipital joint

Joint capsule

2. Atlanto-axial joint

Fig. III-55 - Ox - Cran. cervical region - dors. view

4. Nuchal lig.

5. Supraspinous lig.

3. Joints of the vertebral articular process

Fig. III-56 - Dog - Cervical region - lat. view

Radiography: pg. 613

JOINTS of the VERTEBRAL COLUMN: typical **intervertebral articulations** consist of two types of joints - cartilaginous and synovial. Symphyseal (cartilaginous) joints are formed by intervertebral discs joining adjacent vertebral bodies. Synovial joints are formed by caudal and cranial articular processes of adjacent vertebrae. The atlanto-occipital and atlanto-axial joints are atypical intervertebral articulations.

1. ATLANTO-OCCIPITAL JOINT (the "yes" joint): the condylar joint acting as a modified hinge type of synovial joint between the occipital condyles and the cranial articular surfaces of the atlas. It has a spacious joint capsule strengthened by three membranes (dorsal, ventral, and lateral atlanto-occipital).

2. ATLANTO-AXIAL JOINT (the "no" joint): the pivot type of synovial joint between the dens and cranial articular surface of the atlas and axis. It has a loose joint capsule. The apical ligament of the dens connects the apex of the dens to the occipital bone. The transverse atlantal ligament connects to the two arches of the atlas, crosses over the dens of the axis, thus holding the dens against the ventral arch of the atlas.

3. Joints of the vertebral articular processes: the synovial articulations between the caudal and cranial articular processes of adjacent vertebrae.

4. Nuchal ligament (lig. nuchae, ligament of the nape): the

yellow-elastic connective tissue connecting the upper cervical vertebrae or skull with the spinous processes of the thoracic vertebrae. It helps support the head.

5. Supraspinous ligament: the heavy band of connective tissue running over the tops of the spinous processes from the first thoracic vertebra to the caudal vertebrae. It prevents abnormal separation of the vertebral spines during flexion of the vertebral column. It is the direct continuation of the funicular part of the nuchal ligament.

SPECIES DIFFERENCES

Nuchal ligament: in the **dog**, a paired band of connective tissue extending from the spinous process of the axis to the spinous process of the 1st thoracic vertebra. It is absent in the **cat**. In the **horse** and **ox** it consists of two paired parts. The **funicular** (cord) **part** resembles that of the dog, but is paired and arises from the skull and inserts on spines of the thoracic vertebrae of the withers. The **lamellar** (sheet) **part** (b) consists of two sheets of connective tissue arising from the second and third thoracic spines and the funicular part, and inserting on cervical spines C2-C6.

Bursas of the nuchal ligament in horses: positioned between the bony processes and the funicular part. The **atlantal bursa**

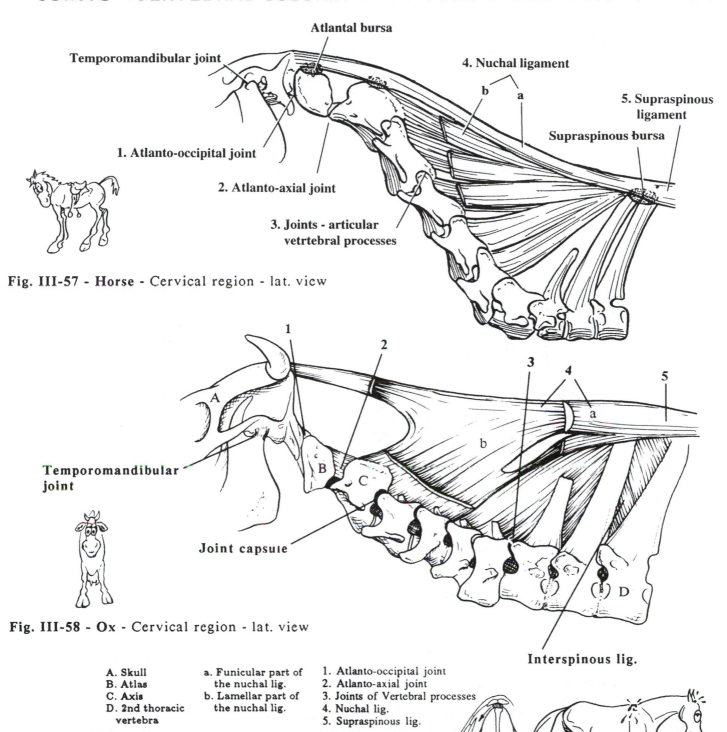

Fig. III-57 - Horse - Cervical region - lat. view

Atlantal bursa

Temporomandibular joint

4. Nuchal ligament

1. Atlanto-occipital joint

2. Atlanto-axial joint

3. Joints - articular vetrtebral processes

5. Supraspinous ligament

Supraspinous bursa

Fig. III-58 - Ox - Cervical region - lat. view

Temporomandibular joint

Joint capsule

Interspinous lig.

A. Skull	a. Funicular part of the nuchal lig.	1. Atlanto-occipital joint
B. Atlas		2. Atlanto-axial joint
C. Axis	b. Lamellar part of the nuchal lig.	3. Joints of Vertebral processes
D. 2nd thoracic vertebra		4. Nuchal lig.
		5. Supraspinous lig.

(cranial nuchal bursa) is constantly found over the atlas. An inconstant bursa (caudal nuchal bursa) is sometimes found over the axis. A constant **supraspinous bursa** is over the most prominent spines of the withers.

Dorsal scapular ligament: the thickening of the thoracolumbar fascia in the withers region. It interdigitates with the origin of the serratus ventralis muscle on the deep surface of the scapula.

CLINICAL

"Poll-evil": inflammation of the atlantal bursa.

"Fistulous withers": inflammation of the supraspinous bursa. Special care should be taken because *Brucella spp.*, which is transmissible to humans (zoonosis), have been isolated. Rupture of this inflamed bursa may migrate down the dorsal scapular ligament and be trapped deep to the scapula.

129

JOINTS - VERTEBRAL COLUMN

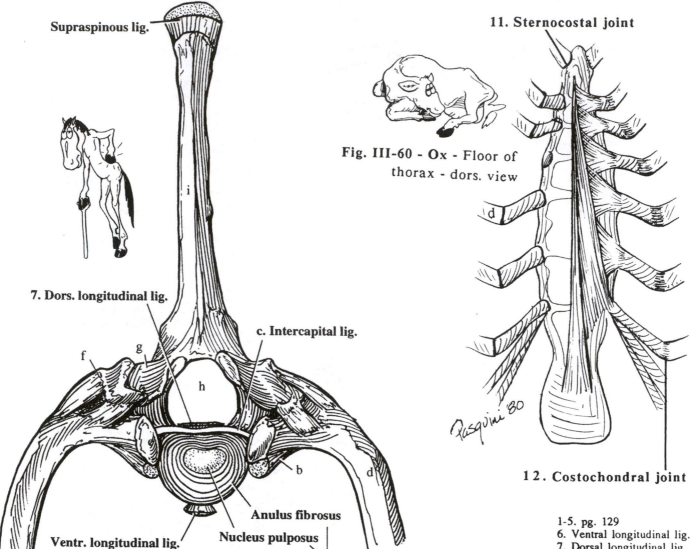

Supraspinous lig.

7. Dors. longitudinal lig.

c. Intercapital lig.

f g h

Ventr. longitudinal lig.

Anulus fibrosus

Nucleus pulposus

8. Intervertebral disc

Fig. III-59 - Horse - 3rd & 4th thoracic
vertebrae - craniolat. view

11. Sternocostal joint

Fig. III-60 - Ox - Floor of
thorax - dors. view

Pasquini 80

1 2. Costochondral joint

1-5. pg. 129
6. Ventral longitudinal lig.
7. Dorsal longitudinal lig.
8. Intervertebral discs
9. Interspinous lig.
10. Costovertebral joint
11. Sternocostal joints
12. Costochondral joints

Other joints and ligaments of the vertebral column:

6. Ventral longitudinal ligament: the tendinous band lying on the ventral surfaces of the vertebrae from the midthoracic region to the sacrum. Cranially its function is performed by the longus colli m. They prevent overextension of the spine.

7. Dorsal longitudinal ligament: the tendinous band on the floor of the vertebral canal from the axis to the sacrum. It prevents hyperflexion of the spine.

8. Intervertebral discs: the layers of fibrocartilage between the bodies of adjacent vertebrae, each consisting of an outer fibrous ring and an inner pulpy nucleus.

• **Anulus fibrosus** (fibrous ring): consists of bands of parallel fibers connecting adjacent vertebral bodies. It is thin dorsally and thick ventrally.

• **Nucleus pulposus** (pulpy nucleus): the semi-fluid remnant of the notochord surrounded by the fibrous ring. It serves to absorb shock.

9. Interspinous ligament: the fibers connecting the spines of adjacent vertebrae along the entire length of the vertebral column.

Interarcuate ligaments or **yellow ligaments** (Fig. III-62): the elastic ligaments filling the dorsal spaces between the arches of adjacent vertebrae.

10. Costovertebral joints: the two distinct articulations between most ribs and the vertebral column. The head of each rib forms a ball-and-socket type of synovial joint with the caudal and cranial costal facets of adjacent vertebrae. The tubercle of each rib forms a plane type of synovial joint with the transverse process of the corresponding vertebra. Each articulation has a joint capsule and corresponding ligaments (radiate ligament of the head, intercapital

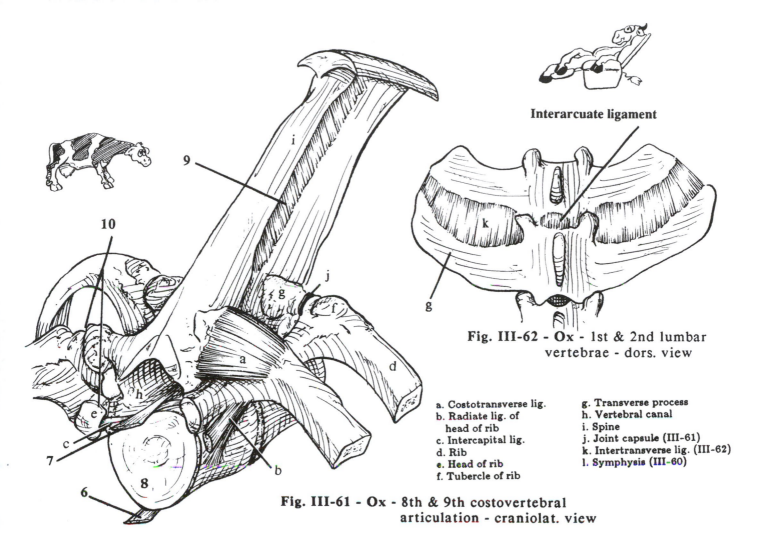

Interarcuate ligament

Fig. III-62 - Ox - 1st & 2nd lumbar
vertebrae - dors. view

a. Costotransverse lig.
b. Radiate lig. of
  head of rib
c. Intercapital lig.
d. Rib
e. Head of rib
f. Tubercle of rib

g. Transverse process
h. Vertebral canal
i. Spine
j. Joint capsule (III-61)
k. Intertransverse lig. (III-62)
l. Symphysis (III-60)

Fig. III-61 - Ox - 8th & 9th costovertebral
articulation - craniolat. view

ligament, costotransverse ligament, and ligament of the neck).

Intercapital ligament: connects the heads of a pair of opposite ribs. It crosses through the intervertebral foramen and over the dorsal part of the vertebral disc. They are not present between the first pair and last two pairs of ribs.

11. Sternocostal joints: the pivot type of synovial articulations between the first eight costal cartilages and the sternum. Each has a joint capsule and ligaments (dorsal and ventral sternocostal radiate ligaments, costoxiphoid ligaments and sternal ligament).

Interchondral joint of the asternal ribs of the costal arch is a slightly movable fibrous joint (synchondrosis). Intersternal joints between the sternebrae are immovable cartilaginous joints (synchondrosis).

12. Costochondral junction or **joints**: the fibrous (syndesmosis) joints between the ribs and the costal cartilages. They have no synovial cavities since they are not synovial joints.

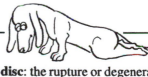

CLINICAL:

Rupture of an intervertebral disc: the rupture or degeneration of the fibrous ring allowing the pulpy nucleus to bulge or "explode" out of the disc. Because the anulus fibrosus is thinnest dorsally, the rupture usually happens dorsally or dorsolaterally into the vertebral canal. This can put pressure on the spinal cord, causing pain or paralysis. This is most common at the thoracolumbar junction (T11 - L2) or the neck region. Rarely does it happen in the thoracic region because of the **intercapital ligaments,** which reinforce the disc dorsally.

Hemilaminectomies: the removal of the right or left dorsal vertebral arch to relieve pressure in the spinal canal.

Disc fenestration: the removal of the remaining nucleus pulposus from a ruptured disc.

"Wobbler": a horse with cervical vertebral instability which impinges on the spinal cord, resulting in different degrees of ataxia.

131

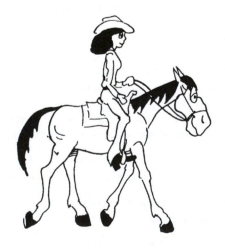

Chapter IV
Muscles

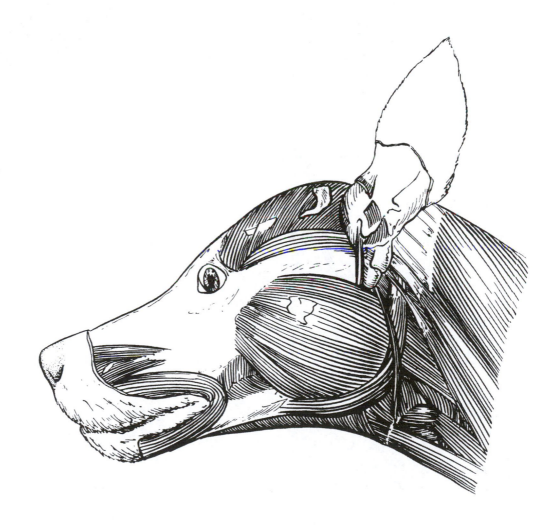

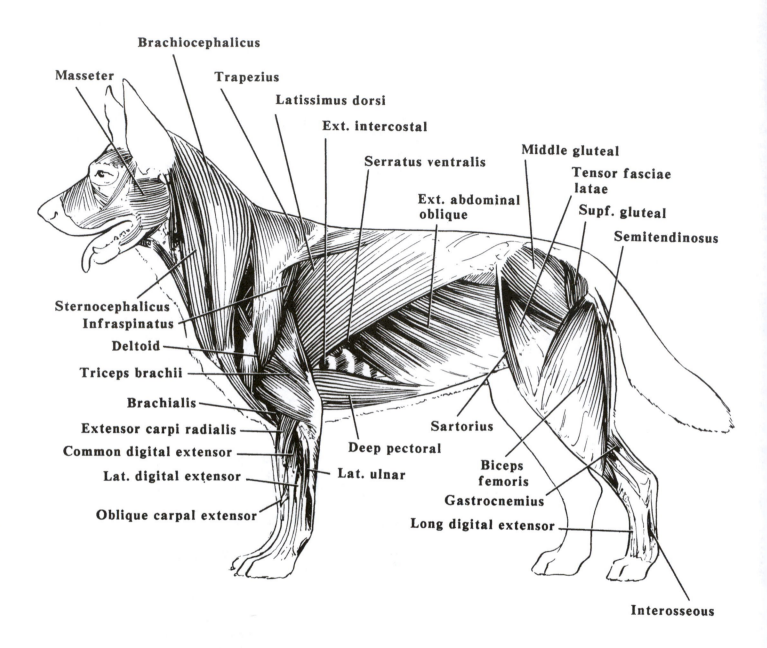

Brachiocephalicus

Masseter

Trapezius

Latissimus dorsi

Ext. intercostal

Serratus ventralis

Middle gluteal

Tensor fasciae latae

Ext. abdominal oblique

Supf. gluteal

Semitendinosus

Sternocephalicus
Infraspinatus

Deltoid

Triceps brachii

Brachialis

Extensor carpi radialis

Common digital extensor

Lat. digital extensor

Oblique carpal extensor

Deep pectoral

Lat. ulnar

Sartorius

Biceps femoris

Gastrocnemius

Long digital extensor

Interosseous

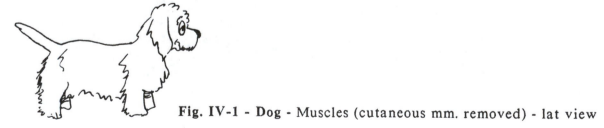

Fig. IV-1 - Dog - Muscles (cutaneous mm. removed) - lat view

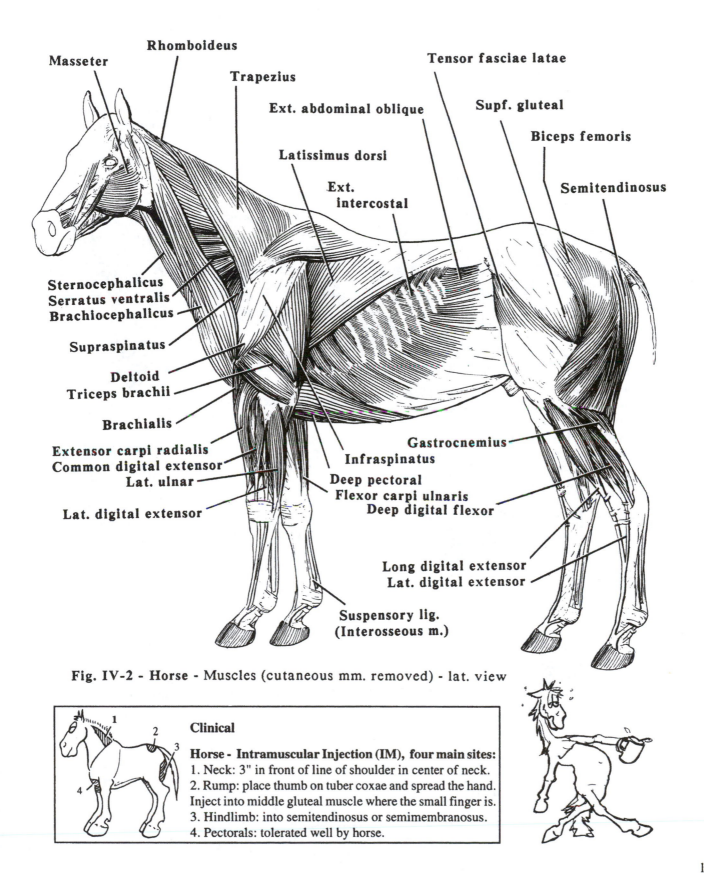

Fig. IV-2 - Horse - Muscles (cutaneous mm. removed) - lat. view

Clinical

Horse - Intramuscular Injection (IM), four main sites:
1. Neck: 3" in front of line of shoulder in center of neck.
2. Rump: place thumb on tuber coxae and spread the hand. Inject into middle gluteal muscle where the small finger is.
3. Hindlimb: into semitendinosus or semimembranosus.
4. Pectorals: tolerated well by horse.

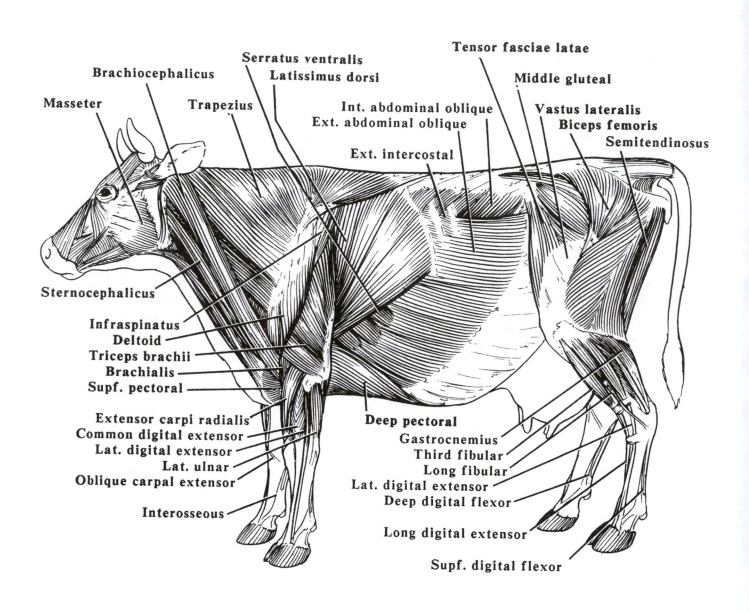

Masseter

Brachiocephalicus

Trapezius

Serratus ventralis
Latissimus dorsi

Tensor fasciae latae

Middle gluteal

Int. abdominal oblique
Ext. abdominal oblique

Vastus lateralis
Biceps femoris
Semitendinosus

Ext. intercostal

Sternocephalicus

Infraspinatus
Deltoid
Triceps brachii
Brachialis
Supf. pectoral

Extensor carpi radialis
Common digital extensor
Lat. digital extensor
Lat. ulnar
Oblique carpal extensor

Interosseous

Deep pectoral
Gastrocnemius
Third fibular
Long fibular
Lat. digital extensor
Deep digital flexor

Long digital extensor

Supf. digital flexor

Fig. IV-3 - Ox - Muscles (cutaneous mm. removed) - lat. view

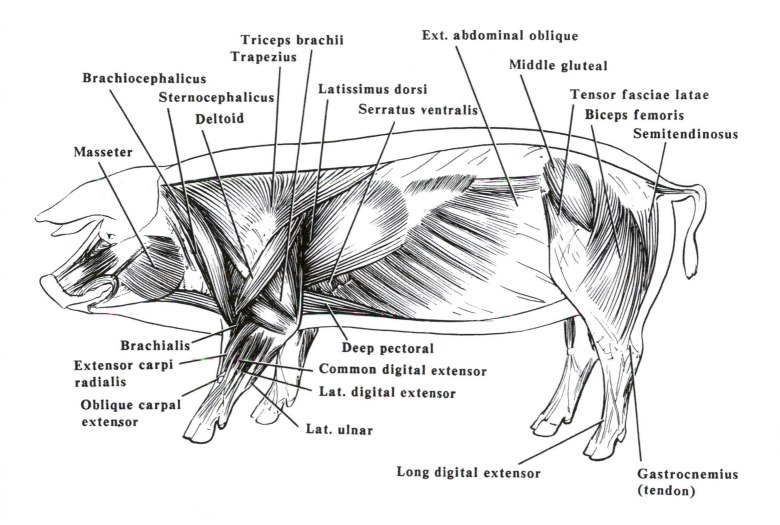

Fig. IV-4 - Pig - Muscles (cutaneous mm. removed) - lat. view

Fig. IV-5 - Cat - Muscles (cutaneous mm. removed) - lat. view

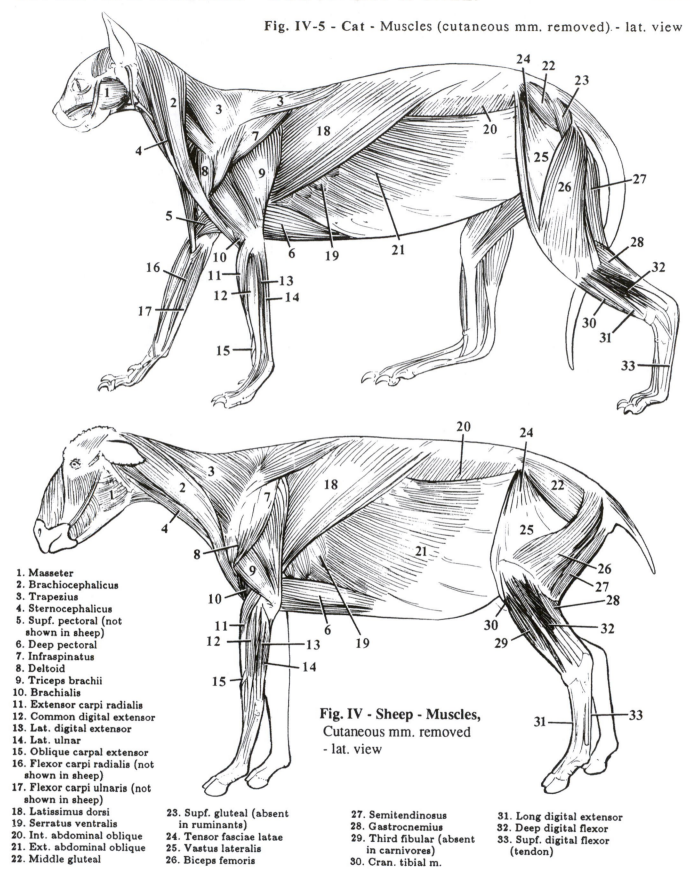

Fig. IV - Sheep - Muscles,
Cutaneous mm. removed
- lat. view

1. Masseter
2. Brachiocephalicus
3. Trapezius
4. Sternocephalicus
5. Supf. pectoral (not shown in sheep)
6. Deep pectoral
7. Infraspinatus
8. Deltoid
9. Triceps brachii
10. Brachialis
11. Extensor carpi radialis
12. Common digital extensor
13. Lat. digital extensor
14. Lat. ulnar
15. Oblique carpal extensor
16. Flexor carpi radialis (not shown in sheep)
17. Flexor carpi ulnaris (not shown in sheep)
18. Latissimus dorsi
19. Serratus ventralis
20. Int. abdominal oblique
21. Ext. abdominal oblique
22. Middle gluteal

23. Supf. gluteal (absent in ruminants)
24. Tensor fasciae latae
25. Vastus lateralis
26. Biceps femoris

27. Semitendinosus
28. Gastrocnemius
29. Third fibular (absent in carnivores)
30. Cran. tibial m.

31. Long digital extensor
32. Deep digital flexor
33. Supf. digital flexor (tendon)

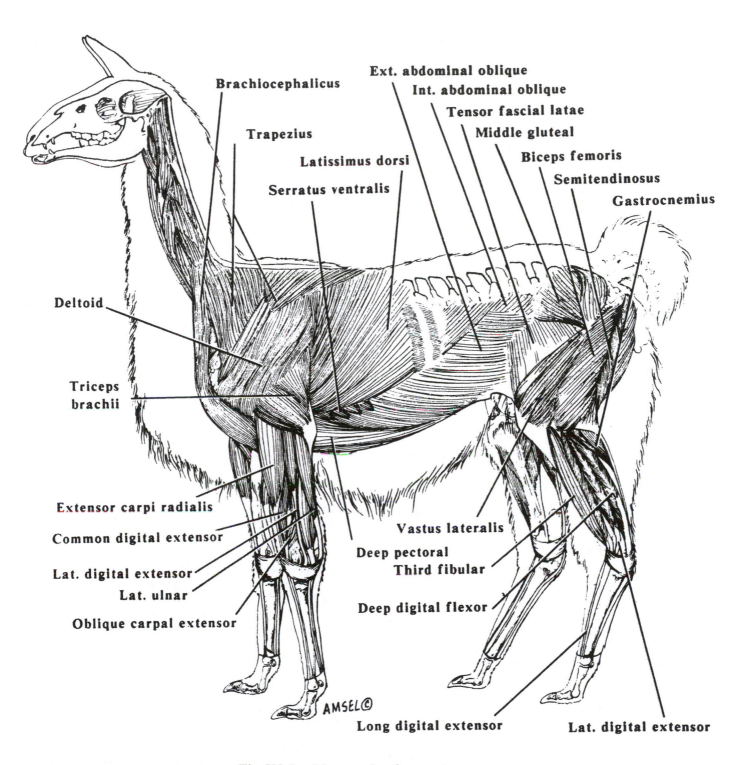

Brachiocephalicus

Ext. abdominal oblique

Int. abdominal oblique

Tensor fascial latae

Trapezius

Middle gluteal

Latissimus dorsi

Biceps femoris

Serratus ventralis

Semitendinosus

Gastrocnemius

Deltoid

Triceps brachii

Extensor carpi radialis

Common digital extensor

Lat. digital extensor

Lat. ulnar

Oblique carpal extensor

Vastus lateralis

Deep pectoral

Third fibular

Deep digital flexor

Long digital extensor

Lat. digital extensor

AMSEL©

Fig IV-7 - Llama - Supf. muscles

MUSCLE

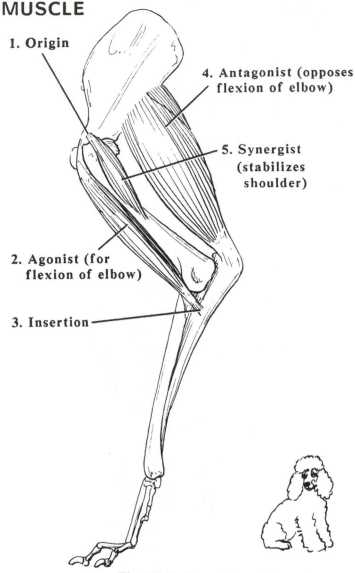

1. Origin

4. Antagonist (opposes flexion of elbow)

5. Synergist (stabilizes shoulder)

2. Agonist (for flexion of elbow)

3. Insertion

Fig. VI-8 - Dog - Muscle functions and attachments - thoracic limb

MUSCLES: the contractile organs responsible for movement in an animal. The two varieties of muscle are **striated** (striped), which includes skeletal and cardiac muscle, and **unstriated** or smooth muscle. Muscles are either **involuntary** or **voluntary**. Involuntary **smooth** and **cardiac** muscles are responsible for breathing, heart beat, peristaltic movements of the intestines, constriction of blood vessels and many other vital functions. Voluntary or **skeletal muscles** are of primary concern in this section. They allow movement from one place to another (location), movement of one part of the body in relation to another, and the maintenance of body posture.

ORIGIN and INSERTION: the attachments of a muscle, usually to bones.

1. Origin (OR-i-jin): the <u>less movable</u> of the two attachme. In the limbs this is usually the more proximal attachment.

2. Insertion: the <u>more movable</u> of the two attachments. In the limbs this is usually the more distal attachment.

MUSCLE ATTACHMENTS:

Fleshy attachments: the apparent direct attachment of muscles to bone, e.g., scapular muscles. In reality, they attach to the periosteum of the bone by very short tendons.

Tendinous attachments: the dense connective tissue connecting spindle-shaped or pennate muscles to bone.

Aponeurotic attachments: the flat, tendinous sheets associated with flat muscles such as those of the abdominal wall.

MUSCLE CONTRACTION: shortening of a muscle, causing a change in the alignments of bones around a joint.

Muscle function: the movement of parts of the body. For each movement a number of muscles contract to produce a smooth controlled movement. Muscles are grouped into prime movers, antagonists, synergists, or fixators. The same muscle may be any of the above, depending on the movement produced.

3. Prime mover or agonist (AG-o-nist) (G. *agon*, a contest): produces the characteristic movement at a joint. The biceps brachii muscle is the prime mover for <u>flexion</u> of the elbow joint.

4. Antagonist: opposes the movement of a prime mover. It aids the prime mover by slowly relaxing so the movement produced is smooth and controlled. The triceps brachii muscle, the prime mover for <u>extension</u> of the elbow joint, is the antagonist to the biceps brachii muscle during flexion of the elbow.

Synergist (G. *syn*, together + *ergon*, work): a muscle that indirectly aids the action of a prime mover.

Fixator: a muscle that stabilizes the proximal end of a limb while the distal end moves.

MUSCLE ACTIONS: depend on how they cross a joint, number of joints crossed and the shape of the joints. The resulting movements (muscle actions) are extension, flexion, rotation, abduction, adduction and circumduction. When visualizing a muscle, imagine what happens to the bones of the joint when the muscle contracts (shortens). For most joints (hinge) there is a flexor side and an extensor side. Note the side of the joint the muscle crosses. Those crossing the flexor surface will cause flexion of the joint upon contraction.

5. Extension: an increase in the angle between bones (moves bones further apart).

6. Flexion: a decrease in the angle between bones (brings bones closer together).

7. Adduction (spelled with a "d", it "adds" to the body): the movement of a limb or structure toward the median plane (toward the body) or, in the digits, toward the limb's axis.

8. Abduction (spelled with a "b"): the movement of a limb away from the body (or median plane), or in the digits, away from the axis of the limb.

9. Rotation: the movement of a part around its long axis.

10. Circumduction: the movement of an extremity that describes the surface of a cone. This is produced by successive flexion, abduction, extension, and adduction.

Supination: the movement of the forearm so the palmar side is rotated upward or forward (as when a cat laps milk from its paw).

Pronation: the movement of the palmar side of the paw or foot downward or backward.

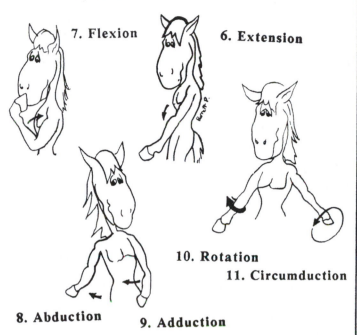

7. Flexion

6. Extension

10. Rotation

11. Circumduction

8. Abduction

9. Adduction

Fig. IV-9 - Cartoons of muscle actions
- inked by Barrett Pasquini

CLINICAL

Rhabdomyolysis, "Monday morning disease": horse given a couple of days off exercise (weekend), maintained on full ration then followed by strenuous exercise (Monday morning).
- Tying up: mild cases with stiff, stilted hindlimb gait.
- Azoturia: severe cases with muscle fasciculations, cramping, sweating, possibly dark urine (myoglobin from muscle breakdown) with kidney damage a sequela.

Exhaustion & post exercise fatigue: common in endurance horses, resulting in depression, lethargy and muscle cramping.

Hyperkalemic periodic paralysis (HYPP) - horse: hereditary condition traced to one Quarterhorse, halter class sire ("Impressive"). His offspring are known for their well developed hindquarters and muscular forearms. Offspring may or may not show signs of HYPP, which manifests as episodes of muscle fasciculations, weakness and possible collapse and death. During an episode there is a marked elevation of blood potassium which returns to normal between episodes. Being an autosomal dominant gene it is possible to decrease or eliminate this condition. This has not happened since the connection to "Impressive" was revealed in the popular press in 1992. Two years later "Impressive" sires were 10 of the top 12.

MUSCULAR ARRANGEMENTS: the muscle fibers (cells) are grouped together into fascicles (bundles) that in turn are grouped together to form the muscle.

Parallel muscle: the muscle bundles (fascicles) run parallel to each other the entire length of the muscle (e.g., sartorius and abdominal muscles). This allows greatest shortening of the muscle, but less strength of contraction.

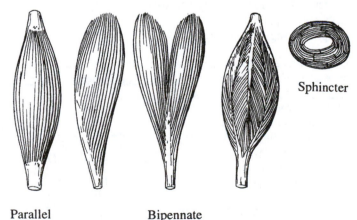

Sphincter

Parallel

Unipennate

Bipennate

Multipennate

Fig. IV-9a - Muscular arrangements

Pennate muscle (penna, feather): the muscle bundles converge on a tendon at an angle. This arrangement allows more bundles, thus, stronger contractions, but less shortening because of the shorter length of the muscle bundles (e.g., gastrocnemius muscle).

- **Unipennate muscle:** a pennate muscle whose tendon runs along one side.

- **Bipennate muscle:** a pennate muscle whose muscle bundles converge on a tendon from two directions.

- **Multipennate muscle**: a pennate muscle whose tendons branch inside the muscle.

Sphincter (SFINK-ter): a muscle whose fibers encircle an opening. Contraction of its fibers close the opening. This type of muscle is found at the entrance and exit of a passageway (e.g., urinary and digestive systems).

MUSCLES - THORACIC LIMB

EXTRINSIC MUSCLES of the THORACIC LIMB (thoracic girdle muscles): the muscles that attach to the thoracic limb and some other part of the body, i.e., to the head, neck, or trunk. The brachiocephalicus (5), trapezius (2), omotransversarius (a), latissimus dorsi (9) and superficial pectoral (11) muscles form the **superficial layer** of the extrinsic muscles. The rhomboid (4), serratus ventralis (8) and deep pectoral (13) muscles form the **deep layer**.

Syssarcosis (sis'sar-KOH-sis): the muscle connection, as opposed to a bone to bone joint, between the thoracic limb and the body.

INTRINSIC MUSCLES: the muscles having both attachments (origin and insertion) on the thoracic limb bones.

INTRINSIC MUSCLES OF THE SHOULDER: act primarily on the shoulder - the deltoid (7), supraspinatus (1), infraspinatus (3), teres major (c), teres minor (b), subscapularis (6) coracobrachialis (d) and biceps brachii (14) muscles.

INTRINSIC MUSCLES OF THE ARM: act primarily on the elbow joint, and are divided into flexor and extensor groups. The flexor group consists of the biceps brachii (14) and brachialis (12) muscles. They are located cranially and innervated by the musculocutaneous nerve. The extensor group, triceps brachii (10), tensor fasciae antebrachii (e) and anconeus (f) muscles, are all located caudally and innervated by the radial nerve.

CRANIOLATERAL FOREARM (ANTEBRACHIAL) MUSCLES: extend the digits and carpus, and supinate the paw – extensor carpi radialis (15), common digital extensor (16), lateral digital extensor (17), lateral ulnar (18) (actually a flexor), oblique carpal extensor (19), and supinator (pg. 160 [#20]) muscles. Most arise directly or indirectly from the lateral (extensor) epicondyle of the humerus and are innervated by the radial nerve.

CAUDAL ANTEBRACHIAL MUSCLES: the flexors of the carpus and digits and pronators of the forearm. Most of them originate on or around the medial (flexor) epicondyle of the humerus and are innervated by the median and ulnar nerves. They include the flexor carpi radialis (22), flexor carpi ulnaris (20), superficial digital flexor (23), and deep digital flexor (25) muscles. The **pronators** include the pronator teres (21) and pronator quadratus muscles in carnivores. Supination and pronation occur in carnivores and pigs, but not other domestic species due to fusion of the ulna and radius and loss of the pronator muscles.

INTRINSIC MUSCLES OF THE MANUS: except for the interosseous muscle (24) which supports the metacarpophalangeal joint, the rest are relatively insignificant.

EXTRINSIC MUSCLES of the THORACIC LIMB

Superficial layer
- Brachiocephalicus (5)
- Trapezius (2)
- Omotransversarius (a)
- Latissimus dorsi (9)
- Superficial pectoral (11)

Deep layer
- Rhomboid (4)
- Serratus ventralis (8)
- Deep pectoral (13)

INTRINSIC MUSCLES:

Intrinsic muscles of the shoulder:
- Deltoid (7)
- Supraspinatus (1)
- Infraspinatus (3)
- Teres major (c)
- Teres minor (b)
- Subscapularis (6)
- Coracobrachialis (d)
- Biceps brachii (14)
- Triceps brachii, long head

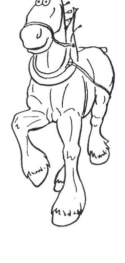

Intrinsic muscles of the arm: flexors and extensors of the elbow.

Flexor group – musculocutaneous nerve
- Biceps brachii (14)
- Brachialis (12)
Extensor group – radial nerve
- Triceps brachii (10)
- Tensor fasciae antebrachii (e)
- Anconeus (f)

Craniolateral forearm muscles – extend the digits and carpus, and supinate the paw – radial nerve – lateral (extensor) epicondyle
- Extensor carpi radialis (15)
- Common digital extensor (16)
- Lateral digital extensor (17)
- Lateral ulnar (18) (actually a flexor)
- Oblique carpal extensor (19)
- Supinator (pg. 160 [#20])

Caudal forearm muscles: flexors of the carpus & digits & pronators of the forearm – median & ulnar nerves – medial (flexor) epicondyle
- Flexor carpi radialis (22)
- Flexor carpi ulnaris (20)
- Superficial digital flexor (23)
- Deep digital flexor (25)
- Pronator teres (21)
- Pronator quadratus

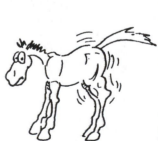

Intrinsic muscles of the manus:
- Interosseous muscle (24)

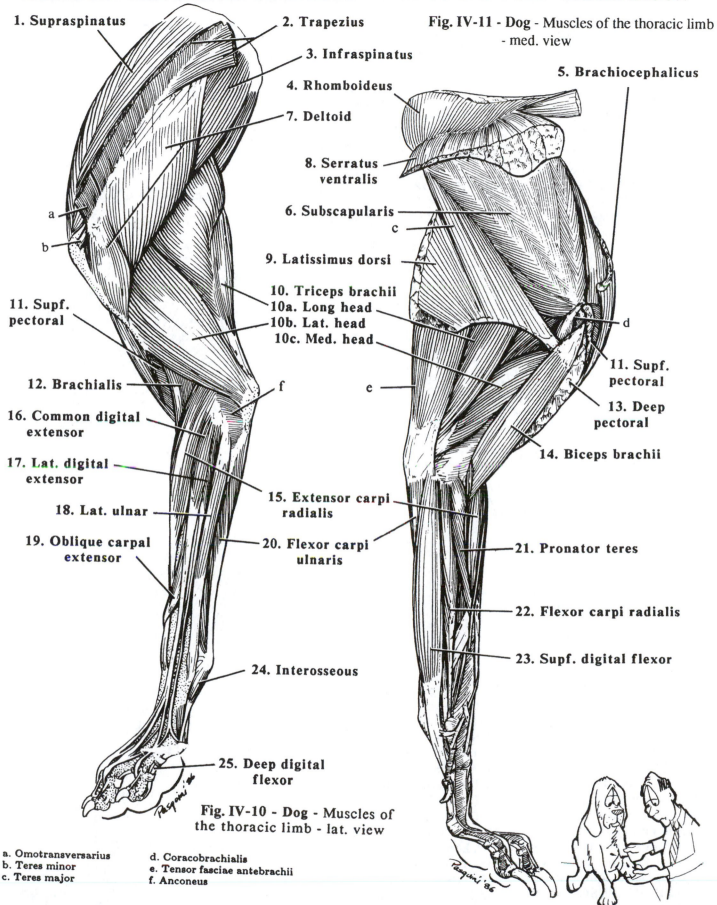

1. Supraspinatus
2. Trapezius
3. Infraspinatus
4. Rhomboideus
7. Deltoid

Fig. IV-11 - Dog - Muscles of the thoracic limb - med. view

5. Brachiocephalicus

8. Serratus ventralis
6. Subscapularis
9. Latissimus dorsi
10. Triceps brachii
10a. Long head
10b. Lat. head
10c. Med. head

11. Supf. pectoral
12. Brachialis
16. Common digital extensor
17. Lat. digital extensor
18. Lat. ulnar
19. Oblique carpal extensor

15. Extensor carpi radialis
20. Flexor carpi ulnaris

24. Interosseous

25. Deep digital flexor

11. Supf. pectoral
13. Deep pectoral
14. Biceps brachii
21. Pronator teres
22. Flexor carpi radialis
23. Supf. digital flexor

Fig. IV-10 - Dog - Muscles of the thoracic limb - lat. view

a. Omotransversarius
b. Teres minor
c. Teres major

d. Coracobrachialis
e. Tensor fasciae antebrachii
f. Anconeus

143

CAT - THORACIC LIMB MUSCLES 1

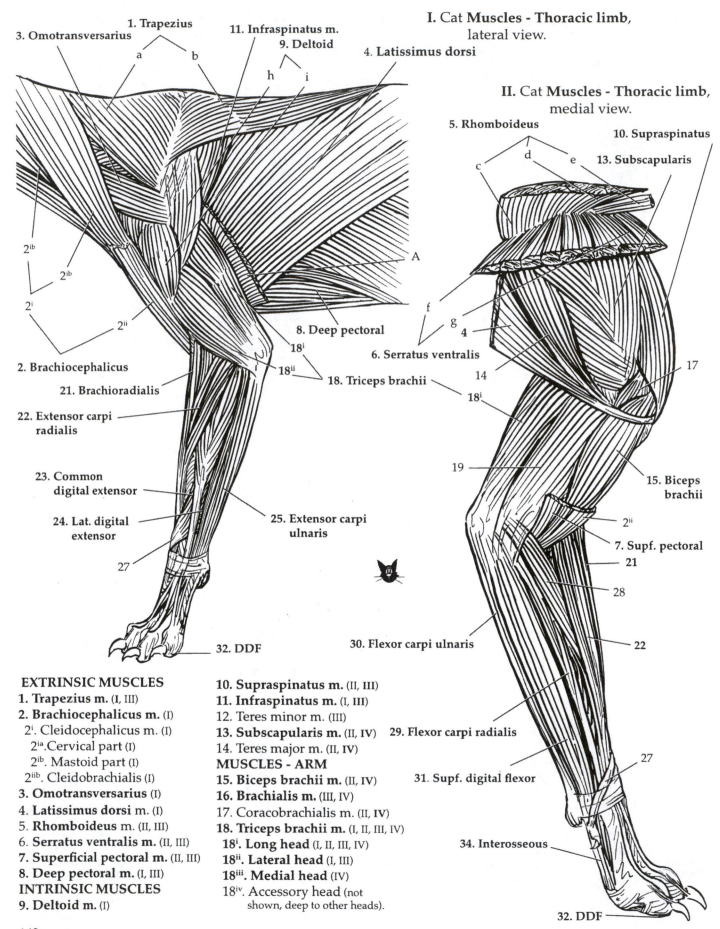

3. Omotransversarius

1. Trapezius
a   b

11. Infraspinatus m.
9. Deltoid
h   i

4. Latissimus dorsi

I. Cat **Muscles - Thoracic limb,** lateral view.

II. Cat **Muscles - Thoracic limb,** medial view.

5. Rhomboideus
c   d   e

10. Supraspinatus

13. Subscapularis

2^{ib}

2^{ib}

2^{i}

2^{ii}

f   g   **4**

6. Serratus ventralis

14

A

8. Deep pectoral

18^{i}
18^{ii}

18. Triceps brachii

18^{i}

17

2. Brachiocephalicus

21. Brachioradialis

22. Extensor carpi radialis

23. Common digital extensor

24. Lat. digital extensor

27

25. Extensor carpi ulnaris

32. DDF

19

15. Biceps brachii

2^{ii}

7. Supf. pectoral
21

28

22

30. Flexor carpi ulnaris

29. Flexor carpi radialis

31. Supf. digital flexor

27

34. Interosseous

32. DDF

EXTRINSIC MUSCLES
1. Trapezius m. (I, III)
2. Brachiocephalicus m. (I)
 2^{i}. Cleidocephalicus m. (I)
  2^{ia}.Cervical part (I)
  2^{ib}. Mastoid part (I)
  2^{iib}. Cleidobrachialis (I)
3. Omotransversarius (I)
4. Latissimus dorsi m. (I)
5. Rhomboideus m. (II, III)
6. Serratus ventralis m. (II, III)
7. Superficial pectoral m. (II, III)
8. Deep pectoral m. (I, III)
INTRINSIC MUSCLES
9. Deltoid m. (I)

10. Supraspinatus m. (II, III)
11. Infraspinatus m. (I, III)
12. Teres minor m. (III)
13. Subscapularis m. (II, IV)
14. Teres major m. (II, IV)
MUSCLES - ARM
15. Biceps brachii m. (II, IV)
16. Brachialis m. (III, IV)
17. Coracobrachialis m. (II, IV)
18. Triceps brachii m. (I, II, III, IV)
18^{i}. Long head (I, II, III, IV)
18^{ii}. Lateral head (I, III)
18^{iii}. Medial head (IV)
 18^{iv}. Accessory head (not shown, deep to other heads).

CAT - THORACIC LIMB MUSCLES 1

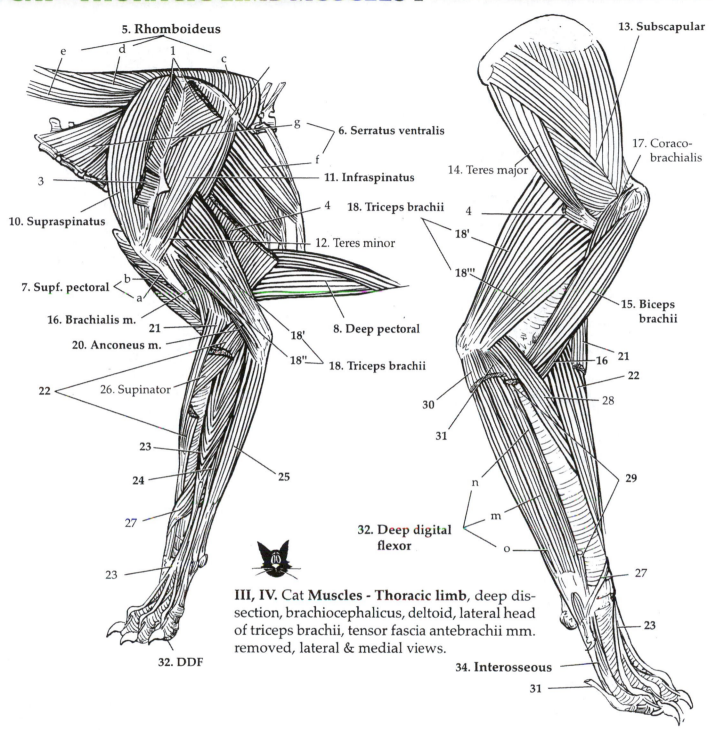

5. Rhomboideus

e d 1 c

13. Subscapular

g

6. Serratus ventralis

f

11. Infraspinatus

3

17. Coraco-brachialis

14. Teres major

10. Supraspinatus

4 **18. Triceps brachii**

4

18'

12. Teres minor

18'''

7. Supf. pectoral b
a

15. Biceps brachii

16. Brachialis m.

21

20. Anconeus m.

8. Deep pectoral

16 21

22 28

22 **26. Supinator** 18'

18" **18. Triceps brachii**

30

23 31

24

25

29

27

n

m

32. Deep digital flexor

o

23 27

23

32. DDF

III, IV. Cat Muscles - Thoracic limb, deep dissection, brachiocephalicus, deltoid, lateral head of triceps brachii, tensor fascia antebrachii mm. removed, lateral & medial views.

34. Interosseous

31

19. Tensor fascia antebrachii m. (II).
20. Anconeus m. (III).
MUSCLES FOREARM
21. Brachioradialis m. (I, II, III, IV).
22. Extensor carpi radialis m. (I, II, III, IV).
23. Common digital extensor m. (I, III, IV).
24. Lateral digital extensor m. (I, III).
25. Extensor carpi ulnaris (ulnaris lateralis) m. (I, III).
26. Supinator m. (III).
27. Oblique carpal extensor / abductor pollicis longus m. (I, **II**, III, IV).
28. Pronator teres m. (II, **IV**).

29. Flexor carpi radialis m. (II, IV).
30. Flexor carpi ulnaris m. (II).
31. Superficial digital flexor (SDF) m. (II).
32. Deep digital flexor m. (DDF)(I, II, III, IV)
33. Pronator quadratus m. (not shown, deep to DDF).
34. Interosseous mm. (II, IV).

A. Cutaneous trunci (I).

a. Thoracic part (trapezius thoracis m.).
b. Cervical part (trapezius cervicis m.).

c. Thoracic head (rhomboideus thoracic m.).
d. Cervical part (rhomboideus cervicis m.).
e. Capital part (rhomboideus captitis m.).
f. Thoracic part (serratus ventralis thoracis m.).
g. Cervical part (serratus ventralis cervicis m.).
h. Spinous part (deltoideus m.).
i. Acromial part (deltoideus m.).
j. Descending part (superficial pectoral m.).
k.Transverse part (superficial pectoral m.).
m. Humeral head (DDF m.).
n. Radial head (DDF m.).
o. Ulnar head (DDF m.).

MUSCLES - THORACIC LIMB - HORSE

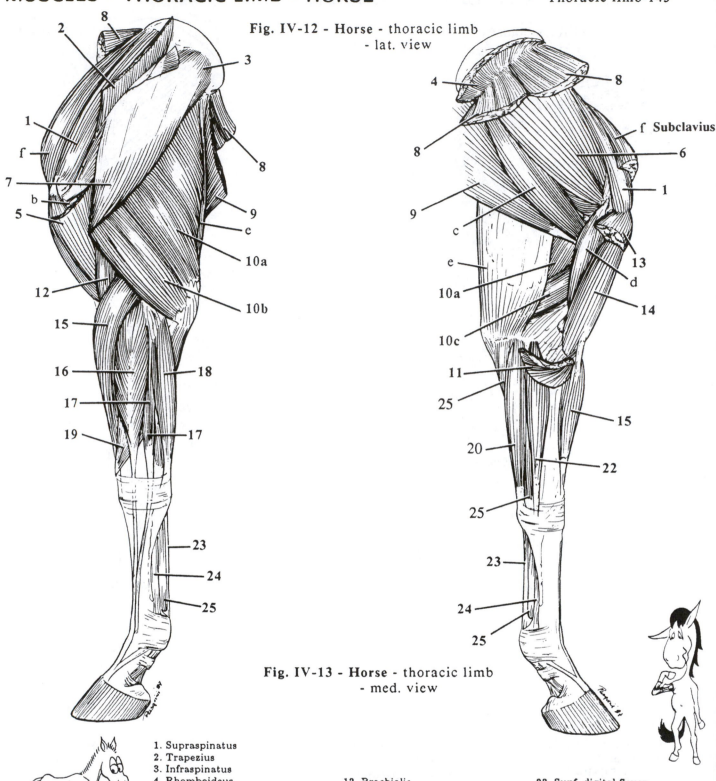

Fig. IV-12 - Horse - thoracic limb - lat. view

f Subclavius

Fig. IV-13 - Horse - thoracic limb - med. view

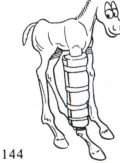

144

1. Supraspinatus
2. Trapezius
3. Infraspinatus
4. Rhomboideus
5. Brachiocephalicus
6. Subscapularis
7. Deltoid
8. Serratus ventralis
9. Latissimus dorsi
10. Triceps brachii
   10a. Long head
   10b. Lat. head
   10c. Med. head
11. Supf. pectoral

12. Brachialis
13. Deep pectoral
14. Biceps brachii
15. Extensor carpi radialis
16. Common digital extensor
17. Lat. digital extensor
18. Lat. ulnar
19. Oblique carpal extensor
20. Flexor carpi ulnaris (IV-13)
21. Pronator teres (absent - horse)
22. Flexor carpi radialis

23. Supf. digital flexor
24. Interosseous
25. Deep digital flexor

a. Omotransversarius (not
   shown in horse)
b. Teres minor
c. Teres major
d. Coracobrachialis
e. Tensor fasciae antebrachii
f. Subclavius

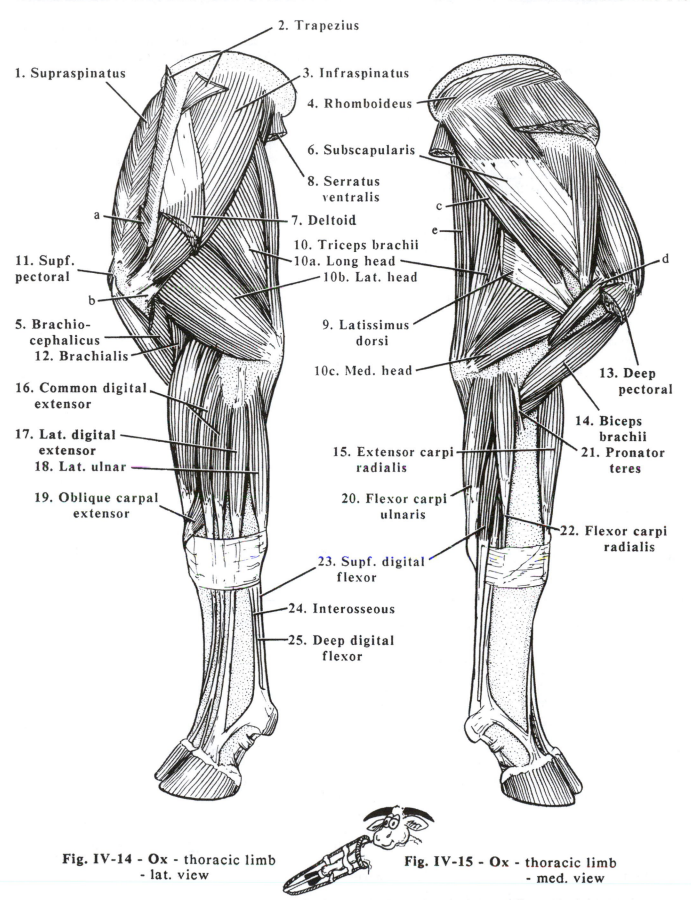

1. Supraspinatus
2. Trapezius
3. Infraspinatus
4. Rhomboideus
6. Subscapularis
8. Serratus ventralis
7. Deltoid
a
c
e
10. Triceps brachii
10a. Long head
10b. Lat. head
11. Supf. pectoral
b
9. Latissimus dorsi
d
5. Brachio-cephalicus
12. Brachialis
10c. Med. head
13. Deep pectoral
16. Common digital extensor
14. Biceps brachii
17. Lat. digital extensor
18. Lat. ulnar
15. Extensor carpi radialis
21. Pronator teres
19. Oblique carpal extensor
20. Flexor carpi ulnaris
22. Flexor carpi radialis
23. Supf. digital flexor
24. Interosseous
25. Deep digital flexor

Fig. IV-14 - Ox - thoracic limb - lat. view

Fig. IV-15 - Ox - thoracic limb - med. view

EXTRINSIC MUSCLES: connect the thoracic limb to the body (head, neck, and trunk).

1. Trapezius (G. *trapezion,* an irregular, four-sided figure): the triangular muscle extending from the dorsomedial neck and thorax to the spine of the scapula. It elevates the scapula, thus, the forelimb. It has two heads – the cervical part (trapezius cervicis) and the thoracic part (trapezius thoracis).

2. Latissimus dorsi (L. widest of the back): the broad, flat, fan-shaped muscle extending from the dorsal thoracolumbar region to the medial side of the humerus. It flexes the shoulder.

3. Brachiocephalicus (brak'ee-oh-se-FAL-ik-us): the wide muscle extending from the head and neck to the arm. The **clavicular intersection** divides this muscle into the cleidocephalicus (b) and the cleidobrachialis (c) muscle. The cleidocephalicus is further divided in all species, except the horse, where it is called the cleidomastoideus. The brachiocephalicus acts to advance the limb or draw the head laterally.

Clavicular (klah-VIK-yoo-lar) (tendon) **intersection** (d): the fibrous remnant of the clavicle located cranial to the shoulder, transversing the brachiocephalicus muscle.

Omotransversarius (a): extends from the shoulder region to the cervical vertebrae. In the horse it is fused with the brachiocephalicus and doesn't attach to the scapular spine, possibly because it has no acromion.

SPECIES DIFFERENCES		
Brachiocephalicus: all its heads are named for their attachments. The value of memorizing the species differences is doubtful.		
• Cleidobrachialis and cleidocephalicus are present in all species.		
• Cleidocephalicus is further divided in all, but the horse.		
Ruminant & pig	Cleidobrachialis	Cleidocephalicus Cleidomastoideus Cleidooccipitalis
Carnivores	Cleidobrachialis	Cleidocephalicus Cleidomastoideus Cleidocervicalis
Horse	Cleidobrachialis	Cleidocephalicus Cleidomastoideus

MUSCLE	ORIGINS	INSERTION	ACTION	NERVE
Trapezius		Spine of scapula	Elevate shoulder & draw it forward or backward	Accessory
Cervical part	Median fibrous raphe of neck			
Thoracic part	Spines of vertebrae $T_{3-8 \text{ or } 9}$			
Omotransversarius	Wing of atlas	Dist. scapular spine	Draw limb forward	Accessory & cervical
Latissimus dorsi	Thoracolumbar fascia	Humerus (teres major tubercle)	Flex shoulder or advance body	Thoraco-dorsal
Brachiocephalicus	Clavicular intersection		Pull limb forward or flex neck laterally	Accessory & axillary
Cleidocephalicus		Skull (neck & skull/mastoid process in carnivores)		
Cleidobrachialis		Humerus		

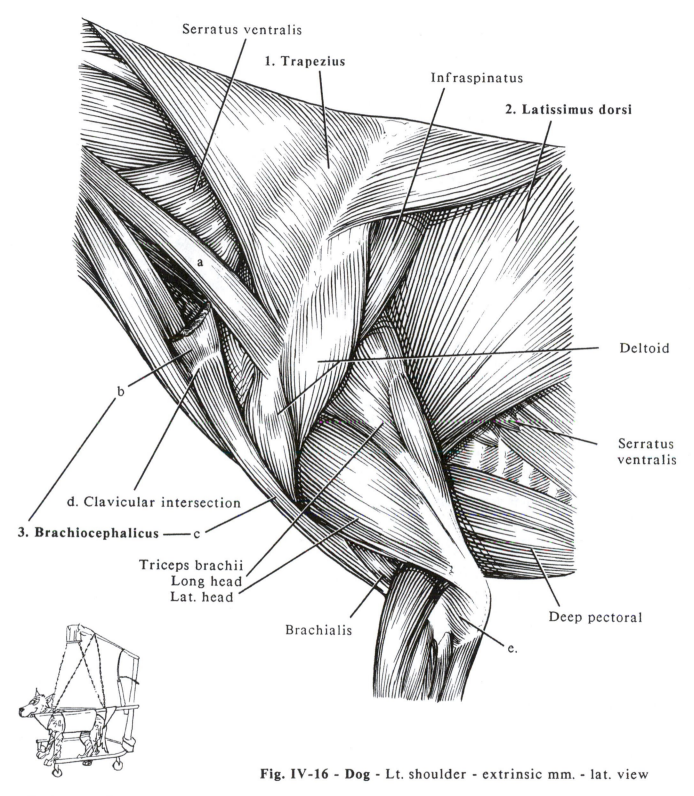

Serratus ventralis

1. Trapezius

Infraspinatus

2. Latissimus dorsi

a

Deltoid

b

Serratus
ventralis

d. Clavicular intersection

3. Brachiocephalicus — c

Triceps brachii
Long head
Lat. head

Brachialis

Deep pectoral

e.

Fig. IV-16 - Dog - Lt. shoulder - extrinsic mm. - lat. view

a. Omotransversarius
b. Cleidocephalicus
c. Cleidobrachialis
d. Clavicular intersection
e. Anconeus

EXTRINSIC MUSCLES - SHOULDER

4. Rhomboid (ROM-boid) or **rhomboideus**: the extrinsic muscle lying deep to the trapezius. It extends from the median raphe of the neck, the thoracic vertebral spines, and the skull to the dorsal border of the scapula and scapular cartilage. It is divided into <u>cervical</u> and <u>thoracic parts</u> in all species; the <u>carnivores</u> and <u>pig</u> have a small <u>capital part</u>. It elevates the forelimb.

5. Serratus ventralis (ser-RAY-tus) (L. *serratus*, a saw): the serrated, fan-shaped muscle extending from the last five cervical vertebrae and first seven or eight ribs to the medial surface of the scapula. It supports the trunk.

6. Superficial pectoral: the flat muscle extending from the sternum to the cranial surface of the humerus. It is divided into two parts, a superficial <u>descending pectoral</u> and a deeper <u>transverse pectoral</u>, based on their fiber direction. It adducts and advances the limb.

7. Deep (ascending) pectoral: the broad muscle extending from the sternum to the greater and lesser tubercles of the humerus. It functions to draw the limb caudally and adduct it.

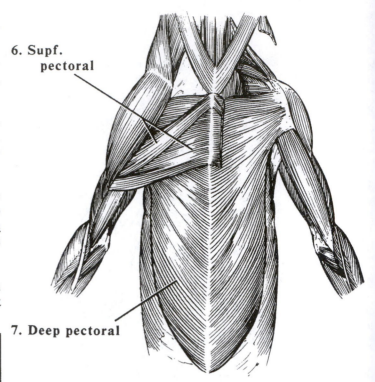

6. **Supf. pectoral**

7. **Deep pectoral**

SPECIES DIFFERENCES

Subclavius (Fig. IV-23, c): pectoral muscle over the cranial border of the supraspinatus muscle in the **horse** and goat. It is small in the ox and absent in the carnivores.

Fig. IV-17 - Dog Thorax - ventr. view

MUSCLE	ORIGINS	INSERTION	ACTION	NERVE
Rhomboideus Cervical part Thoracic part Capital part (carnivores)	Dors. neck and thorax Nuchal crest of skull	Dors. border of scapula & scapular cartilage	Draw shoulder dorsocranially	Dors. br. of spinal nn. (cerv. & thoracic)
Serratus ventralis Cervical part Thoracic part	 Vertebrae C3-7 (transverse processes) Ribs 1-7 or 8	Scapula (serrated face) " "	Raise thorax (both), shift weight to contralateral limb (singly), support trunk (both)	Long thoracic
Supf. pectoral Descending Transverse	Sternum " "	Cran. surface of humerus " "	Adduct & advance limb (extend shoulder)	Pectoral
Deep pectoral (ascending)	Sternum	Humerus (greater & lesser tubercles)	Adduct & retract limb (flex shoulder)	Pectoral & lat. thoracic

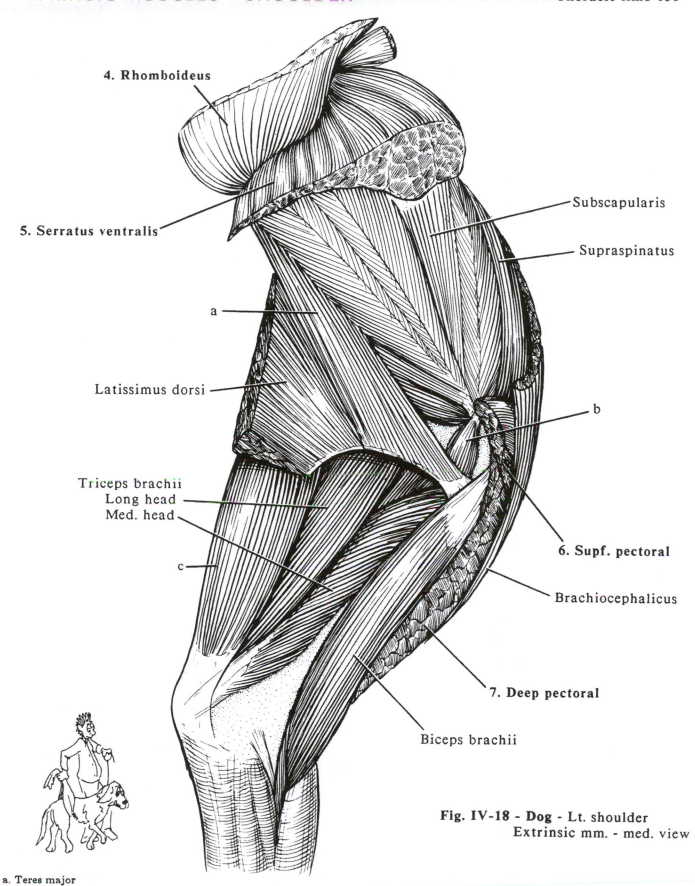

4. Rhomboideus

5. Serratus ventralis

Subscapularis

Supraspinatus

a

Latissimus dorsi

b

Triceps brachii
Long head
Med. head

c

6. Supf. pectoral

Brachiocephalicus

7. Deep pectoral

Biceps brachii

Fig. IV-18 - Dog - Lt. shoulder
Extrinsic mm. - med. view

a. Teres major
b. Coracobrachialis
c. Tensor fasciae antebrachii

INTRINSIC MUSCLES: arise and insert on the thoracic limb bones.

MUSCLES of the SHOULDER and ARM:

8. Supraspinatus (soop-ra-SPY-nayt-us): a shoulder extensor, it originates from and fills the supraspinous fossa. Curving over the shoulder joint, it inserts on the greater tubercle of the humerus. It acts as the shoulder's lateral collateral ligament.

9. Deltoid (G. letter delta) (Fig. IV-16): extends from the scapular spine over the shoulder joint to the deltoid tuberosity of the humerus. Its aponeurosis covers the infraspinatus muscle. It acts to flex the shoulder.

10. Infraspinatus: lies deep to the aponeurosis of the deltoid muscle, originating from and filling the infraspinous fossa. Its strong tendon crosses the shoulder joint to insert on the greater tubercle of the humerus. It flexes the shoulder joint and acts with the supraspinatus muscle as the joint's lateral collateral ligament. There is an infraspinatus bursa between the tendon of insertion and the greater tubercle.

11. Brachialis (BRAY-kee-al-is) (G. *brachium*, arm): arising from the caudal part of the humerus, it curves laterally in the brachial groove. It crosses the cranial (flexor) surface of the elbow to insert on the radius. It flexes the elbow joint with the biceps brachii muscle. The musculocutaneous nerve innervates both the brachialis and biceps brachii muscles.

Teres minor (d): the small muscle ventral to the tendon of insertion of the infraspinatus muscle. It crosses the lateral surface of the shoulder.

Anconeus (c): crosses the lateral aspect of the elbow joint under the triceps brachii muscle. A lateral approach to the elbow is through this muscle.

SPECIES DIFFERENCES:

Deltoid (9): divided into acromial and spinous parts in all domestic animals, except the horse and pig. The horse and pig lack an acromion.

MUSCLE	ORIGINS	INSERTION	ACTION	NERVE
Deltoid		Deltoid tuberosity	Flex shoulder	Axillary
Scapular part	Spine of scapula			
Acromial part (absent in horse & pig)	Acromion process			
Supraspinatus	Supraspinous fossa of scapula	Humerus (greater & lesser tubercles)	Stabilize & extend shoulder	Supra-scapular
Infraspinatus	Infraspinous fossa of scapula	Humerus (greater tubercle)	Stabilize, flex & extend shoulder	Supra-scapular
Teres minor	Caud. border of scapula	Teres minor tuberosity of humerus	Flex shoulder	Axillary
Brachialis	Brachial groove of humerus	Radius	Flex elbow	Musculo-cutaneous
Anconeus	Olecranon fossa	Olecranon	Extend elbow	Radial

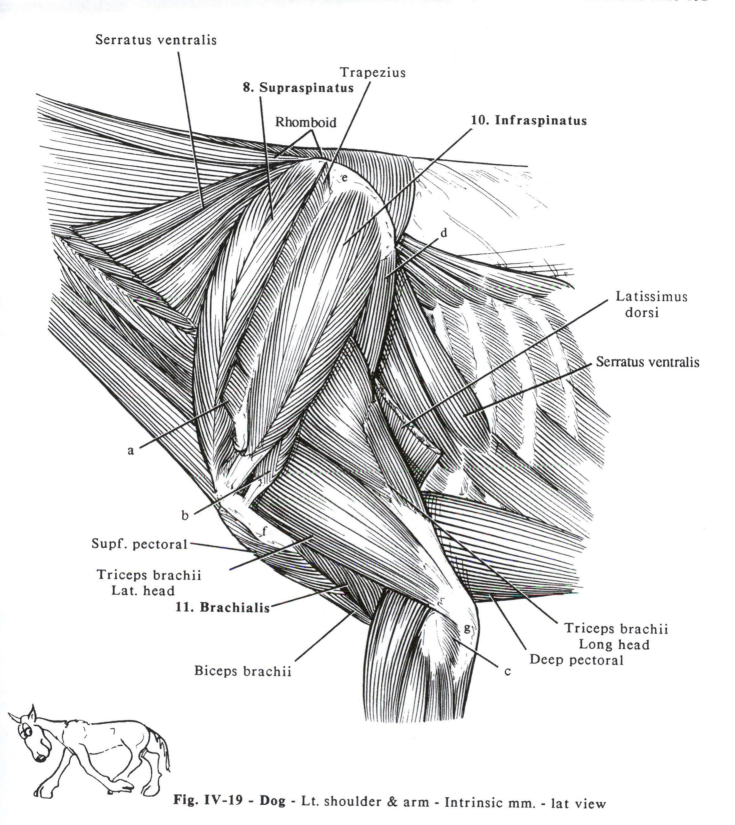

Serratus ventralis

Trapezius

8. Supraspinatus

Rhomboid

10. Infraspinatus

Latissimus dorsi

Serratus ventralis

a

b

f

Supf. pectoral

Triceps brachii Lat. head

11. Brachialis

Biceps brachii

g

c

Triceps brachii Long head

Deep pectoral

Fig. IV-19 - Dog - Lt. shoulder & arm - Intrinsic mm. - lat view

a. Omotransversarius   e. Scapula
b. Teres minor   f. Humerus
c. Anconeus   g. Olecranon (ulna)
d. Teres major

INTRINSIC MUSCLES – SHOULDER & ARM

12. Subscapularis: the large muscle originating from the subscapular fossa. It crosses the shoulder joint and inserts on the lesser tubercle of the humerus. It adducts the shoulder and serves as the shoulder's medial collateral ligament.

13. Triceps brachii (L. *tri,* three + *ceps,* heads): composed of three or four heads. Its long head crosses the shoulder, and all heads cross the elbow joint to insert on the olecranon. It extends the elbow and its long head flexes the shoulder.

14 . Biceps brachii (L. *bi,* two + *ceps,* head): arises from the supraglenoid tubercle, crosses the shoulder and elbow, and inserts on the radial tuberosity of the radius. It extends the shoulder, and more importantly, with the brachialis muscle, flexes the elbow joint.

Coracobrachialis (b): the small muscle extending from the coracoid process over the shoulder to the humerus on the medial side of the axilla.

Teres major (a): arises from the caudal border of the scapula and inserts with the latissimus dorsi muscle on the medial side of the humerus.

Tensor fasciae antebrachii (Fig. IV-18,c): the thin, insignificant muscle arising from the latissimus dorsi muscle and covering the medial surface of the triceps brachii muscle.

SPECIES DIFFERENCES:

Triceps brachii (13): the long, lateral, and medial heads are found in all species. An accessory head occurs in all species, except the horse.

CLINICAL

High radial nerve paralysis: damage to the radial nerve proximal to its innervation of the triceps brachii muscle. This results in a "dropped elbow". Inability to extend the elbow results in the inability to support weight on the affected limb. The loss of innervation to the extensors of the digits also results in knuckling over.

MUSCLE	ORIGINS	INSERTION	ACTION	NERVE
Biceps brachii	Supraglenoid tubercle of scapula	Radial tuberosity	Flex elbow & extend shoulder	Musculo-cutaneous
Coracobrachialis	Coracoid process of scapula	Lesser tubercle of humerus	Flex shoulder	Musculo-cutaneous
Teres major	Caud. border of scapula	Teres major tuberosity of humerus	Flex shoulder	Axillary
Subscapularis	Subscapular fossa	Lesser tubercle of humerus	Adduct & extend shoulder joint	Subscapular
Triceps brachii **Long head**	Caud. edge of scapula	Olecranon	Extend elbow	Radial
Lat. head	Humerus	"		
Med. head	"	"		
Accessory head (absent in horse)	"	"		
Tensor fasciae antebrachii (Fig. IV-18,c)	Latissimus dorsi	Olecranon & antebrachial fascia	Extend elbow	Radial

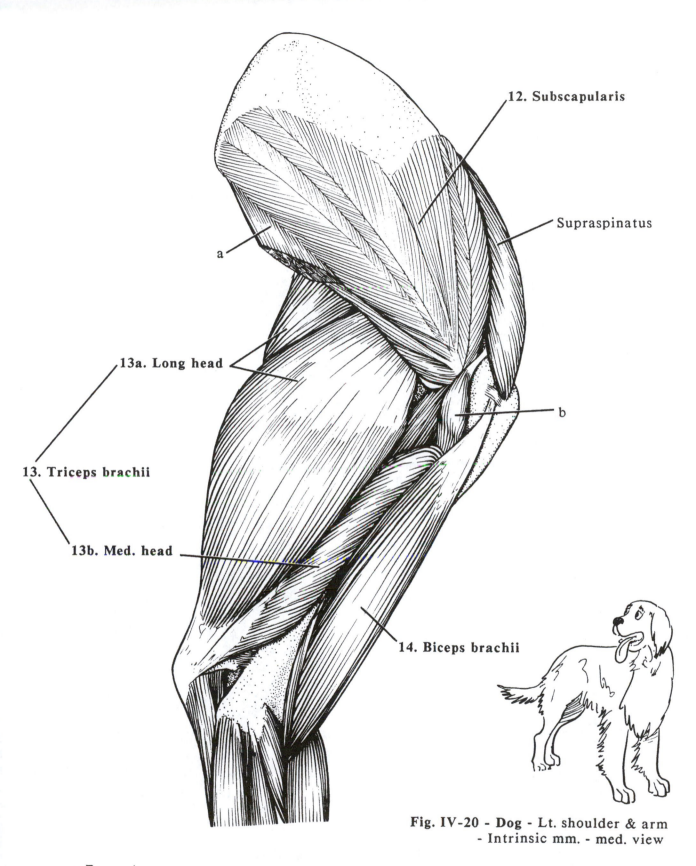

12. Subscapularis

Supraspinatus

13a. Long head

13. Triceps brachii

13b. Med. head

14. Biceps brachii

a

b

Fig. IV-20 - Dog - Lt. shoulder & arm
- Intrinsic mm. - med. view

a. Teres major
b. Coracobrachialis

153

MUSCLES – SHOULDER

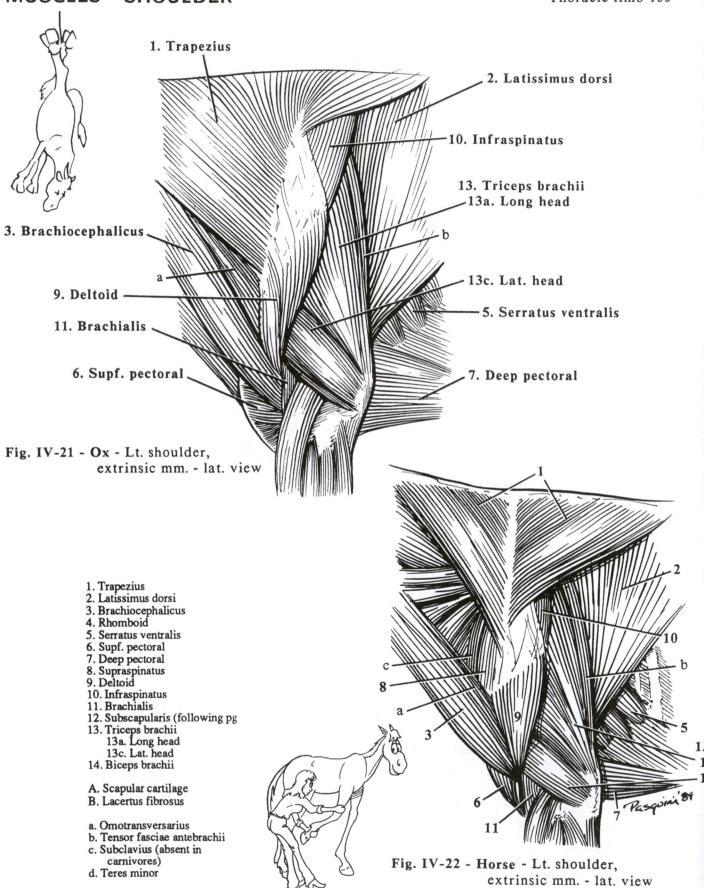

1. Trapezius

2. Latissimus dorsi

10. Infraspinatus

13. Triceps brachii
13a. Long head

b

3. Brachiocephalicus

a

13c. Lat. head

9. Deltoid

5. Serratus ventralis

11. Brachialis

6. Supf. pectoral

7. Deep pectoral

Fig. IV-21 - Ox - Lt. shoulder,
extrinsic mm. - lat. view

1. Trapezius
2. Latissimus dorsi
3. Brachiocephalicus
4. Rhomboid
5. Serratus ventralis
6. Supf. pectoral
7. Deep pectoral
8. Supraspinatus
9. Deltoid
10. Infraspinatus
11. Brachialis
12. Subscapularis (following pg
13. Triceps brachii
   13a. Long head
   13c. Lat. head
14. Biceps brachii

A. Scapular cartilage
B. Lacertus fibrosus

a. Omotransversarius
b. Tensor fasciae antebrachii
c. Subclavius (absent in
   carnivores)
d. Teres minor

Fig. IV-22 - Horse - Lt. shoulder,
extrinsic mm. - lat. view

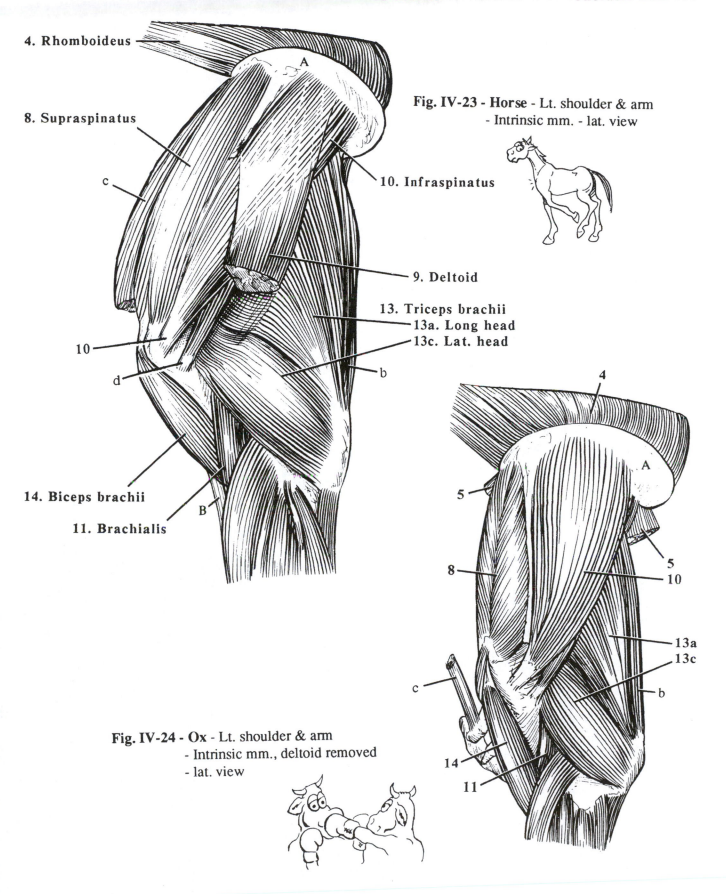

4. Rhomboideus

8. Supraspinatus

c

10

d

14. Biceps brachii

11. Brachialis

B

A

Fig. IV-23 - Horse - Lt. shoulder & arm
- Intrinsic mm. - lat. view

10. Infraspinatus

9. Deltoid

13. Triceps brachii
13a. Long head
13c. Lat. head

b

4

5

A

8

5

10

13a
13c

b

c

14

11

Fig. IV-24 - Ox - Lt. shoulder & arm
- Intrinsic mm., deltoid removed
- lat. view

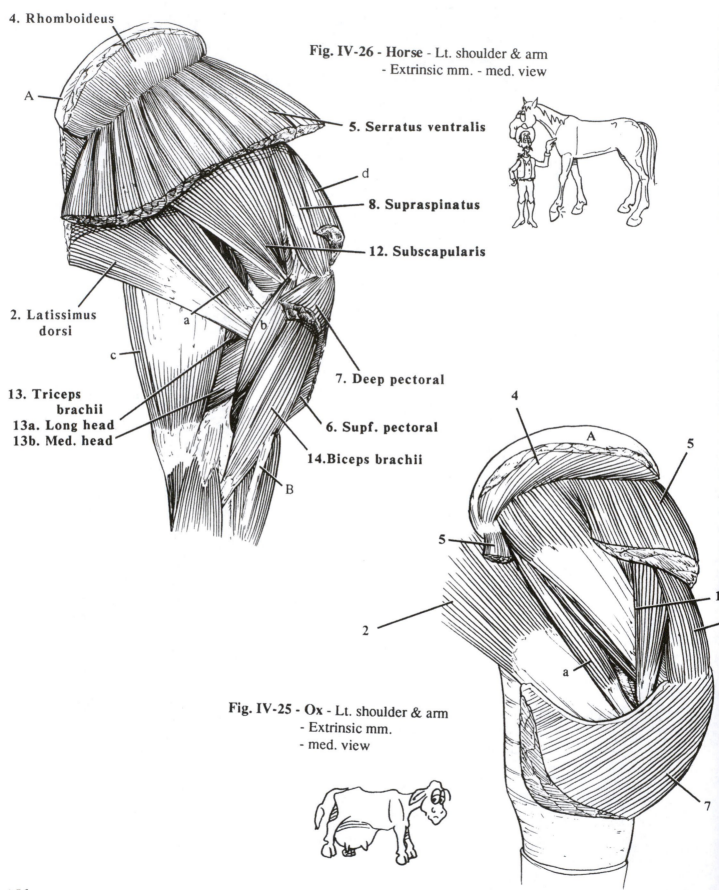

4. Rhomboideus

A

Fig. IV-26 - **Horse** - Lt. shoulder & arm
- Extrinsic mm. - med. view

5. **Serratus ventralis**

d

8. **Supraspinatus**

12. **Subscapularis**

2. Latissimus
dorsi

c

7. **Deep pectoral**

13. Triceps
brachii
13a. Long head
13b. Med. head

6. **Supf. pectoral**

14.Biceps brachii

B

7. Deep pectoral

4

A

5

5

2

1

a

Fig. IV-25 - **Ox** - Lt. shoulder & arm
- Extrinsic mm.
- med. view

7

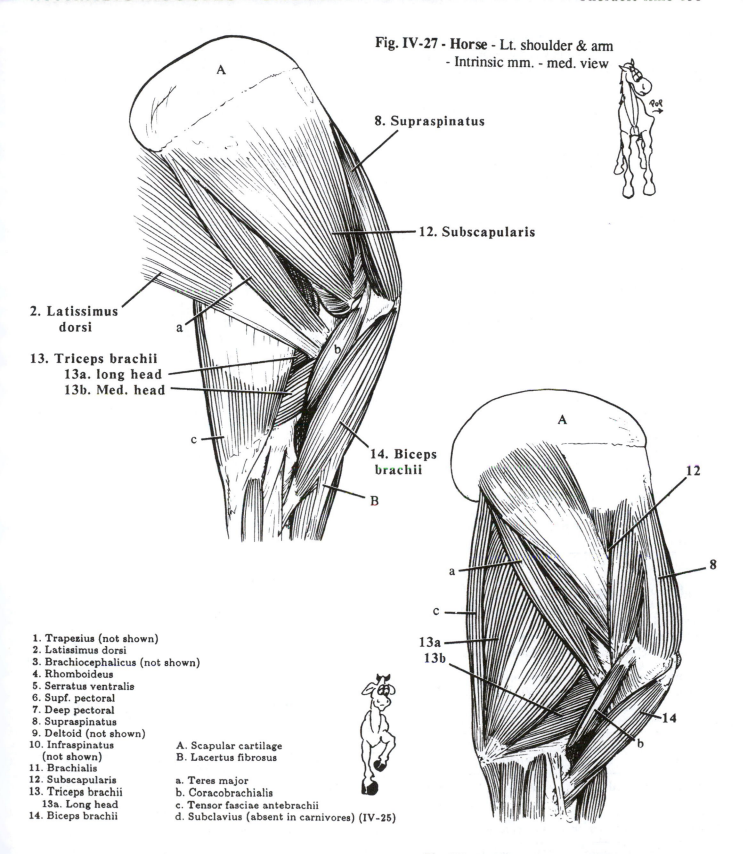

Fig. IV-27 - **Horse** - Lt. shoulder & arm
- Intrinsic mm. - med. view

8. Supraspinatus

12. Subscapularis

2. Latissimus
   dorsi

a

b

13. Triceps brachii
    13a. long head
    13b. Med. head

c

14. Biceps
    brachii

B

A

12

8

a

c

13a

13b

14

b

1. Trapezius (not shown)
2. Latissimus dorsi
3. Brachiocephalicus (not shown)
4. Rhomboideus
5. Serratus ventralis
6. Supf. pectoral
7. Deep pectoral
8. Supraspinatus
9. Deltoid (not shown)
10. Infraspinatus
    (not shown)
11. Brachialis
12. Subscapularis
13. Triceps brachii
    13a. Long head
14. Biceps brachii

A. Scapular cartilage
B. Lacertus fibrosus

a. Teres major
b. Coracobrachialis
c. Tensor fasciae antebrachii
d. Subclavius (absent in carnivores) (IV-25)

Fig. IV-28 - **Ox** - Lt. shoulder & arm
- Intrinsic mm. - med. view

MUSCLES - FOREARM

DORSOLATERAL FOREARM (antebrachial) MUSCLES: extensors of the digits and carpus, and supinators of the paw. Most arise on or near the lateral (extensor) epicondyle of the humerus and are innervated by the <u>radial nerve</u>.

15. Extensor carpi radialis: the largest extensor muscle, it inserts on the metacarpal tuberosity. It extends the carpus and flexes the elbow.

16. Common digital extensor: the long muscle inserting on the extensor process of the third phalanx (phalanges). It extends the digit(s) and carpus.

17. Lateral digital extensor: originating on or near the lateral epicondyle of the humerus and inserting on the phalanges of the lateral digits. It extends the digits and carpus.

18. Ulnaris lateralis (lateral ulnar, extensor carpi ulnaris): the most caudal extensor muscle. It inserts on the proximal part of a metacarpal bone and the accessory carpal bone. Grouped with the extensors, in reality it flexes the carpus in most positions. This is an interesting anatomical point, but clinically of no importance.

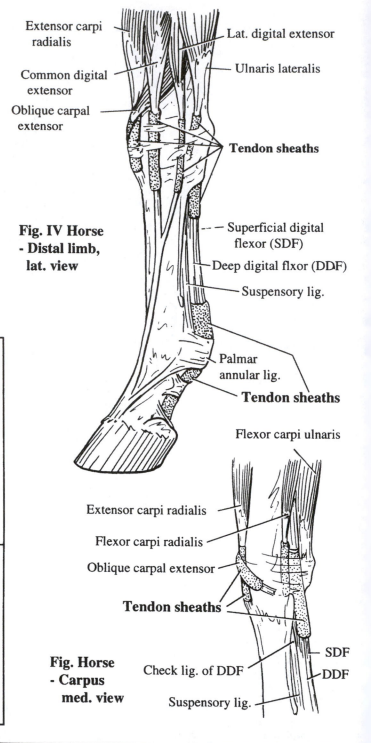

Fig. IV Horse - Distal limb, lat. view

Fig. Horse - Carpus med. view

SPECIES DIFFERENCES

Common digital extensor (16): horse - 1 tendon of insertion for its one digit; Other domestic species - tendon of insertion for each digit (carnivores -5, ruminants - 2 and pigs - 4).

Medial digital extensor: in ruminants and pigs, the medial head of the common/long digital extensor passes to the med. digit(s) balancing the lat. digital extensor. (pg 166, 195)

Lateral digital extensor (17): Horse: lateral side of the proximal phalanx; Other species: inserts on prox., middle & distal phalanges (ruminants: digit IV; Dog: digits 3, 4 and 5; cat: digits 2, 3, 4 and 5).

Clinical

Rupture of common digital extensor: present at birth in foals as part of a congenital complex and are often associated with flexural deformities. There is swelling over the dorsolateral carpus.

Extensor tenosynovitis: uncommon condition in horses due to trauma to the synovial sheaths of the extensor tendons crossing the carpus.

MUSCLE	ORIGINS	INSERTION	ACTION	NERVE
Extensor carpi radialis	Lat. epicondyle (humerus)	Metacarpus	Extend carpal joint, flex elbow	Radial
Common digital extensor	Lat. epicondyle (humerus)	Dors. portion of phalanges	Extend digits	Radial
Lateral digital extensor	On or near lat. epicondyle	Middle phalanges	Extend digits	Radial
Lateral ulnar	Lat. epicondyle (humerus)	Prox. end of Mc V	Flex carpal joint	Radial

Fig. IV-29 - Dog - Lt. forearm
- lat. view

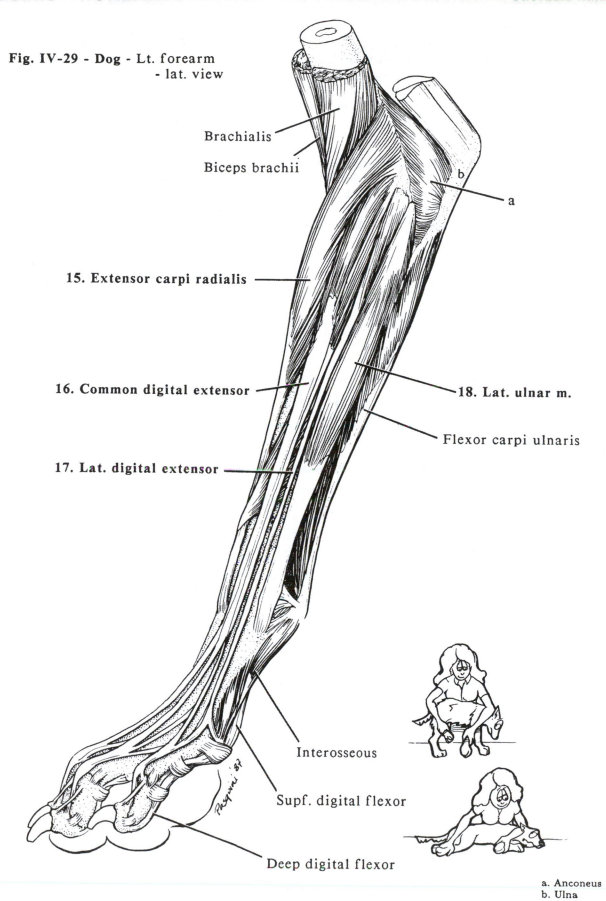

Brachialis

Biceps brachii

b

a

15. Extensor carpi radialis

16. Common digital extensor

18. Lat. ulnar m.

Flexor carpi ulnaris

17. Lat. digital extensor

Interosseous

Supf. digital flexor

Deep digital flexor

a. Anconeus
b. Ulna

159

MUSCLES - FOREARM

19. Pronator teres (PROH-nayt-or TEE-reez, [most people say TER-eez]) (L. *teres*, round): the small muscle in carnivores extending from the medial epicondyle of the humerus obliquely to the radius. It pronates the paw (rotates the palmar side downward). In other domestic species, whose capacity to pronate the forelimb is lost or reduced because of fusion of the ulna and radius, the pronator teres is at best vestigial.

20. Supinator (SYOO-pi-nayt-or, SOO-pi-nayt-or): present in carnivores and occasionally in the pig. It extends from the lateral (extensor) epicondyle to the radius under the extensor carpi radialis muscle. It supinates the paw (rotates the palmar side upward, as when the cat drinks milk with its paw). It is absent from the other domestic species, because their radius and ulna fuse; negating the possibility of supination.

Brachioradialis (d): the small muscle in the superficial fascia over the extensor carpi radialis muscle in carnivores.

Oblique carpal extensor (b): also known as the abductor pollicis (digiti I) longus. (Pollicis refers to thumb, which none of the domestic animals have.) The carnivores have digit I, but none of the other species do. For comparative purposes, we use the anglicization of the NAV permitted extensor carpi obliquus. In the carnivores it has a small sesamoid bone in its tendon on the medial side of the carpus.

Pronator quadratus: a wide, short muscle bridging the length of the interosseous space between the ulna and radius. It is deep to the deep digital flexor muscle.

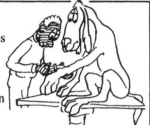

> **CLINICAL**
>
> **Brachioradialis** (d): in carnivores runs with the cephalic vein on the cranial aspect of the forearm. It is roughly the same size as the vein for which it may be mistaken in venipuncture.

MUSCLE	ORIGINS	INSERTION	ACTION	NERVE
Pronator teres	Med. epicondyle of humerus	Med. surface of radius	Pronates paw	Median
Supinator (carnivores)	Lat. epicondyle of humerus	Radius	Supinates paw	Radial
Oblique carpal extensor (long digital I abductor) (abductor digiti I [pollicis] longus)	Cran. surface of forearm	Prox. metacarpus	Extend carpus & abduct carnivore's 1st digit	Radial
Extensor pollicis longus et indicis proprius (carnivores)	Ulna	Metacarpals I & II	Extend digits I & II	Radial
Pronator quadratus (carnivores)	Dist. ulna	Dist. radius	Pronates paw	Median
Brachioradialis (long supinator) (carnivores)	Lat. condyloid crest of humerus	Cran. surface of radius	Supinates paw	Radial

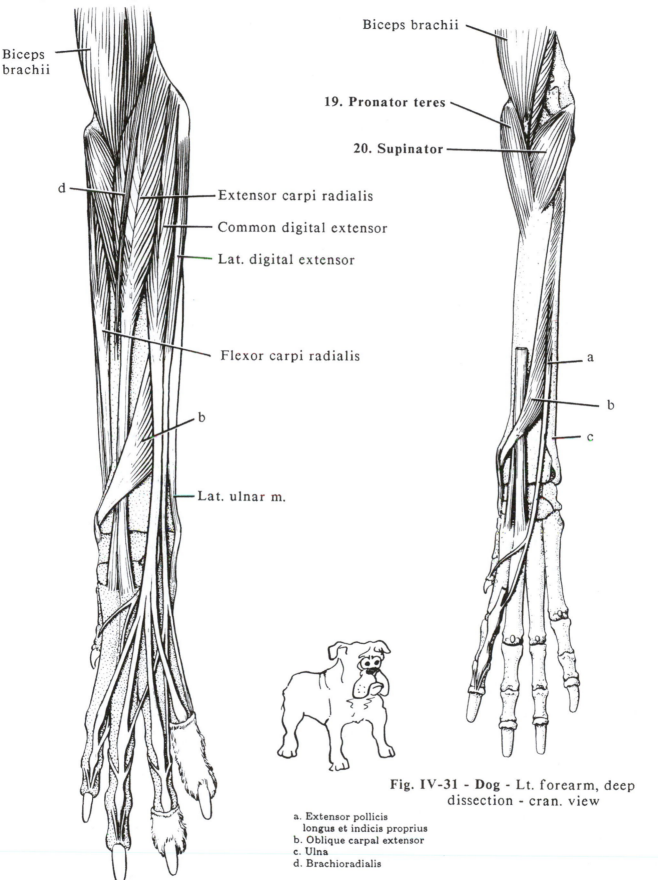

Fig. IV-30 - Dog - Lt. forearm - cran. view

Biceps brachii

Biceps brachii

19. Pronator teres

20. Supinator

d

Extensor carpi radialis

Common digital extensor

Lat. digital extensor

Flexor carpi radialis

a

b

b

c

Lat. ulnar m.

Fig. IV-31 - Dog - Lt. forearm, deep dissection - cran. view

a. Extensor pollicis
   longus et indicis proprius
b. Oblique carpal extensor
c. Ulna
d. Brachioradialis

CAUDAL ANTEBRACHIAL MUSCLES: the flexors of the carpus and digits, and pronators of the paw. They originate from or near the medial (flexor) epicondyle of the humerus, and are innervated by the median and/or ulnar nerves. They include the flexor carpi radialis (21), flexor carpi ulnaris (22), superficial digital flexor (23), deep digital flexor (24) and pronator teres (19).

21. Flexor carpi radialis: the long muscle inserting on the proximal metacarpus. It flexes the carpus.

22. Flexor carpi ulnaris: a two-headed muscle inserting on the accessory carpal bone. It has an ulnar and a humeral head and flexes the carpus. The humeral head can be mistaken for the superficial digital flexor. To differentiate them, follow them to their terminations.

23. Superficial digital flexor (SDF): arises from the medial (flexor) epicondyle of the humerus and inserts on the middle phalanx. It flexes the carpus and digits.

Manica flexoria: the sleeve of the superficial digital flexor tendon located at the metacarpophalangeal joints in all species. It allows the deep digital flexor tendon to pass through and attach distally to the attachment of the superficial digital flexor.

SPECIES DIFFERENCES

Superficial digital flexor (24): has tendons to each digit (carnivore - 5; horse - 1; ruminants - 2), except in the pig which has only 2 for its 4 digits. In the horse it inserts on the proximal end of the middle phalanx and the distal end of the proximal phalanx. These two insertions may prevent "dorsal buckling" (hyperflexion) of the proximal interphalangeal joint. The ruminant has two tendons, the deep one passing through the carpal canal and the superficial one passing through the flexor retinaculum.

Accessory ligament of the superficial digital flexor: a tendinous band that connects the tendon of the superficial digital flexor to the radius. This plays a part in the stay apparatus (pg. 196). It is also known as the "radial head", "proximal check ligament", "superior check ligament" and "radial check ligament".

CLINICAL

Flexural deformities or **contracted tendons**: a congenital or acquired defect in foals involving the flexor tendons of the front and/or hind limb. Flexural deformities is a better name because tendons can't contract. These can effect the fetlock, coffin and carpus (least common). In mild cases conservative treatment of diet, trimming feet and exercise to stretch the ligaments may be enough. Often the distal and/or proximal accessory ("check") ligaments are resected (cut) to help straighten out the distal limb.

• **Fetlock flexural deformity (SDF)**: due mainly to a shortened superficial digital flexor tendon and possibly deep digital flexor tendon. The SDF attaches on either side of the proximal interphalangeal joint (pastern). Shortening results in the the proximal and middle phalanges being pulled back in alignment with the metacarpal bone. Proximal (SDF) check ligament desmotomy and possibly distal (DDF) check ligament desmotomy may be necessary in moderate cases. Severe cases may require cutting the SDF (SDF tenotomy) or the suspensory ligament (suspensory ligament desmotomy).

Club foot, DDF contracture of the DIP joint: caused by a short deep digital flexor tendon (DDF) which pulls the toe back. The DDF passes the DIP (distal interphalangeal) joint to insert on the distal phalanx. Severing the distal (DDF) check ligament may be necessary in moderate cases. Severe cases may require a DDF tenotomy.

Flexural deformities of the carpus: the most uncommon form of flexural deformities. Physical therapy and splints are used in correctable cases.

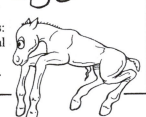

MUSCLE	ORIGINS	INSERTION	ACTION	NERVE
Flexor carpi radialis	Med. (flexor) epicondyle (humerus)	Prox. metacarpus	Flex carpus	Median n.
Flexor carpi ulnaris		Accessory carpal bone	Flex carpus	Ulnar n.
• Ulnar head	Olecranon			
• Humeral head	Med. epicondyle (humerus)			
Supf. digital flexor	Med. epicondyle (humerus)	Palm. surface of middle phalanges	Flex digits & carpus	Ulnar n.

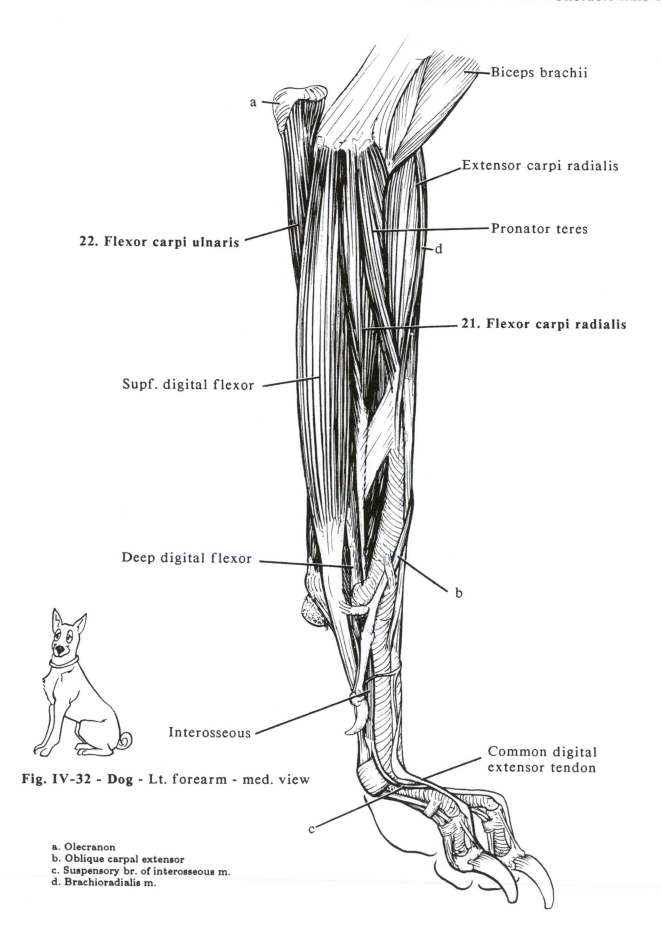

Biceps brachii

Extensor carpi radialis

Pronator teres

a

22. Flexor carpi ulnaris

d

21. Flexor carpi radialis

Supf. digital flexor

Deep digital flexor

b

Interosseous

Common digital
extensor tendon

c

Fig. IV-32 - Dog - Lt. forearm - med. view

a. Olecranon
b. Oblique carpal extensor
c. Suspensory br. of interosseous m.
d. Brachioradialis m.

24. Deep digital flexor: the three-headed muscle arising from the humerus, radius, and ulna and inserting on the <u>distal phalanx</u> (phalanges). It flexes the carpus and digits.

25. Interosseous (in'ter-OS-ee-us) (L. *interosseus, inter,* between + *os,* bone): a muscle of the manus, arising from the proximal palmar surface of the metacarpal bones. It extends distally and splits into two tendons. The tendons insert on the sesamoid bones of the respective metacarpophalangeal joints.
• Extensor branch, joins the common digital extensor muscle's tendon of insertion.

SPECIES DIFFERENCES

Accessory ligament of the deep digital flexor: a tendinous band from the palmar carpal ligament to the tendon of the deep digital flexor. It can be reached from the lateral side. It plays a part in the stay apparatus (pg. 196). Popular synonyms are: "distal check ligament", "carpal check ligament", and "inferior check ligament".

Interosseous (25): horse -3 muscles (2 are insignificant); dog and cat - 4; in the ruminants the 2 interosseous muscles are fused.

Suspensory ligament (Fig. IV-35): another term for the interosseous muscle in the horse. It is completely tendinous upon maturity and plays a role in the stay apparatus and locomotion.
• **Branches of suspensory ligament (horse):** distal end of suspensory ligament that attach to the two proximal sesamoid bones

---

CLINICAL

Bowed tendons (tenosynovitis): a torn tendon in horses, usually resulting from racing stress. The superficial digital flexor of the thoracic limb is most commonly affected, and most commonly in the middle of the metacarpus. Depending on where they are in the metacarpal region they are classified as low, middle, or high.

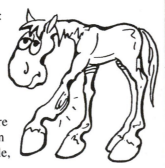

• Low bow: bowed tendon at the fetlock or below is usually the deep digital flexor tendon.

Suspensory desmitis: strain and tearing of the suspensory ligament similar to bowed tendons. This can occur in 3 sites:
• **Suspensory branches:** #1 site, the distal end of the suspensory ligament that attach to the proximal sesmoids.
• **Body of the suspensory ligamant:** often secondary to "splints" or fractures of the splint bones.
• **Origin of suspensory ligament:** least common site, but the hardest to diagnose. Blocking the deep branch of the lateral palmar nerve helps localize this problem.

Ultrasound: use of sound waves to image internal body parts is especially useful for bowed tendons and suspensory desmitis.

Septic tenosynovitis (horse): infection of digital synovial sheaths. This often leads to a permanent debilitating injury.

Severed flexor tendons: common problems. Diagnosis of the tendon severed can be helped by the deformity of the limb.
• **SDF** (superficial digital flexor): dropped fetlock, toe on ground.
• **DDF** (deep digital flexor): Toe off ground, fetlock dropped.
• **SDF + DDF + Suspensory ligament:** fetlock on ground, toe in air.

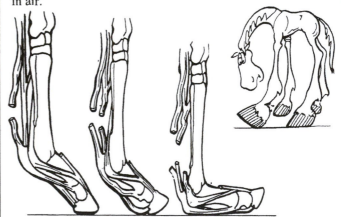

MUSCLE	ORIGINS	INSERTION	ACTION	NERVE
Deep digital flexor	Humerus, radius & ulna (Humeral, radial & ulnar heads)	Dist. phalanges	Flex digits & carpus	Median & ulnar nn.
Interosseous	Prox. end of Mc II, III, IV & V	Prox. sesamoid bones	Part of suspensory apparatus - support fetlock	Deep br. of ulnar

Fig. IV-33 - Dog - Lt. forearm - caud. view

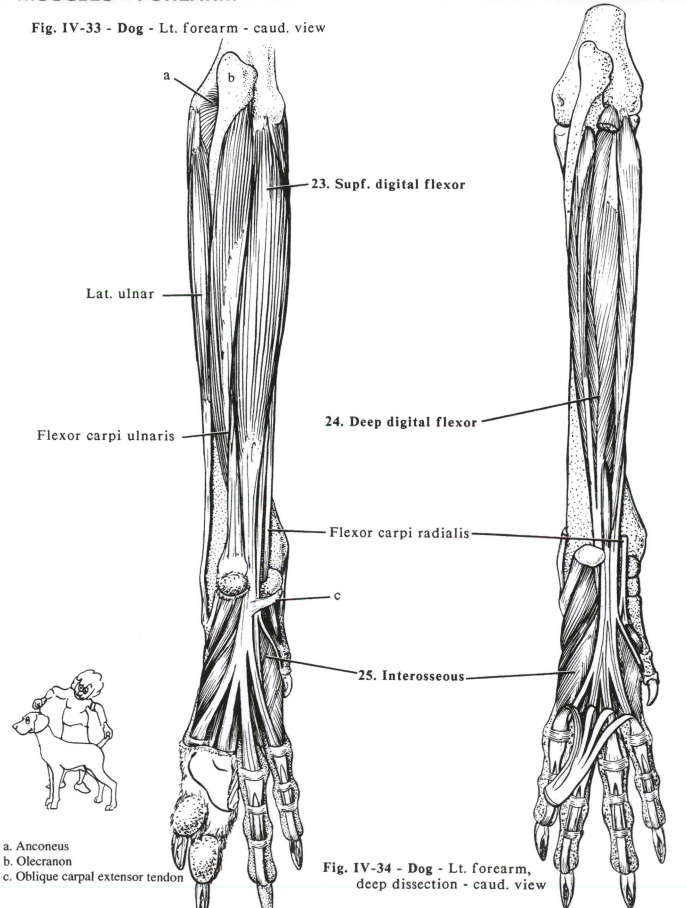

a

b

23. Supf. digital flexor

Lat. ulnar

24. Deep digital flexor

Flexor carpi ulnaris

Flexor carpi radialis

c

25. Interosseous

a. Anconeus
b. Olecranon
c. Oblique carpal extensor tendon

**Fig. IV-34 - Dog - Lt. forearm,
deep dissection - caud. view**

MUSCLES - FOREARM

Fig. IV-35 - Horse - Lt. forearm - lat. view

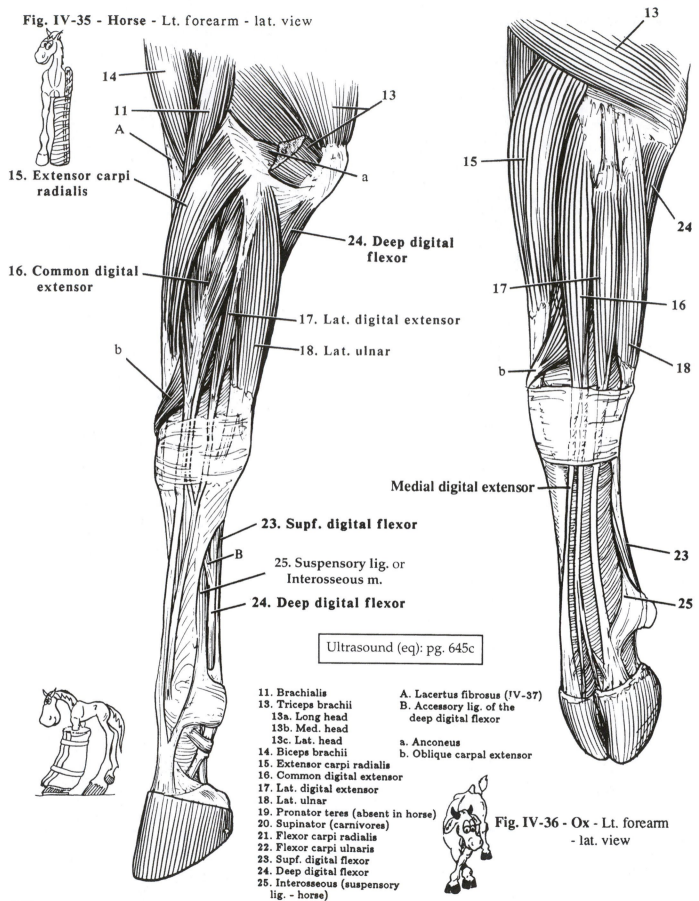

14

11

A

15. Extensor carpi radialis

13

a

24. Deep digital flexor

16. Common digital extensor

b

17. Lat. digital extensor

18. Lat. ulnar

23. Supf. digital flexor

25. Suspensory lig. or Interosseous m.

24. Deep digital flexor

B

15

24

17

16

18

b

Medial digital extensor

23

25

Ultrasound (eq): pg. 645c

11. Brachialis
13. Triceps brachii
   13a. Long head
   13b. Med. head
   13c. Lat. head
14. Biceps brachii
15. Extensor carpi radialis
16. Common digital extensor
17. Lat. digital extensor
18. Lat. ulnar
19. Pronator teres (absent in horse)
20. Supinator (carnivores)
21. Flexor carpi radialis
22. Flexor carpi ulnaris
23. Supf. digital flexor
24. Deep digital flexor
25. Interosseous (suspensory lig. - horse)

A. Lacertus fibrosus (IV-37)
B. Accessory lig. of the deep digital flexor

a. Anconeus
b. Oblique carpal extensor

Fig. IV-36 - Ox - Lt. forearm - lat. view

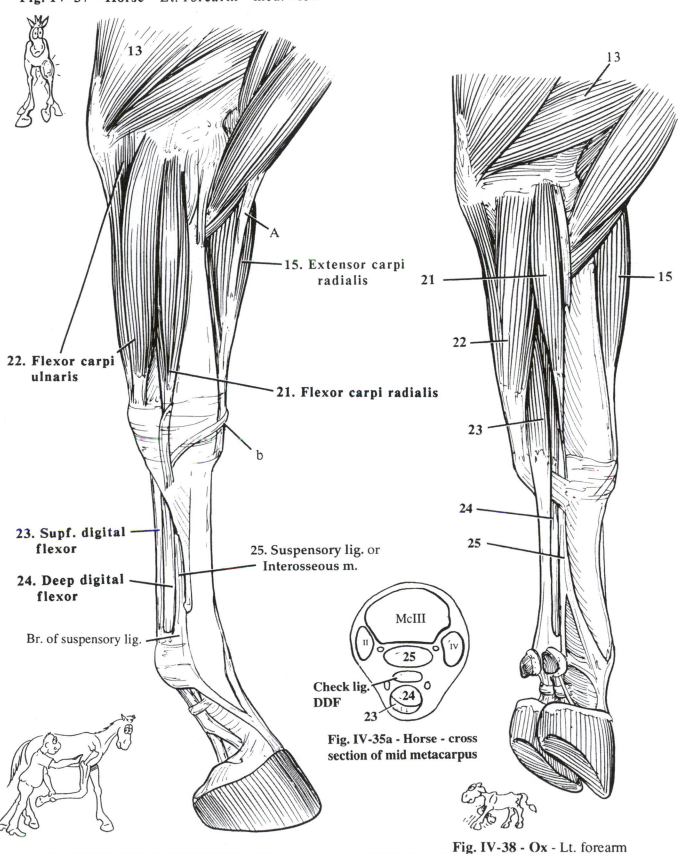

Fig. IV-37 - Horse - Lt. forearm - med. view

13

A

15. **Extensor carpi radialis**

22. **Flexor carpi ulnaris**

21. **Flexor carpi radialis**

b

23. **Supf. digital flexor**

24. **Deep digital flexor**

Br. of suspensory lig.

25. Suspensory lig. or Interosseous m.

13

21

15

22

23

24

25

McIII

II

IV

25

Check lig. DDF

24

23

Fig. IV-35a - Horse - cross section of mid metacarpus

Fig. IV-38 - Ox - Lt. forearm - med. view

MUSCLES – PELVIC LIMB

MUSCLES of the LOIN, HIP and THIGH: The **hip** is the region between the crest of the ilium and greater trochanter of the femur. The **thigh** is the region between the greater trochanter and the stifle. The **loin** is the proximal craniomedial region of the thigh. The **rump** (gluteal region) is the prominence formed by the gluteal muscles.

• **Loin and hip muscles:** divided into three groups: sublumbar, rump, and inner pelvic muscles.

• **Sublumbar muscles:** include the psoas minor, iliopsoas (psoas major and iliacus) and quadratus lumborum muscles. They originate from the ventral surface of the caudal thoracic and lumbar vertebrae and insert on the os coxae and femur. These muscles flex the hip and lumbar vertebral column and fix the lumbar vertebral column. The ventral branches of the lumbar nerves innervate the sublumbar muscles.

• **Rump muscles:** the superficial gluteal, medial gluteal, deep gluteal, and tensor fasciae latae muscles, all originating from the ilium and inserting on the femur. The rump muscles mainly extend the hip joint, except the tensor fasciae latae which, by tensing the fascia of the thigh (fasciae latae), flexes the hip joint and extends the stifle. The cranial and caudal gluteal nerves innervate the rump muscles.

• **Pelvic association:** the internal and external obturators, gemelli, and quadratus femoris mm. (carnivore [car.] & equine [eq]). All originate caudomedial to the hip joint and insert in or near the trochanteric fossa (pg. 96, j). They outward rotate and adduct the limb. They are innervated by the ischiatic n. except the external obturator (obturator n.).

• **Thigh muscles:** divided according to their position: cranial, caudal, and medial:

  • **Cranial thigh muscles:** The extensors of the stifle, innervated by the femoral nerve, they are the four-headed quadriceps femoris and the sartorius muscles. They cover the cranial, lateral, and medial surfaces of the femur, originating from the os coxae and femur and inserting on the tibial tuberosity. They extend the stifle joint and flex the hip.

  • **Medial thigh muscles** (adductor group): They are the sartorius, gracilis, adductor, pectineus, and external obturator muscles. They originate from the os coxae and insert on the bones of the limb. They are innervated by the obturator nerve.

  • **Caudal muscles of the thigh** (hamstring muscles): innervated by the ischiatic nerve, the biceps femoris, caudal crural abductor, semitendinosus, and semimembranosus muscles arise from the ischiatic tuberosity and insert on the medial and lateral sides of the stifle joint. The caudal thigh muscles have varied actions on the hip, stifle, and tarsus.

MUSCLES of the CRUS: the true leg, shank, or gaskin is covered with muscles on the craniolateral and caudal surfaces. There are no muscles on the medial surface, the tibia being directly under the skin. The muscle groups of the crus are not grouped as in the thoracic limb because the angles of the tarsal joint and the digits are opposite. The muscles either extend the digit and flex the tarsus, or flex the digit and extend the tarsus.

• **Craniolateral muscles:** extensors of the digits and flexors of the tarsus, innervated by the peroneal (fibular) nerve. They are the cranial tibial, peroneus longus (long fibular*), long digital extensor, lateral digital extensor, and peroneus tertius (third fibular*) muscles. Located on the craniolateral side of the leg, they originate from the proximal part of the tibia and fibula, except the long digital extensor and peroneus tertius (third fibular) muscles which originate from the extensor fossa of the femur (96, j).

• **Caudal muscles:** flexors of the digits and extensors of the tarsus, innervated by the tibial nerve. They are the gastrocnemius, caudal tibial, popliteus, and superficial and deep digital flexor muscles, originating from the caudal surfaces of the femur and tibia.

MUSCLES of the PES: There is little difference between the muscles of the pes and the manus of the forelimb and they are of the same significance in all the different species, except the interosseous muscle (suspensory ligament) of the horse.

* Fibular may be used instead of peroneal to aid learning by associating muscles with the fibular side of the leg. This option is allowed by the N.A.V.

LOIN & HIP MUSCLES:	
• **Sublumbar muscles:** - ventr. br. of lumbar nn. 　　Psoas minor 　　Iliopsoas 　　　　Psoas major 　　　　Iliacus	Adductor 　　Pectineus 　　External obturator
• **Rump muscles:** cran. & caud. gluteal nn. 　　Superficial gluteal 　　Middle gluteal 　　Deep gluteal 　　Tensor fasciae latae	• **Caudal muscles** (hamstring mm.) - ischiatic n. 　　Biceps femoris 　　Gluteobiceps (rum.) 　　Caud. crural abductor (cam.) 　　Semitendinosus 　　Semimembranosus
• **Inner pelvic muscles:** ischiatic nerve 　　Internal obturator 　　Gemelli 　　Quadratus femoris	**MUSCLES OF THE CRUS:**
THIGH MUSCLES:	• **Craniolateral muscles:** extesors of the digits & flexors of the tarsus - peroneal n. 　　Cranial tibial 　　Peroneus longus (cam. & rum.) 　　Long digital extensor 　　Lateral digital extensor 　　Peroneus tertius (eq. & rum.)
• **Cranial thigh muscles:** extensors of the stifle - femoral n. 　　Quadriceps femoris 　　Sartorius	• **Caudal muscles:** flexors of digits & extensors of tarsus - tibial n. 　　Gastrocnemius 　　Soleus (eq. & cat) 　　Caudal tibial 　　Popliteus 　　Superficial digital flexor 　　Deep digital flexor
• **Medial thigh muscles** (adductor group) - obturator n. 　　Sartorius 　　Gracilis	

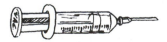

MUSCLES - PELVIC LIMB

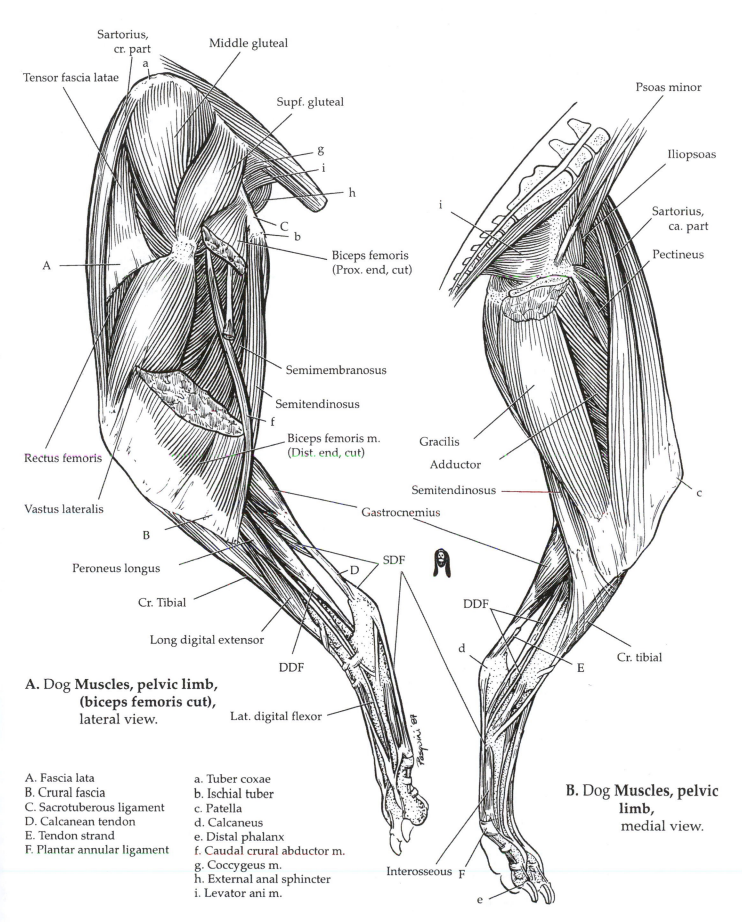

Sartorius, cr. part
Middle gluteal
Tensor fascia latae
a
Supf. gluteal
g
i
h
C
b
Biceps femoris (Prox. end, cut)
A
Semimembranosus
Semitendinosus
f
Biceps femoris m. (Dist. end, cut)
Rectus femoris
Vastus lateralis
B
Peroneus longus
Cr. Tibial
Long digital extensor
DDF
D
SDF
Lat. digital flexor

Psoas minor
Iliopsoas
Sartorius, ca. part
Pectineus
i
Gracilis
Adductor
Semitendinosus
Gastrocnemius
c
DDF
d
E
Cr. tibial
Interosseous F
e

A. Dog **Muscles, pelvic limb,**
   (biceps femoris cut),
   lateral view.

B. Dog **Muscles, pelvic**
   limb,
   medial view.

A. Fascia lata
B. Crural fascia
C. Sacrotuberous ligament
D. Calcanean tendon
E. Tendon strand
F. Plantar annular ligament

a. Tuber coxae
b. Ischial tuber
c. Patella
d. Calcaneus
e. Distal phalanx
f. Caudal crural abductor m.
g. Coccygeus m.
h. External anal sphincter
i. Levator ani m.

MUSCLES - PELVIC LIMB

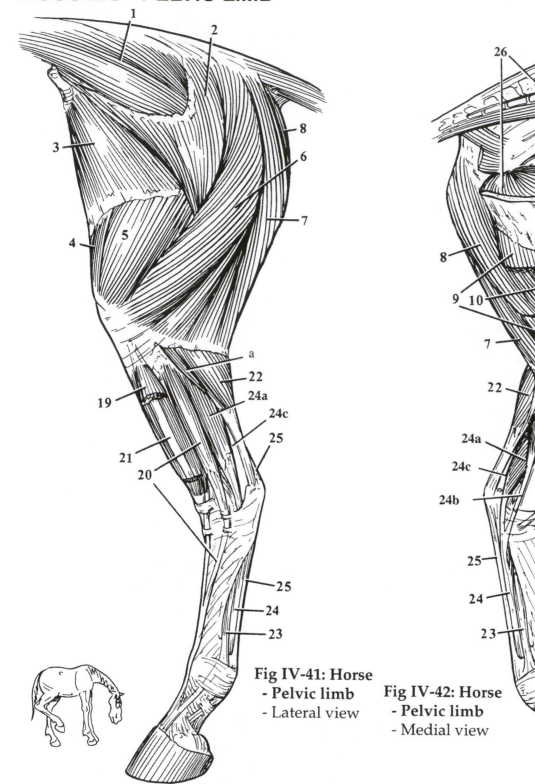

Fig IV-41: Horse
- **Pelvic limb**
- Lateral view

Fig IV-42: Horse
- **Pelvic limb**
- Medial view

1. Middle gluteal (IV-41)
2. Superficial gluteal m.
3. Tensor fasciae latae m.
4. Rectus femoris m.
5. Vastus lateralis m.
6. Biceps femoris m.
7. Semitendinosus m.
8. Semimembranosus m.
9. Gracilis m. (IV-42)

10. Adductor m.
11. Sartorius m.
12. Vastus medialis m.
13. Pectineus m.
14. Iliopsoas m. (psoas major + iliacus mm.)
15. Psoas minor m.
16. Psoas major m.
17. Iliacus m.

18. Cranial tibial m.
19. Long digital extensor m.
20. Lateral digital extensor m. (IV-41)
21. Peroneus tertius m. (third fibular)
22. Gastrocnemius m.
23. Suspensory ligament (Interosseous m.)
24. Deep digital flexor m. (DDF)

24a.Lateral head of DDF
24b Medial head of DDF
24c. Caudal tibial m. of DDF
25. Superficial digital flexor (SDF)
26. Internal obturator m.

a. Soleus m.
b. Popliteal m.

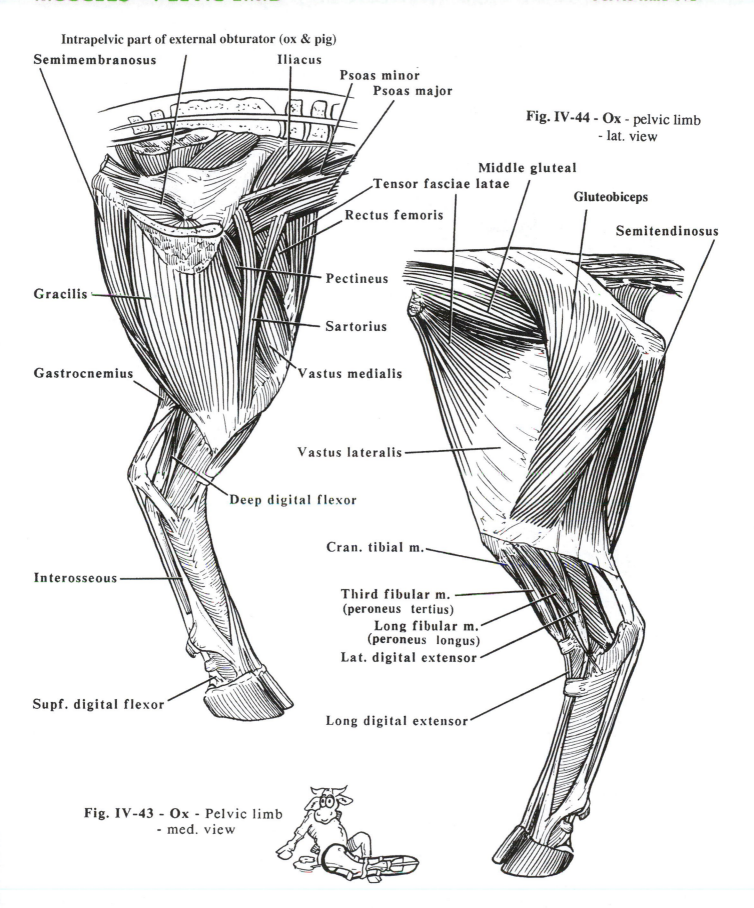

Intrapelvic part of external obturator (ox & pig)

Semimembranosus

Iliacus

Psoas minor

Psoas major

Fig. IV-44 - Ox - pelvic limb
- lat. view

Middle gluteal

Tensor fasciae latae

Gluteobiceps

Rectus femoris

Semitendinosus

Pectineus

Gracilis

Sartorius

Gastrocnemius

Vastus medialis

Vastus lateralis

Deep digital flexor

Cran. tibial m.

Interosseous

Third fibular m.
(peroneus tertius)

Long fibular m.
(peroneus longus)

Lat. digital extensor

Long digital extensor

Supf. digital flexor

Fig. IV-43 - Ox - Pelvic limb
- med. view

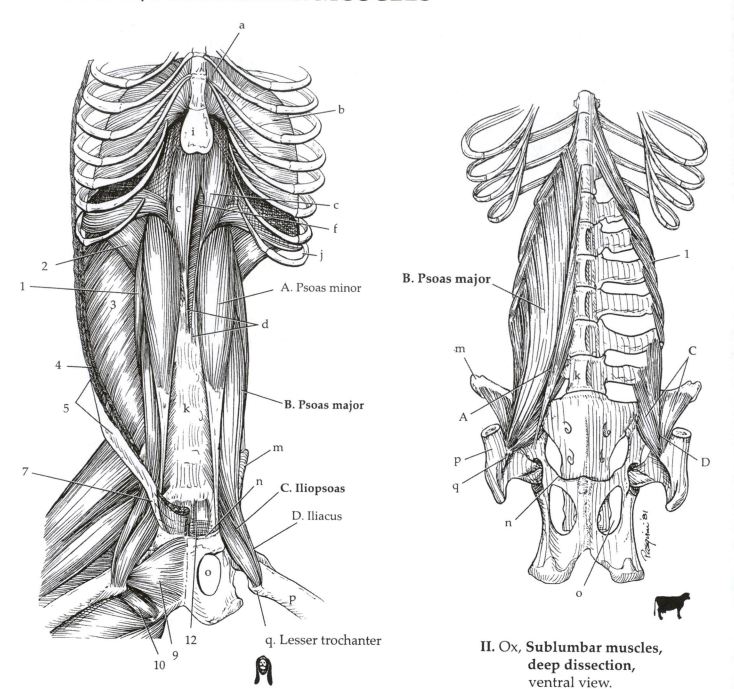

I. Dog, Sublumbar muscles, ventral view.

II. Ox, Sublumbar muscles, deep dissection, ventral view.

A. Psoas minor
B. Psoas major
C. Iliopsoas
D. Iliacus
q. Lesser trochanter

MUSCLE	ORIGINS	INSERTION	ACTION	NERVE
Psoas minor	Thoracolumbar vertebral bodies	Hip bone (psoas minor tubercle)	Stabilize back	Thoracic & lumbar nn. (ventr. brs.)
Iliopsoas		**Lesser trochanter**	**Flex hip**	Lumbar (ventr. brs.) & femoral nn.
Psoas major	Lumbar vertebrae (transverse processes & bodies)	"		
Iliacus	Wings of ilium and sacrum	"	"	Lumbar and femoral n.
Quadratus lumborum	Ribs & lumbar transverse processes	Transverse processes & wing of ilium	Stabilize loin	Thoracic & lumbar nn.

SUBLUMBAR MUSCLES

Sublumbar mm.: muscles below the transverse processes of the lumbar vertebrae (thus, hypaxial mm.), which include the following:

A. **Psoas minor m.** (I, II, III): the thin, glistening muscle located on either side of the aorta and caudal vena cava. It inserts on the "rim" of the pelvis (arcuate line and iliopectineal eminence).

B. **Psoas major m.** (I, II, III): the large m. located dorsal and lateral to the psoas minor m.

C. **Iliopsoas m.** (I, II, III): the combined **psoas major** and **iliacus** mm., it inserts on the lesser trochanter of the femur and is the major flexor of the hip.

D. Iliacus m. (I, II, III): arises from the ilium and fuses with the distal end of the psoas major m. to form the iliopsoas m.

III. Cat, Sublumbar muscles,
ventral view.

1. Quadratus lumborum m. (I, II, III): located under the lateral edge of the psoas major m. extending from the first three thoracic vertebrae and all the lumbar vertebrae to the tips of the transverse processes of the lumbar vertebrae and the medial side of the ilium.
2. Retractor costae m. (I, III): seen from the inside of the abdomen, it extends from the transverse processes of the first three or four lumbar vertebrae to the last rib.
3. Transversus abdominis m. (I, III).
4. Internal abdominal oblique m. (IAO)(I, III).
5. External abdominal oblique m. (EAO)(I, III).
   6. Aponeurosis of EAO / #5 (III).
   7. Inguinal ligament (I, III).
8. Rectus abdominis m. (III).
9. External obturator m. (I, III).
10. Quadratus femoris m. (I, III).
11. Quadriceps femoris m. (III).
12. Ventral sacrocaudalis m. (I, III).

a-h. Diaphragm (I, III).
  a. Costal part (I, III).
  b. Sternal parts (I, III).
  c. Crura, right and left (I, III).
  d. Tendons of the crus (I, III).
  e. Tendinous center (II).
  f. Aortic hiatus (I, III).
  g. Esophageal hiatus (III).
  h. Caval foramen (III).
i. Xiphoid cartilage (I).
j. Ribs (I).
k. Body of lumbar vertebrae (I, II, III).
m. Ilium (I, II, III).
n. Pelvic brim (I, II, III).
o. Obturator foramen (I, II, III).
p. Femur (I, II, III).
q. Lesser trochanter (I, II, III).

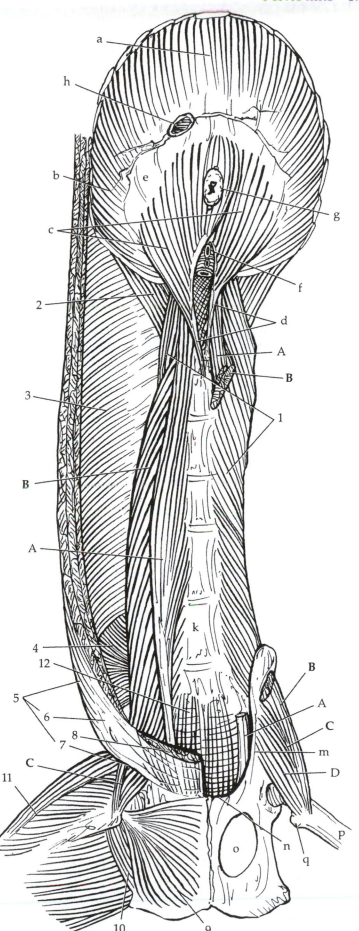

PELVIC ASSOCIATION

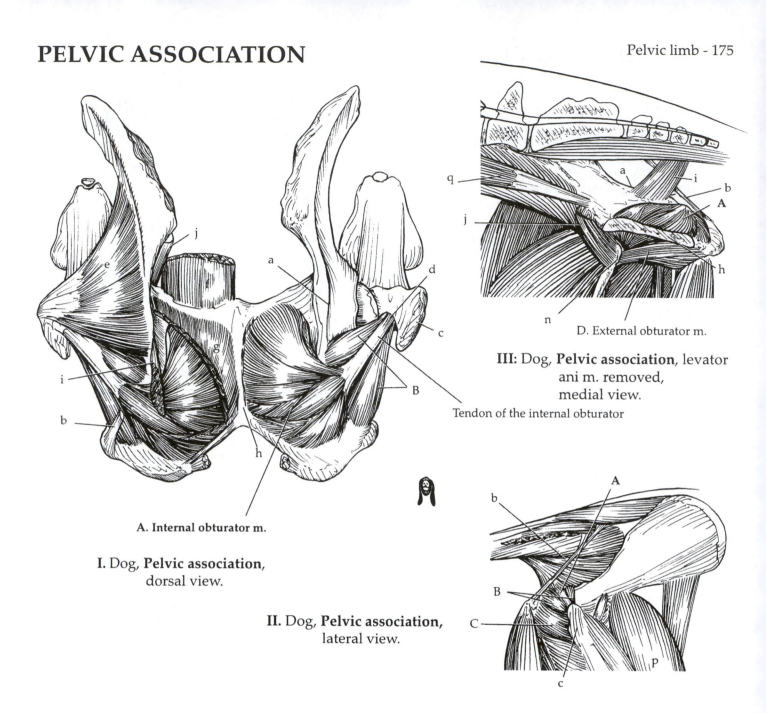

A. Internal obturator m.

I. Dog, **Pelvic association**, dorsal view.

II. Dog, **Pelvic association**, lateral view.

D. External obturator m.

III: Dog, **Pelvic association**, levator ani m. removed, medial view.

Tendon of the internal obturator

Caudal hip muscles: the four muscles arising from the pelvis, passing caudal to the hip joint to insert on or near the trochanteric fossa. They consist of the pelvic association plus the external obturator m.

Pelvic association: consists of the internal obturator, gemelli and quadratus lumborum mm. Along with the external obturator m., all rotate the femur laterally (outward/ supinate) at the hip, thus, opposing the medial rotation of the gluteals, thus, keeping the thigh moving in a sagittal plane. They are innervated by the ischiatic n. which crosses over them.

A. Internal obturator m.*(I, II, III, IV): the fan-shaped muscle arising from the floor (inside) of the pelvis around the obturator foramen. Its shiny tendon crosses the lesser ischiatic notch ventral to the sacrotuberous ligament to reach the trochanteric fossa. It is partially buried in the fused gemelli m.

B. Gemelli m. (I, II, IV, V)): two small, fused muscles passing from the hip bone to the trochanteric fossa. They are grooved dorsally by the tendon of the internal obturator m.
- Bursa: between the tendon of the internal obturator m. and the lesser ischiatic spine.

C. Quadratus femoris m. (II, IV, V, VI): the short, thick muscle just caudoventral to the gemelli, it attaches just distal to the trochanteric fossa.

D. External obturator m. (III, IV, V): the fan-shaped muscle arising from the ventral surface of the hip bones (outside the pelvic cavity); it covers the obturator foramen. Although not part of the pelvic association, its tendon also inserts in the trochanteric fossa, and thus, has the same action.

***Internal obturator**: found only in the horse and carnivores. Its tendon passes over the lesser ischiatic notch to reach the trochanteric fossa. In the pig and ruminants, the similarly-placed muscle is known as the <u>intrapelvic part of the external obturator m</u>. Its tendon passes through the obturator foramen to reach the trochanteric fossa.

PELVIC ASSOCIATION

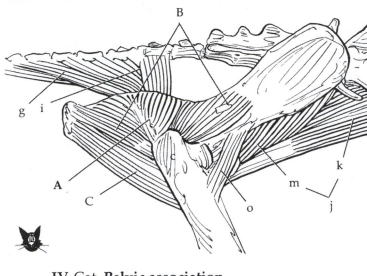

IV. Cat, **Pelvic association,**
lateral view.

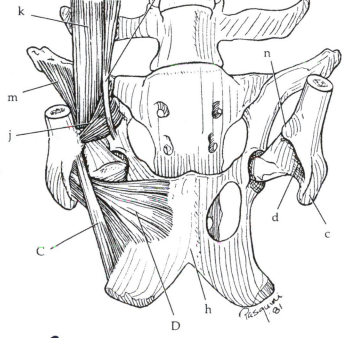

VI. Ox, **Pelvic muscles,**
ventral view.

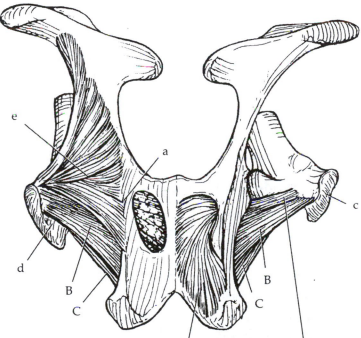

D. External obturator m.,
intrapelvic part in ox and pig.

V. Ox, **Pelvic muscles,**
dorsal view.

a. Ischiatic spine (I, III, V).
b. Sacrotuberous ligament
   (absent in cat)(I, II, III).
c. Greater tubercle (I, II, VI, V, VI).
d. Trochanteric fossa (I, VI, V).
e. Deep gluteal m. (I, V).
f. Prepubic tendon (insertion of the
   rectus abdominis m.)(I).
g. Levator ani m. (I, IV).

h. Pelvic symphysis (I, III, VI, IV).
i. Coccygeus m. (I, III, IV).
j. Iliopsoas m. (I, III, VI).
   k. Psoas major m. (III, IV, VI).
   m. Iliacus m. (III, VI).
n. Lesser trochanter (III, VI).
o. Articularis coxae m. (IV).
p. Quadriceps femoris m. (II).
q. Psoas minor m. (III, VI).

CAUDAL HIP MUSCLES				
MUSCLE	ORIGINS	INSERTION	ACTION	NERVE
Internal obturator	Pelvic floor around obturator foramen	Trochanteric fossa (femur)	Rotate limb laterally	Ischiatic n.
Gemelli	Spine of ischium	"	"	"
Quadratus femoris	Ventral ischium	Near trochanteric fossa	"	"
External obturator	Ventral pelvis	Trochanteric fossa (femur)	"	Obturator n.

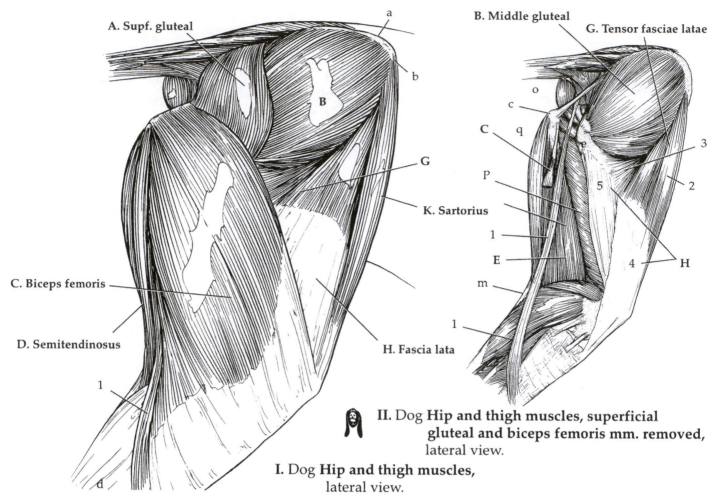

A. Supf. gluteal

a

b

B

G

K. Sartorius

C. Biceps femoris

D. Semitendinosus

1

H. Fascia lata

d

B. Middle gluteal

G. Tensor fasciae latae

o

c

C

q

e

3

P

2

1

5

E

4

H

m

1

II. Dog Hip and thigh muscles, superficial gluteal and biceps femoris mm. removed, lateral view.

I. Dog Hip and thigh muscles, lateral view.

A. Superficial gluteal m. (I, III, IV): small muscle dorsal and slightly caudal to the hip joint. It inserts on the third trochanter of the femur, covering the caudal part of the middle gluteal m.

B. Middle gluteal m. (I, II, III, IV): the large rump muscle arising from the wing of the ilium (gluteal surface) and inserting on the greater trochanter.

"Hamstring muscles": consist of the biceps femoris, semitendinosus and semimembranosus mm. from lateral to medial.

C. Biceps femoris m. (I, II, III): the huge muscle on the caudolateral side of the thigh arising from the sacrotuberous ligament and ischiatic tuberosity. It attaches by the fascia lata and crural fascia to either side of the stifle, and by a strong strand of fascia to the hock (calcanean tuber by way of the calcanean tendon).

D. Semitendinosus m. (I, III): the hamstring muscle arising lateral to the semimembranosus m. It also inserts on the medial side of the limb and, by way of the crural fascia, to the calcaneus.

E. Semi"M"embranosus m. (II, IV): the more "m"edial hamstring m. located adjacent to the adductor m. Its two bellies insert on the medial sides of the femur and the tibia.

F. Popliteal lymph node (IV): the large lymph node in the popliteal region.

G. Tensor fasciae latae m. (I, II, III, IV): the triangular muscle

in the angle formed by the sartorius and middle gluteal mm. It can be divided into two parts (cranial and caudal).

H. Fascia lata (I, II, III, IV): the lateral deep fascia of the thigh. The aponeurosis of the tensor fasciae latae m., it consists of superficial and deep layers.

1. Caudal crural abductor ("fire hydrant") m. (I, II, IV): the thin, strap-like muscle deep to the biceps femoris m. It has been referred to as the "fire hydrant muscle" (who says anatomists have no sense of humor?).

2. Cranial superficial part of the tensor fascia latae m. (I, II, IV): inserts on the superficial fascia latae that blends with the insertion of the biceps femoris m.

3. Caudal deep part of the tensor fascia latae m. (II, IV): inserts on the deep fascia latae that passes caudoventrally deep to the biceps femoris m.

4. Superficial leaf of the fascia lata (II, IV): the aponeurosis of the cranial part of the tensor fascia latae m., it passes over the quadriceps femoris m.

5 Deep leaf of the fascia lata (II, IV): the aponeurosis of the caudal part of the tensor fascia latae m.; it passes caudoventrally deep to the biceps femoris m.

6. Gluteofemoralis m. (cranial crural abductor)(fe) (III, IV): found in the cat caudal to the superficial gluteal m.; extending from the first few caudal vertebrae to the fascia cranial to the biceps femoris m.

7. Tendinous strands (III): from the biceps femoris, semitendinosus and gracilis mm. to the calcanean tendon, and thus, to the calcanean tuberosity.

a. Crest of ilium
b. Coxal tuber
c. Ischial tuber
d. Crural fascia
e. Greater trochanter
f. Distal femur
g. Gastrocnemius m.
h. Soleus m. (not dog)
i. Lateral collateral ligament
j. Fibula
k. Patella (IV)
l. Patellar tendon
m. Tibial tuberosity
n. Long digital extensor m.
o. Internal obturator m.
p. Gemelli m.
q. Quadratus femoris m.
r. Coccygeus m.
s. Levator ani m.
t. External abdominal oblique m.
u. Anus

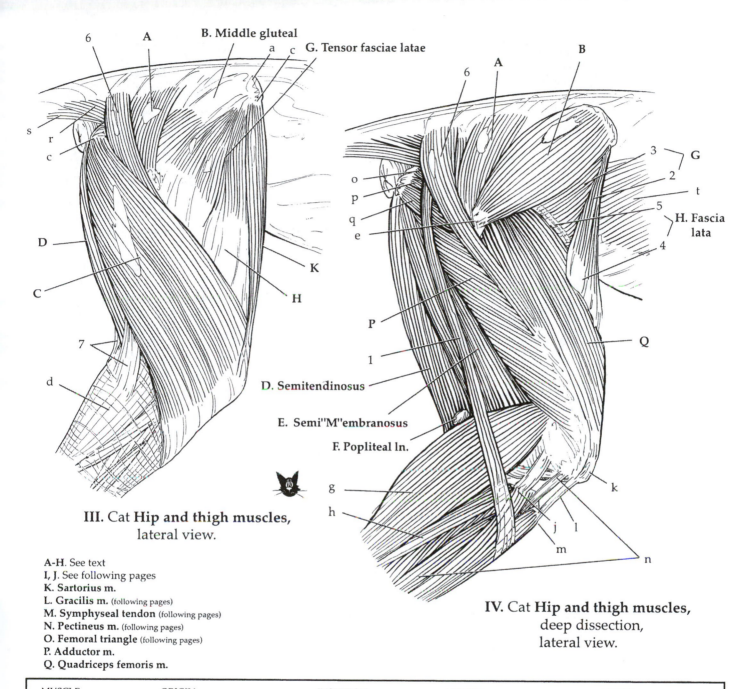

III. Cat **Hip and thigh muscles,** lateral view.

D. Semitendinosus

E. Semi"M"embranosus

F. Popliteal ln.

A-H. See text
I, J. See following pages
K. Sartorius m.
L. Gracilis m. (following pages)
M. Symphyseal tendon (following pages)
N. Pectineus m. (following pages)
O. Femoral triangle (following pages)
P. Adductor m.
Q. Quadriceps femoris m.

IV. Cat **Hip and thigh muscles,** deep dissection, lateral view.

MUSCLE	ORIGIN	INSERTION	ACTION	NERVE
Superficial gluteal	Sacrum, Ca1 & sacrotuberous ligament.	Third trochanter.	Extend hip, abduct limb.	Ca. gluteal n.
Middle gluteal	Wing of ilium.	**Greater trochanter** (crest & gluteal surface).	**Extend hip**, abduct limb & rotate pelvic limb medially.	Cr. gluteal n.
Deep gluteal	Body of ischium.	Greater trochanter.	Abduct limb, extend hip, rotate pelvic limb medially.	Cr. gluteal n.
Caudal crural abductor Gluteofemoralis (fe) (cranial crural abductor)	Sacrotuberous ligament. First few caudal vertebrae.	Lat. crural fascia. Fascia lata.	Abduct limb (fine aim at firehydrant). Abduct limb, extend hip.	Ca. gluteal n.
Tensor fasciae latae	Tuber coxae.	Fascia lata.	Flex hip, extend stifle.	Cr. gluteal n
Biceps femoris	Ischiatic tuber & sacrotuberous ligament.	Patella, tibia & calcaneus.	Extend hip, stifle & tarsus; flex stifle (caudal part of m.).	Ca. gluteal n. & ischiatic n.
Semitendinosus	Ischiatic tuberosity.	Tibial crest, calcaneus.	Extend hip & tarsus, **flex stifle.**	Ischiatic n.
Semimembranosus	Ischiatic tuber (tuberosity).	Med. femur & tibia.	Extend hip & stifle, **flex stifle.**	Ischiatic n.

RUMP & HIP MUSCLES - 2

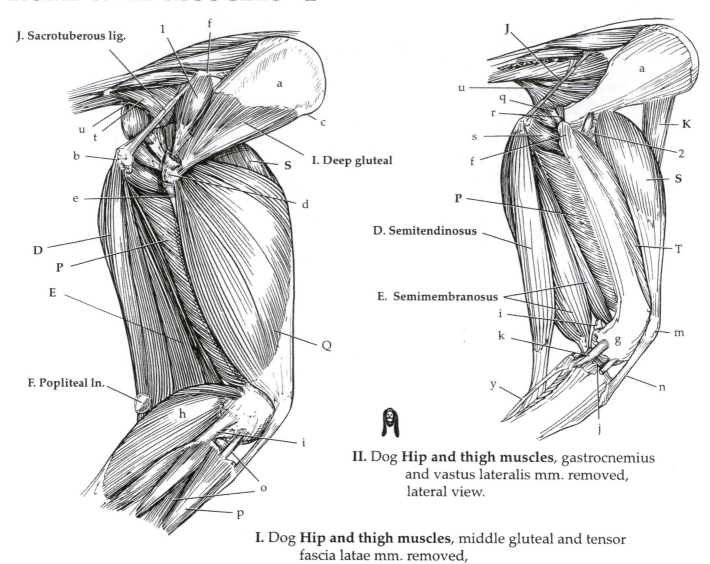

J. Sacrotuberous lig.

I. Deep gluteal

D. Semitendinosus

E. Semimembranosus

F. Popliteal ln.

II. Dog **Hip and thigh muscles**, gastrocnemius and vastus lateralis mm. removed, lateral view.

I. Dog **Hip and thigh muscles**, middle gluteal and tensor fascia latae mm. removed, lateral view.

I. Deep gluteal m.: the small, fan-shaped muscle deep to the middle gluteal m., it extends from the ilium and ischium to the greater trochanter.

J. Sacrotuberous ligament: see species differences.

SPECIES DIFFERENCES:

• **Gluteobiceps muscle**: the fusion of the superficial gluteal and the biceps femoris mm. in ruminants. Therefore, the superficial gluteal m. and the third trochanter are absent in ruminants.

• **Sacrotuberous ligament**: the strong band of connective tissue extending between the caudal sacrum and first caudal vertebra to the ischiatic tuberosity in the dog. It is lacking in the cat. Note that the superficial gluteal, biceps femoris

and caudal crural abductor mm. arise from it.

• Broad sacrotuberous ligament: a sheet of connective tissue forming the lateral pelvic wall (see pages 119 and 185).

CLINICAL:

• **Whorlbone disease (trochanteric bursitis)**: a rare inflammation of the bursa between the middle gluteal muscle and the greater trochanter of the femur in the **horse**. Pain in this bursa causes the horse to "dog trot" (move its rear end to the side and cranially, away from the pain.)

• **Sacrotuberous ligament**: softening to disappearance prior to birthing, it is used as an indictor of impending birth in small ruminants.

MUSCLE	ORIGIN	INSERTION	ACTION	NERVE
Deep gluteal	Body of ischium.	Greater trochanter.	Abduct limb, extend hip, rotate pelvic limb medially.	Cr. gluteal n.
Piriformis	Sacrum & caudal vertebra.	Greater trochanter.	Like middle gluteal m.	Cr. gluteal n.
Articularis coxae	Ilium.	Hip joint capsule & femur.	Prevents pinching of capsule by joint.	

RUMP & HIP MUSCLES - 2

J. No Sacrotuberous lig. in the cat

I. Deep gluteal m.

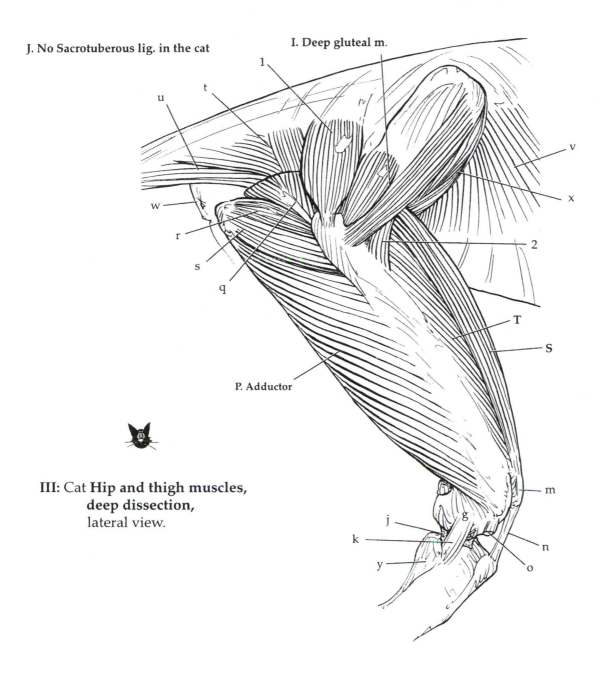

P. Adductor

**III: Cat Hip and thigh muscles,
 deep dissection,
 lateral view.**

A- C. See preceding pages.
D. Semitendinosus m (I, II)
E. Semimembranosus m. (I, II)
F. Popliteal lymph node (I)
G-H. Fascia lata see preceding pages.
I, J. See text
K. Sartorius m. (II)
L-O. See following pages.
P. Adductor m. (I, II, III)
Q-U. Quadriceps femoris m.
Q. Vastus lateralis m. (I)
R. Vastus medialis mm. (see next page)
S. Rectus femoris m. (I, II, III)
T. Vastus intermedius m. (II, III)
U. See following pages.

1. Piriformis m. (I, II, III): only in carnivores, it is deep and caudal to the middle gluteal m. from which it is easily separated. Fused with the middle gluteal, until recently it was considered part of this muscle and need not be considered separately. It extends from the sacrum and caudal vertebra to the major trochanter under cover of the superficial gluteal m.

2. Articularis coxae (II, III): the tiny spindle-shaped m. on the craniolateral side of the hip joint capsule covered by the deep gluteal m. Clinically, it is used as a surgical landmark for opening the joint capsule.

a. Wing of ilium
b. Ischial tuber
c. Coxal tuber
d. Greater trochanter
e. Third trochanter
f. Sacrum
g. Distal femur
h. Gastrocnemius m.
i. Sesamoid bone of the gastrocnemius m. (Fabella)
j. Meniscus
k. Lateral collateral ligament
m. Patella
n. Patellar tendon
o. Long digital extensor m.

p. Cranial tibial m.
q. Internal obturator m.
r. Gemelli m.
s. Quadratus femoris m.
t. Coccygeus m.
u. Levator ani m.
v. Internal abdominal oblique m.
w. Anus
x. Iliopsoas m.
y. Fibula

179

MEDIAL THIGH MUSCLES - 3

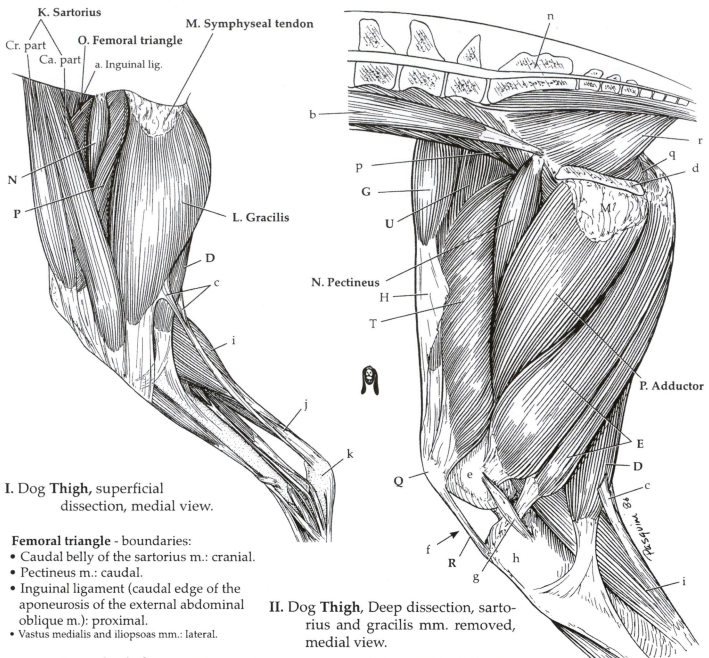

I. Dog Thigh, superficial dissection, medial view.

Femoral triangle - boundaries:
• Caudal belly of the sartorius m.: cranial.
• Pectineus m.: caudal.
• Inguinal ligament (caudal edge of the aponeurosis of the external abdominal oblique m.): proximal.
• Vastus medialis and iliopsoas mm.: lateral.

II. Dog Thigh, Deep dissection, sartorius and gracilis mm. removed, medial view.

K. Sartorius m. (I, II): the strap-like muscle passing from the tuber coxae to the tibia.

L. Gracilis m. (I, III): the thin muscle on the caudomedial surface of the thigh which inserts by an aponeurosis.

M. Symphyseal tendon (I, II): the thick, flat connective tissue arising from the ventral surface of the pelvic symphysis. It provides the origin of the gracilis and adductor mm.

N. Pectineus m. (I, II): the small, spindle-shaped muscle arising from the cranial part of the pelvis.

O. Femoral triangle (I, II): the shallow space through which the vessels of the limb pass.

P. Adductor m.* (I, II, III, IV): the large muscle just caudal to the pectineus m. and deep to the gracilis.

SPECIES DIFFERENCES:

• **Sartorius m.**: in the **dog** is divided into a cranial belly that forms the cranial border of the thigh and a caudal belly that passes on the medial side of the thigh. In the **ruminant** and **pig** it is divided proximally, and undivided in the **cat** and **hor,se.**

CLINICAL:

• **Femoral triangle**: the area bounded by the sartorius muscle cranially, the pectineus muscle caudally and the body wall dorsally. It is a good place to take the pulse as the femoral artery passes through it in carnivores. It is not advised to try this in the larger animals. (Ouch!)

• **Pectineal tenotomy**: cutting the pectineus m. to relieve the pain of hip dysplasia in dogs.

---

* Adductor muscle consists of two heads which are not clearly divisible:
Adductor magnus et brevis m.: large part of the adductor m.
Adductor longus m.: smaller deep part of the adductor m.

MEDIAL THIGH MUSCLES - 3

K. **Sartorius** (not divided in the cat)

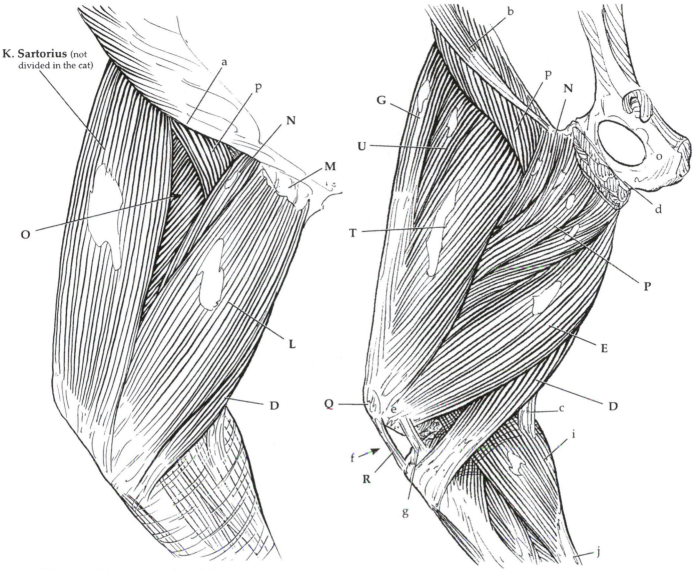

III. Cat **Thigh,** superficial dissection, medial view.

IV. Cat, **Thigh**, Deep dissection, sartorius & gracilis mm. removed, medial view.

A-C. See preceding pages
D. Semitendinosus m. (I, II, III).
E. Semimembranosus m. (II, IV).
F. See preceding pages
G. Tensor fasciae latae m. (II, IV).
H. Fascia lata (II).
I-J. See preceding pages.
K-P: See text.
Q-V. Quadriceps femoris m.
 Q. Patella (II, IV).

R. Patellar ligament (II, IV).
S. Vastus lateralis m. (see preceding pages)
T. Vastus medialis m. (II, IV).
U. Rectus femoris m. (II, IV).
V. Vastus intermedius m. (see preceding pages)

a. Inguinal ligament (III).: caudal edge of the aponeurosis of the external abdominal oblique m.
b. Psoas minor m.
c. Tendon strands from gracilis & semitendinous mm. to calcanean tendon
d. Pelvic symphysis
e. Femur
f. Stifle joint
g. Medial collateral ligament
h. Tibia

i. Gastrocnemius m.
j. Calcanean tendon
k. Calcaneus
m. Coccygeus m.
n. Sacrum
o. Ischium
p. Iliopsoas m.
q. Internal obturator m.
r. Levator ani m.

MEDIAL MUSCLES OF THE THIGH - ADDUCTOR MUSCLES				
MUSCLE	ORIGINS	INSERTION	ACTION	NERVE
Sartorius (cr. & ca parts in dog)	Ilium (iliac fascia - eq).	**Med.** side of stifle.	**Flex hip**, extend stifle, **abduct** thigh.	Femoral n. (saphenous br.)
Gracilis	Pelvic symphysis.	**Med.** stifle & calcaneus.	**Adduct** limb, flex stifle, extend hip & hock.	**Obturator n.**
Pectineus	Pubic bone & prepubic tendon.	**Med.** femur.	**Adduct** limb.	"
Adductor	Pelvis (ventral).	**Med.** femur & stifle.	**Adduct** limb.	"

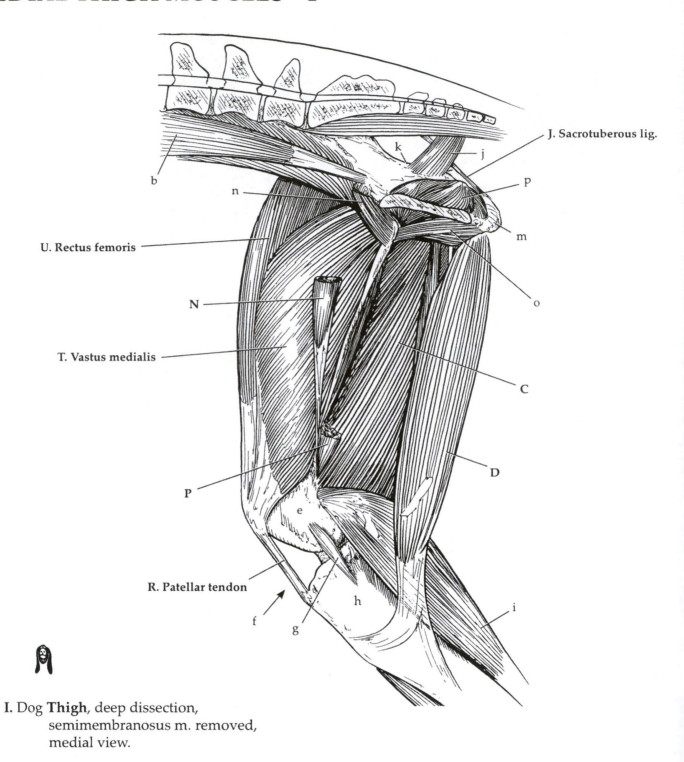

J. Sacrotuberous lig.

U. Rectus femoris

N.

T. Vastus medialis

P.

R. Patellar tendon

I. Dog Thigh, deep dissection,
semimembranosus m. removed,
medial view.

A. Superficial gluteal m.
B. Middle gluteal m.
"Hamstring muscles"
C. Biceps femoris m. (III)
D. Semitendinosus m. (I, II, III)
E. Semi"M"embranosus m. (III)
F-I. (see preceding pages).
J. Sacrotuberous ligament (I).
K. Sartorius m. (III)
L. Gracilis m. (III)

M. Symphyseal tendon (see preceding pages).
N. Pectineus m. (I, III)
O. Femoral triangle (see preceding pages).
P. Adductor m. (I)
Q-V. See text.

a. Sacrum
b. Psoas minor m.
c. Tendon strands from gracilis and semitendinous mm. to calcanean tendon
d. Pelvic symphysis
e. Femur
f. Stifle joint
g. Medial collateral ligament
h. Tibia
i. Gastrocnemius m.

j. Coccygeus m.
k. Ischiatic spine
m. Ischium
n. Iliopsoas m.
o. External obturator m.
p. Internal obturator m.
q. Quadratus femoris m.
r. Cranial head (sartorius m.)
s. Caudal head (sartorius m.)

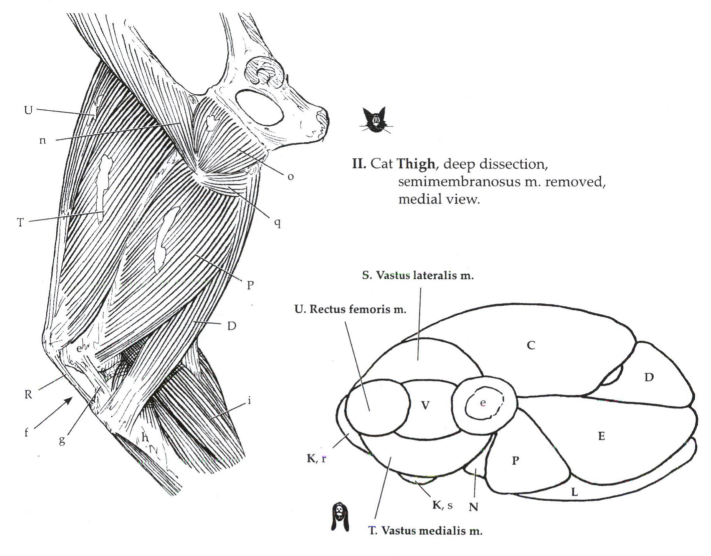

II. Cat Thigh, deep dissection, semimembranosus m. removed, medial view.

S. Vastus lateralis m.

U. Rectus femoris m.

K, r

K, s   N

T. Vastus medialis m.

II. Dog, Cross section of the thigh.

Q-V. Quadriceps femoris m.: the four-headed muscle making up the bulk of the cranial thigh. It inserts on the tibial tuberosity. The major extensor of the stifle, its function is required for the limb to bear weight.

Q. Patella: the large sesamoid bone buried in the tendon of insertion of the quadriceps femoris m.; it articulates with the trochlea of the femur.

R. Patellar ligament: the part of the tendon of insertion of the quadriceps femoris m., from the patella to the tibial tuberosity.

S, T. Vastus lateralis and **vastus medialis mm.**: the two

heads of the quadriceps femoris m. on the lateral and medial sides, respectively.

U. Rectus femoris m.: the straight, round head of the quadriceps femoris m., between the two vasti heads. It extends over the hip joint as well as the stifle joint, thus, affecting both joints (flexes hip).

V. Vastus intermedius m.: located on the cranial aspect of the femur, it is surrounded by the other heads of the quadriceps femoris m. and the femur. It is fused with the two vasti mm.

STIFLE EXTENSOR MUSCLES				
MUSCLE	ORIGIN	INSERTION	ACTION	NERVE
Quadriceps femoris		**Tibial tuberosity**		**Femoral n.**
Rectus femoris	Hip bone (ilium)	"	**Extend stifle** & flex hip	"
Vastus lateralis	Proximal femur	"	**Extend stifle**	"
Vastus medialis	"	"	"	"
Vastus intermedius	"	"	"	"

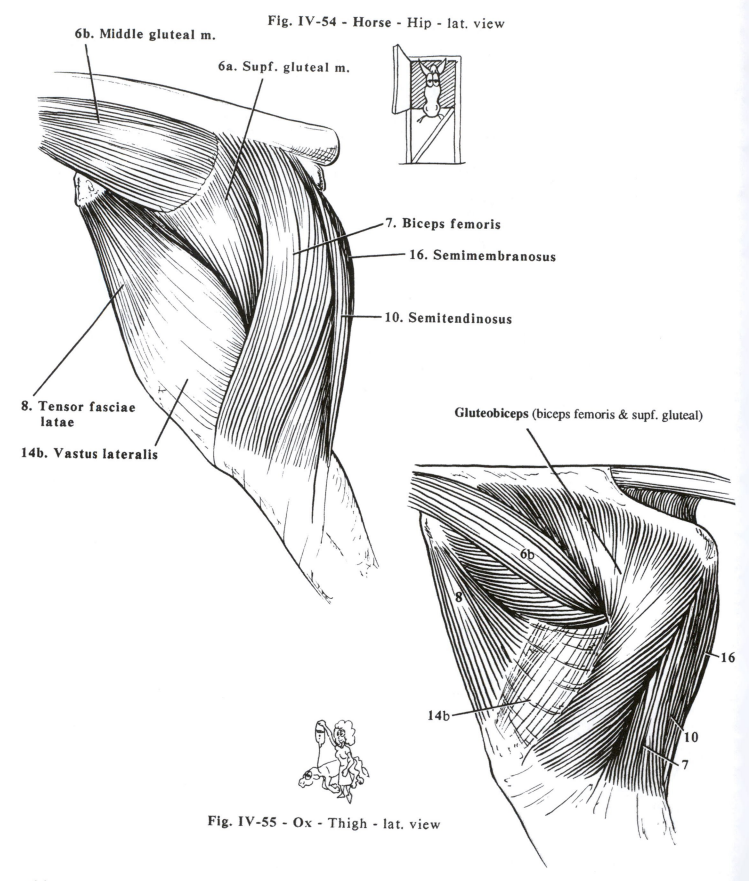

Fig. IV-54 - Horse - Hip - lat. view

6b. Middle gluteal m.

6a. Supf. gluteal m.

7. Biceps femoris

16. Semimembranosus

10. Semitendinosus

8. Tensor fasciae latae

14b. Vastus lateralis

Gluteobiceps (biceps femoris & supf. gluteal)

6b

8

16

14b

10

7

Fig. IV-55 - Ox - Thigh - lat. view

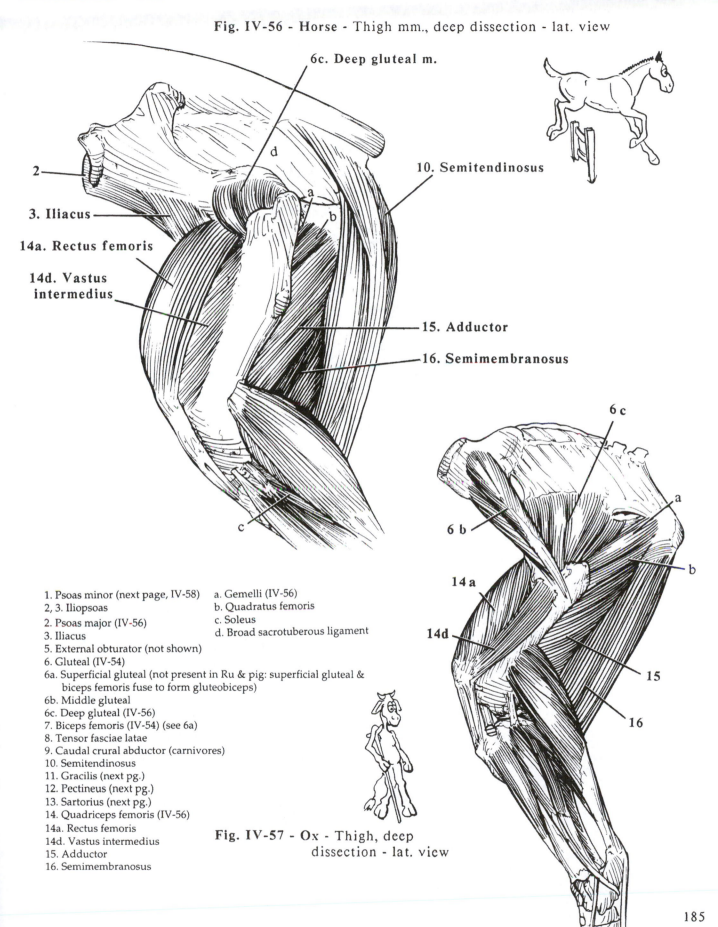

Fig. IV-56 - Horse - Thigh mm., deep dissection - lat. view

6c. Deep gluteal m.

2

3. Iliacus

14a. Rectus femoris

14d. Vastus intermedius

d

a

b

10. Semitendinosus

15. Adductor

16. Semimembranosus

c

6 c

6 b

a

b

14 a

14 d

15

16

Fig. IV-57 - Ox - Thigh, deep dissection - lat. view

1. Psoas minor (next page, IV-58)
2, 3. Iliopsoas
2. Psoas major (IV-56)
3. Iliacus
5. External obturator (not shown)
6. Gluteal (IV-54)
6a. Superficial gluteal (not present in Ru & pig: superficial gluteal & biceps femoris fuse to form gluteobiceps)
6b. Middle gluteal
6c. Deep gluteal (IV-56)
7. Biceps femoris (IV-54) (see 6a)
8. Tensor fasciae latae
9. Caudal crural abductor (carnivores)
10. Semitendinosus
11. Gracilis (next pg.)
12. Pectineus (next pg.)
13. Sartorius (next pg.)
14. Quadriceps femoris (IV-56)
14a. Rectus femoris
14d. Vastus intermedius
15. Adductor
16. Semimembranosus

a. Gemelli (IV-56)
b. Quadratus femoris
c. Soleus
d. Broad sacrotuberous ligament

Fig. IV-58 - Horse - Thigh - med. view

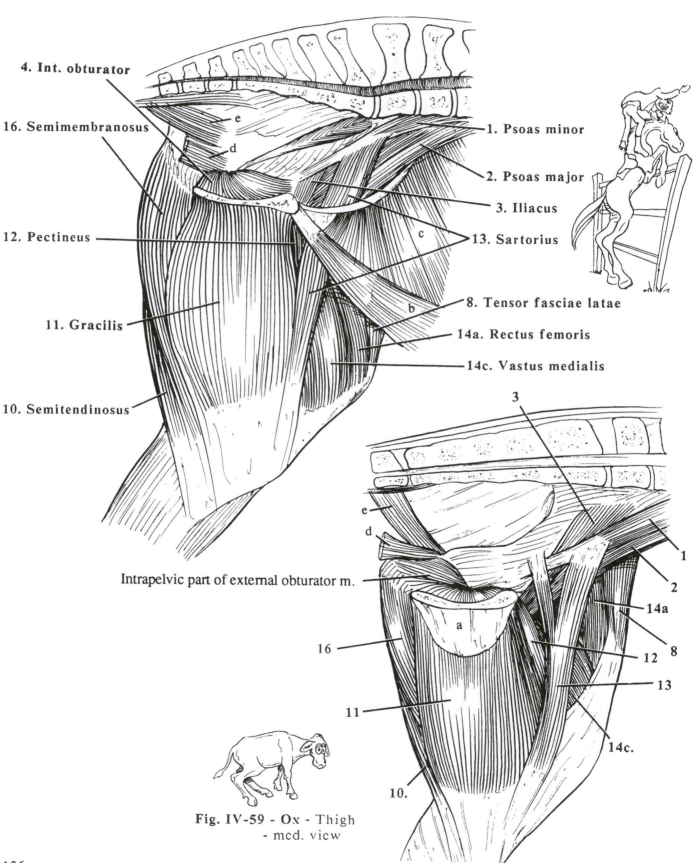

4. Int. obturator

16. Semimembranosus

12. Pectineus

11. Gracilis

10. Semitendinosus

1. Psoas minor

2. Psoas major

3. Iliacus

13. Sartorius

8. Tensor fasciae latae

14a. Rectus femoris

14c. Vastus medialis

Intrapelvic part of external obturator m.

Fig. IV-59 - Ox - Thigh
- med. view

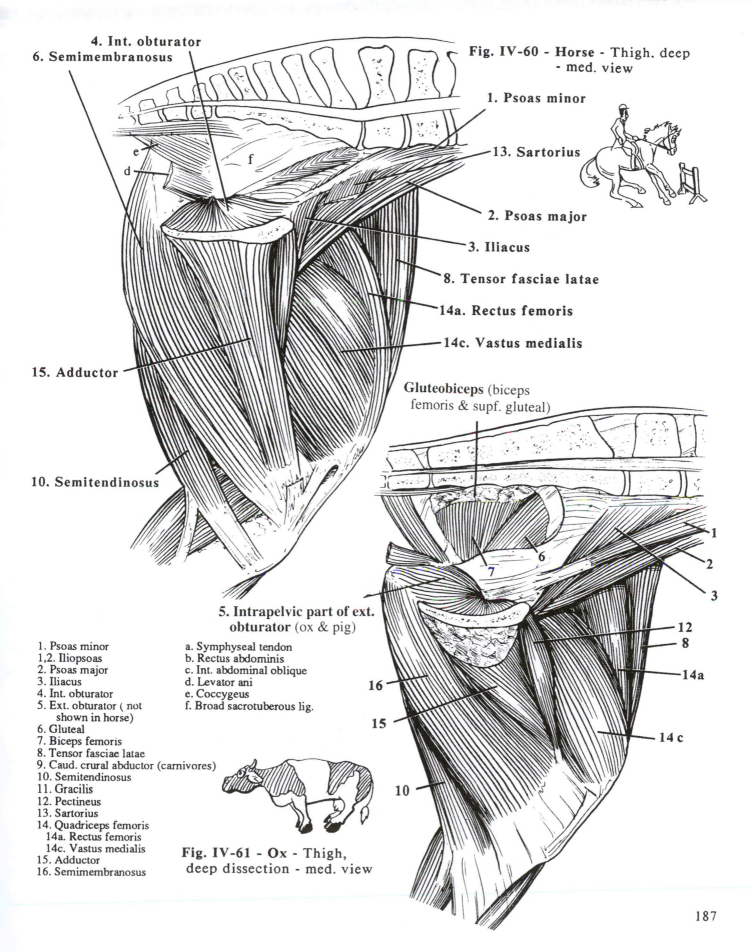

4. Int. obturator
6. Semimembranosus

Fig. IV-60 - Horse - Thigh. deep - med. view

1. Psoas minor

13. Sartorius

2. Psoas major

3. Iliacus

8. Tensor fasciae latae

14a. Rectus femoris

14c. Vastus medialis

e

f

d

15. Adductor

10. Semitendinosus

Gluteobiceps (biceps femoris & supf. gluteal)

7

6

1

2

3

12

8

14a

16

15

14 c

10

5. Intrapelvic part of ext. obturator (ox & pig)

1. Psoas minor
1,2. Iliopsoas
2. Psoas major
3. Iliacus
4. Int. obturator
5. Ext. obturator (not shown in horse)
6. Gluteal
7. Biceps femoris
8. Tensor fasciae latae
9. Caud. crural abductor (carnivores)
10. Semitendinosus
11. Gracilis
12. Pectineus
13. Sartorius
14. Quadriceps femoris
   14a. Rectus femoris
   14c. Vastus medialis
15. Adductor
16. Semimembranosus

a. Symphyseal tendon
b. Rectus abdominis
c. Int. abdominal oblique
d. Levator ani
e. Coccygeus
f. Broad sacrotuberous lig.

Fig. IV-61 - Ox - Thigh, deep dissection - med. view

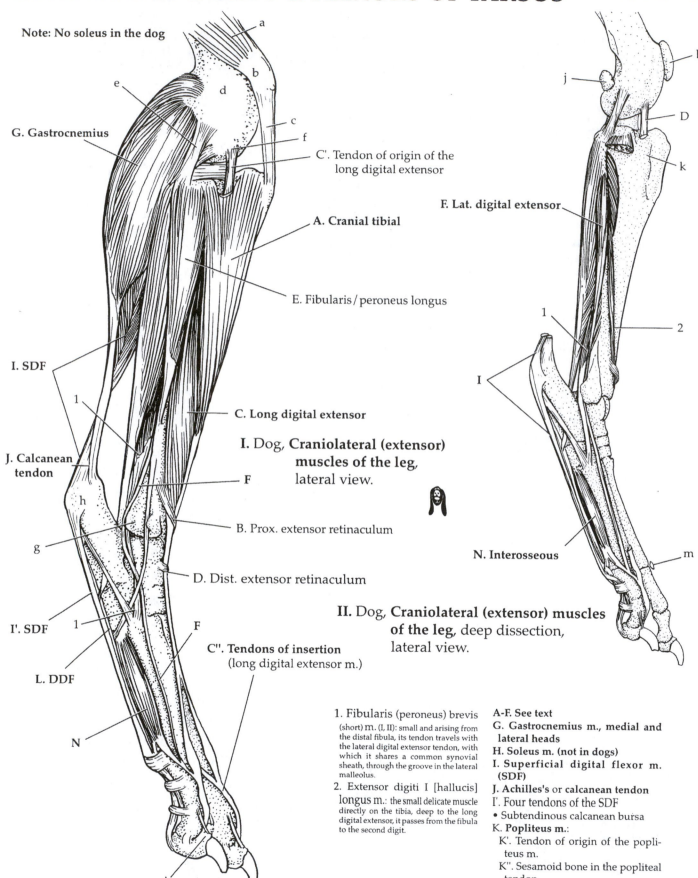

Note: No soleus in the dog

G. Gastrocnemius

C'. Tendon of origin of the long digital extensor

A. Cranial tibial

E. Fibularis / peroneus longus

F. Lat. digital extensor

I. SDF

C. Long digital extensor

I. Dog, **Craniolateral (extensor) muscles of the leg,** lateral view.

J. Calcanean tendon

F

B. Prox. extensor retinaculum

D. Dist. extensor retinaculum

II. Dog, **Craniolateral (extensor) muscles of the leg,** deep dissection, lateral view.

I'. SDF

F

L. DDF

C". Tendons of insertion (long digital extensor m.)

N

N. Interosseous

1. Fibularis (peroneus) brevis (short) m. (I, II): small and arising from the distal fibula, its tendon travels with the lateral digital extensor tendon, with which it shares a common synovial sheath, through the groove in the lateral malleolus.

2. Extensor digiti I [hallucis] longus m.: the small delicate muscle directly on the tibia, deep to the long digital extensor, it passes from the fibula to the second digit.

A-F. See text
G. **Gastrocnemius m., medial and lateral heads**
H. **Soleus m. (not in dogs)**
I. **Superficial digital flexor m. (SDF)**
J. **Achilles's** or **calcanean tendon**
I'. Four tendons of the SDF
• Subtendinous calcanean bursa
K. **Popliteus m.:**
  K'. Tendon of origin of the popliteus m.
  K". Sesamoid bone in the popliteal tendon
L. **Deep digital flexor m. (DDF)**
M. Flexor retinaculum (see next pages)
N. **Interosseous m.**

III. Cat Craniolateral (extensor) muscles of the leg, lateral view.

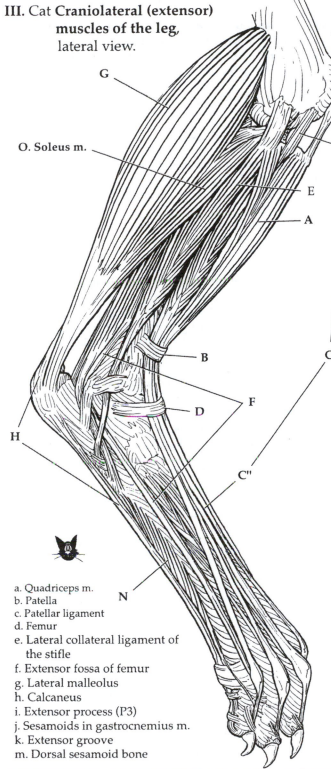

a. Quadriceps m.
b. Patella
c. Patellar ligament
d. Femur
e. Lateral collateral ligament of the stifle
f. Extensor fossa of femur
g. Lateral malleolus
h. Calcaneus
i. Extensor process (P3)
j. Sesamoids in gastrocnemius m.
k. Extensor groove
m. Dorsal sesamoid bone

MUSCLES OF THE CRUS: muscles covering the craniolateral and caudal surfaces of the leg (between the stifle and hock). The craniolateral group of muscles <u>extends</u> the digits and <u>flexes</u> the tarsus and are innervated by the common peroneal (fibular) nerve. This is different from the similarly-placed craniolateral group of the forelimb which extends the digits and the next most proximal joint, the carpus. The caudal group of muscles in the hindlimb <u>flexes</u> the digits and <u>extends</u> the tarsus. The caudal group in the forelimb flexes the digits and the next proximal joint, the tarsus.

A. Cranial tibial m. (I, III): the most cranial of the craniolateral mm., it is also superficial. Contraction results in flexion of the tarsus and supination of the pes. Note: there is no effect on the digits.

B. Proximal extensor retinaculum (crural extensor retinaculum) **(I, III):** a thickening of the crural fascia holding the tendons of the long digital and cranial tibial mm. down to the distal tibia.

C. Long digital extensor m. (I, III): deep to the cranial tibial m., it extends to the digits to flex the tarsus and extend the digits. The **tendon of origin of the long digital extensor m. (C')** arises from the extensor fossa of the femur and crosses the stifle to pierce the cranial tibial m. The four **tendons of insertion of the long digital extensor (C")** continue to the weight-bearing digits to insert on the extensor process of each distal phalanx.

D. Distal extensor retinaculum (tarsal extensor retinaculum) **(I, III):** a thickening of the crural fascia dorsal to the tarsus.

E. Fibularis / peroneus longus m. **(I, III):** the short triangular muscle just caudal to the proximal end of the cranial tibial m.

F. Lateral digital extensor m. (I, III): the thin, weak muscle arising from the fibula between the peroneus longus and the deep digital flexor mm. Its thin tendon passes through the caudal groove on the lateral malleolus to insert on the fifth digit. It extends and abducts digit five.

SPECIES DIFFERENCES:

• **Long digital extensor tendon:** one to each digit (therefore horse has only one), as in the common digital extensor in the front limb.

• **Peroneus longus m.:** absent in the horse.

• **Peroneus tertius m.:** absent in carnivores, fleshy in the ox, and entirely tendinous in the horse where it passively flexes the tarsal joint whenever the stifle joint is flexed (part of the reciprocal apparatus). The cranial tibial muscle passes through the peroneus tertius at the tarsus.

• **Lateral digital extensor** insertions: **carnivores** – digit V; **ox** – digit IV; **pig** - digit IV and V and **horse** – unites with the long digital extensor m.

(For cunean tendon, cunean bursa, reciprocal apparatus see page 194.)

DIGITAL EXTENSOR & TARSAL FLEXORS				
MUSCLE	ORIGIN	INSERTION	ACTION	NERVE
Cranial tibial	Proximal tibia	Mt 1 & 2 (plantar side)	**Flex tarsus, supinate paw**	**Fibular/peroneal n.**
Long digital extensor	Extensor fossa (femur)	Extensor process (P3, digits 2-5)	**Extend digits, flex tarsus**	"
Peroneus longus	Prox. tibia & fibula	4th tarsal bone, plantar metatarsals.	Flex tarsus, rotate paw medially	"
Lat. digital extensor	Fibula	Extensor process P3, digit 5	Extend & abduct digit 5	"
Peroneus brevis	Dist. tibia & fibula	Mt 5	Flex tarsus	"
Extensor digiti 1 [hallicus] longus	Fibula	Metatarsophalangeal joint 2, hallus (digit 1) if present	Extend digit 2 & possibly 1	"

CAUDAL CRURAL MUSCLES: extend the tarsus and flex the digits. They are innervated by the tibial nerve.

22. Gastrocnemius (gas'trok-NEE-mee-us): the large, two-bellied muscle arising from the distocaudal surface of the femur. Its heads enclose the proximal end of the superficial digital flexor. Distally, it inserts on the calcanean tuberosity as part of the calcanean tendon. It extends the tarsal joint and flexes the stifle joint.

Soleus (Fig. IV-64, g): an insignificant muscle, except in the pig and man. It is absent in the dog, but present in the cat. It arises from the fibula and joins the lateral head of the gastrocnemius muscle. The two heads of the gastrocnemius and the soleus are collectively called the triceps surae.

23. Deep digital flexor: a large muscle composed of two or three muscle bellies (species dependent) extending from the caudal surface of the tibia and fibula to the distal phalanx. It flexes the digits and extends the tarsus.

24. Superficial digital flexor: arises from the caudal aspect of the distal femur, deep to the heads of the gastrocnemius muscle. Extending distally, its tendon wraps medially around the gastrocnemius tendon and attaches superficially to the calcanean tuberosity. It then continues on the plantar aspect of the limb to the middle phalange to flexe the digits and extend the tarsus.

25. Interosseous (interossei) (suspensory ligament in the horse): similar to the muscle in the front limb.

• **Calcanean tendon, Achilles' tendon**: tendon of insertion of triceps surae (gastrocnemius & soleus) onto the calcaneus.

• **Calcanean tendon (common)**: the tendon formed by the triceps surae (gastrocnemius and soleus) plus the superficial digital flexor muscles and slips from other muscles (biceps femoris, semitendinosus; and, in the carnivores, the gracilis).

• **Calcanean bursa**: an extensive bursa lying between the superficial digital flexor tendon and the calcanean tuberosity.

SPECIES DIFFERENCES

Long digital extensor tendon (s) of insertion (20): one in the horse; one to each digit in the other species; the same is true of the common digital extensor in the thoracic limb.

Fabellae: sesamoid bones embedded in the tendons of origin of both heads of the gastrocnemius muscle of the **carnivore**.

Accessory ("check") ligament of deep digital flexor: a tendinous slip connecting the tendon of the deep digital flexor to the Mt III in the **horse**. Part of the stay apparatus (pg. 196), it takes tension off the fleshy part of the deep digital flexor tendon. There is not a check ligament of the superficial digital flexor as in the thoracic limb because of the attachment to the calcaneus.

Deep and **superficial digital flexors** (23, 24): have the same distribution as in the thoracic limb of the different species.

Cat – superficial digital flexor: between the calcaneus and digits it has a muscular part (short digital flexor muscle.)

MUSCLE	ORIGINS	INSERTION	ACTION	NERVE
Gastrocnemius	Distocaud. surface of femur	Calcanean tuberosity	Extend tarsus & flex stifle	Tibial
Popliteus	Dist. end of femur	Prox. tibia	Flex stifle	Tibial
Deep digital flexor	Tibia & fibula	Dist. phalanges		Tibial
Supf. digital flexor	Femur	Calcanean tuberosity & middle phalanges	Flex stifle & digits, extend tarsus	Tibial
Interosseous	Prox. metatarsal, med. metacarpals	Prox. sesamoid & digital extensor tendon		Tibial
Soleus (absent in dogs)	Head of fibula (femur in pigs)	Tendon of lat. head of gastrocnemius	Extends tarsus	Tibial

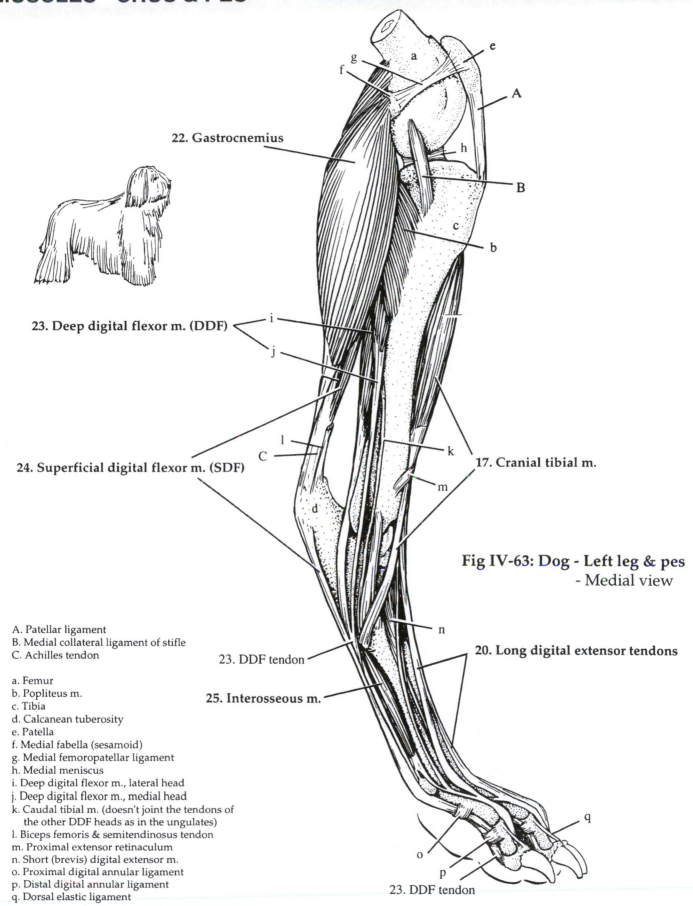

22. Gastrocnemius

23. Deep digital flexor m. (DDF)

24. Superficial digital flexor m. (SDF)

17. Cranial tibial m.

Fig IV-63: Dog - Left leg & pes
- Medial view

20. Long digital extensor tendons

23. DDF tendon

25. Interosseous m.

23. DDF tendon

A. Patellar ligament
B. Medial collateral ligament of stifle
C. Achilles tendon

a. Femur
b. Popliteus m.
c. Tibia
d. Calcanean tuberosity
e. Patella
f. Medial fabella (sesamoid)
g. Medial femoropatellar ligament
h. Medial meniscus
i. Deep digital flexor m., lateral head
j. Deep digital flexor m., medial head
k. Caudal tibial m. (doesn't joint the tendons of
   the other DDF heads as in the ungulates)
l. Biceps femoris & semitendinosus tendon
m. Proximal extensor retinaculum
n. Short (brevis) digital extensor m.
o. Proximal digital annular ligament
p. Distal digital annular ligament
q. Dorsal elastic ligament

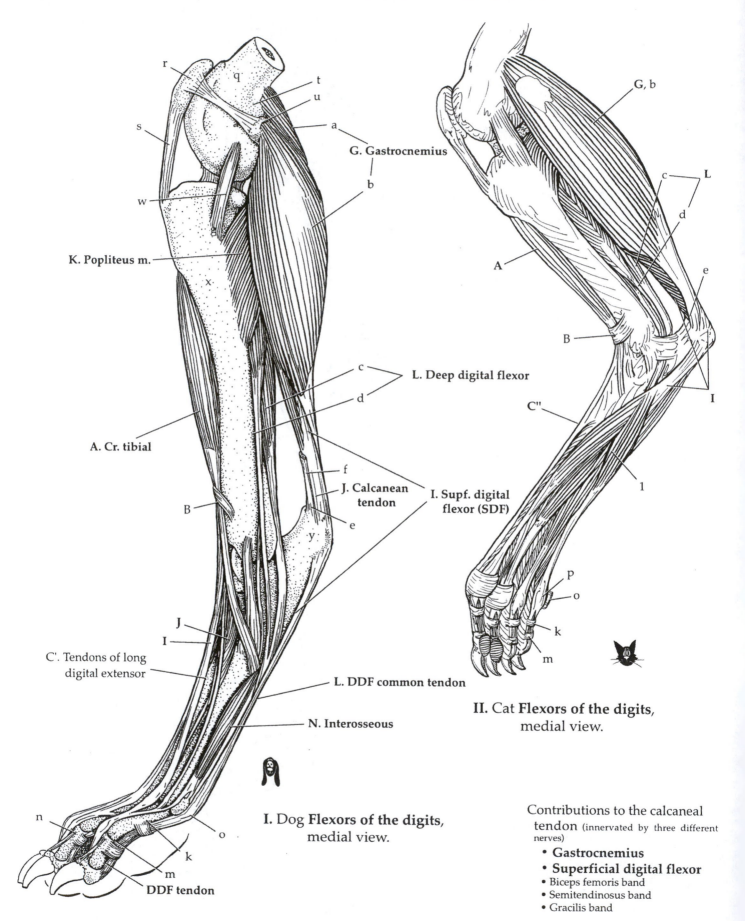

G. Gastrocnemius

K. Popliteus m.

L. Deep digital flexor

A. Cr. tibial

J. Calcanean tendon

I. Supf. digital flexor (SDF)

C'. Tendons of long digital extensor

L. DDF common tendon

N. Interosseous

DDF tendon

I. Dog Flexors of the digits, medial view.

II. Cat Flexors of the digits, medial view.

G, b

L

C"

Contributions to the calcaneal tendon (innervated by three different nerves)
- **Gastrocnemius**
- **Superficial digital flexor**
- Biceps femoris band
- Semitendinosus band
- Gracilis band

CAUDAL CRURAL MUSCLES: extend the tarsus and flex the digits. They are innervated by the tibial nerve.

G. Gastrocnemius m., medial and lateral heads (gas'trok-NEE-mee-us)(**I, II**): the large, two-headed muscle forming the bulk of the caudal crus (the calf muscle in humans). Distally, it inserts on the calcanean tuberosity as part of the calcanean tendon. It extends the tarsal joint and flexes the stifle joint.

H. Soleus m. (see 189 III): not present in the dog, but present in the other domestic species and well developed in the cat. It passes from the fibula to join the tendon on the lateral head of the gastrocnemius. The two heads of the gastrocnemius and the soleus are collectively called the triceps surae.

I. Superficial digital flexor m. (SDF)(I, II): runs deep to the two heads of the gastrocnemius. Distally its belly can be seen on the lateral side, beneath the gastrocnemius m. It switches from deep to superficial by passing medially around the gastrocnemius tendon to reach and cap (attach to) the calcaneus before continuing distally on the plantar aspect of the pes to the digits. The four tendons of the SDF: attach on the middle phalanx of the weight bearing digits (2-5).

J. Achilles or **calcanean tendon (I, II)**: the large connective tissue structure attaching to the calcaneus, it is primarily formed by the SDF and the gastrocnemius mm. The soleus m., in all but the dog, and strands/slips from the biceps femoris, semitendinosus and, in the carnivores, the gracilis mm. also contribute to its formation.

• Subtendinous calcanean bursa: an extensive bursa lying between the SDF and the calcanean tuberosity.

SPECIES DIFFERENCES:

• Long digital extensor tendon(s) of insertion: one in the horse; one to each digit in the other species; the same as the common digital extensor in the thoracic limb.

• Sesamoid bone (fabella): in the origin of each head of the gastrocnemius m. in carnivores that articulates with the condyles of the femur.

• Accessory ("check") ligament of deep digital flexor m.: a tendinous slip connecting the tendon of the deep digital flexor to Mt III in the horse. Part of the stay apparatus (pg. 196), it takes tension off the fleshy part of the deep digital flexor tendon. There is not a check ligament of the superficial digital flexor as in the thoracic limb because of the SDF attachment to the calcaneus.

• Deep and superficial digital flexors: have the same distribution as in the thoracic limb of the different species.

SPECIES DIFFERENCES:

• **"Cunean tendon"**: the common name for the horse's medial insertion of the cranial tibial m..

• **Cunean bursa**: associated with the medial insertion of the cranial tibial muscle in the horse.

• **Reciprocal apparatus in the horse**: consists of two tendinous cords, the superficial digital flexor on the caudal aspect of the crus, and the peroneus tertius muscle on the cranial aspect. Flexion or extension of the stifle or tarsus causes a similar (reciprocal) movement in the other joint due to these two cords.

CLINICAL:

Capped hock or **subcutaneous calcanean bursa**: an acquired bursa between the skin and the superficial digital flexor tendon due to trauma to the area.

MUSCLE	ORIGIN	INSERTION	ACTION	NERVE
Gastrocnemius	Dist. femur (med. & lat. supracondylar tuberosities)	Calcaneus	**Extend hock**	**Tibial n.**
Soleus	Head of fibula	Gastrocnemius (lat.)	Assist gastrocnemius	"
SDF	Caudodist. femur (lat. supracondylar tuberosity)	Calcaneus, P2	**Flex digits**	**Tibial n.**

A. Cranial tibial m.
B. Proximal extensor retinaculum
C. **Long digital extensor m.**
  C". Four tendons of insertion of long digital extensor
D. Distal extensor retinaculum
E. **Fibularis/peroneus longus** m.
F. **Lateral digital extensor m.**
G-I. See text
K. **Popliteus m.**
L. **Deep digital flexor m. (DDF)**
M. Flexor retinaculum (see next pages)
N. Ineroseeous m.

1. Short digital flexor (cat)(II): the muscular part of the superficial digital flexor between the calcaneus and the digits.
2. Quadratus plantae m.
3. Interflexoria m.
4. Lumbricales m.

a. Lateral head of the gastrocnemius m.
b. Medial head of the gastrocnemius m.
c. Lateral head (DDF)
d. Medial head (DDF)
e. Location of subtendinous calcanean bursa
f. Tendon strands from biceps femoris, semitendinosus and gracilis mm. to calcanean tendon
g. Caudal tibial m.: in carnivores doesn't join the tendon of the other DDF heads as it does in ungulates (hoofed animals)
h. Metatarsal bone
i. Short digital extensor m.
k. Proximal digital annular ligament
m. Distal digital annular ligament

n. Dorsal elastic ligament
o. Palmar annular ligament
p. Manica flexoria
q. Femur
r. Patella
s. Patellar ligament
t. Medial femoropatellar ligament
u. Medial sesamoid (fabella)
v. Medial meniscus
w. Medial collateral ligament
x. Tibia
y. Calcaneus

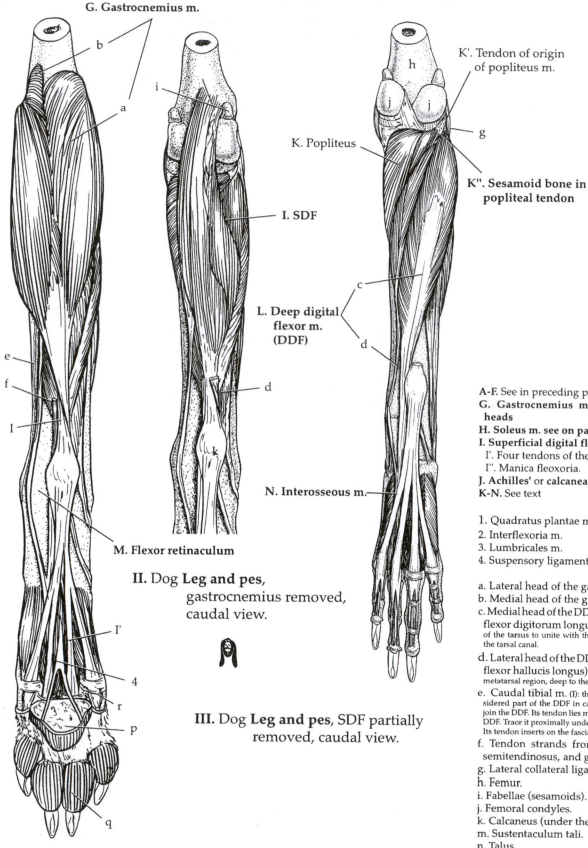

G. Gastrocnemius m.

b

a

i

K'. Tendon of origin
of popliteus m.

h

K. Popliteus

g

K". Sesamoid bone in
popliteal tendon

I. SDF

e

f

I

c

L. Deep digital
flexor m.
(DDF)

d

d

M. Flexor retinaculum

N. Interosseous m.

I'

4

r

p

q

II. Dog Leg and pes,
gastrocnemius removed,
caudal view.

III. Dog Leg and pes, SDF partially
removed, caudal view.

I. Dog Leg and pes, caudal view.

A-F. See in preceding pages.
**G. Gastrocnemius m., medial and lateral
heads**
H. Soleus m. see on page 189
I. Superficial digital flexor m. (SDF)
  I'. Four tendons of the SDF.
  I". Manica fleoxoria.
J. Achilles' or calcanean tendon.
K-N. See text

1. Quadratus plantae m.
2. Interflexoria m.
3. Lumbricales m.
4. Suspensory ligament of metatarsal pad.

a. Lateral head of the gastrocnemius m.
b. Medial head of the gastrocnemius m.
c. Medial head of the DDF (medial digital flexor,
  flexor digitorum longus) m.: crosses the medial side
  of the tarsus to unite with the tendon of the DDF distal to
  the tarsal canal.
d. Lateral head of the DDF (lateral digital flexor,
  flexor hallucis longus) m.: the bulk of the DDF in the
  metatarsal region, deep to the SDF tendon.
e. Caudal tibial m. (I): the small muscle that is not considered part of the DDF in carnivores as its tendon doesn't
  join the DDF. Its tendon lies medial to the medial head of the
  DDF. Trace it proximally under this muscle to its small body.
  Its tendon inserts on the fascia near the tarsus.
f. Tendon strands from the biceps femoris,
  semitendinosus, and gracilis mm.
g. Lateral collateral ligament.
h. Femur.
i. Fabellae (sesamoids).
j. Femoral condyles.
k. Calcaneus (under the SDF).
m. Sustentaculum tali.
n. Talus.
o. Manica flexoria.
p. Metatarsal pad.
q. Digital pad.
r. Palmar annular ligament.

K. Popliteus m.: the triangular muscle deep to the SDF and gastrocnemius mm.; it lies caudally on the proximal tibia.

K'. Tendon of origin of the popliteus m.: arises from the lateral condyle and separates the lateral collateral ligament from the lateral meniscus. This is not the case on the medial side where the medial collateral ligament is attached to the medial meniscus.

K". **Sesamoid bone in the popliteal tendon**: articulates with lateral condyle of the tibia (present in the majority of dogs > 80%).

L. **Deep digital flexor m. (DDF)**: the large muscle on the caudal aspect of the tibia. Its main tendon passes through the tarsal groove, over the sustentaculum tali, and on to split into four tendons to the distal phalanges of the main digits (2-5).

M. **Flexor retinaculum**: a thickening of the tarsal fascia that, with the calcaneus and sustentaculum tali, holds the main tendon of the DDF in the tarsal groove.

N. **Interosseous** (interossei) (suspensory ligament in the horse): similar to the muscle (s) in the front limb.

O. **Tarsal groove**: the passage on the plantar surface of the tarsus over the sustentaculum tali which holds the tendon of the lateral head of the DDF.

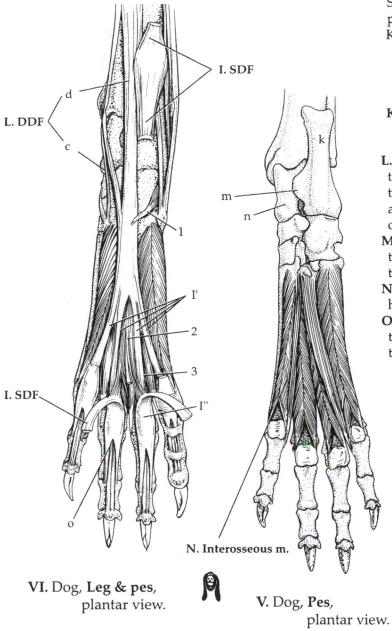

VI. Dog, **Leg & pes**, plantar view.

V. Dog, **Pes**, plantar view.

N. Interosseous m.

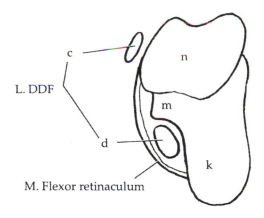

VI. Tarsal groove, schematic.

M. Flexor retinaculum

MUSCLE	ORIGIN	INSERTION	ACTION	NERVE
Popliteus	Lateral condyle (femur)	Proximocaudal tibia	Controversy if flex or extend stifle, medial rotate leg.	Tibial n.
DDF	Caudoprox. tibia & fibula	**Distal phalanges** (P3)	**Flex digits, extend hock.**	Tibial n.
Lateral head (flexor hallucis longus)				
Med. head (flexor digitorum longus)				
Interosseous (suspensory lig. [eq])	Prox. Metacarpal (s)	Prox. **sesamoid bones**	Flex metatarsophalangeal joint, supports the fetlock.	Tibial n.

MUSCLES - CRUS

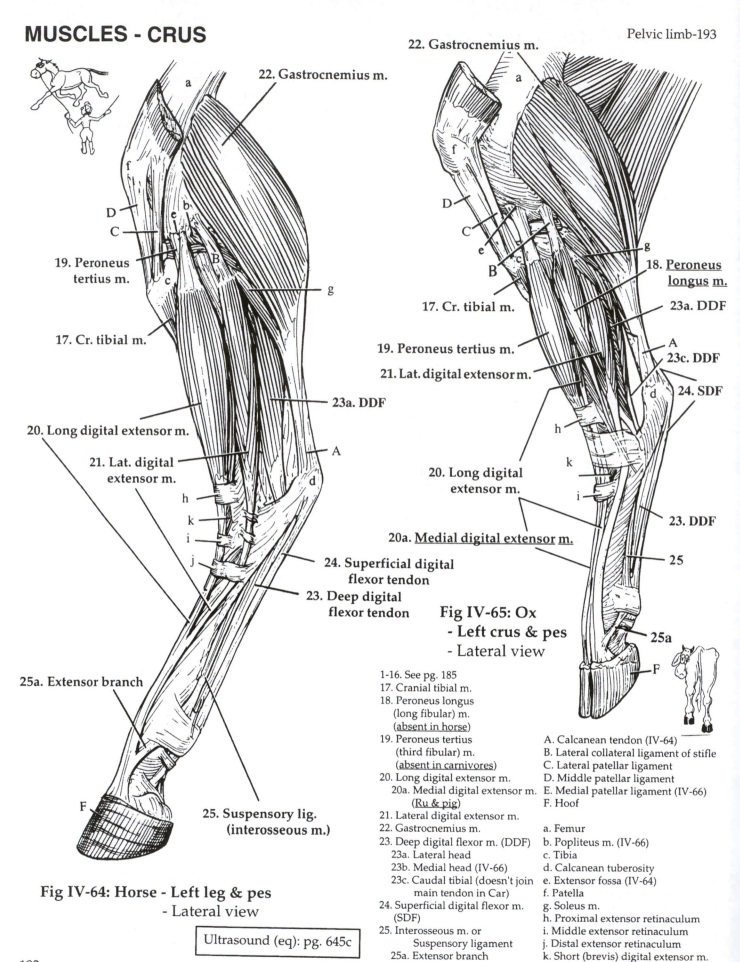

22. Gastrocnemius m.

D

C

19. Peroneus tertius m.

17. Cr. tibial m.

20. Long digital extensor m.

21. Lat. digital extensor m.

h

k

i

j

23a. DDF

A

d

24. Superficial digital flexor tendon

23. Deep digital flexor tendon

25a. Extensor branch

F

25. Suspensory lig. (interosseous m.)

Fig IV-64: Horse - Left leg & pes
- Lateral view

Ultrasound (eq): pg. 645c

22. Gastrocnemius m.

D

C

B

17. Cr. tibial m.

19. Peroneus tertius m.

21. Lat. digital extensor m.

20. Long digital extensor m.

20a. Medial digital extensor m.

18. Peroneus longus m.

23a. DDF

A

23c. DDF

24. SDF

d

23. DDF

25

Fig IV-65: Ox
- Left crus & pes
- Lateral view

25a

F

1-16. See pg. 185
17. Cranial tibial m.
18. Peroneus longus (long fibular) m. (absent in horse)
19. Peroneus tertius (third fibular) m. (absent in carnivores)
20. Long digital extensor m.
  20a. Medial digital extensor m. (Ru & pig)
21. Lateral digital extensor m.
22. Gastrocnemius m.
23. Deep digital flexor m. (DDF)
  23a. Lateral head
  23b. Medial head (IV-66)
  23c. Caudal tibial (doesn't join main tendon in Car)
24. Superficial digital flexor m. (SDF)
25. Interosseous m. or Suspensory ligament
  25a. Extensor branch

A. Calcanean tendon (IV-64)
B. Lateral collateral ligament of stifle
C. Lateral patellar ligament
D. Middle patellar ligament
E. Medial patellar ligament (IV-66)
F. Hoof

a. Femur
b. Popliteus m. (IV-66)
c. Tibia
d. Calcanean tuberosity
e. Extensor fossa (IV-64)
f. Patella
g. Soleus m.
h. Proximal extensor retinaculum
i. Middle extensor retinaculum
j. Distal extensor retinaculum
k. Short (brevis) digital extensor m.

Ultrasound: pg. 645c

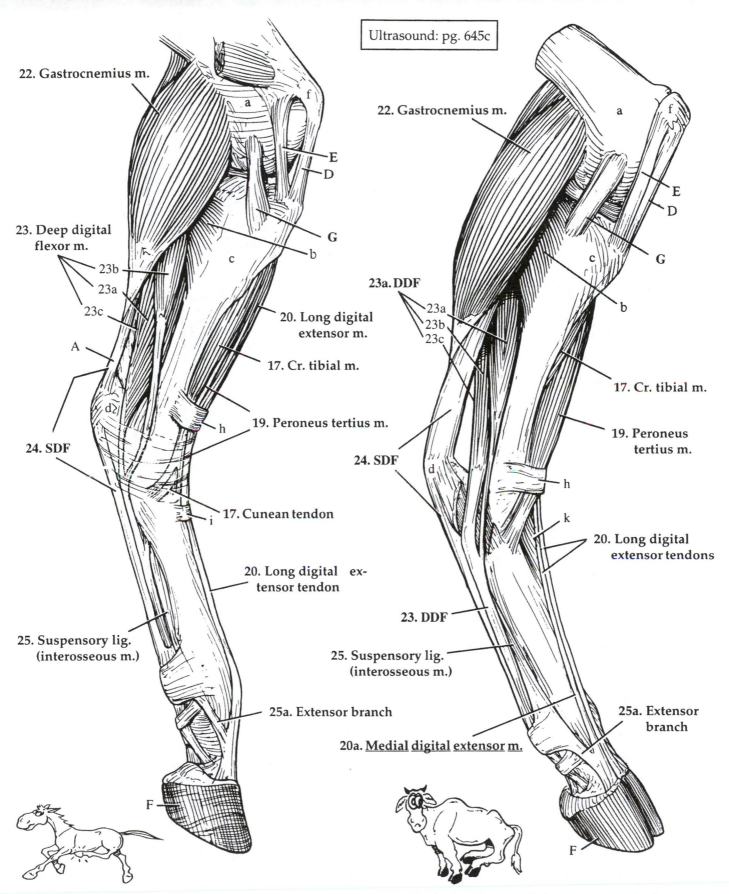

22. Gastrocnemius m.

a

f

E

D

G

b

23. Deep digital flexor m.

23b

23a

23c

c

A

d

24. SDF

h

20. Long digital extensor m.

17. Cr. tibial m.

19. Peroneus tertius m.

17. Cunean tendon

i

20. Long digital ex-tensor tendon

25. Suspensory lig. (interosseous m.)

25a. Extensor branch

F

22. Gastrocnemius m.

a

f

E

D

G

c

b

23a. DDF

23a

23b

23c

17. Cr. tibial m.

19. Peroneus tertius m.

24. SDF

d

h

k

20. Long digital extensor tendons

23. DDF

25. Suspensory lig. (interosseous m.)

25a. Extensor branch

20a. Medial digital extensor m.

F

Fig IV-66: Horse - Left crus & pes - Medial view

Fig X-67: Ox - Left leg & pes - Medial view

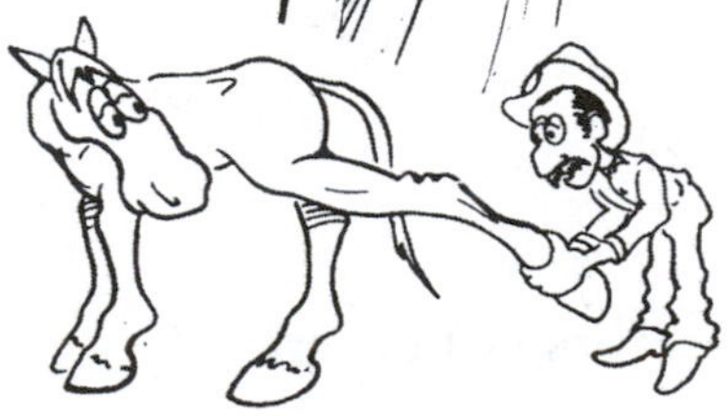

Fig. IV-68 - Horse
- Lt. hindlimb
- cran. view

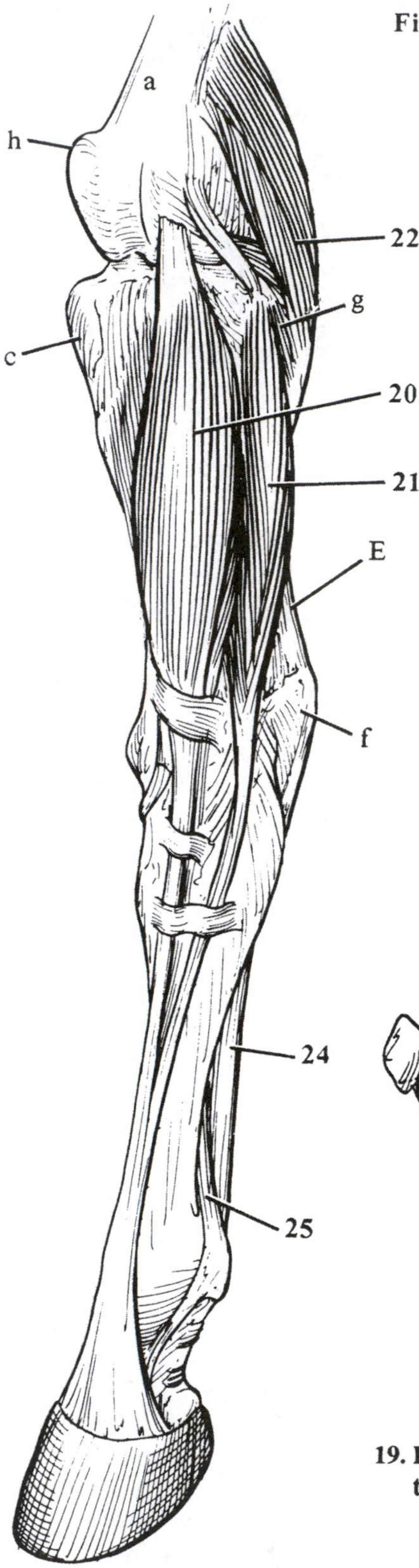
a
h
22
g
c
20. Long digital extensor
21
E
f
24
25

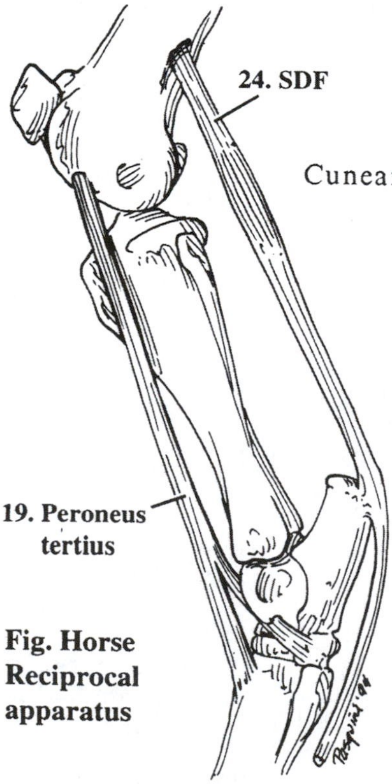
24. SDF
19. Peroneus tertius

Fig. Horse Reciprocal apparatus

Ultrasound: pg. 645c

Fig. IV-69 - Horse - Lt. hindlimb, deep dissection - cran. view

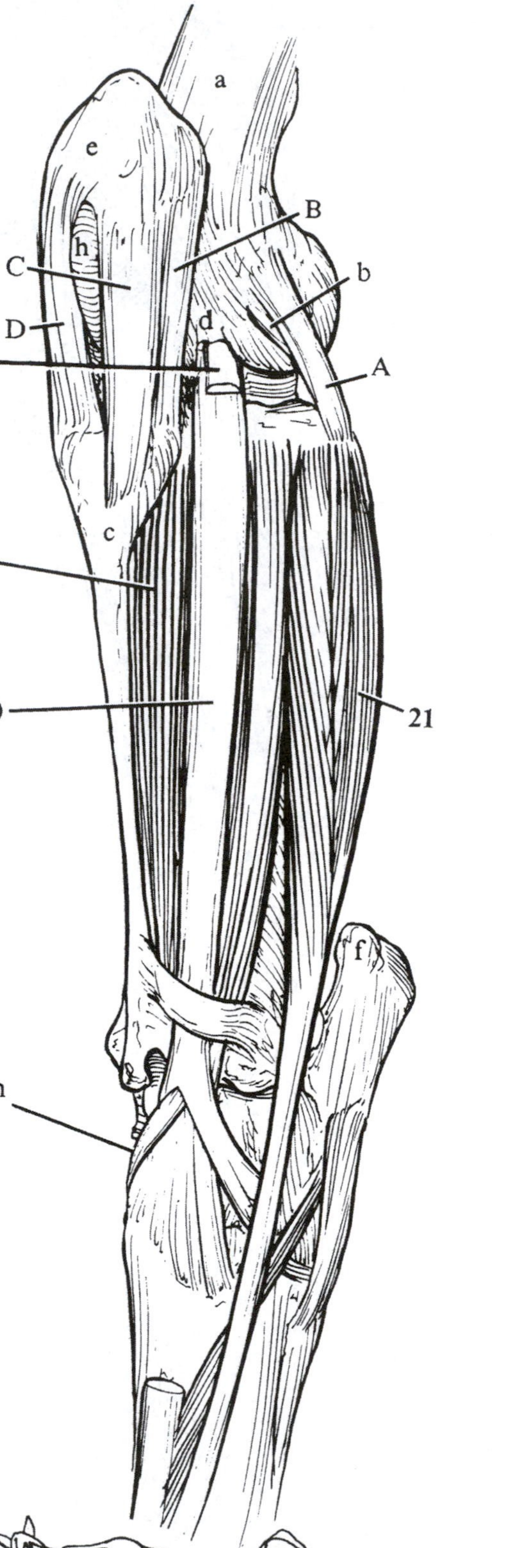
a
e
B
h
C
b
D
d
A
c
17. Cranial tibial m.
19. Peroneus tertius (3rd fibular)
21
f
Cunean tendon

Fig. IV-70 - Ox - Lt. hindlimb - cran. view

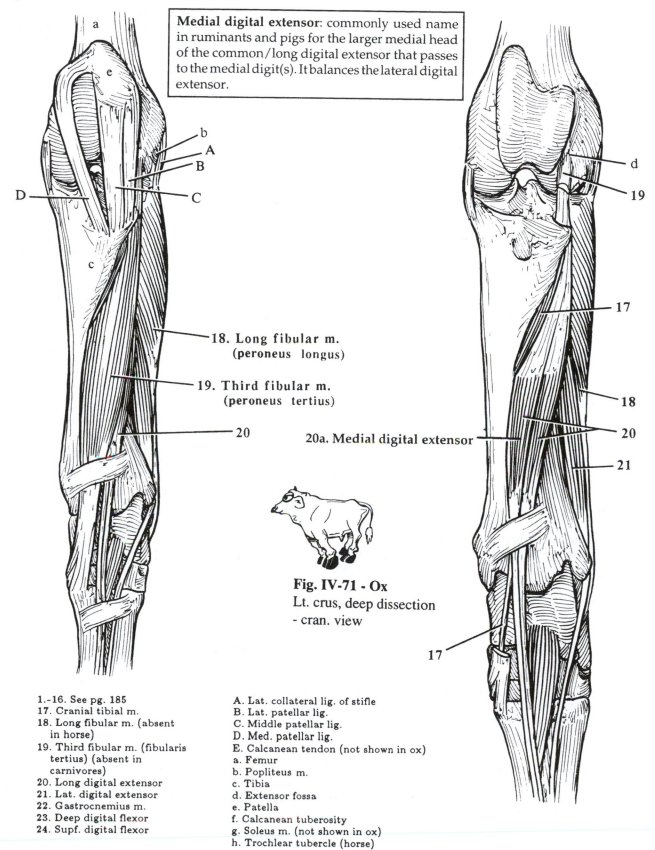

Medial digital extensor: commonly used name in ruminants and pigs for the larger medial head of the common/long digital extensor that passes to the medial digit(s). It balances the lateral digital extensor.

18. Long fibular m.
(peroneus longus)

19. Third fibular m.
(peroneus tertius)

20

20a. Medial digital extensor

Fig. IV-71 - Ox
Lt. crus, deep dissection
- cran. view

d

19

17

18

20

21

17

1.-16. See pg. 185
17. Cranial tibial m.
18. Long fibular m. (absent in horse)
19. Third fibular m. (fibularis tertius) (absent in carnivores)
20. Long digital extensor
21. Lat. digital extensor
22. Gastrocnemius m.
23. Deep digital flexor
24. Supf. digital flexor

A. Lat. collateral lig. of stifle
B. Lat. patellar lig.
C. Middle patellar lig.
D. Med. patellar lig.
E. Calcanean tendon (not shown in ox)
a. Femur
b. Popliteus m.
c. Tibia
d. Extensor fossa
e. Patella
f. Calcanean tuberosity
g. Soleus m. (not shown in ox)
h. Trochlear tubercle (horse)

The **stay apparatus** allows a horse to rest while standing with little muscular activity or fatigue. This ability allows instant action when danger threatens. The horse can then use its evolutionary speed to move away from the threat.

Mechanically, the structures of the stay apparatus bypass tension from the muscle bellies over "non-tiring" connective tissue elements, tendons and ligaments, to bones. This overcomes the tendency of the joints to collapse with minimal energy expenditure.

In the thoracic limb, the **body weight** is suspended from the two scapulae by **tendinous tissue** in the serratus ventralis muscles. The body weight pulls down on the scapula, flexing the shoulder until the **tendons** running through the **biceps brachii** stretch taut. The lacertus fibrosus (4), connecting the tendons of the biceps brachii (2) and extensor carpi radialis (5), transmits the rigidity from shoulder to carpi in an unbroken line (of force). The elbow is locked in extension by the collateral ligaments' placement behind the joint's rotational axis. The suspensory apparatus and the superficial and deep digital flexor tendons and their accessory ligaments prevent hyperextension of the fetlock and digital joints.

To understand the stay apparatus, first understand how the animal's weight would collapse each joint. Then determine what prevents this from happening at each joint. The shoulder would tend to flex, elbow – flex, carpus – flex or extend, fetlock – hyperextend, and pastern – hyperflex or buckle.

STAY APPARATUS of the THORACIC LIMB

SHOULDER FLEXION – prevented by the tendon of the biceps brachii muscle.

1. Serratus ventralis: Fibrous tissue in this muscle suspends the body from the scapulae, like a sling, when the horse is at rest. This causes the shoulder to flex.

2. Tendon of the biceps brachii: runs the entire length of the biceps brachii muscle. Flexion of the shoulder ceases when this tendon is stretched taut. The molded tendon of the biceps brachii over the intermediate tubercle plays a part in stabilizing the shoulder joint.

ELBOW FLEXION – prevented by placement of collateral ligaments behind (caudal to) the axis of the joint.

3. Collateral ligaments of the elbow: the two ligaments on either side of the elbow joint located **caudal to** the axis of rotation. Once the triceps brachii extends the elbow, an active counterforce is required to stretch the ligaments before flexion can occur. This passively maintains the elbow in extension.

CARPUS FLEXION – prevented by the combination of the tendon of the biceps brachii, the lacertus fibrosus, and the tendon of the extensor carpi radialis cranially, and by the flexor tendons and their accessory ligaments caudally.

4. Lacertus fibrosus: the tendinous band connecting the tendon of the biceps brachii muscle to the tendon of the extensor carpi radialis muscle, creating an unbroken line of force from shoulder to metacarpus. When the tendon of the biceps brachii is pulled tight, it pulls on the lacertus fibrosus, which in turn directs the tension past the fleshy part to the tendon of insertion of the extensor carpi radialis muscle.

5. Tendon of the extensor carpi radialis muscle: crosses the carpus and inserts on the proximal metacarpus. When pulled by the lacertus fibrosus, it maintains the carpus in extension.

Superficial and deep digital flexor tendons and their accessory ligaments: pull on the caudal aspect above and below the carpus to help hold it in extension.

CARPUS HYPEREXTENSION – prevented by the block shape of the carpal bones and the palmar carpal ligament.

Block shape of the carpal bones: prevents the carpal joints from hyperextension.

Palmar carpal ligament: holds the palmar aspect of the carpal bones together, preventing hyperextension of the carpal joints.

FETLOCK HYPEREXTENSION – prevented by the suspensory apparatus, the extensor branches of the suspensory ligament, and the flexor tendons and their accessory ligaments.

6,7,8. Suspensory apparatus: consists of the suspensory ligament, proximal palmar sesamoid bones, and the sesamoidean ligaments. These three subunits act as one structure, preventing hyperextension of the fetlock joint at rest. Interruption of any of these three components will result in dropping of the fetlock joint.

• **6. Suspensory ligament** (interosseous muscle): the entirely tendinous muscle extending from the proximal metacarpus to the proximal sesamoid bones. The suspensory ligament has **extensor branches** (12) crossing either side of the fetlock to join the extensor (common) tendon. This junction transfers the tension of the extensor tendon to the suspensory ligament.

• **7. Proximal palmar sesamoid bones:** located in the middle of the suspensory apparatus.

• **8. Sesamoidean ligaments:** a number of ligaments running between the sesamoid bones and the proximal and middle phalanges. These counteract the proximal pull of the suspensory ligament and stabilize the fetlock joint as part of the suspensory apparatus. They consist of "X, Y, V" ligaments: the straight (Y), oblique (V), and cruciate (X) sesamoidean ligaments.

9, 11. Superficial and **deep flexor tendons** and the common digital extensor muscle (long digital extensor muscle in the rear limb) (13): support the digital joints, and with the suspensory apparatus, support the fetlock in the resting animal.

10. Accessory ligament of the superficial digital flexor: the short tendon arising from the distal radius and joining the **tendon** of the superficial digital flexor. During rest, this ligament transfers tension in the tendon to the radius before it reaches the muscle belly. Other names for this ligament are the "radial check ligament", "superior check ligament", "proximal check ligament" or "radial head" of the superficial digital flexor muscle.

12. Accessory check ligament of the deep digital flexor: a short tendon arising from the palmar carpal ligament (the ligament covering the palmar side of the carpus) and joining the tendon of the deep digital flexor. It transfers the tension in the deep digital flexor tendon to the cannon bone before the tension reaches its muscle belly. It is also called the "distal check ligament" or "inferior check ligament".

PASTERN JOINT HYPEREXTENSION – prevented by palmar ligaments, the straight sesamoidean ligament, and the flexor tendons and their accessory ligaments.

Palmar ligaments: short ligaments on the palmar aspect of the pastern. Hyperextension is prevented when they are maximally extended.

Straight sesamoidean ligament: passes from the proximal sesamoid bones across the pastern joint to the middle phalanx.

PASTERN JOINT-"DORSAL BUCKLING" (FLEXION) – prevented by the double attachment of the superficial digital flexor tendon.

Insertion of the superficial digital flexor tendon: attaches to the distal part of the proximal phalanx as well as the proximal part of the middle phalanx. This double attachment on either side of the joint prevents flexion or "dorsal buckling" of this joint.

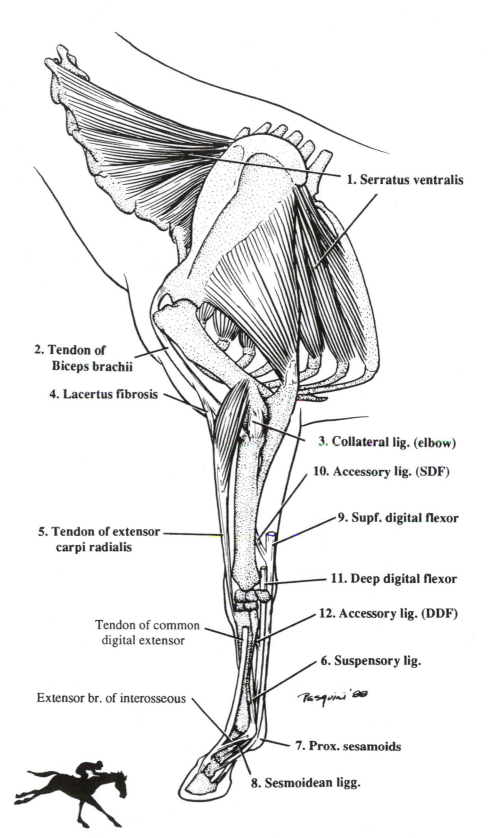

1. Serratus ventralis
2. Tendon of Biceps brachii
4. Lacertus fibrosis
3. Collateral lig. (elbow)
10. Accessory lig. (SDF)
9. Supf. digital flexor
5. Tendon of extensor carpi radialis
11. Deep digital flexor
12. Accessory lig. (DDF)
Tendon of common digital extensor
6. Suspensory lig.
Extensor br. of interosseous
7. Prox. sesamoids
8. Sesmoidean ligg.

Pasquini '88

Fig. IV-72 - Horse - Stay apparatus of thoracic limb (schematic)

STAY APPARATUS

In the pelvic limb, the **stifle** is stabilized by locking of the patella over the trochlear tubercle of the femur. This patellar lock also indirectly stabilizes the **hip joint**. The **tarsus** is held in extension by the connection of the tendinous superficial digital flexor to the femur and calcanean tuberosity. The **digits** are supported by structures similar to those of the thoracic limb.

STIFLE FLEXION – prevented by the "patellar lock".

Patellar lock: a mechanism that passively immobilizes the stifle joint. Extension of the stifle and contraction of lateral muscles cause the patella (A) and medial patellar tendon to move over the trochlear tubercle (medial ridge of the patellar surface) (B) of the femur. The trochlear tubercle projects between the medial (C) and intermediate (middle) patellar ligaments (D). The weight of the animal then flexes the stifle until the medial patellar tendon is stretched to its limit. This locks the patella over the trochlear tubercle, and immobilizes the stifle. The patellar lock can be accomplished only in one limb at a time. The horse must unlock the rested limb, shift its weight to the opposite tiring limb, and lock the patella.

HIP FLEXION – prevented by the "patellar lock".

Once the patella is locked, the weight of the animal flexes the hip and stifle joints until the medial patellar ligament stops these actions. Thus, the stifle and hip joints are stabilized.

TARSUS FLEXION – prevented by the superficial digital flexor.

Superficial digital flexor (5): Largely tendinous, its proximal part is a **fibrous band** (3) connected between the distal end of the femur and the calcanean tuberosity. With the patella "locked", the fibrous band is pulled taut by flexion of the tarsus, keeping the tarsus in extension.

The **digital joints** are stabilized by similar structures to those in the forelimb. The attachments of the superficial digital flexor to the calcaneus eliminates the need for an accessory ligament.

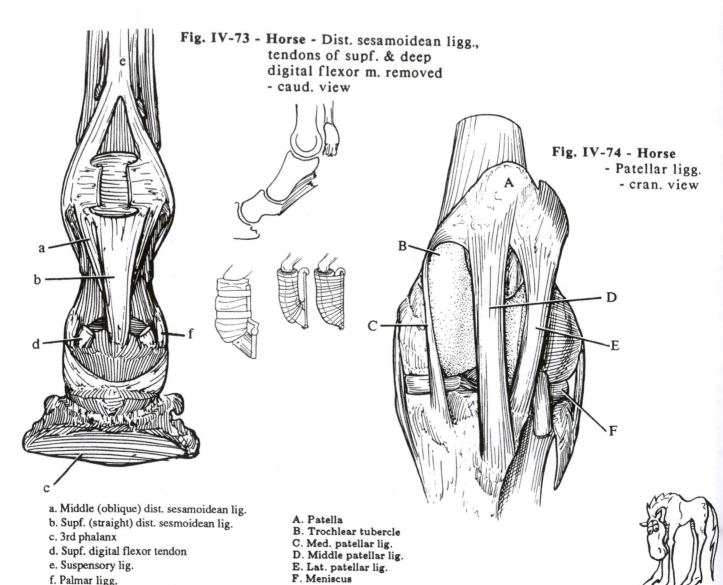

Fig. IV-73 - Horse - Dist. sesamoidean ligg., tendons of supf. & deep digital flexor m. removed - caud. view

Fig. IV-74 - Horse - Patellar ligg. - cran. view

a. Middle (oblique) dist. sesamoidean lig.
b. Supf. (straight) dist. sesmoidean lig.
c. 3rd phalanx
d. Supf. digital flexor tendon
e. Suspensory lig.
f. Palmar ligg.

A. Patella
B. Trochlear tubercle
C. Med. patellar lig.
D. Middle patellar lig.
E. Lat. patellar lig.
F. Meniscus

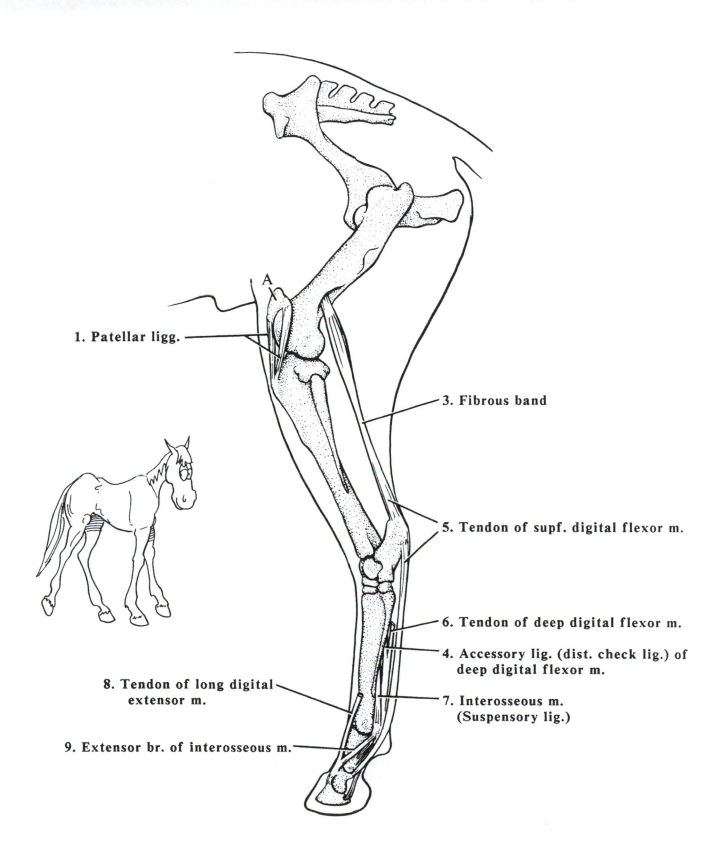

1. Patellar ligg.

3. Fibrous band

5. Tendon of supf. digital flexor m.

6. Tendon of deep digital flexor m.

4. Accessory lig. (dist. check lig.) of deep digital flexor m.

8. Tendon of long digital extensor m.

7. Interosseous m. (Suspensory lig.)

9. Extensor br. of interosseous m.

Fig. IV-75 - Horse - Stay apparatus of the pelvic limb (schematic)

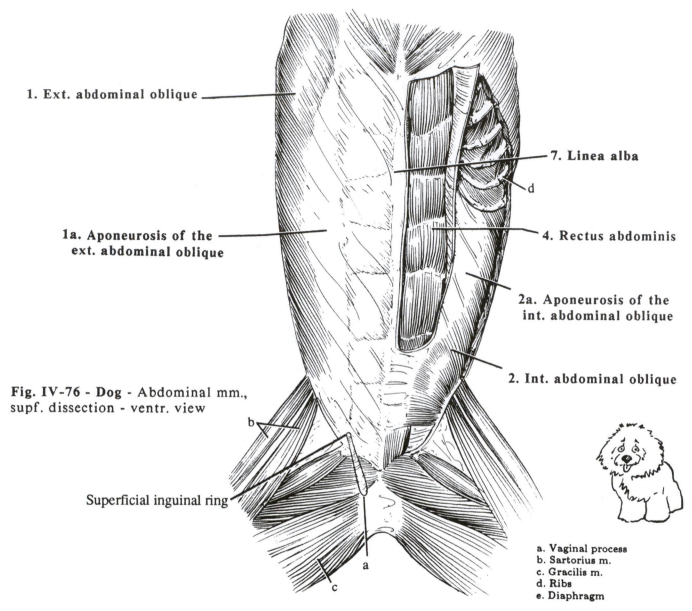

1. Ext. abdominal oblique

7. Linea alba

d

1a. Aponeurosis of the ext. abdominal oblique

4. Rectus abdominis

2a. Aponeurosis of the int. abdominal oblique

2. Int. abdominal oblique

Fig. IV-76 - Dog - Abdominal mm., supf. dissection - ventr. view

b

Superficial inguinal ring

a

c

a. Vaginal process
b. Sartorius m.
c. Gracilis m.
d. Ribs
e. Diaphragm

Abdominal muscles: four muscles forming the ventrolateral abdominal wall. Three are flat muscles (external abdominal oblique, internal abdominal oblique, and transversus abdominis) ending in aponeurotic tendons inserting on the linea alba (white line). These aponeurotic tendons form a sheath around the fourth strap-like muscle, the rectus abdominis. All are innervated by ventral branches of the caudal intercostal and lumbar nerves.

1. External abdominal oblique: the sheet-like muscle extending from the ribs and thoracolumbar fascia obliquely, <u>caudoventrally</u> to the ventral midline (linea alba), by a wide aponeurosis (ap'oh-nyoo-ROH-sis) (1a).

Inguinal ligament: the caudal free edge of the aponeurosis of the external abdominal oblique that extends from the tuber coxae around the iliopsoas muscle to the prepubic tendon.

2. Internal abdominal oblique: the sheet-like layer deep to the external abdominal oblique muscle, arising from the tuber coxae and thoracolumbar fascia. Most of its fibers pass obliquely cranioventrally, crossing the fibers of the external abdominal oblique muscle at approximately right angles. It inserts on the last rib and the linea alba by an aponeurosis (2a).

Cremaster muscle (male): the caudal slip of the internal abdominal oblique muscle. It passes, along with the spermatic cord, out the inguinal canal (pg. 202) and attaches to the vaginal tunic around the spermatic cord and testicle.

3. Transversus abdominis (trans-VERS-us ab-DOM-i-nus): the deepest abdominal muscle; arising from the costal arch, ribs, and by an aponeurosis, from the thoracolumbar fascia. Its muscle fibers run transversely (dorsoventrally). It terminates in an aponeurosis (3a) on the linea alba. Its muscular part **does not** extend

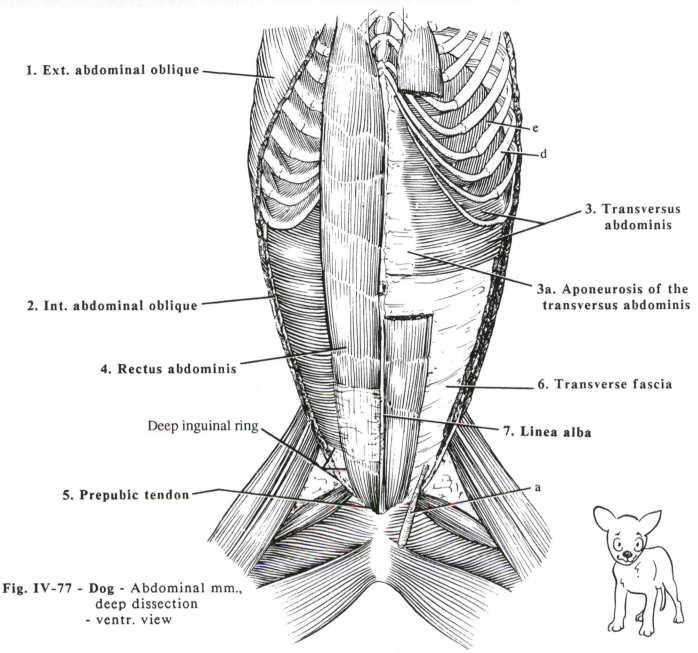

1. Ext. abdominal oblique

e

d

3. Transversus abdominis

3a. Aponeurosis of the transversus abdominis

2. Int. abdominal oblique

4. Rectus abdominis

6. Transverse fascia

Deep inguinal ring

7. Linea alba

5. Prepubic tendon

a

Fig. IV-77 - Dog - Abdominal mm., deep dissection - ventr. view

caudally to the inguinal ring.

4. Rectus abdominis (REK-tus): the two long, straight muscles extending from the sternum along the ventral abdomen on either side of the linea alba to the prepubic tendon (5). The aponeuroses of the other abdominal muscles ensheath the rectus abdominis on both its dorsal and ventral surfaces (external and internal rectus sheaths).

SPECIAL:

5. Prepubic tendon: the tendinous connective tissue mass across the cranial side of the pubic bones serving as the insertion of the rectus abdominis muscles.

6. Transversalis fascia (Fig. IV-83): covers the inner surface of

the transversus abdominis and the rectus abdominis muscles. It extends beyond the caudal edge of the transversus abdominis muscle to form the medial wall of the inguinal canal.

7. Linea alba: the fibrous cord formed by the joining of the aponeuroses of the abdominal muscles from both sides. It is on the ventral midline, extending from the xiphoid cartilage to the pelvic symphysis.

CLINICAL

8. Rectus sheath: formed by the aponeuroses of the flat abdominal muscles as they pass on either side of the rectus abdominis muscle. Clinically the **external rectus sheath**, because of its connective tissue, is the holding layer when closing the abdomen after surgery.

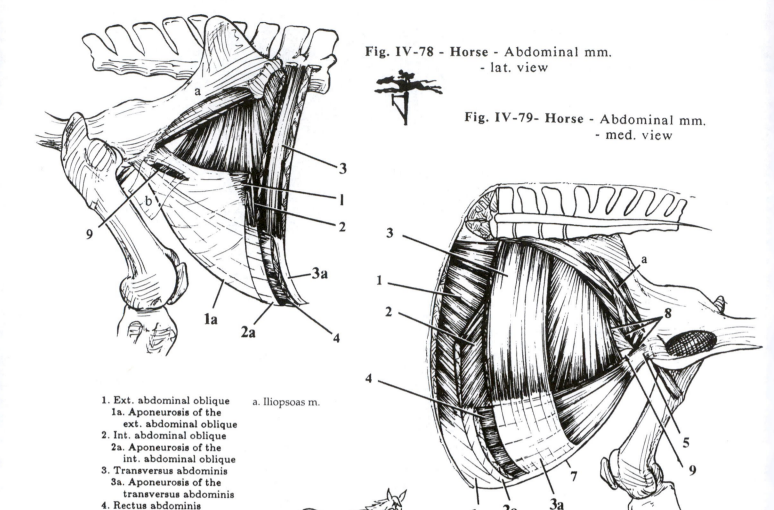

Fig. IV-78 - Horse - Abdominal mm.
- lat. view

Fig. IV-79- Horse - Abdominal mm.
- med. view

1. Ext. abdominal oblique
   1a. Aponeurosis of the
       ext. abdominal oblique
2. Int. abdominal oblique
   2a. Aponeurosis of the
       int. abdominal oblique
3. Transversus abdominis
   3a. Aponeurosis of the
       transversus abdominis
4. Rectus abdominis
5. Prepubic tendon
6. Transverse fascia
7. Linea alba
8. Deep inguinal ring
9. Supf. inguinal ring

a. Iliopsoas m.

INGUINAL CANAL (ING-gwi-nal): the passageway for abdominal structures out of the abdomen. It is a collapsed canal between the deep and superficial inguinal rings. The testicle descends through the inguinal canal just before or just after birth (depending on the species) to reach the scrotum.

8. Deep inguinal ring: the internal opening of the inguinal canal. Its boundaries:
• Cranially - caudal border of the internal abdominal oblique
• Caudolaterally - inguinal ligament
• Medially - lateral border of the rectus abdominis muscle

9. Superficial inguinal ring: the external opening of the inguinal canal. It is a slit in the aponeurosis of the external abdominal oblique muscle.

Lateral wall of the inguinal canal: the aponeurosis of the external abdominal oblique muscle.

Medial wall of the inguinal canal: the transversalis fascia and a little of the internal abdominal oblique muscle.

Structures passing in/out of the inguinal canal:
• External pudendal artery and vein
• Genitofemoral nerve
• Vaginal process (female)
• Spermatic cord (male)
• Cremaster muscle (male).

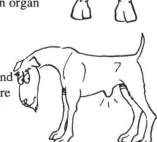

CLINICAL

Hernia: a protrusion of part of an organ through the abdominal wall.

Inguinal hernias: the inguinal canal, a perforation in the abdominal wall, is a weak spot and possible site for hernias. These are common in the <u>horse</u> and <u>pig</u>.

Umbilical hernias: common in young animals.

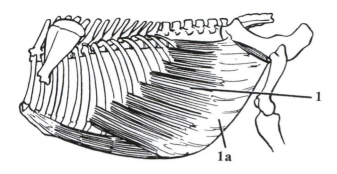

Fig. IV-80 - Ox - Abdominal mm. - lat. view

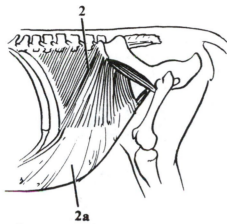

Fig. IV-81 - Ox - Abdominal mm.,
ext. abdominal oblique m. removed

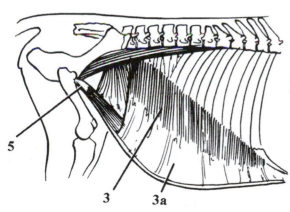

Fig. IV-83 - Ox - Cross section
through 4th lumbar vertebra

Fig. IV-82 - Ox - Abdominal mm., peritoneum
& transverse fascia removed

1. Ext. abdominal oblique	3. Transversus abdominis
1a. Aponeurosis for the ext. abdominal oblique	3a. Aponeurosis for the transversus abdominis
2. Int. abdominal oblique	4. Rectus abdominis
2a. Aponeurosis for the int. abdominal oblique	5. Prepubic tendon
	6. Transversalis fascia
	7. Linea alba

ABDOMINAL SURGICAL APPROACHES:

Ventral midline incision: made through the avascular linea alba.

Paramedian incision: made lateral and parallel to the midline through the rectus abdominis m.

Paracostal incision: made caudal to the last rib and costal arch.

Paralumbar incision: made in the paralumbar fossa.

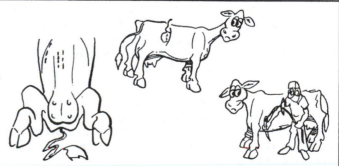

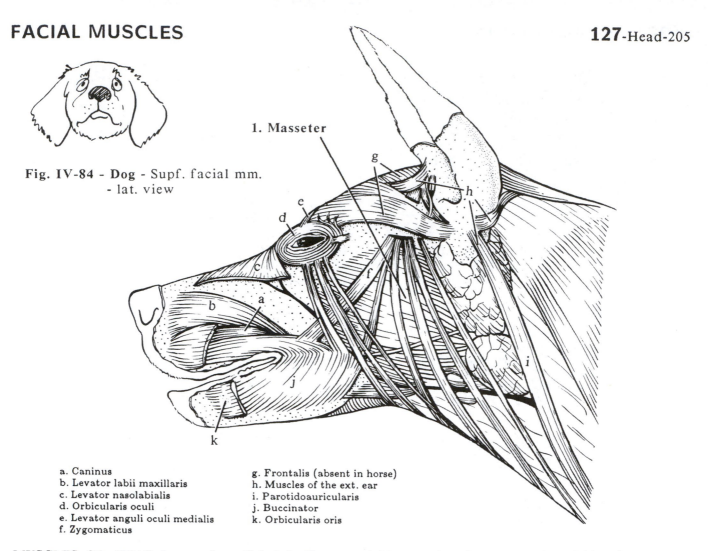

1. Masseter

Fig. IV-84 - **Dog** - Supf. facial mm.
- lat. view

a. Caninus
b. Levator labii maxillaris
c. Levator nasolabialis
d. Orbicularis oculi
e. Levator anguli oculi medialis
f. Zygomaticus

g. Frontalis (absent in horse)
h. Muscles of the ext. ear
i. Parotidoauricularis
j. Buccinator
k. Orbicularis oris

MUSCLES of the HEAD: few are of any clinical significance. Some of interest are given below in the different subdivisions of the muscles of the head.

MUSCLES of FACIAL EXPRESSION: innervated by motor fibers in the facial nerve (Cn VII). These muscles are mentioned in passing because of their relative clinical insignificance. If the facial nerve (motor nerve) is paralyzed these muscles will be affected and cause distortion to the face. The muscles of the cheek and the lips include the orbicularis oris, caninus, levator nasolabialis, buccinator, mentalis and zygomaticus. The muscles of the orbit, forehead and rostral portion of ear can be considered a muscle complex (orbicularis oculi, frontalis, retractor anguli oculi lateralis et medialis, levator nasolabialis) and are of little clinical significance. The muscles of the external ear are divided into four groups: rostral, dorsal, caudal and ventral. Also of passing interest is the scutulum to which many ear muscles attach. The parotidoauricular muscle (i) of the ventral group is noticeable in all lateral views of the head musculature.

MUSCLES of MASTICATION: muscles receiving motor innervation from the mandibular branch of the trigeminal nerve (CN V). They are responsible for chewing (masseter, temporalis, and medial and lateral pterygoid muscles close the jaw; digastricus opens the mouth).

1. Masseter (mas-SEE-ter, mas-SE-ter) (G. *maseter* masticator or chewer): the most powerful muscle closing the jaw, covering the ramus of the mandible.

EXTRINSIC MUSCLES of EYE: innervated by the oculomotor (Cn III), trochlear (Cn IV) and abducent (Cn VI) nerves. (See pg. 550)

MUSCLES of the TONGUE: innervated by the hypoglossal nerve (Cn XII). They are the styloglossus, genioglossus and hyoglossus.

MUSCLES of the PHARYNX and SOFT PALATE: innervated by glossopharyngeal (Cn IX) and vagus (Cn X) nerves. These include the muscles in the pharyngeal wall and the two small muscles to the soft palate.

MUSCLES of the HYOID APPARATUS and LARYNX: most of intrinsic muscles of the larynx are innervated by the vagus (Cn X) nerve. The strap muscles of the neck (pg. 210) are innervated by the ventral branches of the cervical nerves.

Dorsal cricoarytenoideus (FIG. VI-26, 4): the muscle opening the cleft between the vocal folds is innervated by the termination of the recurrent laryngeal nerve (a branch of the vagus nerve).

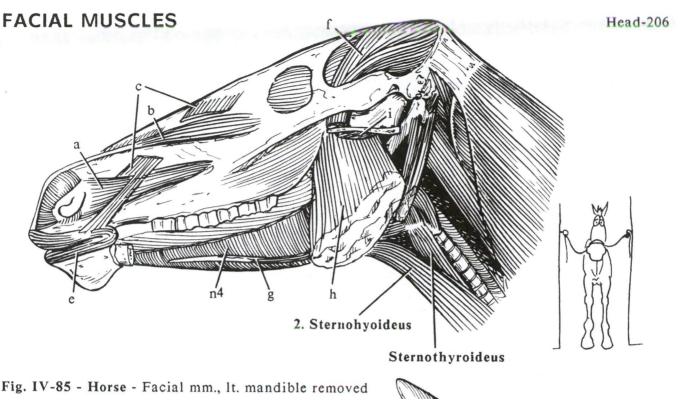

2. Sternohyoideus

Sternothyroideus

Fig. IV-85 - Horse - Facial mm., lt. mandible removed

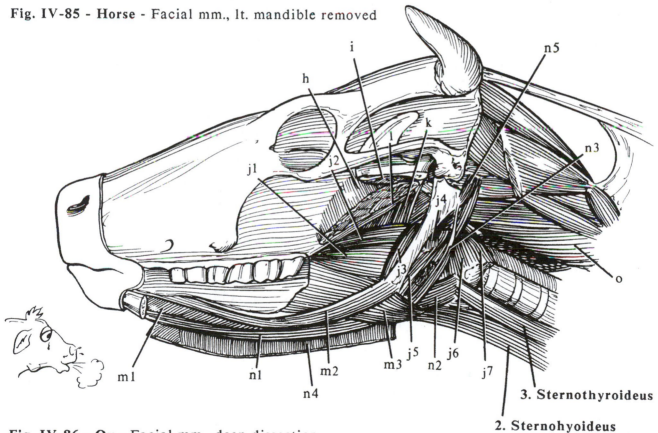

3. Sternothyroideus

2. Sternohyoideus

Fig. IV-86 - Ox - Facial mm., deep dissection

a. Caninus	i. Lat. pterygoid	j7. Cricopharyngeus	n. Hyoid apparatus mm.
b. Levator labii superioris	j. Pharyngeal mm.	k. Levator veli palatini	n1. Geniohyoid
c. Levator nasolabialis	j1. Pterygopharyngeus	l. Tensor veli palatini	n2. Thyrohyoid
d. Frontalis (absent in horse)	j2. Palatopharyngeus	m. Tongue mm.	n3. Stylohyoid
e. Orbicularis oris	j3. Stylopharyngeus rostralis	m1. Genioglossus	n4. Mylohyoid
f. Temporalis	j4. Stylopharyngeus caudalis	m2. Styloglossus	n5. Occipitohyoid
g. Digastricus	j5. Hyopharyngeus	m3. Hyoglossus	o. Longus capitis
h. Med. pterygoid	j6. Thryopharyngeus		

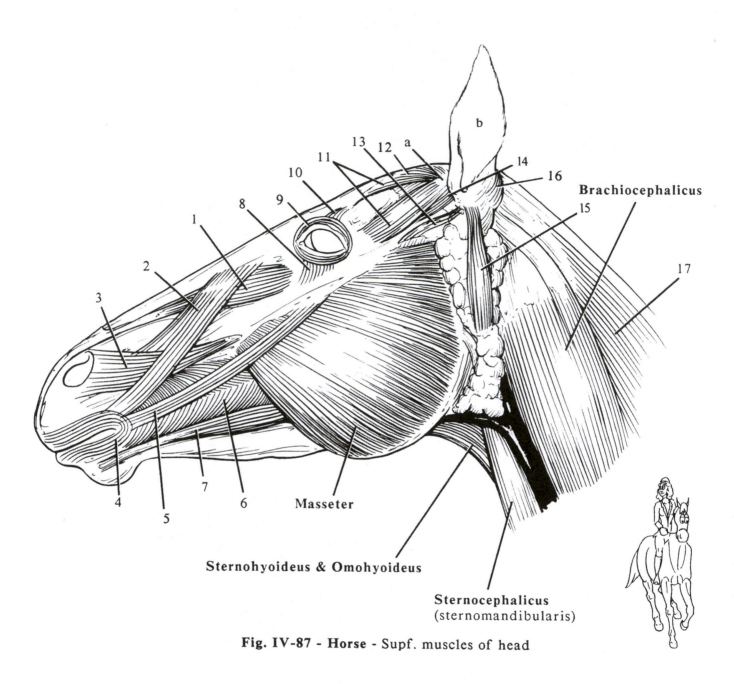

Brachiocephalicus

Masseter

Sternohyoideus & Omohyoideus

Sternocephalicus
(sternomandibularis)

Fig. IV-87 - Horse - Supf. muscles of head

1. Levator labii superioris
2. Levator nasolabialis
3. Caninus
4. Orbicularis oris
5. Zygomaticus
6. Buccinator, buccal part
(supf. part)
6' Molar part (deep part)
7. Depressor labii inferioris
8. Malaris
9. Orbicularis oculi
10. Levator anguli oculi medialis
11. Frontoscutularis
12. Interscutularis

13. Zygomaticoauricularis
14. Scutuloauricularis superficialis
15. Parotidauricularis
16. Cervicoauricularis profundus
17. Splenius
18. Occipitohyoideus
19. Digastricus m., caud. belly, lat. part
(occipitomandibular)
19'. Caud. belly, med. part
19". Rostr. belly
20. Thyropharyngeus
21. Thyrohyoideus
22. Mylohyoideus
23. Temporalis

24. Stylohyoideus
25. Longus capitis
26. Styloglossus
27. Genioglossus
28. Hyoglossus
29. Geniohyoideus
30. Tensor veli palatini
31. Levator veli palatini
32. Pterygopharyngeus
33. Palatopharyngeus
34. Stylopharyngeus caudalis
35. Hyopharyngeus
36. Cricopharyngeus

a. Scutiform cartilage
b. Auricular cartilage
c. Stylohyoid bone
d. Trachea
e. esophagus
f. Tongue
g. Nasal cartilage

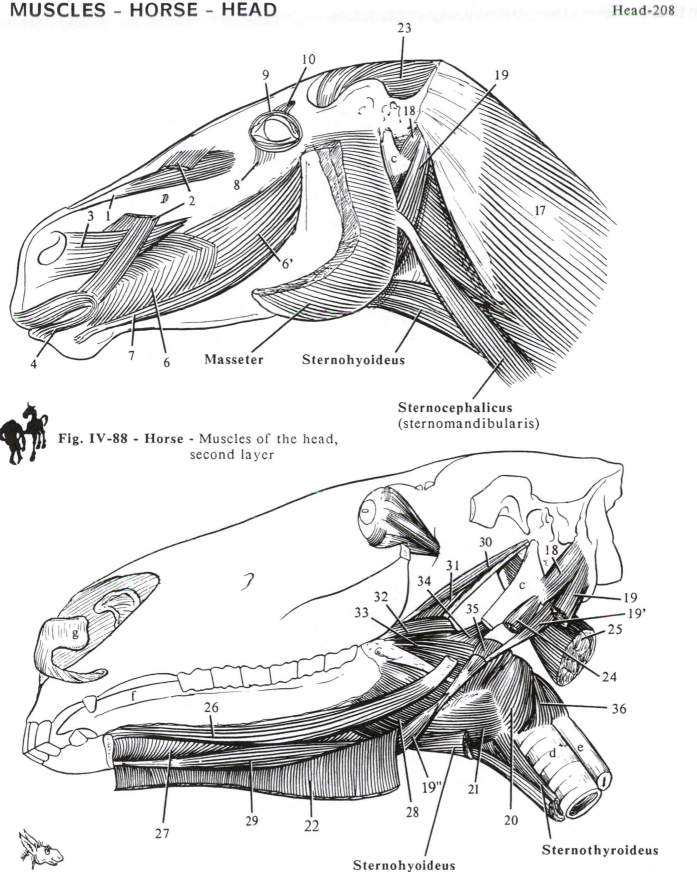

Fig. IV-88 - Horse - Muscles of the head, second layer

Masseter

Sternohyoideus

Sternocephalicus (sternomandibularis)

Fig. IV-89 - Horse - Muscles of head. deep dissection

Sternohyoideus

Sternothyroideus

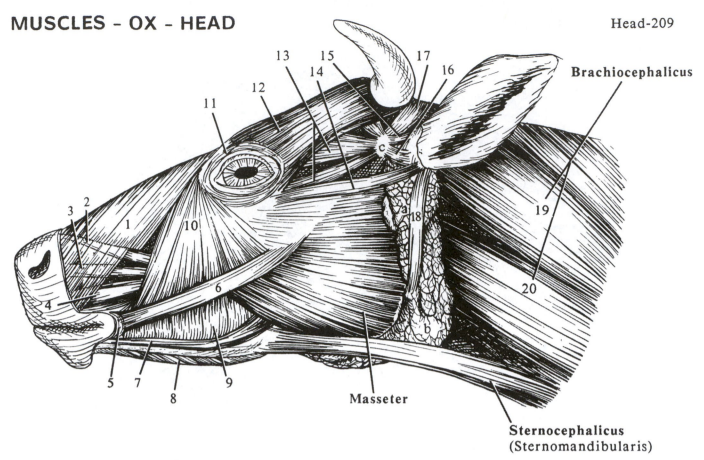

Brachiocephalicus

Masseter

Sternocephalicus
(Sternomandibularis)

Fig. VI-90 – Ox – Supf. muscles of head – lat. view

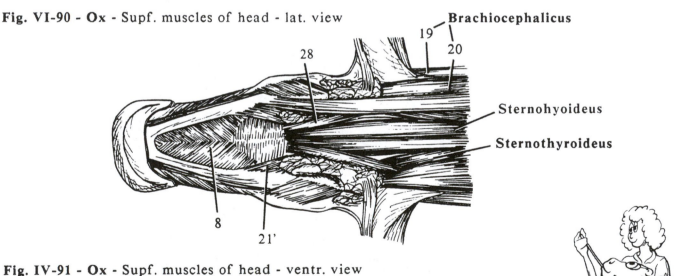

Brachiocephalicus

Sternohyoideus

Sternothyroideus

Fig. IV-91 – Ox – Supf. muscles of head – ventr. view

1. Levator nasolabialis
2. Levator labii superioris
3. Caninus
4. Depressor labii superioris
5. Orbicularis oris
6. Zygomaticus
7. Depressor labii inferioris
8. Mylohyoideus
9. Buccinator, buccal part
   9' Molar part
10. Malaris
11. Orbicularis oculi

12. Frontalis
13. Frontoscutularis
14. Zygomaticoauricularis
15. Scutuloauricularis
    superficialis
16. Scutuloauricularis
    profundus
17. Cervicoscutularis
18. Parotidoauricularis
19. Cleidomastoideus
20. Cleidooccipitalis
21. Digastricus, caud. belly

21' Digastricus, rostral belly
22. Stylohyoideus
23. Omohyoideus
24. Splenius
25. Cricopharyngeus
26. Thyropharyngeus
27. Longus capitis
28. Thryohyoideus
29. Temporalis
30. Lat. pterygoideus
31. Med. pterygoideus
32. Occipitohyoideus

33. Rectus capitis lateralis
34. Obliquus capitis cranialis
35. Longissimus capitis
36. Semispinalis

a. Parotid salivary gl.
b. Mandibular salivary gl.
c. Scutiform cartilage
d. Facial tuberosity
e. Stylohyoid bone
f. Trachea
g. Wing of atlas

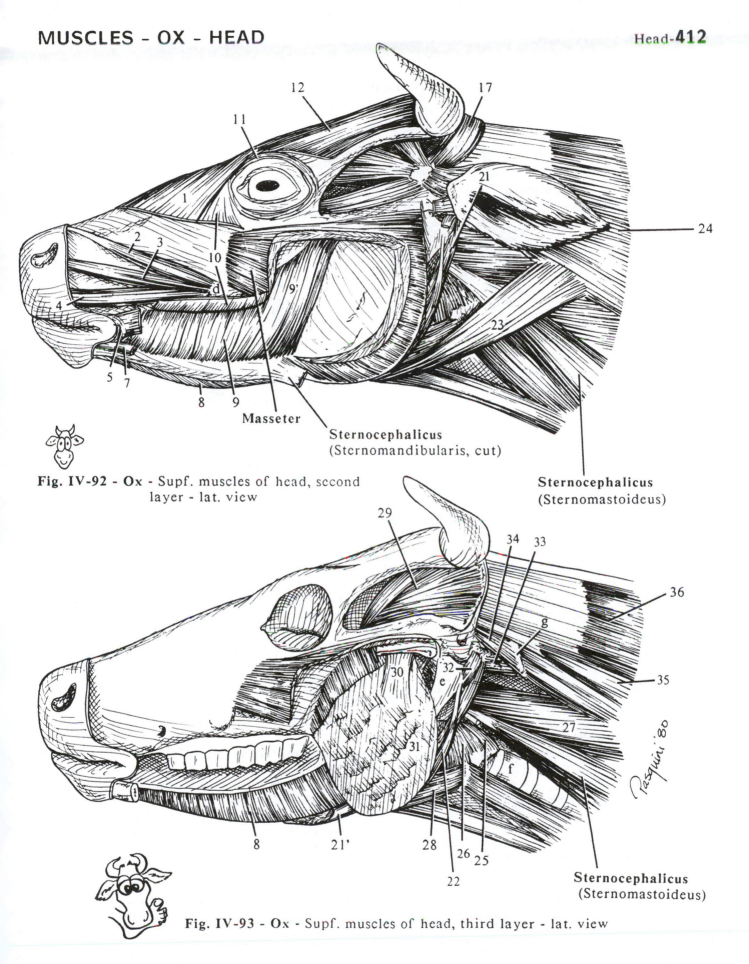

Fig. IV-92 - Ox - Supf. muscles of head, second layer - lat. view

Masseter

Sternocephalicus
(Sternomandibularis, cut)

Sternocephalicus
(Sternomastoideus)

Fig. IV-93 - Ox - Supf. muscles of head, third layer - lat. view

Sternocephalicus
(Sternomastoideus)

Fig. IV-94 - Dog - Supf. mm. of neck - lat. view

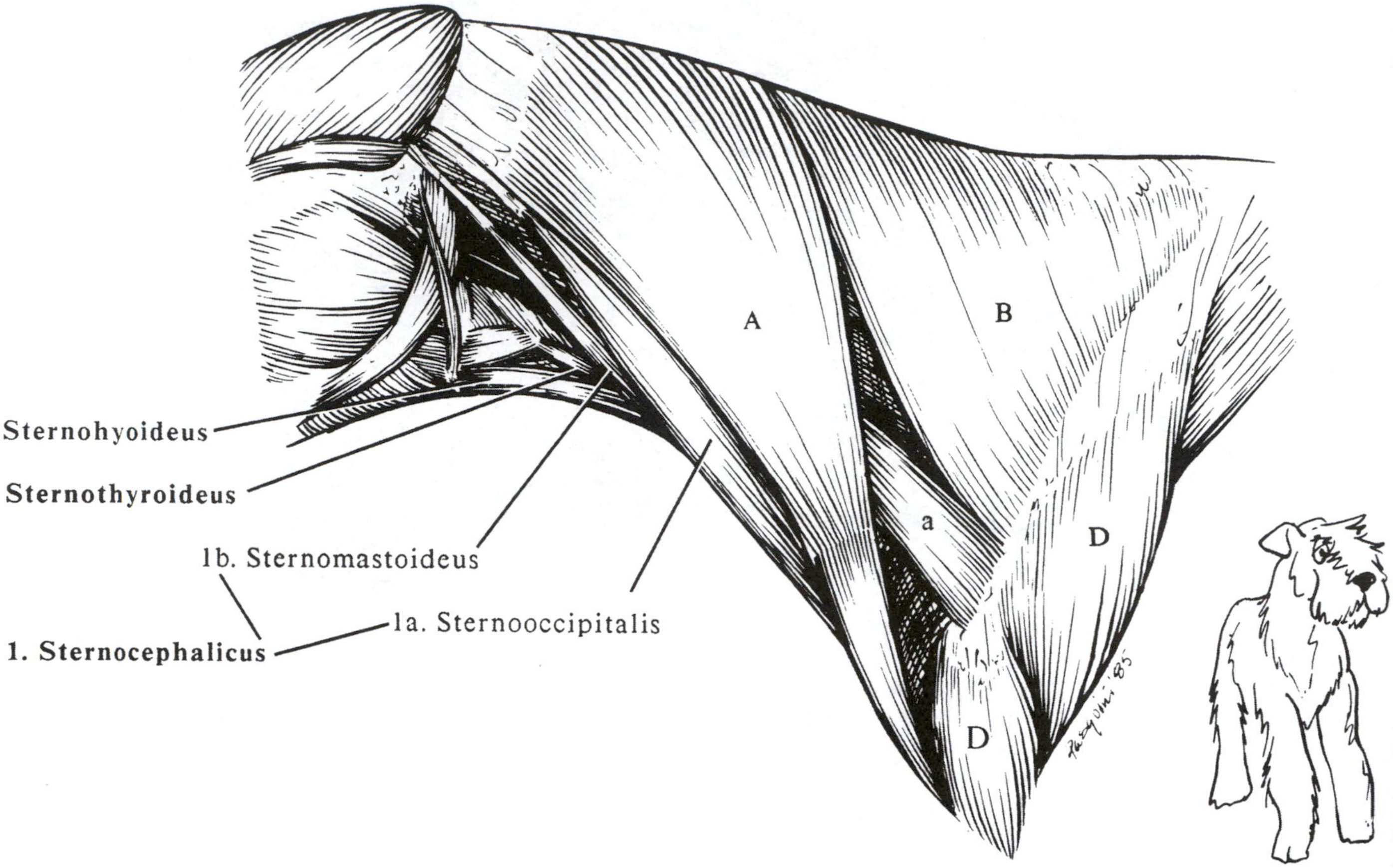

Sternohyoideus

Sternothyroideus

1b. Sternomastoideus

1a. Sternooccipitalis

1. Sternocephalicus

MUSCLES OF THE NECK: consist of a number of superficial muscles (platysma, sternothyroid, sternohyoid, trapezius, omotransversarius, serratus ventralis, and brachiocephalicus) and a number of deep muscles (rhomboid, longus colli, longus capitis, rectus capitis, scalenus, semispinalis, longissimus, splenius, and intertransversarii and the omohyoideus in the horse and ruminants).

1. Sternocephalicus: extends from the sternum to the head. It is divided in the **carnivores, ox** and **goat**; undivided in the **pig, sheep**, and **horse**. In each species they are named for their cephalic (head) attachment. In the goat the sternomandibular head attaches to the zygomatic arch and is sometimes called sternozygomaticus.

Carnivores -	sternomastoid (1b) sternooccipitalis (1a)
Ox and goat -	sternomastoid (1b) sternomandibularis (1c)
Pig and sheep -	sternomastoid (1b)
Horse -	sternomandibularis (1c)

Strap muscles of the neck: consist of the ventrally located sternohyoid and sternothyroid muscles. They cover the ventral surface of the trachea and are separated in an emergency tracheostomy approach.

2. Sternohyoid: the strap-like muscle extending from the first sternebra (manubrium) and first costal cartilage up the neck to insert on the hyoid apparatus (basihyoid bone).

Sternothyroid: arises with the sternohyoid and inclines laterally to insert on the thyroid cartilage of the larynx.

Omohyoideus (Fig. IV-101, 110): a thin muscle found in the cranial neck of the horse and ox. It is absent in the carnivores. In the horse it separates the external jugular vein from the common carotid artery in the cranial neck, but probably doesn't protect the common carotid from unskilled venipuncture.

CLINICAL

Jugular groove: between the brachiocephalicus and sternocephalicus muscles in the horse and ruminants. The deep wall of the jugular groove is formed by the sternomastoid in the ruminants and the omohyoideus in the cranial part of the neck in horses.

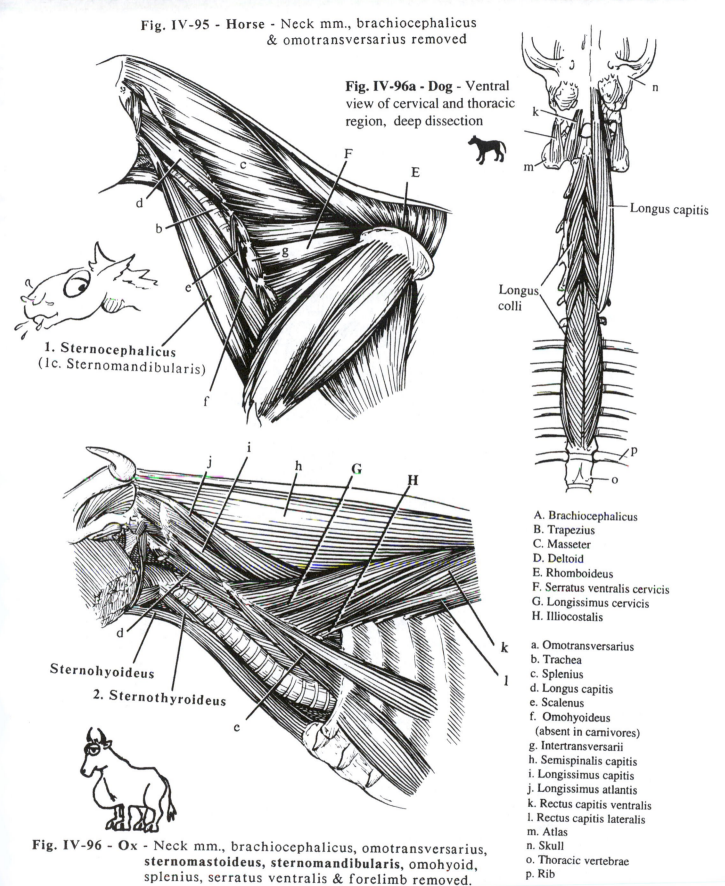

Fig. IV-95 - Horse - Neck mm., brachiocephalicus
& omotransversarius removed

Fig. IV-96a - Dog - Ventral
view of cervical and thoracic
region, deep dissection

Longus capitis

Longus
colli

1. Sternocephalicus
(1c. Sternomandibularis)

Sternohyoideus

2. Sternothyroideus

Fig. IV-96 - Ox - Neck mm., brachiocephalicus, omotransversarius,
sternomastoideus, sternomandibularis, omohyoid,
splenius, serratus ventralis & forelimb removed.

A. Brachiocephalicus
B. Trapezius
C. Masseter
D. Deltoid
E. Rhomboideus
F. Serratus ventralis cervicis
G. Longissimus cervicis
H. Illiocostalis

a. Omotransversarius
b. Trachea
c. Splenius
d. Longus capitis
e. Scalenus
f. Omohyoideus
  (absent in carnivores)
g. Intertransversarii
h. Semispinalis capitis
i. Longissimus capitis
j. Longissimus atlantis
k. Rectus capitis ventralis
l. Rectus capitis lateralis
m. Atlas
n. Skull
o. Thoracic vertebrae
p. Rib

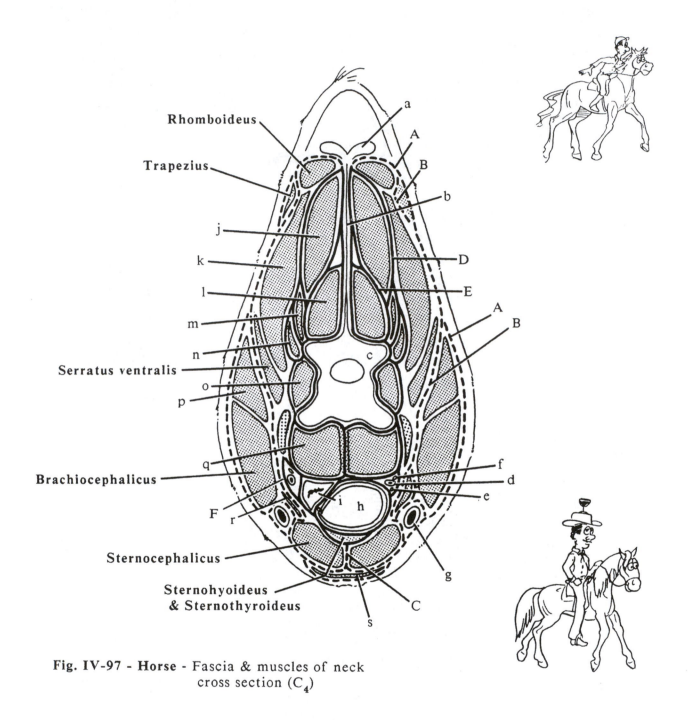

Fig. IV-97 - Horse - Fascia & muscles of neck
cross section (C$_4$)

A-C. Supf. fascia	a. Nuchal lig.	h. Trachea	o. Intertransversarii m.
A. Supf. layer	b. Lamina nuchae	i. Esophagus	p. Omotransversarius m.
B. Deep layer	c. Vertebra C$_4$	j. Semispinalis m.	q. Longus colli m.
C. Fibrous raphe	d. Common carotid a.	k. Splenius m.	r. Omohyoideus m.
D-F. Deep fascia	e. Recurrent laryngeal n.	l. Multifidus m.	s. Cutaneus colli m.
D. Supf. layer	f. Vagosympathetic trunk	m. Longissimus capitis m.	
E. Deep layer	g. Ext. jugular v.	n. Longissimus atlantis m.	
F. Carotid sheath			

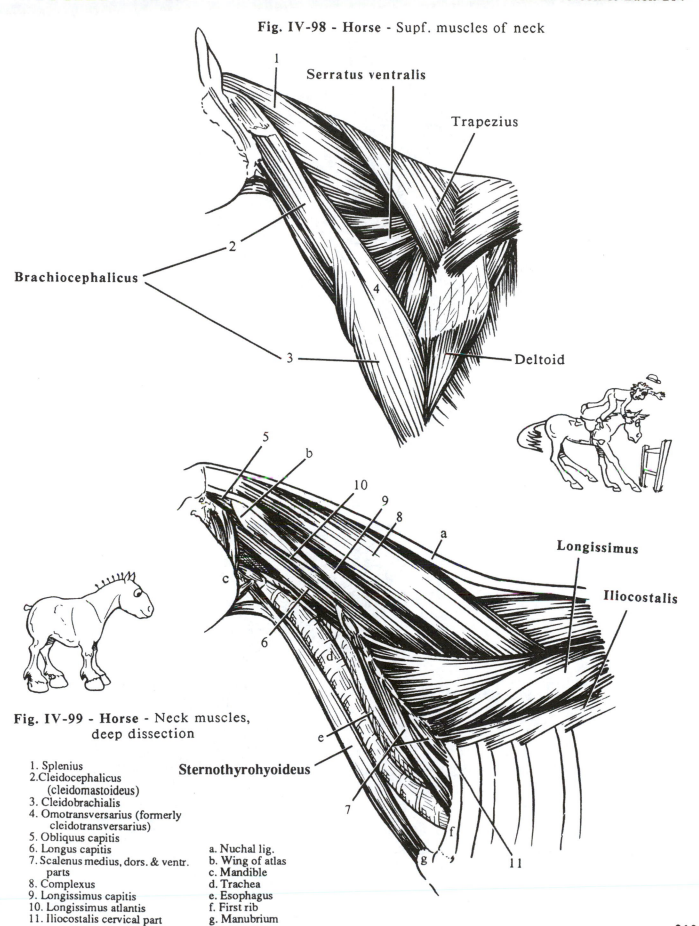

Fig. IV-98 - **Horse** - Supf. muscles of neck

Serratus ventralis

Trapezius

Brachiocephalicus

Deltoid

Fig. IV-99 - **Horse** - Neck muscles,
deep dissection

Longissimus

Iliocostalis

Sternothyrohyoideus

1. Splenius
2. Cleidocephalicus
   (cleidomastoideus)
3. Cleidobrachialis
4. Omotransversarius (formerly
   cleidotransversarius)
5. Obliquus capitis
6. Longus capitis
7. Scalenus medius, dors. & ventr.
   parts
8. Complexus
9. Longissimus capitis
10. Longissimus atlantis
11. Iliocostalis cervical part

a. Nuchal lig.
b. Wing of atlas
c. Mandible
d. Trachea
e. Esophagus
f. First rib
g. Manubrium

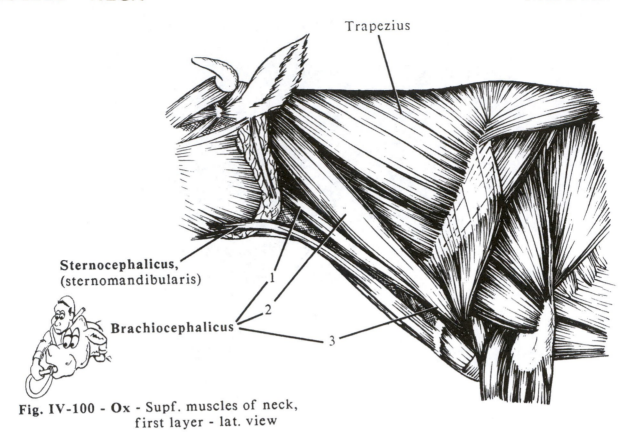

Trapezius

Sternocephalicus,
(sternomandibularis)

Brachiocephalicus

1
2
3

Fig. IV-100 - Ox - Supf. muscles of neck,
first layer - lat. view

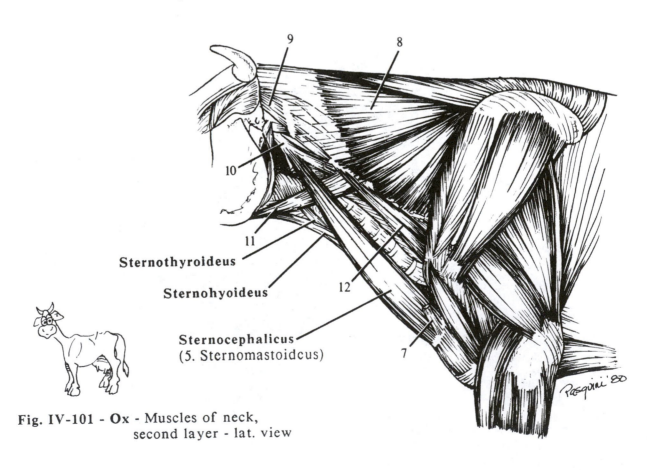

9
8
10
11
12
7

Sternothyroideus

Sternohyoideus

Sternocephalicus
(5. Sternomastoidcus)

Fig. IV-101 - Ox - Muscles of neck,
second layer - lat. view

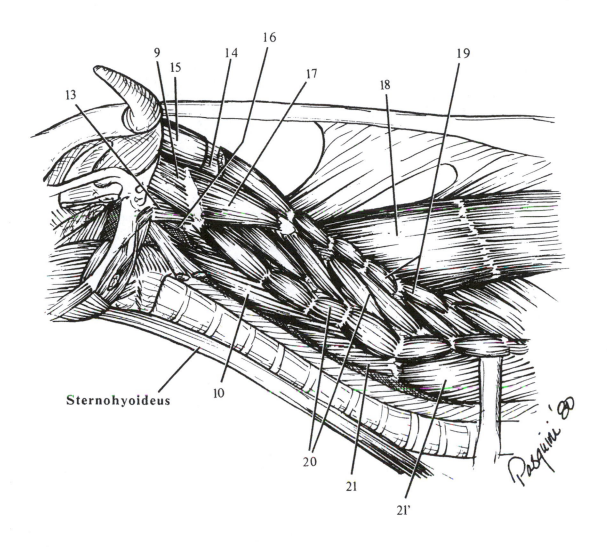

Sternohyoideus

Fig. IV-102 - Ox - Muscles of neck, deep layer
- lat. view

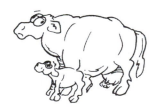

1. Cleidooccipitalis	9. Obliquus capitis cranialis	17. Obliquus capitis caudalis
2. Cleidomastoideus	10. Longus capitis	18. Spinalis et semispinalis dorsi
3. Cleidobrachialis	11. Omohyoideus	19. Multifidus cervicis
4. Sternomandibularis	12. Scalenus	20. Dors. & ventr. intertransversarii
5. Sternomastoideus	13. Rectus capitis lateralis	21. Longus colli, cervical part
6. Omotransversarius	14. Rectus capitis dorsalis minor	21'. Thoracic part
7. Subclavius	15. Rectus capitis dorsalis major	
8. Splenius	16. Rectus capitis ventralis	

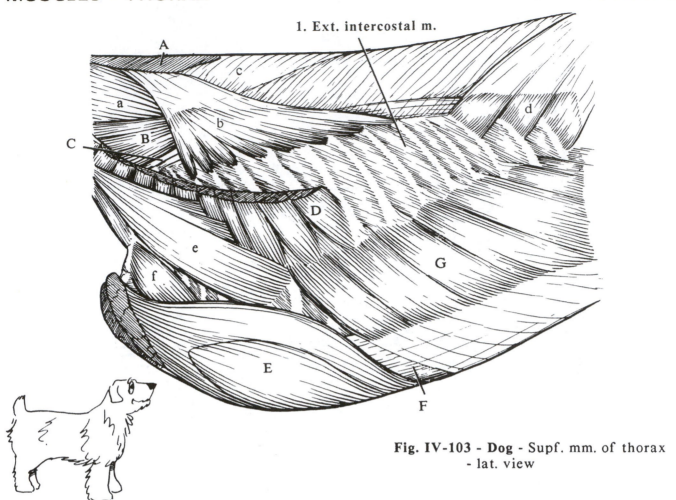

1. Ext. intercostal m.

Fig. IV-103 - Dog - Supf. mm. of thorax
- lat. view

MUSCLES of the THORAX: the muscles associated with the ribs, concerned with breathing. They are the internal and external intercostals, levatores costarum, subcostal, rectus thoracis, retractor costae, transversus thoracis, serratus dorsalis, scalenus muscles, and most importantly the muscles of the <u>diaphragm</u> (see pg. 224).

Breathing:

Inspiration: increasing the volume of the thorax, allowing expansion of the lungs. This is facilitated by pulling the ribs forward and displacing the diaphragm caudally into the abdomen. The external intercostals, levatores costarum, rectus thoracis, cranial serratus dorsalis, scalenus and the diaphragm work in inspiration.

Expiration: opposite from inspiration, the ribs are drawn caudally, decreasing the transverse diameter and volume of the thorax. The internal intercostals, caudal serratus dorsalis and the diaphragm work in expiration.

Muscles:

1. External intercostal muscles: located in the intercostal spaces, their fibers run <u>caudoventrally</u> between adjacent ribs. They act to expand the thorax (inspiration) by pulling the ribs forward.

2. Internal intercostal: the muscles deep to the external intercostal muscles, extending <u>cranioventrally</u> between adjacent ribs, roughly perpendicular to the fibers of the external intercostal muscles. They pull the preceding rib caudally, reducing the transverse diameter of the thorax (expiration).

Transversus thoracis muscle: located on the floor of the thorax dorsal to the sternum. It can be considered morphologically the continuation of the transversus abdominis muscle in the thorax.

Rectus thoracis muscle (f): located on the lateral thorax from the third to the first rib. It is the direct continuation of the rectus abdominis muscle.

Serratus dorsalis cranialis muscle (b): an insignificant muscle over the dorsal part of the ribs. It pulls the ribs forward during inspiration.

Serratus dorsalis caudalis muscle(d): located over the dorsal part of the caudal most ribs, this insignificant muscle pulls the ribs caudally during expiration.

Scalenus muscle (c): extends from the cervical vertebrae to the first ribs. It is an inspiratory muscle.

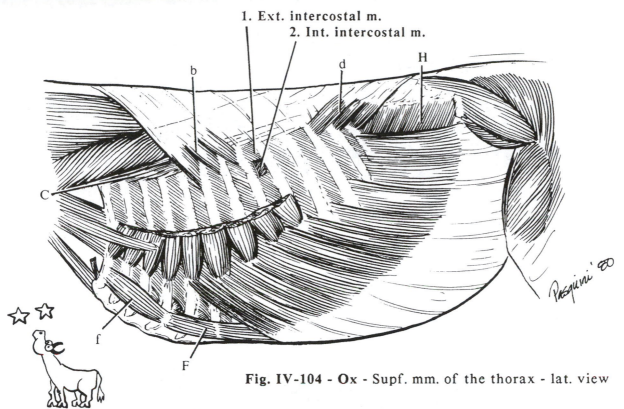

1. Ext. intercostal m.
2. Int. intercostal m.

Fig. IV-104 - Ox - Supf. mm. of the thorax - lat. view

Fig. IV-105 - Horse - Thoracic mm., serratus dorsalis removed &
ext. abdominal oblique cut

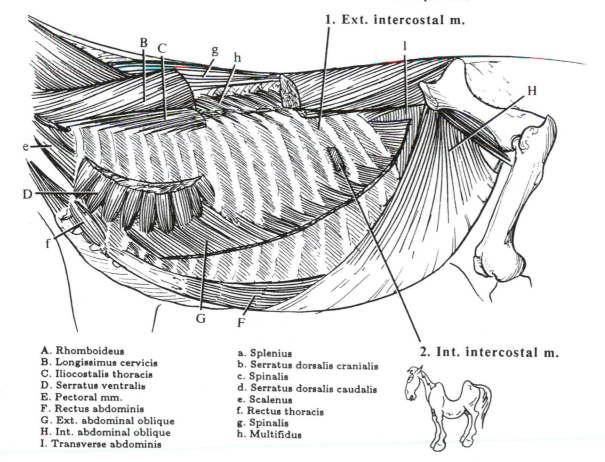

1. Ext. intercostal m.

2. Int. intercostal m.

A. Rhomboideus
B. Longissimus cervicis
C. Iliocostalis thoracis
D. Serratus ventralis
E. Pectoral mm.
F. Rectus abdominis
G. Ext. abdominal oblique
H. Int. abdominal oblique
I. Transverse abdominis

a. Splenius
b. Serratus dorsalis cranialis
c. Spinalis
d. Serratus dorsalis caudalis
e. Scalenus
f. Rectus thoracis
g. Spinalis
h. Multifidus

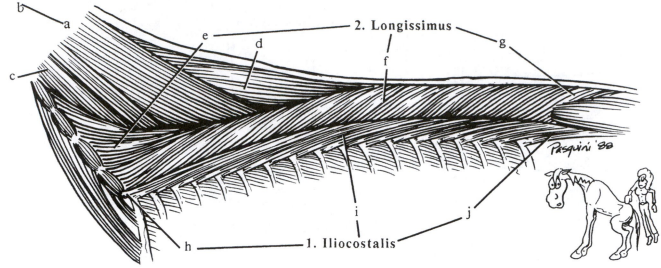

Fig. IV-106 - Horse - Muscles of the back

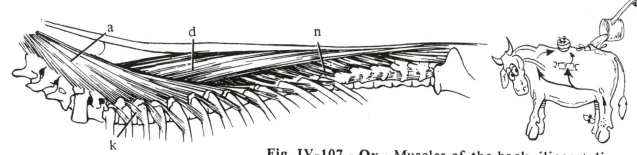

**Fig. IV-107 - Ox - Muscles of the back, iliocostalis
& longissimus removed**

MUSCLES OF THE VERTEBRAL COLUMN (back): flex (bend forward), extend (bend backward), abduct (bend to the side), adduct (return to midline), and rotate (twist) the backbone. Back muscles can be divided into epaxial and hypaxial muscles.

Epaxial muscles: muscles of the back dorsal to the transverse processes of the vertebrae.

Hypaxial muscles: muscles below the transverse processes of the vertebrae.

Flexors of the spine: the rectus abdominis and the hypaxial muscles (the major and minor psoas and iliacus) flex the spine.

Extensors of the spine: the epaxial muscles, including the iliocostalis, longissimus, spinalis et semispinalis, spinalis capitis, multifidi, and intertransversarius muscles.

1. Iliocostalis: the most <u>lateral</u> column of the epaxial muscles, extending in overlapping bundles from the crest of the ilium to the transverse processes of the lumbar vertebrae, the ribs (L. costae) and the transverse processes of the cervical vertebrae. They act together to fix or extend the vertebral column. Alone, they move the column laterally. They also aid in inspiration by pulling the ribs caudally.

2. Longissimus (lon-JIS-i-mus) (L. longest): the intermediate column of epaxial muscles extending in overlapping bundles from the iliac crest to the head. It is divided into thoracolumbar, cervical, atlantal and capital parts. It extends the back and neck and the atlantooccipital joint. Alone, they move the back, neck, and head laterally.

3. Transversospinalis system: the most <u>medial</u> column of epaxial muscles. Its muscle bundles span one or two vertebrae up and down the spinal column.

CLINICAL

Dorsal laminectomies: removal of the dorsal part of the vertebral arch (laminae) to increase room for the spinal cord. To reach the vertebral arch understanding of the epaxial muscles is important.

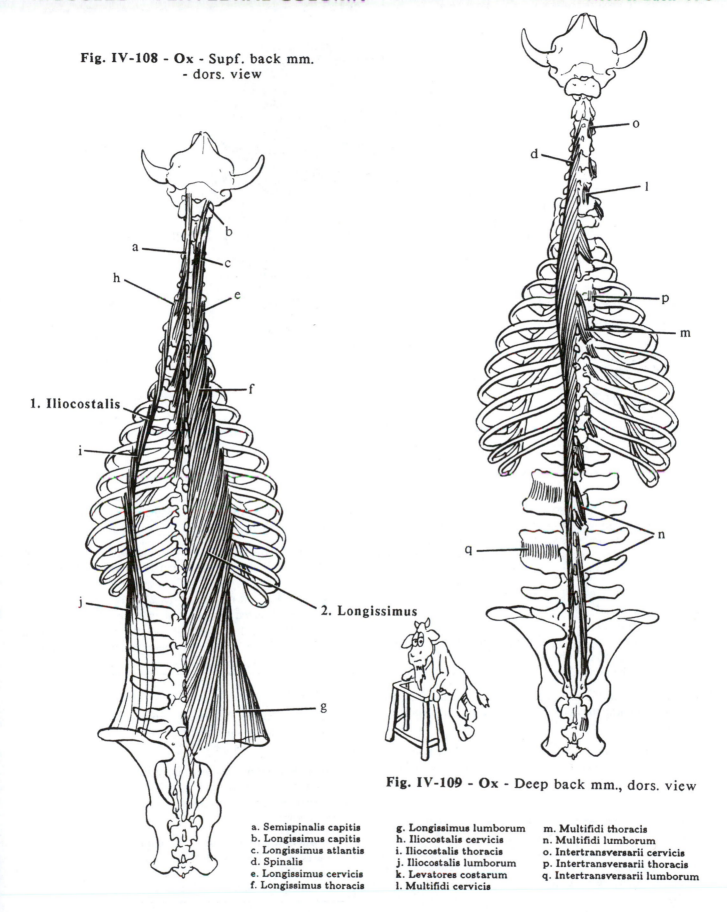

Fig. IV-108 - **Ox** - Supf. back mm.
- dors. view

1. Iliocostalis

2. Longissimus

Fig. IV-109 - **Ox** - Deep back mm., dors. view

a. Semispinalis capitis
b. Longissimus capitis
c. Longissimus atlantis
d. Spinalis
e. Longissimus cervicis
f. Longissimus thoracis

g. Longissimus lumborum
h. Iliocostalis cervicis
i. Iliocostalis thoracis
j. Iliocostalis lumborum
k. Levatores costarum
l. Multifidi cervicis

m. Multifidi thoracis
n. Multifidi lumborum
o. Intertransversarii cervicis
p. Intertransversarii thoracis
q. Intertransversarii lumborum

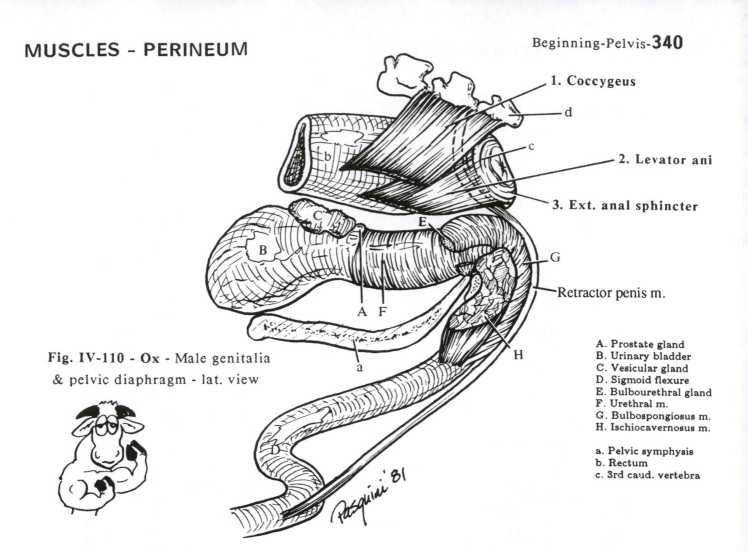

Fig. IV-110 - **Ox** - Male genitalia
& pelvic diaphragm - lat. view

1. Coccygeus
2. Levator ani
3. Ext. anal sphincter
Retractor penis m.

A. Prostate gland
B. Urinary bladder
C. Vesicular gland
D. Sigmoid flexure
E. Bulbourethral gland
F. Urethral m.
G. Bulbospongiosus m.
H. Ischiocavernosus m.

a. Pelvic symphysis
b. Rectum
c. 3rd caud. vertebra

Pasquini '81

PERINEUM (per'i-NEE-um): the wall and associated structures closing the pelvic outlet and surrounding the anal and urogenital canals. The deep boundaries are the same as those for the pelvic outlet: dorsal – 3rd or 4th caudal vertebrae, lateral – sacrotuberous ligament, ventral – ischiatic tuberosity and ischiatic arch.

Superficial boundaries of the perineum:
• Dorsal – base of tail
• Lateral – sacrotuberous ligament
• Ventral – below vulva (base of udder in ruminants) or base of scrotum (in cats and pigs the scrotum, which is below the anus, is included in the perineum).

Pelvic diaphragm: the main muscular component of the perineum for containing the pelvic viscera. It consists of coccygeus and levator ani muscles.

1. Coccygeus muscle (kok-SIJ-ee-us): lateral muscle of the pelvic diaphragm extending from the ischiatic spine to the tail. Along with the levator ani, it pulls the dogs tail between the rear legs.

2. Levator ani muscles: more medial of the muscles of the pelvic diaphragm arising from the floor of the pelvic cavity. In the dog it inserts mainly on the root of the tail to form a sling around the rectum in the dog. They act to compress the rectum, initiating defecation. In ungulates it attaches mainly to the external anal sphincter.

3. External anal sphincter: the striated muscle under voluntary control encircling the anal canal.

Perineal body (per'i-NEE-al): the aggregate of fibrous and muscular tissue between the anus and the vulva or the bulb of the penis.

Ischiorectal fossa: the pyramidal space on either side of the anus with its apex directed cranially. It is bounded by the pelvic diaphragm, floor of the pelvis and the sacrotuberous ligament. Usually filled with fat, it is where fingers and thumbs are pressed when expressing anal sacs.

CLINICAL

Perineal laceration: the tearing of the perineum (which often may include the perineal body) during foaling.

Perineal hernia: protrusion of an organ or tissue through the perineum. This can be caused by rents in the muscles of the pelvic diaphragm.

Prolapse of the rectum or of the vagina and uterus: the protrusion of the rectal mucosa through the anus; or of the vagina and/or uterus through the vulva.

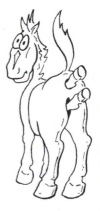

CUTANEOUS MUSCLES

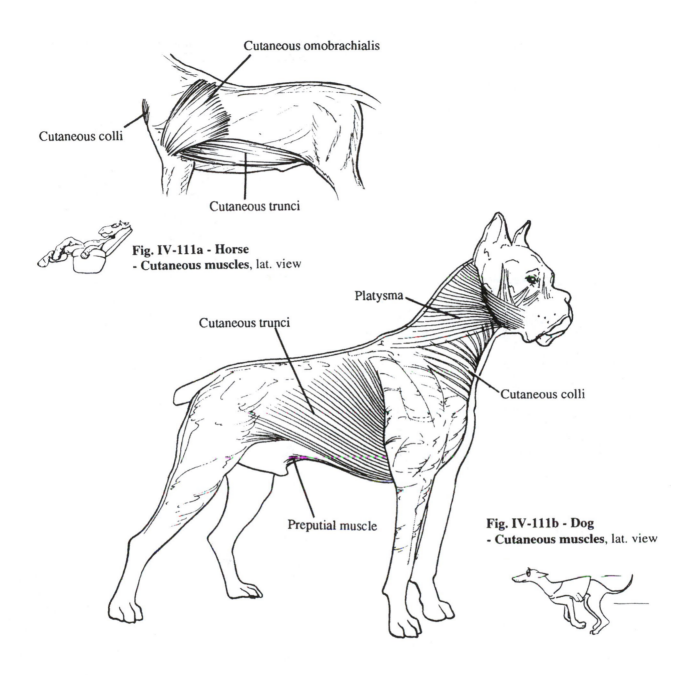

Cutaneous omobrachialis

Cutaneous colli

Cutaneous trunci

Fig. IV-111a - Horse
- Cutaneous muscles, lat. view

Cutaneous trunci

Platysma

Cutaneous colli

Preputial muscle

Fig. IV-111b - Dog
- Cutaneous muscles, lat. view

CUTANEOUS MUSCLES: the thin, interrupted sheets spread over the body in the superficial fasciae (platysma, cutaneous omobrachialis, cutaneous trunci, and preputial muscles). These muscles twitch the skin (to remove flies).

Platysma: the cutaneous muscle over the neck and face.

Frontalis: found in man, ruminants, and pigs, over the frontal bone.

Cutaneous colli: Best developed in the **horse,** it arises from the sternum and spreads up the neck over the caudal part of the external jugular vein.

Cutaneous trunci: covers the side of the trunk and is present in all domestic species, but absent in man.

Cutaneous omobrachialis: a continuation of the cutaneous trunci muscle over the shoulder and arm of horses and ruminants.

Preputial muscles: cutaneous muscles found in carnivores, ruminants and pigs. All have cranial preputial muscles on the ventral midline connecting to the prepuce. The bull also has caudal preputial muscles.

FASCIAE

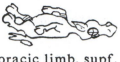

Fig. IV-112 - **Ox** - Thoracic limb, supf. fascia
- lat. view

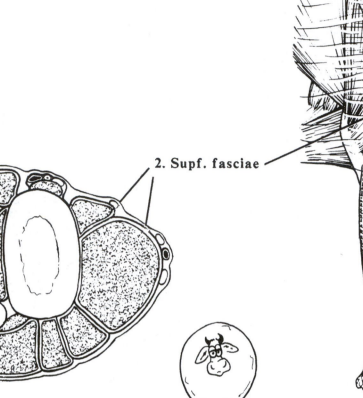

2. Supf. fasciae

1. Deep fasciae

Fig. IV-113 - **Ox** - Prox. forearm, deep fascia
- cross section

FASCIA (FASH-ee-ah) (pl=fasciae [FASH-ee-ee]): a sheet or layer of fibrous connective tissue that lies deep to the skin or around muscles and various organs of the body.

1. Superficial fascia or **subcutis**: the loose connective tissue lying deep to the skin covering the entire body. Functionally, it provides a storehouse of water and fat, and insulates and protects the body. It allows structures to move easily against each other.

2. Deep fascia: the dense connective tissue under the superficial fascia, investing most of the body. Septa, extensions of the deep fascia, extend between muscles to bones, thus, compartmentalize muscles or groups of muscles.

• **Retinaculum** (ret'i-NAK-yoo-lum) pl. retinacula [L. "a rope, cable"]: local thickenings of the deep fascia that hold tendons in place.

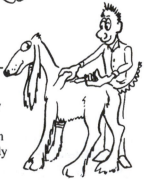

CLINICAL

Subcutaneous injections: easily made into the superficial fascia. Because of its looseness, the skin can be pulled away from the body and the injection given.

Facial planes: formed by the deep fascia around muscles, these dictate which way pus or fluid will flow. Pus in one region can migrate down the fascial planes to break out at a distant site, e.g., an infection in the deep neck running along the fascial planes to enter the thorax.

Surgery: fascial planes can be used as cleavage planes to reach deep structures relatively free of blood.

Chapter V
Digestive System

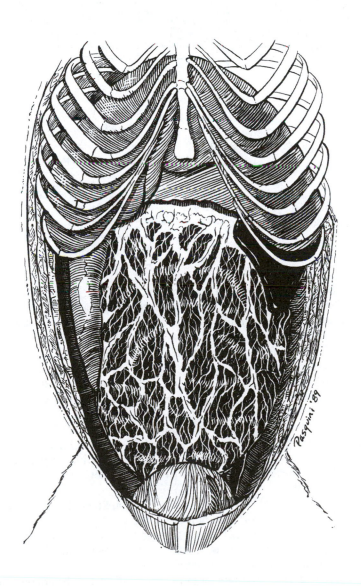

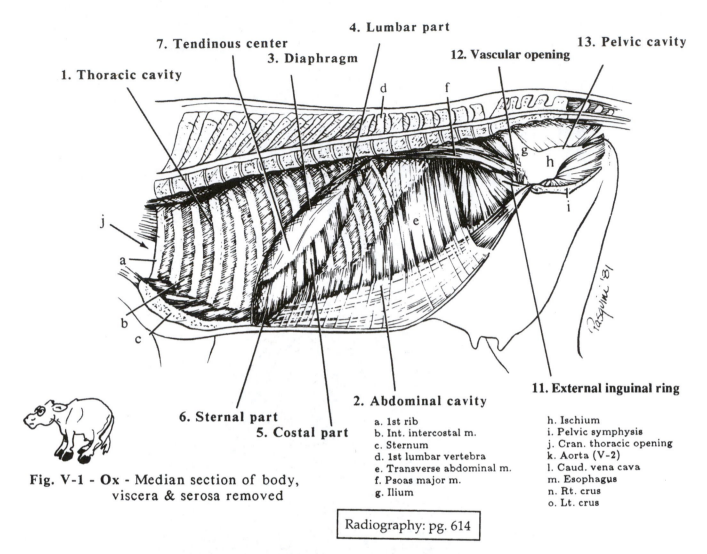

Fig. V-1 - Ox - Median section of body, viscera & serosa removed

2. Abdominal cavity

a. 1st rib
b. Int. intercostal m.
c. Sternum
d. 1st lumbar vertebra
e. Transverse abdominal m.
f. Psoas major m.
g. Ilium

11. External inguinal ring

h. Ischium
i. Pelvic symphysis
j. Cran. thoracic opening
k. Aorta (V-2)
l. Caud. vena cava
m. Esophagus
n. Rt. crus
o. Lt. crus

6. Sternal part
5. Costal part

Radiography: pg. 614

BODY CAVITIES: the compartments of the body – thoracic, abdominal, and pelvic. The diaphragm separates the thoracic cavity from the abdominal and pelvic (abdominopelvic) cavities.

1. THORACIC CAVITY (thoh-RAS-ik): the space within the thorax containing the thoracic organs, the pleura and pleural cavities, the pericardium and pericardial cavity. The **cranial thoracic opening** (thoracic inlet) (j) is the entrance into the thoracic cavity. It is formed by the first pair of ribs and the vertebrae and sternebrae to which they connect. The diaphragm closes the **caudal thoracic opening.**

2. ABDOMINAL CAVITY: the space within the trunk between the diaphragm and the pelvic cavity.

3. DIAPHRAGM (DY-a-fram) (G. *phren*): the dome-shaped muscle separating the thoracic and abdominal cavities, innervated by the phrenic nerve. It is the principal muscle concerned with respiration. Moving cranially or caudally decreases or increases the volume of the thorax during expiration or inspiration, respectively. The diaphragm projects as a dome into the bony

thorax. Therefore, the caudal bony thorax is filled with abdominal viscera. The diaphragm has three major openings between the thorax and the abdomen: the aortic hiatus, the esophageal hiatus, and the caval foramen.

4. Crura or **lumbar part:** the dorsal part of the diaphragm consisting of the right and left crura (sing. = crus). The crura connect to the ventral side of the lumbar vertebral bodies and form the aortic hiatus.

5. Costal part: the lateral muscular part of the diaphragm, extending between the thoracic (costal) wall and the tendinous center.

6. Sternal part: the ventral muscular part.

7. Tendinous center: the V-shaped aponeurotic (tendinous) center of the diaphragm.

Cupula: the cranial part of the dome of the diaphragm.

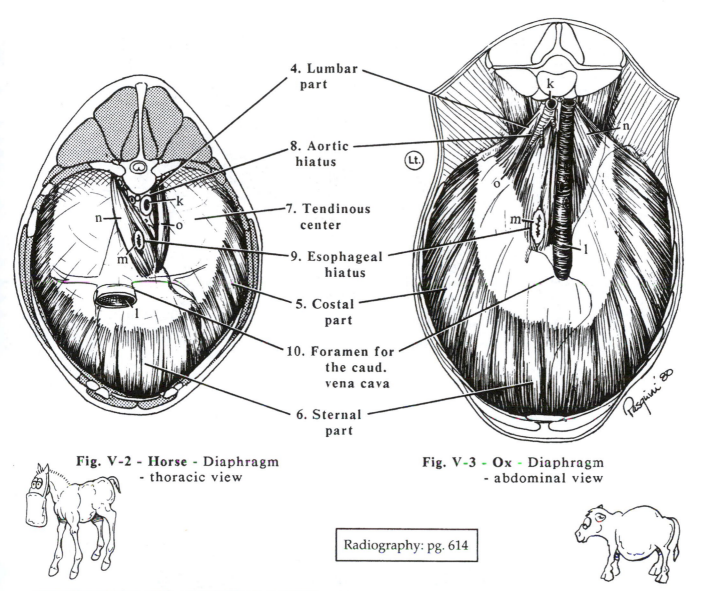

4. Lumbar part

8. Aortic hiatus

7. Tendinous center

9. Esophageal hiatus

5. Costal part

10. Foramen for the caud. vena cava

6. Sternal part

Fig. V-2 - **Horse** - Diaphragm
- thoracic view

Fig. V-3 - **Ox** - Diaphragm
- abdominal view

Radiography: pg. 614

OPENINGS INTO THE ABDOMINAL CAVITY:

8. Aortic hiatus (hy-AY-tus) (L. general term for a gap, cleft or opening): the opening in the dorsal part of the diaphragm for the passage of the abdominal aorta (also the azygos vein and the thoracic duct). It is formed between the crura and the lumbar vertebrae.

9. Esophageal hiatus: located ventral to the aortic hiatus through the crura. The esophagus, the ventral and dorsal vagal trunks, and the esophageal vessels enter the abdomen here.

10. Caval foramen: the opening in the center of the diaphragm (tendinous center) for the caudal vena cava.

Pelvic inlet: the communication between the abdominal and pelvic cavities.

Abdominal opening of the uterine tube: the opening to the outside of the abdominal (peritoneal) cavity in the female (pg. 340). In the male the abdominal cavity is closed.

11. Inguinal canal: the cleft through the abdominal wall that allows blood vessels, nerves, and the spermatic cord to pass through the abdominal wall.

12. Vascular (lacunae) opening into femoral canal: the opening out of the abdominal cavity to the pelvic limb for passage of nerves and vessels.

13. PELVIC CAVITY (PEL-vik) or pelvis (L. basin): the space bounded by the two hip bones, the sacrum, and the first two caudal vertebrae. It contains the rectum, the anal canal, and the pelvic parts of the reproductive and urinary viscera.

Peritoneal part of the pelvic cavity: the cranial portion lined by pouches of the abdominal peritoneum.

Retroperitoneal part: the caudal portion not lined by abdominal peritoneum.

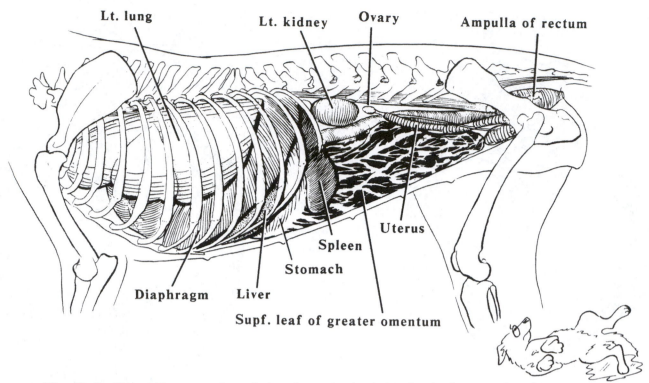

Fig. V-4 - Dog - Topography of the thoracic & abdominal viscera - lt. view

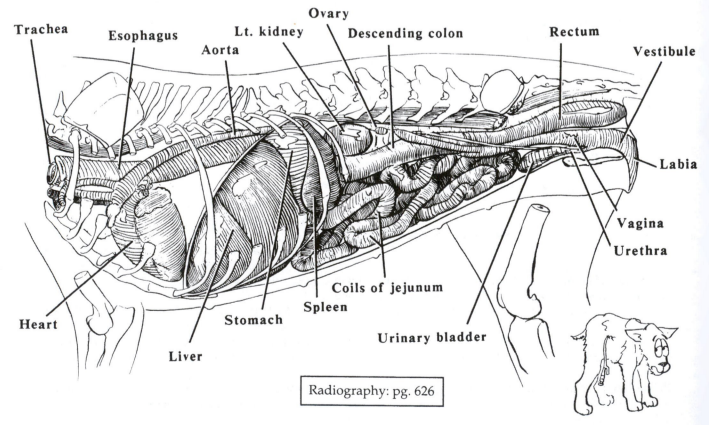

Radiography: pg. 626

Fig. V-5 - Dog - Topography of the deep thoracic & abdominal viscera - lt. view

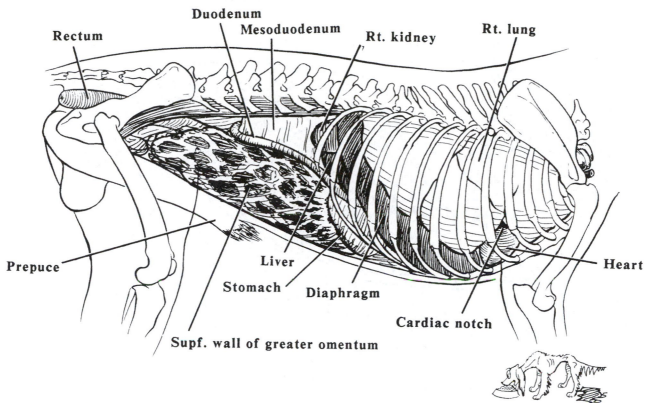

Rectum

Duodenum

Mesoduodenum

Rt. kidney

Rt. lung

Prepuce

Liver

Heart

Stomach

Diaphragm

Cardiac notch

Supf. wall of greater omentum

Fig. V-6 - Dog - Topography of the thoracic & abdominal viscera - rt. view

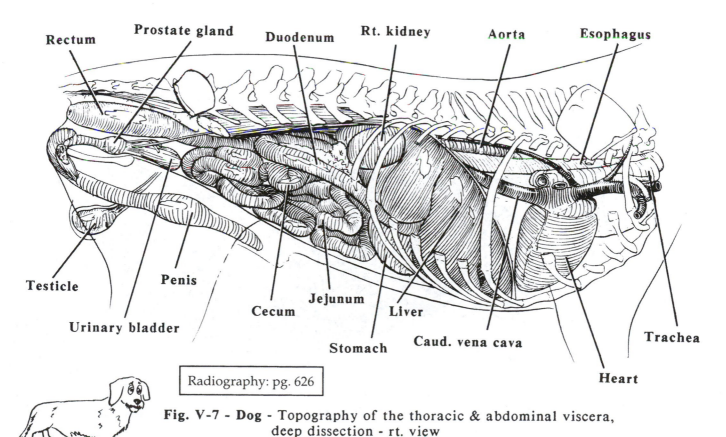

Rectum

Prostate gland

Duodenum

Rt. kidney

Aorta

Esophagus

Testicle

Penis

Urinary bladder

Cecum

Jejunum

Liver

Stomach

Caud. vena cava

Heart

Trachea

Radiography: pg. 626

Fig. V-7 - Dog - Topography of the thoracic & abdominal viscera, deep dissection - rt. view

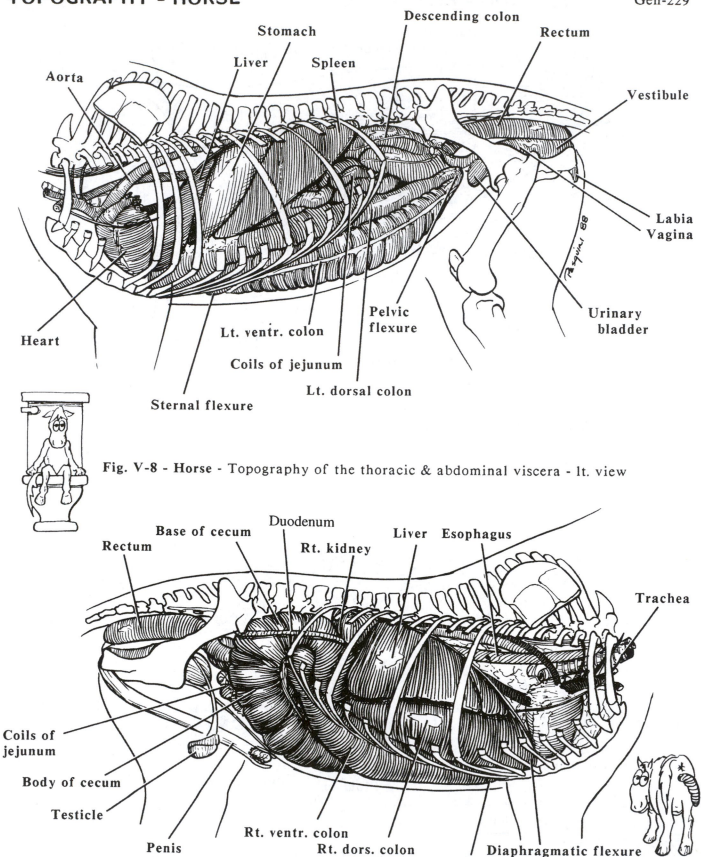

Fig. V-8 - Horse - Topography of the thoracic & abdominal viscera - lt. view

Fig. V-9 - Horse - Topography of the thoracic & abdominal viscera - rt. view

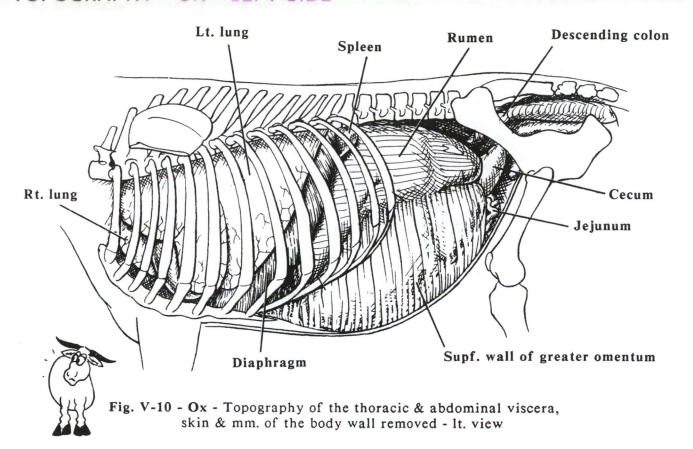

Fig. V-10 - Ox - Topography of the thoracic & abdominal viscera, skin & mm. of the body wall removed - lt. view

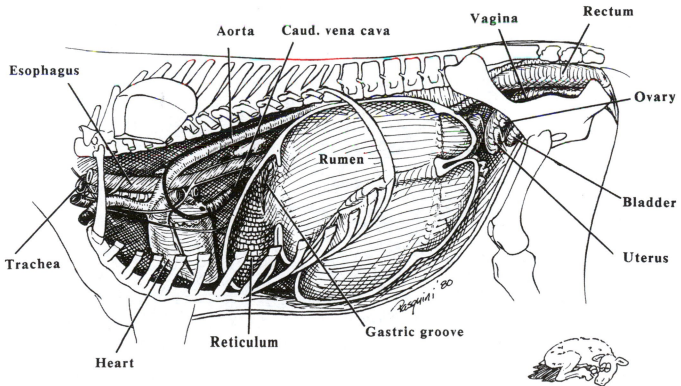

Fig. V-11 - Ox - Topography of the thoracic & abdominal viscera, lungs & diaphragm removed, rumen & reticulum opened - lt. view

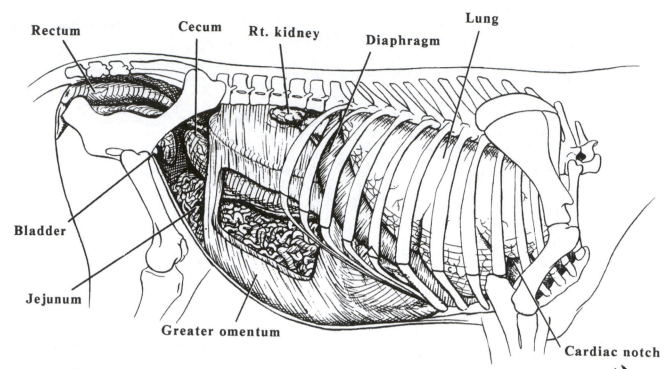

Fig. V-12 - Ox - Topography of the thoracic & abdominal viscera, skin & mm. of the body wall removed - ɪt. view

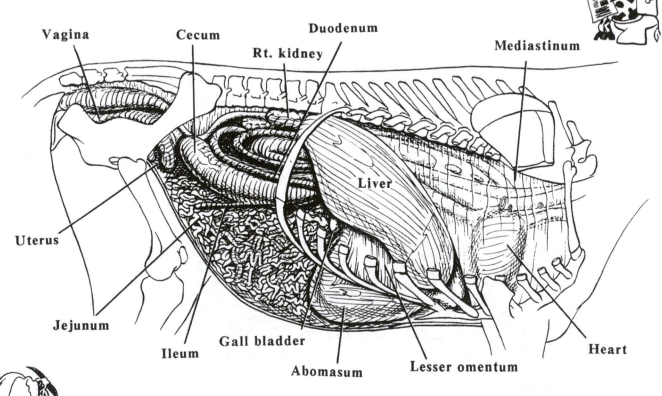

Authors note: Terrible drawings of small intestines, way too small & long!

Fig. V-13 - Ox - Topography of the thoracic & abdominal viscera, lungs, diaphragm, greater omentum & mesoduodenum removed - rt. view

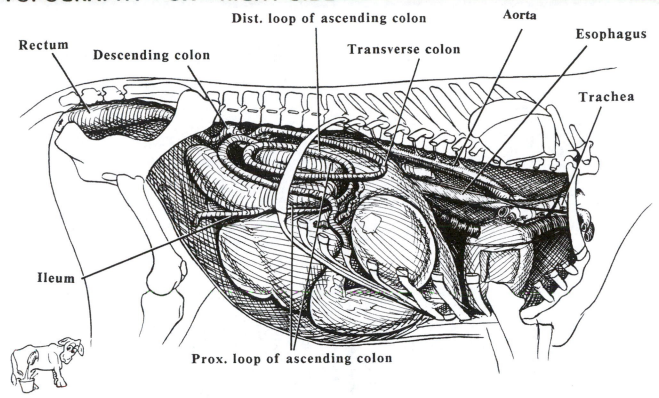

Fig. V-14 - Ox - Topography of the thoracic & abdominal viscera, mediastinum, liver, lesser omentum, rt. kidney, jejunum & reproductive tract removed - rt. view

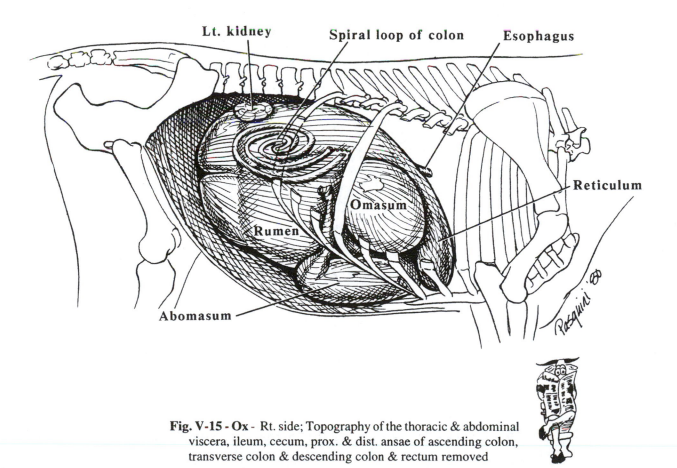

Fig. V-15 - Ox - Rt. side; Topography of the thoracic & abdominal viscera, ileum, cecum, prox. & dist. ansae of ascending colon, transverse colon & descending colon & rectum removed

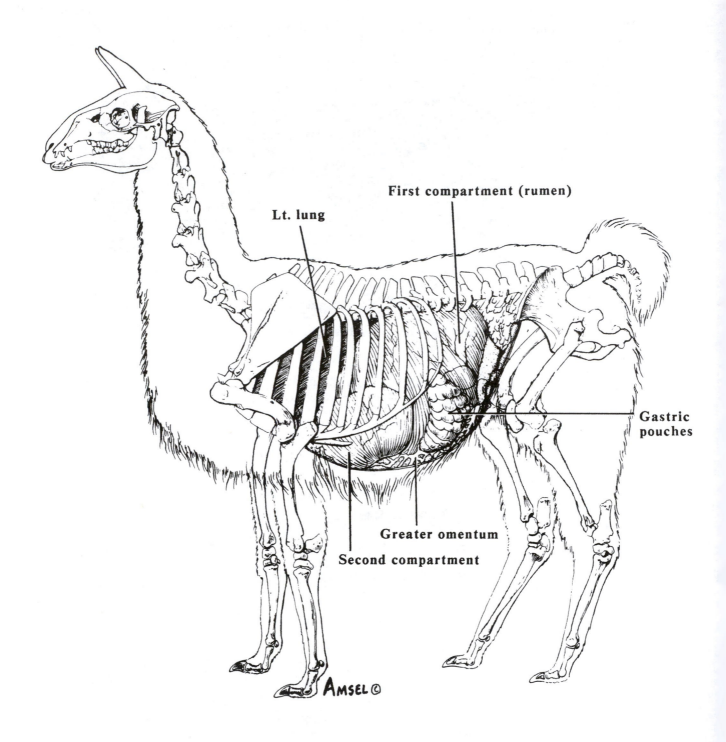

Fig. V-16 - Llama - Topography of the thoracic & abdominal viscera - lt. view

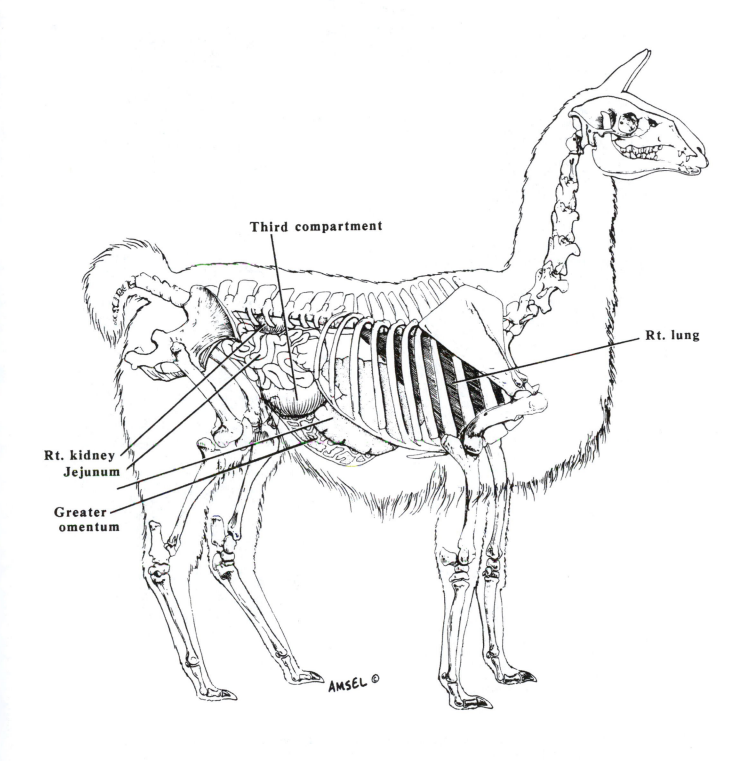

Third compartment

Rt. lung

Rt. kidney
Jejunum

Greater
omentum

AMSEL ©

Fig. V-17 - Llama - Topography of the thoracic & abdominal viscera - rt. view

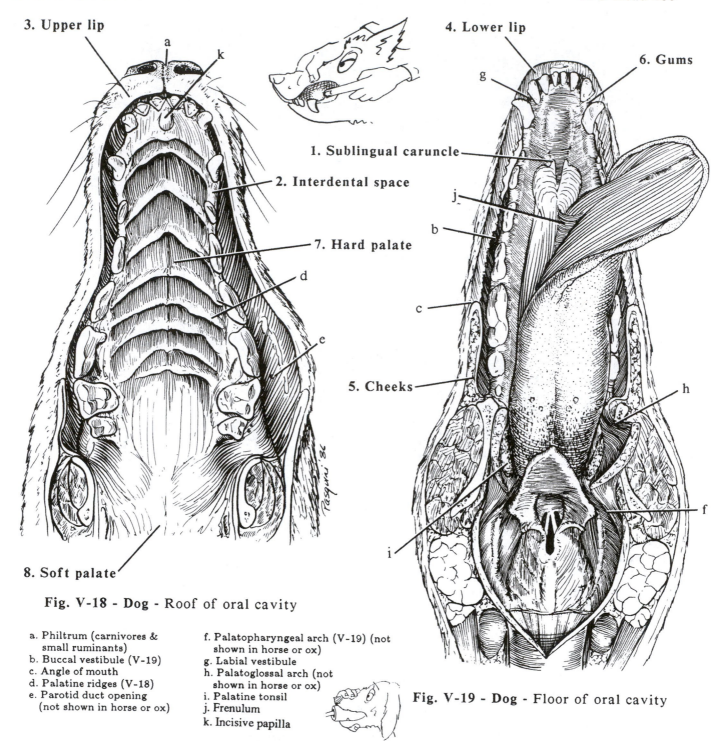

3. Upper lip

a

k

4. Lower lip

6. Gums

g

1. Sublingual caruncle

2. Interdental space

j

b

7. Hard palate

d

c

e

5. Cheeks

h

8. Soft palate

i

f

Fig. V-18 - Dog - Roof of oral cavity

a. Philtrum (carnivores & small ruminants)
b. Buccal vestibule (V-19)
c. Angle of mouth
d. Palatine ridges (V-18)
e. Parotid duct opening (not shown in horse or ox)
f. Palatopharyngeal arch (V-19) (not shown in horse or ox)
g. Labial vestibule
h. Palatoglossal arch (not shown in horse or ox)
i. Palatine tonsil
j. Frenulum
k. Incisive papilla

Fig. V-19 - Dog - Floor of oral cavity

MOUTH (os): a term designating either the opening between the lips (oral fissure, cleft) or the whole oral cavity.

ORAL CAVITY: the space extending from the lips to the pharynx, bounded laterally by the cheeks. It is divided into the oral cavity proper and the vestibule.

Labial vestibule (g): the space between the incisors and the lips.

Buccal vestibule (b): the space between the cheek teeth and the cheeks.

Frenulum (j): the central fold of mucous membrane connecting the floor of the oral cavity and the ventral surface of the tongue.

1. Sublingual caruncles: the mucosal elevations on the floor of the oral cavity, under the tongue just caudal to the incisors. The

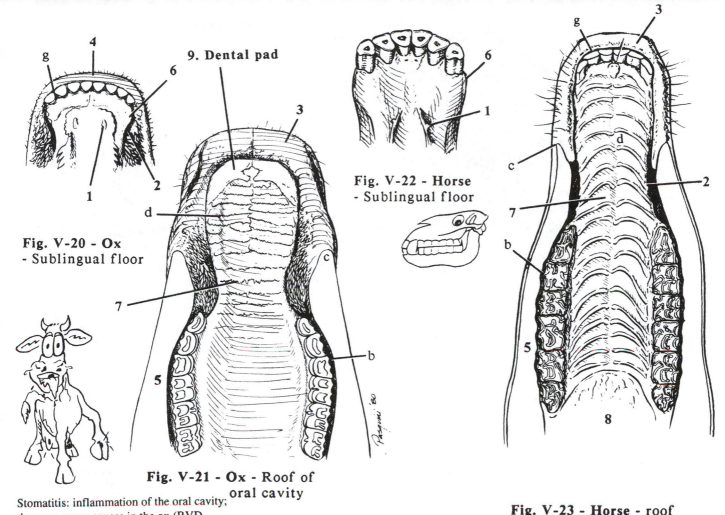

Fig. V-20 - Ox - Sublingual floor

9. Dental pad

Fig. V-21 - Ox - Roof of oral cavity

Fig. V-22 - Horse - Sublingual floor

Fig. V-23 - Horse - roof of oral cavity

Stomatitis: inflammation of the oral cavity; there are many causes in the ox (BVD, foot and mouth, Blue tongue, etc.)

mandibular and sublingual salivary ducts open on the caruncles (pg. 259).

2. Interdental spaces (diastemata, sin. = diastema): the spaces between the teeth.

3, 4. LIPS (L. *labium*, sin. = *labia*): the structures bounding the oral fissure. They possess long, tactile hair, and regular hair.

Philtrum (a): the median cleft of the upper lip in carnivores and small ruminants.

Angle of the mouth (c): where the upper and lower lips unite.

5. CHEEK (L. *mala, bucca*): the caudolateral wall of the oral cavity.

6. GUMS or gingivae (jin-JI-vee): the oral mucosa over the jaws, enclosing the necks of the teeth.

PALATE: the roof of the oral cavity and oropharynx composed of a rostral bony part (the hard palate) and a caudal musculomembranous part (the soft palate). The palate separates

the respiratory and the digestive passages in the head.

7. Hard palate (L. *palatum durum*): the osseous plate and its highly vascular mucosal covering that separates the oral and nasal cavities. The osseous plate is formed by processes of the palatine, maxillary and incisive bones. The hard palate is bounded rostrally and laterally by the upper dental arch and continues caudally as the soft palate. Just behind the incisors is the incisive papilla (k) onto which the incisive ducts open. The ducts connect the nasal and oral cavity, absent in the horse.

Palatine ridges: six to ten paired elevations crossing the hard palate transversely.

8. Soft palate (L. *palatum molle*): the caudal extension of the hard palate, dividing the rostral region of the pharynx into oral and nasal parts.

SPECIES DIFFERENCES

9. Dental pad: replaces the upper incisors and canines in ruminants. It provides a heavily cornified epithelium against which the lower incisors grind food.

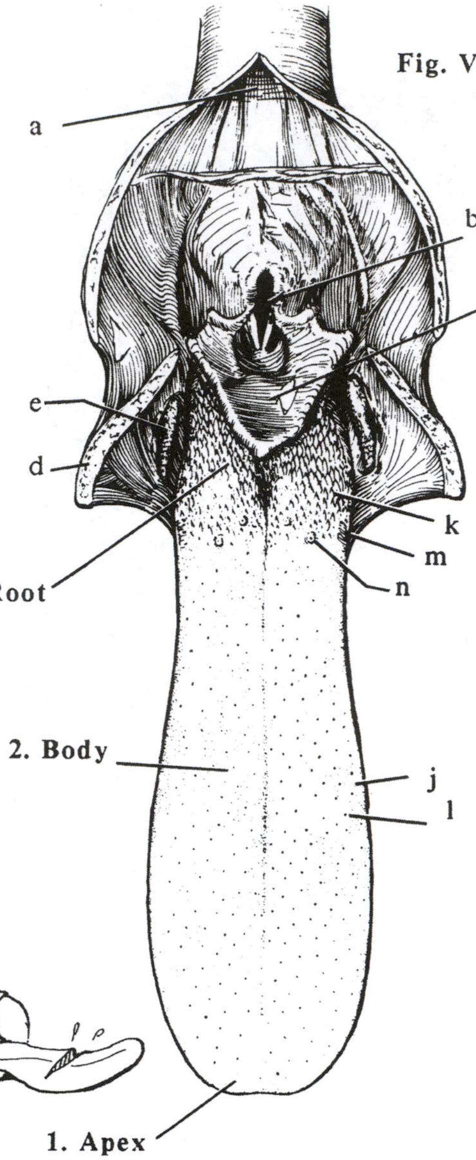

TONGUE

Fig. V-24 - **Dog** - Tongue & opened pharynx - dors. view

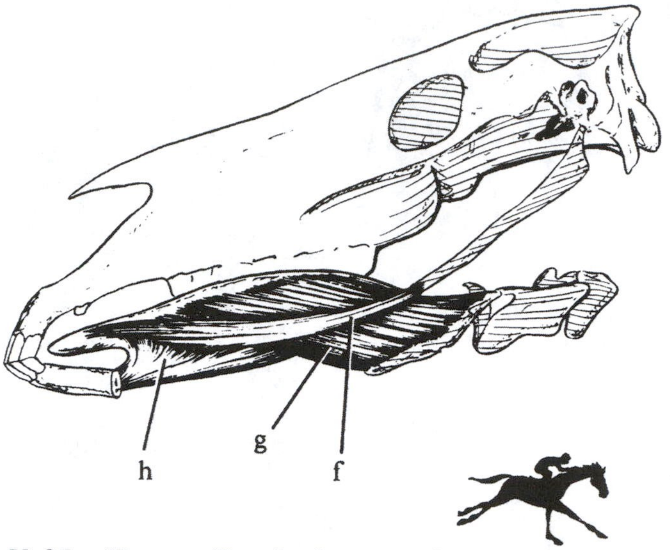

3. Root

2. Body

1. Apex

Fig. V-25 - **Horse** - Extrinsic mm. of the tongue

a. Esophagus
b. Laryngeal opening
c. Epiglottis
d. Soft palate
e. Palatine tonsil (carnivores)
f. Styloglossal m.
g. Hyglossal m.
h. Genioglossal m.

i. Tonsillar fossa (ox)
j. Filiform papillae
k. Conical papillae
l. Fungiform papillae
m. Foliate papillae (absent in ruminants)
n. Vallate papillae
o. Lenticular papillae (ruminants)

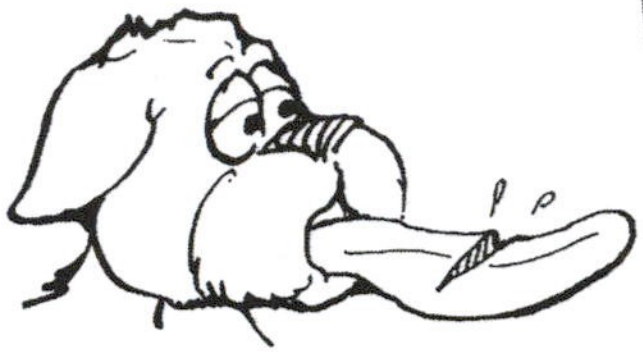

TONGUE (L. *lingua*, G. *glossa*): the muscular organ filling the oral cavity. The many papillae (pa-PIL-ee) on its dorsal surface are named according to their shape. These papillae have a mechanical or gustatory (GUS-ta-toh-ree) (taste) function, or both. Filiform (FIL-i-form) papillae (j), covering the tongue's dorsum, are thorn-shaped structures serving the mechanical function of directing food caudally. In the ox and cat they are heavily cornified. Conical (k) and lenticular papillae (o), cone-shaped papillae located on the caudal third of the tongue's dorsum also have a mechanical function. The mushroom-shaped fungiform (FUN-ji- form) papillae (l), scattered among the more numerous filiform papillae, have taste buds and are therefore gustatory as well as mechanical. Foliate papillae (m), a series of leaf-shaped ridges separated by furrows (crypts) on the lateral border of the tongue, are gustatory (absent in the ox). **Vallate papillae** (n), the largest and least numerous of the papillae, are rostral to the root of the tongue. They are circled by a cleft filled with taste buds. Marginal papillae along the edge of the rostral half of the newborn puppy's tongue function in suckling, helping to prevent milk from spilling over the tongue's sides. They disappear when the diet

changes from milk to solids. The papillae, although interesting, are of little clinical significance (Doc, my dog can't taste sweets anymore!). They, especially the vallate papillae, shouldn't be mistaken for pathology. The tongue, especially in the dog, aids in temperature control through heat loss by panting. The ox's tongue is a prehensile structure for gathering grass.

1. Apex: the rostral free end of the tongue.

2. Body: the major part of the tongue attaching to the mandible.

3. Root: the caudal end of the tongue, attaching to the hyoid apparatus.

INNERVATION OF THE TONGUE:

Taste (special sense): the sense of taste to the rostral two thirds of the tongue is carried over the chorda tympani nerve, a branch of the facial nerve (Cn VII). Taste from the caudal third of the tongue passes by the glossopharyngeal (Cn IX) and vagus (Cn X) nerves.

Sensation (pain, temperature and tactile): carried over the lingual branch of the mandibular nerve (Cn V).

Motor innervation: via the hypoglossal nerve (Cn XII).

TONGUE

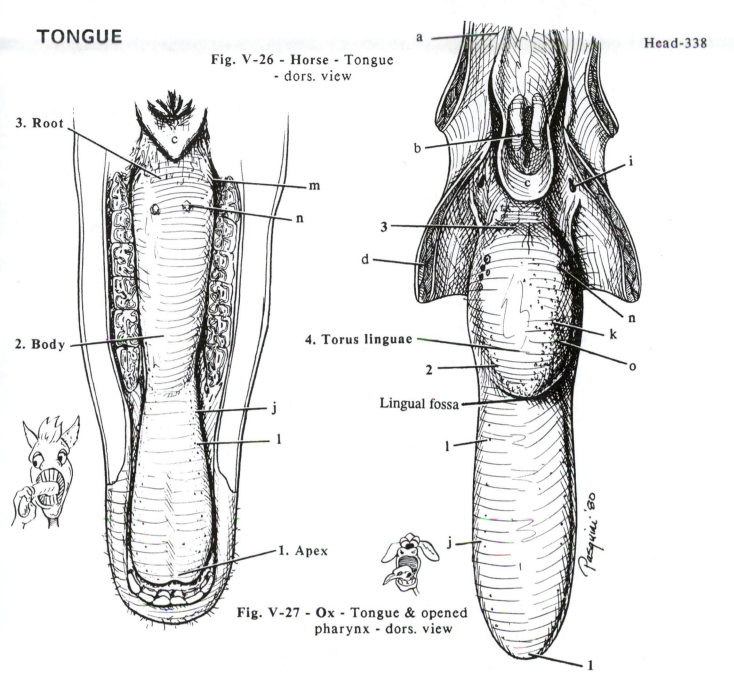

Fig. V-26 - Horse - Tongue - dors. view

3. Root

m

n

2. Body

j

l

1. Apex

a

b

c

i

3

d

n

k

4. Torus linguae

2

Lingual fossa

l

o

j

1

Pasquini '80

Fig. V-27 - Ox - Tongue & opened pharynx - dors. view

MUSCLES of the TONGUE can be divided into intrinsic and extrinsic lingual muscles. The intrinsic muscles of the tongue or the lingual muscles proper are the many muscular bundles running in diverse directions to form the bulk of the tongue. They cause subtle changes in the shape of the tongue during swallowing, chewing, and vocalization. The extrinsic muscles of the tongue, anchoring it to the skeleton, are the paired styloglossal (f), hyoglossal (g) and genioglossal (h) muscles; they are responsible for its gross movements. In addition, because the tongue is attached to the hyoid apparatus, the muscles attaching to the hyoid bone (-hyoideus) also move the tongue.

SPECIES DIFFERENCES

4. Torus linguae (L. *torus* swelling): a round swelling of the caudodorsal surface of the ox's tongue.

5. Lingual fossa or fossa linguae: depression in front of the ox's

torus linguae. This is a site of penetration of foreign objects.

Tongue cartilage: the dog has a bar of cartilage (lyssa) embedded in the ventral surface of the apex. The **horse** has a similar structure embedded in the median plane of the dorsal surface.

CLINICAL

Bovine tongue: a prehensile organ, therefore, its amputation should be avoided.

Tongue trauma: common in indiscriminately eating cattle. Foreign body penetration common in transverse groove in front of torus linguae.

Wodden tongue: infection of Actinobacillosis bacteria causing swelling and hardening of tongue in cattle

TEETH

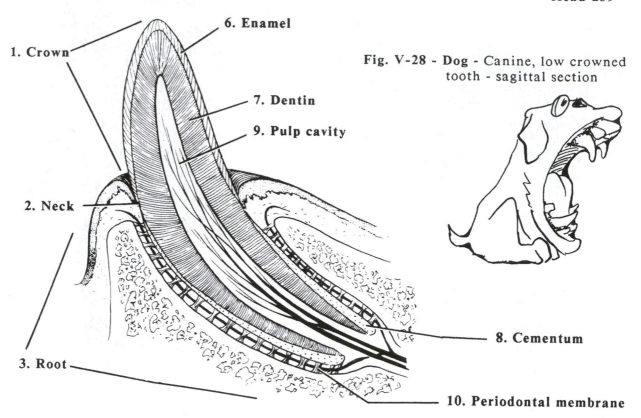

1. Crown
6. Enamel
7. Dentin
9. Pulp cavity
2. Neck
3. Root
8. Cementum
10. Periodontal membrane

Fig. V-28 - Dog - Canine, low crowned tooth - sagittal section

TEETH or dentes (sin. = dens): perform the principle function of mastication, but also aid in food gathering (prehension) and are formidable weapons in some species.

Dental arches: arrangement of teeth into two opposing superior (upper) and inferior (lower) arches. The domestic species have two types of teeth – brachydont and hypsodont.

Low-crowned or **brachydont teeth** (Gr. *brachys* short + *odous* tooth): the simple teeth of man, carnivores, pig, ruminant's incisors and horse's deciduous incisors. They consist of a crown, neck and root.

1. Crown: the part projecting above the gum line covered with enamel.

2. Neck: the constriction between the crown and the root at the gum line.

3. Root: the part below the gum line embedded in the alveoli (bony sockets) of the incisive, mandible or maxillary bones.

High-crowned or **hypsodont teeth** (HIP-so-dont)(Gr. *hypsos* height + *odous* tooth) (evergrowing): the teeth having no distinct neck, as seen in all permanent horse teeth, the ruminant cheek teeth and the tusks of pigs. With the exception of the horse's canine teeth, they continue to erupt throughout life.

4. Body: different from low-crowned teeth because of the absence of a neck. Some anatomists divide the body into a **crown** (the exposed part of the tooth above the gum line) and a **body** (the embedded part below the gum line).

5. Root: the short, proximal part of the tooth.

STRUCTURE of TEETH: composed of three substances from outward in – cementum, enamel, and dentin.

6. Enamel (ee-NAM-el): the hardest substance in the body.
• Low-crowned (brachydont) teeth: the enamel covers only the crown.
• High-crowned (hypsodont) teeth: enamel envelops the body (crown & body), but not the root.

7. Dentin (ivory): a hard substance similar to bone forming the bulk of the tooth and surrounding the pulp cavity.

8. Cementum (see-MEN-tum): a thin, bone-like covering.
• Low-crowned (brachydont) teeth: the cementum covers the root only.
• High-crowned (hypsodont) teeth: covers the entire tooth, superficial to the enamel.

9. Pulp cavity: the central space of the tooth containing the pulp.

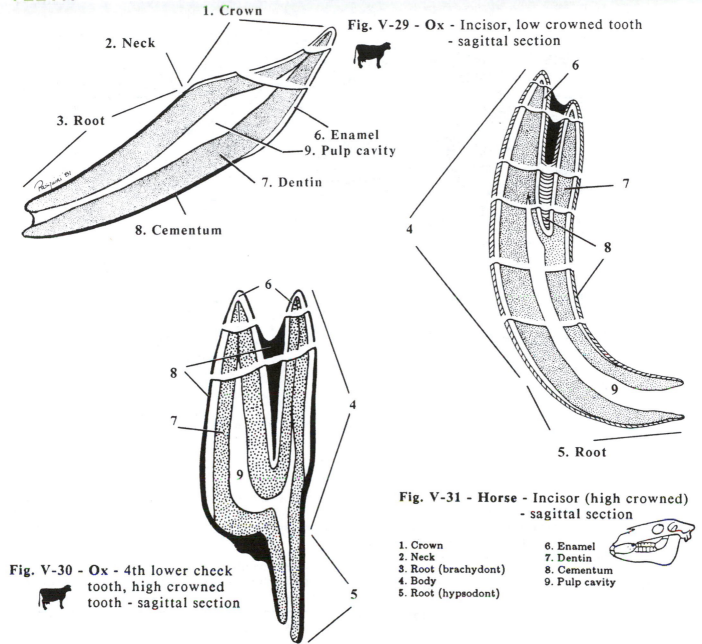

Fig. V-29 - Ox - Incisor, low crowned tooth
- sagittal section

1. Crown
2. Neck
3. Root
6. Enamel
9. Pulp cavity
7. Dentin
8. Cementum
6
7
4
8
9
5. Root

Fig. V-30 - Ox - 4th lower check
tooth, high crowned
tooth - sagittal section

6
8
7
9
4
5

Fig. V-31 - Horse - Incisor (high crowned)
- sagittal section

1. Crown
2. Neck
3. Root (brachydont)
4. Body
5. Root (hypsodont)

6. Enamel
7. Dentin
8. Cementum
9. Pulp cavity

PULP: the soft tissue filling the pulp cavity, including sensory nerves, arteries, veins, lymphatics, and primitive connective tissue.

CUSPS (L. points): the individual bumps on the occlusal (chewing) surface of teeth.

ALVEOLI (al-VEE-oh-ly) (sin.= alveolus hollow): the bony sockets of the incisive, mandible, and maxillary bones in which the roots of teeth are embedded.

• Lamina dura: the thin shell of dense bone lining the alveoli. It shows up radiographically separated from the tooth roots by the radiolucent periodontal membrane. Radiographic loss of the lamina dura indicates problems.

10. PERIODONTAL MEMBRANE (per-ee-oh-DON-tal): the dense fibrous connective tissue connecting the wall of the alveoli and the cementum covering the teeth.

GOMPHOSIS (gom-FOH-sis): the proper name for the implantation of teeth in the alveoli. This is not a true joint because the teeth are not part of the skeleton.

"OVERSHOT" (prognathia): an elongated jaw (mandible).

"UNDERSHOT" (brachygnathia [brak-ig-NAY-thee-ah]): a shortened jaw (mandible).

TEETH

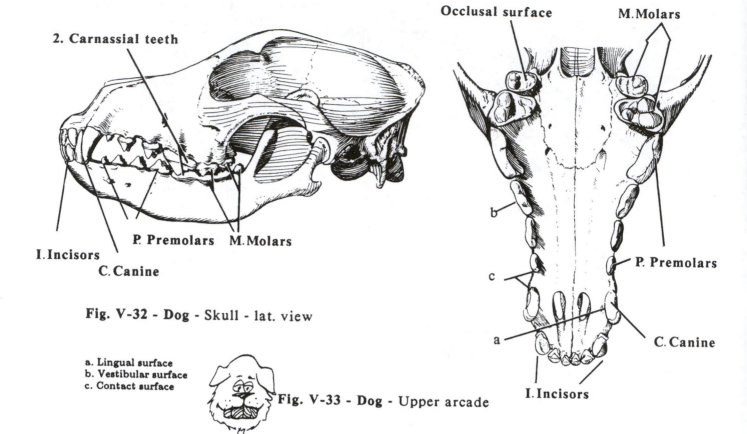

Fig. V-32 - Dog - Skull - lat. view

a. Lingual surface
b. Vestibular surface
c. Contact surface

Fig. V-33 - Dog - Upper arcade

INCISORS, CANINES, PREMOLARS and **MOLARS**: The teeth are divided into groups by their location and function: incisors, canines, premolars and molars. Each tooth has a number of surfaces. The **vestibular surface** (b) faces the lips or cheeks. The **lingual surface** (a) faces the tongue. **The contact surface** (c) is the side adjacent to the next tooth. The **mesial contact surface** faces the median plane on the incisors, and rostrally on the canine and cheek teeth. The **distal contact surface** faces away from the median plane on the incisors, and caudally on the canine and cheek teeth.

Occlusal or **masticatory surface** (L. *occlusio* to close up): faces the opposite dental arch and is where "chewing" takes place.

I. Incisors (I) (cutters): the rostral-most teeth embedded in the incisive bone (upper) and the mandible's incisive part (lower).

C. Canine (C) (L. *canis* dog) (piercers): the large tooth between the incisors and the cheek teeth.

Cheek teeth (grinders): a general term for the teeth caudal to the canine and incisors in the maxillary

  P. Premolars (P): the rostral cheek teeth.

  M. Molars (M): the caudal cheek teeth.

DECIDUOUS and **PERMANENT TEETH**: the two sets of teeth in all the domestic species. The eruption of both groups is orderly and may be used to estimate the animal's age.

Deciduous dentition: the "baby teeth" ("milk teeth") developing early in life, giving the young animal a functional set of teeth. They are smaller and fewer in number than the permanent dentition.

Permanent dentition: the second set of teeth replacing the deciduous dentition as the jaw lengthens. They must last the life of the animal.

SPECIES DIFFERENCES

Carnassial (sectorial) teeth: the large, shearing teeth of both the **dog** and **cat**. They are the upper 4th premolar (P4) and the lower 1st molar (Ml).

Tusks (Fig. V-43): the canine teeth of the pig. The lower tusks are larger than the upper, and the boar's are larger than the sow's.

"Wolf teeth": the horse's rudimentary upper first premolars. They are usually absent.

CLINICAL

Carnassial tooth abscess (Upper P4): results in swelling or draining (pus) below the carnivore's eye. Since it has three roots in both dogs and cats it should be split when extracted. If not, because the roots diverge, a root may break off.

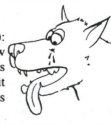

TEETH

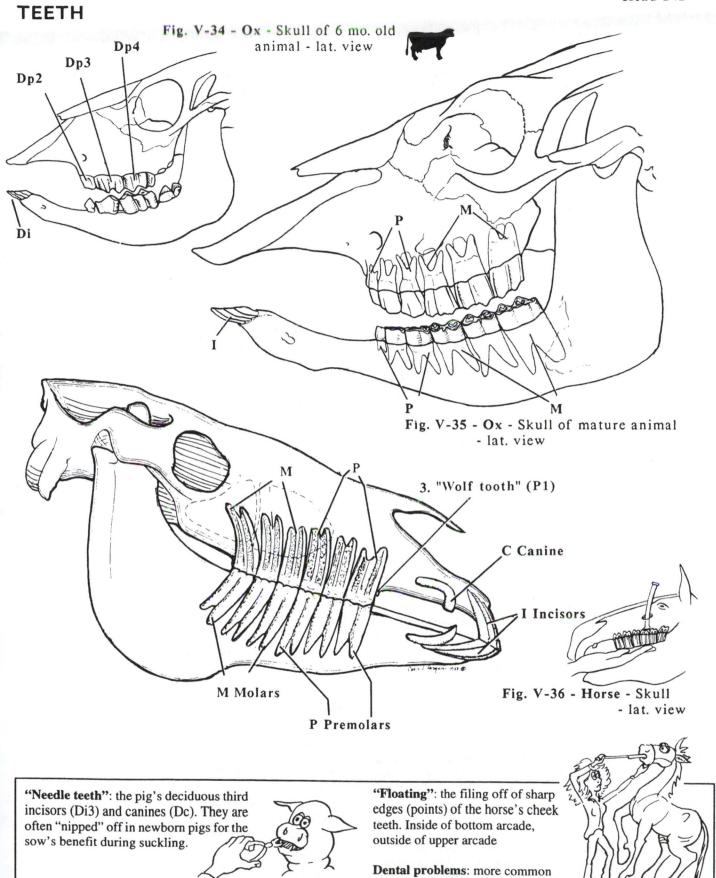

Fig. V-34 - Ox - Skull of 6 mo. old animal - lat. view

Dp2
Dp3
Dp4
Di

P   M

I

Fig. V-35 - Ox - Skull of mature animal - lat. view

P   M

M   P

3. "Wolf tooth" (P1)

C Canine

I Incisors

M Molars

P Premolars

Fig. V-36 - Horse - Skull - lat. view

"Needle teeth": the pig's deciduous third incisors (Di3) and canines (Dc). They are often "nipped" off in newborn pigs for the sow's benefit during suckling.

"Floating": the filing off of sharp edges (points) of the horse's cheek teeth. Inside of bottom arcade, outside of upper arcade

Dental problems: more common in horses than in cattle.

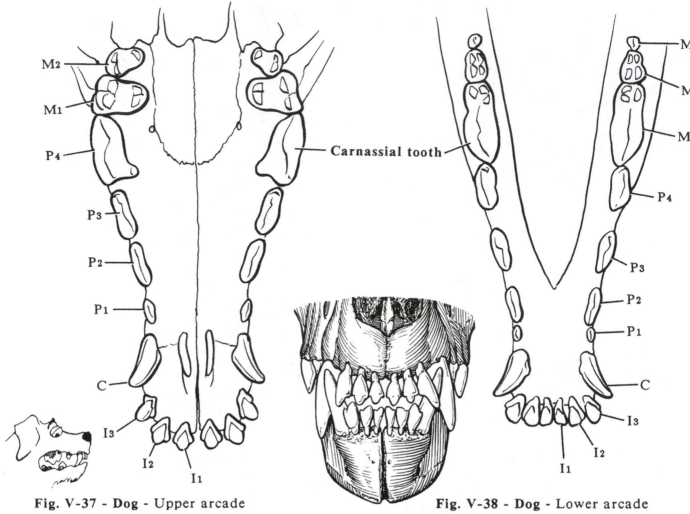

Fig. V-37 - Dog - Upper arcade

Fig. V-38 - Dog - Lower arcade

DENTAL FORMULA: a shorthand representation indicating the number of teeth of an animal. Due to bilateral symmetry, only half of each dental arcade is numbered in the formula's parenthesis. The total number in the parentheses multiplied by the "2" gives the total number of teeth. The permanent teeth are represented by capital letters (Incisors=I, Canines=C, Premolars=PM or P and Molars=M). In the fraction following each letter, the numerator represents half the number of upper jaw teeth and the denominator half those in the lower jaw.

DECIDUOUS DENTAL FORMULA: identical to the permanent formula except the premolar one (Pm1) and the molars have no predecessors. Deciduous teeth are represented by lower case letters following a "D".

SPECIES DIFFERENCES: The generalized pattern of 44 permanent teeth is seen only in the pig. The other domestic species have fewer teeth due to reduction in the number of cheek teeth, except the ruminants which are also missing the

upper incisors and canines. If premolars are missing, the more rostral ones are affected; if molars, the more caudal ones are affected (**P4 is always next to M1**).

Pig: has a full mouth of 44 permanent teeth.

Dog: missing upper M3 and therefore, has 42 teeth. Brachiocephalic breeds may be missing more teeth, so the dental formula for dogs is not constant, as it is in cats.

Horse: usually missing the upper P1 (wolf tooth) and always missing lower P1. In the mare, the canines often are small and may not erupt. With all these variations, the horse may possess from 36 to 42 permanent teeth. Deciduous canines are usually vestigial and seldom erupt, thus, only 24 deciduous teeth.

Ruminants: missing the upper incisors and canines; replaced by a dental pad. They also lack upper and lower P1, giving them 32 permanent teeth.

TEETH

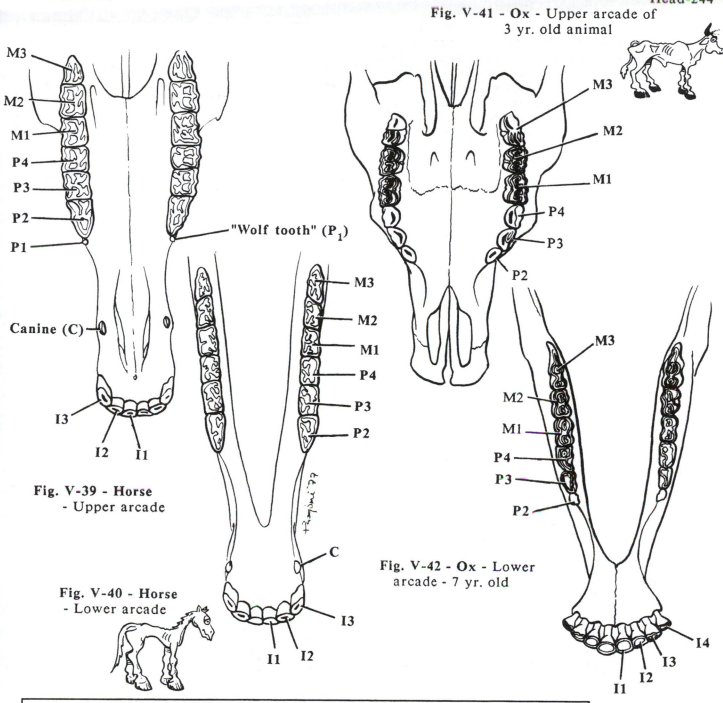

Fig. V-41 - Ox - Upper arcade of 3 yr. old animal

Fig. V-39 - Horse - Upper arcade

Fig. V-40 - Horse - Lower arcade

Fig. V-42 - Ox - Lower arcade - 7 yr. old

Species	Permanent	Deciduous
PIG	2(I 3/3 C 1/1 P 4/4 M 3/3) = 44	2(I 3/3 C 1/1 P 3/3) = 28
DOG	2(I 3/3 C 1/1 P 4/4 M 2/3) = 42	2(I 3/3 C 1/1 P 3/3) = 28
HORSE	2(I 3/3 C 1(0)/1(0) P 3(4)/3 M3/3) = 36-42	2(I 3/3 C 0/0 P 3/3) = 24
RUMINANT	2(I 0/4 P 3/3 M 3/3) = 32	2(I 0/4 P 3/3) =20
CAT	2(I 3/3 C1/1 P 3/2 M 1/1) =30	2(I 3/3 C 1/1 P 3/2) = 26

Different diets of the domestic species have resulted in evolution of different forms of teeth. The carnivores tear and bolt their fleshy food with little chewing. Their teeth reflect this in being sharp, tearing structures. The molars of the dog, which do more chewing than the cat, have a flattened occlusal surface. For the horse and ruminant's grazing diet (herbivores), the cheek teeth have enlarged and merged into a continuous occlusal surface. This accommodates the continuous grinding mastication with considerable wear.

Pig - aging teeth	Eruption
Di3	**Before birth**
Dc	**Before birth**
Remaining deciduous teeth	4 days - 7 wk.
Permanent	
P1	5 mo.
M1	4-6 mo.
Remaining permanent teeth	8-20 mo.

Fig. V-43 - Pig - Upper arcade

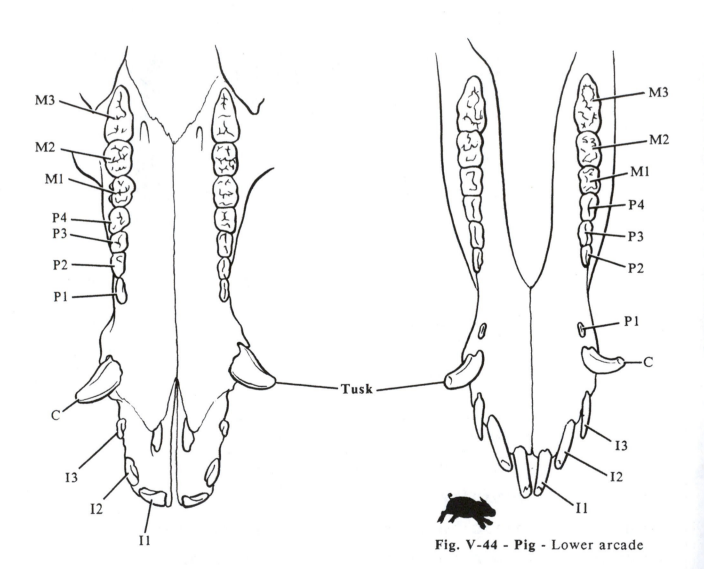

Fig. V-44 - Pig - Lower arcade

Dog – Aging teeth	Age
Deciduous teeth erupt	**By 6 weeks**
Permanent teeth erupt	**By 6 months**
Cusps worn off incisors	
Lower I1	1 1/2 yrs.
Lower I2	2 1/2 yrs.
Upper I1	3 1/2 yrs.
Upper I2	4 1/2 yrs.
Lower I3	6 yrs.
Incisors absent	16 yrs.
Canines absent	20 yrs.

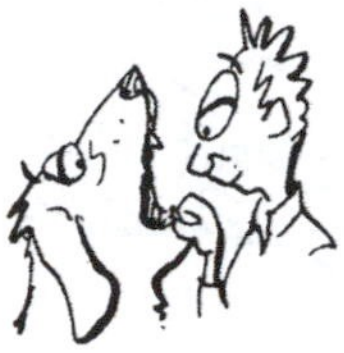

CANINE DECIDUOUS DENTITION: For the first 3 weeks of life, the puppy has no teeth. By 6 weeks all its deciduous teeth have erupted. As the puppy's jaw grows the permanent teeth begin to replace the deciduous teeth and have all erupted by 6-7 months. This is useful information because puppy shots are usually given around 6 weeks and around 6 months dogs are spayed. There are no deciduous premolars for P1 and the molars.

Fig. V-46 - Cat - Lower arcade

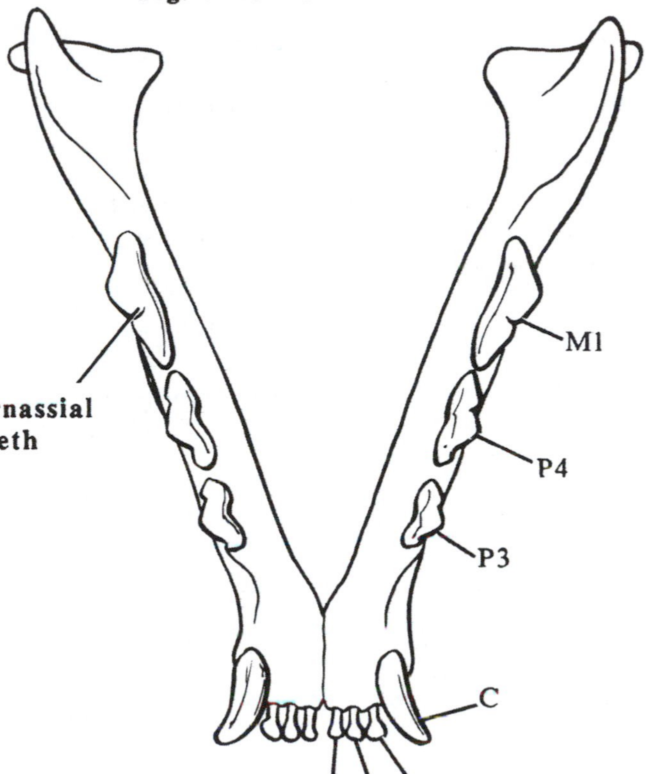

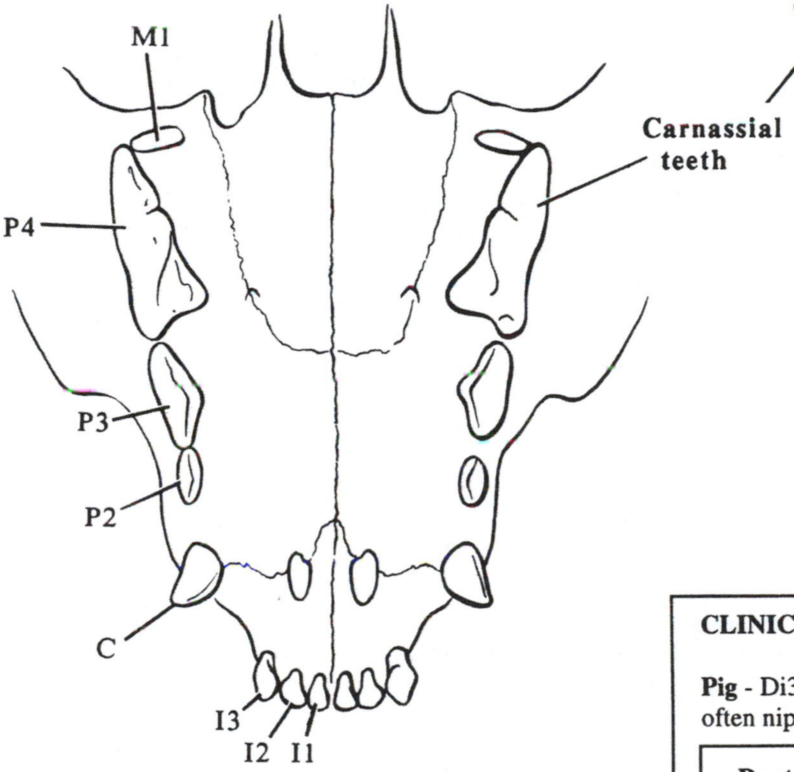

Carnassial teeth

M1

P4

P3

C

I1 I2 I3

M1

P4

P3

P2

C

I3

I2 I1

Fig. V-45 - Cat - Upper arcade

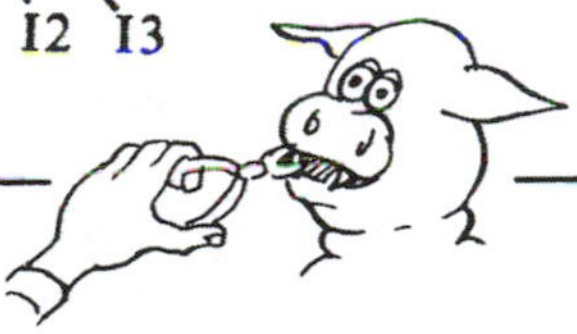

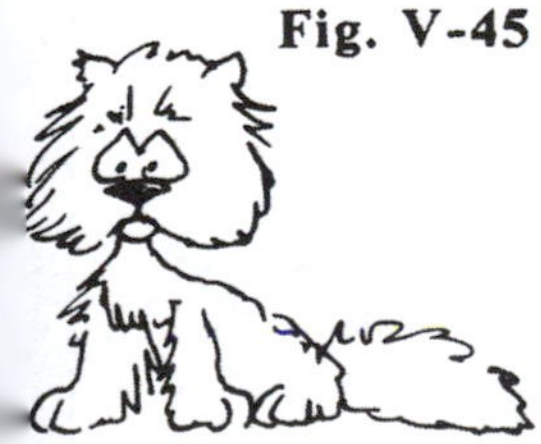

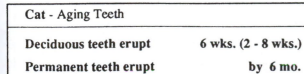

Cat - Aging Teeth	
Deciduous teeth erupt	6 wks. (2 - 8 wks.)
Permanent teeth erupt	by 6 mo.

CLINICAL

Pig - Di3 and Dc ("needle teeth") erupt before birth and are often nipped off to prevent injuries to others.

Roots of cheek teeth:

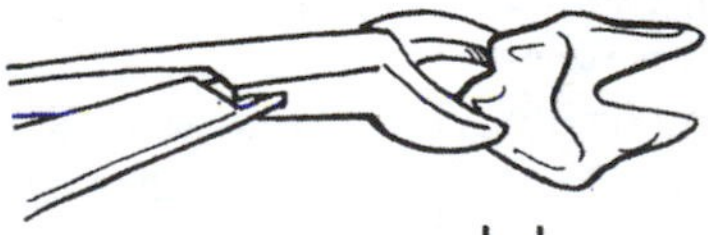

Dog - This is important in teeth extractions.
Upper
1st 1 has 1
Next 2 have 2
Last 3 have 3
Lower
First and last has 1
The rest have 2

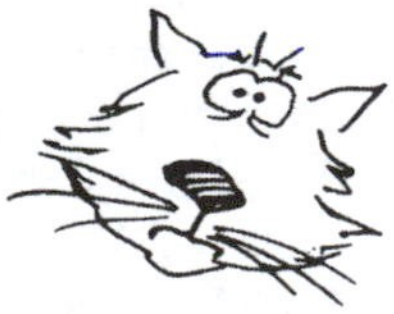

Cat - three roots are found in upper P4 (carnassial tooth) and in upper Dp3 and Dp4.

HORSE TEETH

HORSE TEETH (adult): typically herbivorous (grass eating) dentition with high crowned (hypsodont) teeth that, except for the canines, grow throughout life.

HORSE INCISORS: are numbered I1, I2 and I3 or central, intermediate, and corner incisors respectively. Each incisor is curved with the concavity on its lingual side.

I1. Central incisor: the 1st incisor, closest to the median plane.

I2. Intermediate incisor: the 2nd incisor.

I3. Corner incisor: the 3rd, most lateral incisor.

STRUCTURE: the horse's incisors are composed of three substances - dentin, enamel and cementum. With wear, the different structures on the occlusal surface of the teeth appear, giving clues to the age of the animal.

Eruption: the emergence of a tooth through the gum line.

1. Cup, infundibulum or **"mark"**: the deep depression in the occlusal surface, lined by cementum and enamel. The cup is usually filled with black decaying material.

2. Enamel spot: the enamel at the bottom of the cup. When the cup is worn away, the spot remains for a while. Harder than the surrounding dentin, it is raised above the dentin.

3. Dental star: the darker, secondary dentin filling the pulp cavity as the occlusal surface nears it. The star first appears rostral to the enamel spot. As the spot disappears, the star becomes centrally located.

In wear: the removal of enamel due to contact of opposing teeth. A small area of yellow dentin surrounded by white enamel results.

Level: the flattening of the occlusal surface, showing the formation of two enamel rings separated by dentin. The outer enamel ring surrounds the entire tooth and the inner ring the infundibulum (cup).

SHAPE OF THE OCCLUSAL SURFACE - INCISORS: changes with age due to the long, curved, pyramidal shape of the incisors. The distal end is flattened rostrocaudally. The base is flattened from side to side. As the teeth wear, the shape of the occlusal surface changes. The young animal has a transverse oval surface. With wear it becomes round, then triangular, and finally longitudinally oval or rectangular.

CHEEK TEETH: premolar and molar teeth. They are rectangular with infoldings of enamel on their occlusal surface. Together they form a continuous grinding surface. They continue to grow after they come into wear. Isolated cheek teeth are indistinguishable from each other, except for the wolf tooth, P2 and M3. The upper arcade is wider than the lower causing wear to occur on the inside (lingual edge) of the upper teeth and on the outside (labial edge) of the lower teeth resulting in "points" on the outside edge of the upper teeth and inside edge of lower teeth. The occlusal surface slants down and out (ventrobuccally).

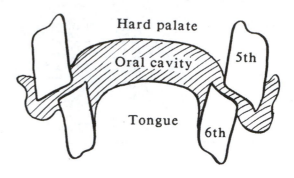

Fig. V-47 - Horse - Cross section through 5th upper cheek tooth & 6th lower cheek tooth

Horse - Cheek teeth	
Teeth	**Eruption**
P1	**5-6 months**
P2	**2-2 1/2 years**
P3	**3 years**
P4	**4 years**
M1	**1 year**
M2	**2 years**
M3	**3 1/2-4 years**

CLINICAL

"Floating": the periodic filing off of the points of a horse's cheek teeth.

Points:
- Outside edge of the upper teeth
- Inside edge of the lower teeth

Cap: a deciduous tooth remaining attached to its permanent replacement. The only teeth affected are Dp2, Dp3 and Dp4.

Memory aid - Since the deciduous premolars are roughly replaced the year corresponding to their number, expect to see caps at those times.	
Dp2 cap	**2 to 2 1/2 years**
Dp3 cap	**3 years**
Dp4 cap	**4 years**

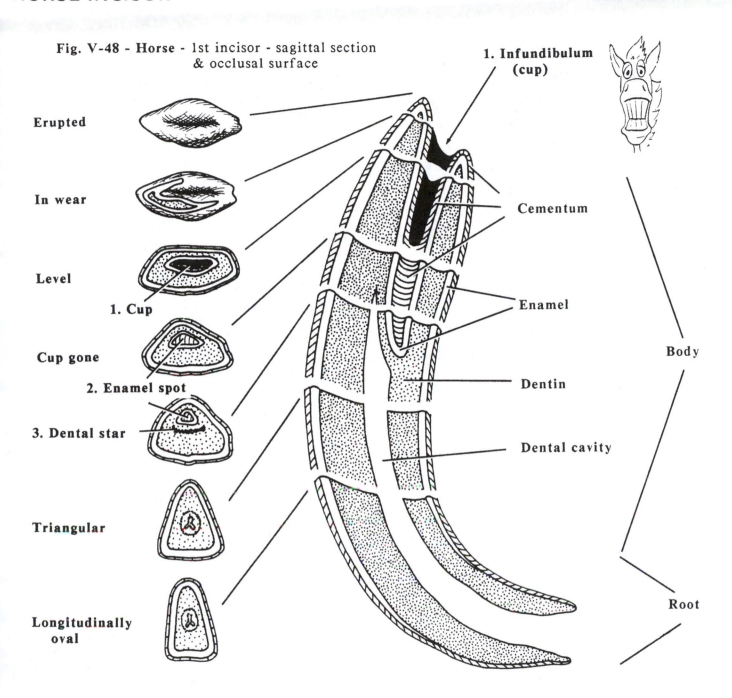

Fig. V-48 - Horse - 1st incisor - sagittal section
& occlusal surface

1. **Infundibulum (cup)**

Erupted

In wear

Level

1. Cup

Cup gone

2. Enamel spot

3. Dental star

Triangular

Longitudinally oval

Cementum

Enamel

Dentin

Dental cavity

Body

Root

HORSE TEETH - TERMS

Scissor mouth: when viewed from the front, an oblique angle to the incisors' occlusal surface due to uneven wear.

Shear mouth: a narrow lower dental arch requiring frequent floating (knocking off of points).

Step mouth: an uneven occlusal plane of the cheek teeth due to lack of wear of one or more of the teeth.

Wave mouth: a subtle form of step mouth.

Sow mouth: an elongated mandible ("overshot" or prognathia).

Parrot mouth: a shortened mandible ("undershot" or brachygnathia).

Bishoping: the altering of an older horse's teeth to make it look younger. A common technique is drilling and staining false cups.

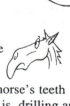
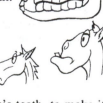

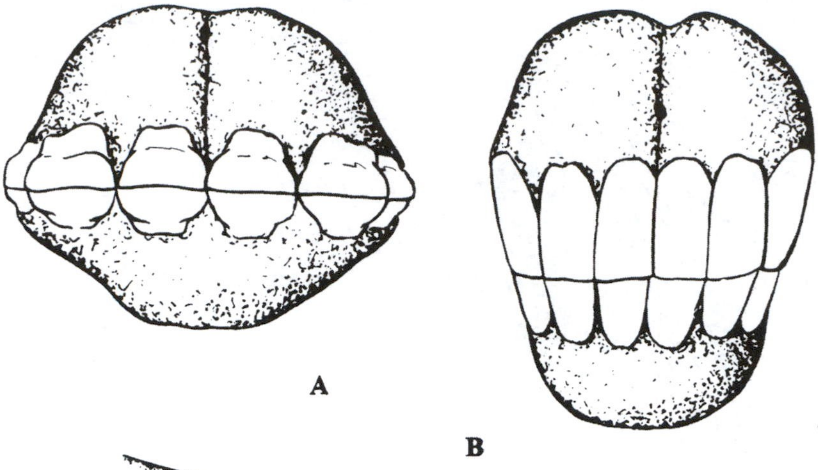

Fig. V-49 - Horse - Incisors - rostr. view

A. Two year old, deciduous incisors
B. Five year old, permanent incisors

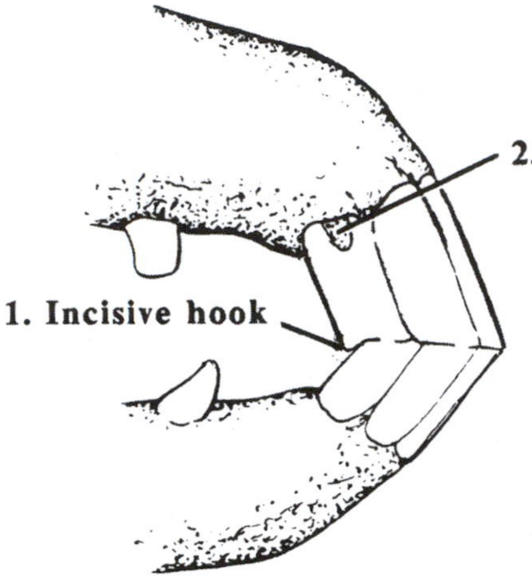

A

B

Pasquini '78

2. Galvayne's groove

1. Incisive hook

Fig. V-50 - **Horse** - Incisors of 11 yr.
old animal - lat. view

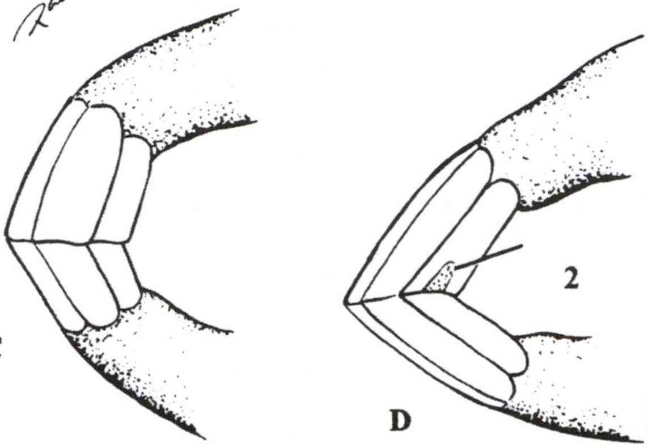

C

D

2

Fig. V-51 - **Horse** - Incisors - lat. view

C. Five year old
D. Twenty-five year old

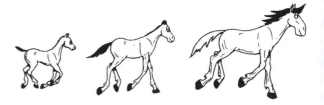

ROUGH ESTIMATE of a HORSE'S AGE: Certain structures and appearances can give an estimate of the horse's age. They are **unreliable** and should be used in conjunction with eruption and wear times.

Angle of the permanent incisors: the angle the upper and lower incisors meet when viewed from the side. Because of the incisor's curved shape, more pronounced on its proximal end, the angle formed by opposing incisors is roughly 180° in a young animal. With age, wear makes this angle more and more acute (< 180°).

1. Seven year (incisive) **hook**: the bulge on the caudal end of the upper corner incisor. It forms because the bottom corner incisor doesn't wear the entire occlusal surface of the upper one. The hook is said to appear at 7 years, disappear at 9 years and reappear at 11 years of age. It may or may not be present. If present, all that can be said is that the horse is probably older than 7 years (unreliable).

2. Galvayne's groove: a long groove on the middle of the upper corner incisor's labial surface. Wear from the lips removes the cementum of the tooth, except in the groove, leaving the white enamel surrounding the darker cementum in the groove. The groove is said to appear under the gum line at 10 years of age, half way down the tooth at 15, reaches the occlusal surface at 20, and disappears at 30. If present, the horse is probably over 10 years old. (Very subjective and unreliable.)

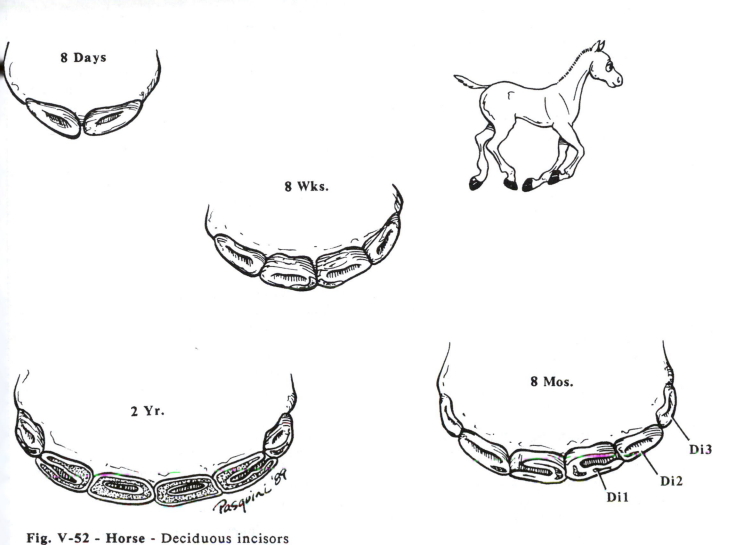

Fig. V-52 - Horse - Deciduous incisors
- occlusal surface

DECIDUOUS INCISORS			
	Di$_1$ (central)	Di$_2$ (intermediate)	Di$_3$ (corner)
Erupts	8 days	8 weeks	8 months
In Wear	1 year	1 year	2 years

AGE of the NEWBORN HORSE: deciduous incisors, smaller than permanent incisors, have a definite **neck** (low crowned - brachyodont teeth). A horse with deciduous incisors is less than 2 1/2 years of age. For easy recall, 8 days, 8 weeks, and 8 months or 7-7-7 can be used for eruption of Di1, Di2 and Di3, respectively (1 week, 1 month and 8 months is more correct). At 1 year, Di1 and Di2 come into wear. At 2 years, Di3 is in wear.

AGING a HORSE by the LOWER INCISORS: The most definitive age of a horse is its **birthday**. If unknown, use eruption and wear of the lower incisors to estimate its age. The lower incisors are used because of accessibility (the upper incisors only increase difficulty without increasing accuracy). Due to individual variation and feed types, you must avoid being definitive. Thus, a horse should be said **"to have the teeth of a horse of a certain age"**, not that the horse is so many years old. The major student pitfall is wanting to give the minute of birth and the phase of the moon. The following scheme will allow you to give valuable information to the horse owner. You will be able to tell him that the four year old horse he just bought is over ten. It will not make you a expert, but even a small animal practitioner can remember and use it at a Texas barbecue. To become an expert requires aging many horses and developing a feel (the art of aging). The *Official Guide for Determining the Age of the Horse* edited by Davis is a must to the expert.

DECIDUOUS or PERMANENT: Spread the horse's lips to see the incisors. First determine if the incisors are permanent or deciduous. If no permanent incisors have erupted, the horse has the teeth of a horse under 2 1/2 years old (see pg. 249). Students have the most problem with differentiating deciduous from permanent incisors. Deciduous incisors have a distinct neck, are smaller and usually lack the longitudinal ridges found on the labial surface of permanent incisor.

NO PERMANENT INCISORS - UNDER 2 1/2

ERUPTION TIME: The tooth breaking through the gum to become visible is the **most accurate** "estimate" of age. A common student pitfall is ignoring a tooth that has <u>just</u> broken through (can't be a "little" erupted or a "little" pregnant). Newly erupted permanent incisors will be covered by yellow cementum, lack a neck and be much larger than their deciduous counterparts.

ERUPTION - I1 - 2 1/2 years
I2 - 3 1/2 years
I3 - 4 1/2 years

Once the upper and lower incisors are in contact, the mouth must be gently opened to view the occlusal surface. Hold the lower lip and jaw and place a finger in the space behind the incisors (interdental space).

IN WEAR: when the occlusal surfaces are in contact, rubbing off the cementum and enamel to show dentin. This occurs approximately 6 months after eruption. If all the lower incisors are erupted and I3 is in wear (dentin seen on its occlusal surface), the horse has the mouth of a 5 year old. If all lower incisors are not erupted, then add 6 months to the eruption times of those present.

IN WEAR - I1 - 3 yrs
I2 - 4 yrs.
I3 - 5 yrs.

LEVEL: wear has flattened the occlusal surface, indicated when there are two enamel rings separated by dentin. Since this is hard to see in a live, moving horse, use the disappearance of cups rather than level times.

CUP GONE: disappearance of the infundibulum. It is **unreliable** due to variability in depth. I3 is very unreliable. The ease of seeing the cup gone (no black decayed material in it) makes it preferable to leveling times.

CUP GONE - I1 - 6 yrs.
I2 - 7 yrs.
I3 - 8 yrs.

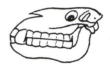

Eruption, in wear, and cup gone times are the **most accurate indicators of age, in that order**. The data below is less accurate and should be disregarded if they conflict with the above.

DENTAL STAR: appearance is unreliable, a dental star (or what appears to be a dental star - staining) may appear at any age. Instead, next use cup gone for the upper incisors or rounding of the occlusal surface which occur at the same time.

ROUND: refers to the shape of the occlusal surface, which actually appears triangular. "Round" means the transverse diameter equals the longitudinal diameter. This is hard to determine, so for ease, check the disappearances of the cups in the upper incisors.

CUP GONE - UPPER INCISORS: are easily detected because the disappearance of the dark mark is apparent.

CUP GONE **I1 - 9 yrs.**
UPPER INCISORS **I2 - 10 yrs.**
I3 - 11 yrs.

TRIANGULAR: when the longitudinal dimension becomes greater than the transverse dimension of the occlusal surface (unreliable). This occurs at 16 and 17 years for I1 and I2, respectively. (I3 is very unreliable).

TRIANGULAR I1 - 16 yrs.
I2 - 17 yrs.

ENAMEL SPOT: supposed to disappear from the occlusal surfaces between 13 and 16 years (unreliable).

RECTANGULAR (longitudinally oval): when the longitudinal direction is much larger than the transverse diameter.

RECTANGULAR - over 18 yrs.

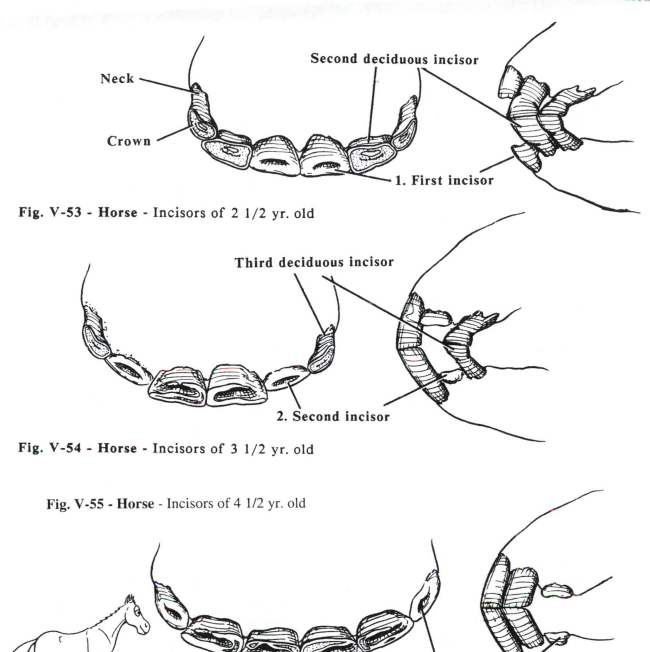

Fig. V-53 - Horse - Incisors of 2 1/2 yr. old

Fig. V-54 - Horse - Incisors of 3 1/2 yr. old

Fig. V-55 - Horse - Incisors of 4 1/2 yr. old

Note: These are all estimates in order of their reliability. When you are first stopped by any eruption or wear data, do not check later age indicators. For example, if I3 is not in wear (not 5 years yet) but the cup is gone from I1 (6 years), the horse is not yet 5 years old, much less 6. Most students want to look at the teeth for a minute and come up with a number (e.g., 13 years, 5 months, 4 days, 2 hours, 5 minutes and 3 seconds under a full moon). Aging over 10 is really an art and should be given in ranges (e.g., a horse with all cups gone, but no triangular teeth has the mouth of a horse between 11 and 16). I have my students count out loud as they go through the aging indicators. Though you may feel silly, the numbers will start to flow in order and repetition will make it second nature. As a practitioner when a teenage horse owner asks what you are counting, explain and attempt to teach them the method. They will appreciate your effort and have their dad call you back next time "Flicka" has a problem.

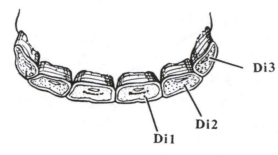

Fig. V-56 - Horse - 2 yrs.
- all deciduous in wear

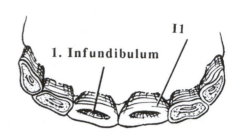

Fig. V-57 - Horse - 2 1/2 yrs.
- I1 erupted

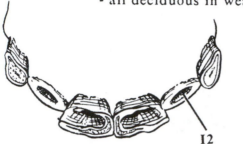

Fig. V-58 - Horse - 3 1/2 yrs.
- I2 erupted

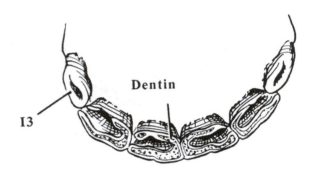

Fig. V-59 - Horse - 4 1/2 yrs.
- I3 erupted

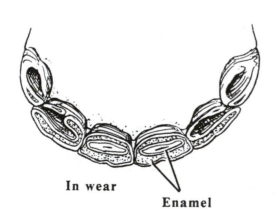

Fig. V-60 - Horse - 5 yrs.
- I3 in wear

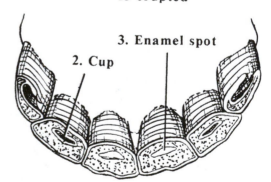

Fig. V-61 - Horse - 6 yrs.
- I1 cup gone

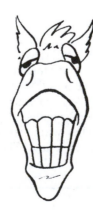

Counting and aging

- Deciduous - under 2 1/2 yrs.
- Deciduous - erupted, 8 days, 8 weeks 8 months
- Deciduous - in wear, 1, 1, 2 years
- Permanent - erupted, **2 1/2, 3 1/2, 4 1/2**
- Wear, **3, 4, 5**
- Cups gone, lower, **6,7,8**
- Upper cups gone, **9,10, 11**
- Triangular, **16, 17**
- Rectangular, **over 18**
- Older, count on a crystal ball.

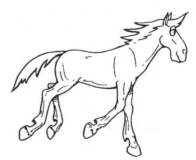

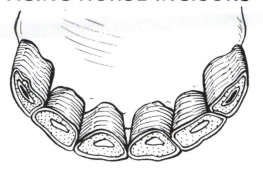

Fig. V-62 - Horse - 7 yrs.
- I2 cup gone

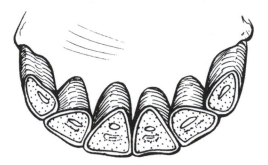

Fig. V-63 - Horse - 9 yrs.
- I1 round

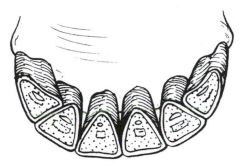

Fig. V-64 - Horse - 10-11 yrs.
- I2 round

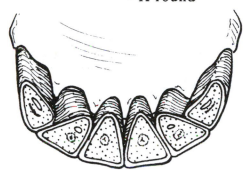

Fig. V-65 - Horse - 16 yrs.
- I1 triangular

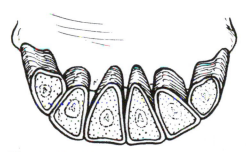

Fig. V-66 - Horse - 18 yrs. - rectangular

The Age Of A Horse

To tell the age of any horse,
Inspect the lower jaw, of course;
The six front teeth the tale will tell,
And every doubt and fear dispel.

Two middle nippers you behold
Before the foal is eight days old;
Before eight weeks, two more will come.
Eight months the corners cut the gum.

The outside enamel will disappear
From the middle two in just one year;
Also one year for the second pair -
In two years corners too will wear.

At two and a half the middle nippers drop;
At three and a half the second pair can't stop;
When four and a half the third pair goes,
At five a new worn set he shows.

The deep black spots will pass from view
At six years, from the middle two;
The second pair at seven years,
At eight the spot each corner clears.

From middle nippers upper jaw,
At nine the black spots will withdraw;
The second pair at ten are bright,
Eleven finds the corners light.

As time goes on the horsemen know
The oval teeth three-sided grow;
They longer get, project before,
Till twenty - when we know no more.

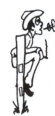

ANONYMOUS (modified)

HORSE – AGING - PERMANENT INCISORS			
	Center incisor	Middle incisor	Corner incisor
Eruption	2 1/2	3 1/2	4 1/2
In wear	3	4	5
Level	5	6	7
Cup gone (lower)	6	7	8
Dental star	8	9	10
Cup gone (upper), or **round** (lower)	9	10	11
Enamel spot gone	13	–	16
Triangular	16	17	16-17
Rectangular	18	19	20-21

OX INCISORS

RUMINANT INCISORS (low crowned [brachydont] teeth): There are four lower incisors (the canine being considered an incisor). The upper incisors are absent, replaced by the dental pad.

I4. Canine: looks like and located with the incisors, is considered the 4th incisor (I4).

Dental pad: a cornified connective tissue elevation replacing the upper incisors. It serves to oppose the lower incisors.

SHAPE: The incisors have a crown with a distinct neck and a round root (low-crowned [brachydont] teeth).

SURFACES:

1. Longitudinal ridges: serrations marking the lingual surface.

2. Occlusal surface: contacting the dental pad, and appearing when the teeth come into wear. Its lingual border is at first wavy due to longitudinal ridges.

LEVEL: when the occlusal surface is not wavy, due to wear past the longitudinal ridges.

AGING the OX by its INCISORS:
• Deciduous incisors
  - Birth: all of the ox's deciduous incisors have erupted by birth. They may still be covered by a thin pink membrane.
  - Two weeks: the gums have receded to the neck of Di1.
  - One month: all the incisors' crowns are exposed.
• Eruption of permanent incisors
  - I1: 1.5-2 years
  - I2: 2-2.5 years
  - 13: 3 years
  - I4: 4 years
• All in wear: 5 years
• Leveling of peramanent incisors
  - I1: 6 years
  - I2: & years
  - I3: 8 years
  - I4: 9 years
ª Round "pegs": 15 years (those that remain)

"Pegs": the roots of the incisors when the crowns have been completely worn away.

"Broken mouth": when the crowns of the incisors are worn off leaving the pegs (roots) or some incisors are missing. This reduces the cattle's grazing efficiency, and often result in their being culled (removal from the herd).

"Pearls": the roots of the incisors worn down to the gums.

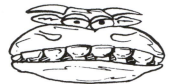

RUMINANT – AGING PERMANENT INCISORS	
I1	1yr.
I2	2 yrs.
I3	3yrs.
I4	4 yrs.

Clinical:
Dental disorders are common in cattle, but less so than in horses
• Dental caries, premature dental attrition, fractured teeth, periodontal diseases, osteodystrophy fibrosa

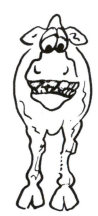

SHEEP and GOAT: the eruption of the numbered permanent incisors roughly corresponds to their age. I1 – 1 to 1 1/2 yrs.; I2 – 1 1/2 to 2 yrs.; I3 – 2 1/2 to 3 yrs.; I4 – 3 to 4 yrs. For a rough estimate of the age of sheep and goats in years, count the erupted permanent incisors.

SUMMARY: To roughly estimate the age of ruminants (cattle, sheep and goats) count the number of erupted permanent incisors for age in years. To be more correct with cattle, add one year to the first incisor – I1- 2, I2-2, I3-3 and I4 - 4 years. If all incisors have erupted and are in wear, say 5 years. (see chart pg. 257)

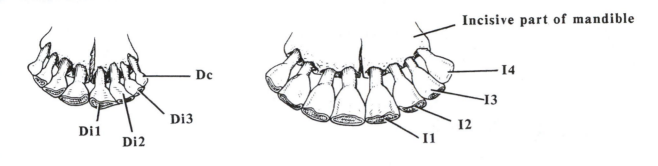

Fig. V-67 - Ox
 - Deciduous incisors

Fig. V-68 - Ox
 - Permanent incisors

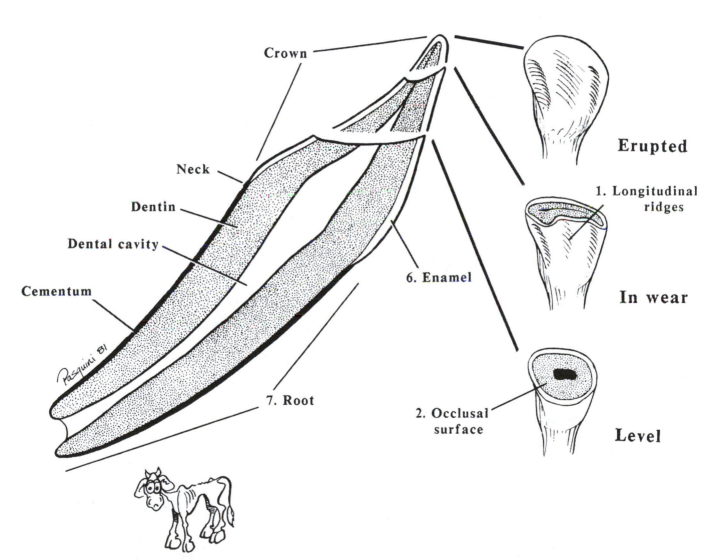

Fig. V-69 - Ox - 4th lower cheek tooth - sagittal section & occlusal surface

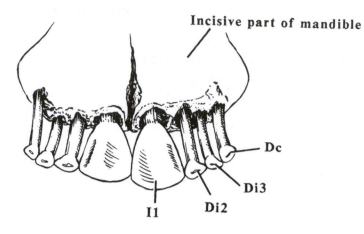

Incisive part of mandible

Dc

Di3

Di2

I1

Fig. V-70 - Ox - 1 1/2-2 yrs. - I1 erupted

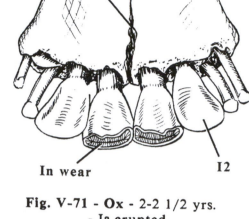

Intermandibular symphysis

In wear

I2

Fig. V-71 - Ox - 2-2 1/2 yrs. - I2 erupted

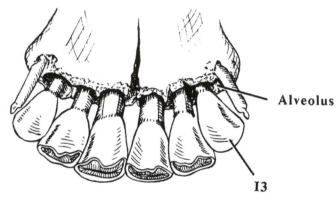

Alveolus

I3

Fig. V-72 - Ox - 3 yrs. - I3 erupted

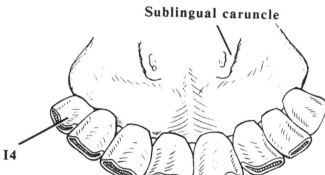

Sublingual caruncle

I4

Fig. V-73 - Ox - 4 yrs. - I4 erupted

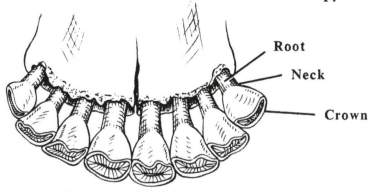

Root

Neck

Crown

Fig. V-74 - Ox - 5 yrs. - all in wear

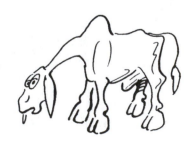

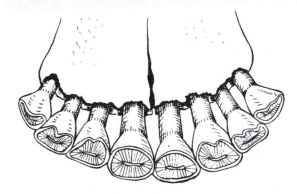

Fig. V-75 - Ox - 6 yrs. - I1 level

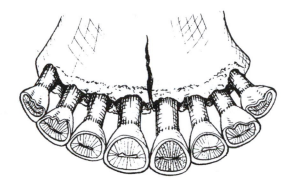

Fig. V-76 - Ox - 7 yrs. - I2 level

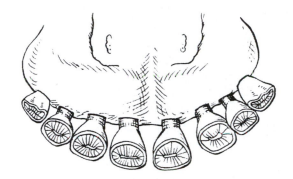

Fig. V-77 - Ox - 8 yrs. - I3 level

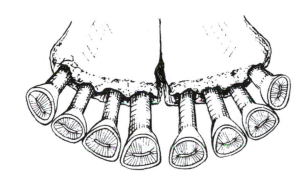

Fig. V-78 - Ox - 9 yrs. - I4 level

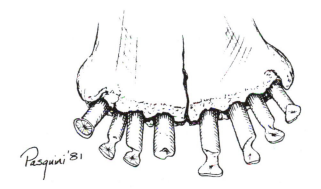

Fig. V-79 - Ox - 15 yrs. - missing or pegs

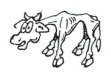

Teeth	Eruption	In wear	Level & Neck Emerged from Gum	Incisors Not Missing Reduced to Pegs
First Incisor (I_1)	1 1/2 - 2 yrs.		6 yrs.	
Second Incisor (I_2)	2 - 2 1/2 yrs.	All at 5 yrs.	7 yrs.	15 yrs.
Third Incisor (I_3)	3 yrs.		8 yrs.	
Fourth Incisor (canine)(I_4)	3 1/2 - 4 yrs.		9 yrs.	

SALIVARY GLANDS

6. Parotid ln.

1. Parotid salivary gland

Fig. V-80 - Dog - Head - lat. view

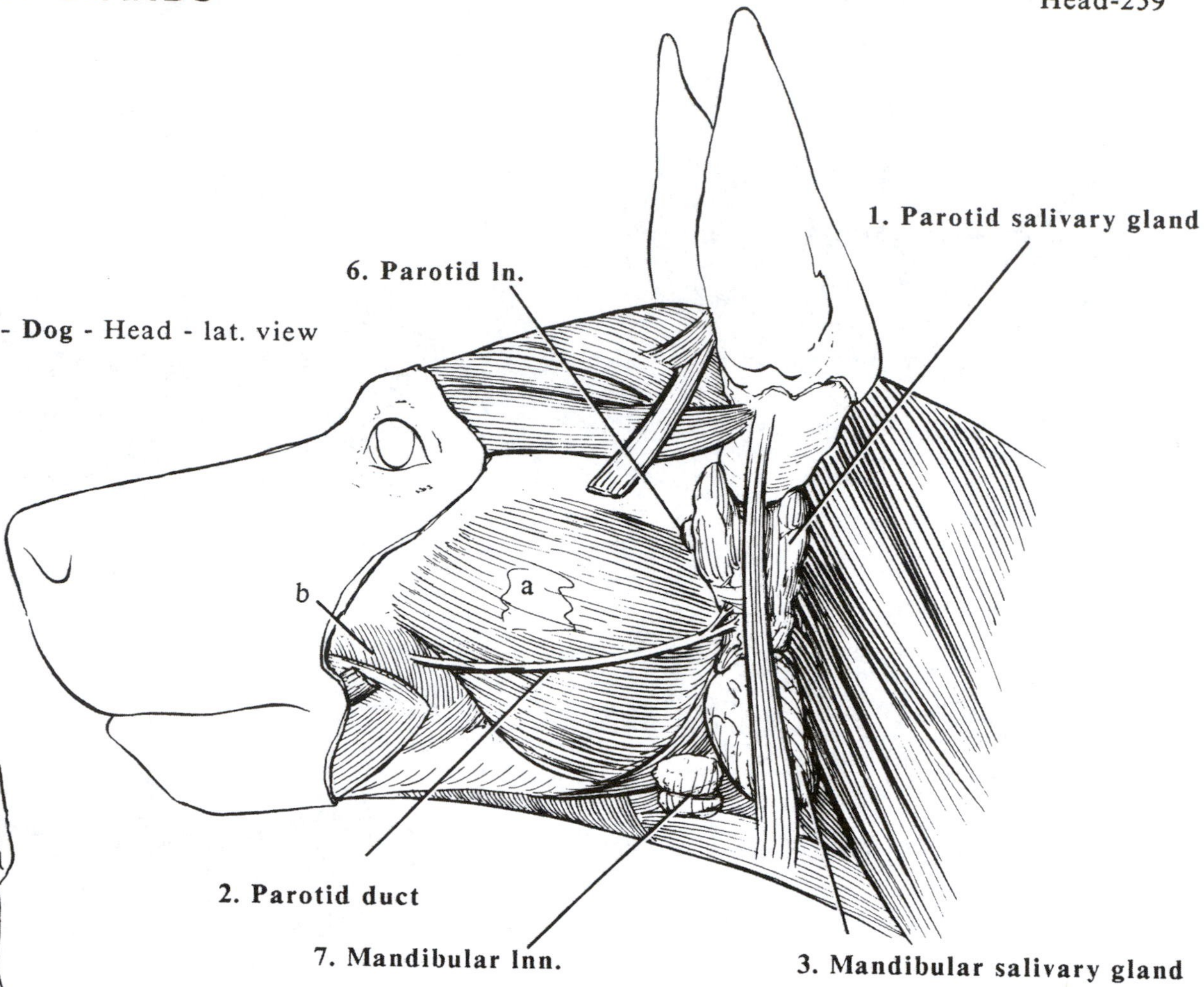

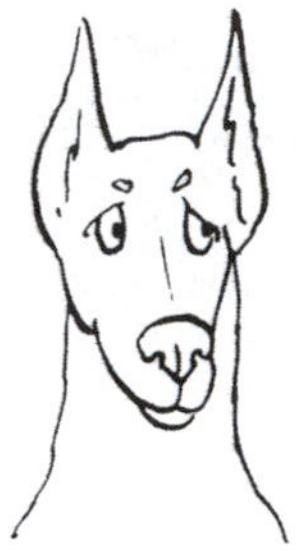

b

a

2. Parotid duct

7. Mandibular lnn.

3. Mandibular salivary gland

SALIVARY GLANDS: the extramural glands (glands outside the wall of the digestive system) emptying into the digestive system via ducts. The preparation of food (ingesta) for swallowing begins with lubrication and wetting by salivary secretions, saliva (sa-LY-va). Saliva consists primarily of water, some protein, glycoprotein, a significant amount of electrolytes, and antibodies (IgA). Salivary glands are classified by size, duct length, and by secretions. Secretions can be serous, mucous (MYOO-kus), or mixed (both). The parotid salivary gland has predominantly a serous secretion; the mandibular and sublingual are mixed. Parasympathetic and sympathetic ANS nerve fibers innervate the salivary glands.

MINOR SALIVARY GLANDS: located in the wall of the oral cavity and oral pharynx, having very <u>short</u> ducts. They are named based on location, i.e., labial, buccal and lingual (lips, cheek, and tongue). The minor salivary glands are only locally important.

MAJOR SALIVARY GLANDS: located some distance from the oral cavity and empty their secretions via <u>long</u> ducts.

1. Parotid (pa-ROT-id) (G *para*, near +*eotis*, ear) **salivary gland:** the unencapsulated, lobular gland below the auricular (ear) carti-

lage.

2. Parotid duct: pierces the cheek mucosa to drain its serous fluid into the buccal vestibule.

3. Mandibular salivary gland: the encapsulated, round or oval gland located caudal to the angle of the jaw. It is a mixed gland.

4. Mandibular duct: runs rostrally with the major sublingual duct, medial to the mandible under the floor of the mouth. It opens on or near the sublingual caruncle.

5. Sublingual salivary gland: the gland under the tongue having polystomatic and monostomatic parts. The **polystomatic part** (c) consists of diffuse clusters of glandular tissue on either side of the tongue, each cluster with its own duct. The **monostomatic part** (d) is caudal to the polystomatic sublingual gland, and rostral to the mandibular salivary gland. The monostomatic part and the mandibular salivary gland share a common capsule in the carnivores. The major sublingual duct accompanies the mandibular duct to the sublingual caruncle, where they open either together or separately.

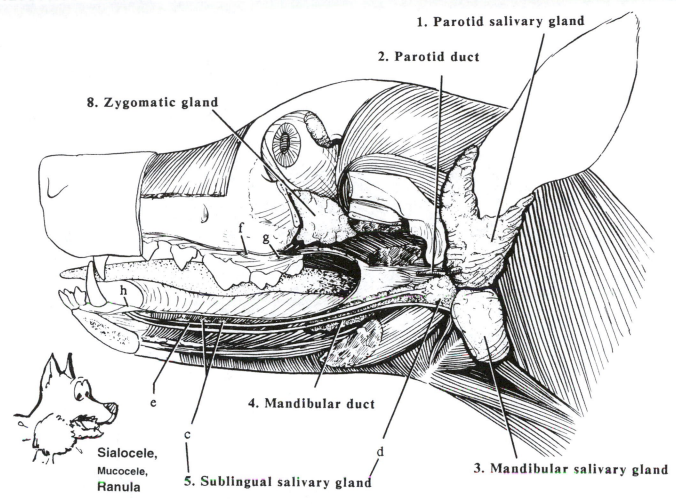

1. Parotid salivary gland

2. Parotid duct

8. Zygomatic gland

f

g

h

e

c

4. Mandibular duct

d

5. Sublingual salivary gland

3. Mandibular salivary gland

Sialocele,
Mucocele,
Ranula

Fig. V-81 - **Dog** - Head, deep dissection of
mandibular & sublingual glands
- lat. view

a. Masseter m.
b. Buccal m.
c. Polystomatic part (V-81)
d. Monostomatic part
e. Major sublingual duct

f. Parotid duct opening
g. Zygomatic duct opening
   (carnivores)
h. Sublingual caruncle

LYMPH NODES: lymphoid tissue often associated with the salivary glands of the same name.

6. Parotid lymph node: a small node near the rostral edge of the parotid gland. These drain the orbit and dorsal structures of the head.

7. Mandibular lymph nodes: two to four palpable nodes rostroventral to the mandibular salivary gland. These drain the ventral structures of the head.

Retropharyngeal lymph nodes: consist of medial and lateral groups of nodes. The medial retropharyngeal ones are located on the roof of the pharynx; the lateral (inconstant in dog) in the atlantal fossa (depression below atlas). They drain the head (deep structures and the parotid and mandibular lymph nodes) and adjacent neck, including the pharynx and larynx.

SPECIES DIFFERENCES

8. Zygomatic gland: the large buccal glands medial to the zygomatic arch in **carnivores**. Its duct opens caudal to the parotid duct opening.

Sublingual glands: The **dog** and **cat** have a caudally-located monostomatic part and a rostrally-located polystomatic part. The **horse** has only a polystomatic part. The **ruminants** have both parts, but they have reversed positions, the monostomatic part being rostral to the polystomatic part.

Parotid duct opening:
• **Dog** – across from the upper carnassial tooth (P4)
• **Ox** – across from the last or 5th upper cheek tooth
• **Horse, goat** and **pig** – across from the 3rd upper cheek tooth
• **Cat** – across from the 2nd upper cheek tooth

Parotid duct's path:
• **Carnivores** and usually **small ruminants**: crosses the lateral surface of the masseter muscle.
• **Horse, ox** and **pig**: courses ventrally to the inside of the mandible and then onto the cheek with the facial vessels.

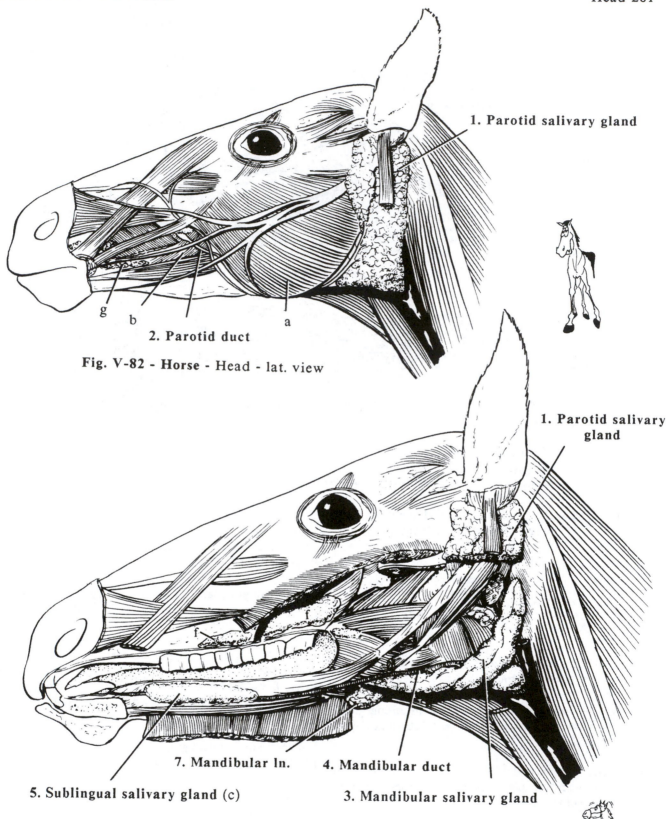

1. Parotid salivary gland

g b

2. Parotid duct

a

Fig. V-82 - Horse - Head - lat. view

1. Parotid salivary gland

7. Mandibular ln.

4. Mandibular duct

5. Sublingual salivary gland (c)

3. Mandibular salivary gland

Fig. V-83 - Horse - Head, deep dissection of mandibular
& sublingual glands - lat. view

SALIVARY GLANDS

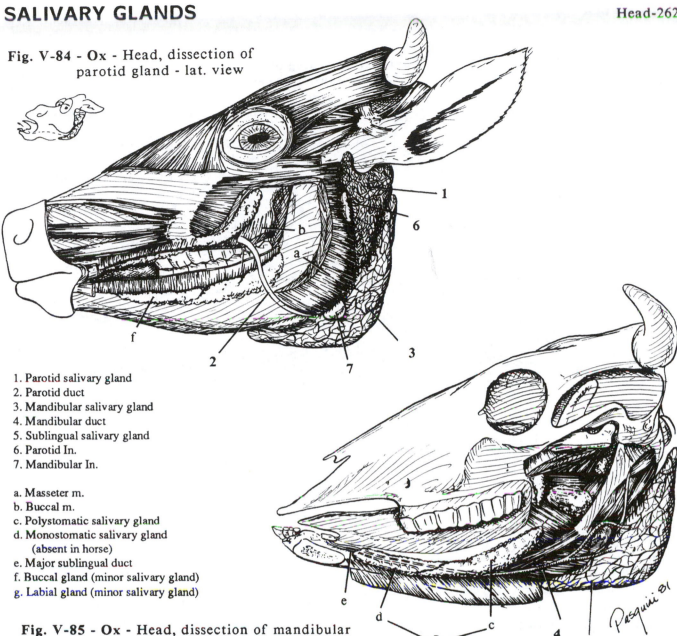

Fig. V-84 - Ox - Head, dissection of parotid gland - lat. view

1. Parotid salivary gland
2. Parotid duct
3. Mandibular salivary gland
4. Mandibular duct
5. Sublingual salivary gland
6. Parotid ln.
7. Mandibular ln.

a. Masseter m.
b. Buccal m.
c. Polystomatic salivary gland
d. Monostomatic salivary gland
   (absent in horse)
e. Major sublingual duct
f. Buccal gland (minor salivary gland)
g. Labial gland (minor salivary gland)

Fig. V-85 - Ox - Head, dissection of mandibular & sublingual glands - lat. view

---

CLINICAL:

Palpation of the dog's mandibular lymph nodes and salivary gland: Grasp the skin and deep structures at the angle of the jaw. Let them slip through your fingers, and feel a big lump (the mandibular gland) and a few small lumps (mandibular lymph nodes).

Mandibular or **sublingual ducts**: may become blocked due to trauma or inflammation, resulting in an accumulation of saliva producing a swelling (mucocele). Mucoceles are named for their location: under the tongue - <u>ranula</u> or <u>salivary cyst (sialocele)</u>; the neck - <u>cervical mucocele</u>. The gland itself may become blocked. Surgical removal of the glands and as much of the ducts as possible in the dog may be required to relieve either condition. Both the mandibular and the sublingual sali-

vary glands are removed together because they share a capsule, thus, one can't be removed without damaging the other.

Lymph nodes: the differentiation of an enlarged lymph node from a salivary gland is useful in diagnosis.

Ox's parotid lymph node: drains the orbit and is checked during slaughter because of cancer eye in cattle.

Translocation of the parotid duct: the surgical dissection of the parotid duct and its movement to the lateral canthus of the eye to treat dry eye (keratoconjunctivitis sicca) in the dog. Whenever a dog sees food it then salivates ("spits") onto its eyes.

PHARYNX

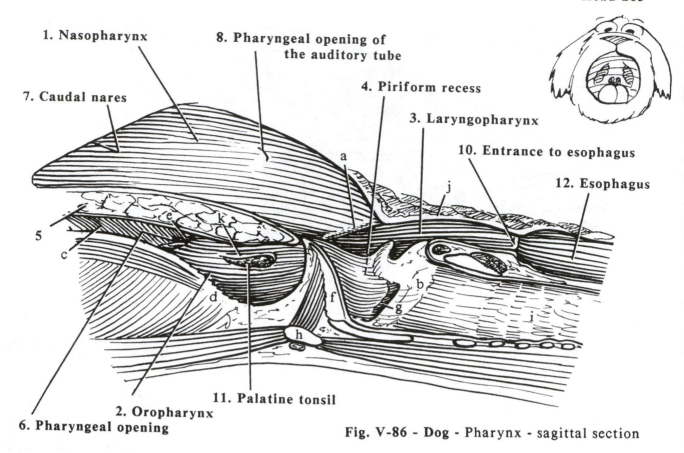

1. Nasopharynx

7. Caudal nares

8. Pharyngeal opening of the auditory tube

4. Piriform recess

3. Laryngopharynx

10. Entrance to esophagus

12. Esophagus

11. Palatine tonsil

2. Oropharynx

6. Pharyngeal opening

Fig. V-86 - Dog - Pharynx - sagittal section

PHARYNX (FAR-inks): acts as the common passageway for the digestive and respiratory systems. It connects the nasal and oral cavities with the trachea and esophagus respectively, serving to direct the intake of food and air into their proper channels. The soft palate (5) divides the rostral portion of the pharynx into the oropharynx and the nasopharynx. The common caudal portion is the laryngopharynx.

1. Nasopharynx (nay'zoh-FAR-inks): a part of the respiratory channel located dorsal to the soft palate and extending from the caudal nares to the laryngopharynx. The caudal free edge of the soft palate and the palatopharyngeal arches (a) demarcate the nasopharynx from the laryngopharynx.

2. Oropharynx (or'oh-FAR-inks): a part of the digestive channel ventral to the soft palate, extending from the oral cavity to the base of the epiglottis. The palatoglossal arches (e) demarcate the oropharynx from the oral cavity.

3. Laryngopharynx (layr-in'joh-FAR-inks): the part of the pharynx where air from the nasopharynx crosses to reach the larynx, and food and water from the oropharynx crosses into the esophagus. Thus, it is part of both the respiratory and digestive channels. The laryngopharynx is between the base of the epiglottis and the esophageal entrance. The rostral portion of the larynx projects into the laryngopharynx.

• **4. Piriform recess**: the continuation of the floor of the oropharynx on either side of the larynx. It is part of the laryngopharynx.

5. SOFT PALATE : the caudal musculomucosal continuation of the hard palate that divides the rostral part of the pharynx into oropharynx and nasopharynx.

MUSCLES of the PHARYNX: make up the walls of the pharynx. All are constrictors, except the caudal stylopharyngeal muscle that dilates the pharynx. The constrictor muscles (pterygopharyngeus, palatopharyngeus, stylopharyngeus rostralis, hyopharyngeus, thyropharyngeus and cricopharyngeus) act in an undulating fashion to move food toward the esophagus.

OPENINGS of the PHARYNX:

6. Pharyngeal opening (aditus pharyngis or isthmus faucium): the opening from the oral cavity to the oropharynx formed by the soft palate, the tongue and the palatoglossal arches.

7. Caudal nares or **choanae** (KOH-ay-nee) (sin.= choana): the osseous opening between the caudal nasal cavity and the nasopharynx.

8. Pharyngeal openings of the auditory tubes: the slits in the lateral walls of the nasopharynx leading into the auditory tubes, thus, to the middle ear.

9. Laryngeal opening (aditus laryngis): the opening into the larynx surrounded by the rostral laryngeal cartilages.

10. Esophageal opening (aditus esophagi): opening at the caudal end of the laryngopharynx into the esophagus.

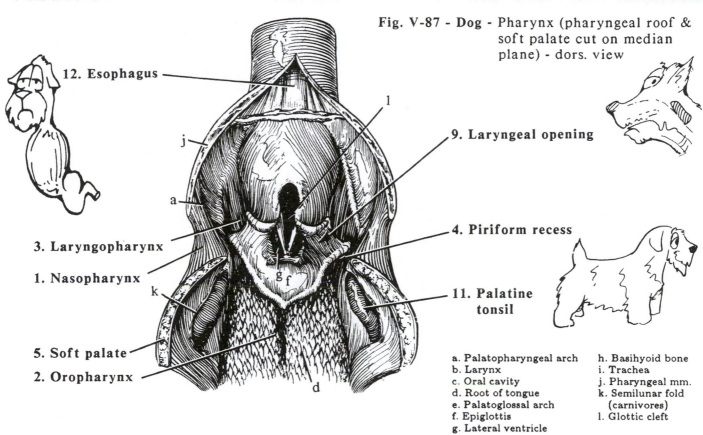

Fig. V-87 - Dog - Pharynx (pharyngeal roof & soft palate cut on median plane) - dors. view

12. Esophagus

l

9. Laryngeal opening

3. Laryngopharynx

1. Nasopharynx

4. Piriform recess

11. Palatine tonsil

5. Soft palate

2. Oropharynx

a. Palatopharyngeal arch
b. Larynx
c. Oral cavity
d. Root of tongue
e. Palatoglossal arch
f. Epiglottis
g. Lateral ventricle

h. Basihyoid bone
i. Trachea
j. Pharyngeal mm.
k. Semilunar fold (carnivores)
l. Glottic cleft

TONSIL: aggregation of lymphatic tissue in the pharyngeal mucosa. Some are distinct accumulations and others are diffuse and difficult to see. Named according to their locations (lingual, palatine, pharyngeal, tubal [around the entrance of the auditory tube], tonsil of the soft palate). They help to protect the openings of the pharynx against microorganisms and toxic substances.

11. Palatine tonsil: the lymphoid aggregation in the oropharynx. In carnivores it is a long cylindrical structure placed in a tonsilar fossa and covered medially by a semilunar fold (k).

12. ESOPHAGUS (ee-SOF-a-gus): the first part of the alimentary canal. It is a muscular tube that transports food from the oral cavity and pharynx down the neck and through the thorax to the stomach. It has cervical, thoracic and abdominal parts. Cornified, stratified squamous epithelium lines and protects the esophagus. The esophagus passes down the neck at first dorsal to the trachea, and then shifts to the left of the trachea. Inside the thorax, it returns to a position dorsal to the trachea, passing over the tracheal bifurcation to the right of the aorta. The esophagus pierces the esophageal hiatus of the diaphragm and terminates in the short abdominal portion at the cardia of the stomach.

CLINICAL:

Pyriform recess in the dog: the site where bones may become lodged and shut off the laryngeal opening of the airway. Its wall is the site where the incision for a pharyngostomy tube is placed.

Stomach tube - horse: can be seen passing in the esophagus of a horse on the left side of the neck.

Pharyngostomy: surgical incision of the pharynx.

Pharyngostomy tube: passed through the pharyngeal wall and down the esophagus to the stomach to feed dogs that can't take food through their mouth. The pyriform recess is located, a hemostat is pushed against its wall, and the wall is incised over the hemostat.

Choke: common in greedy eating cattle; serious because rapidly develops life threatening bloat. The four primary locations for choke: pharyngeal inlet, thoracic inlet, base of heart and cardia of rumen. Choke is less serious in the horse.

Pharyngeal trauma/abscesses: common in cattle and pigs during medication with a balling gun or long dose syringe.

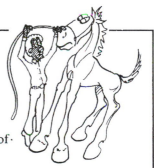

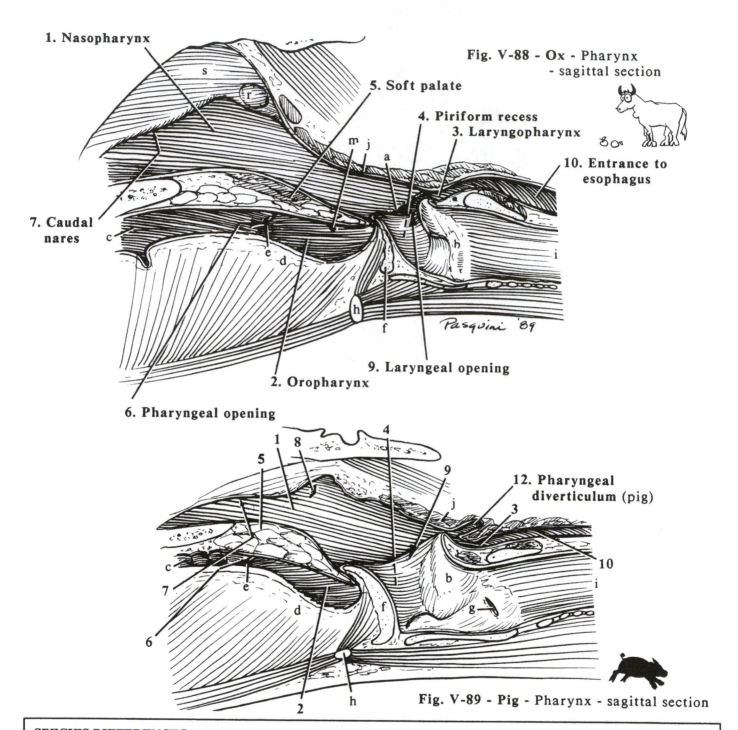

1. Nasopharynx

5. Soft palate

4. Piriform recess

3. Laryngopharynx

Fig. V-88 - Ox - Pharynx - sagittal section

10. Entrance to esophagus

7. Caudal nares

9. Laryngeal opening

2. Oropharynx

6. Pharyngeal opening

Pasquini '89

1 8 4

5

9

12. Pharyngeal diverticulum (pig)

3

10

7

6

2

Fig. V-89 - Pig - Pharynx - sagittal section

SPECIES DIFFERENCES

tonsils are.

Pharyngeal (FAR-in-jee-al) **diverticulum:** the blind, mucosal pouch in the roof of the nasopharynx of pigs. Directed caudally above the opening of the esophagus, it is often fatally mistaken for the esophagus when "pilling" pigs.

Tonsilar opening of the palatine tonsil in the ox: opening in the wall of the oropharynx leading into a space where the palatine

Horse: the soft palate is extremely long. It lies ventral to and in front of the tip of the epiglottis. The horse, unable to voluntarily raise its soft palate, exclusively breathes through its nose. This also explains why horses vomit through their nose. Displacement of the soft palate over the epiglottis interferes with breathing as it is sucked into the larynx.

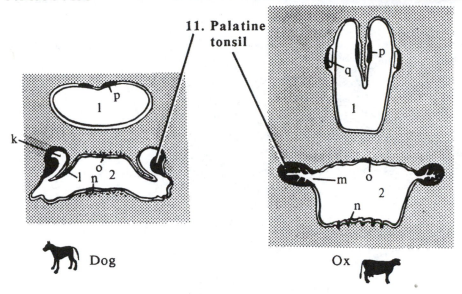

11. Palatine tonsil

Dog   Ox   Horse

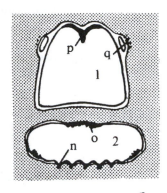

Fig. V-90 - Pharynx - Schematic cross section showing lymphatic tissue
(modified from Nickel, et al, The Viscera of the Domestic
Animals, Verlag, Paul, Parley, 1973)

1. Nasopharynx	a. Palatopharyngeal arch	k. Tonsilar fossa (carnivores)
2. Oropharynx	b. Larynx	l. Semilunar fold (carnivores)(V-90)
3. Laryngopharynx	c. Oral cavity	m. Tonsilar opening of
4. Piriform recess	d. Root of tongue	palatine tonsil (ox) (V-88)
5. Soft palate	e. Palatoglossal arch	n. Lingual tonsil (V-90)
6. Pharyngeal opening	f. Epiglottis	o. Tonsil of soft palate
(aditis pharyngis)	g. Lateral ventricle (absent	p. Pharyngeal tonsil (V-88)
7. Caudal nares (choanae)	in carnivores & cat)	q. Tubal tonsil (V-90)
8. Pharyngeal opening of	h. Basihyoid bone	r. Retropharyngeal ln. (V-88)
auditory tube	i. Trachea	s. Pharyngeal septum
9. Laryngeal opening	j. Pharyngeal mm.	
(aditis laryngis)		
10. Entrance to esophagus		
11. Palatine tonsil		
12. Pharyngeal diverticulum (pig)		

Type	Carnivores	Pig	Ruminants	Horse
Lingual tonsil	*	*	+	+
Palatine tonsil	+	-	+[1]	+
Tonsil of soft palate	*	+	*	+
Pharyngeal tonsil	+	+	+	+
Tubal tonsils (around pharyngeal opening of auditory tubes)	-	+	+	*
Paraepiglottic tonsil	*	+	+,-[2]	-

+ Identifiable
* Diffuse, difficult to identify
- Absent
1 Tonsillar opening is seen in the oropharynx of the ox
2 Absent in ox, present in small ruminants

Adapted from Veterinary Anatomy,
M.J. Shively,

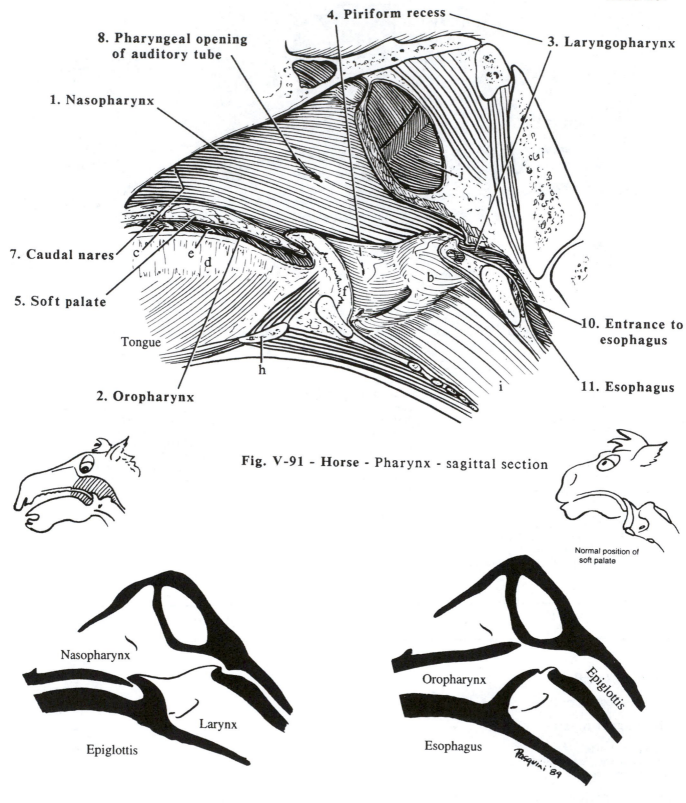

4. Piriform recess

3. Laryngopharynx

8. Pharyngeal opening of auditory tube

1. Nasopharynx

7. Caudal nares

5. Soft palate

Tongue

2. Oropharynx

10. Entrance to esophagus

11. Esophagus

Fig. V-91 - Horse - Pharynx - sagittal section

Normal position of soft palate

Nasopharynx

Larynx

Epiglottis

Oropharynx

Epiglottis

Esophagus

A. Breathing

B. Swallowing

Fig. V-92 - Horse - Pharynx cavity (schematic)

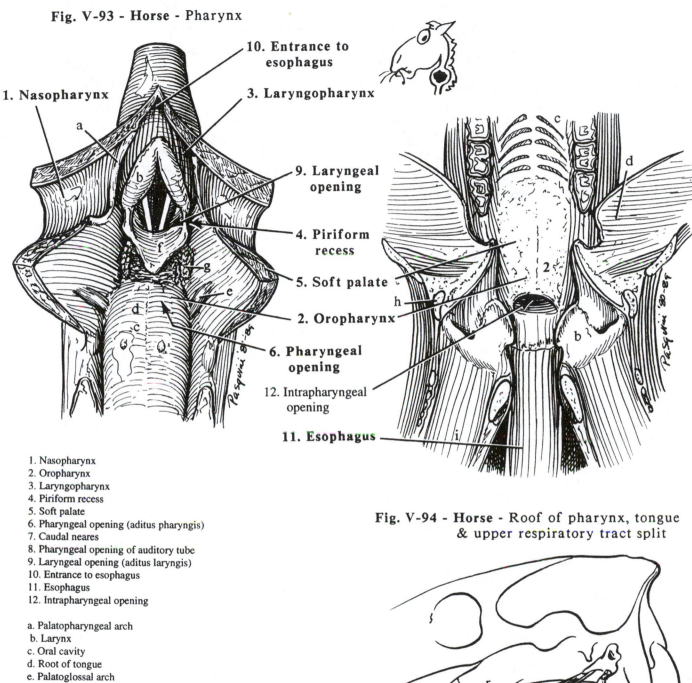

Fig. V-93 - Horse - Pharynx

1. Nasopharynx

10. **Entrance to esophagus**

3. **Laryngopharynx**

9. **Laryngeal opening**

4. **Piriform recess**

5. **Soft palate**

2. **Oropharynx**

6. **Pharyngeal opening**

12. Intrapharyngeal opening

11. **Esophagus**

1. Nasopharynx
2. Oropharynx
3. Laryngopharynx
4. Piriform recess
5. Soft palate
6. Pharyngeal opening (aditus pharyngis)
7. Caudal neares
8. Pharyngeal opening of auditory tube
9. Laryngeal opening (aditus laryngis)
10. Entrance to esophagus
11. Esophagus
12. Intrapharyngeal opening

a. Palatopharyngeal arch
b. Larynx
c. Oral cavity
d. Root of tongue
e. Palatoglossal arch
f. Epiglottis
g. Lingual tonsil
h. Hyoid apparatus
i. Trachea
j. Guttural pouch (horse)
k-q. Pharyngeal constrictors
k. Pterygopharyngeus m.
l. Palatopharyngeus m.
m. Stylopharyngeus rostralis m.
n. Hyopharyngeus m.
o. Thyropharyngeus m.
p. Cricopharyngeus m.
q. Stylopharyngeus caudalis m.
r. Levator palatini
s. Retractor veli paltini

Fig. V-94 - Horse - Roof of pharynx, tongue & upper respiratory tract split

Stylohyoid bone

Fig. V-95 - Horse - Pharyngeal mm.

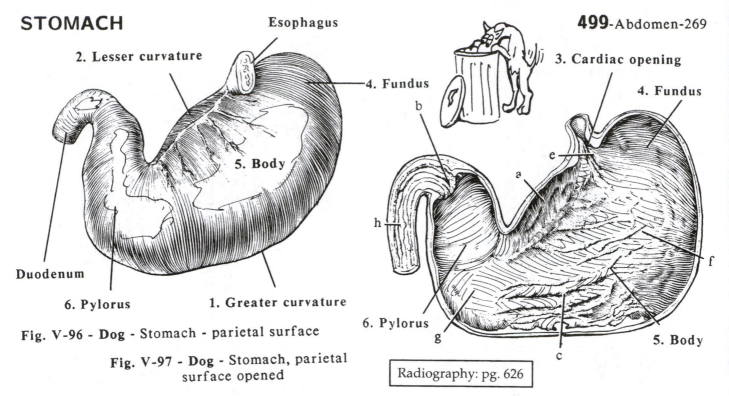

Fig. V-96 - **Dog** - Stomach - parietal surface

Fig. V-97 - **Dog** - Stomach, parietal surface opened

Radiography: pg. 626

STOMACH (G. *gaster*): the dilation in the GI tract caudal (aboral) to the esophagus receiving ingesta from the esophagus and temporarily storing it. Gastric enzymes, chiefly pepsin, rennin, and hydrochloric acid, are secreted by the glands in the stomach wall. Muscular movements of the stomach mix ingesta and enzymes and slowly move them into the duodenum. Stomachs are lined by glandular epithelium, nonglandular epithelium or both. The **nonglandular lining** is a continuation of the stratified squamous epithelium of the esophagus. The **glandular lining** is a simple columnar epithelium that continues into the duodenum. Carnivores have a **glandular stomach lining**. A **composite stomach** is lined by nonglandular and glandular epithelium and is found in the ruminants, horse and pig. The wall of the stomach consists of an inner mucous membrane, a muscular coat and a serosal coat. The muscular coat is unique in having an extra layer, the internal oblique layer, in addition to the outer longitudinal and the inner circular layers. It is present only over the expandable fundus and body of the stomach. At the cardia its fibers are thicker and form the cardiac loop (ansa cardiaca).

Simple stomach: the single compartment stomach found in the carnivores, horse and pig. It has been incorrectly called monogastric, implying the complex stomach is polygastric (having more than one stomach).

Complex stomach: the four compartment stomach found in the ruminants. The additional three compartments are called the forestomachs and may be the source of the incorrect four stomach concept. The complex stomach is still only one stomach.

PARTS of the SIMPLE STOMACH

1. Greater curvature (curvatura major): the long, convex surface of the stomach extending from the cardia to the pylorus. The superficial leaf of the greater omentum attaches to the greater curvature externally.

2. Lesser curvature (curvatura minor): the short, concave sur-

face of the stomach, also extending from the cardia to the pylorus. It is the attachment site of the caudal edge of the lesser omentum externally.

Parietal surface: the side of the stomach in contact with the liver.

Visceral surface: the side of the stomach in contact with the remaining the abdominal viscera.

3. Cardia (KAR-dee-ah)(Gr. *kardia* heart): the opening or the part of the stomach around the opening. The **cardiac opening** (ostium cardiacum) is the opening of the esophagus into the stomach. **The cardiac part** (pars cardiaca) is the portion of the stomach around the esophagus. It is the "fixed" point (doesn't move) of the stomach. Do not confuse it with the cardiac gland region which may or may not correspond to this location in the different species. The fundic and pyloric gland regions of the stomach mucosa also don't necessarily correspond to the external fundic and pyloric regions.

4. Fundus (L. bottom): the blind, expanded portion of the stomach's left side, immediately adjacent to the cardia. It is often filled with gas that can be seen in radiographs.

5. Body (corpus): the largest part of the stomach, extending from the cardia to the pyloric part.

6. Pylorus: (py-LOR-us) (G. *pyloros*, gatekeeper): the distal opening of the stomach, surrounded by a strong band of circular muscle, and through which the stomach contents are emptied into the duodenum. This term is variously used to mean the pyloric part of the stomach, pyloric antrum, pyloric canal, pyloric opening and pyloric sphincter.

Pyloric part: portion of stomach distal to the body.
Pyloric antrum: wide proximal portion of the pyloric part.
Pyloric canal: narrow distal part of the pyloric part terminating at the pyloric opening.
Pyloric opening (ostium pyloricum): opening of the stomach into the duodenum through which ingesta leave.

STOMACH

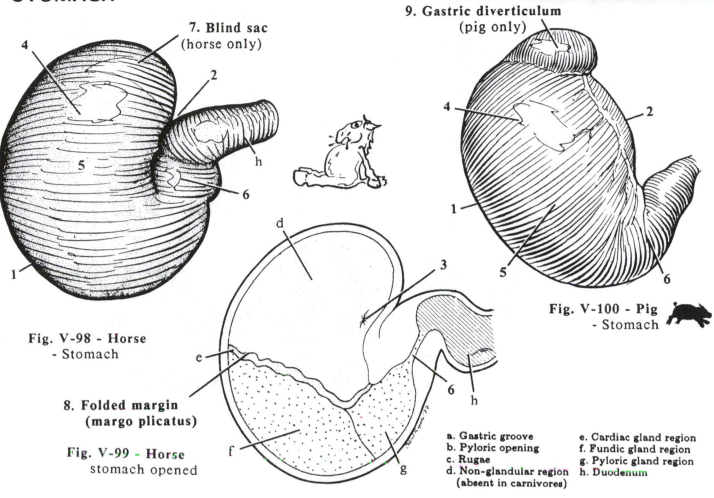

7. Blind sac
(horse only)

Fig. V-98 - Horse
- Stomach

8. Folded margin
(margo plicatus)

Fig. V-99 - Horse
stomach opened

9. Gastric diverticulum
(pig only)

Fig. V-100 - Pig
- Stomach

a. Gastric groove
b. Pyloric opening
c. Rugae
d. Non-glandular region
   (absent in carnivores)
e. Cardiac gland region
f. Fundic gland region
g. Pyloric gland region
h. Duodenum

SPECIES DIFFERENCES

HORSE: a simple composite stomach.

- **7. Blind sac** (saccus cecus): the extensive fundus of the horse's stomach lined by nonglandular mucosa. It is homologous to the forestomach found in ruminants.

- **8. Folded margin** or **margo plicatus**: the grossly visible, internal, irregular, raised line separating the stomach's nonglandular and glandular portions in the **horse.**

PIG: a simple composite stomach with a small nonglandular part around the cardia.

- **9. Gastric diverticulum** (diverticulum ventriculi): the extension of the pig's fundus.

- **Torus pyloricus**: the round swelling of the pylorus in the lumen of the pyloric canal, also present in the ruminants.

CARNIVORES: a simple glandular stomach.

RUMINANTS: a complex composite stomach consisting of four compartments (see pg. 270).

CLINICAL

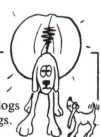

Gastric dilatation/volvulus complex: emergency situation in large and giantbreed dogs with deepchests, rarely occurring in small dogs.

Gastritis: inflammation of stomach.

Gastric ulcers: more pathogenic in foals than adults. They also occur in dogs and cats, pigs and abomasal ulcers in cattle.

Pyloric stenosis: constriction of the pyloric canal in carnivores. The serosa and muscular layer (but not the mucosa) can be cut to enlarge the pyloric canal.

Gastric dilatation - horses: due to grain overload resulting in violent colic and gastric reflux.

"Bots": the larva of *Gastrophilus* spp. flies found attached to the interior of the horse's stomach.

Stomach worms - horse: Draschia, Habronema and Trichostrongylus spp. are all controlled by ivermectin deworming.

Ox - exploratory laparotomy: pg 646

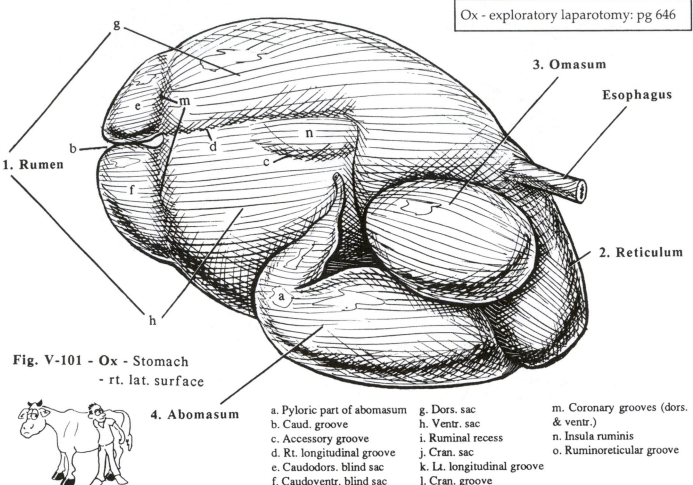

Fig. V-101 - Ox - Stomach
- rt. lat. surface

4. Abomasum

3. Omasum

Esophagus

2. Reticulum

1. Rumen

a. Pyloric part of abomasum
b. Caud. groove
c. Accessory groove
d. Rt. longitudinal groove
e. Caudodors. blind sac
f. Caudoventr. blind sac

g. Dors. sac
h. Ventr. sac
i. Ruminal recess
j. Cran. sac
k. Lt. longitudinal groove
l. Cran. groove

m. Coronary grooves (dors. & ventr.)
n. Insula ruminis
o. Ruminoreticular groove

RUMINANT STOMACH: a complex, composite stomach consisting of four compartments. The first (proximal) three compartments, forestomach (proventriculus) (the rumen, reticulum and omasum) are nonglandular and lined with stratified squamous epithelium. The distal compartment, the abomasum, is the glandular stomach.

1. RUMEN (ROO-men): the largest of the four compartments, filling most of the abdomen's left half. The rumen is divided into dorsal and ventral sacs by right and left longitudinal grooves and cranial and caudal grooves. The rumen is a fermentation vat for microorganisms to break down cellulose into metabolizable components. The rumen fills the left half of the abdomen, displacing the other organs to the right side.

Grooves: the external depressions in the rumen (longitudinal, cranial, caudal and coronary).

Dorsal sac (g): the upper part of the rumen.

Ventral sac (h): the lower part of the rumen.

• **Ruminal recess** or **recessus ruminis** (i): the cranial end of the ventral sac.

Atrium or **cranial sac** (j): the ventral part of the rumen, between the cranial pillar and the ruminoreticular fold.

2. RETICULUM (re-TIK-yoo-lum): the most cranial compartment of the ruminant stomach, located on the median plane against the diaphragm.

3. OMASUM (oh'MAY-sum): the spherical compartment caudal to the reticulum.

4. ABOMASUM (ab'oh-MAY-sum): the elongated "true stomach" lined by glandular tissue, located on the right side in contact with the ventral abdominal wall.

CLINICAL

Bloat: excessive accumulation of gas in the rumen and reticulum.

Stomach tube: a long tube passed through the mouth and down the esophagus into the rumen to relieve bloat. If a stomach tube fails, then a trocar can be used to relieve gas build up.

Trocarization: the placement of a hollow tube (trocar) through the left paralumbar fossa and rumen wall to release gas from the rumen.

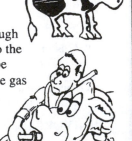

RUMINANT STOMACH

Fig. V-102 - Ox - Stomach - lt. lat. side

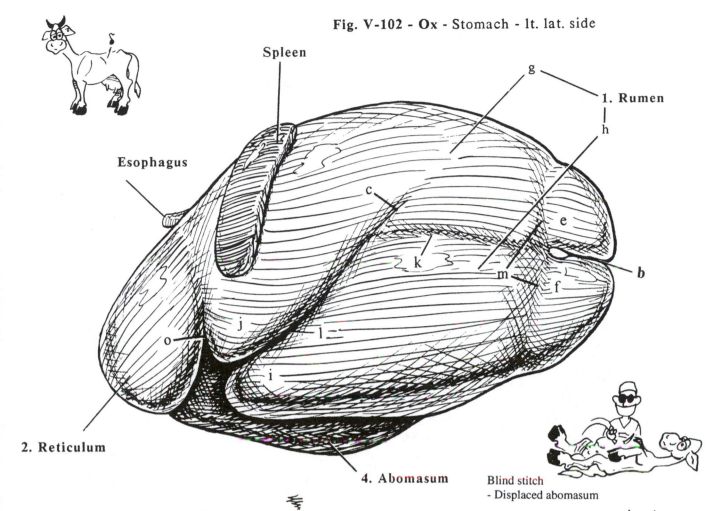

Spleen

Esophagus

g

1. Rumen

h

c

e

k

m

b

f

j

l

o

i

2. Reticulum

4. Abomasum

Blind stitch
- Displaced abomasum

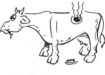

Grain overload: problem in cattle and horses.

Abomasal impaction: accumulation of feed in abomasum and failure of transport to distal GI tract.

Rumen palpation: the steady pressure against the left paralumbar fossa to feel the contractions of the rumen, which normally occur 2-3 times per minute.

"Hardware disease": a common term for traumatic reticulitis caused by perforation of the reticular wall by a sharp object. Due to its weight, metal entering the cardia falls into the reticulum. Normal contraction can force the metal through the reticular wall and into other structures (commonly the liver, occasionally the pericardium). Often a magnet is placed in the reticulum to gather "hardware" and prevent migration.

Displaced abomasum: the relocation of the abomasum to the right (RDA) or left (LDA) causing disturbances in digestion that may be life threatening. The abomasum may be repositioned and sutured in the correct position.

• **LDA, left displaced abomasum**: passes under the rumen and up its left side to become positioned between the rumen and the left abdominal wall. Auscultation and percussion will reveal abnormal gas sounds on left.

Rumenotomy: the surgical opening of the rumen. This is done through the left paralumbar fossa and dorsal sac of the rumen. If performed to relieve "hardware disease", the reticulum can be found by palpating along the dorsal wall of the rumen until the reticulum is reached. The cranial sac can be differentiated from the reticulum by its absence of a "honey comb" mucosa.

Ruminal fistula: a permanent opening of the rumen to the outside used to study rumen physiology. The left paralumbar fossa and the dorsal sac of the rumen are opened. The edges of the opening of the dorsal sac of the rumen are sutured to the edges of the paralumbar skin incision, and a removable artificial plug is left in place.

RUMINANT STOMACH

Fig. V-103 - Ox - Stomach, reticulum & rumen opened

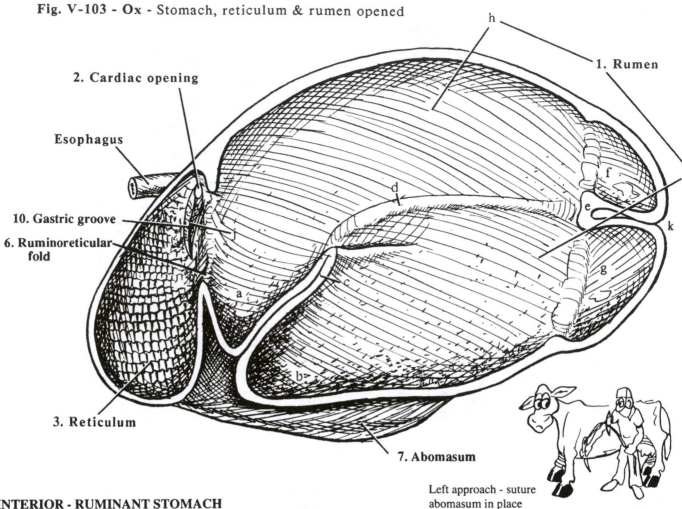

2. Cardiac opening

Esophagus

10. Gastric groove

6. Ruminoreticular fold

3. Reticulum

7. Abomasum

1. Rumen

Left approach - suture abomasum in place

INTERIOR - RUMINANT STOMACH

1. RUMEN: the interior of the rumen has pillars representing the exterior grooves. Many papillae (peg-like mucosal projections) give the surface a "pile rug" appearance.

• **Pillars:** the internal representations of the external grooves (longitudinal, cranial, caudal and coronary). The intralumenal opening (ostium) is between the dorsal and ventral sac formed by the longitudinal, cranial, and caudal pillars.

• **Dorsal sac** (g): the upper part of the rumen.

• **Ventral sac** (h): the lower part of the rumen.

  - **Recessus ruminis** (b): the cranial end of the ventral sac.

  - **Atrium or cranial sac** (a): the ventral part of the rumen between the cranial pillar and the ruminoreticular fold.

•**2. Cardiac opening** or **cardia:** the esophageal entrance into the rumen. Heavy material (grain and metal) entering the rumen usually falls through the cranial part of the rumen into the reticulum, directly below the cardiac opening.

3. RETICULUM: the interior has a honeycomb appearance due to its intersecting mucosal crests.

4. OMASUM: the third compartment, sometimes called the "Butchers bible" or "Book" because of the page appearance of its muscular laminae.

  • **5. Omasal laminae:** Covered with short papillae, they are parallel, leaf-like structures projecting into the interior from the wall of the omasum.

6. Ruminoreticular fold: the inner septum corresponding to the external ruminoreticular groove. It separates the rumen from the reticulum.

7. ABOMASUM: the compartment lined with glandular mucosa similar to the simple stomach of the carnivore.

• **8. Pylorus:** the part of the abomasum opening into the duodenum.

• **9. Torus pyloricus:** a round elevation of the pylorus into the pyloric canal; similar to the pig.

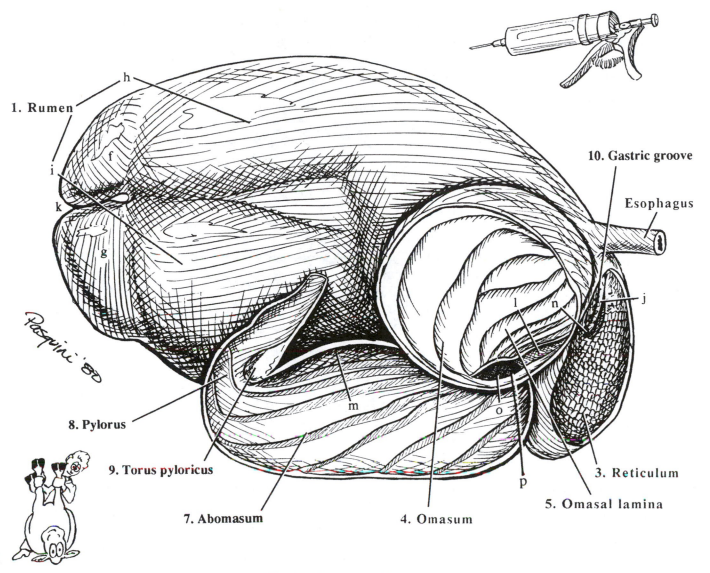

1. Rumen

10. Gastric groove

Esophagus

8. Pylorus

9. Torus pyloricus

7. Abomasum

4. Omasum

5. Omasal lamina

3. Reticulum

Fig. V-104 - Ox - Stomach, omasum & abomasum opened

a. Cran. sac (atrium)	g. Caudoventr. blind sac	m. Abomasal groove
b. Ruminal recess	h. Dors. sac	n. Reticuloomasal opening
c. Cran. pillar	i. Ventr. sac	o. Omasoabomasal opening
d. Rt. longitudinal pillar	j. Reticular groove	p. Velum abomasacum
e. Caud. pillar	k. Caud. groove	
f. Caudodors. blind sac	l. Omasal groove	

10. GASTRIC GROOVE: the channel through the stomach following its lesser curvature, found in all the domestic species, but of greatest importance in suckling ruminants. Suckling with the head up causes the lips of this groove to close. This forms a tube from the cardiac opening to the abomasum. Through this tube milk bypasses the rumen, reticulum and omasum to empty directly into the abomasum. This reflex disappears in the adult, except in response to some liquid salts. The gastric groove is divided into the reticular groove (esophageal, milk groove) (j), the omasal groove (I) and the abomasal groove (m).

Clinical:

Ostertagia ostertagi: #1 parasite of cattle. These roundworms overwinter (hibernate) in the gastric glands of the abomasum. As they emerge in the spring they cause major problems.

Ruminal/vagal indigestion: common group of diseases of dysfunction of the ruminant stomach.

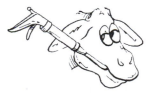

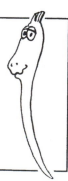

SMALL INTESTINE

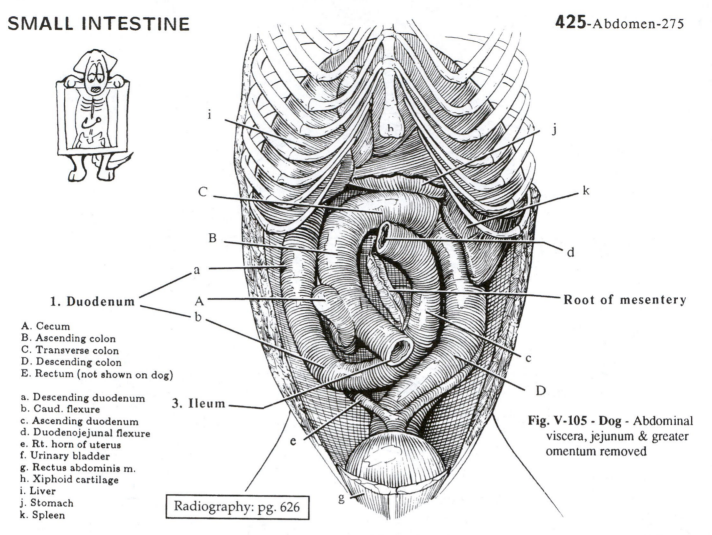

1. Duodenum

A. Cecum
B. Ascending colon
C. Transverse colon
D. Descending colon
E. Rectum (not shown on dog)

a. Descending duodenum
b. Caud. flexure
c. Ascending duodenum
d. Duodenojejunal flexure
e. Rt. horn of uterus
f. Urinary bladder
g. Rectus abdominis m.
h. Xiphoid cartilage
i. Liver
j. Stomach
k. Spleen

3. Ileum

Root of mesentery

Fig. V-105 - Dog - Abdominal viscera, jejunum & greater omentum removed

Radiography: pg. 626

SMALL INTESTINE: the principal site of digestion and absorption, extending from the pylorus of the stomach to the large intestine and divided into duodenum, jejunum and ileum.

1. DUODENUM (dyoo'-OD-e-num or dyoo-oh-DEE-num) (L. *duodeni*, twelve): receives ingesta from the stomach.

• Cranial part: extends cranially from the pylorus. It then turns caudally at the cranial duodenal flexure.

• **Descending duodenum** (a): continues caudally on the abdomen's <u>right</u> side, in contact with the right abdominal wall. The bile and pancreatic ducts empty into the descending duodenum.

• Caudal flexure (b): the bend where the descending duodenum becomes the **ascending duodenum** (c).

• **Ascending duodenum**: travels on the right side of the root of the mesentery (pg. 284) and terminates in the duodenojejunal flexure (d). The **duodenocolic ligament** connects the caudal flexure of the duodenum and the ascending duodenum to the descending colon.

2. JEJUNUM (je-JOO-num) (L. *jejunus*, empty): the longest part of the small intestine. Beginning at the duodenojejunal flexure (d), the jejunum runs ventrally and caudally, forming many coils and loops and occupying the ventral abdominal cavity. The

jejunum has a long mesentery, allowing great range of motion.

3. ILEUM (IL-ee-um) (L. rolled up, twisted): the short, terminal portion of the small intestine. It is indistinguishable grossly from the jejunum. Arbitrarily, it can be said to start at the end of the ileocecal fold (connecting peritoneum between the ileum and colon) or end of the antimesenteric ileal artery. It empties into the large intestine.

SPECIES DIFFERENCES

Small intestines: grossly similar in all the domestic species.

Sigmoid loop: the "s" shaped curve of the cranial part of the duodenum in the horse, ruminant and pig. It is located against the visceral side of the liver.

Duodenal ampulla: the dilated cranial part of the horse's duodenum.

Flange of the bovine small intestine: the part of the small intestine with the longest mesentery. The proximal and middle parts of the jejunum have a short mesentery. The flange, consisting of the distal end of the jejunum and the proximal end of the ileum, has a long mesentery, thus, great mobility. The ruminants have a proximal convoluted part and a distal straight part to their ileum.

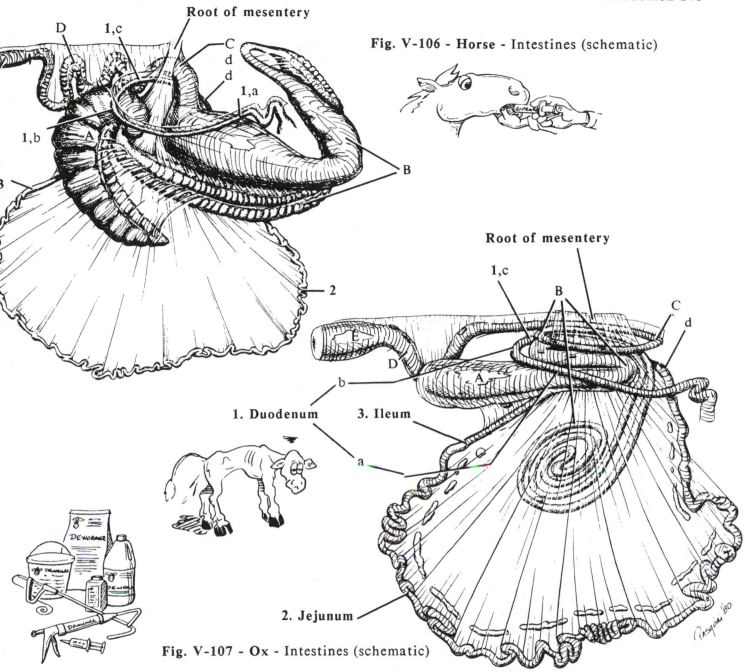

Root of mesentery

D   1,c

C

C

d

d

1,a

1,b   A

3

2

B

Fig. V-106 - Horse - Intestines (schematic)

Root of mesentery

1,c

B

C

d

E

D

b   A

1. Duodenum   **3. Ileum**

a

2. Jejunum

Fig. V-107 - Ox - Intestines (schematic)

Ileocecal opening - into the cecum of the <u>horse</u>

Ileocolic opening - into the ascending colon of <u>carnivores</u> and <u>ruminants</u>. Some consider the ruminant to have an ileocecocolic opening (a "T" junction into cecum and ascending colon).

CLINICAL

Torsion of the intestine: the turning or twisting of the intestine, cutting off its blood supply.

Intussuception (in'tus-sus-SEP-shun)**:** the condition in which a segment of intestine inverts ("telescopes") into the lumen of the adjacent segment.

Intestinal resection and anastomosis: the cutting out of a damaged section of intestine and reconnection of healthy bowel. To ensure the vascular supply, cut the mesenteric border longer than the antimesenteric border of the two ends to be rejoined.

Volvulus: the specific term for a torsion of the intestine, causing obstruction.

Enteropathy: any disease of the intestine.

Enterotomy: an incision into the intestine. This is often done to remove foreign bodies.

LARGE INTESTINE

LARGE INTESTINE: the cecum, colon, rectum and anal canal. It extends from the ileum to the anus, and functions to dehydrate fecal contents by absorbing water.

1. CECUM (SEE-kum) (L. *caccus*, blind): the blind diverticulum at the beginning of the colon.

2. Cecocolic orifice: the opening from the cecum into the colon.

Ileocecal (il'-ee-oh-SEE-kal) **fold:** the fold of connecting peritoneum between the cecum and the ileum.

COLON (KOH-lon) (G. *kolos*, large intestine, hollow): ascending, transverse and descending segments of the large intestine fixed in the dorsal abdomen by a short mesentery.

3. Ascending colon: the first part of the colon. In the carnivores, it is the **right colon,** extending cranially on the right side of the dorsal abdomen, medial to the descending duodenum.

4. Ileocolic orifice: ileal opening into colon, except in the horse.

5. Transverse colon: the middle colon arching cranially around the mesenteric root from <u>right to left</u> in all domestic species.

6. Descending colon: the longest segment of the large intestine. It extends from the transverse colon caudally on the <u>left</u> side of the dorsal abdomen to the pelvic inlet. Here it continues without demarcation as the rectum.

7. Rectum (REK-tum) (L. *rectus*, straight): the large intestine within the pelvic cavity, extending from the descending colon to the anal canal.

Anal canal: the short termination of the alimentary canal, opening to the exterior as the **anus.**

8. Anus (L. ring): the external opening of the intestine.

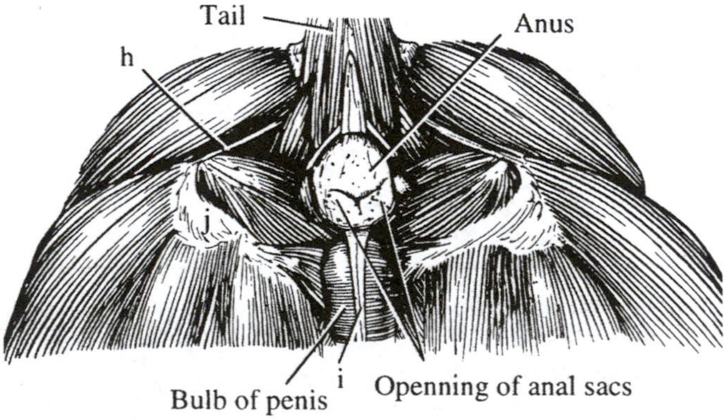

SPECIES DIFFERENCES

Ascending colon: most species differences of the large intestine are due to modification of the ascending colon.

• **Carnivores:** have a short, straight ascending colon.

• **Pig** and **ruminants:** forms a coil, the spiral colon.

• **Horse:** forms a double horseshoe-shaped loop.

Cecum: located on the abdomen's <u>right</u> side except in the pig, where it is on the left.

Openings into the cecum: the horse has two openings of the cecum, the **iliocecal** and **cecocolic.** The other domestic species have the cecocolic opening; while the ileum opens into the colon by the **ileocolic** opening.

Anal sacs: pouches located between the inner smooth and outer striated sphincter muscles of the **carnivore's** anus (cats as well as dogs). The anal sacs open into the anal canal at positions comparable to 4 and 8 o'clock.

Bands (teniae): the smooth muscle bands on the **horse** and **pig** cecum, the horse's colon and part of the pig's ascending colon. These bands cause the sacculations (haustra) of the gut wall.

Rectal ampulla (c): the dilated terminal part of the rectum in the horse, dog and ox.

CLINICAL

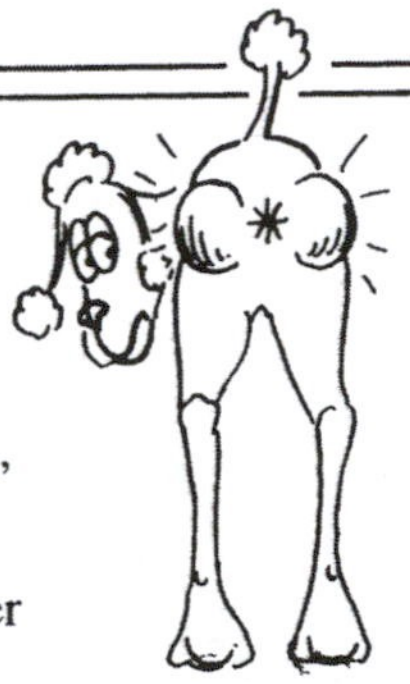

Colitis: inflammation of the colon.

Typhlitis: inflammation of the cecum

Anal sacs: their ducts can become plugged, causing discomfort (scooting).

Rectal prolapse: the protrusion of the inner surface of the rectum through the anus.

Fig. 107a - Dog - Caud. view of anal region

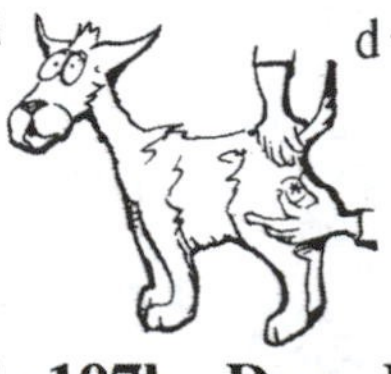

Labels: Tail, Anus, h, j, Bulb of penis, i, Openning of anal sacs

a. Anorectal line
b. Columnar zone
c. Anocutaneous line or intermediate zone
d. Cutaneous zone
e. Retococcygeus m.
f. Lymph follicles
g. Circumanal glands
h. Sacrouberous lig.
i. Retractor penis m.
j. Ischiatic tuberosity

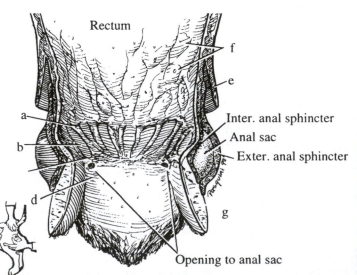

Fig 107b - Dog - Rectum & anal canal, opened on mid-dorsal line

Labels: Rectum, f, e, Inter. anal sphincter, Anal sac, Exter. anal sphincter, a, b, d, g, Opening to anal sac

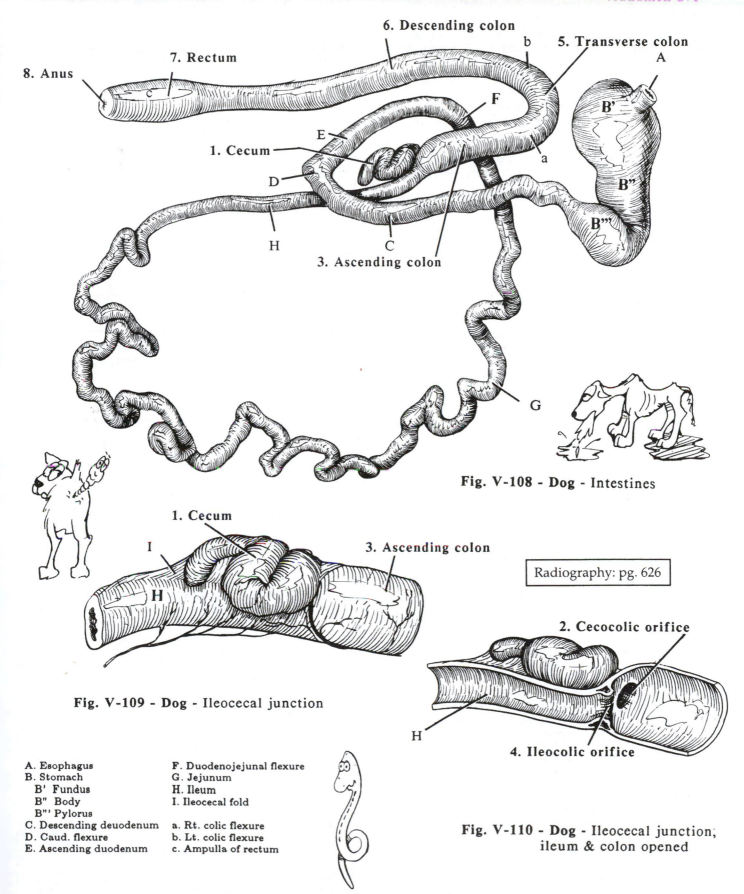

6. Descending colon

5. Transverse colon

7. Rectum

8. Anus

E

1. Cecum

D

F

A

B'

B"

B'''

a

b

H

C

3. Ascending colon

G

Fig. V-108 - Dog - Intestines

1. Cecum

I

H

3. Ascending colon

Radiography: pg. 626

2. Cecocolic orifice

H

4. Ileocolic orifice

Fig. V-109 - Dog - Ileocecal junction

Fig. V-110 - Dog - Ileocecal junction;
ileum & colon opened

A. Esophagus
B. Stomach
  B' Fundus
  B" Body
  B''' Pylorus
C. Descending deuodenum
D. Caud. flexure
E. Ascending duodenum

F. Duodenojejunal flexure
G. Jejunum
H. Ileum
I. Ileocecal fold

a. Rt. colic flexure
b. Lt. colic flexure
c. Ampulla of rectum

CECUM: a huge, comma-shaped structure occupying much of the right abdominal cavity. It consists of a base, body and apex.
- **1. Base**: the bulbous beginning of the cecum in the **right** paralumbar fossa.
- **2. Body**: the continuation of the base cranially along the right wall and floor of the abdominal cavity.
- **3. Apex**: the tapered end of the cecum on the floor of the abdominal cavity, caudal to the xiphoid cartilage. The ventral colon wraps around it.

4. Ileocecal opening: the ileal opening into the base of the cecum. In the other domestic species, the ileum opens into the colon.

5. Cecocolic opening: the opening at the base of the cecum to the ascending colon.

COLON: a highly modified structure with great capacity in the horse.

Ascending colon: due to its size, also called the **great colon**. Imagine the generalized short ascending colon grasped in its middle and stretched out. The formed loop then is folded on itself. This gives the double horseshoe loop of the horse's ascending colon. The two loops lie on top of each other, with the front of the loops toward the diaphragm, and the turn between the two loops at the pelvic inlet. The different portions of the ascending colon listed as they receive food are – right ventral colon – sternal flexure – left ventral colon – pelvic flexure – left dorsal colon – diaphragmatic flexure and right dorsal colon.

- **6. Right ventral colon**: the beginning of the ascending colon at the cecocolic opening and extending cranially on the right abdominal floor to the sternum.

- **7. Sternal flexure**: the connection between the right and left ventral colons curving around the apex of the cecum.

- **8. Left ventral colon**: the continuation of the sternal flexure that ends in the pelvic flexure.

- **9. Pelvic flexure**: the connection of the left ventral and left dorsal colons in the left paralumbar fossa, near the pelvic inlet.

- **10. Left dorsal colon**: the continuation the pelvic flexure cranially on top of the left ventral colon, and against the left abdominal wall.

- **11. Diaphragmatic flexure**: the continuation of the left dorsal colon on top of the sternal flexure.

- **12. Right dorsal colon**: the greatly expanded continuation of the diaphragmatic flexure caudally to the transverse colon. The ampulla coli ("stomach-like" dilatation) is the expanded terminal portion of the right dorsal colon.

13. Transverse colon: the segment of colon curving from right to left cranial to the root of the mesentery.

14. Descending colon: the continuation of the transverse colon to the rectum. Smaller than the ascending colon, the descending colon is called the **small colon**. Compared to the other domestic species, the horse's descending colon is long with a long mesocolon, allowing it a wide range of motion.

RECTUM: the terminal part of the intestines located in the pelvic cavity. In the horse, as in the dog and ox, it has a terminal dilation, the **rectal ampulla.**

Mesocolon: the connecting peritoneum arising from the abdominal roof and extending between the dorsal and ventral colons.

Bands or **teniae** (TEE-nee ah) sin. tenia (L. "a flat band"): the variable number of longitudinal smooth muscle cords on the cecum and the different segments of the colon. Some of these are hidden in the mesentery attached to the different segments. On the ventral colon there are two bands in the mesocolon and two free bands. The band on the pelvic flexure and the left dorsal colon is in the mesocolon. One of the bands of the right dorsal colon is in the mesocolon and two are free. The small colon has a mesocolic and a free band. The cecocolic fold connects the right ventral colon to the lateral band of the cecum. The ileocecal fold connects the ileum to the dorsal band of the cecum.

Sacculations or **haustra**: the series of pouches in the walls of the cecum and ventral colon formed by the bands of these intestinal segments.

CLINICAL

Bands and **segment identification**: the teniae are used to distinguish between parts of the large intestine and, indirectly, the small intestine. The most significant segments to be differentiated are the descending colon (two bands), the pelvic flexure (one band) and the small intestine (no bands). These need to be distinguished because of their similar size and because they are all located in the left paralumbar fossa.

Impaction: tightly wedged intestinal contents so as to be immovable.
- Common impaction sites due to diameter changes from large to small:
  - Pelvic flexure
  - Cecum
  - Transverse colon

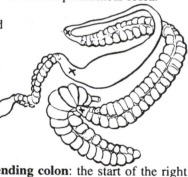

Displacement of the ascending colon: the start of the right ventral colon is connected to the base of the cecum and the end of the right dorsal colon is attached to the transverse colon. The rest of the ascending colon is free to move and possibly twist on itself. These usually can be diagnosed by rectal palpation.

- **Right dorsal displacement**: the ascending colon twists in the right abdomen; the pelvic flexure points cranially.

- **Nephrosplenic entrapment**: left dorsal displacement, the colon slides up the left side of the abdomen between the spleen and left body wall and becomes entrapped

Enteroliths: mineral concretions that can obstruct the start of the transverse colon.

Tapeworms: *Anoplocephala perfolata, A. magna,* and *Paranoplocephala mamillana,* located in the intestines; not proven to cause clinical disease.

Rectal tears: easily done in a horse during rectal palpation (#1 cause of lawsuits).

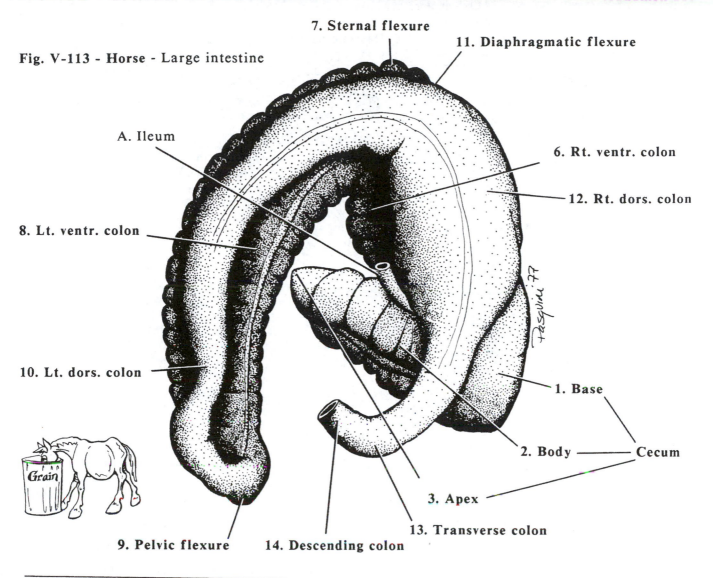

Fig. V-113 - Horse - Large intestine

7. Sternal flexure
11. Diaphragmatic flexure
A. Ileum
6. Rt. ventr. colon
12. Rt. dors. colon
8. Lt. ventr. colon
10. Lt. dors. colon
1. Base
2. Body — Cecum
3. Apex
13. Transverse colon
9. Pelvic flexure
14. Descending colon

NUMBER OF BANDS ON HORSE INTESTINES

Small intestine	0
Cecum and ventr. colon including sternal flexure	4
Pelvic flexure	1
Lt.dors. colon	1
Rt. dors.colon	3
Small colon	2

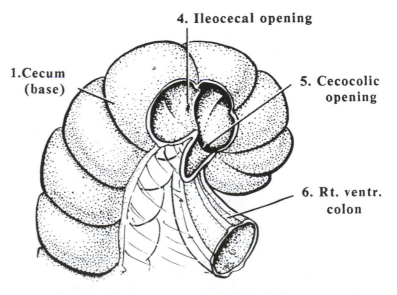

4. Ileocecal opening
1.Cecum (base)
5. Cecocolic opening
6. Rt. ventr. colon

Fig. V-114 - Horse - Cecum & ventr. colon opened - rt. side

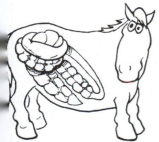

Rt. dors. displacement

Rectal tears

Ox - exploratory laparotomy: pg 646

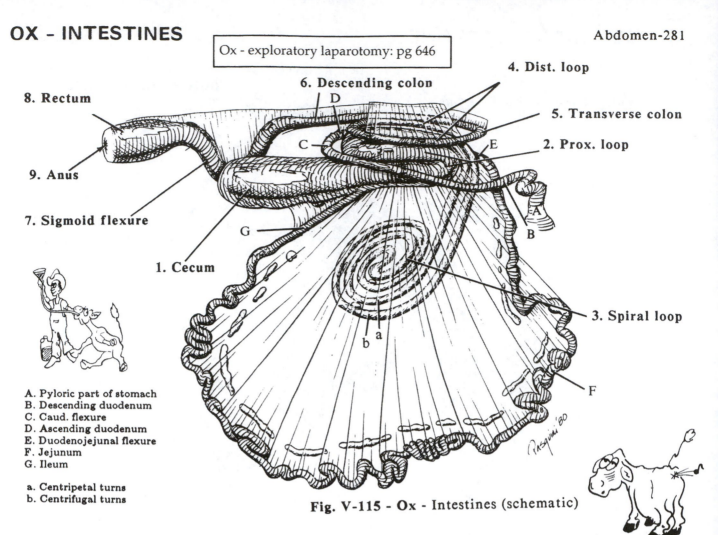

8. Rectum

9. Anus

7. Sigmoid flexure

6. Descending colon

4. Dist. loop

5. Transverse colon

2. Prox. loop

1. Cecum

3. Spiral loop

A. Pyloric part of stomach
B. Descending duodenum
C. Caud. flexure
D. Ascending duodenum
E. Duodenojejunal flexure
F. Jejunum
G. Ileum

a. Centripetal turns
b. Centrifugal turns

Fig. V-115 - Ox - Intestines (schematic)

1. CECUM - OX: the large, blind tube extending caudally from the ileocecocolic junction on the right side of the mesentery.

COLON - OX

Ascending colon: the part of the large intestine divided into proximal, spiral and distal loops.

• **2. Proximal loop:** the S-shaped loop continuing the cecum cranially. It doubles back caudally on the right side of the mesentery, and then cranially on the left side of the mesentery to continue as the spiral loop.

• **3. Spiral loop:** the segment rolled up on itself, forming a flat disc attached to the left side of the mesentery. Usually two centripetal turns (a) spiral toward the central flexure. Two centrifugal turns (b) spiral away from the central flexure and continue as the distal loop.

Sheep and goat: the last centrifugal coil separates from the spiral loop and passes in the greater mesentery very near the jejunal coils before continuing as the distal loop.

• **4. Distal loop:** U-shaped, it runs first caudally on the left side of the mesentery, and then cranially on the right side of the mesentery to become the transverse colon. It is attached high in the abdomen with the transverse colon and start of the descending colon.

5. Transverse colon: arches from right to left in front of the mesenteric root to become descending colon.

6. Descending colon: the continuation of the transverse colon caudally on the abdomen's left side next to the ascending duodenum.

• **7. Sigmoid flexure:** the region of the descending colon with a long mesocolon hanging down into the abdomen; it allows great range of motion during rectal palpation.

8. RECTUM: the continuation of the descending colon into the pelvic cavity to terminate in the **anal canal** and **anus** (9).

Clinical:

Cecal dilation and volvulus: twisting of the cecum and its filling with gas. This results in distention of the right paralumbar fossa and a large area of resonance.

Rectal prolapse: a common condition in cattle caused by tenesmus (straining).

Proctitis: inflammation of the rectum.

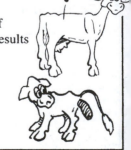

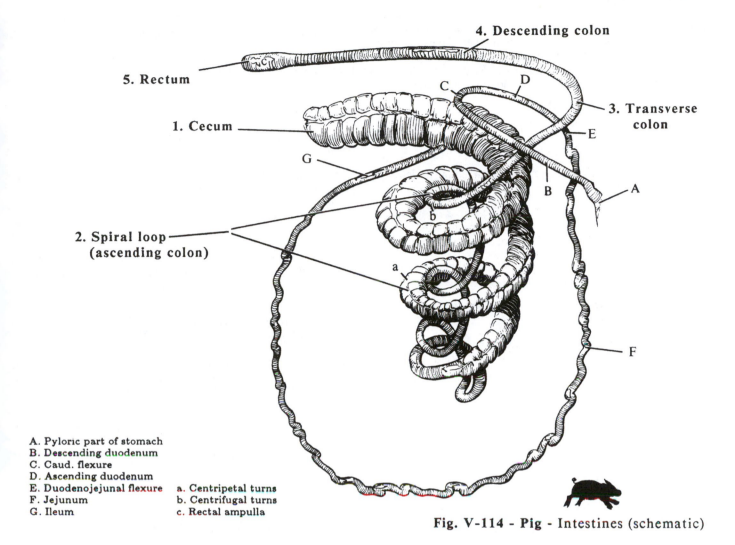

4. Descending colon

5. Rectum

1. Cecum

G

**2. Spiral loop
(ascending colon)**

C

D

**3. Transverse
colon**

E

A

B

b

a

F

A. Pyloric part of stomach
B. Descending duodenum
C. Caud. flexure
D. Ascending duodenum
E. Duodenojejunal flexure
F. Jejunum
G. Ileum

a. Centripetal turns
b. Centrifugal turns
c. Rectal ampulla

Fig. V-114 - Pig - Intestines (schematic)

1. CECUM - PIG: the blind sac extending caudally from the ileocolic junction. It has tendinous bands that form rows of sacculations as in the horse. Unlike the other domestic species, in the pig it is on the <u>left</u> side of the abdomen.

COLON - PIG: divided into ascending, transverse and descending parts.

Ascending colon: the highly modified part of the colon responsible for the pig's unique intestinal pattern.

2. Spiral loop: the coiling loop of the ascending colon forming a cone-shaped structure. The large first part makes centripetal turns clockwise (when viewed dorsally) on the outside of the cone to the cone's apex (central flexure). The thinner, second part makes centrifugal turns counterclockwise inside the centripetal turns and then continues as the transverse colon. The centripetal turns have tendinous bands and sacculations.

3. Transverse colon: the continuation of the ascending colon from right to left around the front of the mesentery.

4. Descending colon: the continuation of the transverse colon in a straight line to the pelvic cavity.

5. RECTUM: the continuation of the descending colon through the pelvic cavity to terminate as the anal canal. The **rectal ampulla** (ampulla recti) (c) is the flask-like dilation of the terminal rectum.

SEROUS MEMBRANES

SEROUS MEMBRANE or **SEROSA**: a thin continuous membrane lining the closed cavity of the body and covering the cavity's organs. The serosa consists of a layer of mesothelium* backed by connective tissue. The serosa secretes a lubricating fluid, allowing movement of the organs without friction. The serous membranes of the abdominal and thoracic cavities are the peritoneum and pleura respectively.

Parietal (pa-RY-e-tal) **serosa**: lines a cavity wall, intimately.

Visceral serosa: invests the organs within a cavity.

Connecting serosa: the two layers of serosa uniting parietal and visceral serosal layers or two visceral serosal layers.

PERITONEUM (per'i-toh-NEE-um): the serosa lining the abdomen and covering its organs. It consists of parietal and visceral peritoneum that are continuous at folds of connecting peritoneum.

A. Parietal peritoneum: the serosa lining the inner wall of the abdominal, pelvic and scrotal cavities.

B. Visceral peritoneum: the serosa covering the organs of the abdominal and pelvic cavities.

C. Connecting peritoneum: the double-layered serosa connecting parietal and visceral peritoneum, or between visceral peritoneum. It includes the mesenteries, omentum, ligaments and folds.

• **1. Mesenteries**: see pg. 284

• **2. Omentum**: see pg. 286

• **Ligaments**: connecting peritoneum between visceral peritoneum surrounding some organs and parietal peritoneum, or between visceral peritoneum of two organs.

  - **3. Ligaments of the liver**: the connecting peritoneum (right and left triangular and coronary ligaments) between the liver and diaphragm.

  - **Falciform ligament**: a fold of connecting peritoneum extending from the liver to the ventral abdominal wall as far caudally as the umbilicus. In young animals the **round ligament** of the liver, the remnant of the fetal umbilical vein, is found in the free edge of the falciform ligament.

  - **Ligaments of the urinary bladder** (Fig. VII-10): the connecting peritoneum (median and lateral ligaments) between the bladder and pelvic wall.

• **4. FOLD**: a connecting peritoneum between two visceral organs (e.g., ileocecal fold).

D. PERITONEAL CAVITY: the potential space between the parietal and visceral peritoneum. This potential cavity contains no organs, only a small amount of lubricating fluid. Entirely closed in the male, it is open in the female at the abdominal end of the oviduct. This opening leads to the outside of the body cavity through the urogenital tract. The **ovarian bursa** (pg. 348) and **omental bursa** (pg. 286) are subdivisions of the peritoneal cavity. The **vaginal cavity** (pg. 362) of the spermatic cord is a diverticulum of the peritoneal cavity.

*Mesothelium: a layer of cells derived from mesoderm that lines the body cavities of the embryo. In the adult, it forms the epithelium of all serous membranes.

Pouches of the peritoneal cavity: formed by the caudal reflection of the peritoneum between organs in the pelvic cavity.

• **Rectogenital pouch** (a): the reflection of the peritoneal cavity between the rectum and the reproductive organs.

  – **Pararectal fossa** (b): the part of the rectogenital pouch on either side of the rectum.

• **Vesicogenital pouch** (c): the reflection of the peritoneal cavity between the urinary bladder and the internal genitalia.

• **Vesicopubic pouch** (d): the reflection of the peritoneal cavity between the ventral wall of the pelvic cavity (pubis of the ossa coxarum) and the urinary bladder.

E. Retroperitoneal (re'-troh-per-i-toh-NEE-al): the term used for a structure between the peritoneum and cavity wall, thus, having no connecting peritoneum (e.g. kidneys). It also applies to the portion of the pelvic organs not covered by peritoneum.

CLINICAL

Peritonitis (per'-i-toh-NY-tis): inflammation of the peritoneum.

Colic: a manifestation of abdominal pain. A common symptom in horses to many conditions.

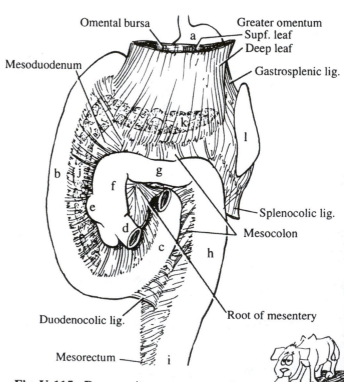

Fig. V-115 - Dog - peritoneum - ventr. view

a. Stomach	g. Transverse colon
b. Descending duodenum	h. Descending colon
c. Ascending duodenum	i. Rectum
d. Ilium	j. Pancreas, rt. lobe
e. Cecum	k. Pancreas, lt lobe
f. Ascending colon	l. Spleen

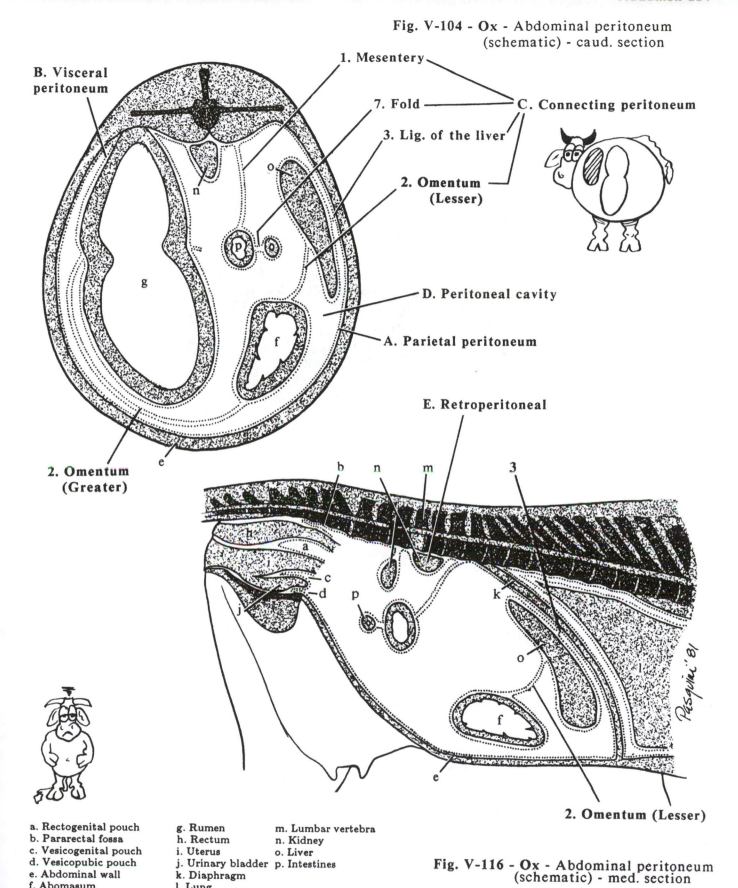

Fig. V-104 - **Ox** - Abdominal peritoneum
(schematic) - caud. section

B. **Visceral**
peritoneum

1. Mesentery

7. Fold ——— C. **Connecting peritoneum**

3. Lig. of the liver

2. **Omentum**
(Lesser)

D. Peritoneal cavity

A. Parietal peritoneum

E. Retroperitoneal

2. **Omentum**
(Greater)

2. **Omentum (Lesser)**

Fig. V-116 - **Ox** - Abdominal peritoneum
(schematic) - med. section

a. Rectogenital pouch	g. Rumen	m. Lumbar vertebra
b. Pararectal fossa	h. Rectum	n. Kidney
c. Vesicogenital pouch	i. Uterus	o. Liver
d. Vesicopubic pouch	j. Urinary bladder	p. Intestines
e. Abdominal wall	k. Diaphragm	
f. Abomasum	l. Lung	

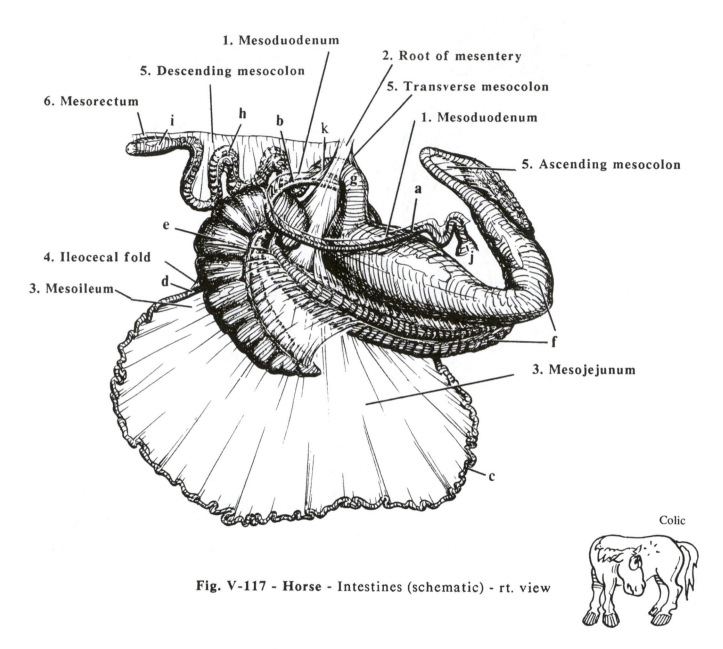

1. Mesoduodenum

5. Descending mesocolon

6. Mesorectum

2. Root of mesentery

5. Transverse mesocolon

1. Mesoduodenum

5. Ascending mesocolon

e

4. Ileocecal fold

3. Mesoileum

d

f

3. Mesojejunum

c

Colic

Fig. V-117 - Horse - Intestines (schematic) - rt. view

MESENTERIES (MEZ-en-ter-eez): a type of <u>connecting peritoneum</u> between the intestinal and reproductive tracts to the abdominal wall. They are the expansive, double-layered serosal folds between the visceral peritoneum and the parietal peritoneum. They contain the blood vessels, lymphatics and nerves supplying their respective organs. They are named according to the organs they suspend by adding the name of the organ to meso- (mesoduodenum, mesoileum, mesocolon, etc.). The "broad ligament" (mesovarian, mesometrium, etc.) is described in the chapter on reproduction (pg. 348).

1. Mesoduodenum: the peritoneal fold suspending the duodenum from the dorsal body wall. The descending mesoduodenum

encloses the right lobe of the pancreas.

Duodenocolic ligament (k): a peritoneal fold connecting the ascending duodenum to the descending colon.

2. Root of the mesentery: the narrow attachment of the long mesojejunum and mesoileum to the dorsal wall of the abdominal cavity. Located at the level of the second lumbar vertebra, it is thick because it contains the cranial mesenteric artery, intestinal lymphatics, and the mesenteric plexus of autonomic nerves. It is continuous toward the mouth (orad) with the mesoduodenum and away from the mouth (aborad) with the mesocolon.

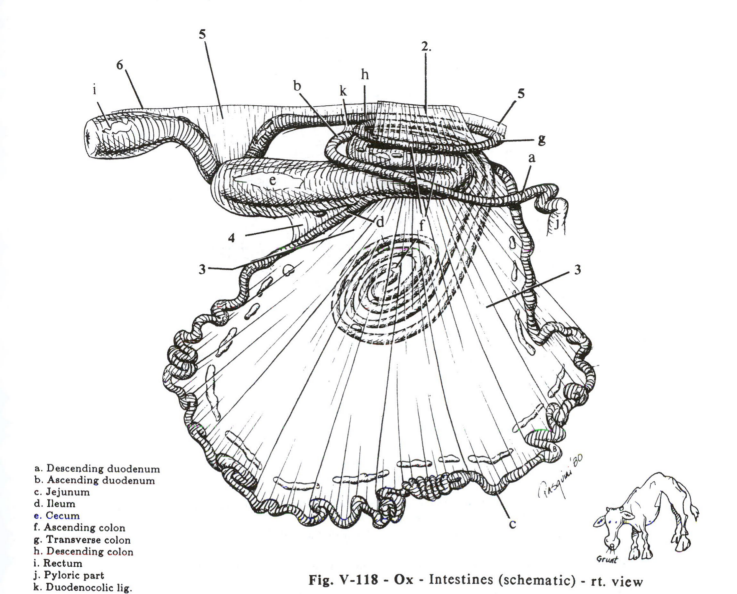

a. Descending duodenum
b. Ascending duodenum
c. Jejunum
d. Ileum
e. Cecum
f. Ascending colon
g. Transverse colon
h. Descending colon
i. Rectum
j. Pyloric part
k. Duodenocolic lig.

Fig. V-118 - Ox - Intestines (schematic) - rt. view

3. Mesojejunum and **mesoileum**: the continuation of the mesoduodenum that is very long and wide to support the jejunum and ileum.

4. Ileocecal fold: a fold of connecting peritoneum between the ileum and cecum. The jejunum and ileum are grossly indistinguishable. Use the proximal extent of this fold to roughly determine the beginning of the ileum. The proximal end of the antimesenteric ileal artery can also be used to roughly determine the junction of the ileum and jejunum.

5. Mesocolon: the serosal fold suspending the colon. It can be divided into ascending, transverse and descending mesocolons.

6. Mesorectum: the short mesentery suspending the rectum from the dorsal wall of the pelvic cavity.

SPECIES DIFFERENCES

Bovine mesentery: short when compared to other species. This makes exteriorizing parts of the intestine difficult. The mesentery in young calves and emaciated adults is filled with fat which, during surgery, obscures parts lying deep to them. The mesenteries of the ascending duodenum, the distal loop of the ascending colon, the transverse colon and the cranial part of the descending colon are fused together into a "conjoined tendon". The "conjoined tendon" anchors these structures high in the abdomen, making them difficult to distinguish from each other.

Bovine "flange": the most mobile part of the small intestine due to its long mesentery. It consists of the distal part of the jejunum and the proximal part of the ileum.

6. Omental vestibule

1. Lesser omentum

Fig. V-119 - Dog - Abdominal peritoneum
- med. section (schematic)

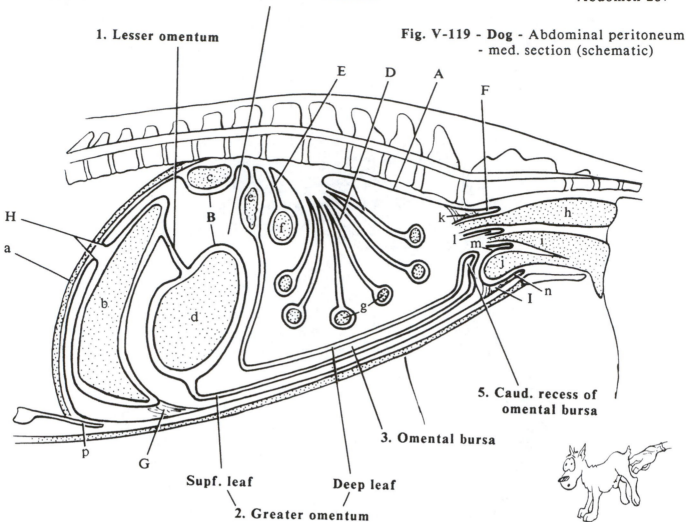

5. Caud. recess of omental bursa

3. Omental bursa

Supf. leaf

Deep leaf

2. Greater omentum

OMENTUM (oh-MEN-tum) (pl.= omenta) (Gr. *epiploon*): a double-layered connecting peritoneum between the stomach and abdominal organs or abdominal wall.

1. Lesser omentum: connects the lesser curvature of the stomach and first part of the duodenum to the porta of the liver. It is continuous aborad (away from the mouth) with the mesoduodenum.

• Gastrohepatic ligament: that portion of the lesser omentum connecting the lesser curvature of the stomach with the liver.

• Hepatoduodenal ligament: that portion of the lesser omentum connecting the liver to the duodenum.

2. Greater omentum: connects the greater curvature of the stomach to the dorsal abdominal wall. Greatly elongated in the dog, the greater omentum folds over itself. This results in a deep and a superficial leaf (four layers of peritoneum) between the viscera and the ventral abdominal wall.

• **Superficial leaf**: extends from the stomach caudally to the pelvic inlet where it reflects and returns cranially as the deep leaf.

• **Deep leaf**: attaches to the dorsal abdominal wall and contains the

left lobe of the pancreas between its peritoneal layers.

• Gastrophrenic ligament: connects the stomach to the diaphragm.

• **Gastrosplenic ligament**: connects the stomach to the spleen.

• Phrenicosplenic ligament: connects the spleen to the diaphragm.

3. Omental bursa: the potential space between the two leaves of the greater omentum and the structures to which they attach. It is a subdivision of the peritoneal cavity.

4. Omental (epiploic) foramen: the opening between the general peritoneal cavity and the omental bursa. It is located dorsally in the right side of the abdominal cavity between the caudal vena cava and the portal vein. It can be found by lifting the caudate lobe of the liver and placing a finger between these two vessels.

6. Omental vestibule: the cranial part of the omental bursa. The omental foramen opens into the omental vestibule.

5. Caudal recess of the omental bursa: the caudal part of the potential space between the two leaves of the greater omentum.

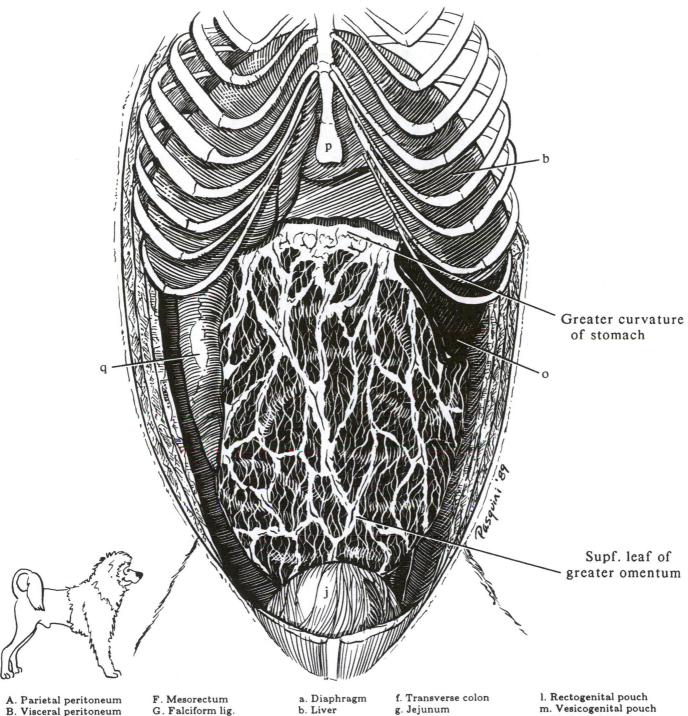

b

p

Greater curvature
of stomach

q

o

Pasquini '89

Supf. leaf of
greater omentum

j

A. Parietal peritoneum
B. Visceral peritoneum
C. Root of mesentery
D-F. Connecting peritoneum
D. Mesojejunum
E. Mesocolon

F. Mesorectum
G. Falciform lig.
H. Lig. (coronary)
   of liver
I. Lig. (median) of
   urinary bladder

a. Diaphragm
b. Liver
c. Kidney (retro-
   peritoneal)
d. Stomach
e. Pancreas

f. Transverse colon
g. Jejunum
h. Rectum
i. Uterus
j. Urinary bladder
k. Pararectal fossa

l. Rectogenital pouch
m. Vesicogenital pouch
n. Vesicopubic pouch
o. Spleen (V-120)
p. Xiphoid cartilage
q. Descending duodenum

**Fig. V-120 - Dog - Abdominal
wall removed**

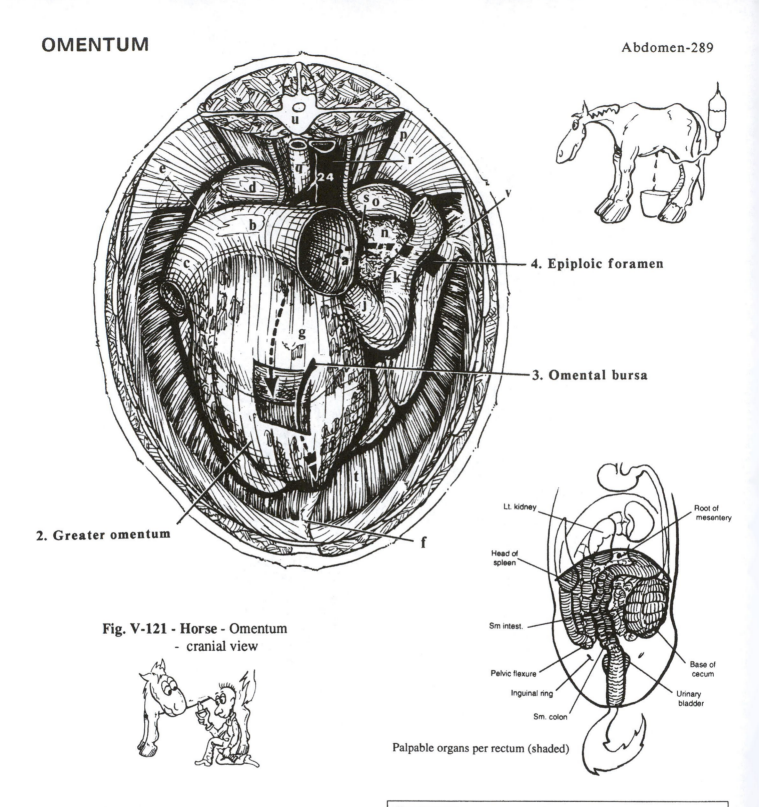

Fig. V-121 - Horse - Omentum
- cranial view

4. **Epiploic foramen**

3. **Omental bursa**

2. **Greater omentum**

Lt. kidney

Root of mesentery

Head of spleen

Sm intest.

Base of cecum

Pelvic flexure

Urinary bladder

Inguinal ring

Sm. colon

Palpable organs per rectum (shaded)

SPECIES DIFFERENCES

Greater omentum: as described above for animals with simple stomachs such as the carnivores, pig and horse. The ruminant, having several stomach compartments, has a different arrangement (pg. 290).

CLINICAL

Peritoneum: should not be sutured separately when closing an abdominal incision (laparotomy). It can be included in other sutured layers. The less trauma to the peritoneum, the better the closure.

Intestinal herniation or entrapment through the omental (epiploic) foramen: rare.

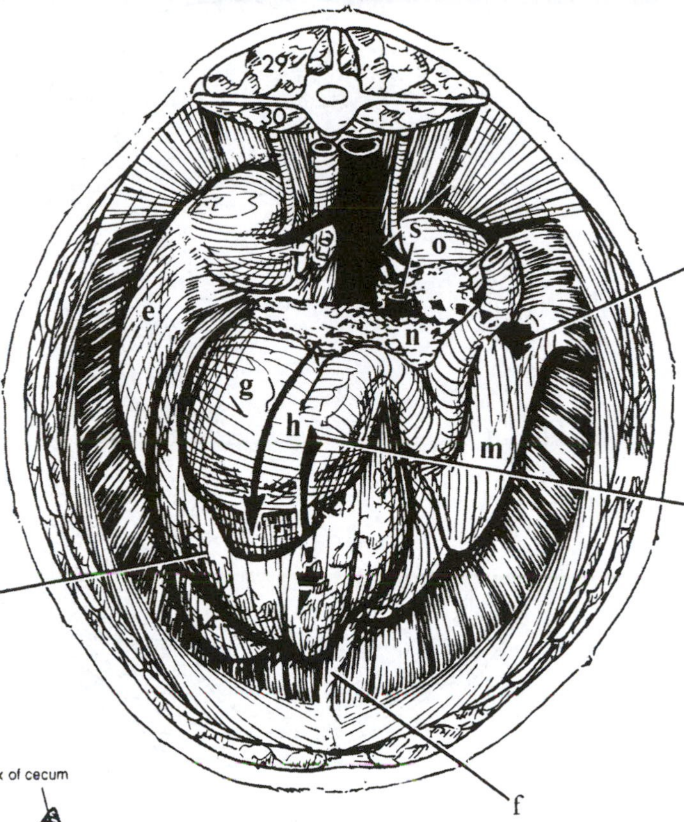

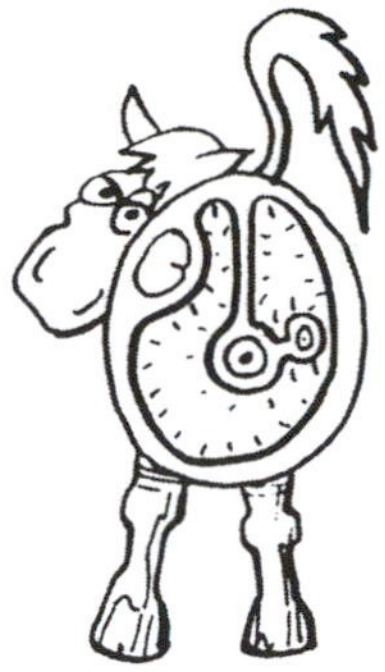

Fig. V-122 - Horse - Omentum & epiploic foramen, transverse colon removed

4. Omental foramen

3. Omental bursa

1. Greater omentum

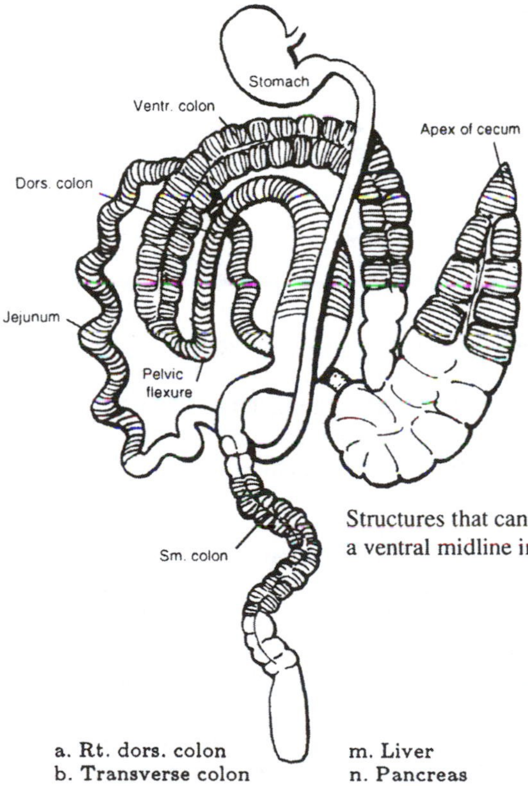

Structures that can be exteriorized through a ventral midline incision (shaded)

Stomach
Ventr. colon
Dors. colon
Jejunum
Pelvic flexure
Sm. colon
Apex of cecum

a. Rt. dors. colon
b. Transverse colon
c. Descending colon
d. Lt. kidney
e. Spleen
f. Falciform lig.
g. Body of stomach
h. Lesser curvature
i. Greater curvature
j. Pylorus
k. Cran. duodenum
l. Descending duodenum

m. Liver
n. Pancreas
o. Rt. kidney
p. Ureter
q. Aorta
r. Caud. vena cava
s. Portal v.
t. Diaphragm
u. 4th lumbar vertebra
v. Rt. triangular lig. of liver

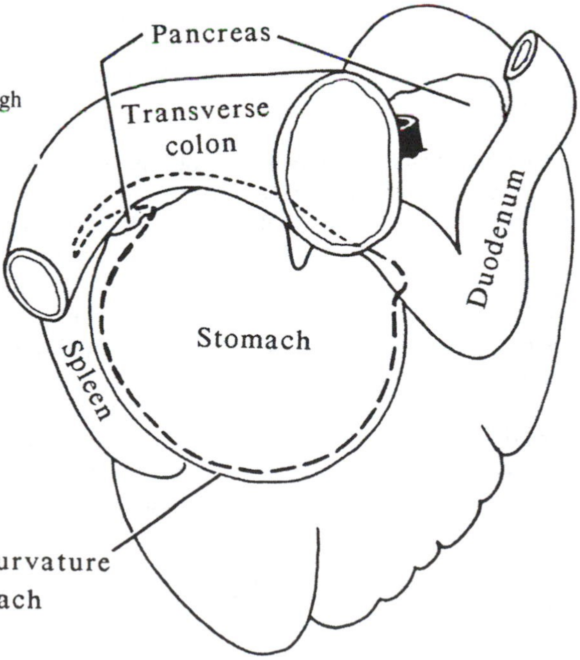

Pancreas

Transverse colon

Duodenum

Spleen

Stomach

Greater curvature of stomach

Fig. V-123 - Horse - Line of attachment of greater omentum

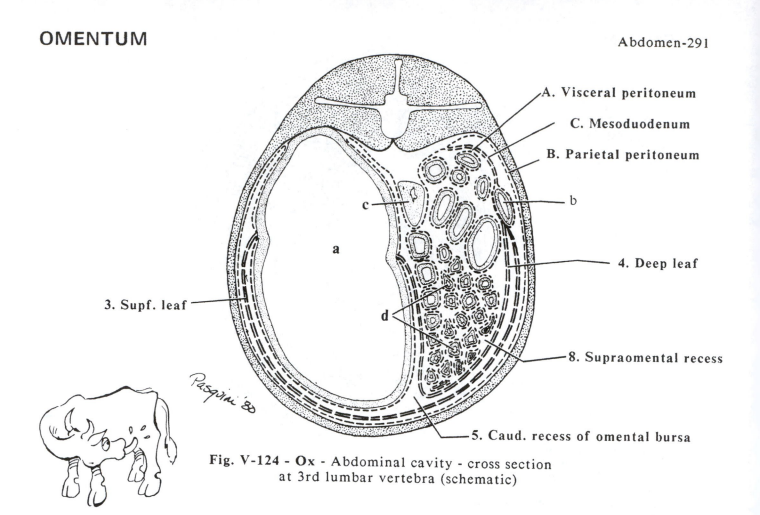

Fig. V-124 - Ox - Abdominal cavity - cross section
at 3rd lumbar vertebra (schematic)

A. Visceral peritoneum
C. Mesoduodenum
B. Parietal peritoneum
b
4. Deep leaf
8. Supraomental recess
5. Caud. recess of omental bursa
3. Supf. leaf

OMENTUM - RUMINANT: the omenta of the ruminants, because of their complex stomachs, are arranged differently than animals with simple stomachs.

1. Lesser omentum: the connecting peritoneum between the liver and the omasum, the lesser curvature of the abomasum, and the cranial duodenum. It covers the right side of the omasum.

2. Greater omentum: has two leaves as in the other species. The superficial leaf arises from the left side of the rumen, and the deep leaf from the right side of the rumen. Both leaves extend ventrally and to the right, forming a sling for the intestines to the right of the rumen. Both leaves ascend together along the right abdominal wall to attach to the descending duodenum. The two leaves are continuous around the caudal end of the rumen as the **caudal edge** of the greater omentum.

3. Superficial leaf: attaches to the greater curvature of the abomasum and the descending duodenum. It extends along the ventral abdominal wall to the left side to attach to the left longitudinal groove of the rumen.

4. Deep leaf: extends from the right longitudinal groove of the rumen to the descending duodenum.

5. Omental bursa: the space, as in the other domestic species, between the superficial and deep leaves of the greater omentum.

It is divided into a vestibule and a caudal recess.

6. Omental (epiploic) foramen: the opening between the omental bursa and the general peritoneal cavity. It is medial to the caudate lobe of the liver and between the caudal vena cava and the portal vein.

7. Caudal edge of the greater omentum: the joining of the superficial and deep leaves of the greater omentum at the caudal edge of the rumen. The caudal edge is attached on the right to the descending duodenum. On the left, it attaches to the caudal groove of the rumen where the superficial and deep leaves join.

8. Supraomental recess: the space above the deep leaf of the greater omentum. It is open caudally and contains the intestines.

CLINICAL

Omentum: when opening the right paralumbar fossa of the ruminant, the greater omentum ("omental curtain"), the descending duodenum and mesoduodeum only are seen. The superficial and deep leaves of the greater omentum extend from the descending duodenum forming a sling under the intestines. To visualize the intestines in the supraomental recess, grasp the caudal edge of the greater omentum and move it cranially like a shower curtain.

Fig. V-125 - Ox - Omentum & abdominal viscera - rt. side

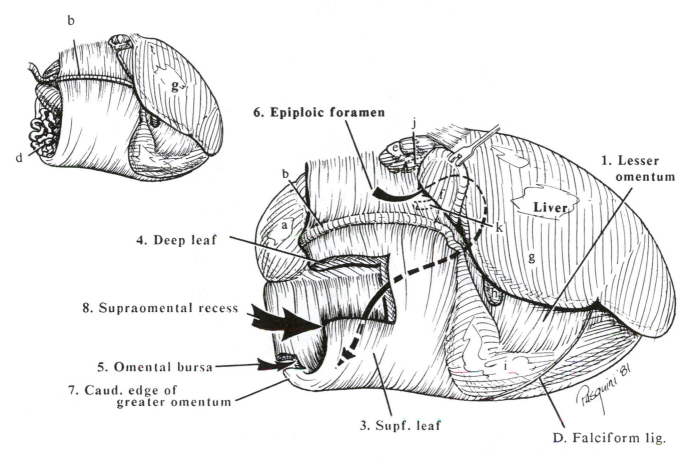

6. Epiploic foramen

1. Lesser omentum

Liver

4. Deep leaf

8. Supraomental recess

5. Omental bursa

7. Caud. edge of greater omentum

3. Supf. leaf

D. Falciform lig.

Pasquini '81

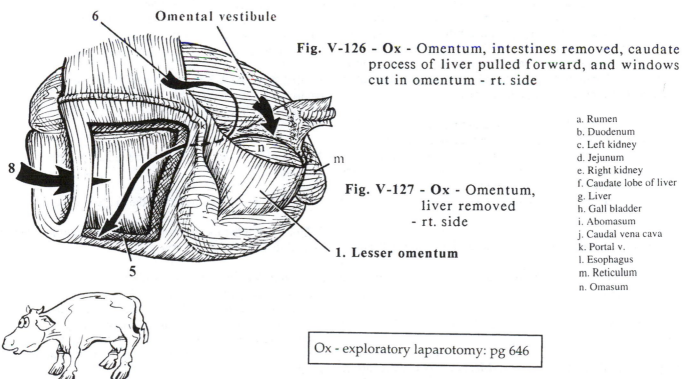

6
Omental vestibule

8

5

Fig. V-126 - Ox - Omentum, intestines removed, caudate process of liver pulled forward, and windows cut in omentum - rt. side

a. Rumen
b. Duodenum
c. Left kidney
d. Jejunum
e. Right kidney
f. Caudate lobe of liver
g. Liver
h. Gall bladder
i. Abomasum
j. Caudal vena cava
k. Portal v.
l. Esophagus
m. Reticulum
n. Omasum

Fig. V-127 - Ox - Omentum, liver removed - rt. side

1. Lesser omentum

Ox - exploratory laparotomy: pg 646

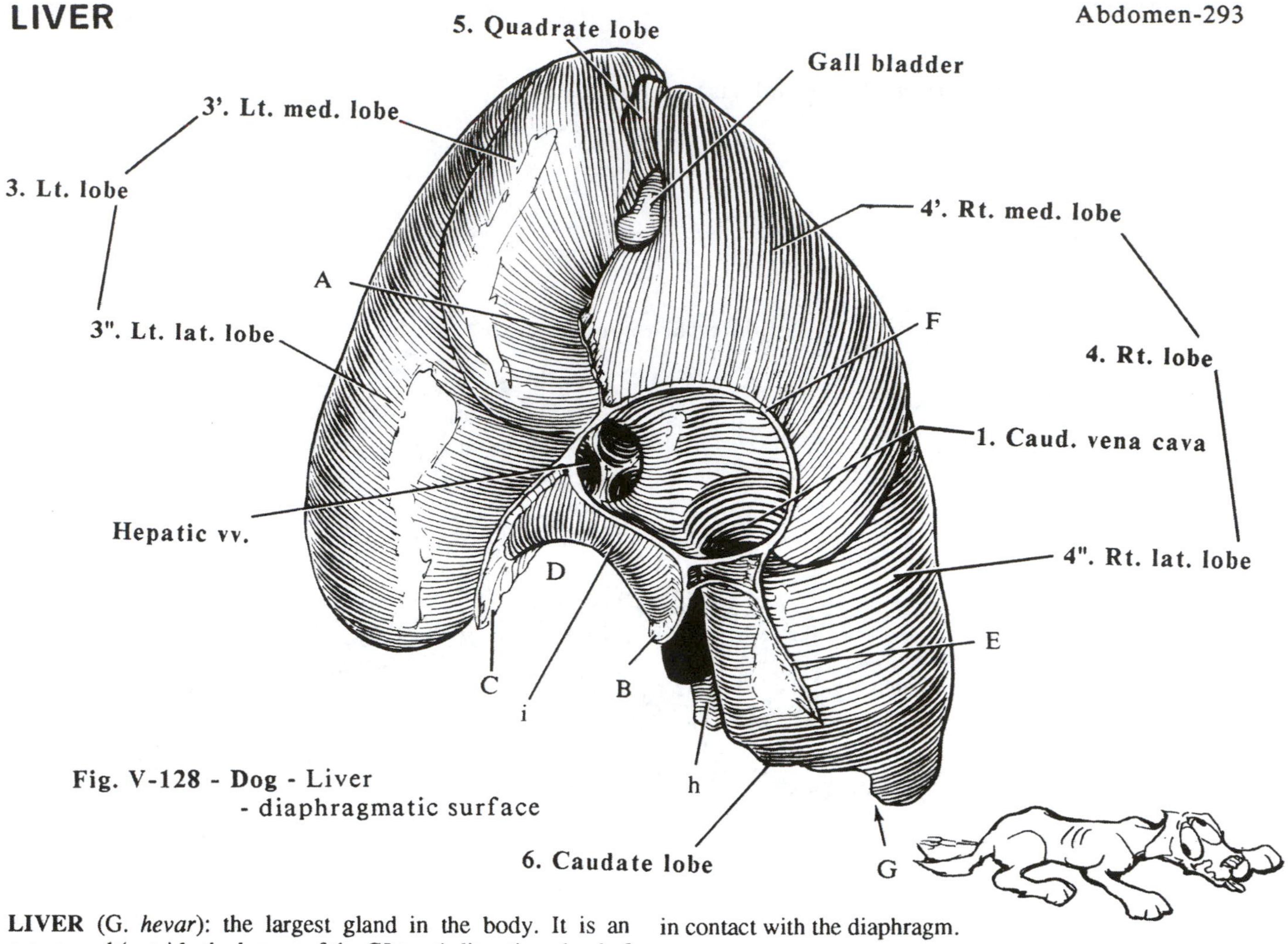

LIVER

5. Quadrate lobe

Gall bladder

3'. Lt. med. lobe

3. Lt. lobe

4'. Rt. med. lobe

A

F

3". Lt. lat. lobe

4. Rt. lobe

1. Caud. vena cava

Hepatic vv.

4". Rt. lat. lobe

D

E

C

B

i

h

Fig. V-128 - Dog - Liver
- diaphragmatic surface

6. Caudate lobe

G

LIVER (G. *hevar*): the largest gland in the body. It is an extramural (outside the lumen of the GI tract) digestive gland of substantial importance in metabolism. Situated between the vessels draining the intestines and the general circulation, the liver has many complex functions, e.g., detoxification of drugs and toxins, formation and secretion of bile, metabolism of carbohydrates and fats, plasma protein production, urea formation, inactivation of polypeptide hormones, and reduction and conjugation of adrenal and gonadal steroid hormones.

The liver is in the abdominal cavity, abutting the diaphragm. The caudate process encloses the cranial pole of the right kidney in the right dorsal abdomen. The stomach and first part of the descending duodenum lie against the liver's visceral surface. Three distinct landmarks are used to orient the liver once it is removed from the body cavity – caudal vena cava, porta, and renal impression.

1. Caudal vena cava: runs through the <u>dorsal</u> portion of the liver.

2. Porta: the area where the vessels and nerves enter the organ on the <u>visceral</u> surface.

3. Renal impression: the indentation for the right kidney on the liver's <u>right</u> side.

Diaphragmatic surface (dy-a-fra-MAT-ik): the convex surface

in contact with the diaphragm.

Visceral surface: the side in contact with the abdominal viscera. The right kidney, stomach, duodenum, colon and jejunum produce impressions on the liver's visceral surface when the organ is hardened <u>in situ.</u>

LOBES and PROCESSES of the LIVER: deep fissures divide the liver into four basic lobes, and two processes. The right and left lobes may be divided into medial and lateral lobes, depending on the species.

3. Left lobe: lies to the left of the median plane except in the ruminants.

4. Right lobe: lies to the right of the median plane.

5. Quadrate lobe: located between the right and left lobes and ventral to the porta of the liver.

6. Caudate lobe: located dorsal to the porta of the liver, consisting of caudate and papillary processes. The **papillary process** (i) is the part of the caudate lobe to the left of the median plane lying in the lesser curvature of the stomach. The **caudate process** (h) is the most caudal region of the liver. It has a renal impression that cups the cranial end of the right kidney in all domestic species, except the pig.

LIVER

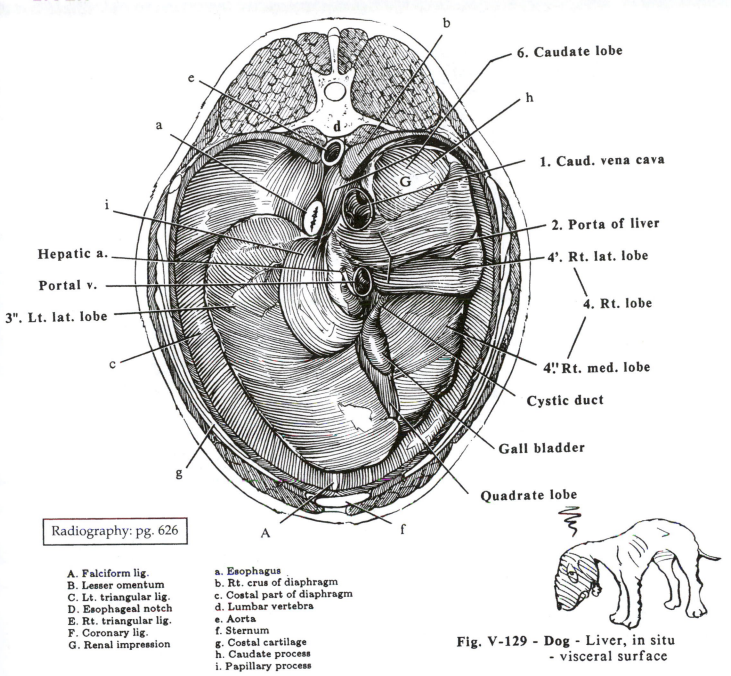

6. Caudate lobe

h

1. Caud. vena cava

2. Porta of liver

4'. Rt. lat. lobe

4. Rt. lobe

4'' Rt. med. lobe

Cystic duct

Gall bladder

Quadrate lobe

Hepatic a.

Portal v.

3". Lt. lat. lobe

Radiography: pg. 626

A. Falciform lig.
B. Lesser omentum
C. Lt. triangular lig.
D. Esophageal notch
E. Rt. triangular lig.
F. Coronary lig.
G. Renal impression

a. Esophagus
b. Rt. crus of diaphragm
c. Costal part of diaphragm
d. Lumbar vertebra
e. Aorta
f. Sternum
g. Costal cartilage
h. Caudate process
i. Papillary process

Fig. V-129 - Dog - Liver, in situ - visceral surface

SPECIES DIFFERENCES:

Carnivores: the right and left lobes are divided into <u>medial</u> and <u>lateral</u> lobes. The caudate lobe is divided into a <u>caudate</u> process and <u>papillary</u> process as in the ox.

Pig: similar to the carnivores, except for the <u>lack of the papillary process</u> of the caudate lobe.

Horse: resembles the carnivores, except the <u>right lobe is undivided</u> and the <u>papillary process is also missing</u>, as in the pig. The horse's liver is located obliquely across the diaphragm with the left lobe ventral and the right lobe dorsal.)Some authors based on branching of ducts and vessels within the liver say the left lobe is also not divided.)

Ruminants: resembles the carnivores, except that <u>neither right nor left lobe is divided</u>. The rumen has moved the <u>liver to the right</u> side of the abdominal cavity. The liver is also rotated, with the right lobe dorsal and the left lobe ventral.

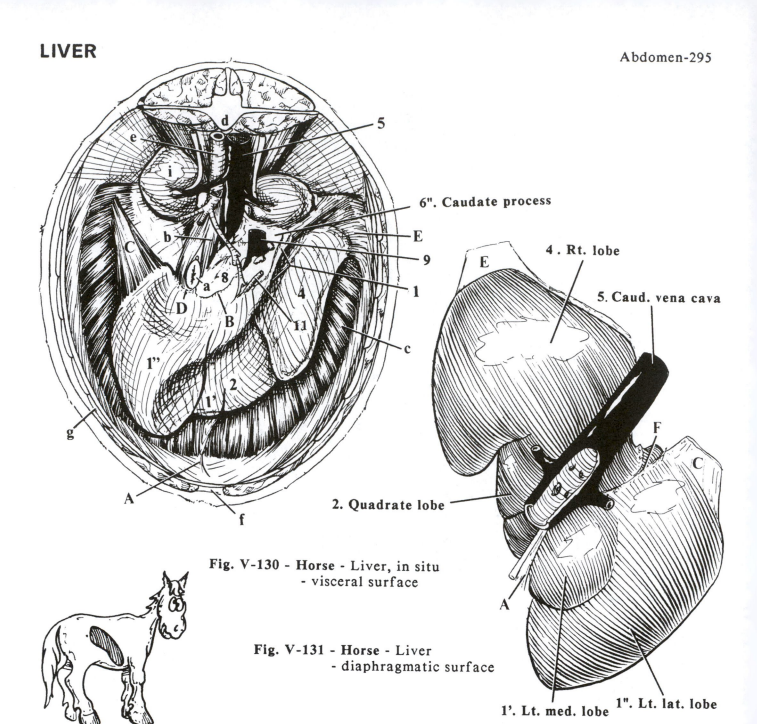

Fig. V-130 - Horse - Liver, in situ
- visceral surface

Fig. V-131 - Horse - Liver
- diaphragmatic surface

6". Caudate process

E

9

1

c

4. Rt. lobe

5. Caud. vena cava

F

C

2. Quadrate lobe

1'. Lt. med. lobe

1". Lt. lat. lobe

LIVER ATTACHMENTS: The **fibrous capsule** is the strong, mainly collagenous, tissue layer closely investing the liver's surface and interior vascular and nervous elements. The liver is covered with visceral peritoneum.

Coronary ligament of the liver (F): the reflection of peritoneum from the diaphragmatic surface of the liver onto the diaphragm. It forms a circular area of reflection (corona means crown, thus, its name) around the caudal vena cava. The coronary ligament comes together in three places to form the two triangular and falciform ligaments.

Right triangular ligament (E): attaches the dorsal part of the right lateral lobe to the right crus of the diaphragm.

Left triangular ligament (C): attaches the dorsal part of the left lateral lobe to the left crus and tendinous center of the diaphragm.

Falciform ligament (L. *falx*, sickle + *forma*, form) (A): connects the ventral liver to the sternal part of the diaphragm and ventral abdomen.

Round ligament of the liver: contained in the free border of the falciform ligament, is a vestige of the umbilical vein of the fetus.

Lesser omentum (B): extends from the porta of the liver to the lesser curvature of the stomach and the cranial portion of the duodenum. It can be divided into hepatoduodenal and gastrohepatic parts.

LIVER

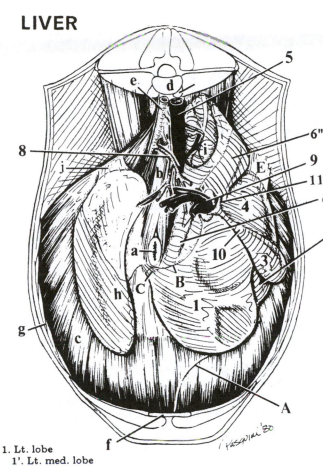

Ox - exploratory laparotomy: pg 646

Fig. V-132 - Ox - Liver, spleen & rt. kidney

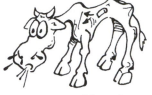

Liver abscesses

6". Caudate process

9

11

6'. Papillary process

2. Quadrate lobe

Fig. V-133 - Ox - Liver
- diaphragmatic surface

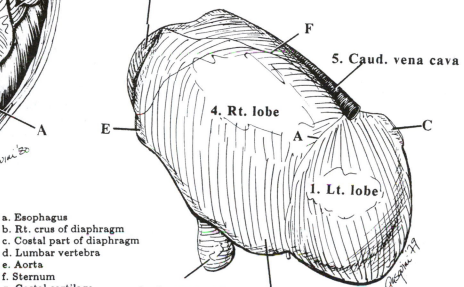

6. Caudate lobe

5. Caud. vena cava

4. Rt. lobe

1. Lt. lobe

3. Gall bladder

2. Quadrate lobe

1. Lt. lobe
  1'. Lt. med. lobe
  1". Lt. lat. lobe
2. Quadrate lobe
3. Gall bladder
4. Rt. lobe
5. **Caud. vena cava**
6. Caudate lobe
  6'. Papillary process
  6". Caudate process
7. Hepatic vv.
8. Hepatic a.
9. Portal v.
10. Cystic duct
  (absent in horse)
11. Bile duct

A. Falciform lig.
B. Lesser omentum
C. Lt. triangular lig.
D. Esophageal notch
E. Rt. triangular lig.
F. Coronary lig.

a. Esophagus
b. Rt. crus of diaphragm
c. Costal part of diaphragm
d. Lumbar vertebra
e. Aorta
f. Sternum
g. Costal cartilage
h. Spleen
i. Rt. kidney
j. Splenophrenic lig.

CLINICAL

Liver abscesses: common in beef feedlot operations.

Hepatitis (hep-a-TY-tis): inflammation of the liver.

Liver flukes: migrate through the liver and reside in bile ducts in sheep and cattle.

Black leg: fatal *Clostridium novyi* infection secondary to liver flukes in sheep.

Tyzzer's disease: fatal bacterial hepatitis in foals caused by <u>Bacillus piliformis</u> (bacteria).

Serum hepatitis/Theiler's disease: hepatitis in horses due to biologics such as tetanus antitoxin.

Pyrrolizidine alkaloid toxicity: poisonous plant liver toxicity and photosensatization.

LIVER BIOPSY SITES

Horse:
• **Rt. 12th ICS** (intercostal space) on a line between the tuber coxae and point of the shoulder.
• **Lt. 8th ICS** (intercostal space) at the level of the deltoid tuberosity. Direct needle medially, dorsally and cranially.

Ox: Rt. 10th or 11th ICS about 1/4th of the length of the bony rib, ventral to the vertebral column.

Dog: Laparotomy incision caudal to the xiphoid process, hold the left lobe of liver with your finger and insert the needle through a separate stab incision into the liver.

LIVER

| Lobes | Species | | | |
	Carnivores	Ruminants	Horse	Pig
Left lobe	+	+	+	+
Lt. lat.	+	-	+	+
Lt. med.	+	-	+	+
Quadrate	+	+	+	+
Right lobe	+	+	+	+
Rt. med.	+	-	-	+
Rt. lat.	+	-	-	+
Caudate lobe	+	+	+	+
Caudate process	+	+	+	+
Papillary process	+	+	-	-

HISTOLOGY OF THE LIVER: The structural unit of the liver is the lobule. It consists of cords of hepatic cells (1) radiating out from a central vein (3). Sinusoids between the cords receive blood from branches of the hepatic arteries and portal vein passing on the periphery of the lobule. The sinusoids empty into a central vein in the middle of the liver lobule.

BLOOD SUPPLY: the liver has a dual blood supply. **Functional blood,** to be processed by the organ itself, comes to the liver via the portal system, bringing nutrients freshly absorbed from the gut. It accounts for about 3/4 of the blood flow to the liver. **Nutrient blood** (oxygenated) comes from the hepatic artery to keep the hepatocytes alive. Both types of blood empty into the liver sinusoids. Blood in the sinusoids empties into central veins, then into hepatic veins that empty into the caudal vena cava.

Lobule: structural unit of the liver.

1. Hepatic cells: liver cells, arranged radially around a central vein.

Portal vein: the large vein carrying nutrient rich (functional) blood from the stomach, intestines, pancreas and spleen into the liver at the porta of the liver.

Proper hepatic arteries: carry oxygenated (nutritional) blood to cells of the liver, also via the porta. They are branches of the common hepatic artery (a branch of the celiac artery).

2. Liver sinusoids: spaces where blood received from both the hepatic arteries and portal vein interacts with hepatic cells, then exits via central veins.

3. Central veins: course from the center of each liver lobule, receiving blood from liver sinusoids and carrying it to the hepatic veins.

4. Hepatic veins: the veins located inside the liver and emptying into the caudal vena cava. The central veins join to form the hepatic veins.

BILE: the liquid secretion of the liver cells into the duct system of the liver.

6. Bile canaliculi: small tubes immediately surrounding and collecting bile from the hepatic cells. They travel to the periphery of the lobule opposite the direction of blood flow, where they join to form interlobular ducts.

7. Interlobular ducts: ducts passing in the interstitial tissue between the lobules. They unite to form lobular ducts that course to the porta, joining to form the hepatic ducts.

Hepatic ducts: the 3 to 5 ducts that leave the porta to join with the cystic duct.

GALL BLADDER or **cholecyst** (KOH-lee-sist)[Gr. *chole* bile + *kystis* bladder]: the sac storing and concentrating bile. Bile aids in digestion and lubrication of food entering the duodenum from the stomach. The gall bladder is located in the fossa between the quadrate and the right medial lobes of the liver. The horse does not have a gall bladder.

Cystic duct: connects the gall bladder with the hepatic ducts. Together, these make the bile duct. The cystic duct is a two way street, bile can pass through it for storage in the gall bladder. When needed, the stored bile can pass through the cystic duct to the bile duct and into the duodenum. Bile is discharged through the cystic and bile ducts into the duodenum.

Bile duct: the duct formed by the junction of the hepatic ducts and, in species with a gall bladder, the cystic duct. It travels in the lesser omentum (hepatoduodenal ligament) to enter the duodenum. It is joined by the pancreatic duct, and both open on the major duodenal papillae.

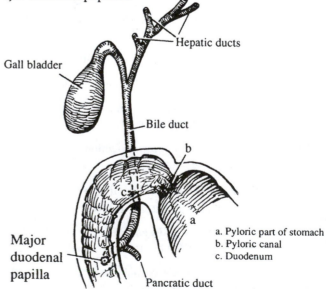

Hepatic ducts
Gall bladder
Bile duct
b
Major duodenal papilla
a. Pyloric part of stomach
b. Pyloric canal
c. Duodenum
Pancratic duct

296

LIVER

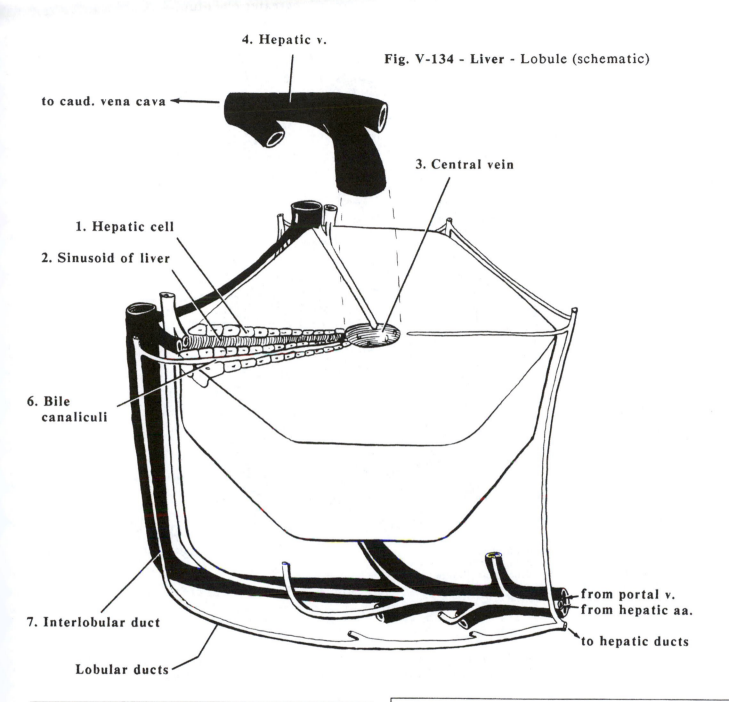

4. Hepatic v.

Fig. V-134 - Liver - Lobule (schematic)

to caud. vena cava ←

3. Central vein

1. Hepatic cell

2. Sinusoid of liver

6. Bile canaliculi

from portal v.
from hepatic aa.

7. Interlobular duct

to hepatic ducts

Lobular ducts

SPECIES DIFFERENCES:

Horse: has no gall bladder and thus no cystic duct. Its hepatic ducts join to form the bile duct.

CLINICAL

Cholecystectomy (koh'lee-sis-TEK-toh-mee): surgical removal of the gall bladder.

Cholecystitis (koh'lee-sis-TY-tis): inflammation of the gall bladder.

Cholecystoduodenostomy (koh'lee-sis'toh-dyoo'oh-de-NOS-toh-mee): surgical anastomosis of the gall bladder to the duodenum.

PANCREAS

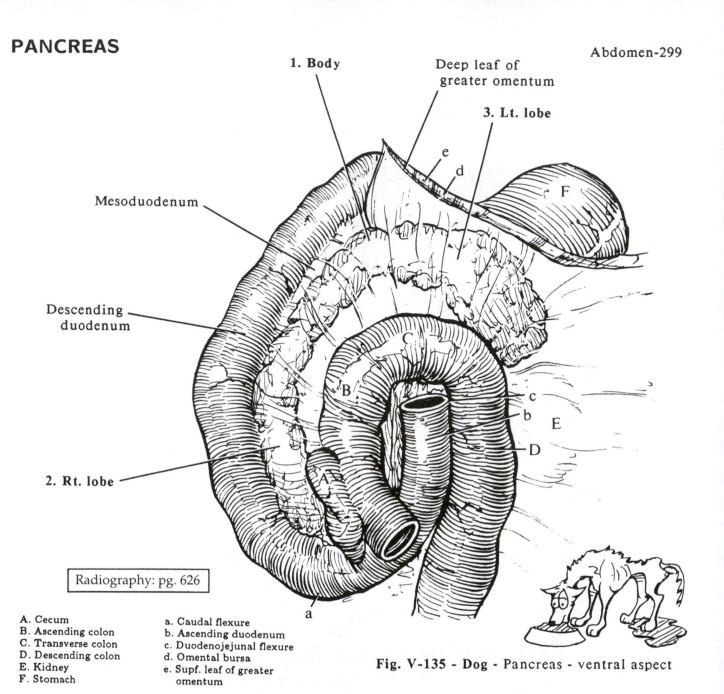

1. Body

Deep leaf of greater omentum

3. Lt. lobe

Mesoduodenum

Descending duodenum

2. Rt. lobe

Radiography: pg. 626

A. Cecum
B. Ascending colon
C. Transverse colon
D. Descending colon
E. Kidney
F. Stomach

a. Caudal flexure
b. Ascending duodenum
c. Duodenojejunal flexure
d. Omental bursa
e. Supf. leaf of greater omentum

Fig. V-135 - Dog - Pancreas - ventral aspect

PANCREAS (PAN-kree-as)[Gr. *pan* all + *kreas* flesh]: the V-shaped gland composed of two lobes joined by a body. It has both exocrine and endocrine functions.

Endocrine: the islet cells of the pancreas secrete insulin and glucagon into the blood, which keep the sugar concentrations of the blood at a constant level.

Exocrine (EK-soh-krin): pancreatic enzymes that aid in the digestion of carbohydrates, fats and proteins are carried to the descending duodenum by pancreatic ducts.

1. Body: the middle portion of the pancreas connecting the two lobes. It lies in contact with the pyloric part of the stomach.

2. Right lobe: the right portion of the pancreas in the mesoduodenum next to the descending duodenum.

3. Left lobe: lies in the deep leaf of the greater omentum. Extending from the body of the pancreas caudally and to the left, it lies along the dorsal abdomen toward the cranial pole of the left kidney.

DUCTS OF THE PANCREAS

4. Pancreatic (Wirsung's) **duct**: the tube opening with the bile duct on the major duodenal papilla (6).

5. Accessory pancreatic (Santorini's) **duct**: the tube opening into the duodenum on the minor duodenal papilla (7).

PANCREAS

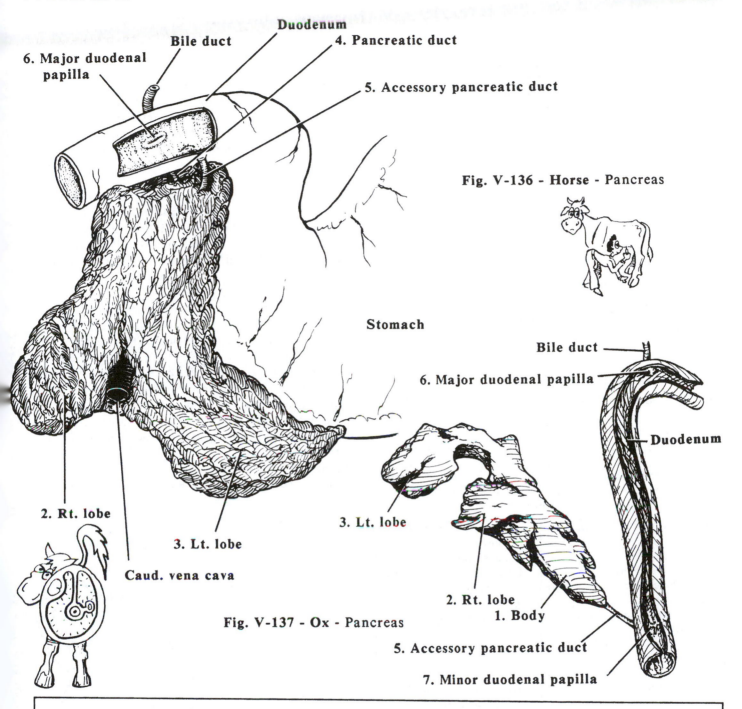

6. Major duodenal papilla

Bile duct

Duodenum

4. Pancreatic duct

5. Accessory pancreatic duct

Fig. V-136 - Horse - Pancreas

Stomach

Bile duct

6. Major duodenal papilla

Duodenum

3. Lt. lobe

2. Rt. lobe

3. Lt. lobe

2. Rt. lobe

1. Body

Caud. vena cava

Fig. V-137 - Ox - Pancreas

5. Accessory pancreatic duct

7. Minor duodenal papilla

SPECIES DIFFERENCES - DUCTS

Horse: both

Dog: accessory (always); **pancreatic** (usually, but always smaller of the two)

Ox: accessory (always) & pancreatic (occasionally)

Cat: pancreatic (always) & accessory (occasionally)

Pig: accessory (only)

Small ruminants: pancreatic (only)

	Dog	Cat	Pig	Horse	Ox	Sheep & goat
Pancreatic duct	+ (-)	+	-	+	-(+)	+
Accessory pancreatic duct	+	- (+)	+	+	+	-

Location of the minor duodenal papilla: Horse - same level as the major, but on opposite wall; Carnivores and pig - a few centimeters away from the major; Ox - a foot distal to the major papilla. Small ruminants and most cats don't have one because they don't have an accessory pancreatic duct

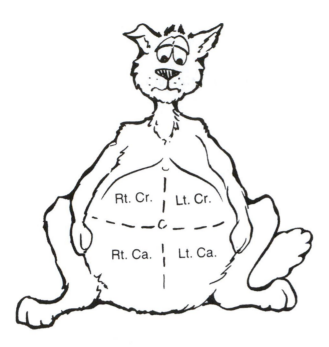

Quadrants of the Abdominal Cavity: are defined by 2 imaginary lines, one on the ventral midline crossed by a transverse one through the umbilicus. Knowing the contents of the quadrants helps when viewing radiographs and in visualizing where different structures are. The greatest number of individual structures are located in the cranial quadrants.

• **Both cranial quadrants**: body of stomach - transverse colon - left limb of pancreas - liver - diaphragm	
• **Right cranial quadrant**: diaphragm epiploic foramen caudal lobe of liver right lobe & body of pancreas pylorus & pyloric antrum descending duodenum right adrenal cranial lobe of right kidney	• **Left cranial quadrant**: diaphragm left liver lobes fundus & body of stomach cranial pole of left kidney spleen left limb of pancreas
• **Right caudal quadrant**: descending duodenum cecum right uterine horn right ovary caudal pole of right kidney right ductus deferens right vaginal ring right ureter	• **Left caudal quadrant**: descending colon left ureter caudal mesenteric artery mesocolon left uterine horn left ovary left ductus deferens left vaginal ring left ureter
• **Both caudal quadrants**: uterine body - urinary bladder - prostate (if enlarged) - terminal branches of aorta - caudal flexure of duodenum - ileum	

Divisions of the Abdominal Cavity

The abdomen can be divided into 9 regions by 2 imaginary transverse lines crossed by two imaginary longitudinal lines as shown in the cartoon. The transverse lines pass through the caudal extent of the costal arch and the tuber coxae. The cranial abdominal region extends from the front (summit) of the diaphragm (6th or 7th intercostal space) to the caudal part of the costal arch. It is divided into right and left hypochondriac regions (covered by the costal arch) and the xiphoid region between the costal arches. The middle abdominal region extends from the caudal end of the costal arch to the tuber coxae and is divided into right and left flank and the umbilical regions. The caudal abdominal region extends from the transverse plane of the tuber coxae to the pelvic inlet. It is divided into the pubic and right and left inguinal regions. Of the above regions the following are commonly used to describe the position of organs, pains or swellings.

- **Umbilical region**: area around the umbilicus (center of abdomen).
- **Flank** (lateral) **regions**: part of middle abdomen lateral to the umbilical region.
- **Paralumbar fossa (right** and **left)**: the dorsal part of the flank. Its boundaries are the transverse processes of the lumbar vertebrae, last rib and the ridge of the internal abdominal oblique muscle extending from the tuber coxae to the last rib.
- **Pubic region**: the midline part of the caudal abdomen cranial to the pubis.
- **Inguinal regions**: the part of the abdomen between the pubic region and the fold of the flank and thigh on each side.

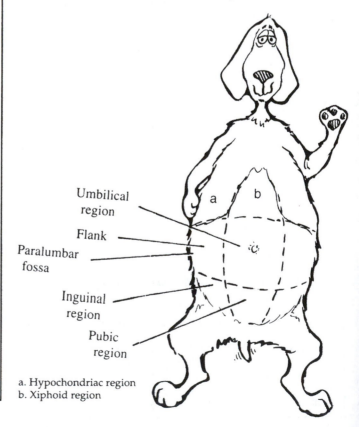

a. Hypochondriac region
b. Xiphoid region

Chapter VI
Respiratory System

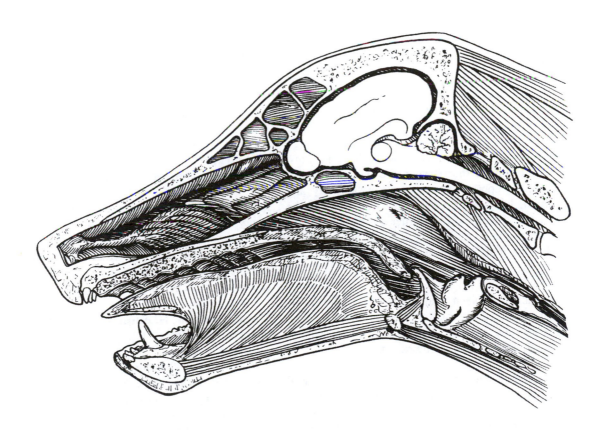

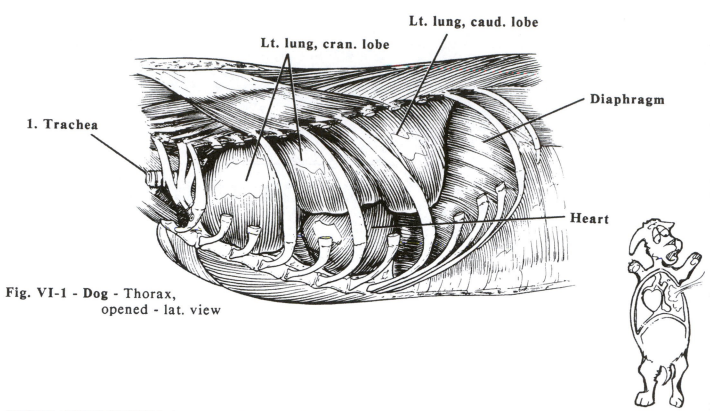

Lt. lung, cran. lobe

Lt. lung, caud. lobe

Diaphragm

1. Trachea

Heart

Fig. VI-1 - **Dog** - Thorax,
opened - lat. view

RESPIRATORY SYSTEM: the connected structures from the nostrils and oral cavity to and including the lungs. It is subdivided at the cranial end of the larynx into upper and lower respiratory tracts. The major function of the respiratory tract is transport and exchange of gaseous oxygen and carbon dioxide into and out of the blood. Oxygen is utilized by the cells for metabolism. Carbon dioxide is the resulting waste product.

The respiratory system is a portal of entry into the body and must be guarded. The tonsils of the pharynx are one part of this protective system. The upper respiratory tract, nasal cavity, and nasopharynx optimally warm or cool the gases brought into the body. Hairs associated with the nares filter out large particles. Smaller particles get stuck in the lining mucosa. Many ciliated lining cells drive the mucous coat back to the oral cavity for elimination.

Phonation: production of sound caused by movement of air across the vocal folds, causing them to vibrate. The associated resonance, changed and modified by the tongue, oral cavity, mouth and lips, produces characteristic sounds.

Olfaction: the sense of smell, perceived in the brain (cerebral cortex), involves receptors (olfactory nerve, CN I) located in the nasal cavity. Gaseous material and airborne particles are inhaled and detected (smelled) once dissolved in the mucous coat lining the nasal cavity.

Heat regulation: by panting, the dog helps control body temperature via evaporation. The lungs also play a role in acid-base balance and regulation of circulating substances in the blood.

NOSE: the external nose, its associated cartilage, and the nasal cavity.

External nose: the rostral structure protruding slightly from the face.

1. Philtrum (G. *philtron* a love charm): the groove in the lip and middle of the nose separating the nostrils.

2. Nostrils (cranial nares): the external openings into the nasal cavity, thus, the respiratory system.

3. Bony nasal aperture: the rostral ends of the nasal bones and the incisive bones, referred to as the immovable nose. The nasal cartilages extend from the opening rostrally.

Movable portion of the nose: the nasal cartilages, their ligaments and skin coverings.

4. Cartilage of the nose: the structures giving the nose its characteristic appearance. The nasal cartilages project rostrally from the bony nasal aperture.

SPECIES DIFFERENCES

Philtrum: deep in the carnivores and small ruminants; shallow or absent in the pig, ox and horse.

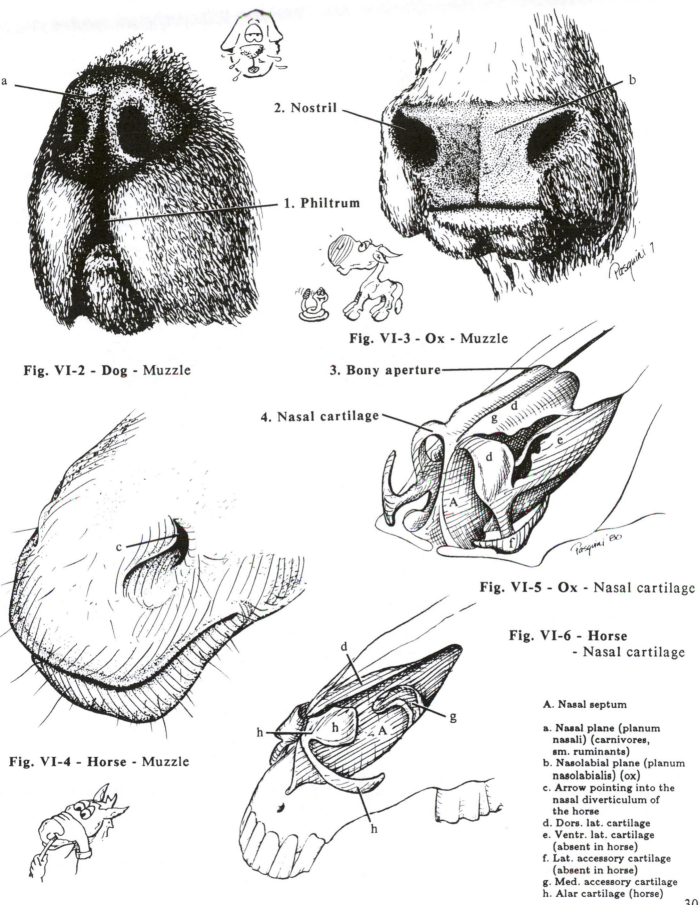

a

2. Nostril

b

1. Philtrum

Fig. VI-3 - Ox - Muzzle

Fig. VI-2 - Dog - Muzzle

3. Bony aperture

4. Nasal cartilage

d

g

e

d

A

f

Fig. VI-5 - Ox - Nasal cartilage

c

Fig. VI-6 - Horse
- Nasal cartilage

d

g

h

h

A

h

Fig. VI-4 - Horse - Muzzle

A. Nasal septum

a. Nasal plane (planum
nasali) (carnivores,
sm. ruminants)
b. Nasolabial plane (planum
nasolabialis) (ox)
c. Arrow pointing into the
nasal diverticulum of
the horse
d. Dors. lat. cartilage
e. Ventr. lat. cartilage
(absent in horse)
f. Lat. accessory cartilage
(absent in horse)
g. Med. accessory cartilage
h. Alar cartilage (horse)

NASAL CAVITY

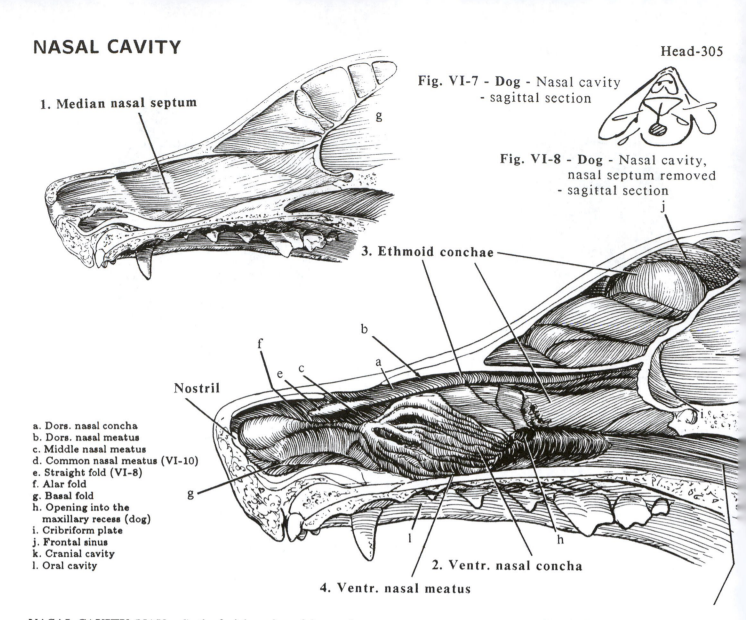

1. Median nasal septum

Fig. VI-7 - Dog - Nasal cavity - sagittal section

Fig. VI-8 - Dog - Nasal cavity, nasal septum removed - sagittal section

3. Ethmoid conchae

Nostril

a. Dors. nasal concha
b. Dors. nasal meatus
c. Middle nasal meatus
d. Common nasal meatus (VI-10)
e. Straight fold (VI-8)
f. Alar fold
g. Basal fold
h. Opening into the maxillary recess (dog)
i. Cribriform plate
j. Frontal sinus
k. Cranial cavity
l. Oral cavity

2. Ventr. nasal concha

4. Ventr. nasal meatus

NASAL CAVITY (NAY-zul): the facial portion of the respiratory tract extending from the <u>nostrils</u> to the <u>caudal nares</u>. It is divided into halves by the <u>median nasal septum</u>. The nasal cavity can be divided into three parts. The vestibule is the rostral part just inside the nostril. The middle part is filled with nasal <u>conchae</u>. These are thin scrolls of bone covered by mucous membrane. Passages between the conchae are called <u>meatuses</u> (meatus). The caudal part contains the numerous ethmoturbinates. The nasal cavity is connected to the paranasal sinuses (pg. 56) and the nasopharynx.

Opening of the nasolacrimal duct: at the junction between the skin and mucous membrane, just inside the nostril.

1. Median nasal septum: the perpendicular partition separating the nasal cavity into left and right halves. It is composed of bony (vomer, nasal and ethmoid bones), cartilaginous, and membranous parts. Its cranial cartilaginous part expands laterally, forming the nasal cartilages for each nostril.

2. Ventral nasal concha: the extensively folded structure filling the middle lumen of the nasal cavity. It is a separate and distinct bone of the skull.

3. Ethmoidal conchae: the delicate, mucosa-covered, bony scrolls known as ethmoturbinates filling the caudal part of the nasal cavity. They are part of the ethmoid bone.

• **Dorsal nasal concha** (a): the upper concha extending from the ethmoid bone's cribriform plate to the rostral nasal cavity.

Nasal conchae (KONG-kee, KONG-kay) (L. shells) (sin.= concha [KONG-ka]): the bony scrolls covered by nasal mucosa that fill each half of the nasal cavity. With the median nasal septum, they divide the cavity into passageways (meatuses).

Nasal meatus (mee-AY-tus) (pl.= meatus or meatuses) (L. a way, path, course): the passageways between the conchae of each half of the nasal cavity.

• Dorsal nasal meatus (b): the narrow passageway between the dorsal nasal concha and the nasal bones leading into the caudal nasal cavity.

NASAL CAVITY

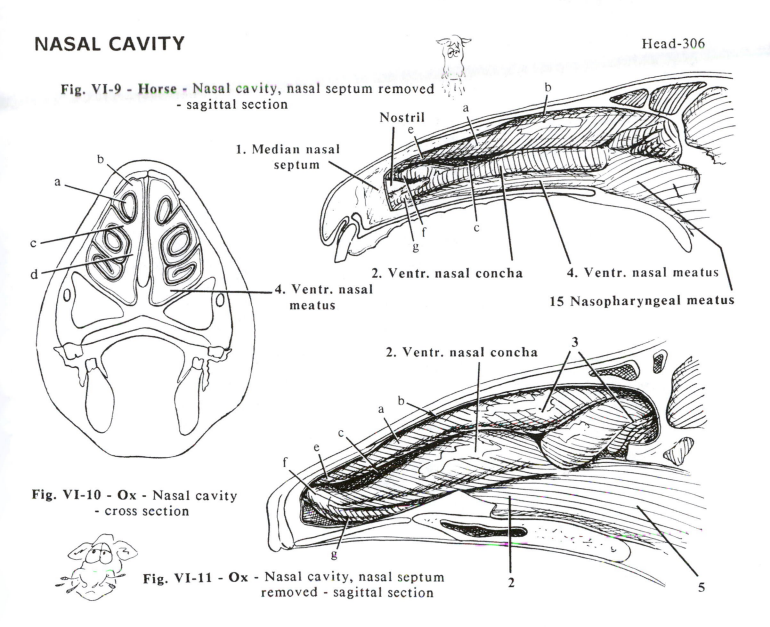

Fig. VI-9 - **Horse** - Nasal cavity, nasal septum removed
- sagittal section

Nostril

1. Median nasal septum

2. Ventr. nasal concha   4. Ventr. nasal meatus

15 Nasopharyngeal meatus

4. Ventr. nasal meatus

Fig. VI-10 - **Ox** - Nasal cavity
- cross section

2. Ventr. nasal concha

Fig. VI-11 - **Ox** - Nasal cavity, nasal septum
removed - sagittal section

• **Middle nasal meatus** (c): the passageway between the dorsal nasal concha and the ventral nasal concha leading into the caudal nasal cavity.

• **Common nasal meatus** (d): the narrow vertical space between the median nasal septum and the conchae, from the roof to the floor of the nasal cavity. Laterally it is continuous with the other meatuses.

• **4. Ventral nasal meatus**: the largest meatus located between the ventral nasal concha and the hard palate. It leads directly into the nasopharynx.

5. Nasopharyngeal meatus: the short passageway connecting the ventral nasal meatus with the caudal naris (choana) on each side.

6. Caudal nares or **choanae** (ko-AY-nee) (sin.= choana): the two openings of the nasopharyngeal meatus into the nasopharynx, separated by the vomer bone.

SPECIES DIFFERENCES

Nasal diverticulum ("false nostril"): the dorsal passage through the horse's nostrils into a blind cutaneous pouch. When "tubing" a horse, a thumb placed in the diverticulum will aid in directing the tube into the ventral nasal meatus.

Rostral bone (os rostrale) (pg. 52,1): the bone in the nose of a pig to help it "root".

CLINICAL

"Nasogastric tubing" in horses: the passage of a stomach tube through the nasal cavity, pharynx, and esophagus to the stomach. The tube must be passed through the **ventral nasal meatus**, nasopharyngeal meatus, and caudal nares to reach the pharynx and the esophagus. Passing the tube in the dorsal or middle nasal meatus would lead into the ethmoturbinates and cause massive hemorrhage.

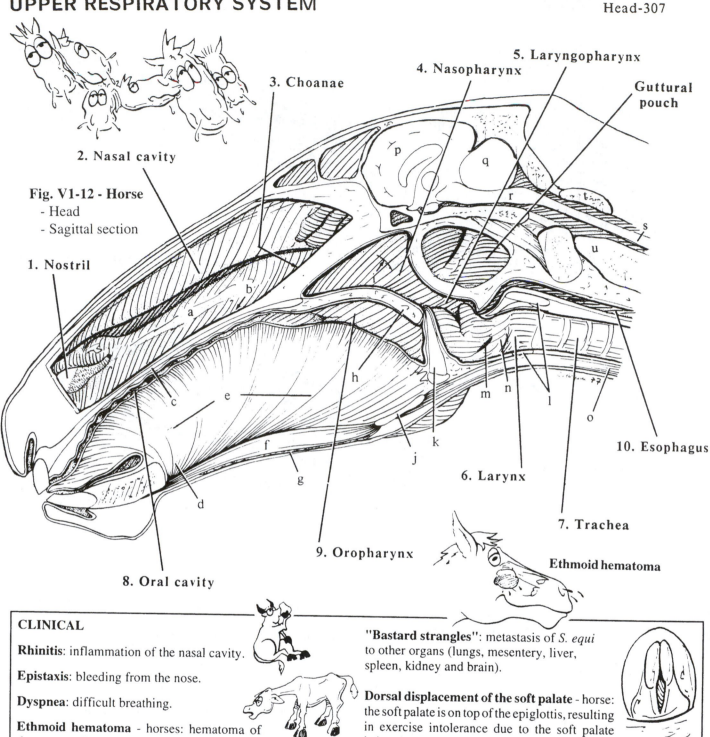

Fig. V1-12 - Horse
 - Head
 - Sagittal section

1. Nostril
2. Nasal cavity
3. Choanae
4. Nasopharynx
5. Laryngopharynx
Guttural pouch
6. Larynx
7. Trachea
8. Oral cavity
9. Oropharynx
10. Esophagus

Ethmoid hematoma

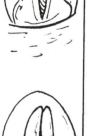

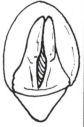

CLINICAL

Rhinitis: inflammation of the nasal cavity.

Epistaxis: bleeding from the nose.

Dyspnea: difficult breathing.

Ethmoid hematoma - horses: hematoma of the mucosa lining ethmoid conchae, resulting in intermittent epistaxis.

Pharyngeal lymphoid hyperplasia: disease of young horses resulting in cough and pharyngeal pain.

"Strangles", horse distemper: *Streptococcus equi* infection of horses causing abscesses and swelling of lymph nodes (submandibular and retropharyngeal). Untreated horses sound like they are strangling, hence the name.

"Bastard strangles": metastasis of *S. equi* to other organs (lungs, mesentery, liver, spleen, kidney and brain).

Dorsal displacement of the soft palate - horse: the soft palate is on top of the epiglottis, resulting in exercise intolerance due to the soft palate being drawn into the larynx during inspiration. Normally the epiglottis overlaps the dorsal side of the soft palate.

Epiglottic entrapment - horse: displacement of subepiglottic tissue over the epiglottis resulting in exercise intolerance. Endoscopic examination through the nose can differentiate entrapment from displacement. In entrapment the margins of the epiglottis, but not the epiglottis itself are obscured, in displacement the epiglottis is obscured.

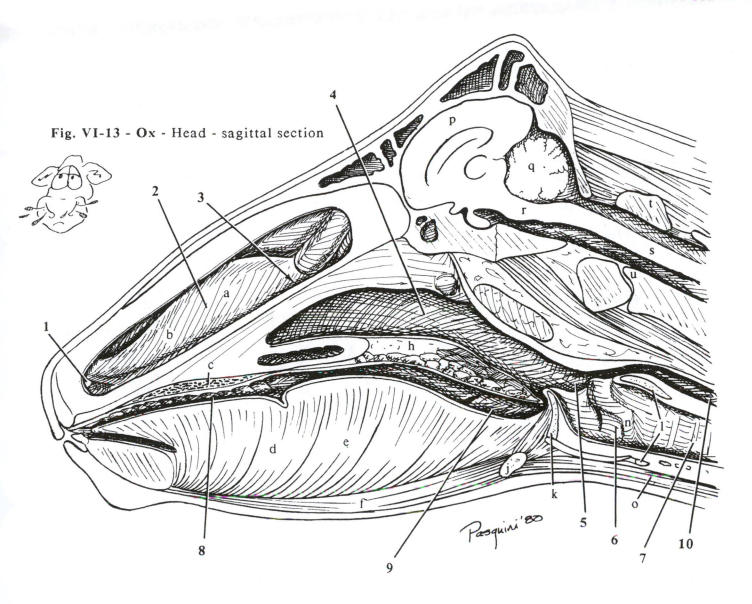

Fig. VI-13 - Ox - Head - sagittal section

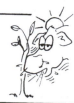

1. Nostril	a. Ventr. nasal concha	h. Soft palate	o. Sternohyoideus m.
2. Nasal cavity	b. Ventr. nasal meatus	i. Opening into auditory tube	p. Cerebral hemisphere
3. Choanae	c. Hard palate	j. Lingual process	q. Cerebellum
4. Nasopharynx	d. Genioglossus m.	k. Epiglottic cartilage	r. Medulla oblongata
5. Laryngopharynx	e. Tongue	l. Cricoid cartilage	s. Spinal cord
6. Larynx	f. Geniohyoid m.	m. Lat. laryngeal ventricle	t. Dors. arch of atlas
7. Trachea	g. Mylohyoid m.	(horse & carnivores)	u. Dens of axis
8. Oral cavity	(not shown in ox)	n. Vocal fold	
9. Oropharynx			
10. Esophagus			

CLINICAL

"Summer snuffles", Allergic rhinitis: type I hypersensitivity in cattle resulting in dyspnea and intense pruritis (itching).

"Rednose": hyperemia of the muzzle in cattle due to infectious bovine rhinotracheitis (IBR) virus.

Pharyngitis. inflammation of the pharynx.

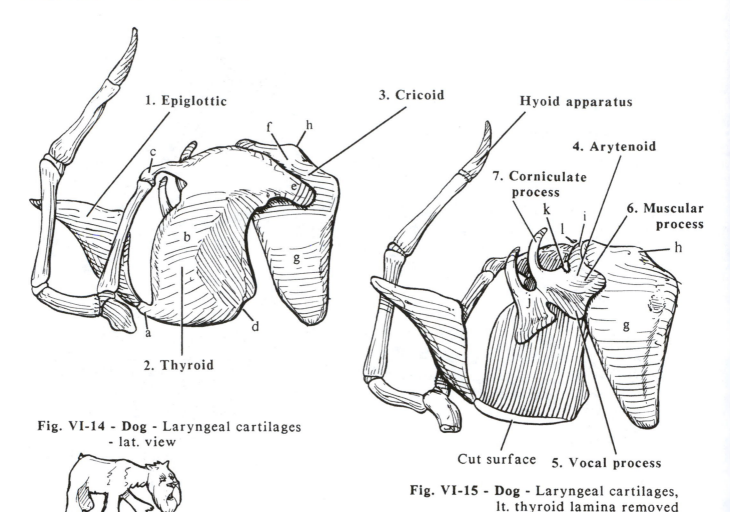

1. Epiglottic

3. Cricoid

Hyoid apparatus

4. Arytenoid

7. Corniculate process

6. Muscular process

2. Thyroid

Cut surface   **5. Vocal process**

Fig. VI-14 - Dog - Laryngeal cartilages - lat. view

Fig. VI-15 - Dog - Laryngeal cartilages, lt. thyroid lamina removed - lat. view

LARYNX (LAR-inks) (G. upper end of windpipe): the musculocartilaginous tube connecting the laryngopharynx with the trachea and containing the vocal cords (the organs of phonation).

LARYNGEAL CARTILAGES (lah-RIN-jee-al): the group of cartilages forming the structure of the larynx. They consist of the single epiglottic, thyroid, cricoid, and paired arytenoid cartilages (and the insignificant sesamoid and interarytenoid cartilages in the dog).

1. Epiglottis or **epiglottic cartilage**: the rostral most cartilage giving structure to the epiglottis which closes the laryngeal opening during deglutition (swallowing), protecting the lungs from foreign bodies.

2. Thyroid cartilage (G. *thyroideus*, resembling a shield): the largest cartilage, single and open dorsally. The laryngeal prominence is the ventral projection of the thyroid cartilage, known as the palpable "Adam's apple" in man.

3. Cricoid cartilage (KRY-koyd) (G. ring): the signet ring-

shaped cartilage connecting the thyroid cartilage and the trachea.

• **4. Arytenoid cartilages** (ar'ee-TEE-noid, ar'e-TE-noid): the paired, irregular, pyramid shaped cartilages articulating medially with the rostrodorsal border of the cricoid cartilage. The arytenoid cartilages have a number of processes - vocal, muscular, corniculate, and cuneiform

• **5. Vocal process**: the ventral projection of the arytenoid cartilage into the cavity of the larynx. It provides the dorsal attachment for the vocal cord. Ventrally the vocal cords attach to the floor of the thyroid cartilage.

• **6. Muscular process**: the <u>lateral</u> process of the arytenoid cartilage, providing a point of insertion of the intrinsic muscles of the larynx, especially the dorsal cricoarytenoideus muscle. The pull of this muscle swings the vocal process of the arytenoid cartilage and vocal cords laterally, thus, opening the space between them (glottic cleft).

• **7. Corniculate process**: the rostral horn-like process that forms the dorsal part of the laryngeal opining. It is absent in the cat.

LARYNX – CARTILAGE

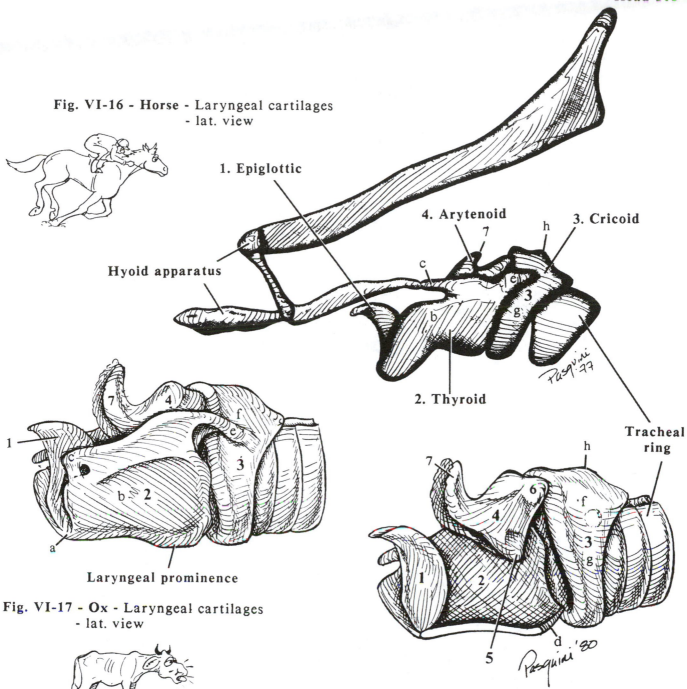

Fig. VI-16 - Horse - Laryngeal cartilages
- lat. view

1. Epiglottic

4. Arytenoid   7   h   3. Cricoid

c   e

Hyoid apparatus   b   3   g

2. Thyroid

Pasquini '77

Tracheal
ring

1   7   4

c   h   6   f

e   4   3

b   2   g   3

a   1   2   g   d

Laryngeal prominence   5   d   '80   Pasquini

Fig. VI-17 - Ox - Laryngeal cartilages
- lat. view

Fig. VI-18 - Ox - Laryngeal cartilages, lt. thyroid
lamina removed - lat. view

a. Petiolus of epiglottic
   cartilage (absent in cat)
b. Lamina (thyroid cartilage)
c. Rostr. cornu (except pig)
d. Thyroid notch (except pig)
e. Caud. cornu
f. Cricoid arch
g. Cricoid lamina

h. Median crest of cricoid
   cartilage
i. Articular process
j. Cuneiform process (dog & horse)
k. Interarytenoid cartilage
   (dog & pig)
l. Sesamoid (dog)

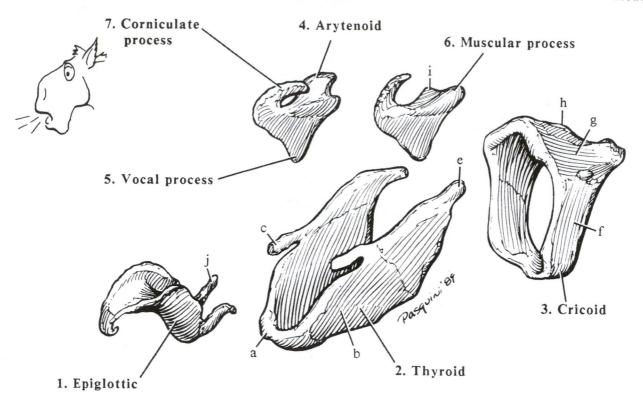

7. Corniculate process

4. Arytenoid

6. Muscular process

5. Vocal process

3. Cricoid

1. Epiglottic

2. Thyroid

Fig. VI-19 - Horse - Laryngeal cartilages
- rostrolat. view

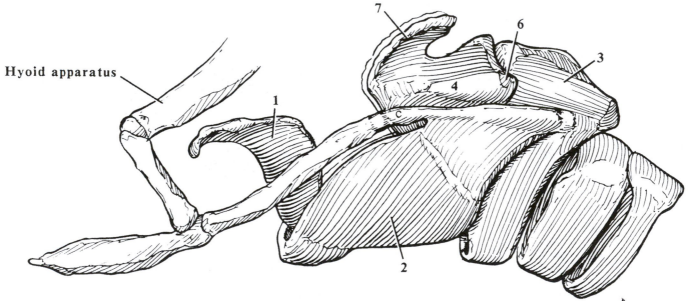

Hyoid apparatus

Fig. VI-20 - Horse - Laryngeal cartilages and part of
hyoid apparatus - lat. view

1. Epiglottic cartilage	a. Petiolus (absent in cat)	f. Cricoid arch
2. Thyroid cartilage	b. Lamina (thyroid cartilage)	g. Cricoid lamina
3. Cricoid cartilage	c. Rostr. cornu (except pig)	h. Median crest
4. Arytenoid cartilage	d. Caud. thyroid notch	i. Articular process
5. Vocal process	(except pig) (VI-23)	j. Cuneiform process
6. Muscular process	e. Caud. cornu (VI-19)	(dog & horse)
7. Corniculate process		

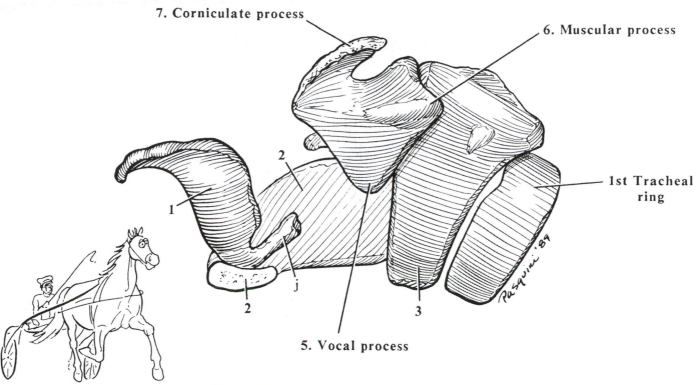

7. Corniculate process

6. Muscular process

1st Tracheal ring

5. Vocal process

Fig. VI-21 - Horse - Laryngeal cartilages, lt. thyroid lamina removed - lat. view

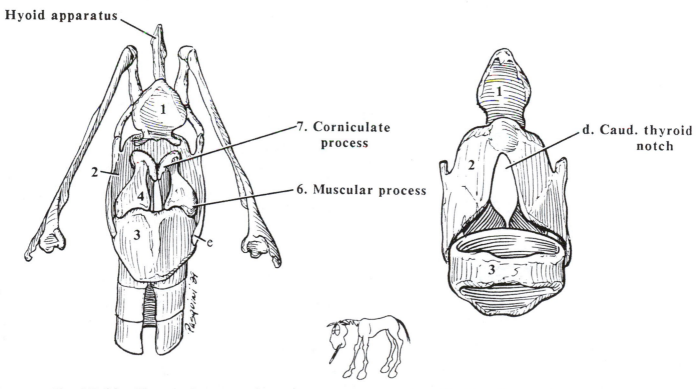

Hyoid apparatus

7. Corniculate process

6. Muscular process

d. Caud. thyroid notch

Fig. VI-22 - Horse - Laryngeal cartilages - dors. view

Fig. VI-23 - Horse - Laryngeal cartilages - ventr. view

LARYNX

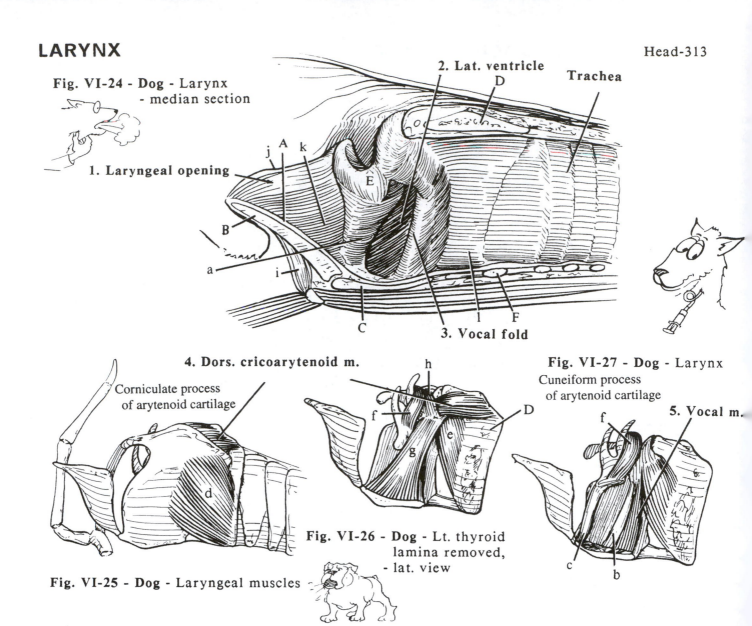

Fig. VI-24 - Dog - Larynx - median section

1. Laryngeal opening

2. Lat. ventricle

Trachea

3. Vocal fold

4. Dors. cricoarytenoid m.

Corniculate process of arytenoid cartilage

Fig. VI-25 - Dog - Laryngeal muscles

Fig. VI-26 - Dog - Lt. thyroid lamina removed, - lat. view

Fig. VI-27 - Dog - Larynx
Cuneiform process of arytenoid cartilage

5. Vocal m.

LARYNGEAL CAVITY: the space enclosed by the laryngeal cartilages, muscles, ligaments, and mucous membrane. The laryngeal cavity is divided into three regions. The part just inside the laryngeal opening is the vestibule. The glottic cleft is the narrow middle part of the larynx. The infraglottic cavity is the part caudal to the glottic cleft.

1. Laryngeal opening (aditus laryngis): the passageway for air from the mouth or nose into the larynx. Its borders are the epiglottis, aryepiglottic fold (j), and the corniculate process of the arytenoid cartilage.

2. Lateral ventricles of the larynx: lateral depressions in the vestibule just cranial to the vocal folds. They allow the vocal fold lateral movement.

3. Vocal fold or vocal cord: the mucosa-covered vocal ligament and muscle caudal to the ventricle. It extends from the vocal process of the arytenoid cartilage to the interior floor of the thyroid cartilage.

4. Glottic cleft (rima glottidis [L. *rima*, cleft]): the narrowest space of the lumen of the larynx located between the structures of the glottis (the vocal cords and two vocal processes of the arytenoid cartilage).

MUSCLES OF THE LARYNX: laryngeal muscles cover the laryngeal cartilages in the undissected larynx. They are subdivided into extrinsic and intrinsic muscles. Extrinsic muscles extend from laryngeal cartilages to other body structures. Intrinsic muscles arise and terminate on laryngeal cartilage and are named according to their attachments: dorsal cricoarytenoid, lateral cricoarytenoid, transverse arytenoid, thyroarytenoid and cricothyroid).

5. Dorsal cricoarytenoid muscle: the only intrinsic muscle abducting (pulling apart) the vocal folds to open the glottis. It is innervated by the caudal laryngeal nerve (the end of the recurrent laryngeal nerve, a branch of the vagus nerve). The other intrinsic muscles either adduct (pull together) or alter the tension of the vocal folds.

6. Vocal (vocalis) muscle: the muscle of the vocal fold extending from the thyroid cartilage to the vocal process of the arytenoid cartilage. It relaxes the vocal fold by pulling the arytenoid

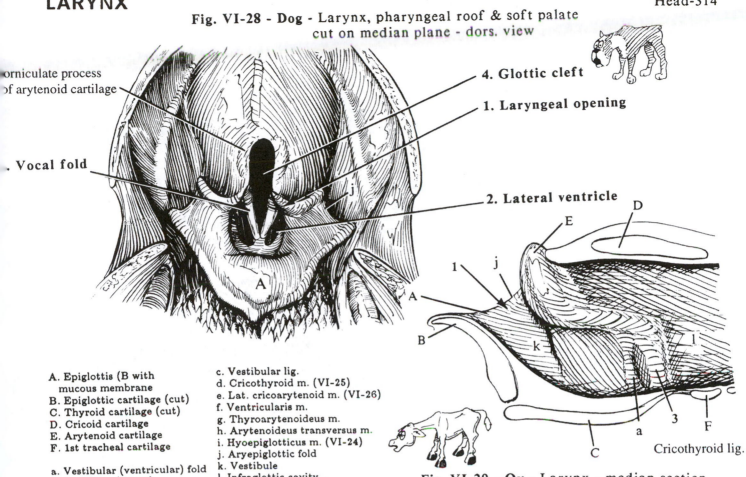

Fig. VI-28 - Dog - Larynx, pharyngeal roof & soft palate cut on median plane - dors. view

orniculate process of arytenoid cartilage

. Vocal fold

4. **Glottic cleft**

1. **Laryngeal opening**

2. **Lateral ventricle**

A. Epiglottis (B with mucous membrane
B. Epiglottic cartilage (cut)
C. Thyroid cartilage (cut)
D. Cricoid cartilage
E. Arytenoid cartilage
F. 1st tracheal cartilage

a. Vestibular (ventricular) fold
b. Vocal lig. (VI-27)

c. Vestibular lig.
d. Cricothyroid m. (VI-25)
e. Lat. cricoarytenoid m. (VI-26)
f. Ventricularis m.
g. Thyroarytenoideus m.
h. Arytenoideus transversus m.
i. Hyoepiglotticus m. (VI-24)
j. Aryepiglottic fold
k. Vestibule
l. Infraglottic cavity

Cricothyroid lig.

Fig. VI-29 - Ox - Larynx - median section

cartilage downward. It is not separate from the general thyroarytenoid muscle in animals lacking a lateral ventricle (cat & ruminants)

Cricothyroid muscles: extend from the ventral side of the cricoid cartilage to the lateral sides of the thyroid cartilage. Ventrally they look like a "bowtie" and can be used to judge midline.

Cricothyroid ligament: between cricoid and thyroid cartilage.

SPECIES DIFFERENCES

Lateral ventricle of the larynx: present in the horse, pig and dog; absent in the cat and ruminant.

CLINICAL

Laryngitis (lar'in-JY-tis): inflammation of the larynx.

Intubation: placement of an endotracheal tube into the larynx and trachea. To intubate a tranquilized dog, open its mouth, grasp the tongue, and gently pull it rostrally. Use the endotracheal tube to push the soft palate up to visualize the epiglottis. Then hold the epiglottis down with the tube and look into the larynx (through the laryngeal opening). See the space between the

vocal folds (glottic cleft). Direct the tube between the vocal folds into the trachea. Inflate the endotracheal tube cuff and tie the tube around the upper jaw with gauze. Attach the tube to the gas anesthesia machine. As long as you see the tube go between the vocal cords you will be in the right place.

"Roarer" - laryngeal hemiplegia in horses: paralysis of the left (usually) recurrent laryngeal nerve to the abductor of the glottic cleft, the dorsal cricoarytenoid muscle. This results in the left vocal fold everting into the lumen of the larynx and causing a characteristic sound ("roar"). This is irritating and interferes with breathing, especially during a race. One corrective surgical procedure replaces the dorsal cricoarytenoideus muscle with a suture. The suture is tied so that the vocal process is permanently pulled laterally, opening the glottic cleft.

Ventral laryngotomy in the horse: opening the larynx. Incise the skin over the laryngeal prominence. Find the midline using the cricothyroid ("bowtie") muscles, then incise through the cricothyroid ligament that fills the caudal thyroid notch. This opens the larynx allowing access to it and the pharynx through the glottic cleft and laryngeal opening.

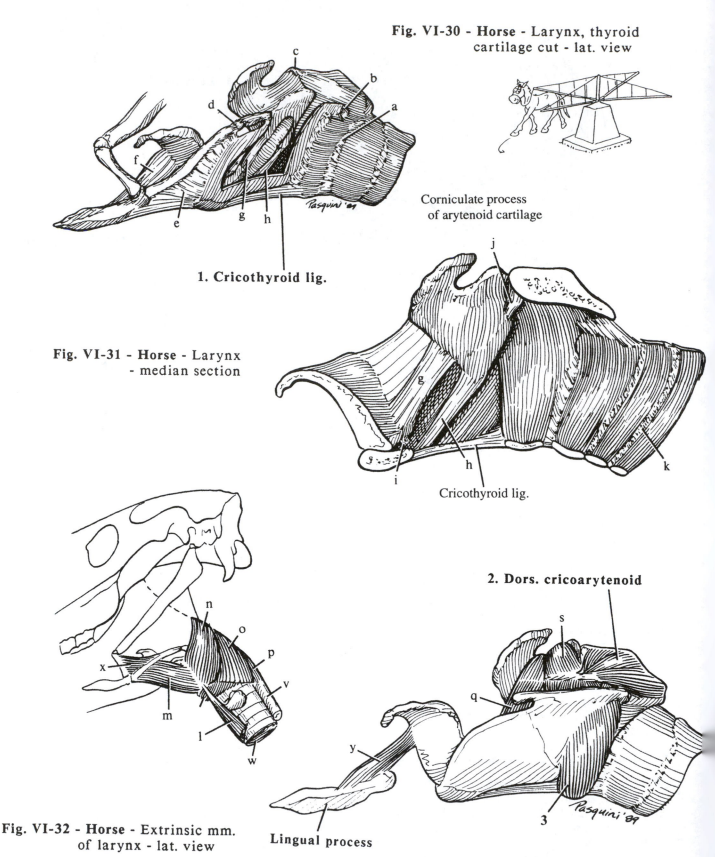

Fig. VI-30 - Horse - Larynx, thyroid cartilage cut - lat. view

Corniculate process
of arytenoid cartilage

1. Cricothyroid lig.

Fig. VI-31 - Horse - Larynx
- median section

Cricothyroid lig.

2. Dors. cricoarytenoid

Fig. VI-32 - Horse - Extrinsic mm.
of larynx - lat. view

Lingual process

Fig. VI-33 - Horse - Intrinsic mm.
of larynx - lat. view

LARYNX - MUSCLES

Fig. VI-34 - Horse - Larynx, lt. thyroid lamina removed - lat. view

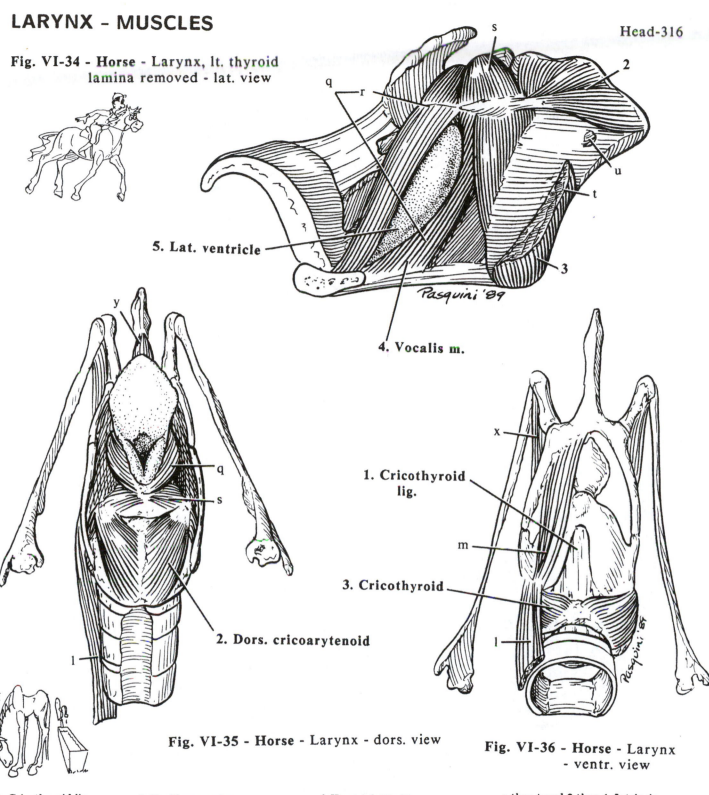

5. Lat. ventricle

4. Vocalis **m.**

Pasquini '89

y

q

s

2. Dors. cricoarytenoid

l

Fig. VI-35 - Horse - Larynx - dors. view

x

1. Cricothyroid lig.

m

3. Cricothyroid

l

Pasquini '85

Fig. VI-36 - Horse - Larynx - ventr. view

1. Cricothyroid lig.
2. Dors. cricoarytenoid m.
3. Cricothyroid m.
4. Vocalis m.

A. Epiglottis (VI-31)
B. Thyroid cartilage
C. Cricoid cartilage
D. Arytenoid cartilage
E. Vocal process
F. Corniculate process
G. Cuneiform process
H. Aryepiglottic fold

I. Hyoid apparatus
J. Lingual process of
   basihyoid bone
K. Muscular process
L. Tracheal ring
M. Caud. thyroid notch

a. Cricotracheal lig.
b. Cricothyroid joint
c. Cricoarytenoid joint
d. Thyrohyoid articulation
   (cartilaginous)
e. Thyrohyoid membrane

f. Hyoepiglottic lig.
g. Vestibular lig. (absent
   in cat)
h. Vocal lig.
i. Thyroepiglottic lig.
j. Dors. cricoarytenoid lig.
k. Anular lig. of trachea
l thru p. Extrinsic mm. of larynx
   l. Sternothyroideus
   m. Thyrohyoideus
   n. Thyropharyngeus
   o. Cricopharyngeus
   p. Cricoesophageus

q thru t and 2 thru 4. Intrinsic
   mm. of larynx
   q. Thyroarytenoideus (ventricularis
     & vocalis m.)
   r. Ventricularis
   s. Arytenoideus transversus
   t. Cricoarytenoideus lateralis
u. Facet for caud. cornual process
   of thyroid cartilage
v. Esophagus
w. Tracheal m.
x. Ceratohyoideus m.
y. Hyoepiglotticus m.

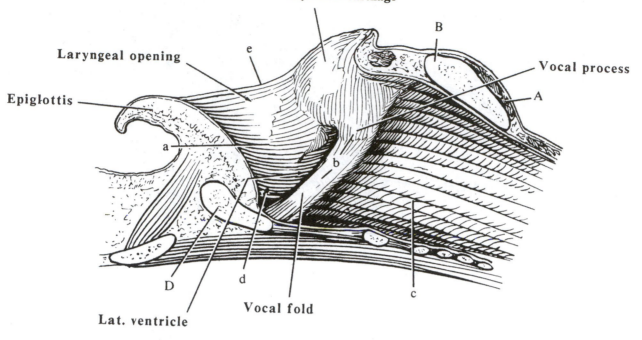

Corniculate process
of arytenoid cartilage

Laryngeal opening

Epiglottis

Vocal process

A

Lat. ventricle

D

d

Vocal fold

c

e

b

a

B

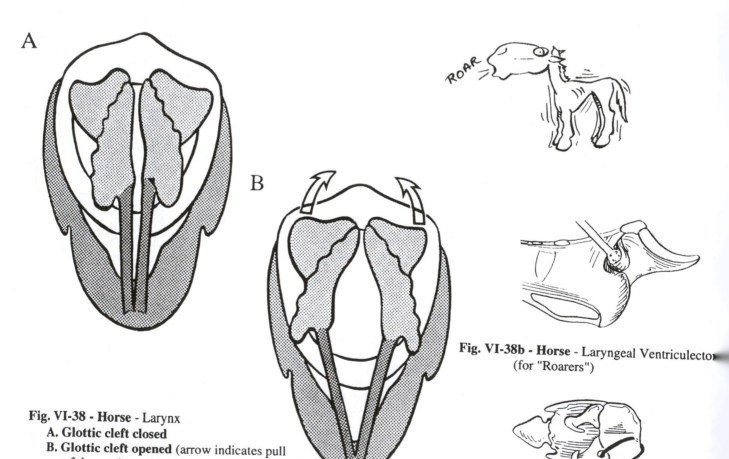

ROAR

Fig. VI-38b - Horse - Laryngeal Ventriculectomy
(for "Roarers")

Fig. VI-38a - Horse - The Prosthetic Laryngoplasty
(suture back arytenoid cartilage to
open glottic cleft)

A

B

Fig. VI-38 - Horse - Larynx
  A. Glottic cleft closed
  B. Glottic cleft opened (arrow indicates pull
   of dors. cricoarytenoid mm. on muscular
   process of the arytenoid cartilage)

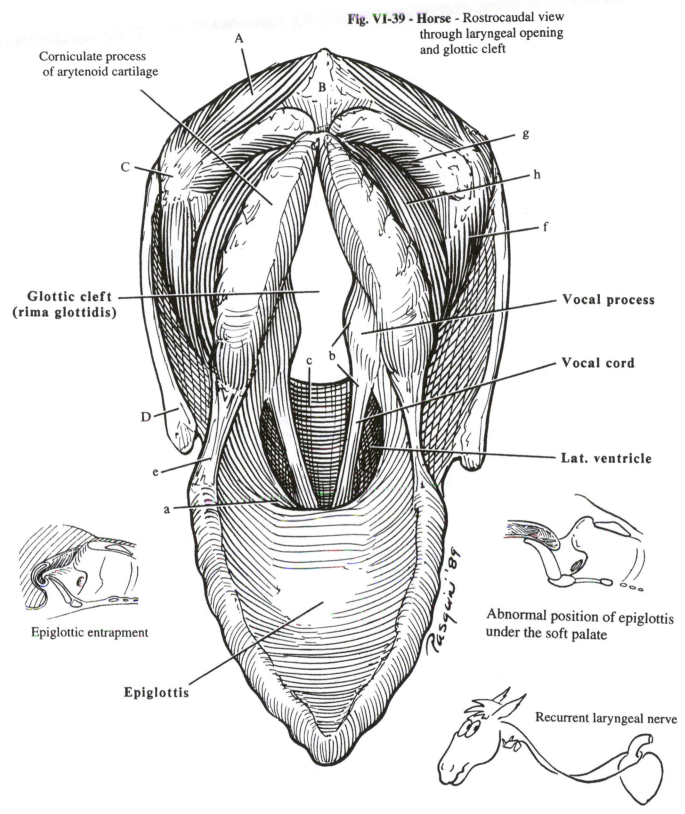

Fig. VI-39 - Horse - Rostrocaudal view
through laryngeal opening
and glottic cleft

Corniculate process
of arytenoid cartilage

Glottic cleft
(rima glottidis)

Vocal process

Vocal cord

Lat. ventricle

Epiglottic entrapment

Abnormal position of epiglottis
under the soft palate

Epiglottis

Recurrent laryngeal nerve

Pasquini '89

A. Dors. cricoarytenoid
B. Cricoid cartilage
C. Muscular process of
   arytenoid cartilage
D. Thyroid cartilage

a. Vestibule
b. Glottis (vocal fold
   & vocal process)
c. Infraglottic cavity
d. Med. ventricle

e. Aryepiglottic fold
f. Cricoarytenoideus lateralis
g. Arytenoideus transversalis
h. Thyroarytenoideus

PLEURA: the serosa* lining the thoracic cavity and the thoracic organs; forming two <u>pleural sacs</u> on either side of the mediastinum.

1. Pulmonary (visceral) pleura: the serosa on the surface of a lung.

Parietal pleura: the serosa lining the walls of the thorax including the mediastinum and diaphragm.

• **2. Mediastinal parietal pleura**: the serosa on the mediastinum.

   3. Pericardial pleura: part of the mediastinal pleura on either side of the pericardium.

• **4. Costal pleura**: the serosa lining the thoracic wall.

• **Diaphragmatic pleura**: the serosa covering the diaphragm's thoracic side.

Connecting pleura: the double layer of serosa connecting visceral pleura and parietal pleura.

• **Pulmonary ligaments**: the connecting pleura between the pulmonary pleura from the left and right caudal lung lobes to the mediastinal parietal pleura.

• **Plica vena cava**: the connecting pleura between the caudal vena cava and the diaphragm, pericardial sac, and floor of the thorax.

6. Mediastinum (mee'dee-as-TY-num): the cleft or wall between the right and left mediastinal pleura. Near the median thoracic plane, it divides the thorax into two cavities. The thoracic organs, other than the lungs, (heart, esophagus, trachea, aorta, and thymus) help form the mediastinum. These organs can be considered to make a wall, the mediastinum, which separates the thorax into two cavities. The wall concept also helps explain why the pleura on the mediastinum is called parietal. In places the mediastinum is just formed by the contact between the two mediastinal pleurae. Such places may be fenestrated (perforated).

Parts of the mediastinum: The heart and its pericardium are located in the mediastinum, dividing it into cranial, middle, and caudal mediastinum. It also can be divided into dorsal (above the base of the heart) and ventral portions (below the top of the heart).

• **Cranial mediastinum**: part of mediastinum cranial to the heart.

• **Middle mediastinum**: part of mediastinum containing the heart.

• **Caudal mediastinum**: part of mediastinum caudal to the heart.

5. PLEURAL CAVITIES: the two cavities inside the pleural sacs, between the visceral and parietal layers of the pleura. Imagine the two pleural sacs as balloons of serosa blown up in the two cavities of the thoracic cavity. The space or wall between

where the two balloons abut each other on the midline is the mediastinum. The lungs grow out of the mediastinum and push the pleura ahead of them, thus, the lungs never enter the pleural cavities.

Pleural cupula: the cranial extent of the pleural cavity extending through the thoracic inlet. It can be mistakenly opened during caudal neck surgeries.

Costodiaphragmatic recess: the potential space between the costal wall and the dome-shaped diaphragm.

Mediastinal recess: the space filled by the accessory lobe of the right lung, between the mediastinum and the plica vena cava.

Line of pleural reflection: where the pleura reflects from the costal wall into the diaphragm. Roughly, this line passes along the eighth costal cartilage and then curves dorsocaudally to the angle of the last rib. This line represents the separation of the thoracic and abdominal cavities. A needle inserted caudoventral to this line will enter the abdomen, one placed craniodorsal will enter the thorax, and if long enough, the abdomen because of the doming of the diaphragm.

Basal borders of the lungs: the caudoventral border of the lungs. It parallels the line of pleural reflection, but is craniodorsal to it because the lungs do not fill the costodiaphragmatic recess. It extends from the 6th costochondral junction to the second to last intercostal space at the border of the epaxial muscles.

Radiography: pg. 614

CLINICAL

Pleuritis: inflammation of the pleura.

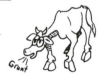

Fenestrations or **perforations in the mediastinum**: normal in the <u>dog</u>, <u>horse</u> and <u>sheep</u>; not found in the <u>ox</u>, <u>goat</u>, <u>pig</u>, or young animals of any species. In theory these could allow a unilateral pneumothorax or pyothorax to become bilateral.

Hyaline membrane disease: parturition before the lungs mature with insufficient surfactant produced.

Pneumothorax: air or gas in the pleural space.

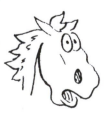

Pyothorax: thoracic empyema (accumulation of pus in a body cavity).

---

*A serosa is any smooth membrane, consisting of a mesothelial layer and a connective tissue layer, lining the cavities of the body.

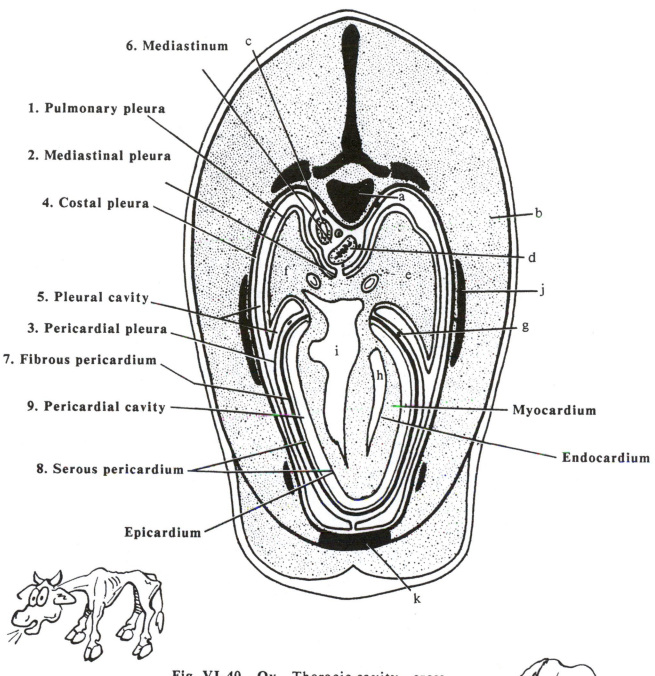

6. Mediastinum

1. Pulmonary pleura

2. Mediastinal pleura

4. Costal pleura

5. Pleural cavity

3. Pericardial pleura

7. Fibrous pericardium

9. Pericardial cavity

8. Serous pericardium

Epicardium

Myocardium

Endocardium

Fig. VI-40 - Ox - Thoracic cavity - cross section through heart

a. Thoracic vertebra
b. Body wall
c. Aorta
d. Esophagus
e. Rt. lung
f. Lt. lung
g. Phrenic n.
h. Rt. ventricle
i. Lt. ventricle
j. Rib
k. Sternebra

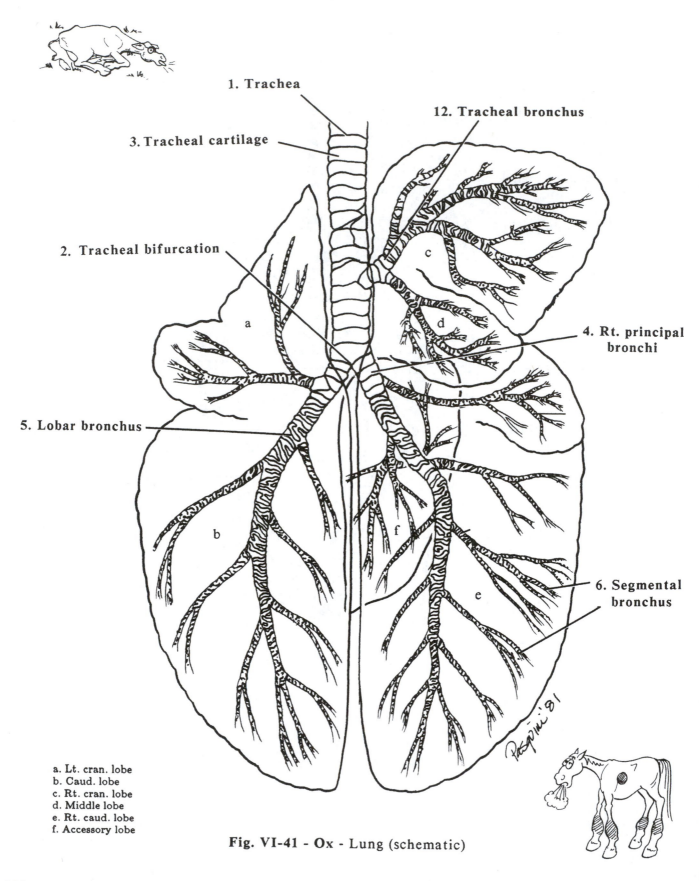

1. Trachea

12. Tracheal bronchus

3. Tracheal cartilage

2. Tracheal bifurcation

4. Rt. principal bronchi

5. Lobar bronchus

6. Segmental bronchus

a. Lt. cran. lobe
b. Caud. lobe
c. Rt. cran. lobe
d. Middle lobe
e. Rt. caud. lobe
f. Accessory lobe

Fig. VI-41 - Ox - Lung (schematic)

BRONCHIAL TREE

1. TRACHEA (TRAY-kee-a) or windpipe: the cylindrical tube extending from the larynx down the neck into the thorax to the lungs. It terminates by bifurcating into the right and left primary bronchi above the base of the heart. The <u>cervical part</u> runs from the larynx to the thoracic inlet. The <u>thoracic part</u> continues to the bifurcation. The trachea, consisting of cartilaginous rings connected by annular ligaments, is covered by adventitia and lined by a mucous membrane.

2. Bifurcation: the splitting of the trachea into right and left primary bronchi above the base of the heart, just to the right of midline.

• **Tracheal carina**: the ridge at the bifurcation between the principle bronchi. Radiologists call the tracheal bifurcation the carina.

3. Tracheal cartilages: the "C"-shaped hyaline cartilage rings, incomplete dorsally. They make up the skeleton of the trachea and keep it open.

Annular ligaments: fibroelastic tissue uniting the tracheal cartilages, making the trachea a flexible tube.

Trachealis muscle: smooth muscle connecting the open, dorsal ends of the tracheal cartilages.

BRONCHIAL TREE

4. Right and **left primary (principal) bronchi** (BRONG-ky) ([Gr. *bronchos,* windpipe] sin.= bronchus): the short, thick segment entering each lung's hilus to divide into lobar bronchi.

5. Lobar ("secondary") bronchi: the divided continuation of the principal bronchi ventilating one lobe and giving rise to segmental bronchi.

6. Segmental ("tertiary") bronchi: the branches of the lobar bronchi ventilating a bronchopulmonary segment.

Bronchopulmonary segment: a self-contained, cone-shaped section of lung tissue within a lobe.

7. Bronchioles: small tubes with no cartilaginous support, arising from segmental bronchi. The bronchioles are the last strictly conductive branches.

8. Respiratory bronchioles (BRONG-kee-ohl-es): terminal bronchioles whose walls contain some alveoli, therefore, conduct and "respire" (allow gas exchange with blood). They are present in dogs, cats, and horses.

9. Alveolar (al-VEE-oh-lar) **ducts**: passages from respiratory bronchioles surrounded by alveoli.

10. Alveolar sacs: terminations of alveolar ducts, surrounded by alveoli.

11. Alveoli (al-VEE-oh-ly) sin.= alveolus: thin walled sacs for gas exchange.

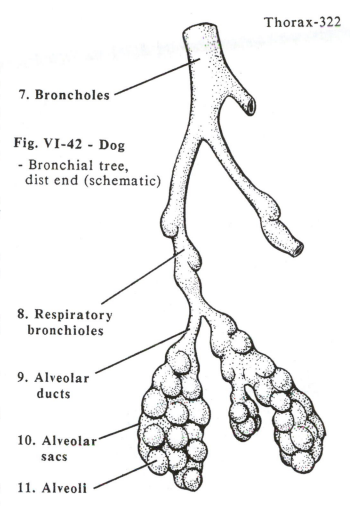

7. Broncholes

Fig. VI-42 - Dog
- Bronchial tree, dist end (schematic)

8. Respiratory bronchioles

9. Alveolar ducts

10. Alveolar sacs

11. Alveoli

SPECIES DIFFERENCES

12. Tracheal bronchus: the bronchus in ruminants and pigs arising cranial to the tracheal bifurcation to supply the right lung's cranial lobe.

Radiography: pg. 618

CLINICAL:

Transtracheal wash (TTW): injection and aspiration of material into and from the trachea for lab work.

Bronchus of the right middle lobe: directed downward, thus, a common site for infection to migrate.

"Honker": tracheal edema in feedlot cattle.

"Husk": lungworm (*Dictycoalus*) disease in cattle.

Tracheostomy (trayk-kee-OS-toh-mee): surgically opening the trachea to the outside. This usually is done in the upper neck, cranial to where the sternocephalic muscles diverge. Here the trachea is covered only by the strap muscles of the neck (sternohyoid and sternothyroid).

LUNGS

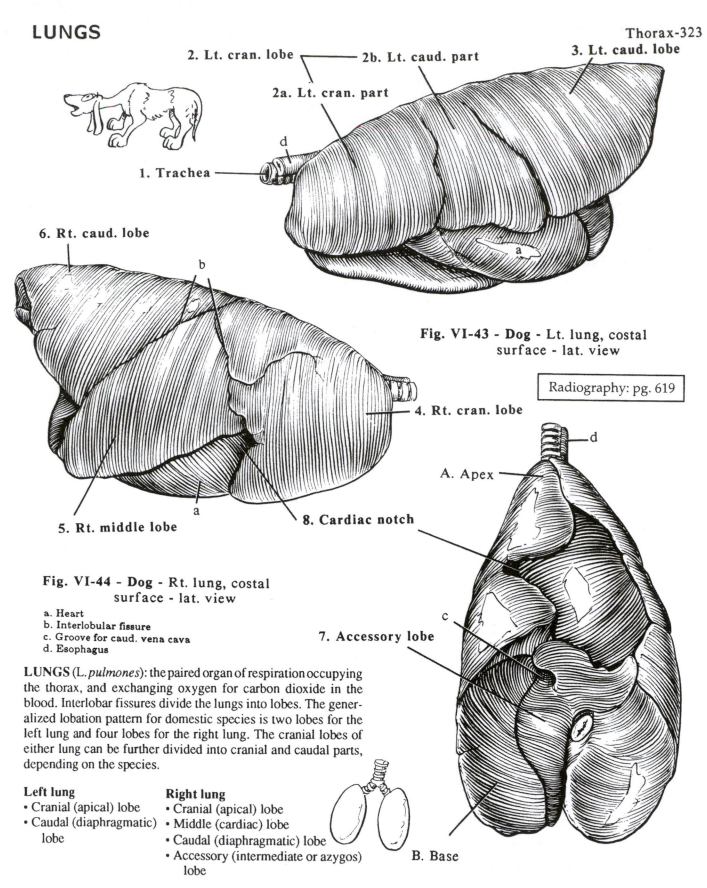

2. Lt. cran. lobe — 2b. Lt. caud. part

2a. Lt. cran. part

3. Lt. caud. lobe

1. Trachea

d

a

Fig. VI-43 - Dog - Lt. lung, costal
surface - lat. view

Radiography: pg. 619

6. Rt. caud. lobe

b

4. Rt. cran. lobe

5. Rt. middle lobe

a

8. Cardiac notch

Fig. VI-44 - Dog - Rt. lung, costal
surface - lat. view

a. Heart
b. Interlobular fissure
c. Groove for caud. vena cava
d. Esophagus

A. Apex

c

7. Accessory lobe

B. Base

d

Fig. VI-45 - Dog - Lungs, diaphragmatic
surface - caudoventr. view

LUNGS (L. *pulmones*): the paired organ of respiration occupying
the thorax, and exchanging oxygen for carbon dioxide in the
blood. Interlobar fissures divide the lungs into lobes. The generalized lobation pattern for domestic species is two lobes for the
left lung and four lobes for the right lung. The cranial lobes of
either lung can be further divided into cranial and caudal parts,
depending on the species.

Left lung
• Cranial (apical) lobe
• Caudal (diaphragmatic)
  lobe

Right lung
• Cranial (apical) lobe
• Middle (cardiac) lobe
• Caudal (diaphragmatic) lobe
• Accessory (intermediate or azygos)
  lobe

A. Apex: the cranial end of the lungs lying in the thoracic inlet.

B. Base: the caudal end of the lungs resting on the diaphragm.

LUNGS

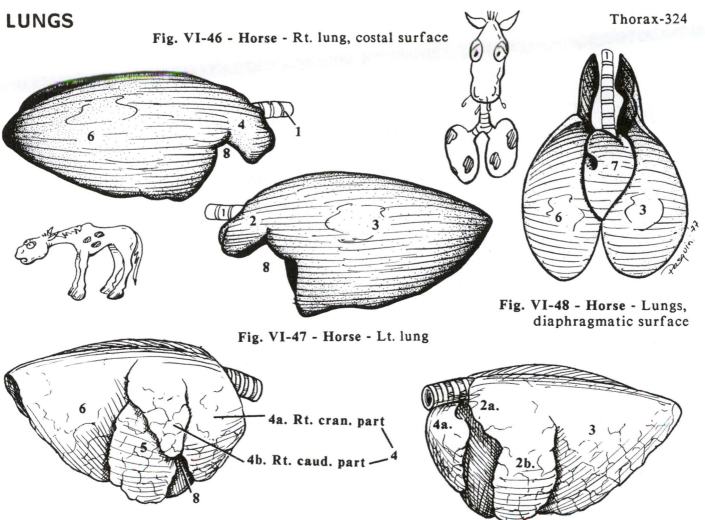

Fig. VI-46 - Horse - Rt. lung, costal surface

Fig. VI-47 - Horse - Lt. lung

Fig. VI-48 - Horse - Lungs, diaphragmatic surface

4a. Rt. cran. part

4b. Rt. caud. part — 4

Fig. VI-49 - Ox - Rt. lung, costal surface

2a.

4a.

3

2b.

Fig. VI-50 - Ox - Lt. lung, costal surface

Fig. VI-51 - Ox - Lungs, diaphragmatic surface

	Left Lung	Right Lung

Generalized	Two lobes
	Cranial lobe
	  Cranial part
	  Caudal part
	Caudal lobe
		Four lobes
		Cranial lobe
		Middle lobe
		Caudal lobe
		Accessory lobe

Carnivores	"	"
Pig	"	"
Ruminants	"	Four lobes, but cran. lobe divided into cran. and caud. parts
Horse	Cran. lobe not divided into cran. and caud. parts	Three lobes, middle lobe missing

1. Trachea
2. Lt. cran lobe
  2a. Lt. cran. part
  2b. Lt. caud. part
3. Lt. caud. lobe
4. Rt. cran. lobe

4a. Rt. cran. part
4b. Rt. caud. part
5. Rt. middle lobe
  (absent in horse)
6. Rt. caud. lobe
7. Accessory lobe
8. Cardiac notch

LUNGS

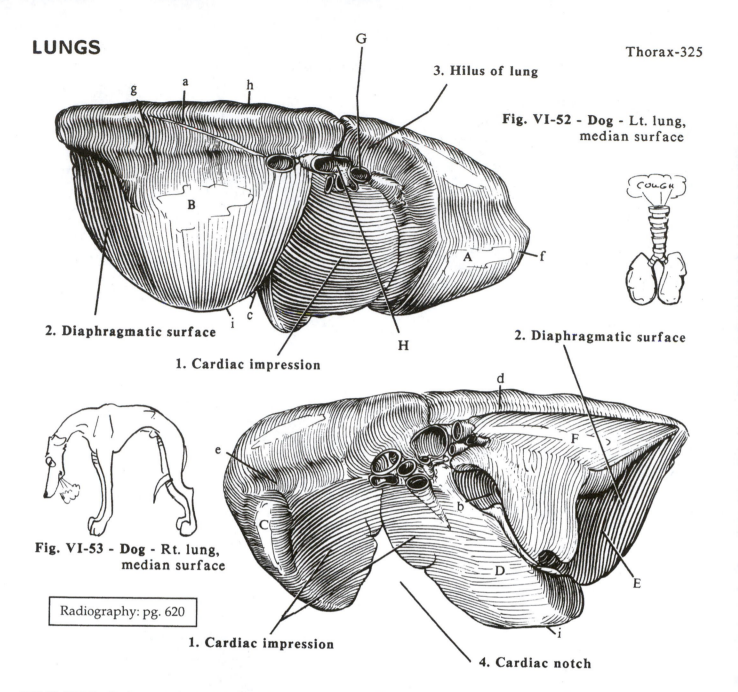

Fig. VI-52 - **Dog** - Lt. lung,
median surface

3. Hilus of lung

2. Diaphragmatic surface

2. Diaphragmatic surface

1. Cardiac impression

COUGH

Fig. VI-53 - **Dog** - Rt. lung,
median surface

Radiography: pg. 620

1. Cardiac impression

4. Cardiac notch

LUNG SURFACES and their IMPRESSIONS:

Costal surface: lies laterally against the thoracic wall.

Medial surface: faces the opposite lung through the mediastinum.

1. Cardiac impression: the impression formed by the heart on the lung's medial surface, between the 3rd and 6th rib.

2. Diaphragmatic surface: the concave surface conforming to the diaphragm.

3. Hilus of the lung: the area on the medial surface where the pulmonary bronchus and the pulmonary and bronchial vessels and nerves enter the lungs.

Root of the lung: the aggregation of structures entering the lung at the hilus.

4. Cardiac notch: the opening between lobes of the lungs where the heart sac comes in contact with the thoracic wall.

PULMONARY VESSELS:

Pulmonary (PUL-moh-ner'ee) **trunk:** the vessel leaving the right ventricle which divides into right and left pulmonary arteries to the lungs. Upon entering the lungs the pulmonary arteries split into smaller and smaller branches parallelling the airways. These vessels <u>do not</u> supply the lung tissue, but exchange gases and return oxygenated blood to the heart via the pulmonary veins.

Bronchial vessels: supply lung tissue with oxygen. They arise from branches of the aorta.

LUNGS

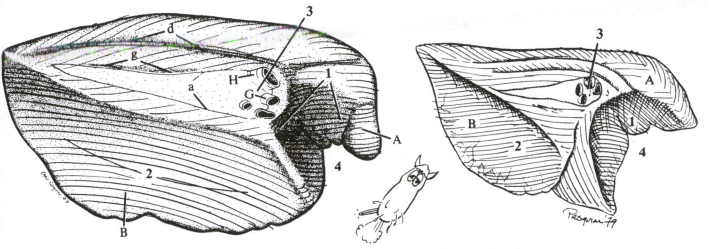

Fig. VI-54 - **Horse** - Lt. lung, median surface

Fig. VI-55 - **Ox** - Lt. lung, median surface

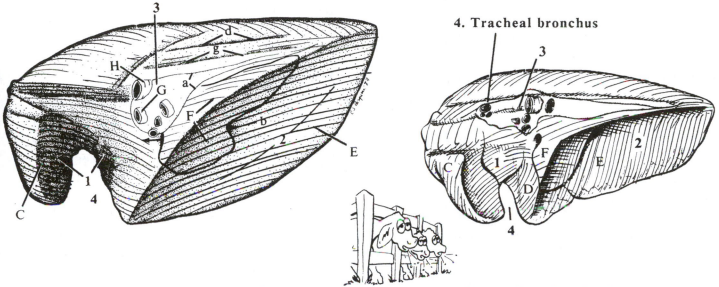

4. Tracheal bronchus

Fig. VI-56 - **Horse** - Rt. lung, median surface

Fig. VI-54 - **Ox** - Rt. lung,
median surface

A. Lt. cran. lobe	E. Rt. Caud. lobe	a. Pulmonary lig.
B. Lt. caud. lobe	F. Accessory lobe	b. Groove for caud.
C. Rt. cran. lobe	G. Pulmonary a.	vena cava
D. Rt. middle lobe	H. Primary bronchi	c. Interlobular fissure

d. Aortic impression	g. Esophageal
e. Impression for	impression
lt. subclavian a.	h. Dors. border
f. Apex	

SPECIES DIFFERENCES

Generalized pattern of lobes: two lobes (cranial and caudal) on the left and four on the right (cranial, caudal, middle, and accessory).

Carnivores, pig, and **ruminants**: have the generalized pattern of lobes.

Ruminants: both right and left cranial lobes are divided into cranial and caudal parts. They also have distinct connective tissue septa in the lung tissue.

Horse: missing the right middle lobe, thus has only three lobes on the right, five total. The lobes are not divided by distinct fissures.

CLINICAL

Cardiac notch: the site for directing a needle into the heart (cardiac puncture) without piercing lung tissue.

LUNGS - CLINICAL

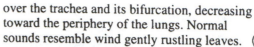

Shipping fever: bronchopneumonia of cattle caused by stress + bacteria + viral infections.

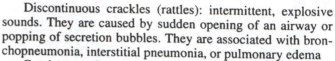

"Snots"/Rhinopneumonitis: common viral cause of respiratory infections in horses.

"Rattles"/ *Rhodococcus equi* lung: bacteria causing suppurative pyogranulomatous pneumonia in foals.

"Bleeders"/Exercise induced pulmonary hemorrhage: horses, bleeding from lungs due to exercise (racing).

"Heaves": hypersensitive reaction causing a chronic cough which results in a "heave line" (hypertrophy of abdominal muscle along the costal arch).

Pneumonia: inflammation of lungs with consolidation.

Aspiration pneumonia: may result from drenching cattle or regurgitation during surgery for any species.

Hyaline membrane disease, Neonatal respiratory stress syndrome: parturition before lungs mature with insufficient surfactant produced.

PERCUSSION: the act of striking a part with short, sharp blows and listening for the sound made. This can aid in diagnosing the condition of the underlying parts. The noise of percussion is produced by three sources: 1) impact noise of a finger or hammer striking intercostal space (it is of little diagnostic value and is diminished by using a rubber hammer or the cushion of the finger); 2) vibration of the body wall; 3) resonance of the underlying air-filled cavity which acts like a drumhead. Solid structures don't resonate. Percuss with light force over an intercostal space to reduce the amount of wall in the vibration (percussion over ribs causes more of the wall to vibrate).

Finger percussion method: always used in small animals and more accurate in large animals. Place the middle finger over the intercostal muscle. Tap a finger just proximal to the fingernail with the tip of the middle finger of the other hand. Allow the finger to recoil. A hammer and pleximeter can be used in large animals.

Basal border of the lungs located by percussion: systematically percuss one intercostal space at a time. Percuss two points; one over the lung and one well below the lung. Continue percussing, reducing the distance between these two points until you find the basal border. This will actually be above the anatomical border of the lung (the lung is very thin at the basal border).

AUSCULTATION OF THE LUNGS: listening to air passing through airways of the lungs with a stethoscope. The normal resting animal will have quiet or inaudible sounds. An excited, panting dog will have loud sounds. Normal lung sounds are louder over the trachea and its bifurcation, decreasing toward the periphery of the lungs. Normal sounds resemble wind gently rustling leaves.

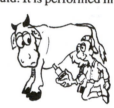

• **Abnormal sounds**:

Discontinuous crackles (rattles): intermittent, explosive sounds. They are caused by sudden opening of an airway or popping of secretion bubbles. They are associated with bronchopneumonia, interstitial pneumonia, or pulmonary edema

Continuous wheezes (rales): caused by air passing through narrowed airways. On expiration these are associated with spasm, neoplasia, mucosal edema, foreign bodies, or tracheobronchial lymphadenopathy. On inspiration they are associated with narrowing (stenosis) of the larynx, trachea, or principal bronchi.

Auscultation of the ox: normal sounds are harsher and louder than in the horse.

Auscultation triangle: a restricted area due to the thoracic limb.
• Cranial - caudal border of triceps brachii
• Dorsal - epaxial muscles
• Caudoventral - curved line from olecranon to next to last intercostal space

LUNG BIOPSY: must be done craniodorsal to the basal border of the lung (obviously!).

PLEUROCENTESIS or thoracocentesis: the surgical puncture of the chest wall for drainage of fluid. It is performed in the dependent (lowest) point on the standing animal. This is caudal to the heart and cranial to the diaphragmatic line of pleural reflection. This varies from side to side and species to species. *General rule*: puncture the middle of an intercostal space (avoid cranial and caudal branches of ventral intercostal vessels), dorsal to the costochondral junction.

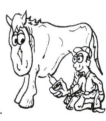

• Ox: 6th or 7th intercostal space above the costochondral junction.
• Horse: 7th intercostal space above the superficial thoracic ("spur") vein.

THORACOTOMIES: surgical opening of the thoracic cavity. These openings can be through an intercostal space, by removal of a rib, or by splitting the sternum (mediastinotomy).

Respiratory assistance during thoracotomies: not needed in standing cattle because of their thick mediastinum. Thus, opening one side will not collapse the opposite lung as it might in the dog.

Vacuum of thorax: necessary for breathing. When closing a thoracotomy, inflate the lungs maximally as the last closing sutures are placed.

LOBECTOMY: the removal of a lung lobe. Trauma and neoplasia are two common indications for this procedure. The bronchi and bronchial vessels must be ligated.

Chapter VII
Urinary System

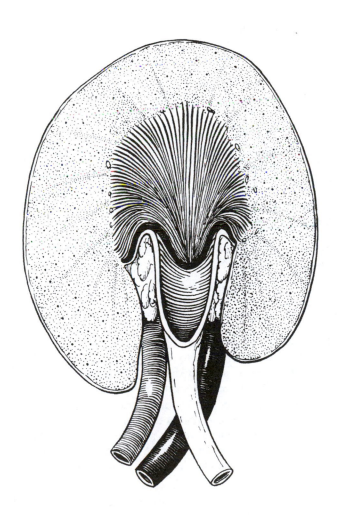

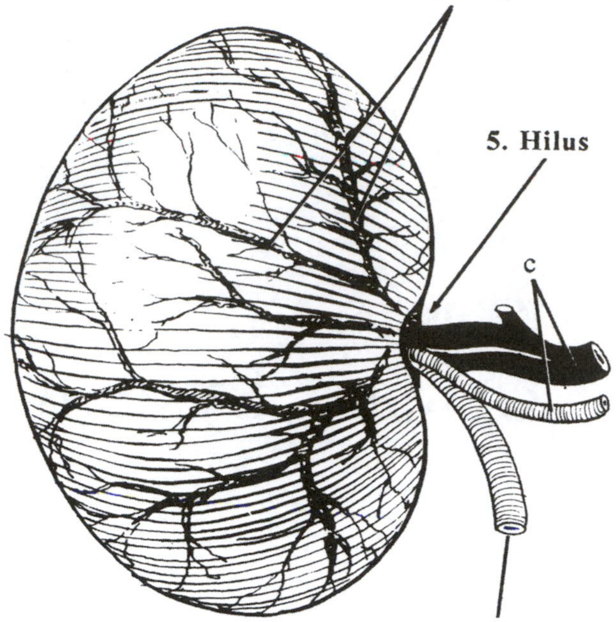

URINARY SYSTEM

3. Capsular veins

5. Hilus

c

B

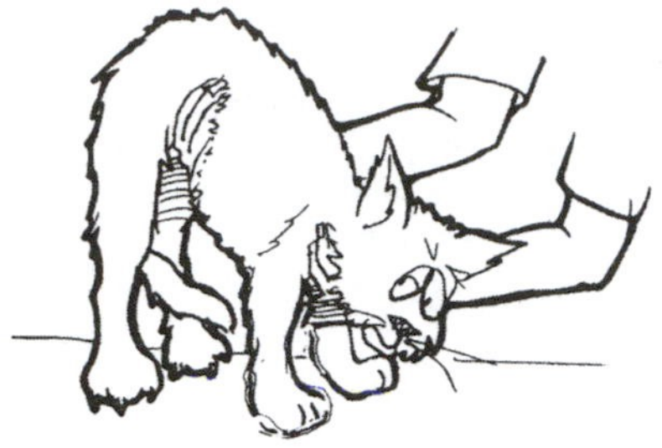

Fig. VII-1 - Cat - Kidney

URINARY SYSTEM: considered part of the urogenital system, the urinary system includes the kidneys, ureters, urinary bladder, and urethra. The **ureters** connect the kidneys to the **urinary bladder,** which empties to the outside through the **urethra.**

KIDNEYS (L. *renes*): functional organs of the urinary system that filter blood and produce urine. Both kidneys are located high in the abdomen's lumbar region at the level of the thoracolumbar junction. They are retroperitoneal (behind the peritoneum) and against the crura of the diaphragm.

1. Right kidney: the more cranial kidney by a half-kidney length. Its cranial end is embedded in the renal impression (recess) of the liver's caudate lobe, except in the pig.

2. Left kidney: the more caudal kidney, except in the pig where both kidneys are at the same level.

PERIRENAL FAT: a mass of protective fat surrounding the kidney and holding it in place.

FIBROUS CAPSULE: the loosely attached (except at the hilus) capsule of collagenous and some elastic fibers. It peels away easily from the healthy kidney.

4. ADRENAL GLANDS (a-DREE-nal): paired glands located against the roof of the abdominal cavity at the thoracolumbar junction. Cranial to the kidneys, except in the horse where they are medial to the kidneys. They are endocrine glands producing mineralocorticoids (cortical, outer zone), glucocorticoids and sex hormones (cortical, inner zone) and norepinephrine and epinephrine (medulla). The adrenal glands are part of the sympathetic autonomic nervous system and participate in the "flight or fight" response by dumping epinephrine into the blood stream.

SPECIES DIFFERENCES

Shape:
- Bean-shaped and smooth (not lobated): **carnivores, small ruminants, pigs** and the **horse's left** kidney.
- Heart-shaped and smooth: **horse's right** kidney.
- Lobated: **ox**

3. Capsular veins: the normal, distinct veins under the capsule of the **cat's** kidney.

Mobile kidneys: the left kidney of the **cat** and **ruminants** hangs down into the abdominal cavity; thus, is not retroperitoneal. The rumen pushes the left kidney to the right of the median plane in **ruminants.**

Location: the right kidney is cranial to the left in all species, except the **pig** where they are at the same level. The cat's kidneys are at a level caudal to the dog's kidneys level.

	Right kidney	Left kidney
Dog	T12-13 to L2-3	**Slightly more caudal**
Cat	L1 to 4	L3 to 5
Ox	T13 to L3	L2-3 to L5
Small ruminants	T13 to L2	L4 to L6
Horse	T15-17 to L1	T16-18 to L2-3
Pig	L1 to L4	L1 to L4

CLINICAL

Nephritis (ne-FRY-tis): inflammation of the kidneys.

Phrenicoabdominal vein: passes over the ventral surface of the adrenal gland. It is used to find the adrenal glands in surgery or at necropsy.

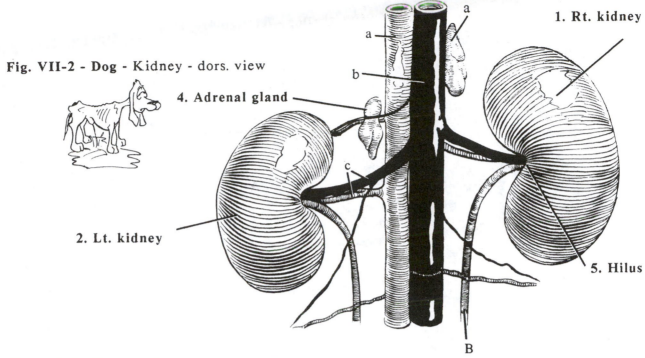

Fig. VII-2 - **Dog** - Kidney - dors. view

4. Adrenal gland

2. Lt. kidney

1. Rt. kidney

5. Hilus

B

Fig. VII-3 - **Horse** - Kidneys - ventr. view

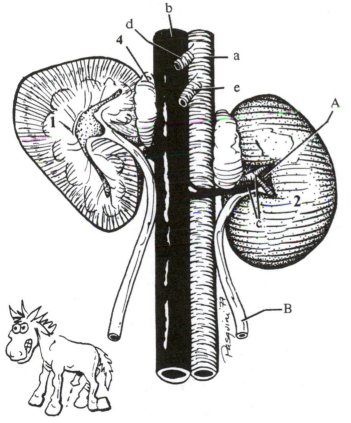

A. Hilus
B. Ureter

a. Aorta
b. Caud. vena cava
c. Renal a. & v.
d. Celiac a.
e. Cran. mesenteric a.

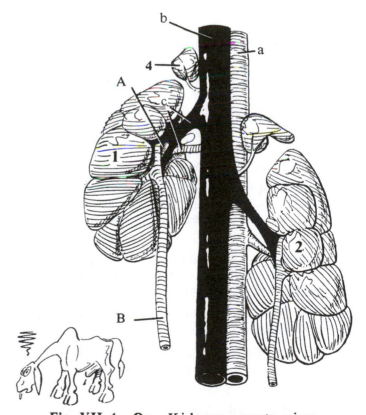

Fig. VII-4 - **Ox** - Kidneys - ventr. view

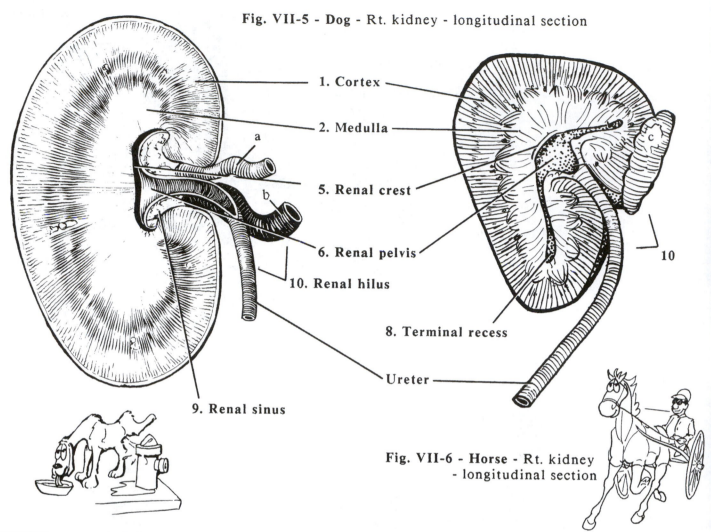

Fig. VII-5 - Dog - Rt. kidney - longitudinal section

1. Cortex
2. Medulla
5. Renal crest
6. Renal pelvis
10. Renal hilus
8. Terminal recess
Ureter
9. Renal sinus

Fig. VII-6 - Horse - Rt. kidney - longitudinal section

KIDNEY: composed of many lobes, each lobe consists of a medullary pyramid capped by cortical tissue. The apex of the pyramid is the renal papilla. Fusion of kidney tissue accounts for the different types of kidneys.

1. Cortex (KOR-teks): the outer layer of the kidney parenchyma beneath the capsule; characterized grossly by its light color and granular appearance. The cortex contains the renal corpuscles and the convoluted parts of the renal tubules (pg. 336).

2. Medulla (me-DUL-ah): the inner layer of the kidney parenchyma, characterized by its striated appearance. It contains collecting ducts and nephric loops.

3. Lobes (Fig. VII-8): the kidney units, obvious in the ox, but not in the other domestic species.

Renal papilla (REE-nal): the apex of a kidney lobule that drips urine into the proximal end of the ureter. The degree of fusion of the lobes results in individual papillae or a renal crest.

• 4. Individual papillae (Fig. VII-7): found in the **ox** and **pig**, as a results of incomplete fusion of the medullary pyramids.

• 5. Renal crest: the ridge resulting from complete fusion of the medullary pyramids, found in **carnivores**, **small ruminants** and **horses**.

PROXIMAL END of the URETER: the part of the ureter receiving urine from the renal papillae. Its shape varies depending on the species.

• 6. Renal pelvis (G. *pyelos*, tub or basin): the expanded proximal end of the ureters in kidneys with a renal crest (carnivores, small ruminants and horses), and in the pig (which has papillae).

• 7. Calyx (KAY-liks) (pl=calyces) (G. *kalyx*, cup of a flower): the cup-shaped structure receiving urine from individual papillae in the ox and pig. In the ox individual calyces (KAL-iseez) empty into two branches of the ureter (sometimes called major calyces). In the pig, calyces empty into a renal pelvis.

9. RENAL SINUS: the potential space occupied by the ureter, branches of the renal artery and vein, and lymphatics and nerves entering the kidney.

10. RENAL HILUS (HY-lus): the opening into the renal sinus where the ureter and renal vessels enter the kidney.

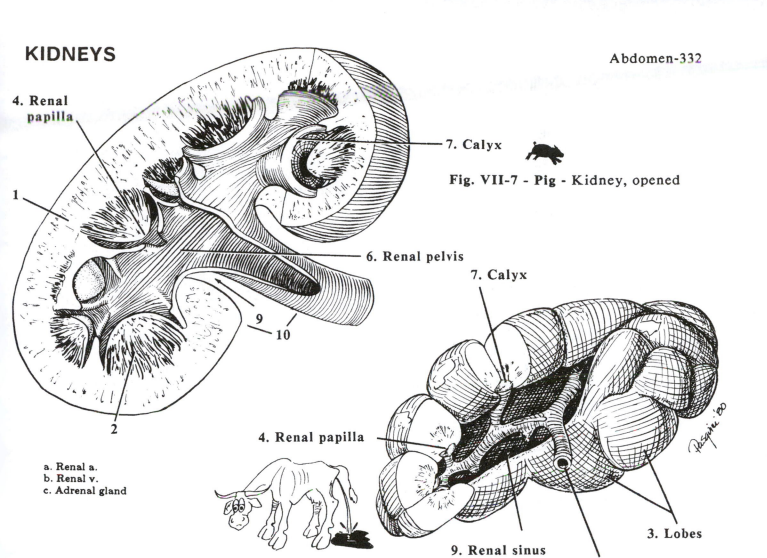

4. Renal papilla

1

2

7. Calyx

Fig. VII-7 - Pig - Kidney, opened

6. Renal pelvis

9
10

a. Renal a.
b. Renal v.
c. Adrenal gland

7. Calyx

4. Renal papilla

9. Renal sinus

3. Lobes

Ureter

Fig. VII-8 - Ox - Lt. kidney, opened

SPECIES DIFFERENCES

	Papillae	Renal crest	Calyces	Pelvis
Carnivores		+		+
Horse		+		+
Small ruminants		+		+
Ox	+		+	
Pig	+		+	+

Smooth kidneys: the appearance resulting from complete fusion of the kidney cortical tissue - **carnivores**, **horse**, **pig** and **small ruminants**. Kidneys of the dog, goat, and sheep are hard to distinguish grossly.

Pig: has a smooth kidney due to fused cortical tissue, but has unfused medullary tissue, resulting in papillae in a smooth kidney. It has no renal crest.

Lobated kidney: found in the ox, resulting from incomplete fusion of kidney lobes. It has calyces and papillae, but no renal pelvis.

8. Terminal recesses - horse (Fig. VII-6): the long tube-like

extensions that collect and carry urine from the kidney poles to the small renal pelvis. Different sources consider them either large collecting ducts or diverticulum of the renal pelvis. (To the student this argument is the least of problems!)

Glands in the wall of the horse's renal pelvis: secrete mucous which gives the horse's urine a turbid (and foamy) appearance.

All these renal terms (sinus, pelvis, hilus, and crest) are confusing for the student. Organize structures into those that are part of the kidney parenchyma, those that are part of the ureter, and those that are neither.

	Kidney	Ureter	Neither
Cortex	+		
Medulla	+		
Papillae	+		
Renal crest	+		
Terminal recess	+?	+?	
Calyces		+	
Renal pelvis		+	
Renal sinus			+
Renal hilus			+

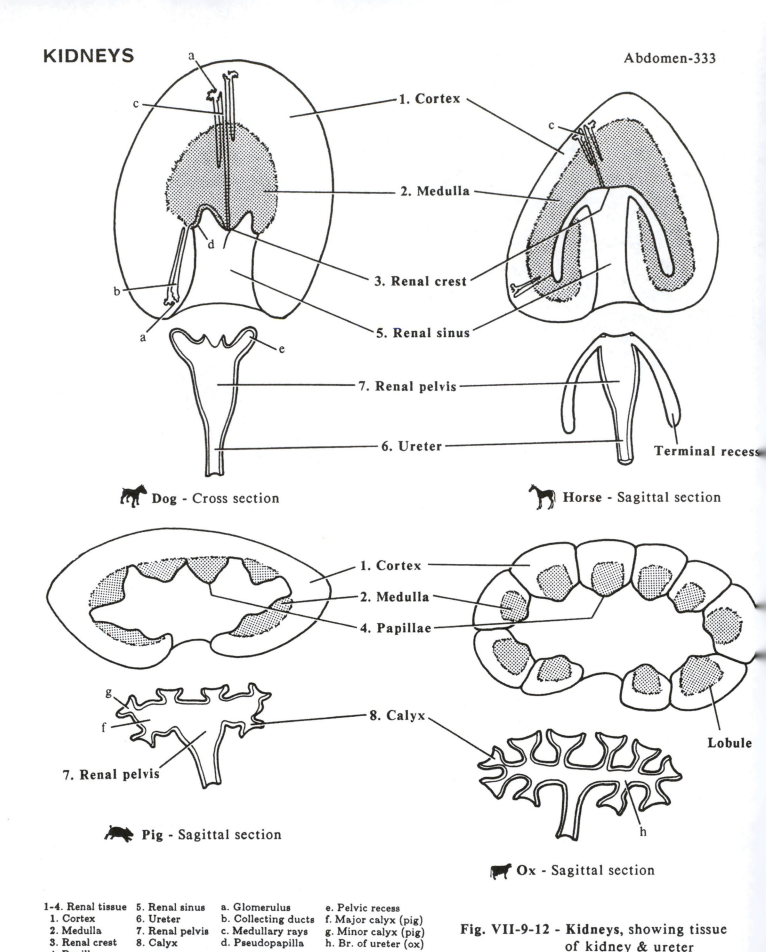

KIDNEYS

Abdomen-333

1. Cortex

2. Medulla

3. Renal crest

5. Renal sinus

7. Renal pelvis

6. Ureter

Terminal recess

🐕 **Dog - Cross section**

🐴 **Horse - Sagittal section**

1. Cortex

2. Medulla

4. Papillae

8. Calyx

Lobule

7. Renal pelvis

🐷 **Pig - Sagittal section**

🐂 **Ox - Sagittal section**

1-4. Renal tissue	5. Renal sinus	a. Glomerulus	e. Pelvic recess
1. Cortex	6. Ureter	b. Collecting ducts	f. Major calyx (pig)
2. Medulla	7. Renal pelvis	c. Medullary rays	g. Minor calyx (pig)
3. Renal crest	8. Calyx	d. Pseudopapilla	h. Br. of ureter (ox)
4. Papillae			

Fig. VII-9-12 - Kidneys, showing tissue of kidney & ureter

332

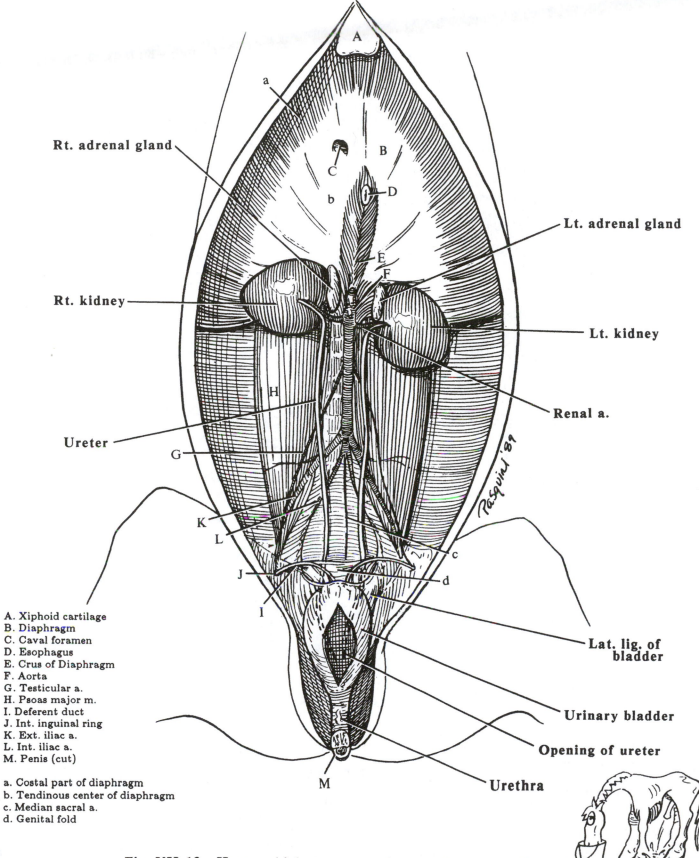

A. Xiphoid cartilage
B. Diaphragm
C. Caval foramen
D. Esophagus
E. Crus of Diaphragm
F. Aorta
G. Testicular a.
H. Psoas major m.
I. Deferent duct
J. Int. inguinal ring
K. Ext. iliac a.
L. Int. iliac a.
M. Penis (cut)

a. Costal part of diaphragm
b. Tendinous center of diaphragm
c. Median sacral a.
d. Genital fold

Rt. adrenal gland
Rt. kidney
Ureter
Lt. adrenal gland
Lt. kidney
Renal a.
Lat. lig. of bladder
Urinary bladder
Opening of ureter
Urethra

Fig. VII-13 - Horse - Abdomen, opened ventrally, viscera & caud.
vena cava removed, urinary bladder opened

KIDNEYS

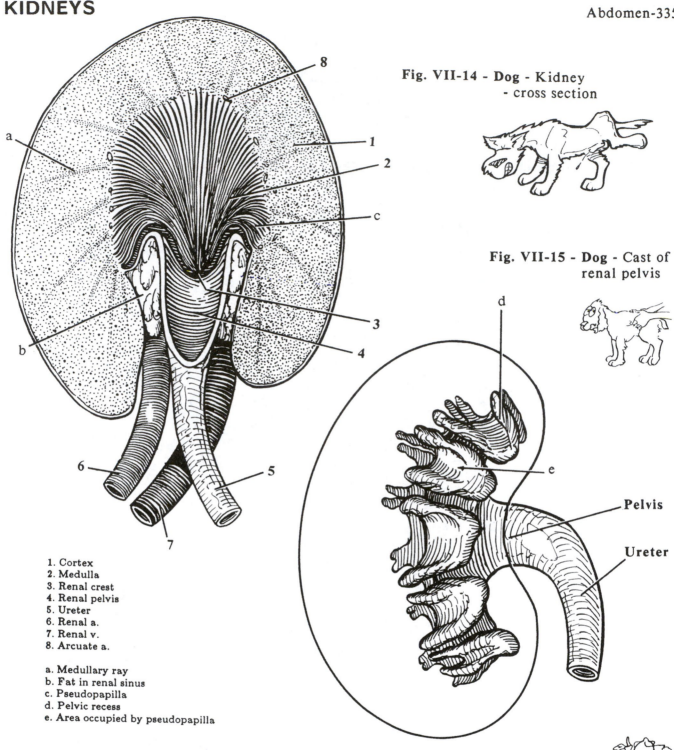

Fig. VII-14 - Dog - Kidney - cross section

Fig. VII-15 - Dog - Cast of renal pelvis

Pelvis

Ureter

1. Cortex
2. Medulla
3. Renal crest
4. Renal pelvis
5. Ureter
6. Renal a.
7. Renal v.
8. Arcuate a.

a. Medullary ray
b. Fat in renal sinus
c. Pseudopapilla
d. Pelvic recess
e. Area occupied by pseudopapilla

Patent (persistent) urachus: connects the urinary bladder to the umbilicus. It usually degenerates after birth. If patent, it causes urine to dribble from the umbilicus; and should be surgically removed.

Urinary calculi (sin.=calculus): an abnormal concretion in any part of the urinary system (kidney pelvis, urinary bladder, urethra).

• Urolithiasis: the formation of urinary calculi.

Cystitis: inflammation of the urinary bladder.

Cystocentesis: tapping of the urinary bladder with a needle to remove urine. This may be necessary to prevent rupture of the bladder in tomcats that have urethral calculi.

Cystotomy: opening of the urinary bladder.

KIDNEY - ARTERIAL SUPPLY

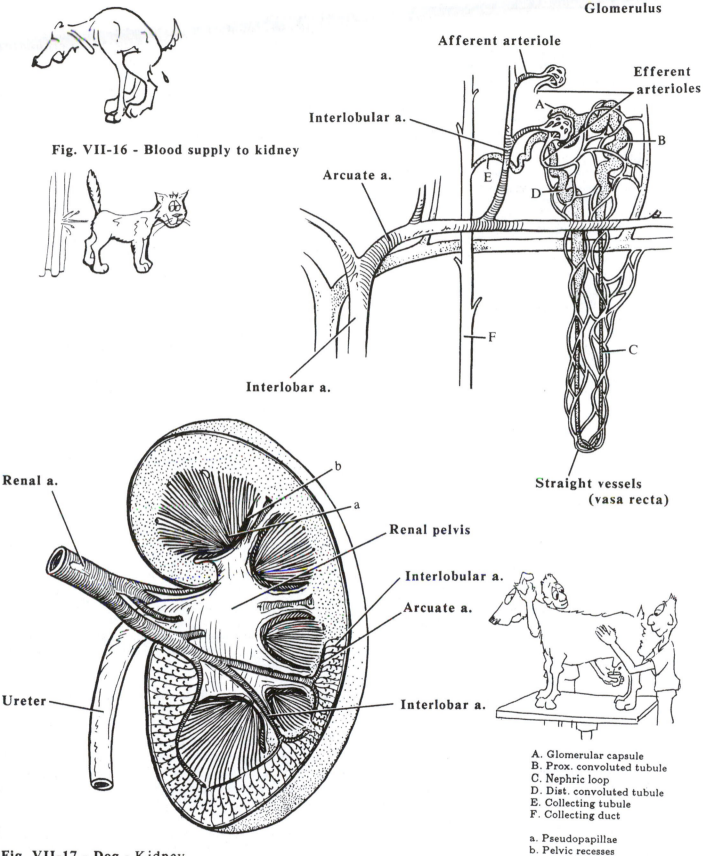

Glomerulus

Afferent arteriole

Efferent arterioles

Interlobular a.

Arcuate a.

Interlobar a.

Straight vessels (vasa recta)

Fig. VII-16 - Blood supply to kidney

Renal a.

b

a

Renal pelvis

Interlobular a.

Arcuate a.

Ureter

Interlobar a.

A. Glomerular capsule
B. Prox. convoluted tubule
C. Nephric loop
D. Dist. convoluted tubule
E. Collecting tubule
F. Collecting duct

a. Pseudopapillae
b. Pelvic recesses

Fig. VII-17 - Dog - Kidney
 - parasagittal section

CLINICAL - KIDNEYS

Nephrectomy (Gr. *nephros*, kidney + *ektome*, excision): removal (excision) of a kidney. Always check that the other kidney is present and functioning first. Also check for double renal arteries.

Nephrotomy (Gr. *nephros* + *tome*, a cutting): surgical incision into a kidney. This can be done to remove a calculus.

Pyelonephritis (py'e-loh-ne-FRI-tis) (Gr. *pyelos*, pelvis + *nephros* + *itis*): inflammation of the kidney and its pelvis.

Renal biopsy: the removal of renal tissue for histopathological evaluation.
• **Horse**: push the left kidney per rectum against the left paralumbar fossa and direct the biopsy needle through the wall.
• **Ox**: as in the horse per rectum, but push the kidney to the right paralumbar fossa.
• **Dog**: oblique incision in the craniodorsal angle of the paralumbar fossa. Hold the kidney against the wall with a finger and insert the needle through a separate puncture site.
• **Cat**: palpate the kidney against the abdominal wall and direct the needle through the wall.
(From *Applied Veterinary Anatomy*, Habel and de Lahunta, 1986).

Rectal palpation of the ureters: possible in **cattle** with calculi or pyelonephritis.

Oak poisoning: common in cattle eating oak leaves or acorns, resulting in renal dysfunction.

Amyloidosis: uncommon accumulation of amyloid (sheets of protein) in multiple systems, including the renal glomerulus. It is associated with chronic inflammation.

Ectopic ureters: a ureter that terminates some place other than the urinary bladder - uterus, vagina, or urethra. This results in urinary incontinence (dribbling urine). This affects toy breeds more than large breeds. Reimplant the ureters by duplicating the oblique path through the wall of the urinary bladder to prevent reflux of urine up the ureter.

Nephrotoxic substances:
• **Aminoglycoside antibiotics**
• **Heavy metals**
• **Antifreeze** (ethylene glycol)

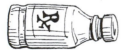
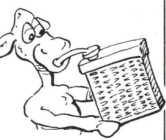

NEPHRON (NEF-ron): the microscopic, functional unit of the kidney, consisting of a urine-producing tubule and a renal corpuscle. Collecting ducts (not a part of the nephron) carry the urine produced by the nephron to the renal pelvis.

1. Renal corpuscle (KOR-pus'l): the glomerulus and the glomerular capsule.

2. Glomerulus (gloh-MER-yoo-lus): a tuft of arterial capillaries associated with the glomerular capsule.

3. Afferent arteriole: the small vessel entering the glomerulus.

4. Efferent arteriole: the small vessel leaving the glomerulus.

5. Vascular pole of the glomerulus: the point at which the afferent and efferent arterioles enter and leave the glomerulus.

6. Glomerular (Bowman's) capsule: the double-walled, cup-shaped, expanded end of the renal tubule surrounding the glomerulus. It has a visceral layer and a parietal layer.

• 7. Visceral layer: surrounds the glomerulus (capillary tuft).

• 8. Parietal layer: surrounds the urinary space, the visceral layer and the glomerulus. It is continuous with the visceral layer at the glomerulus' vascular pole.

• **9. Urinary space** or space of Bowman's capsule: the space between visceral and parietal layers of the glomerular capsule. Fluid is filtered from the glomerulus through the visceral layer of the glomerular capsule, collects in this space, and drains into the lumen of the tubular part of the nephron.

Tubular part of the nephron: consists of the proximal convoluted tubule, the nephric loop, and the distal convoluted tubule.

10. Proximal convoluted tubule: the longest part of the nephron, a twisted tube extending from the glomerular capsule toward the medulla, where it straightens into the nephric loop.

11. Nephric loop or loop of Henle: descends into the medulla and then ascends to continue as the distal convoluted tubule. It has thick and thin parts.

12. Distal convoluted tubule: continues the nephric loop close to the glomerulus and then joins the collecting ducts.

13. COLLECTING DUCTS: the long tubes receiving urine from the distal convoluted tubules. They run through the medulla, joining other collecting ducts to open onto the renal crest or individual papillae as papillary ducts. These are not considered part of the nephron.

14. Papillary ducts: the openings of the collecting duct onto the renal crest or individual papillae, depending on the species.

NEPHRON

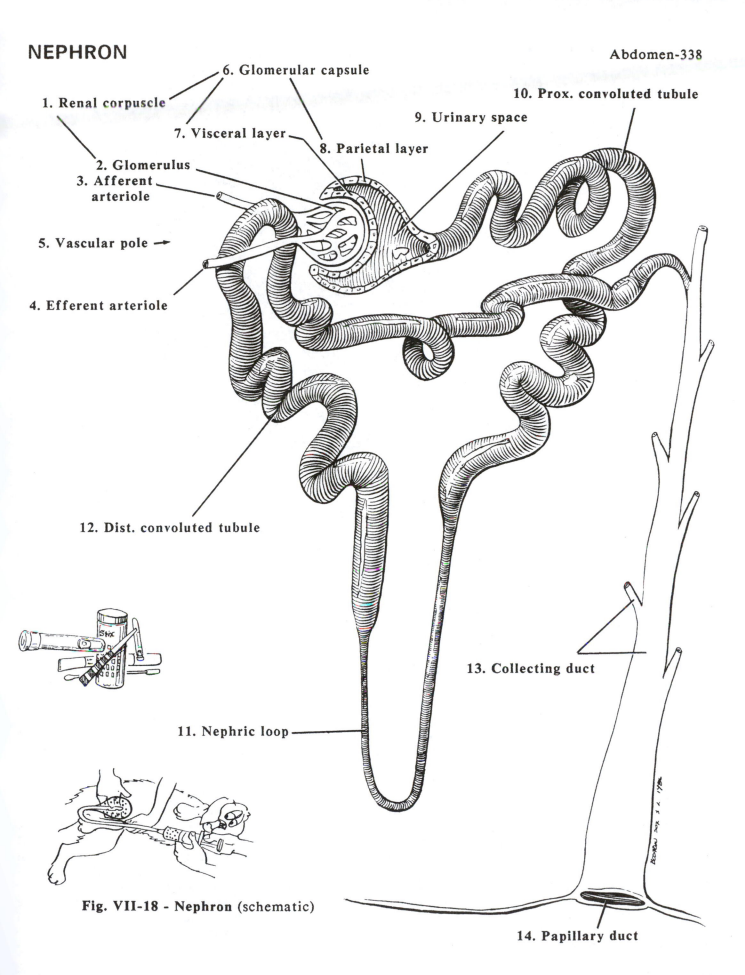

6. Glomerular capsule

1. Renal corpuscle

10. Prox. convoluted tubule

9. Urinary space

7. Visceral layer

8. Parietal layer

2. Glomerulus

3. Afferent arteriole

5. Vascular pole →

4. Efferent arteriole

12. Dist. convoluted tubule

13. Collecting duct

11. Nephric loop

14. Papillary duct

Fig. VII-18 - Nephron (schematic)

URINARY BLADDER

Fig. VII-l9. Horse
- Topographic anatomy
- View of caudal abdomen

6. Rt. kidney

1. Ureter

5. Lt. kidney

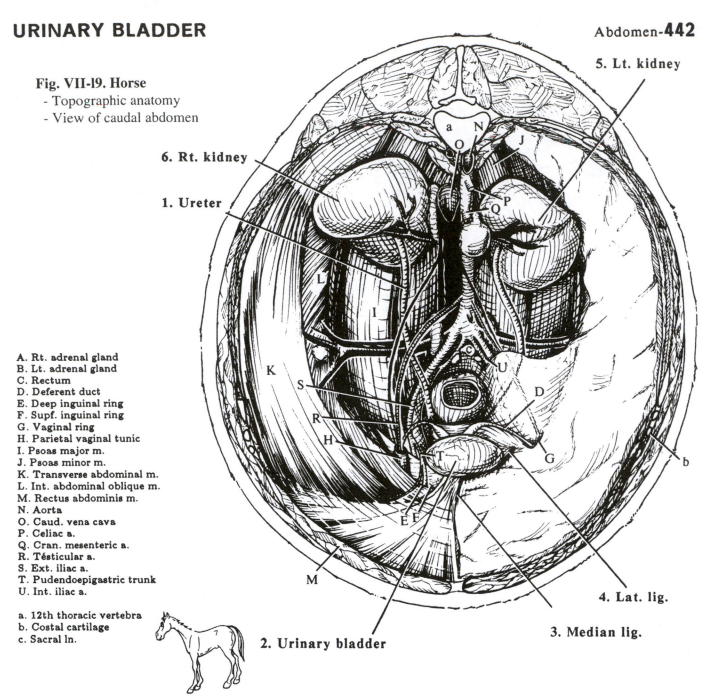

A. Rt. adrenal gland
B. Lt. adrenal gland
C. Rectum
D. Deferent duct
E. Deep inguinal ring
F. Supf. inguinal ring
G. Vaginal ring
H. Parietal vaginal tunic
I. Psoas major m.
J. Psoas minor m.
K. Transverse abdominal m.
L. Int. abdominal oblique m.
M. Rectus abdominis m.
N. Aorta
O. Caud. vena cava
P. Celiac a.
Q. Cran. mesenteric a.
R. Testicular a.
S. Ext. iliac a.
T. Pudendoepigastric trunk
U. Int. iliac a.

a. 12th thoracic vertebra
b. Costal cartilage
c. Sacral ln.

4. Lat. lig.

3. Median lig.

2. Urinary bladder

1. URETER (yoo-REE-ter): the paired fibromuscular tubes carrying urine from the kidneys to the urinary bladder. Located retroperitoneally along the dorsal abdominal wall, each ureter runs caudally to the brim of the pelvis. They pass ventral to the ductus deferens, loop around the rectum and internal genitalia to the reach the urinary bladder's dorsal surface. The ureters pass through the urinary bladder's wall at an acute angle, preventing backflow and still allowing urine to empty into a full bladder by peristaltic action.

2. URINARY BLADDER: the greatly distensible pouch receiving and storing urine from the kidneys for release out the urethra. The empty bladder lies almost entirely within the pelvic cavity, but with distention extends into the abdominal cavity. The bladder has a free **apex**, a **body**, and a **neck**.

Trigone of the urinary bladder: the internal area of the dorsal bladder between the two ureteral openings and the start of the urethra.

Ligaments of the Urinary Bladder: the three connecting peritoneal folds reflected from the urinary bladder onto the abdominal and pelvic walls. The **median** (ventral) **ligament** (3) reflects from the bladder's ventral surface to the pelvic floor and abdominal wall, as far cranially as the umbilicus. The urachus is the vestigial structure from the apex of the bladder to the umbilicus in the medial ligament. The two **lateral ligaments** (4) connect the sides of the bladder to the lateral pelvic wall. The round ligament of the bladder, a remnant of the umbilical arteries of the fetus, travel in the edge of the lateral ligaments.

Chapter VIII
Reproductive System

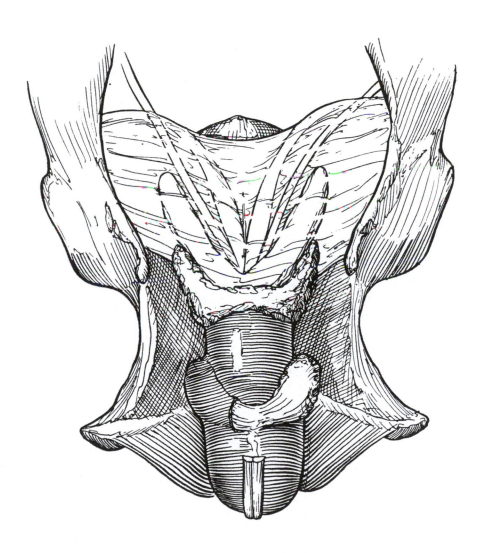

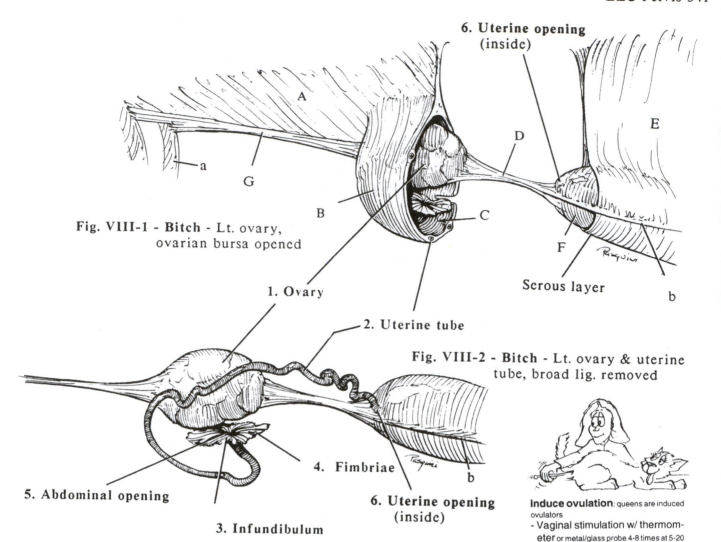

6. Uterine opening
(inside)

Fig. VIII-1 - **Bitch** - Lt. ovary,
ovarian bursa opened

Serous layer

1. Ovary

2. Uterine tube

Fig. VIII-2 - **Bitch** - Lt. ovary & uterine
tube, broad lig. removed

4. Fimbriae

5. Abdominal opening

6. Uterine opening
(inside)

3. Infundibulum

Induce ovulation: queens are induced ovulators
- Vaginal stimulation w/ thermometer or metal/glass probe 4-8 times at 5-20 minute intervals

1. OVARIES (OH-var-ees): the female gonads homologous to the male testicles. The ovaries are round or oval and may be nodular. They function in the maturation of the female germ cells (oocytes) and in hormone production. The visceral peritoneal covering of the ovary is called the superficial epithelium. The tunica albuginea (white tunic) is the condensed connective tissue underlying the epithelium surrounding the ovary.

Cortex: the outer zone of the ovary. It is composed of follicles in various stages of development, corpora lutea, and connective tissue stroma.

Medulla: the central area of the ovary. It contains blood vessels, nerves, lymphatics, smooth muscle fibers and connective tissue fibers.

2. UTERINE TUBE (YOO-ter-in) ("oviduct" or fallopian tube): the duct running from the ovary, between the layers of the mesosalpinx (pg. 348), to the tip of the uterine horn. It conveys the oocytes or fertilized egg from the ovary to the uterus and conveys sperm toward the ovary. It is the site of fertilization of the ootid.

3. Infundibulum (L. funnel): the expanded, funnel-shaped ovarian end of the uterine tube.

4. Fimbriae (L. fringes): the irregular, finger-like projections on the free edge of the infundibulum. At ovulation, they pick up the oocyte from the surface of the ovary and direct it to the infundibulum.

Abdominal opening of the uterine tube: the opening in the center of the infundibulum. It is the only opening of the peritoneal cavity to the outside in the female animal. The male has no such opening.

SPECIES DIFFERENCES

Location of the Ovaries:
• **Bitch, queen** and **mare**: lie caudal to the kidneys in the sublumbar region.
• **Cow, ewe** and **sow**: lie at the pelvic inlet due to caudal migration.
• **Mare**: the cortex and medulla of the ovary are reversed, the cortex being in the center surrounded by the medulla.

7. Ovulation fossa: the central depression in the mares's ovary where ovulation takes place.

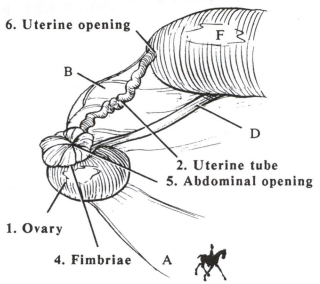

6. Uterine opening

B

F

D

2. Uterine tube
5. Abdominal opening

1. Ovary

4. Fimbriae A

Fig. VIII-3 - Mare - Rt. ovary & uterine tube

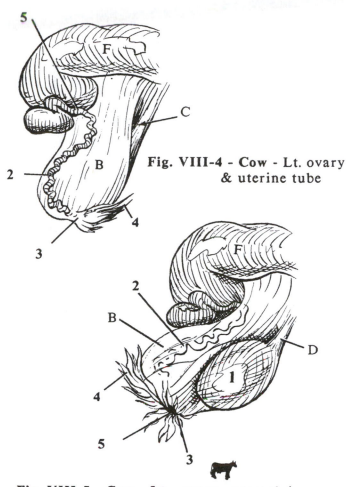

5

F

C

B

2

4

3

Fig. VIII-4 - Cow - Lt. ovary
& uterine tube

2

B

F

D

4

5

3

1

Fig. VIII-5 - Cow - Lt. ovary, mesosalpinx
moved to show ovarian bursa

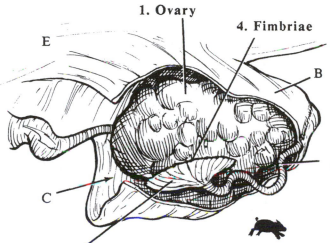

1. Ovary

4. Fimbriae

E

B

C

2. Uterine tube

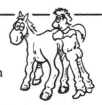

3. Infundibulum   **Fig. VIII-6 - Sow** - Ovary, mesosalpinx cut

A. Mesovarium
B. Mesosalpinx
C. Ovarian bursa
D. Proper lig. of ovary
E. Mesometrium
F. Uterine horn
G. Suspensory lig. (carnivores)

a. Last rib
b. Round lig. of uterus

CLINICAL

Palpation of the ovaries per rectum: to determine the stage of estrus and condition of the ovary in the mare and cow.

Estrus: recurrent, restricted period of sexual receptivity in females (other than humans), marked by intense sexual urge.

Anestrus: the lack of estrus.

Repeat breeders: mares and cows that are bred 3 or more times without becoming pregnant.

Cystic ovarian disease (Nymphomania, buller cow): a cyst on the cow's ovary resulting in anestrus most of the time or nymphomania in some cases. Chronic cases result in masculine characteristics.

Persitent corpus luteum: #1 cause of anestrus during breeding season in <u>mares</u>.

Ovariectomy: the removal of the ovaries.

Ovariohysterectomy: removal of the ovaries and most of the uterus.

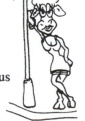

UTERUS

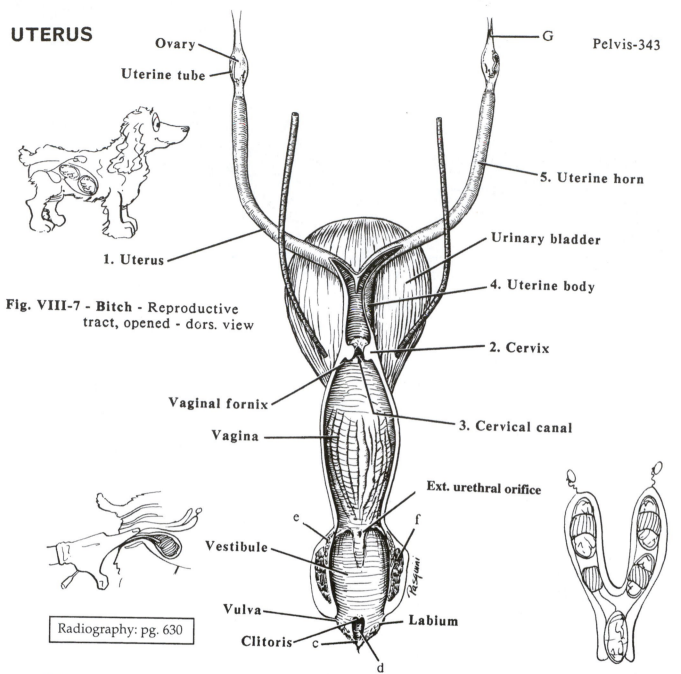

Ovary
Uterine tube
1. Uterus

Fig. VIII-7 - Bitch - Reproductive tract, opened - dors. view

G
5. Uterine horn
Urinary bladder
4. Uterine body
2. Cervix

Vaginal fornix
Vagina

3. Cervical canal

Ext. urethral orifice

e
f

Vestibule

Radiography: pg. 630

Vulva
Clitoris
c
d
Labium

1. UTERUS (YOO-te-rus)(G. *hystera*): the highly expandable, tubular organ where the embryo/fetus develops.

2. Cervix (SER-viks)(L. neck): the constricted caudal part of the uterus joining the uterus to the vagina. It usually is located in the pelvic cavity.

3. Cervical canal: the channel through the cervix. Having openings at both ends (the internal uterine ostium and the external ostium), it is closed, except during estrus and birth.

4. Body: the part of the uterus between the cervix and the uterine horns. It opens into each uterine horn and into the cervix. The body of the uterus lies dorsal to the urinary bladder and ventral to the descending colon and rectum.

5. Uterine horns: the two musculomembraneous extensions of the uterine body which are continuous cranially with the uterine tubes. They are located entirely within the abdomen.

SPECIES DIFFERENCES

Uterine horns and body:
• **Carnivores** and **sow**: very long horns compared to their body, an adaptation for litter bearing (carrying several developing young).
• **Mare**: relatively short horns, of equal length to its uterine body.
• **Cow** and **ewe**: long horns and short bodies like the carnivores and sow. The ends of the uterine horns are coiled up like ram's horns and continue back parallel to each other. They are bound together by the intercornual ligaments, giving the false impression of a long uterine body.

Caruncles (L. *carunculae*, small fleshy masses): the regularly-spaced, circular to ovoid, internal, specialized thickenings of the ruminant's endometrium, making up the maternal com-

UTERUS

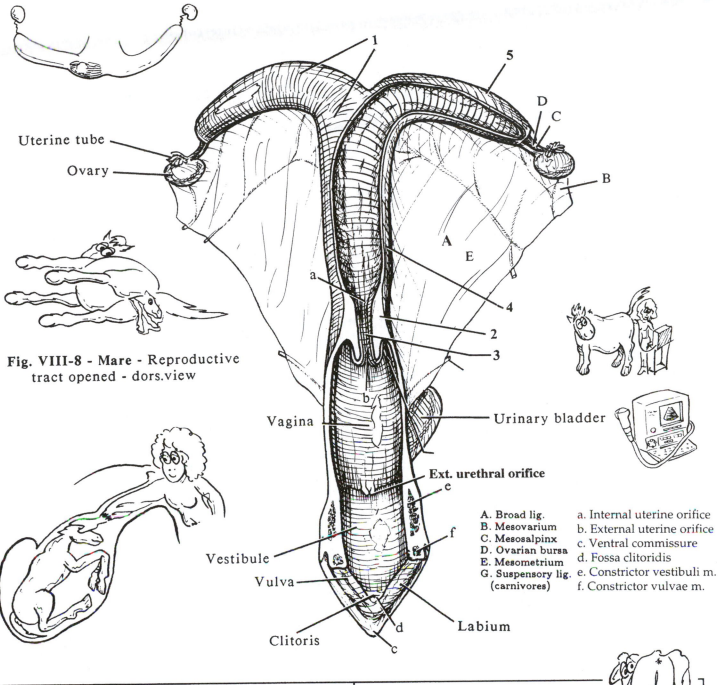

Uterine tube

Ovary

Fig. VIII-8 - Mare - Reproductive tract opened - dors.view

Vagina

Urinary bladder

Ext. urethral orifice

Vestibule

Vulva

Clitoris

Labium

1
5
D
C
B
A
E
4
2
3
a
b
e
f
d
c

A. Broad lig.
B. Mesovarium
C. Mesosalpinx
D. Ovarian bursa
E. Mesometrium
G. Suspensory lig.
  (carnivores)

a. Internal uterine orifice
b. External uterine orifice
c. Ventral commissure
d. Fossa clitoridis
e. Constrictor vestibuli m.
f. Constrictor vulvae m.

ponent of the placenta. The fetal component is the cotyledon. Together the caruncle and the cotyledon make up a placentome. The placentomes enlarge during pregnancy and can be palpated to estimate the stage of pregnancy.

Clinical

Uterine prolapse: turning inside out of the uterus and vagina and their projection through the vulva. Most common in dairy cow and sow. The prolapsed uterus can often be pushed back in and sutured in place until it heals.

Uterine infection: infection of uterus.
• Endometritis (inflammation of. endometrium)
• Metritis (inflammation of all layers)
• Pyometra (accumulation of pus in uterus)

Uterine torsion: twisting of the uterus on its long axis. It may be diagnosed by rectal palpation or vaginal exam. May be corrected in cows or horses with rolling and a plank.

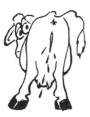

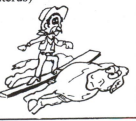

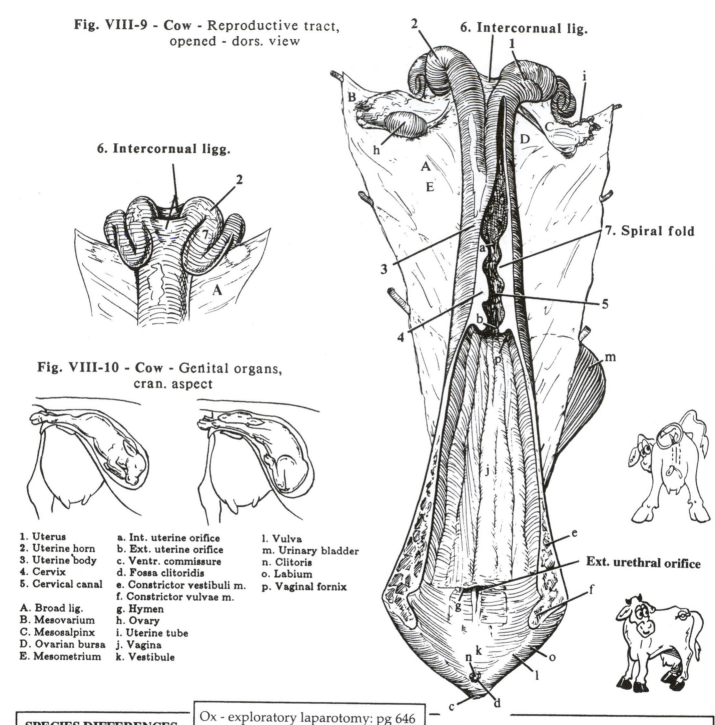

Fig. VIII-9 - Cow - Reproductive tract, opened - dors. view

6. Intercornual lig.

6. Intercornual ligg.

7. Spiral fold

Fig. VIII-10 - Cow - Genital organs, cran. aspect

Ext. urethral orifice

1. Uterus
2. Uterine horn
3. Uterine body
4. Cervix
5. Cervical canal

A. Broad lig.
B. Mesovarium
C. Mesosalpinx
D. Ovarian bursa
E. Mesometrium

a. Int. uterine orifice
b. Ext. uterine orifice
c. Ventr. commissure
d. Fossa clitoridis
e. Constrictor vestibuli m.
f. Constrictor vulvae m.
g. Hymen
h. Ovary
i. Uterine tube
j. Vagina
k. Vestibule

l. Vulva
m. Urinary bladder
n. Clitoris
o. Labium
p. Vaginal fornix

Ox - exploratory laparotomy: pg 646

SPECIES DIFFERENCES

6. Intercornual ligaments: dorsal and ventral ligaments connecting the uterine horns in the <u>cow</u> and <u>ewe</u>.

Cervix:

• **Mare** and **carnivores**: have a simple cervix bulging into the vagina (portio vaginalis) to form a distinct vaginal recess (fornix).

• **7. Spiral folds - cow** and **ewe**: have a very long cervix, characterized by transverse folds that interdigitate with each other to effectively occlude, along with the mucous secretions, the cervical canal. It is open only during estrus and parturition.

• **8. Pulvini** (L. *pulvinus* a cushion): the mounds or cushions in the **sow** that interdigitate with each other, closing the canal.

UTERUS

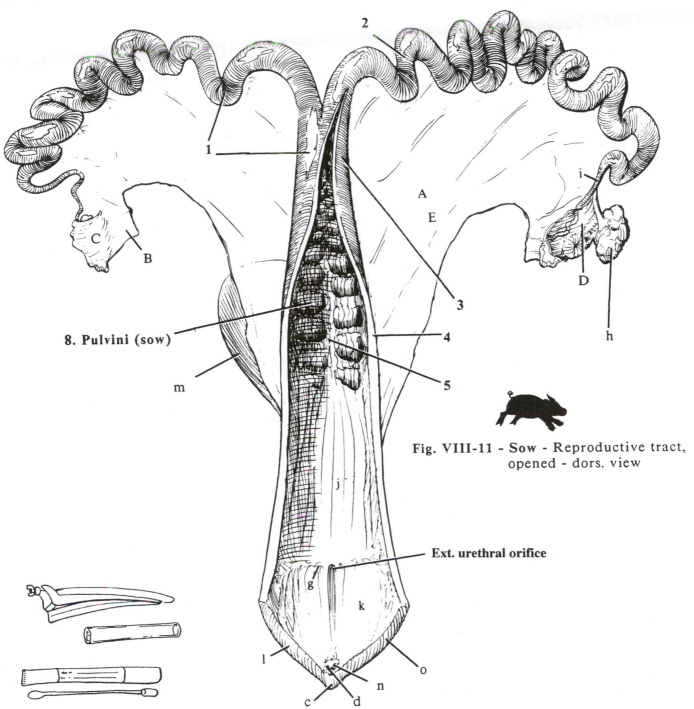

8. Pulvini (sow)

Ext. urethral orifice

Fig. VIII-11 - Sow - Reproductive tract, opened - dors. view

CLINICAL

Pregnancy diagnosis in cattle and horses: palpation of the reproductive tract per rectum to detect pregnancy.

Intercornual ligaments (ox) (6): grasped with a hand in the descending colon when palpating per rectum. Once grasped, it is used to flip the uterus into the pelvis for palpation of the uterus and ovaries.

Cesarean section: removal of the fetus through incisions in the abdominal and uterine walls. It is performed most often on cows and small dogs. After the fetus has been removed the uterus and abdomen are sutured closed.

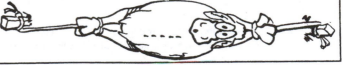

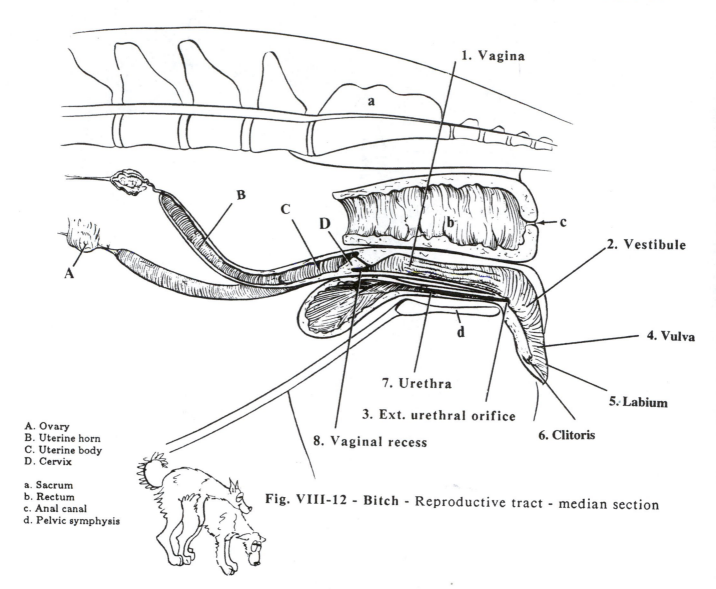

1. Vagina

a

B

C

D

b

c

2. Vestibule

4. Vulva

5. Labium

7. Urethra

3. Ext. urethral orifice

6. Clitoris

8. Vaginal recess

d

A. Ovary
B. Uterine horn
C. Uterine body
D. Cervix

a. Sacrum
b. Rectum
c. Anal canal
d. Pelvic symphysis

Fig. VIII-12 - Bitch - Reproductive tract - median section

1. VAGINA (va-JY-na): the part of the reproductive tract between the cervix and the vulva. With the vestibule and vulva, it is the female's copulatory organ and the birth canal. The **hymen** is the poorly developed, vestigial, mucosal folds at the junction of the vagina and the vestibule.

2. VESTIBULE (VES-ti-byool) (L. *vestibulum*, antechamber): the part of the reproductive tract belonging to both the urinary and the genital systems. It connects the vagina with the external genital opening*, the vulva.

3. External urethral orifice: the urethral opening at the vaginovestibular junction. This opens on a papilla, the <u>urethral tubercle</u> , in the carnivores.

4. VULVA (VUL-va): the external orifice that terminates the genital tract.

*The shallow human vestibule is included in the external genitalia. In quadrupeds, where it is much longer, it is considered an internal rather than an external organ.

5. Labia (LAY-bee-a)(sin.= labium): the right and left lips of the vulva. The **vulvar cleft** is the opening between the labia leading into the vestibule.

6. Clitoris (CLI-to-ris, CLY-to-ris): the partial homologue of the male penis located within the ventral commissure of the vulva. It has left and right crura that attach to the ischiatic arch. The crura come together to form the body. The glans, the only exposed part of the clitoris, is in the clitoral fossa surrounded by the clitoral prepuce.

7. FEMALE URETHRA (yoo-REE-thra): the tube transporting urine from the urinary bladder through the external urethral orifice to the vestibule.

Urethral (urethralis) **muscle**: the skeletal muscle covering the lateral and ventral sides of the urethra. The sphincter formed by the urethral muscle is under voluntary control.

VAGINA - VESTIBULE - VULVA

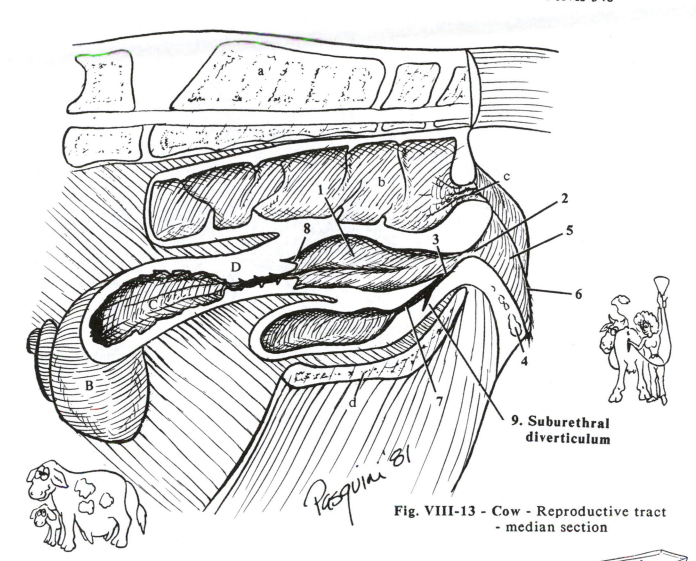

Fig. VIII-13 - Cow - Reproductive tract
- median section

9. Suburethral diverticulum

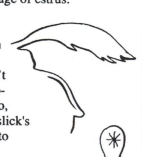

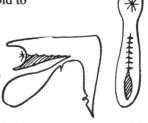

SPECIES DIFFERENCES

8. Vaginal fornix (recess): the cranioventral recess formed by the cervix bulging into the vagina (portio vaginalis) in the <u>mare</u> and <u>bitch</u>. The cow and ewe have a craniodorsal recess.

Vestibular bulbs: the organized erectile venous plexuses in the vestibular walls of the <u>mare</u> and <u>bitch</u>. During the dog's "tie" the bulbs are erect and press against the penis caudal to the enlarged bulb of the glans.

9. Suburethral diverticulum: the blind pocket just cranial and ventral to the external urethral opening in the <u>sow</u> and <u>cow</u>. This is clinically important when catheterizing a cow.

Vestibular glands: open into the vestibule and lubricate the reproductive organs during parturition and copulation. The cow, queen, and sometimes the ewe have major vestibular glands ("glands of Bartholin"); the bitch, ewe, mare and sow have minor vestibular glands.

Os clitoridis: a homologue os penis is found radiographically in some bitches.

CLINICAL

Vaginal smears: the use of microscopic slides of vaginal secretions in the **bitch** to determine the stage of estrus.

"Windsucker" (pneumovagina): a conformational defect in the **mare** in which the vaginal opening is deeply located and the lips of the vulva don't close properly. This becomes a reproduction problem when feces falls into, or urine pools in the vestibule. A Caslick's surgery closes the upper vulvar fold to prevent contamination

Urine pooling: occurs in horses and cows. In horses it is due to an abnormal cranioventral slope to the vagina.

BROAD LIGAMENT

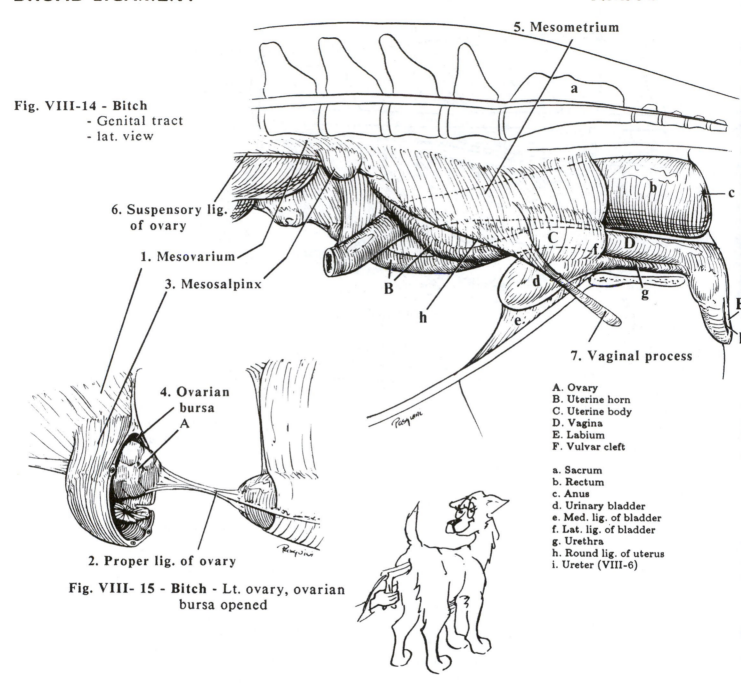

Fig. VIII-14 - Bitch
- Genital tract
- lat. view

5. Mesometrium

6. Suspensory lig. of ovary

1. Mesovarium

3. Mesosalpinx

7. Vaginal process

4. Ovarian bursa
A

2. Proper lig. of ovary

Fig. VIII- 15 - Bitch - Lt. ovary, ovarian bursa opened

A. Ovary
B. Uterine horn
C. Uterine body
D. Vagina
E. Labium
F. Vulvar cleft

a. Sacrum
b. Rectum
c. Anus
d. Urinary bladder
e. Med. lig. of bladder
f. Lat. lig. of bladder
g. Urethra
h. Round lig. of uterus
i. Ureter (VIII-6)

BROAD LIGAMENT: the fold of connecting peritoneum (serosa) connecting the visceral peritoneum of the female reproductive tract to the parietal peritoneum of the abdominal wall. It is subdivided into portions supporting individual parts of the reproductive tract: mesovarium, mesosalpinx and mesometrium.

1. Mesovarium (mes'oh-VAY-ree-um): the cranial part of the broad ligament attaching the ovary to the dorsolateral abdominal wall.

• 2. Proper ligament of the ovary or ovarian ligament: the caudal continuation of the mesovarium's cranial free edge connecting the ovary to the end of the uterine horn.

3. Mesosalpinx (mes'oh-SAL-pinks) (G. *salpin* tube or trumpet): the lateral fold arising from the mesovarium that holds the uterine tube between its two layers. The mesosalpinx is the only portion of the broad ligament not directly attached to the abdominal wall.

4. Ovarian (oh-VAR-ee-an) **bursa:** the small peritoneal cavity formed by the mesosalpinx and mesovarium into which projects the ovary.

Mesometrium (mes'oh-MEE-tree-um): the part of the broad ligament attaching the uterine horns and body to the dorsolateral body wall. The **round ligament of the uterus** (e) is the caudal continuation of the proper ligament of the ovary and is located in

BROAD LIGAMENT

Ovariectomy of a mare through a vaginal
approach (colpotomy) using an ecraseur.

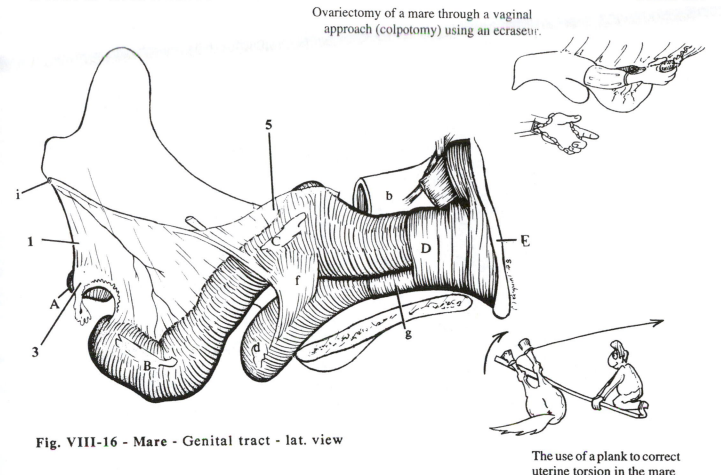

Fig. VIII-16 - Mare - Genital tract - lat. view

The use of a plank to correct
uterine torsion in the mare

the free edge of a secondary fold off the mesometrium. It extends
through the inguinal canal.

Structures associated with the broad ligament:

Ovarian vessels: the blood supply to the ovary traveling in the
mesovarium.

Uterine vessels: the blood supply to the uterus traveling in the
mesometrium. Upon reaching the uterus they course cranially
along the sides of the uterus and uterine horns to anastomoses with
the uterine branches of the ovarian arteries and veins.

SPECIES DIFFERENCES

6. Suspensory ligament of the ovary: the mesovarium's cranial
free edge attaching the ovary to the last rib, present only in the
carnivores.

Mesosalpinx: completely covers the ovary, except for a small
slit in the bitch. In the cow, sow and mare it is less extensive, just
"draping" over the ovary.

Cow: the broad ligament is attached along the pelvic inlet
instead of the dorsolateral body wall. The horns of the uterus coil
back on themselves, placing the ovaries just cranial to the brim

of the pelvis; much farther caudal than the other domestic
species.

7. Vaginal process: the evagination of the parietal and visceral
peritoneum through the inguinal canal (in the carnivores). It
contains the round ligament of the uterus.

CLINICAL:
• **Suspensory ligament of the ovary** (6): broken when
spaying a bitch to bring the ovary to the incision site.
• **Ovariohysterectomy** or **"spay"**: removal of the ovaries,
uterine tubes, and uterus (a small animal veterinarian's
"bread and butter"). A midline incision is made through the
linea alba (make it large, not a "key hole" incision). Find a
uterine horn. Pull this toward the incision. With a finger,
strum the suspensory ligament to break it down so the ovary
can be brought to the skin incision. Ligate the ovarian vessels
in the mesovarium. Follow the uterine horn back to the body
and up the other horn to find the other ovary. Ligate its
ovarian vessels. Break down the broad ligament back to the
uterine body. Clamp and ligate the uterine body and uterine
arteries together or separately. Sever the uterine body and
remove it, the horns, and ovaries. Close the animal.

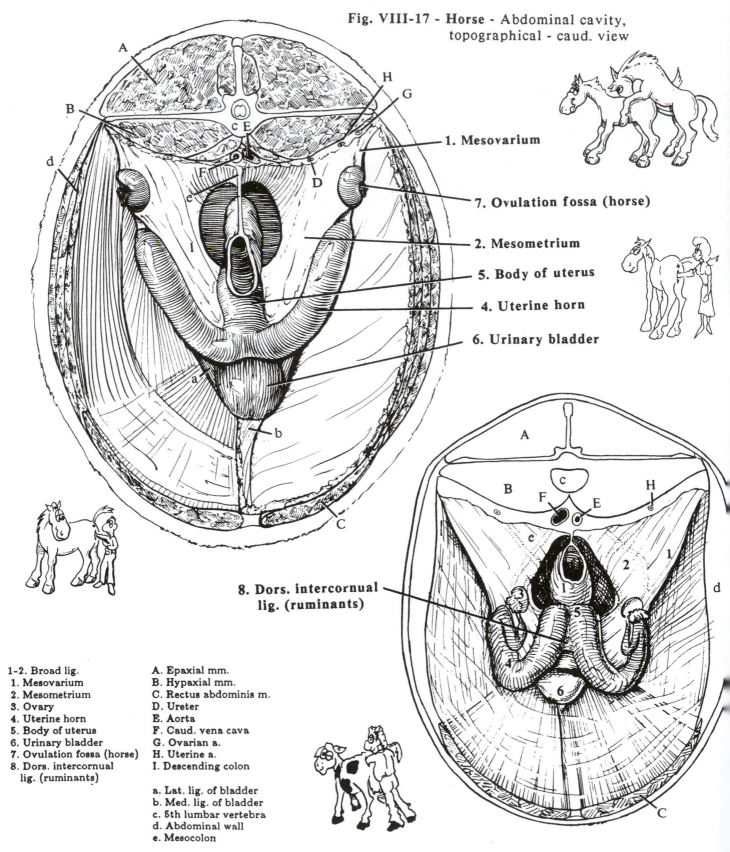

Fig. VIII-17 - Horse - Abdominal cavity, topographical - caud. view

1. Mesovarium

7. Ovulation fossa (horse)

2. Mesometrium

5. Body of uterus

4. Uterine horn

6. Urinary bladder

8. Dors. intercornual lig. (ruminants)

1-2. Broad lig.
1. Mesovarium
2. Mesometrium
3. Ovary
4. Uterine horn
5. Body of uterus
6. Urinary bladder
7. Ovulation fossa (horse)
8. Dors. intercornual lig. (ruminants)

A. Epaxial mm.
B. Hypaxial mm.
C. Rectus abdominis m.
D. Ureter
E. Aorta
F. Caud. vena cava
G. Ovarian a.
H. Uterine a.
I. Descending colon

a. Lat. lig. of bladder
b. Med. lig. of bladder
c. 5th lumbar vertebra
d. Abdominal wall
e. Mesocolon

Fig. VIII-18 - Cow - Abdominal cavity, topographical - caud. view

GENITAL ORGANS - COW

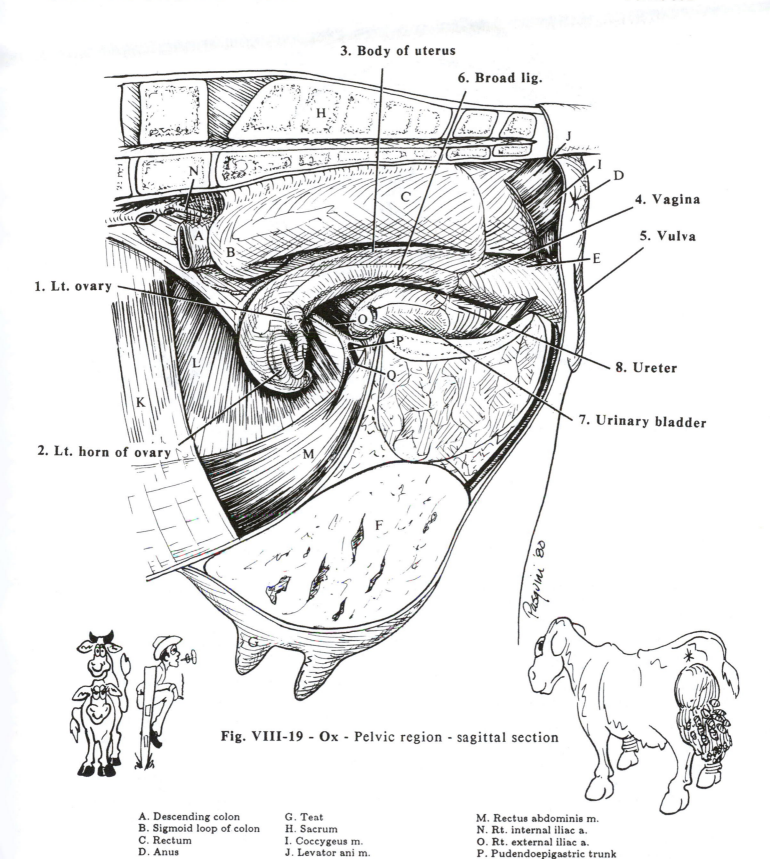

3. Body of uterus

6. Broad lig.

4. Vagina

5. Vulva

1. Lt. ovary

8. Ureter

2. Lt. horn of ovary

7. Urinary bladder

Fig. VIII-19 - Ox - Pelvic region - sagittal section

A. Descending colon
B. Sigmoid loop of colon
C. Rectum
D. Anus
E. Retroperitoneal area
F. Body of udder

G. Teat
H. Sacrum
I. Coccygeus m.
J. Levator ani m.
K. Transverse abdominal m.
L. Int. abdominal oblique m.

M. Rectus abdominis m.
N. Rt. internal iliac a.
O. Rt. external iliac a.
P. Pudendoepigastric trunk
Q. Ext. pudendal a.

EMBRYONIC MEMBRANES

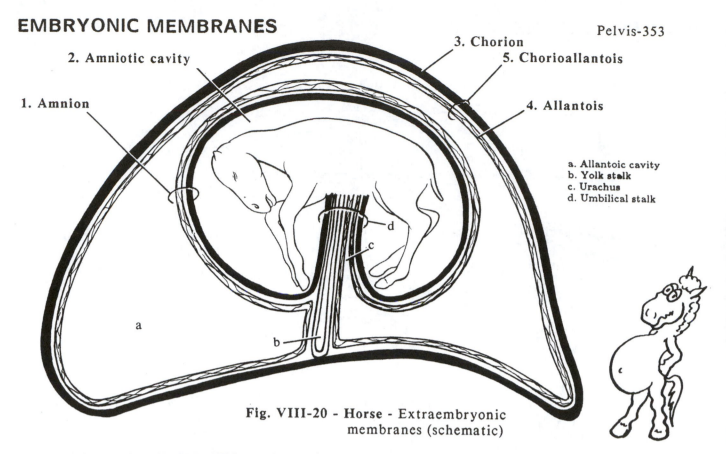

2. Amniotic cavity

3. Chorion

5. Chorioallantois

1. Amnion

4. Allantois

a. Allantoic cavity
b. Yolk stalk
c. Urachus
d. Umbilical stalk

Fig. VIII-20 - Horse - Extraembryonic
membranes (schematic)

EXTRAEMBRYONIC MEMBRANES: membranes formed around the embryo for protection and implantation in the maternal endometrium.

1. Amnion: the inner embryonic membrane surrounding the amnionic cavity and fetus.

2. Amniotic cavity: the cavity encompassed by the amnion and filled with amnionic fluid, providing the fluid environment that protects the fetus.

3. Chorion: the outer embryonic membrane surrounding the allantoic cavity, amnion, amniotic cavity, and fetus. This layer makes up the fetal component of the placenta.

4. Allantois: an evagination from the hindgut. This extraembryonic membrane lines the inside of the chorion, forming the chorioallantoic membrane. It also lines the outside of the amnion, forming the allantoamnion. This layer provides the vasculature to the two membranes (chorion and amnion) it lines.

5. Chorioallantois: the fused chorion and allantois.

PLACENTA: the structure formed by apposition of fetal and maternal tissue. It functions to exchange nutrients and oxygen from the mother to the fetus; and waste products from the fetus to the mother. It also has endocrine functions and forms a barrier between fetal and maternal blood.

Fetal Component: formed by the three layers of the chorioallantoic membrane, as follows:

6. Fetal endothelium: lines the allantoic blood vessels.

7. Fetal connective tissue of the chorioallantois: mesoderm surrounding the blood vessels.

8. Chorionic epithelium: the surface layer of the chorioallantoic membrane.

Maternal Component: consists of three layers of the endometrium (uterine mucosa), as follows:

9. Maternal epithelium of the endometrium (uterine lamina epithelialis).

10. Maternal connective tissue: surrounds the vessels of the endometrium.

11. Maternal endothelium: lines the vessels of the endometrium.

SPECIES DIFFERENCES:

A. Epitheliochorial placenta: has all six layers (three fetal and three maternal), seen in the horse, pig, and ruminants.

• **Adeciduate** (a=not, deciduus=falling off) **placenta**: the maternal component is not sloughed during birth (horse and pig).

• **Partially deciduate placenta**: part of the endometrium (maternal component) is sloughed off (ruminants).

B. Endotheliochorial placenta: found in the carnivores. The maternal epithelium and connective tissue layers are absent, the maternal endothelium being in direct contact with the chorionic epithelium.

• **Deciduate placenta**: found in carnivores, the maternal endometrium is lost during birth.

PLACENTAL TYPES

CLASSIFICATION of the PLACENTA: using shape and vascular arrangement of the apposition of maternal and fetal tissues.

12. Diffuse placenta: **horse** and **pig**; apposition over most of the chorioallantois by villi and microvilli evaginating into the endometrium.

13. Cotyledonary placenta or **placentomes:** found in ruminants where apposition is in discrete areas.

Placentome: the functional, discrete placental part consisting of a connected cotyledon and caruncle found in the <u>ruminants</u>. In the <u>cow</u> it is dome-shaped, in the <u>small ruminant</u> it has a dent in its top.

• **14. Cotyledon:** the **fetal component** of the placenta that forms villous processes that interdigitate with the maternal components.

• **15. Caruncles:** the maternal component consisting of discrete units scattered over the endometrium. They are proliferations of the connective tissue and are also found in non-pregnant animals.

16. Zonary placenta: found in <u>carnivores</u>, a broad band of apposition of maternal and fetal tissue around the transverse circumference of the chorioallantois.

A. EPITHELIOCHORIAL

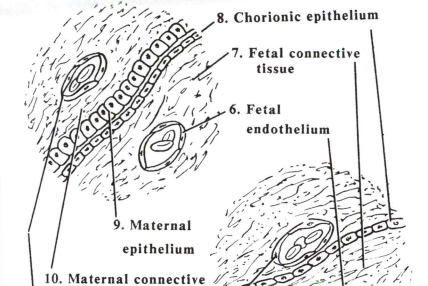

8. Chorionic epithelium
7. Fetal connective tissue
6. Fetal endothelium
9. Maternal epithelium
10. Maternal connective tissue
11. Maternal endothelium

B. ENDOTHELIOCHORIAL

Fig. VIII-21 - Placental components

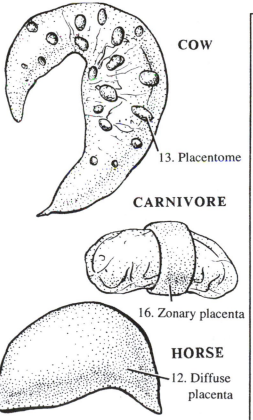

COW

13. Placentome

CARNIVORE

16. Zonary placenta

HORSE

12. Diffuse placenta

Fig. VIII-22 - Placentae

CLINICAL

Retained placenta: common in cattle and less of an emergency than in the mare.

Hydramnios and hydrallantois: excessive accumulation of fluid in amnionic and allantoic sacs; most common in cows, but still fairly rare.

Abortion: expulsion of dead or non-viable fetus.

Mummification: dehydration of a dead, retained fetus.

Hermaphrodites: have a genital tract that can't be easily distinguished as female or male.

Freemartinism: bovine female born co-twin to a male and having a defective genital tract.

Twinning in horses: disastrous to pregnancy, usually resulting in natural abortion.

Dystocia: difficult parturition.
• **Cattle:** common and a major cause of calf loss. Often requires assistance:
   - Mutation: manually correcting position of the fetus
   - Forced extraction
   - Cesarean section
   - Fetotomy: cutting fetus into pieces and removing the pieces.
• **Mare:** less common than in cattle, but a true emergency.
• **Bitch:** common in smaller breeds.

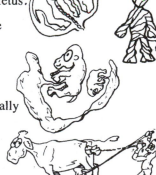

Pseudopregnancy: common in bitches; uncommon in queens

RECTAL PALPATION - COW

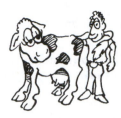

Determining the stage of estrus or pregnancy in cattle is economically very important to the cattleman. This can be done by systematic, gentle, and efficient rectal palpation. To orient yourself, once in the rectum, find the cervix. It is a firm cylinder that may be over the brim of the pelvis or completely in the abdomen, depending on the stage of pregnancy. Sweep your open hand over the brim of pelvis to locate it. Next, retract the uterus into the pelvic cavity of cows open (not pregnant) or less than 90 days pregnant. If over 90 days pregnant, this can't be done. To retract the uterus, move cranially to the cervix to the uterine horns and locate the intercornual ligaments. Grasp the ventral intercornual ligament and flip the uterine horns and ovaries into the pelvic cavity.

Palpate the entire length of the uterine horns for consistency. An empty horn will have a meaty consistency. A pregnant horn will be fluid filled with resiliency and fluctuation.

There are four criteria used to diagnose a positive pregnancy: 1. Palpable amnionic vesicle; 2. Slip of fetal membranes; 3. Palpable fetus and 4. Palpable placetomes.

Amnionic vessel: can be palpated from 30 to 65 days of gestation (after 65 days it is too large and soft to palpate). It is found in the most distended part of the horn with the thinnest wall. It should not be used routinely to diagnose pregnancy because this may cause abortion.

"Membrane slip": chorioallantoic membranes can be felt at 30 to 35 days post breeding (with practice). Grasp the horn with the thumb and finger and let it slip through. The membrane will pass through first, followed by the uterine wall. The membrane "slip" feels like a taut string slipping lengthwise between the finger and thumb.

Placetomes: small ones can be detected at 70 to 75 days. They increase in size as pregnancy continues. Do not mistake one for an ovary!

Fetus: fairly reliable indication of pregnancy! It can be palpated after 65 to 70 days.

Uterine (middle uterine) artery: can be palpated going to the gravid horn at 85 to 90 days of gestation. A "buzzing" sensation, fremitus, can be palpated at 90 to 120 days in the artery. The movable uterine artery travels in the broad ligament to the horns of the uterus. By rectal palpation, run your fingers from the abdominal cavity to the pelvic cavity along the lateral wall. The first artery encountered is the immovable external iliac artery coursing down the cranial edge of the shaft of the ilium. The next artery is the movable uterine artery.

Common errors in pregnancy diagnoses are mistaking the urinary bladder and the rumen for the uterus. Pregnancy diagnosis is important to cattlemen between 35 and 120 days after the bull has been taken away from the herd. If the cow is open (not pregnant), the cattlemen need to know when she will come into heat (estrus) again so she can be covered (bred). If the horns are empty (non-pregnant), palpate the ovaries to determine the stage of estrous.

Palpation of the ovaries and uterus: in conjunction with the chart, can tell the stage of estrous the animal is in. Thus, it can be estimated how long before the cow comes back into heat and will be ready to breed.

The ovaries are located on the ventrolateral margin of the pelvic inlet, just cranial to the external iliac artery. Pregnancy draws the ovaries forward. To palpate the ovaries they should be retracted by grasping the ventral intercornual ligament and flipping the horns and ovaries into the pelvic cavity.

F (Mature follicle): a spherical mass of cells containing a cavity and ovum (egg, female sexual cell). This is a soft, fluctuating structure that can be identified during rectal palpation.

OVD (Ovulation depression): the depression left in the mature follicle after ovulation, usually lasting 24 hours.

CH (Corpus hemorrhagicum): a ruptured follicle filled with blood. It is a soft, but not fluctuating, elevation on the ovary. Depending on its size, it is classified as a CHl (1 cm), CH2 (1-2 cm) or CH3 (larger than 2 cm).

CL (Corpus luteum): results when the blood in a corpus hemorrhagicum is replaced by cells that produce hormones (progesterone). It feels firm to hard and is classified, depending on size, into CL3 (greater than 2 cm and firm), CL2 (1-2 cm and firm) and CLl (1 cm and hard).

S (Static ovary): an ovary in which no follicle, corpus hemorrhagicum or corpus luteum can be felt.

Uterus: palpating the uterus can also indicate the stage of estrus and should be correlated to what is found on the ovaries.

UN - uterus normal
UT - uterus turgid
UE - uterus edematous

Abbreviations used are: **F**, follicle; **OVD**, ovulation depression, **CHl**, corpus hemorrhagicum 1 cm. in diameter (soft); **CH2**, 1-2 cm (soft); **CH3**, 2 cm. (soft) **CL3**, corpus luteum (fully developed); **CL2**, 1-2 cm. (firm); **CL3**, 1 cm. (hard); **S**, static; **UT**, uterus turgid; **UE**, uterus edematous; **UN**, uterus normal.

Chart from R. Zemjanis, "Diagnostic and Therapeutic Techniques in Animal Reproduction" 2nd ed. 1970, Williams & Wilkins-Baltimore

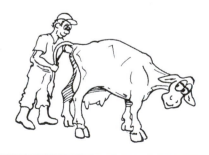

OVARIES & ESTRUS

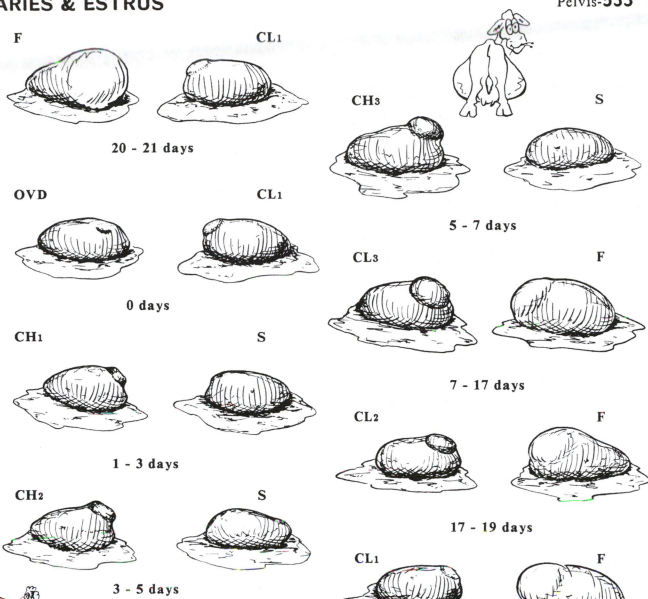

F   CL₁

20 - 21 days

OVD   CL₁

0 days

CH₁   S

1 - 3 days

CH₂   S

3 - 5 days

CH₃   S

5 - 7 days

CL₃   F

7 - 17 days

CL₂   F

17 - 19 days

CL₁   F

20 - 21 days

| Findings in ovaries & uterus | | | Approximate | Days to |
Right ovary	Left ovary	Uterus	estrus cycle	predict estrus
F	CL₁	UT	20 - 21	0
OVD	CL₁	UT	O	18 - 21
CHl	S	UT	1 - 3	19 - 20
CH₂	S	UE	3 - 5	15 - 18
CH₃	S	UN	5 - 7	13 - 17
CL₃	F	UN	7 - 17	6 - 11
CL₂	F	UT	17 - 19	1 - 4
CL₁	F	UT	20 - 21	0 - 1

TESTIS

F. Efferent duct

5. Deferent duct

B. Mediastinum testis

A. Tunica albuginea

G. Epididymal duct

C. Lobules

b

D. Seminiferous
tubules

E. Rete testis

2. Epididymis

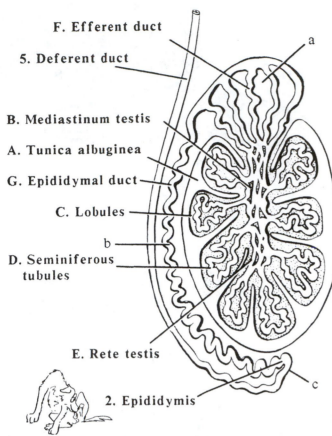

Fig. VIII-20 - Dog - Testicle, epididymis
& deferent duct (schematic)

1. TESTICLE or **TESTIS** (TES-tis) (pl.= testes): the male gonad that produces both testosterone (male sex hormone) and spermatogonia, the male germ cell that differentiates into sperm. The testicles are contained in the scrotum and vary considerably in shape and size among the species.

A. White tunic or **tunica albuginea**: the strong, white, fibrous capsule enveloping the testicle.

B. Mediastinum testis: the cord of fibrous tissue running through the middle of the testicle, containing the rete testis. Septa, webs of connective tissue, radiate from the mediastinum to the tunica albuginea, dividing the testicle into numerous lobules.

C. Lobules: the units of the testicle, each contains a few seminiferous tubules.

D. Seminiferous tubules (sem'i-NI-fer-us TOO-byools): the hollow structures in which germ cells differentiate to spermatozoa. The major part of the tubules are the convoluted seminiferous tubules, where sperm production occurs. The straight seminiferous tubules are the short, straight part near the mediastinum. They do not produce sperm.

E. Rete (REE-tee) **testis**: the network of irregular, interconnecting channels continuing as the straight seminiferous tubules through the mediastinum to the efferent ductules.

F. Efferent ductules: the 8-15 channels leading into the head of the epididymis; they unite to form the epididymal duct.

G. EPIDIDYMAL DUCT (ductus epididymidis): the continuous, coiled channel forming the epididymis between the efferent ductules and the deferent duct.

2. EPIDIDYMIS (Ep'i-DID-i-mis): the structure adjacent to the testicle formed by the epididymal duct. The **head** (a) of the epididymis, consists of the efferent ductules and the first part of the epididymal duct. The **body** (b), the central part, consists of the highly coiled epididymal duct connecting the head and tail of the epididymis. The **tail** (c), the bulbous end of the epididymis, continues on as the ductus deferens. Spermatozoa mature in the head and body of the epididymis and are then transferred to the deferent duct as fertile sperm.

3. PROPER LIGAMENT OF THE TESTICLE: connects the tail of the epididymis to the testicle.

4. SCROTAL LIGAMENT and **LIGAMENT OF THE TAIL OF THE EPIDIDYMIS**: connects the tail of the epididymis to the scrotum. They are divided by the visceral vaginal tunic (pg. 362), into the part outside the tunic, the scrotal ligament; and the part inside the vaginal tunic, the ligament of the tail of the epididymis.

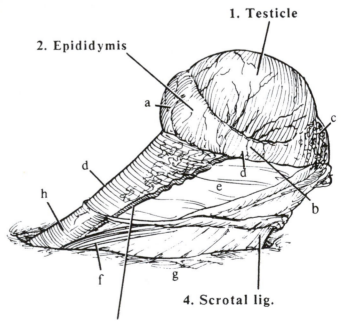

1. Testicle

2. Epididymis

4. Scrotal lig.

5. Deferent duct

Fig. VIII-21 - Dog - Testicle

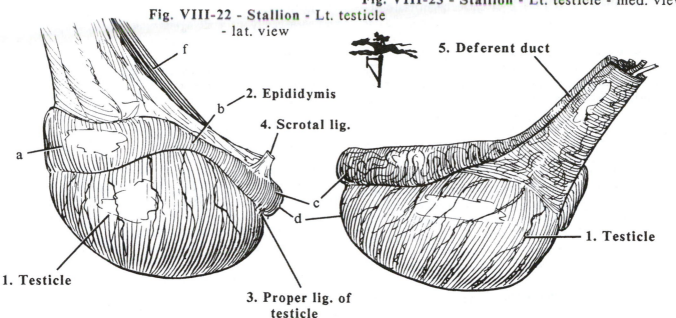

Fig. VIII-22 - Stallion - Lt. testicle - lat. view

f

2. Epididymis

b

4. Scrotal lig.

a

c

d

1. Testicle

1. Testicle

3. Proper lig. of testicle

Fig. VIII-23 - Stallion - Lt. testicle - med. view

5. Deferent duct

1. Testicle

5. DUCTUS DEFERENS, deferent (DEF-er-ent) duct (d) or "vas deferens": the continuation of the epididymal duct at the tail of the epididymis. It travels beside the body of the epididymis, up the spermatic cord, and through the inguinal canal to reach the abdomen. In the abdomen, it arches caudally to the pelvic cavity passing through the prostate gland to open into the pelvic urethra.

•**Ampulla (am-PYOOL-a)**: the enlarged terminal end of the ductus deferens, absent in the <u>boar</u> and <u>tomcat</u>. Its wall is very glandular, causing an increase in the diameter of the duct, but not in the diameter of the lumen.

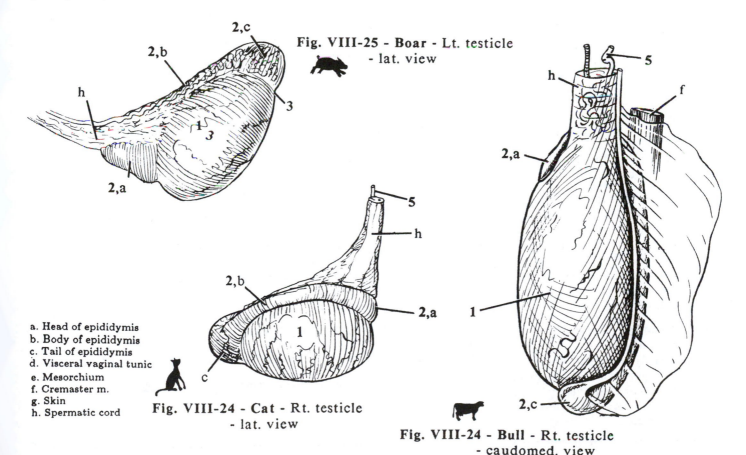

Fig. VIII-25 - Boar - Lt. testicle - lat. view

2,c

2,b

h

2,a

3

1

3

5

h

f

2,a

1

2,c

Fig. VIII-24 - Bull - Rt. testicle - caudomed. view

2,b

2,a

5

h

1

c

a. Head of epididymis
b. Body of epididymis
c. Tail of epididymis
d. Visceral vaginal tunic
e. Mesorchium
f. Cremaster m.
g. Skin
h. Spermatic cord

Fig. VIII-24 - Cat - Rt. testicle - lat. view

DESCENT OF THE TESTICLES

DESCENT of the TESTICLES: The testicles begin fetal development within the abdomen behind the kidneys. The epididymis and deferent duct connect the testicle caudally to the urethra. The gubernaculum, a jelly-like cord, extends from the testicle to the tail of the epididymis and then into the inguinal canal. The testicle, the epididymis, and the ductus deferens develop retroperitoneal-ly, between the peritoneum and the body wall. They are thus, covered by visceral peritoneum, that is continuous with the parietal peritoneum. During development, the knoblike, free end of the gubernaculum, covered with visceral and parietal peritoneum, lies through the inguinal canal of the developing abdominal wall. The testicle and epididymis move caudally, following the gubernaculum through the inguinal canal and into the scrotum. Moving through the inguinal canal, the testicles carry their vis-ceral peritoneum. They also pick up the parietal peritoneum and the fascial layers of the inner and outer abdominal wall. Once out-side the abdominal cavity, the two peritoneal layers become known as the vaginal tunic (vaginal process). The gubernaculum shrinks to become the proper ligament of the testicle, the ligament of the tail of the epididymis, and the scrotal ligament.

Time of descent of the testicles:
- **Ruminants** and **pig**: before birth.
- **Carnivores**: shortly after birth.
- **Horse**: 10-14 days before or after birth.

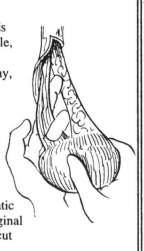

CLINICAL

Inguinal hernia: the protrusion of a loop of organ or tissue through the inguinal canal. Common and hereditary in the **horse** and **pig**, affected animals should not be used for breeding and preferably castrated.

- **Direct inguinal hernia**: when herniated tissue explodes directly through the wall of the abdomen, without bothering to weave down the inguinal canal.

- **Indirect inguinal hernia**: when herniated tissue passes down the inguinal canal.

Castration: the removal of the gonads – testicles (and epididymis) in the male, ovaries in the female. The uterus is usually removed with the ovaries (spay, ovariohysterectomy). "Closed" and "open" castration refer to whether the peritoneal cavity has or has not been opened.

- **"Open technique"**: opens the vaginal cavity and thus, the peritoneal cavity by cutting through the parietal vaginal tunic. The spermatic cord, covered only by the visceral vaginal tunic, is ligated and then the cord is cut distal to the ligation.

- **"Closed technique"**: a castration that does <u>not</u> open the peritoneal cavity (parietal vaginal tunic cut AFTER the spermatic cord is ligated proximally). The parietal and visceral vaginal tunics and the spermatic cord are ligated closing the vaginal cavity proximally. The cord is then transected distal to the ligature, therefore, the peritoneal cavity is never opened.

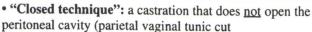

Emasculator: an instrument used in castration of large animals. It has two closely connected parts; one crushes the vessels and spermatic cord and the other, at the same time, cuts the cord distally to the crush. *Memory Aid*: The emasculator's nut and cutting part are on the same side. The saying "nut to nut" when using an emasculator insures the cut will be distal to the crush.

Castration of a calf: "closed technique" at 1-8 weeks of age. The bottom of the scrotum is cut off and the tunic-covered testicles pulled distally. The parietal vaginal tunic is left closed as an emasculator crushes and cuts the spermatic cord.

Castration of a piglet: "open technique" in the first 3 weeks of life. With the piglet held up by its hocks, each testicle is pushed cranially and the skin over it incised. The testicle is pulled through the incision and the scrotal ligament broken. Maintaining traction on the testicle, the tunic-covered cord is scraped until it breaks (thus, opening the vaginal cavity) with a sterile scalpel.

Castration of the cat: "open technique" after 6 months of age. The plucked scrotum is incised over each tunic-covered testicle to free it from the scrotum. Each testicle, inside the unopened vaginal tunic, may be pulled until the cord tears away, opening the tunic ("pull technique"). (For those new veterinarians that don't want to be forced to use this technique by their first employer, develop speed in some other technique.) Alternative opened technique: the parietal vaginal tunic may be incised and the spermatic vessels and deferent duct tied together. Closed technique: all the structures of the cord may be ligated first and then the cord severed distal to ligation.

Castration of the dog: "open or closed technique" after 6 months of age. The testicle is pushed cranially and the skin over it incised. Each testicle is pushed through this incision. The spermatic cord can then be ligated ("closed"). To do an "open" castration, the parietal vaginal tunic is cut and moved proximally off the cord. The mesorchium is then broken; the structures of the cord ligated and severed.

CASTRATION INCISIONS

- **Two scrotal incisions** are used in <u>horses</u>, <u>cats</u> and <u>older pigs</u>.

- **One prescrotal incision** is used in the <u>dog</u>.

- **Amputation of the distal scrotum** or two scrotal incisions are used in the <u>ruminants</u>.

DESCENT OF THE TESTICLES

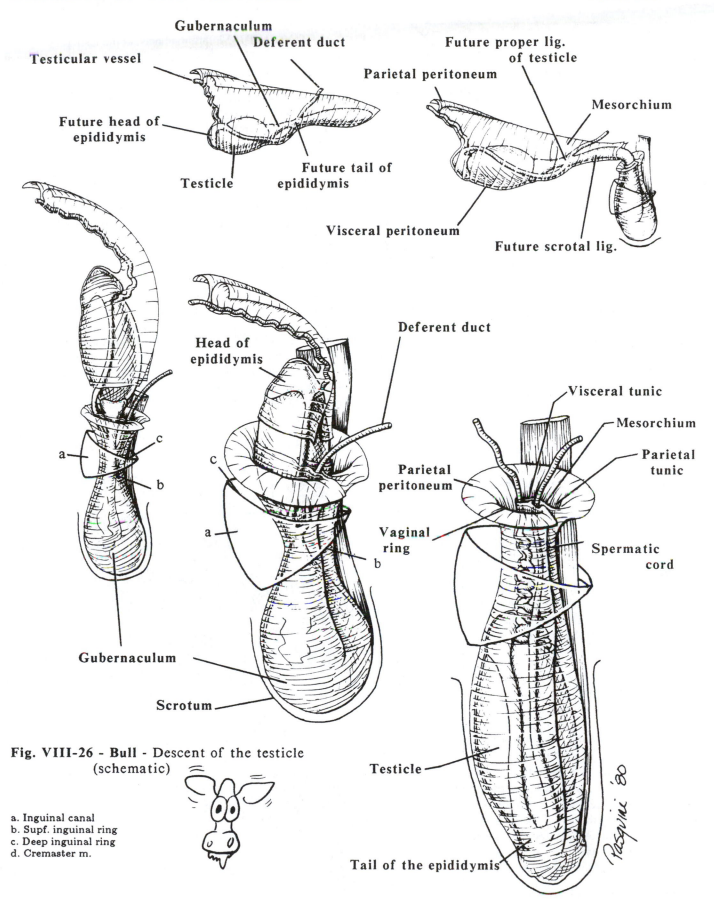

Gubernaculum

Deferent duct

Testicular vessel

Future proper lig. of testicle

Parietal peritoneum

Mesorchium

Future head of epididymis

Testicle

Future tail of epididymis

Visceral peritoneum

Future scrotal lig.

Head of epididymis

Deferent duct

Visceral tunic

Mesorchium

Parietal tunic

Parietal peritoneum

Vaginal ring

Spermatic cord

Gubernaculum

Scrotum

Testicle

Tail of the epididymis

Fig. VIII-26 - Bull - Descent of the testicle (schematic)

a. Inguinal canal
b. Supf. inguinal ring
c. Deep inguinal ring
d. Cremaster m.

CRYPTORCHIDISM

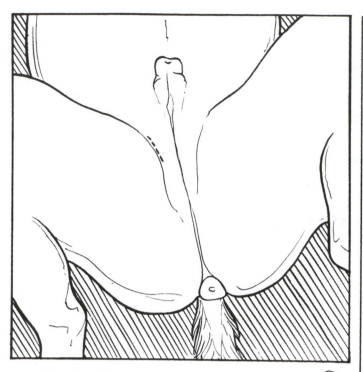

Fig. VIII-27 - Horse, inguinal incision site

CRYPTORCHIDISM: failure of one or both testicles to descend into the scrotum. The retained testicle can be anywhere between the scrotum and the caudal pole of the kidney.

Stallion: cryptorchidism is often called "ridglings"," originals" or "rigs" in the horse.
• **Inguinal cryptorchid**: the most common, has an undeveloped testicle in the canal or just outside the superficial inguinal ring ("high flanker").
• **Descended epididymis**: when the tail of the epididymis and the ductus deferens are located in the inguinal canal and the testicle is in the abdomen, just inside the vaginal ring.
• **Complete abdominal cryptorchid:** when the testicle and the epididymis lie within the abdominal cavity.

The undescended testicle should be removed. As abdominal surgery should be avoided whenever possible in the horse, the best approach is through the skin over the inguinal canal. Palpation of the inguinal region or rectal palpation may locate the cryptorchid. In an inguinal cryptorchid, incise over the inguinal canal, locate and remove the testicle. A descended epididymis can also be found by this approach. Once found it can be used to pull the testicle out. With a complete abdominal cryptorchid, try to find the gubernaculum and follow this through the inguinal canal to the tail of the epididymis and the testicle.

HORSE CASTRATION: usually done between 1 and 2 years of age. Both the "opened" and closed" techniques employ two separate incisions in the scrotum.

"Open technique": pull each testicle through its scrotal incision. Incise the parietal vaginal tunic opening the vaginal cavity and thus the peritoneal cavity. With an emasculator crush the ductus deferens, cremaster muscle, and parietal vaginal tunic. Then crush the spermatic vessels. Enlarge the scrotal skin incisions for drainage.

"Closed technique": should be done in a sterile environment. Pull the tunic-covered testicles through the scrotal incisions. Place a suture knot in the cremaster muscle then bring the suture material around the cord and tie tightly (closing the vaginal tunic proximally). Transect the cord distal to the ligature. Enlarge the scrotal skin incisions for drainage. The ligature is a possible nidus for infection and is why this should be done in a sterile environment. An emasculator is not used in the closed technique for fear of the testicular artery slipping out of the crushed tissue.

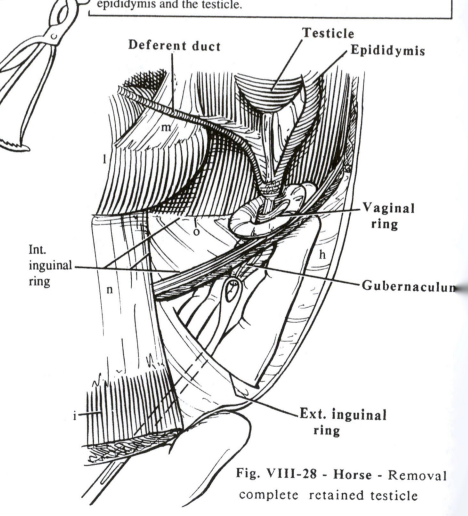

Fig. VIII-28 - Horse - Removal complete retained testicle

Fig. VIII-29 - Horse - Caud. abdomen - cross section

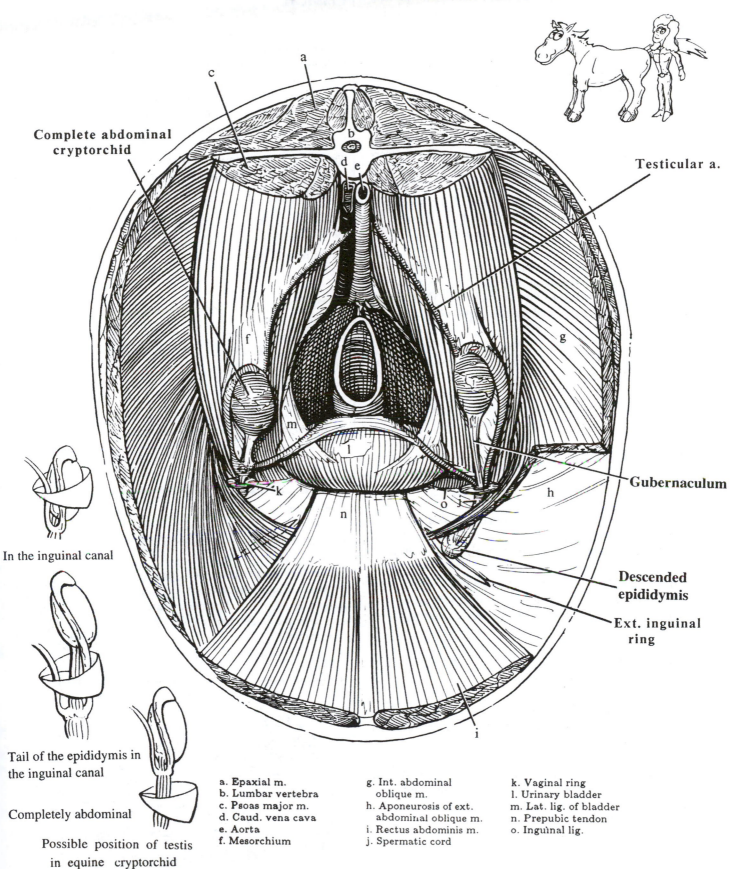

Complete abdominal
cryptorchid

Testicular a.

Gubernaculum

Descended
epididymis

Ext. inguinal
ring

In the inguinal canal

Tail of the epididymis in
the inguinal canal

Completely abdominal

Possible position of testis
in equine cryptorchid

a. Epaxial m.
b. Lumbar vertebra
c. Psoas major m.
d. Caud. vena cava
e. Aorta
f. Mesorchium

g. Int. abdominal
   oblique m.
h. Aponeurosis of ext.
   abdominal oblique m.
i. Rectus abdominis m.
j. Spermatic cord

k. Vaginal ring
l. Urinary bladder
m. Lat. lig. of bladder
n. Prepubic tendon
o. Inguinal lig.

361

SPERMATIC CORD

SPERMATIC CORD: the structure extending from the testicle through the inguinal canal; consisting of the ductus deferens, the testicular vessels and nerves, and the lymphatics and their serous coverings.

Vaginal tunic: the double wall of serous membrane (visceral and parietal) around the spermatic cord and testicle in the male and the round ligament of the uterus in the female.

1. Visceral vaginal tunic: the continuation of the abdominal visceral peritoneum tightly investing the structures of the spermatic cord and the testicle.

2. Parietal vaginal tunic: the continuation of the abdominal parietal peritoneum through the inguinal canal. It surrounds the visceral vaginal tunic-covered spermatic cord and testicle.

3. Mesorchium or **connecting vaginal tunic**: the serosal fold connecting the visceral vaginal tunic with the parietal vaginal tunic. It is similar to the connecting serosa between the parietal peritoneum lining the abdominal walls and the visceral peritoneum covering the gut.

• **Mesoductus**: the fold of connecting vaginal tunic between the mesorchium and the ductus deferens.

• **Mesofuniculus**: the part of the mesorchium between the parietal vaginal tunic and where the mesoductus arises.

4. Vaginal cavity: the potential space between the two vaginal tunic layers. It is continuous with the peritoneal cavity at the vaginal ring.

5. Vaginal ring: the crescent-shaped opening located on the abdominal side of the deep inguinal ring. It is formed by the evagination of the parietal peritoneum through the inguinal canal.

6. Pampiniform plexus: the coils of the testicular veins around the testicular artery, making up the bulk of the spermatic cord. It functions to draw heat from the testicular artery, cooling the blood before it reaches the testicle.

7. Testicular artery: the convoluted artery supplying the testicle and arising from the abdominal aorta.

8. Spermatic fascia: the inner and outer abdominal fascia that, along with the peritoneum, invest the testicle as it passes through the inguinal canal.

Uterus masculinus: the remnant of the paramesonephric duct. It is usually present between the layers of the genital fold and between the ampulla of the ductus deferens in the horse. It is also often found in the bull.

CLINICAL

Each ductus deferens loops dorsally over the ureter. This makes it possible to dislodge the ureters when using the "pull technique" to neuter a tomcat.

Varicocele: abnormally distended and tortuous veins of the pampiniform plexus (appears like a bag of worms).

Torsion of the spermatic cord: excessively long mesorchium predisposes twisting during a horse race.

Orchitis: inflammation of the testicle.

Testicular tumors:
• Older dogs - common
• Older bulls - occurs
• Other species - rare

Epididymitis: inflammation of the epididymis.

Spermatocele: local distention of the epididymis with sperm due to occlusion.

Seminal vesiculitis: inflammation of the seminal vesicle.

Testicular degeneration: due to heat injury resulting from cryptorchid, ectopic testes, inguinal hernias, systemic disease or prolonged high environmental temperature.

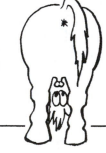

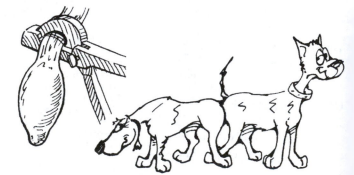

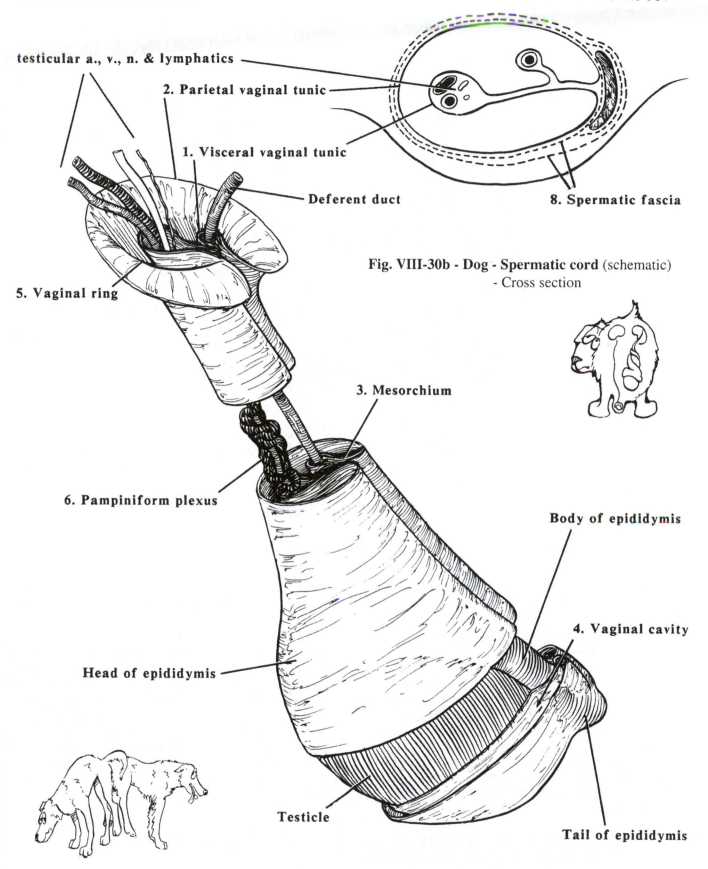

testicular a., v., n. & lymphatics

2. Parietal vaginal tunic

1. Visceral vaginal tunic

Deferent duct

8. Spermatic fascia

Fig. VIII-30b - Dog - Spermatic cord (schematic) - Cross section

5. Vaginal ring

3. Mesorchium

6. Pampiniform plexus

Body of epididymis

4. Vaginal cavity

Head of epididymis

Testicle

Tail of epididymis

Fig. VIII-30a - Dog - Schematic of vaginal tunic

Fig. VIII-31 - Dog - Pelvic cavity, sacrum removed
- Dorsal view

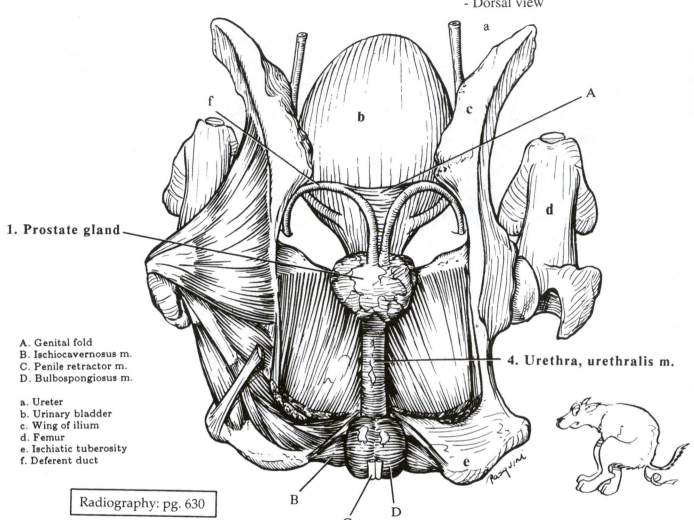

1. **Prostate gland**

A. Genital fold
B. Ischiocavernosus m.
C. Penile retractor m.
D. Bulbospongiosus m.

a. Ureter
b. Urinary bladder
c. Wing of ilium
d. Femur
e. Ischiatic tuberosity
f. Deferent duct

4. **Urethra, urethralis m.**

Radiography: pg. 630

ACCESSORY SEX GLANDS: the glands associated with the urethra that add the liquid portion to the ejaculate. They differ among the species and consist of the prostate, vesicular, and bulbourethral glands. Some consider the ampullae of the deferent ducts an accessory sex gland.

1. Prostate gland (PROS-tayt): adds prostatic secretions to the ejaculate to provide an optimum environment for sperm survival and motility. Present in some form in all the domestic species, it may consist of a visible body, surrounding the neck of the bladder; a disseminate part, consisting of lobules in the wall of the pelvic urethra; or both. The ductus deferens run through the gland to open into a papilla, the colliculus seminalis, in the dorsal part of the pelvic urethra. The prostatic ducts open into the entire length of the pelvic urethra.

2. Vesicular glands: the paired structures located dorsolateral to the neck of the bladder. They are present in the stallion, ruminant, and boar. They secrete an alkaline fluid rich in fructose into the urethra.

3. Bulbourethral ("Cowper's") glands: the paired glands on the dorsocaudal aspect of the pelvic proximal urethra near the bulb of the penis.

MALE URETHRA: the common passageway for sperm and urine extending from the bladder to the external urethral orifice. The pelvic part extends from the neck of the bladder to the pelvic outlet; its cranial portion (prostatic urethra) travels through the prostate, while the urethralis muscle encloses the rest. The **penile** or **cavernous part** (pars spongiosa) begins where the urethra enters the bulb of the spongy body (corpus spongiosum). The spongy body (corpus spongiosum) encircles the urethra to its external opening. The <u>colliculus seminalis</u> is a mound projecting from the dorsal part of the prostatic part of the urethra.

4. Urethral muscle (m. urethralis): the skeletal muscle enclosing the distal part of the pelvic urethra.

External urethral opening: the opening to the outside of the body, located at the tip of the penis.

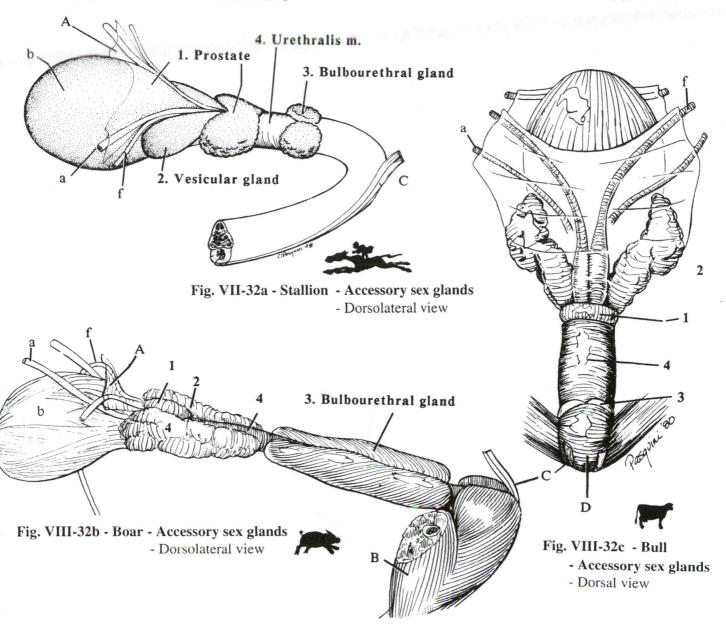

Fig. VII-32a - Stallion - Accessory sex glands
- Dorsolateral view

4. Urethralis m.

1. Prostate

3. Bulbourethral gland

2. Vesicular gland

Fig. VIII-32b - Boar - Accessory sex glands
- Dorsolateral view

3. Bulbourethral gland

Fig. VIII-32c - Bull
- Accessory sex glands
- Dorsal view

SPECIES DIFFERENCES

Stallion, ruminants and **boar**: have all three accessory sex glands.

Dog: has only a prostate gland. It has two lobes completely surrounding the urethra.

Tom cat: has prostate and bulbourethral glands, but no vesicular gland. The prostate does not completely surround the urethra ventrally.

Small ruminants: lack a prostatic body, having only a disseminate part, which can not be seen grossly.

Boar: its bulbourethra are two large cylinders extending cranially along the pelvic urethra covered by bulboglandularis muscle.

Horse: its vesicular gland has a lumen, therefore, is often called the **seminal vesicle**. The prostate does not contain a disseminate part; it has two lobes connected by an isthmus.

Seminal vesicle: the name of the vesicular gland in the **horse** because it has a lumen.

Common excretory duct: the duct of the ductus deferens and the vesicular gland in the horse, ruminant, and possibly the boar, which opens on the colliculus seminalis.

CLINICAL

Inflammation or **hyperplasia of the prostate**: infection or increased growth of the prostate, occuring mainly in dogs.

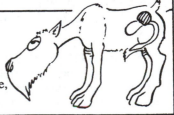

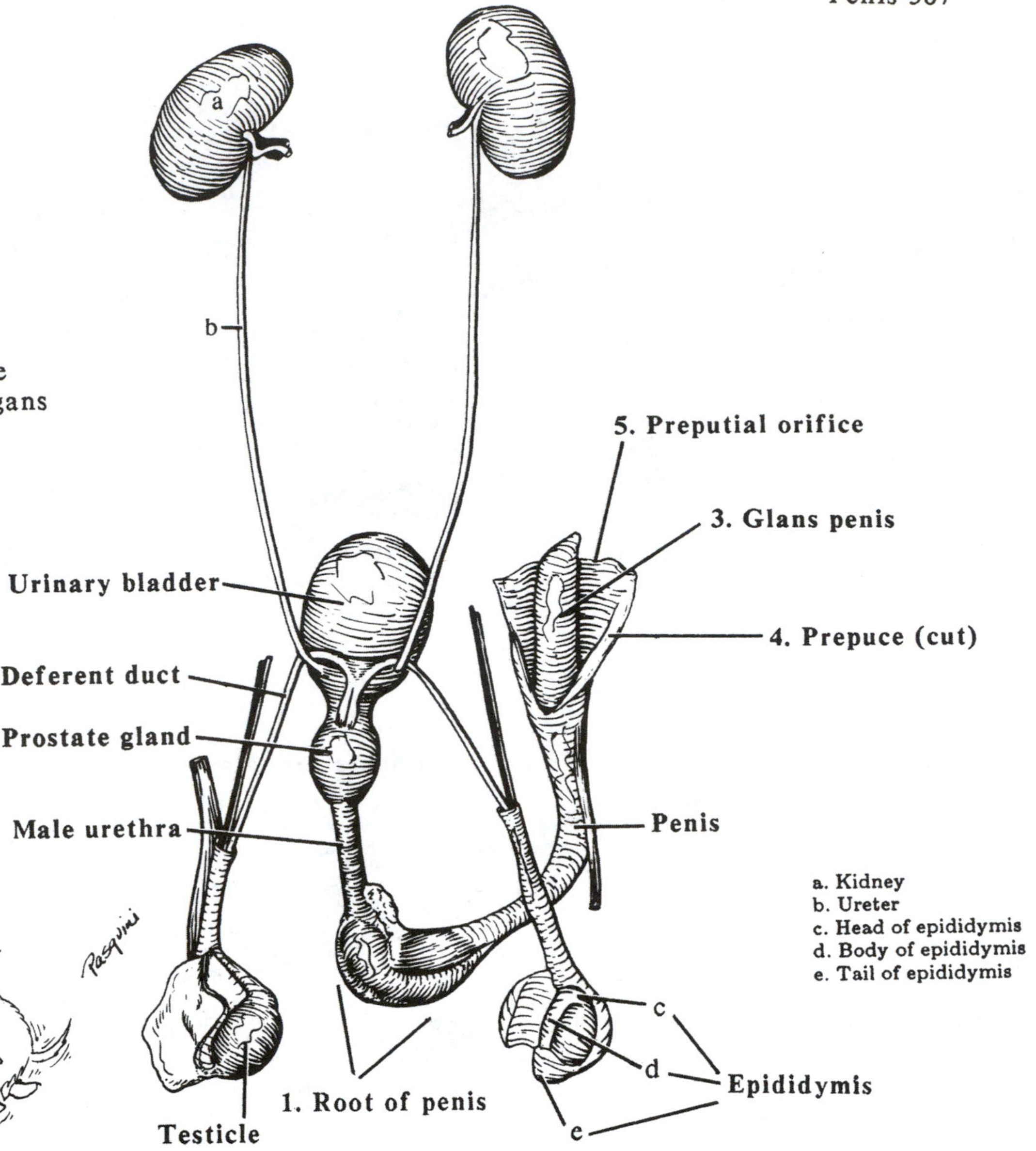

PENIS

Fig. VIII-33 - Dog - Male genital organs

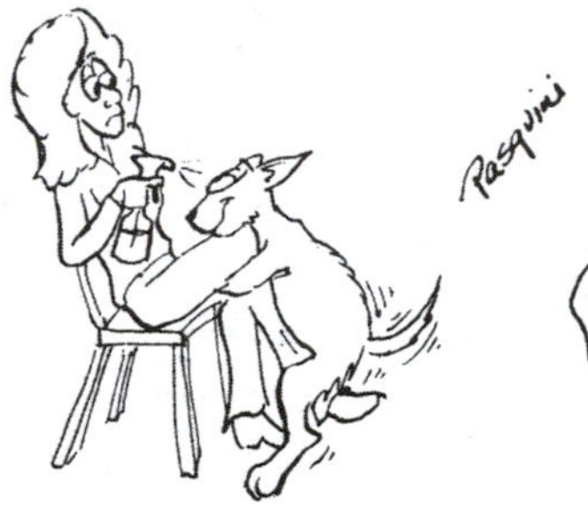

5. Preputial orifice

3. Glans penis

4. Prepuce (cut)

Urinary bladder

Deferent duct

Prostate gland

Male urethra

Penis

a. Kidney
b. Ureter
c. Head of epididymis
d. Body of epididymis
e. Tail of epididymis

c
d
Epididymis
e

1. Root of penis

Testicle

PENIS (L. tail): the male copulatory organ, extending from the ischiatic arch cranially (except in the cat) between the thighs. The penis provides a passageway for semen and urine to the outside of the body, thus, is a part of both the urinary and genital systems.

1. Root: the proximal part of the penis attaching to the ischial arch. The root consists of the bulb of the penis and crura of the penis.

2. Body: the main part of the penis between the root and the glans.

3. Glans: the distal free part of the penis.

CLASSIFICATION: penises are classified according to their connective tissue content into fibroelastic and musculocavernous types.

FIBROELASTIC PENIS: characteristic of **ruminants** and the **boar**. The large connective tissue content causes them to be firm even when they are not erect. Erection is characterized by greatly increasing the length (straightening of the sigmoid flexure) and

stiffening from engorgement with blood, without an increase in diameter.

MUSCULOCAVERNOUS PENIS: characteristic of **carnivores** and the **horse**. The low connective tissue content causes them to be flaccid when not erect. Erection is accomplished by engorgement of erectile tissue with blood, increasing the length and the diameter of the penis, while stiffening it.

4. PREPUCE (PREE-pyoos) (L. *preputuim* foreskin): the cutaneous sheath around the free part of the penis in the quiescent state (nonerect). It has an inner lamina continuous with the skin over the glans penis. Its outer lamina is continuous with the skin on the abdomen.

5. Preputial orifice: the external opening of the prepuce to the outside environment.

Preputial cavity: the space between the prepuce and the glans of the penis in the nonerect state.

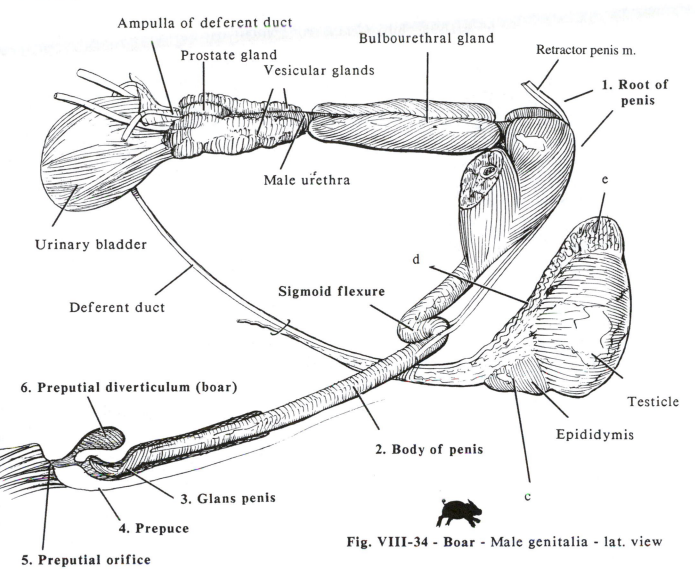

Ampulla of deferent duct

Prostate gland

Vesicular glands

Bulbourethral gland

Retractor penis m.

1. Root of penis

e

Male urethra

d

Urinary bladder

Sigmoid flexure

Deferent duct

Testicle

Epididymis

6. Preputial diverticulum (boar)

2. Body of penis

c

3. Glans penis

4. Prepuce

Fig. VIII-34 - Boar - Male genitalia - lat. view

5. Preputial orifice

Radiography: pg. 630

SPECIES DIFFERENCES

Tom cat's penis: directed caudoventrally when not erect. All the other species are directed cranioventrally. Upon erection it faces cranioventrally like the rest.

Os penis (baculum): the bone found in the penises of **carnivores**. (The os penis of coyotes is sometimes called the "prospector's toothpick"!) In the dog (not the cat) its ventral surface is grooved for the urethra.

6. Preputial diverticulum: a blind pocket in the dorsal wall of the **boar's** prepuce. It is partially divided midsagittally by a septum. Trapped material in this diverticulum gives the boar its characteristic odor.

Horse's prepuce: because of the great length attained on erection of the penis, the prepuce needs to be proportionately long or it would tear from the body whenever the horse gets "excited". Instead of having a long prepuce that would drag the ground, it has an extra fold inside the first.

• **External fold of the prepuce**: corresponds to the prepuce of other animals.

• **External preputial opening**: cranial edge of the external prepuce.

• **Preputial fold** (pg. 378): the second fold of the prepuce inside the preputial sheath of the horse.

• **Preputial ring** (pg. 378,f): the cranial edge of the preputial fold of the horse.

7. Sigmoid flexure: the double curve found in the penis of the ruminant and boar. The straightening of the sigmoid flexure causes the lengthening of the penis during erection.

PENIS

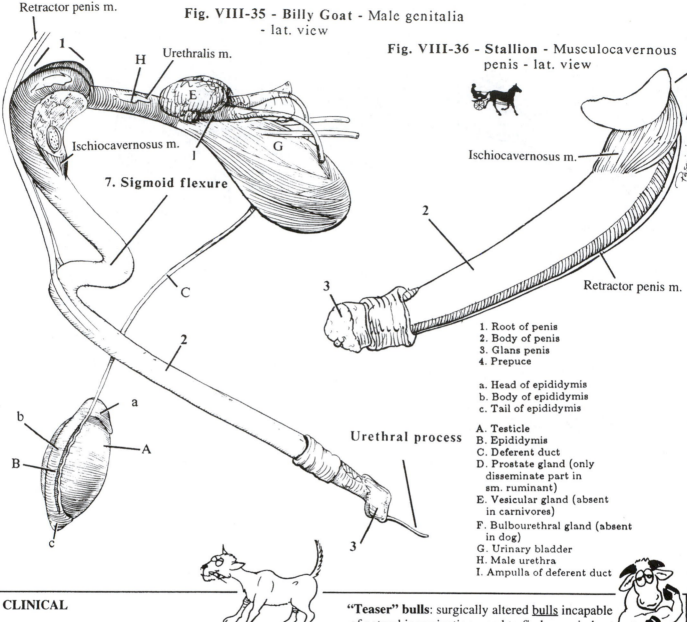

Fig. VIII-35 - Billy Goat - Male genitalia
- lat. view

Retractor penis m.

Urethralis m.

Ischiocavernosus m.

7. Sigmoid flexure

Fig. VIII-36 - Stallion - Musculocavernous
penis - lat. view

Ischiocavernosus m.

Retractor penis m.

Urethral process

1. Root of penis
2. Body of penis
3. Glans penis
4. Prepuce

a. Head of epididymis
b. Body of epididymis
c. Tail of epididymis

A. Testicle
B. Epididymis
C. Deferent duct
D. Prostate gland (only
   disseminate part in
   sm. ruminant)
E. Vesicular gland (absent
   in carnivores)
F. Bulbourethral gland (absent
   in dog)
G. Urinary bladder
H. Male urethra
I. Ampulla of deferent duct

CLINICAL

Urethral calculus (sin. = calculi): a
concretion obstructing the urethra.
The tomcat has a high incidence of urethral obstruction (FUS).
In the dog calculi usually lodge just proximal to the os penis; in
the ox, in the distal part of the sigmoid flexure; in the sheep, in
the sigmoid flexure or the urethral process.

FUS, feline urolithiasis, "plugged-tomcat" syndrome: common in male cats. The tomcat must be unplugged manually or
it may require a catheter. In severe cases cystocentesis (needle
aspiration of urine from the urinary bladder) may be required.

"Broken penis" or hematomas of the penis:
due to trauma causing a "explosion" of
the corpus cavernosum through the tunica
albuginea. It can occur in bulls (rarely in
stallions) during mating or semen collection.

"Teaser" bulls: surgically altered bulls incapable
of natural insemination, used to find cows in heat
(estrus) for artificial insemination (A.I.).

Inability to "extend the penis": the inability to protrude the
penis from the prepuce. This is due to several causes - phimosis,
persistent frenulum, congenital short penis, adhesions and
keratomas.

Persistent frenulum: a fold of tissue which joins the prepuce
and the glans and which should normally break down. It can be
transected so the penis can be extended.

Paralysis of the penis: the inability to
retract the penis into the prepuce. This
is due to several causes. Some
tranquilizers have been reported to cause
paralysis of the penis in the stallion.

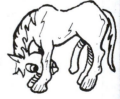

PENIS

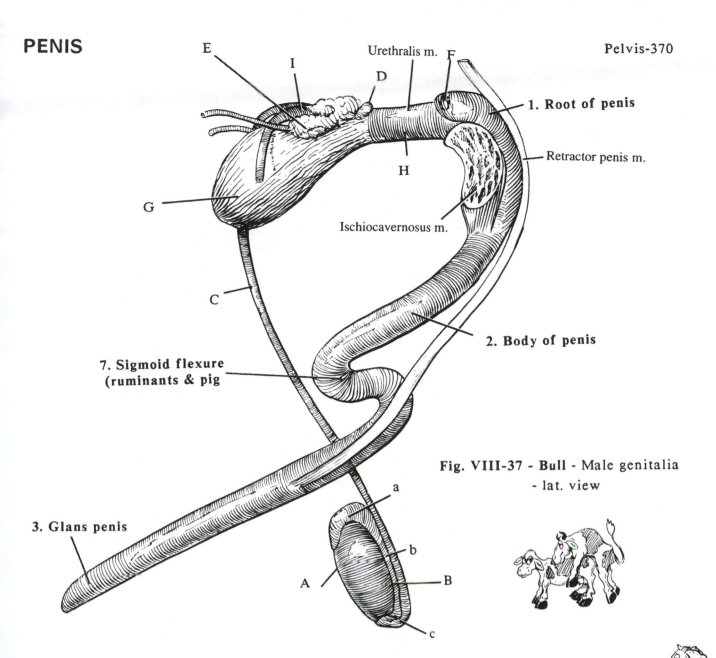

E
I
Urethralis m. F
D
1. **Root of penis**
Retractor penis m.
H
G
Ischiocavernosus m.
C
2. Body of penis
7. Sigmoid flexure (ruminants & pig
a
Fig. VIII-37 - Bull - Male genitalia - lat. view
3. Glans penis
b
A
B
c

Phimosis: stricture of the preputial orifice.

Paraphimosis: protrusion of the penis through a constricted prepucial orifice and the inability to retract it.

Balanoposthitis: inflammation of glans penis (balanitis) and prepuce (posthitis)

Penile deviation: caused by a defect in the dorsal apical ligament in <u>bulls</u>.

"Balling up": masturbation by <u>boars</u> into their preputial diverticulum. Surgically closing the diverticulum stops this "vice"

Prolapse of the prepuce: common in <u>Brahma bulls</u>.

Impotency: lack of desire and/or inability to copulate.

Premature erection: in the <u>stallion</u>, full erection before intromission; flowering or belling of the glans penis makes the penis too large to enter the mare.

"Bean": the smegma (cheesy secretion of the sebaceous glands) and debri that becomes trapped in the urethral sinus of the horse's fossa glandis.

Urethritis: inflammation of the urethra.

Catheterization of the urinary bladder: possible in all species, <u>except the bull</u> where a fold of mucous membrane over the openings of the bulbourethral glans (urethral diverticulum) prevents catheterization. In the <u>boar</u> and <u>small male ruminants</u> the sigmoid flexure must first be straightened out before catheterization.

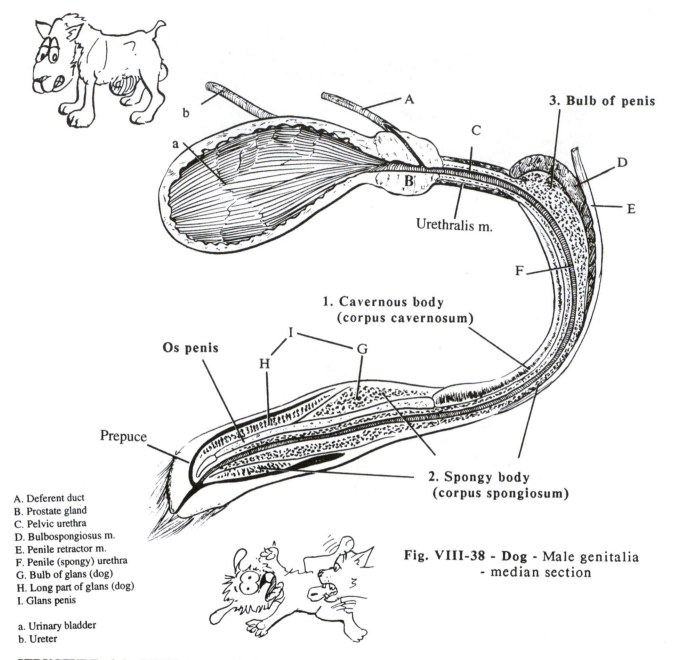

3. Bulb of penis

Urethralis m.

1. Cavernous body (corpus cavernosum)

Os penis

Prepuce

2. Spongy body (corpus spongiosum)

A. Deferent duct
B. Prostate gland
C. Pelvic urethra
D. Bulbospongiosus m.
E. Penile retractor m.
F. Penile (spongy) urethra
G. Bulb of glans (dog)
H. Long part of glans (dog)
I. Glans penis

a. Urinary bladder
b. Ureter

Fig. VIII-38 - Dog - Male genitalia
- median section

STRUCTURE of the PENIS: composed of erectile tissue divided into two cavernous bodies and one spongy body.

1. Corpus cavernosum (cavernous body): the paired erectile tissue with enlarged venous spaces. Proximally, the right and left cavernous bodies separate, forming the two crura. In the carnivores the two bodies are separated by a complete septum, but in the other species perforations in the septum result in one body.

Crura (L. legs)(sin.= crus): the proximal ends of the corpus cavernosum covered by the ischiocavernosus muscle. The right and left cavernous bodies attach separately to their respective sides of the ischial arch. The crura, along with the bulb, make up the root of the penis.

Corpus spongiosum (spongy body): the tube of erectile tissue directly enclosing the urethra. It forms the bulb and the glans of the penis.

3. Bulb of the penis: the expanded, proximal part of the corpus spongiosum at the ischial arch. The bulb is between the crura and is covered by the bulbospongiosus muscle.

4. Tunica albuginea (white tunic): the thick, fibroelastic capsules enclosing the cavernous bodies and the spongy body. **Trabeculae**, a connective tissue framework, runs inwards from the white tunic, supporting the blood spaces in both the cavernous and spongy bodies.

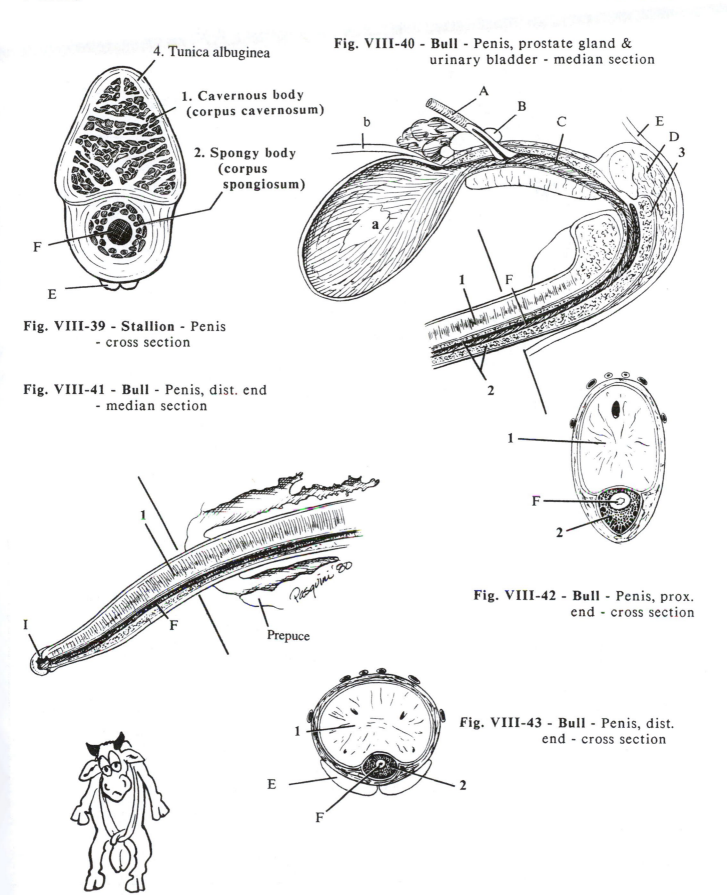

4. Tunica albuginea

1. Cavernous body (corpus cavernosum)

2. Spongy body (corpus spongiosum)

Fig. VIII-39 - Stallion - Penis - cross section

Fig. VIII-41 - Bull - Penis, dist. end - median section

Fig. VIII-40 - Bull - Penis, prostate gland & urinary bladder - median section

Prepuce

Fig. VIII-42 - Bull - Penis, prox. end - cross section

Fig. VIII-43 - Bull - Penis, dist. end - cross section

PENIS

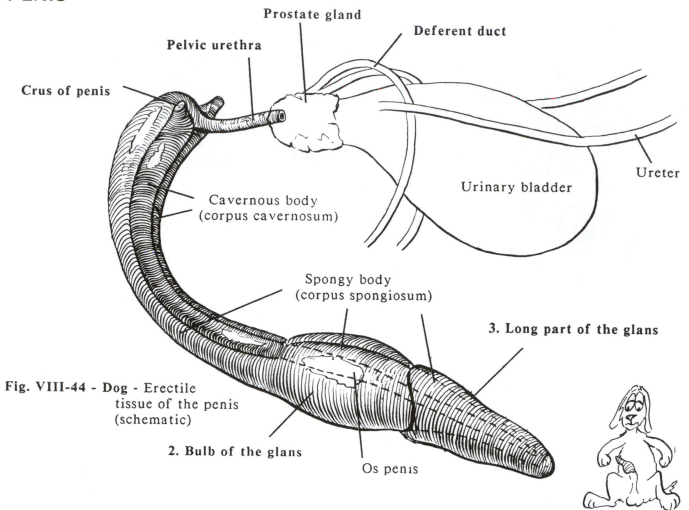

Prostate gland

Pelvic urethra

Deferent duct

Crus of penis

Ureter

Urinary bladder

Cavernous body
(corpus cavernosum)

Spongy body
(corpus spongiosum)

3. Long part of the glans

Fig. VIII-44 - **Dog** - Erectile
tissue of the penis
(schematic)

2. Bulb of the glans

Os penis

1. GLANS PENIS: the distal free end of the penis. It is erectile tissue derived from the corpus spongiosum surrounding the urethra. It differs greatly between the species.

SPECIES DIFFERENCES

Dog: has a large glans penis subdivided into two parts:

• **2. Bulb of the glans** or **bulbus glandis**: the part of the glans surrounding the proximal os penis. The bulb, due to its potential for great expansion, is responsible, along with expansion of the bitch's vestibular bulb and contraction of the vestibular muscles, for the "tie" during copulation.

• **3. Long part of the glans** (pars longa glandis): the distal part of the dog's glans surrounding the os penis.

Cat: has backward projecting cornified spines on its glans. This may explain the queen's (female) scream as the tom (male) withdraws.

Boar: has a twisted "corkscrew" glans.

Ruminants: like the boar, have a twisted glans. They also have an urethral process.

4. Urethral process: the free end of the urethra in ruminants, very long in the ram and goat (resembles a "party favor").

Apical ligament (Lig. apicale penis): seen in <u>bulls</u> arising from the tunica albuginea along the dorsal midline and the left side. It attaches distally to the dorsal surface of the tunica albuginea near the apex of the corpus cavernosum penis. Thinner fibers diverge across the right side and attach close to the right lip of the urethral groove.

Horse:

• **Urethral process** (pg 377): the short, free end of the urethra.

• **Crown of the glans** or **corona glandis** (pg. 377): a ridge surrounding the glans penis of the horse.

• **Fossa of the glans** (fossa glandis) (pg 377-8): the depression around the horse's urethral process.

• **Urethral sinus** (pg 378): the dorsal diverticulum of the fossa of the glans.

• **Collum glandis**: the constriction (neck) caudal to the crown of the glans.

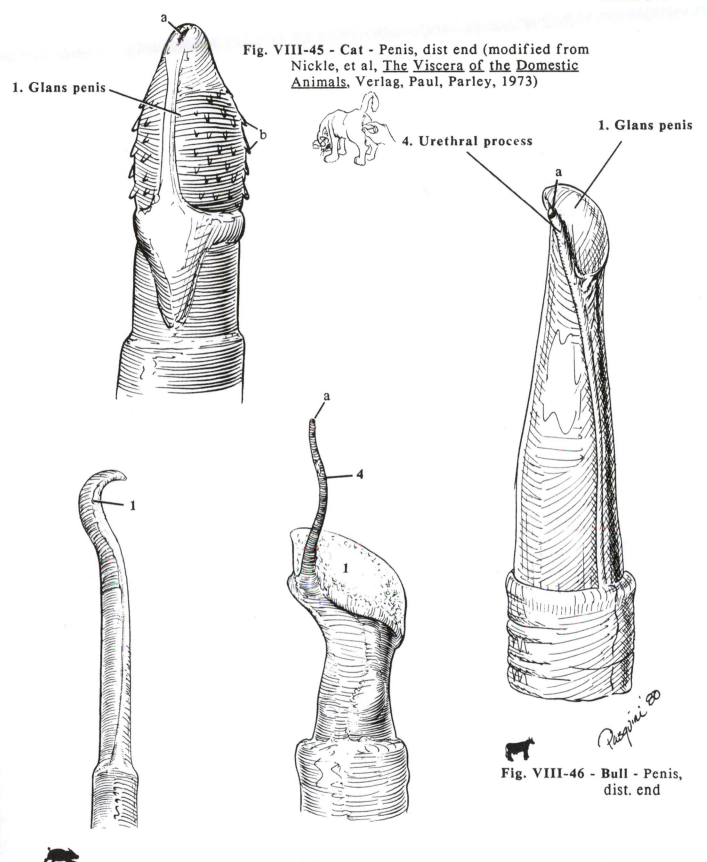

1. Glans penis

Fig. VIII-45 - Cat - Penis, dist end (modified from Nickle, et al, The Viscera of the Domestic Animals, Verlag, Paul, Parley, 1973)

4. Urethral process

1. Glans penis

Fig. VIII-46 - Bull - Penis, dist. end

Fig. VIII-47 - Boar - Penis, dist. end

Fig. VIII-48 - Ram - Penis, dist. end

a. Ext. urethral opening
b. Spines (cat)

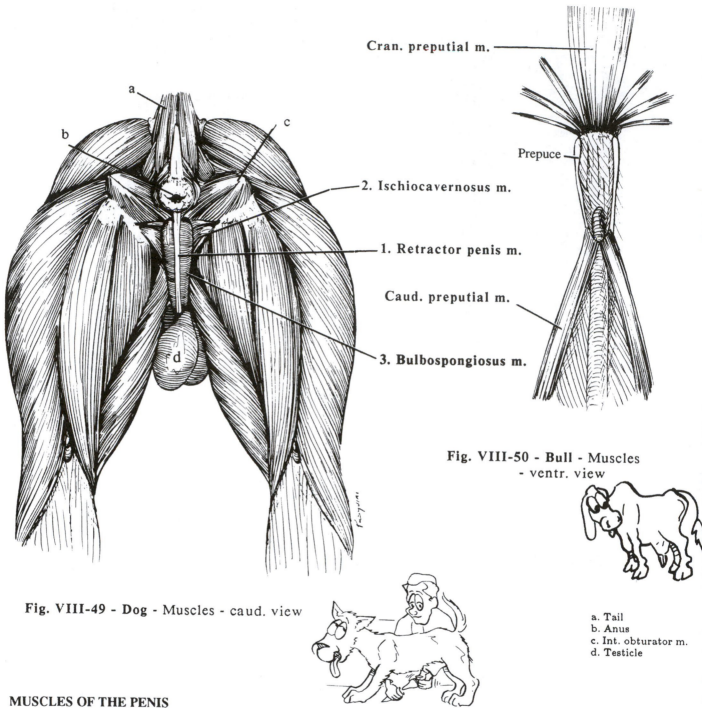

Cran. preputial m.

Prepuce

2. Ischiocavernosus m.

1. Retractor penis m.

Caud. preputial m.

3. Bulbospongiosus m.

Fig. VIII-50 - Bull - Muscles - ventr. view

Fig. VIII-49 - Dog - Muscles - caud. view

a. Tail
b. Anus
c. Int. obturator m.
d. Testicle

MUSCLES OF THE PENIS

1. Retractor penis muscle: the paired <u>smooth</u> muscles originating from the first few caudal vertebrae, They travel laterally around the rectum and then continue side by side over the urethral surface of the penis to attach distally.

2. Ischiocavernosus muscle: the short skeletal muscle covering each crus of the penis, arising from the ischiatic arch and inserting on the cavernous body (corpus cavernosum).

3. Bulbospongiosus muscle: the paired skeletal muscles covering the bulb of the penis (proximal portion of the spongy body) and the bulbourethral glands. In the horse it extends distally all the way to the glans of the penis.

Cranial and caudal preputial muscles: the unimportant skeletal muscles that pull the prepuce cranially over the penis, or caudally to unsheath it.

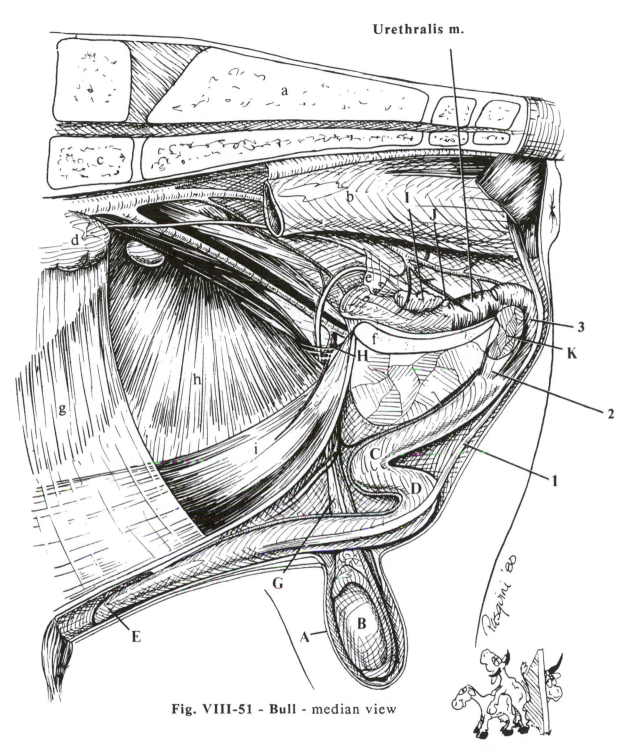

Urethralis m.

Fig. VIII-51 - Bull - median view

A. Scrotum
B. Testicles
C. Body of penis
D. Sigmoid flexure
E. Glans penis
F. Deferent duct

G. Spermatic cord
H. Vaginal ring
I. Vesicular gland
J. Prostate gland
K. Crus of penis

a. Sacrum
b. Rectum
c. Aorta
d. Kidney
e. Genital fold

f. Pelvic symphysis
g. Transverse abdominal m.
h. Int. abdominal oblique m.
i. Rectus abdominis m.

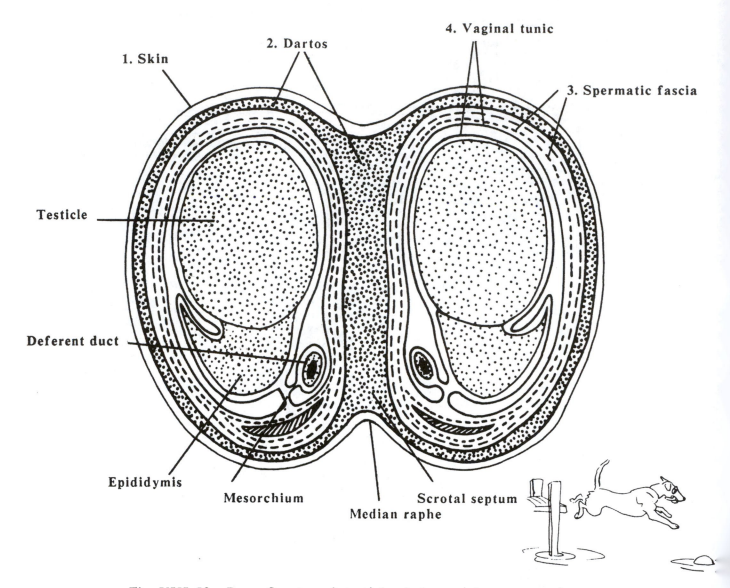

Fig. VIII-52 - Dog - Scrotum & testicles (schematic) - cross section

SCROTUM (SKROH-tum): the pouch containing the testicles and epididymides. It consists of the skin, the dartos, fascia, and the vaginal tunics. In the pig and cat, the scrotum is located directly below the anus. The other domestic species have pendulous scrota a distance below the anus.

1. Skin: the pigmented integument of the scrotum.

2. Dartos (DAR-tohs) (tunica dartos): the fibromuscular layer just below the skin and in the scrotal septum. Contraction of the

dartos draws the testicles closer to the body in cold weather.

3. Spermatic fascia: the continuation of the inner and outer abdominal fascia around the testicle and spermatic cord.

Ligament of the tail of the epididymis and scrotal ligament: connect the tail of the epididymis to the scrotum.

4. Vaginal tunic (pg 362): evagination of the peritoneum through the inguinal canal covering the spermatic cord and testicle (visceral layer) and lining the inside of the scrotum (parietal layer).

GENITALIA - STALLION

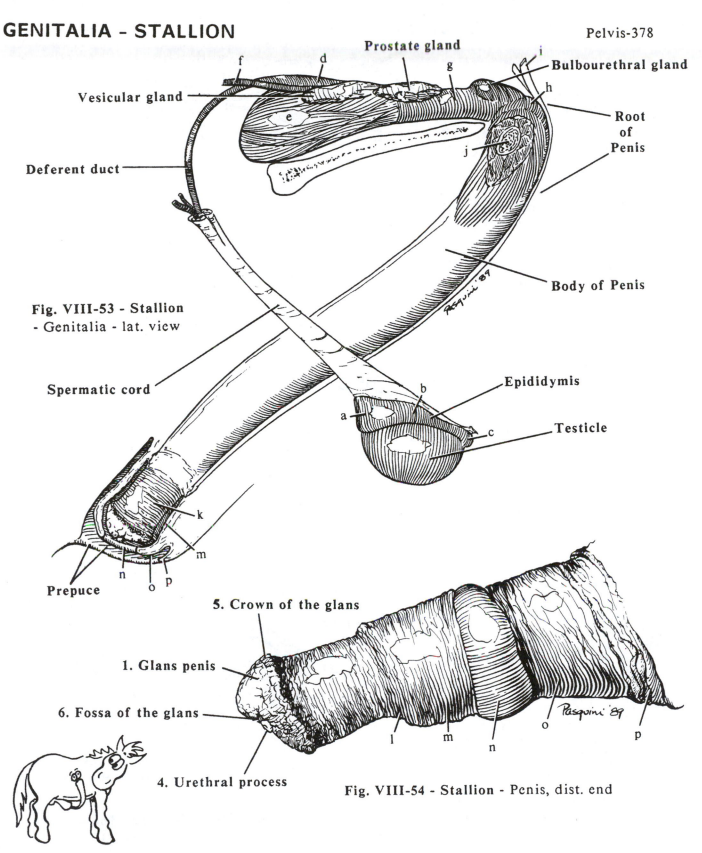

Prostate gland

Bulbourethral gland

Vesicular gland

Deferent duct

Root
of
Penis

Body of Penis

**Fig. VIII-53 - Stallion
- Genitalia - lat. view**

Spermatic cord

Epididymis

Testicle

Prepuce

5. Crown of the glans

1. Glans penis

6. Fossa of the glans

4. Urethral process

Fig. VIII-54 - Stallion - Penis, dist. end

a. Head of epididymis
b. Body of epididymis
c. Tail of epididymis
d. Ampulla of deferent duct
e. Urinary bladder
f. Ureter

g. Pelvic urethra
h. Bulbospongiosus m.
i. Rectractor penis m.
j. Cavernous body
   (corpus cavernosum)
k. Free part of penis

l. Attachment of inner
   layer of prepuce
m. Inner layer of int.
   fold of prepuce
n. Preputial ring
o. Outer layer of int.

fold of prepuce
p. Ext. prepuce

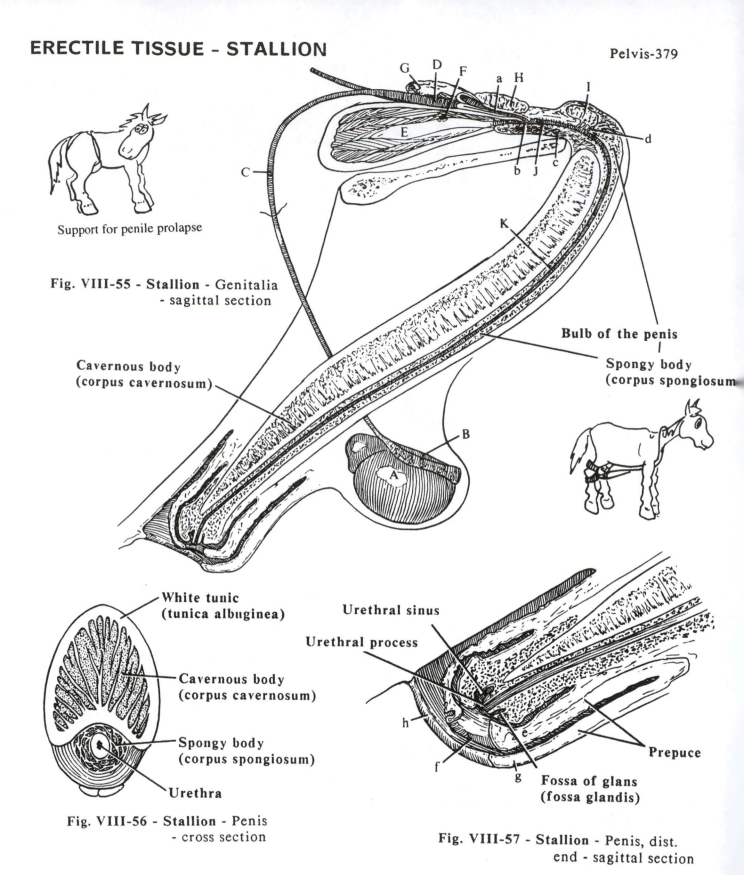

Support for penile prolapse

Fig. VIII-55 - Stallion - Genitalia - sagittal section

Cavernous body (corpus cavernosum)

Bulb of the penis

Spongy body (corpus spongiosum

White tunic (tunica albuginea)

Cavernous body (corpus cavernosum)

Spongy body (corpus spongiosum)

Urethra

Urethral sinus

Urethral process

Prepuce

Fossa of glans (fossa glandis)

Fig. VIII-56 - Stallion - Penis - cross section

Fig. VIII-57 - Stallion - Penis, dist. end - sagittal section

A. Testicle
B. Epididymis
C. Deferent duct
D. Ampulla of deferent duct
E. Urinary bladder
F. Opening of ureter

G. Seminal vesicle
H. Prostate gland
I. Bulbourethral gland
J. Pelvic part of urethra
K. Penile urethra

a. Excretory duct of seminal vescicle
b. Colliculus seminalis
c. Urethralis m.
d. Ducts of bulbourethral gland

e. Int. prepuce (VIII-57)
f. Preputial ring
g. Ext. prepuce
h. Ext. fold of prepuce

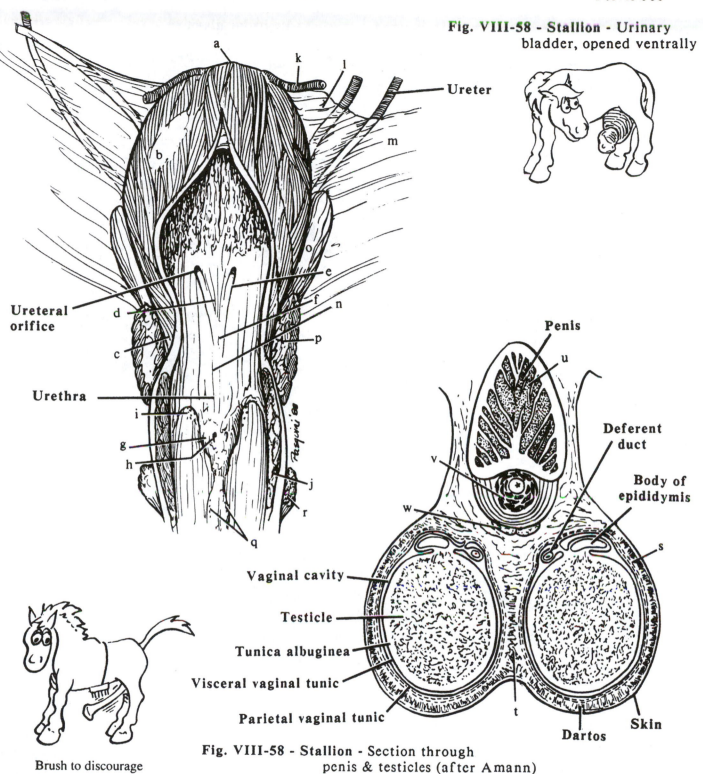

Fig. VIII-58 - Stallion - Urinary
bladder, opened ventrally

Ureter

Ureteral orifice

Urethra

Penis

Deferent duct

Body of epididymis

Vaginal cavity

Testicle

Tunica albuginea

Visceral vaginal tunic

Parietal vaginal tunic

Dartos

Skin

Fig. VIII-58 - Stallion - Section through penis & testicles (after Amann)

Brush to discourage masterbation

a. Apex of bladder	(opening of ductus	(vestige of umbilcal a.)	r. Bulbourethral glands
b. Body	deferens & execretory	l. Genital fold	s. Spermatic fasciae (VIII-58)
c. Neck	duct of seminal	m. Lat. lig. of bladder	t. Scrotal septum
d. Trigone	vesicles)	n. Int. urethral orifice	u. Cavernous body
e. Ureteric fold	i. Opening of prostatic	o. Seminal vesicles	(corpus cavernosus m.)
f. Urethral crest	ductules	p. Prostate gland	v. Spongy body
g. Colliculus seminalis	j. Urethralis m.	q. Openings of ducts of	(corpus spongiosus m.)
h. Ejaculatory orifice	k. Round lig. of bladder	bulbourethral gland	w. Retractor penis m.

379

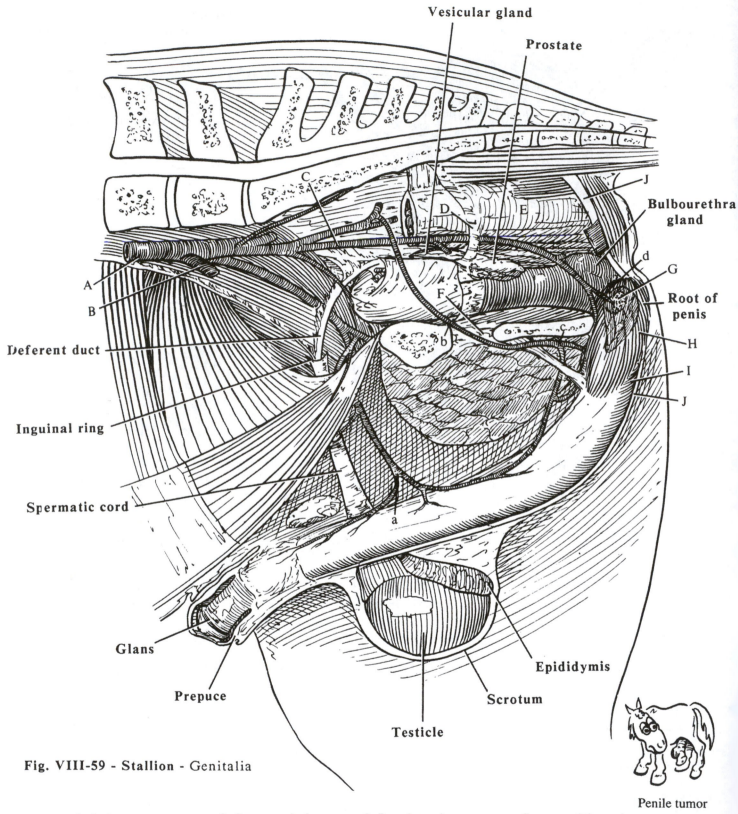

Fig. VIII-59 - Stallion - Genitalia

Vesicular gland

Prostate

Bulbourethra gland

Root of penis

Deferent duct

Inguinal ring

Spermatic cord

Glans

Prepuce

Testicle

Scrotum

Epididymis

Penile tumor

A. Aorta
B. Ext. iliac a.
C. Int. iliac a.
D. Peritoneum
E. Rectum
F. Obturator foramen

G. Cavernous body (corpus cavernosum)
H. Ischiocavernosus m.
I. Bulbospongiosus m.
J. Retractor penis m.
K. Testicular a.

L. Deep femoral a.
M. Pudendoepigastric trunk
N. Ext. pudendal a.
O. Prostatic a.
P. Caud. gluteal a.
Q. Int. pudendal a.

a. Cran. aa. of the penis (br. of ext. pudendal a.)
b. Obturator a.
c. Middle a. of penis (horses)
d. Dors. a. of the penis (br. of int. pudendal a.)

Chapter IX
Circulatory System

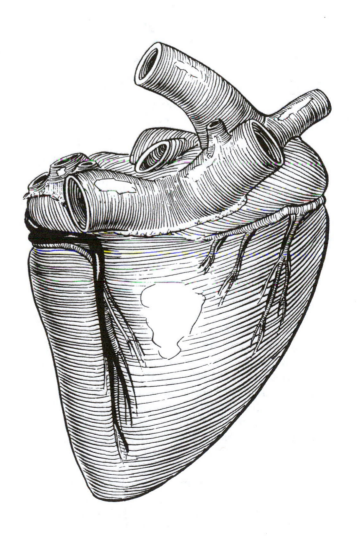

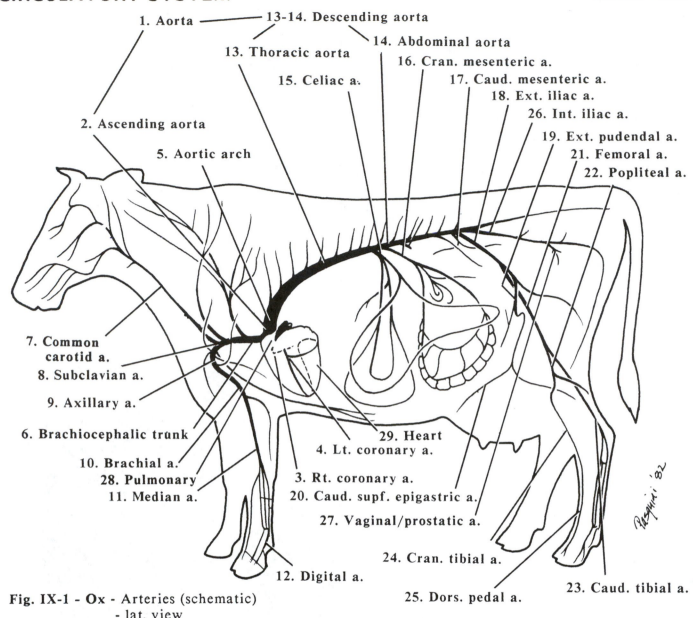

Fig. IX-1 - Ox - Arteries (schematic)
- lat. view

Labels:
1. Aorta
13-14. Descending aorta
14. Abdominal aorta
13. Thoracic aorta
16. Cran. mesenteric a.
15. Celiac a.
17. Caud. mesenteric a.
18. Ext. iliac a.
26. Int. iliac a.
2. Ascending aorta
19. Ext. pudendal a.
21. Femoral a.
5. Aortic arch
22. Popliteal a.
7. Common carotid a.
8. Subclavian a.
9. Axillary a.
6. Brachiocephalic trunk
10. Brachial a.
28. Pulmonary
11. Median a.
29. Heart
4. Lt. coronary a.
3. Rt. coronary a.
20. Caud. supf. epigastric a.
27. Vaginal/prostatic a.
24. Cran. tibial a.
12. Digital a.
25. Dors. pedal a.
23. Caud. tibial a.

CIRCULATORY SYSTEM: consists of the heart, blood vessels and lymphatics. It provides for the metabolic requirements – nutrition, waste removal, protection – of the body's cells via the blood, the interstitial fluid and the lymph. Blood acquires oxygen in the lungs, nutrients from the digestive tract and hormones from the endocrine glands. It then transfers them to the interstitial fluid in exchange for waste products and transports all waste to the lungs, kidneys and sweat glands for elimination from the body or to the liver for detoxification and recycling.

The circulatory system has two principal divisions: the blood vascular system and the lymph vascular system. The blood vascular system includes a powerful pump, the heart. Arteries leave the left side of the heart. They branch into progressively smaller arteries until they form microscopic vessels called capillaries. The permeable capillaries exchange oxygen and nutrients for waste products with the interstitial fluid. Capillaries feed into small veins that join to form larger and larger veins, all carrying oxygen-depleted blood back to the right side of the heart. The heart pumps this blood to the lungs again via arteries, where CO_2 is exchanged for oxygen. Newly oxygenated blood returns through veins to the left side of the heart that pumps it to the rest of the body and heart via the aorta. The lymphatic system removes wastes and bacteria from the interstitial fluid and returns protein-rich fluid to the bloodstream.

Interstitial fluid: the fluid bathing the cells of the body. It carries on the necessary exchange between the cells, blood and lymph.

Lymph vascular system: consists of the lymph, lymph vessels, lymph nodes and lymphatic organs. This system returns protein-rich fluid from the interstitial fluid to the general circulation. It also filters waste and bacteria from the interstitial fluid.

PERICARDIUM

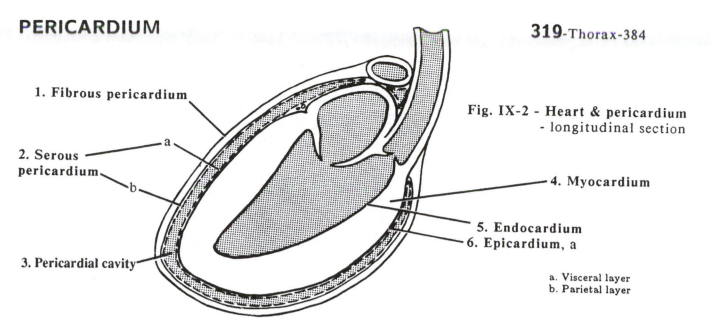

1. Fibrous pericardium

2. Serous pericardium

3. Pericardial cavity

Fig. IX-2 - Heart & pericardium
- longitudinal section

4. Myocardium

5. Endocardium
6. Epicardium, a

a. Visceral layer
b. Parietal layer

Blood vascular system: consists of the blood, heart, arteries, capillaries and veins.

Artery (AR-ter-ee): a vessel carrying blood <u>away</u> from the heart. Arteries are generally thicker and stronger than veins, sustaining their <u>higher pressure.</u>

Capillary (KAP-i-lar'ee): a microscopic vessel that joins others to form an extensive network throughout the body tissue. Positioned between the arteries and veins, the permeable capillaries allow exchange of gases and nutrients between the blood and the interstitial fluid.

Veins: vessels carrying blood <u>back</u> to the heart. They are thinner-walled and carry greater <u>volume</u> than arteries.

PERICARDIUM: the fibroserous sac enclosing the heart; composed of the fibrous and serous* pericardium, covered by mediastinal (pericardiac) pleura.

7. Fibrous pericardium: a tough, fibrous sac surrounding the serous pericardium, the heart and the pericardial cavity. It is closed above by its attachment to the great vessels of the heart. When discussing the pericardial serous membranes, the fibrous pericardium will be considered as a wall.
- **Sternopericardiac ligament**: connects the pericardium to the floor of the thorax.
- **Phrenicopericardiac ligament**: connects the pericardium to the diaphragm.

2. Serous pericardium: a serous* membrane forming a closed cavity. It covers the heart (visceral layer [a]) and lines the inner surface of the fibrous pericardial sac (parietal layer [b]).
- **Parietal layer of the serous pericardium**: lines the inner surface of the fibrous pericardium (considered a wall). It reflects onto the surface of the heart as the visceral layer.
- **Visceral layer of the serous pericardium** (b): covers the myocardium of the heart closely. It is also called the epicardium.

*A serosa is any smooth membrane, consisting of a mesothelial layer and a connective tissue layer, lining the cavities of the body.

3. Pericardial cavity: a potential space between the visceral and parietal layers of serous pericardium. It has approximately one ml. of yellow fluid between the contacting layers, which acts as a lubricant to allow the heart freedom of movement during contraction. Other serous body cavities have almost no fluid.

LAYERS OF THE HEART: the three layers having "-cardium" in their name with prefixes telling the location of each ("epi-" meaning being on top of, "endo-" being inside of, and "myo-" the muscular part of).

4. Myocardium: the muscle layer making up the majority of the thickness of the heart wall. It is between the endocardium and epicardium.

5. Endocardium: a thin, mesothelial layer lining the atria and ventricles. This layer is continuous with the endothelium lining the great vessels entering and leaving the heart.

6. Epicardium: a thin layer of mesothelium covering the surface of the heart. The epicardium is the visceral layer of the serous pericardium.

CLINICAL

Pericarditis: inflammation of the pericardium

"Surgeon's pericardium": the structure a surgeon must incise to reach the pericardial cavity (for open heart surgery). It consists of the mediastinal (pericardial) pleura, the fibrous pericardium and the parietal layer of the serous pericardium. After open heart surgery the pericardium need <u>not</u> be sutured completely closed to prevent cardiac tamponade.

Cardiac tamponade: acute compression of the heart due to fluid effusion or hemorrhage into the pericardium.

Hydrops pericardii: an excessive production and concurrent retarded absorption of pericardial fluid caused by pericarditis.

THE HEART

HEART: a muscular, four-chambered organ that drives the circulatory system. It has specific input channels (veins) and specific output channels (arteries).

PULMONIC CIRCULATION: through the <u>right</u> side of the heart to the lungs. The right (pulmonic) side receives blood from the body and pumps it to the lungs for oxygenation. It returns to the left side of the heart.

SYSTEMIC CIRCULATION: through the <u>left</u> side of the heart to the heart itself and to the rest of the body, delivering oxygenated blood from the lungs.

CIRCULATION through the HEART: Blood enters either atrium by veins, is pumped into the respective ventricles, and on to the lungs or body through the arteries. The <u>right atrium</u> receives deoxygenated venous blood through a number of veins, but primarily the <u>caudal</u> and <u>cranial vena cavae</u>. The blood then enters the right ventricle, which pumps it through the <u>pulmonary trunk</u> into the lungs (pulmonic circulation). <u>Pulmonary veins</u> carry oxygenated blood from the lungs to the <u>left atrium</u>. Blood then descends to the <u>left ventricle</u>. The left ventricle pumps it through the <u>aorta</u> to the rest of the body (systemic circulation).

Major vessels returning blood to the heart:

1. Cranial vena cava: the large vein returning blood from the head, neck and thoracic limbs to the right atrium.

2. Caudal vena cava: the large vein returning blood from part of the thorax, the viscera and the caudal part of the body to the right atrium.

3. Right atrium (AY-tree-um): the chamber of the heart receiving deoxygenated blood from the body.

4. Right ventricle (VEN-tri-kul): the chamber receiving blood from the right atrium and sending it to the lungs. The <u>conus</u> is the funnel-shaped end of the right ventricle leading to the pulmonary trunk.

5. Pulmonary trunk: the large vessel carrying blood from the right ventricle to the pulmonary arteries, thus, to the lungs.

6. Pulmonary arteries: the two branches of the pulmonary trunk carrying blood to the lungs; one to the right lung, one to the left.

Lungs: receive deoxygenated blood through the pulmonary veins. It oxygenates the blood and sends it back to the heart through pulmonary veins.

7. Pulmonary veins: the numerous vessels emptying oxygenated blood from the lungs into the left atrium of the heart.

8. Left atrium: receives oxygenated blood from the lungs via the pulmonary veins.

9. Left ventricle: sends oxygenated blood to the body and heart.

10. Aorta: the major outflow from the left ventricle into the systemic circulation.

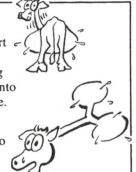

CLINICAL

• Problems in the right side of the heart (pulmonic circulation) cause blood to backup in the caudal vena cava, filling the abdomen with fluid (ascites) and into the jugular, resulting in a jugular pulse.

• Problems in the left side (systemic circulation) cause blood to backup into the lungs (congestion of the lungs).

Conduction system - Heart: consists of three parts

1. Sinoatrial (SA) node (nodus sinuatrialis): modified muscle that initiate the heart beat. It is located in beneath the endocardium of the right atrial wall ventral to the opening of the cranial vena cava

2. Atrioventricular (AV) node (nodus atrioventricularis): located in interatrial septum cranial to coronary sinus opening. It gives rise to the atrioventricular bundle

3. Atrioventricular bundle (fasciculus atrioventricularis): mass of modified muscle cells located within atrioventricular septum. They leave the AV node, penetrate the fibrous skeleton of the heart an then divide into Branches

3a. Right and left branches (limbs, crura): Purkinje fibers (specialized cardiac muscle cells) travel under the endocardium of the interventricular septum to innervate the heart.

3b. Marginal bands (trabecula septomarginalis): bands of muscle tissue that carries Perkinje fibers from the right bundle branch to outer wall.

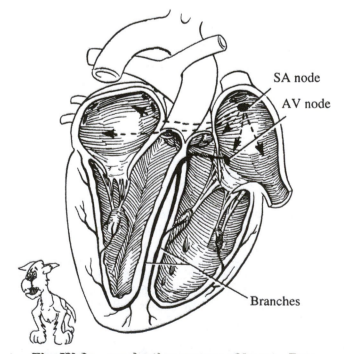

Fig. IX-2a - conduction system of heart - Dog

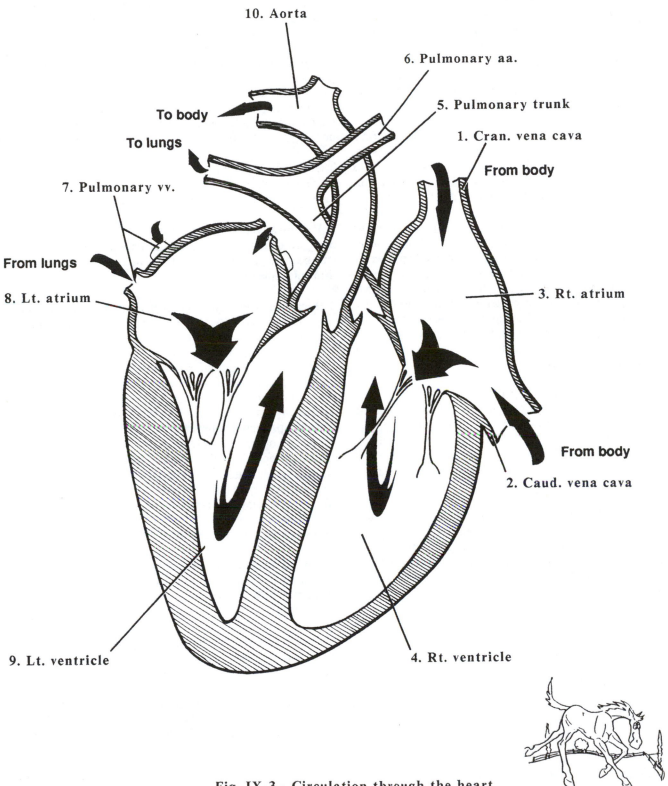

10. Aorta

6. Pulmonary aa.

5. Pulmonary trunk

To body

To lungs

1. Cran. vena cava

From body

7. Pulmonary vv.

From lungs

8. Lt. atrium

3. Rt. atrium

From body

2. Caud. vena cava

9. Lt. ventricle

4. Rt. ventricle

Fig. IX-3 - Circulation through the heart
(schematic)

FETAL CIRCULATION

During fetal development, the placenta functions as the lungs and liver for the fetus, supplying it with oxygen and nutrients and eliminating fetal waste products. The fetal lungs and liver need only enough blood to nourish their growing tissue as they are non-functional. The bulk of the blood is diverted to "functional" tissues (especially the heart and brain) by three shunts in the fetal circulation: the ductus venosus, the foramen ovale and the ductus arteriosus. These shunts bypass structures, creating a dual circulatory system – the one in the fetus shutting down within minutes after birth to allow the other, the adult circulation, to take over.

The umbilical vein brings nutrient- and oxygen-rich blood from the placenta into the fetus. It enters the liver to join the portal vein. The ductus venosus connects the umbilical vein with the caudal vena cava, allowing some of the umbilical blood to bypass the liver sinusoids and empty directly into the caudal vena cava.

The caudal vena cava empties into the right atrium where about three fifths of the oxygen-rich blood is shunted through the foramen ovale to the left atrium. Thus, the blood bypasses the pulmonic circulation and enters the systemic circulation. From the left atrium it passes into the left ventricle and out the aorta to supply the heart via the coronary arteries. Distally, the oxygen-rich blood travels over the brachiocephalic trunk into the arteries that supply the brain (common carotid arteries). Thus, the ductus venosus and the foramen ovale insure that the blood richest in oxygen reaches the heart and brain by the fastest route.

The cranial vena cava returns oxygen-poor blood from the cranial parts of the body to the right atrium to mix with the unshunted, oxygen-rich, caudal vena caval blood in the right ventricle. This mixed blood, although not as rich in oxygen as that shunted through the foramen ovale, is still oxygenated, therefore, is shunted away from the lungs via the right ventricle and pulmonary trunk.

The ductus arteriosus shunts blood from the pulmonary trunk to the aorta before it reaches the non-functional lungs. It enters the aorta distal to the origin of the brachiocephalic trunk, thus, supplying the caudal body without diluting the oxygen content of the blood coursing to the brain via the common carotid arteries (branches of the brachiocephalic trunk).

The umbilical arteries, large branches of the terminal aorta, return the fetal blood via the umbilical cord to the placenta for oxygenation and waste elimination.

At birth the umbilical cord is disrupted, stopping blood traveling over the umbilical vein. The ductus venosus becomes part of the portal liver circulation.

The newborn's first breath expands the lungs with air, relieving the pressure on the vessels and capillaries of the lungs and allowing them to expand for the first time. As the vessels open, resistance to blood flow drops, allowing more blood through pulmonary arteries to reach the lungs. The ductus arteriosus, a muscular artery, begins to close shortly after birth due to the change in oxygen content of the blood flowing through it. It eventually becomes the ligamentum arteriosum. Closure of the ductus arteriosus allows even more blood to reach the lungs.

The greater volume of blood through the lungs returns through the pulmonary veins to the left atrium. This increases the left atrial pressure, functionally closing the "flap valve" of the foramen ovale. With time this functional closure becomes an anatomical closure as the walls of the foramen fibrose, leaving a remnant of the foramen ovale, a depression called the fossa ovale. Blood is no longer shunted from the right to the left atrium.

The closure of the three shunts gives the newborn an "adult circulatory system". Oxygen now comes from the newborn's lungs and nutrients from its intestines via the portal vein.

1. Umbilical veins: vessels carrying oxygen- and nutrient-rich blood from the placenta to the fetus. Paired in the umbilical cord, they become a single umbilical vein in the fetal abdomen, which then enters the liver.

2. Ductus venosus (venous duct): the fetal shunt from the umbilical vein directly through the liver to the caudal vena cava, bypassing the liver sinusoids.

3. Foramen ovale (oval foramen): the opening in the wall separating the two atria (the interatrial septum) allowing blood to shunt from the right to the left atrium. It is a double-walled structure with holes in each wall offset from each other. In the fetus, the pressure is greater in the right atrium, pushing blood through the opening in the right atrial wall, between the two walls, and out the opening in the left atrial wall. With the first breath at birth, blood returning from the lungs raises the pressure in the left atrium above that in the right, pushing the two walls together and effectively closing the foramen ovale.

• **Fossa ovale:** the adult remnant of the foramen ovale.

4. Ductus arteriosus (arterial duct): the shunt between the pulmonary trunk and the aorta, diverting most of the blood from the pulmonary trunk (pulmonic circulation) to the aorta (systemic circulation).

• **Ligamentum arteriosum** (arterial ligament): the adult remnant of the ductus arteriosus between the pulmonary trunk and the aorta.

5. Umbilical arteries: the pathways of oxygen-depleted blood from the fetus to the placenta. They arise from terminal branches of the aorta (internal iliac arteries), and travel via the umbilical cord to reach the placenta.

2. Venous duct

4. Arterial duct

3. Oval foramen

1. Intestines (l)

m

k

f

b h g e

a

c

d

1

5. Umbilical aa.

1. Umbilical vv.

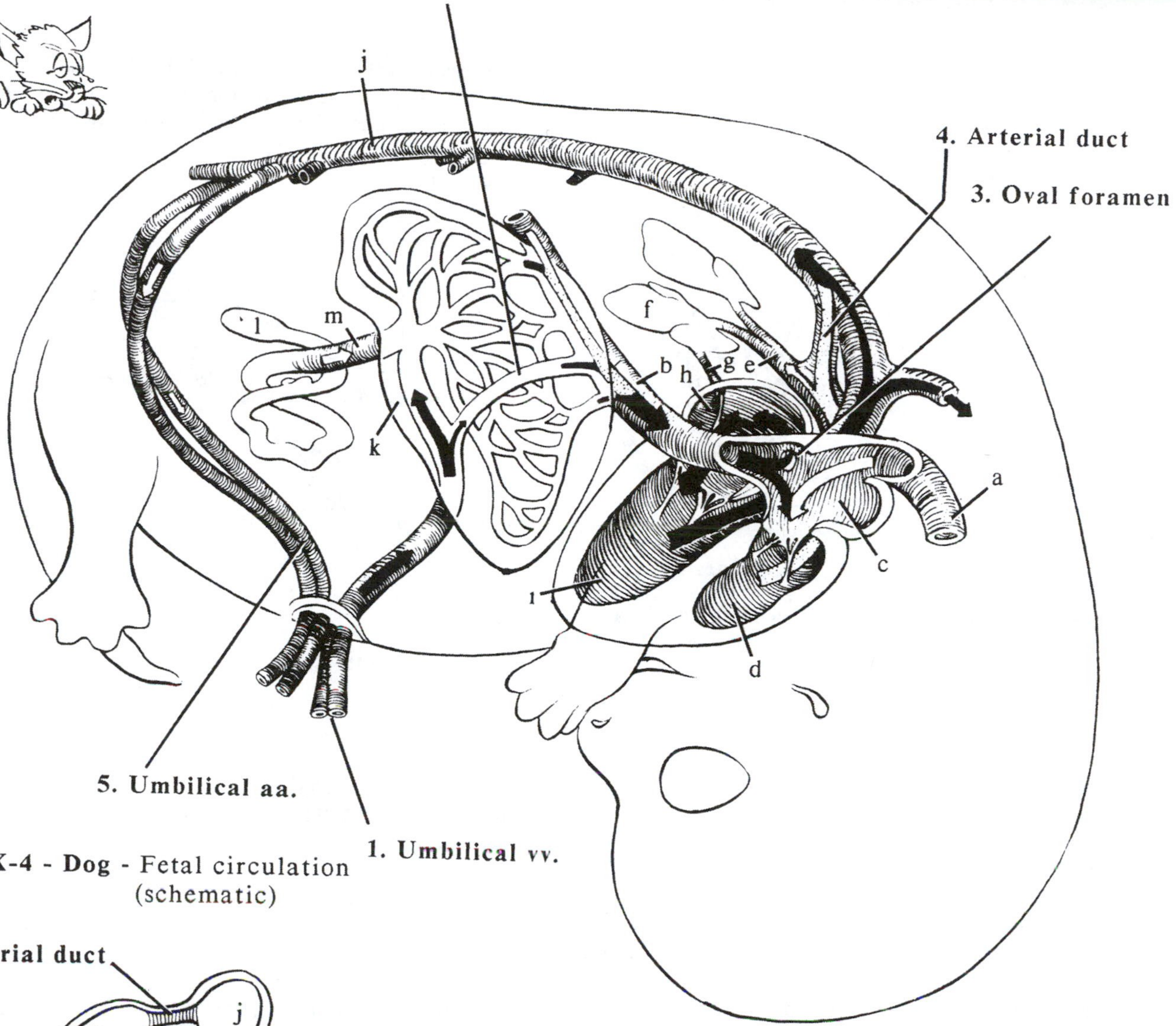

Fig. IX-4 - Dog - Fetal circulation
(schematic)

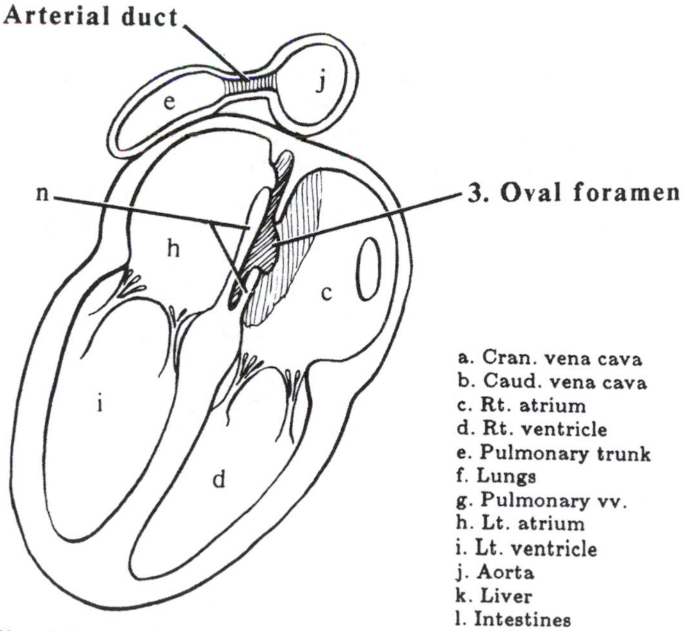

4. Arterial duct

3. Oval foramen

n

h

c

e

j

i

d

**Fig. IX-5 - Section of heart
& oval foramen**

a. Cran. vena cava
b. Caud. vena cava
c. Rt. atrium
d. Rt. ventricle
e. Pulmonary trunk
f. Lungs
g. Pulmonary vv.
h. Lt. atrium
i. Lt. ventricle
j. Aorta
k. Liver
l. Intestines
m. Portal v.
n. Double wall of
   oval foramen

CLINICAL:

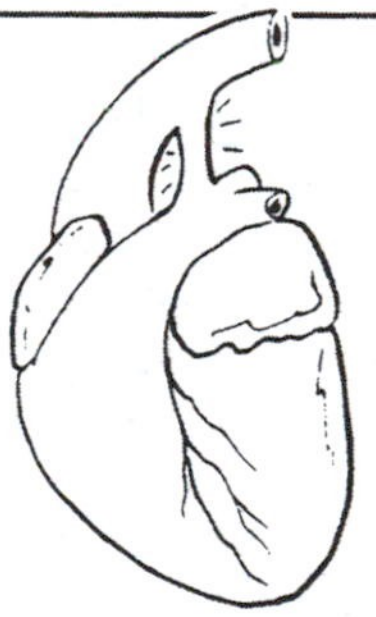

Patent ductus arteriosus: the arterial duct doesn't close after birth. This should be corrected early through a left intercostal incision through the fourth intercostal space. The ductus is carefully isolated and ligated.

Patent foramen ovale (interatrial channel): normal in calves and of no clinical significance if found on necropsy.

Aortic isthmus: the part of a calf's aorta between the brachiocephalic trunk and the entrance of the ductus arteriosus. It is normally smaller than the rest of the aorta and the large ductus arteriosus. Do not mistake the combined pulmonary trunk, the ductus arteriosus and the descending aorta for an aorta coming out of the right ventricle.

DEVELOPMENT OF THE HEART

Primitive heart tube

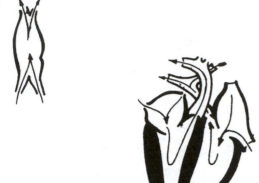

Adult heart

Fig. IX-6 - Development of heart
and blood flow

FORMATION of the HEART TUBE: The primitive embryo is a three-layered structure: the external layer is ectoderm [a], the internal is endoderm [b] and between is a mesoderm layer [c] (lying on the yolk). The <u>mesoderm</u> layer is most concerned with cardiogenesis.

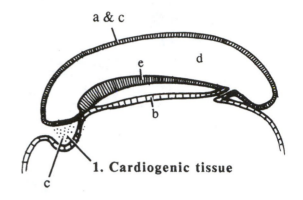

Fig. IX-7 - Presomite embryo
- sagittal section

CARDIOGENESIS: the development of the heart from a simple tube in the embryo (with one inflow and one outflow) to an "adult" four-chambered structure with two separate circulations in series (pulmonary and systemic). While these transformations prepare the fetus for life independent of the placenta (pg. 384), the heart must still meet the unique requirements of the fetus (pg. 386). Understanding the development of the heart makes the function and the anatomy of the adult heart and the fetal heart, and the structure and disability of common heart malformations more understandable.

Changes in the developing heart result from two different processes: one is growth, the other degeneration. Growth is an increase in size and/or number of cells. Degeneration is the death of cells. Both of these processes occur in a focal manner; areas of the heart tube grow while other areas degenerate, resulting in the shape of the adult heart.

As the fetus grows, diffusion becomes insufficient to meet the cellular needs, necessitating a circulatory system. The heart begins pumping primitive blood through a primitive vascular system while developing and changing. Within a matter of minutes after birth the animal must shift from the intrauterine to the extrauterine pattern of circulation. This requires a system that can modify itself as it functions during development.

Stages in heart development:
• 1. Formation of the heart tube.
• 2. Cardiac loop formation.
• 3. Partitioning of the heart and outflow channels.

The <u>mesodermal cardiogenic tissue</u> (1) which gives rise to the heart begins cranial to the head of the embryo. With growth, the cardiogenic tissue is drawn underneath the head into the throat (cervical) region and then into the thorax. As the embryo continues to fold, the cardiogenic tissue comes to be located ventral to the foregut (f) (future esophagus); the relationship found in the adult.

The heart begins as <u>two tubes</u> (2) located laterally. As the embryo folds, the paired tubes are brought together and fuse (3) to form a <u>single tube</u>, the endocardium (5). A thick layer of mesoderm (future myocardium) surrounds the endocardial tube. A thin layer of epicardium (mesothelium) envelopes both the myocardium and endocardium. This single tube develops by fusion progressing cranially to caudally.

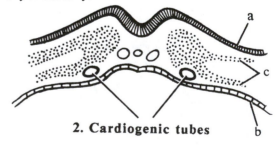

2. Cardiogenic tubes

Fig. IX-8 - Transverse section through cardiac
region of embryo

DEVELOPMENT OF THE HEART

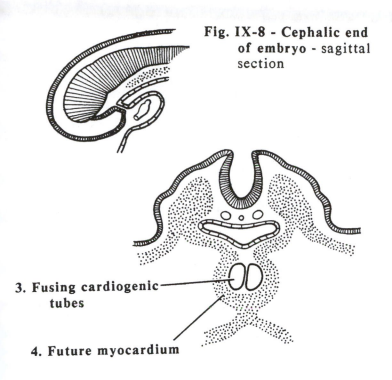

Fig. IX-8 - Cephalic end of embryo - sagittal section

3. Fusing cardiogenic tubes

4. Future myocardium

Fig. IX-9 - Cephalic end of embryo - transverse section

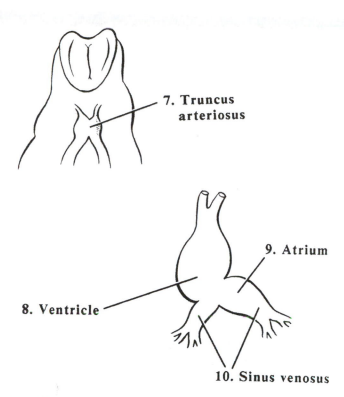

7. Truncus arteriosus

9. Atrium

8. Ventricle

10. Sinus venosus

Fig. IX-11,12 - Developing heart - ventr. views

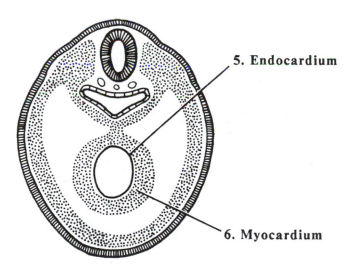

5. Endocardium

6. Myocardium

Fig. IX-10 - 4 somite embryo - transverse section

The first part of the heart to differentiate and start beating is the truncus arteriosus (7) (aortic trunk), the common outflow of the primitive heart. Behind the truncus arteriosus, the tube is still paired and continuing to fuse. As the tube fuses caudally, forming the ventricle (8), the heart rate increases. The atrium (9) then forms and the heart rate again picks up. The last chambers to develop, the right and left sinus venosus (10), remain unfused until much later. They receive venous return from the vessels of the allantois, yolk sac and body of the fetus. With the appearance of each sinus venosus, the heart rate increases to its maximal level.

The increase in rate with the appearance of each new chamber is called the pacemaker phenomenon. Specialized cells of the heart spontaneously depolarize, generating action potentials which spread to the remainder of the heart. The sinus venosus contains the cells with the fastest depolarization rate, thus, become the pacemaker of the heart. In the adult these pacemaker cells are the SA node (the remnant of the right sinus venosus which becomes incorporated into the right atrium.) If the SA node becomes damaged, other parts of the heart can take over as slower pacemakers.

Legend for Fig. IX-6-12

a. Ectoderm
b. Endoderm
c. Mesoderm
d. Amniotic cavity
e. Neural plate
f. Foregut

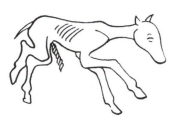

11. Fixed points

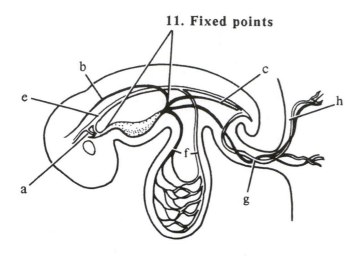

Fig. IX-14 - Early fetal blood flow
(schematic)

FORMATION OF THE CARDIAC LOOP: the primitive, straight-tube heart is anchored at each end by vessels connected to it. Cranially it is anchored where the truncus arteriosus is connected to the <u>ventral aortae</u> (12) (future <u>aortic arches</u> [13]). It is anchored distally where the venous return comes into the sinus venosus. Thus anchored, the tube begins to bulge out to the right side (ventral view) as it lengthens. Continued growth forces the ventricle below and caudally, causing the previously cranially-located ventricle to become caudal and ventral to the atria; the orientation in the adult heart. The truncus pushes into the atrium, prestaging the two adult atria.

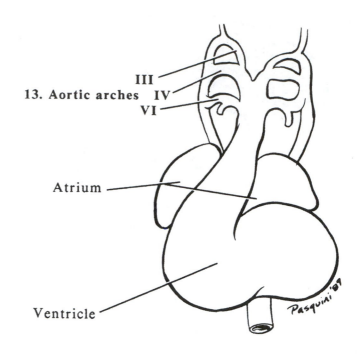

13. Aortic arches

Fig. IX-16 - Fetal heart - ventr. view

PARTITIONING of the HEART: Internally, at this time, the heart is partitioning in preparation for birth. As partitioning continues, shunts form so that fetal circulation can continue to bypass the pulmonic circulation.

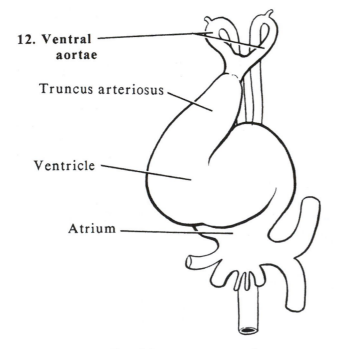

12. Ventral aortae

Truncus arteriosus

Ventricle

Atrium

Fig. IX-15 - Fetal heart - ventr. view

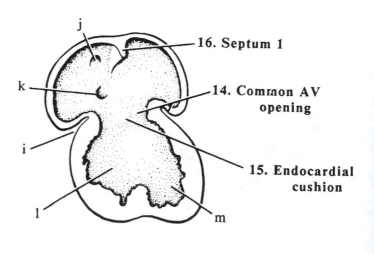

16. Septum 1

14. Common AV opening

15. Endocardial cushion

Fig. IX-17 - Heart - frontal section

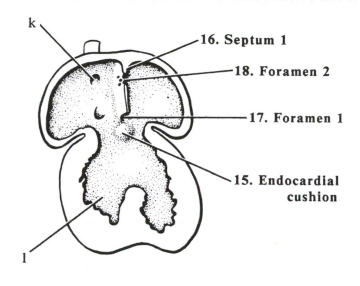

Fig. IX-18 - Fetal heart - frontal section

- k
- 16. Septum 1
- 18. Foramen 2
- 17. Foramen 1
- 15. Endocardial cushion
- l

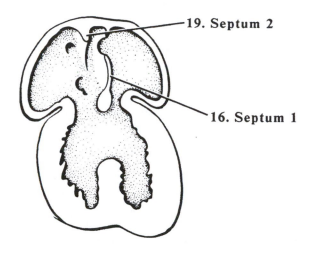

Fig. IX-19 - Fetal heart - frontal section

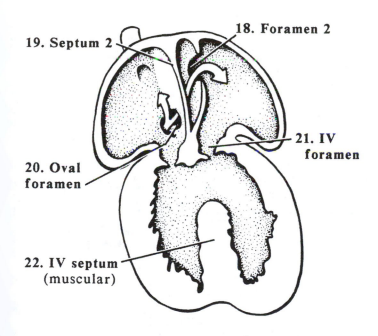

- 19. Septum 2
- 18. Foramen 2
- 21. IV foramen
- 20. Oval foramen
- 22. IV septum (muscular)

Fig. IX-20 - Heart - frontal section

Partitioning of the common atrioventricular passageway: The common atrium is demarcated from the common ventricle by a constriction (i). The common AV opening is subdivided into two passageways by the atrioventricular endocardial cushions (15) which are growing out to meet each other.

Partitioning of the common atrium: Septum 1 (17) (septum primum) grows downward from the dorsal wall of the atrium toward the endocardial cushion to partition the common atrium. The diminishing opening formed by this septum is foramen 1 (20). Before reaching the cushions and completely partitioning the atrium, perforations develop high in the septum and coalesce to form foramen 2 (21). This allows continued communication between the right and left atria.

Septum 2 (19) grows downward, parallel with and to the right of septum 1, to cover foramen 2. It then stops growing, leaving an oval-shaped opening, the foramen ovale (20). During fetal life, the volume of blood coming into the right atrium causes a higher pressure than that in the left atrium. This high pressure forces blood through the foramen ovale, between the two walls of the septum and out foramen 2, bypassing the pulmonic circulation. Septum 1 acts like a flutter valve, thus, a functional partition is formed (which is also an opening). This permits a fetal circulation that is ready to switch immediately to the adult circulation at birth.

Partitioning of the ventricle and the outflow channel: The ventricle is partitioned by the outgrowth of the interventricular (IV) septum (22). The septum extends upward from the ventral side of the heart toward the endocardial cushions, leaving an opening – the interventricular (IV) foramen (21). This closes later as a sequel to the partitioning of the common outflow tract of the ventricle.

DEVELOPMENT OF THE HEART

Partitioning of the truncus arteriosus: The common outflow of the undivided ventricles, the truncus arteriosus, is connected to the ventral aortae. The two ventral aortae fuse to form the aortic sac (a) from which the aortic arches arise. The truncus arteriosus will be partitioned from the aortic arches to the ventricles so that each ventricle has one outflow connecting to the correct aortic arch.

Partitioning begins by the appearance of truncal ridges (23) in the lumen of the truncus arteriosus. The ridges grow toward each other, beginning first at the aortic sac and moving toward the ventricles. They spiral and fuse, forming the spiral septum (24). The two parallel outflow channels (aortic and pulmonary) spiral around each other, connecting the right ventricle to the pulmonary trunk (27) and the left ventricle to the aorta (26).

As the many aortic arches develop, some degenerate and some persist, determining the patterns that result. The 6th aortic arch gives rise to the pulmonary trunk and pulmonary arteries and is connected to the right ventricle in the adult, thus, forming the pulmonic circulation. The systemic circulation is formed by the 3rd and 4th arches. The left 4th aortic arch gives rise to the aorta, and in the adult is connected to the left ventricle. The two 3rd aortic arches give rise to the common carotid arteries. The ductus arteriosus (28) connects the pulmonary trunk to the aorta in the fetus, shunting blood from the pulmonic circulation to the systemic circulation. This duct closes at birth or soon after, becoming the ligamentum arteriosum.

Closure of the interventricular foramen: before closure, the incomplete interventricular (IV) septum (22) (with the interventricular (IV) foramen (21) above it) can be seen in an opened right ventricle (b). The left ventricle (c) can be seen through the interventricular foramen. Both ventricles still have a common outflow, the truncus. Further up, the truncus is partitioned. As partitioning continues, the two edges of the truncal cushions grow together with the endocardial cushions (15), closing off the interventricular septum and finishing the two outflows. The membranous part (25) of the interventricular septum is the last part to close.

CLINICAL

Ectopia cordis: interference with the migration of the heart into the thorax, resulting in the heart being located somewhere other than the thorax (usually in the cervical region).

Atrial septal defect (ASD): One type of ASD results when the foramen ovale and second foramen overlap, allowing blood to flow from left to right, resulting in poor oxygenation of blood which can lead to cyanosis.

Persistent right 4th aortic arch: the right instead of the left 4th aortic arch becomes the aorta. The aorta is then on the right side of the esophagus instead of the left. The aorta, ligamentum arteriosum, and the base of the heart form a ring around the esophagus. This is the most common vascular ring anomaly. When a dog is weaned to solid food, large particles can't get past this constriction and the animal regurgitates undigested food. The ligamentum arteriosum is surgically isolated, ligated twice, and cut between the two ligatures.

Transposition of the great vessels: the correct ventricles do not match up with the correct outflow channels. This is fatal!

Interventricular septal defect (VSD): failure of the interventricular septum to close, involving the membranous part of the septum. The most common cardiac anomaly in large animals, it causes a systolic murmur.

Tetralogy of Fallot: this developmental anomaly has four components:

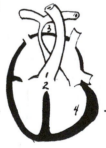

- Pulmonic stenosis
- The aorta over-rides both ventricles
- Ventricular septal defect
- Hypertrophy of the right ventricle

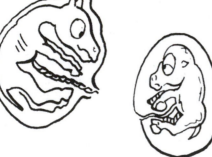

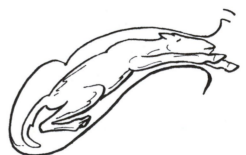

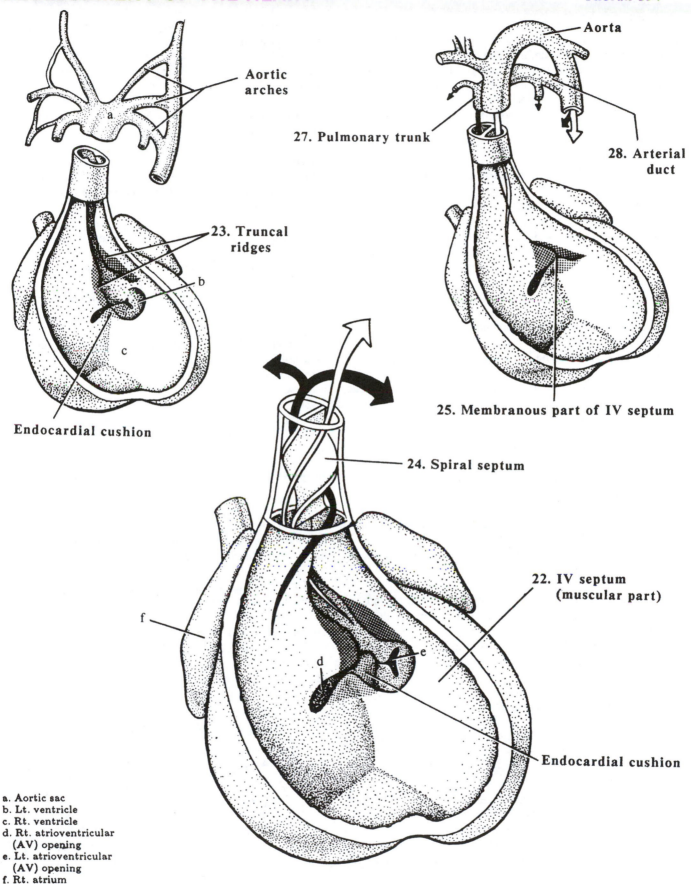

Aortic arches

27. Pulmonary trunk

Aorta

28. Arterial duct

23. Truncal ridges

Endocardial cushion

25. Membranous part of IV septum

24. Spiral septum

22. IV septum (muscular part)

Endocardial cushion

a. Aortic sac
b. Lt. ventricle
c. Rt. ventricle
d. Rt. atrioventricular (AV) opening
e. Lt. atrioventricular (AV) opening
f. Rt. atrium

Fig. IX-21-23 - Fetal heart, rt. ventricle opened - schematic

HEART - EXTERIOR

FREE HEART: to orient a heart that has been removed from the body, first locate the apex which is directed downward (caudoventral) in the live animal. The base (or top of the heart) is opposite the apex. The cranial and caudal sides can be oriented by finding the aorta, which arches caudally; or the auricles, which point to the left, with the pulmonary trunk between them. With the heart oriented thusly, the right and left sides are easily identified.

- Apex – down
- Aorta – arches caudally
- Auricles – beside the pulmonary trunk, point to the left

Since the chambers of the heart are connected by specific vessels, locating vessels helps identify chambers; and identifying chambers helps locate vessels. So many vessels enter the heart, the majority of them pulmonary veins, it is confusing. To simplify identification, locate the great vessels first – the aorta, the pulmonary trunk and the two venae cavae. The remaining vessels are the pulmonary veins.

Find the vessels to locate the chambers they connect:

- **Cranial and caudal vena cava** locate the <u>right atrium</u>.

- **Pulmonary veins** locate the left atrium, where they terminate.

- **Pulmonary trunk** locates the right ventricle.

- **Aorta** locates the left ventricle.

Coronary groove: Partially encircling the heart, it marks the separation of the atria and ventricles.

Interventricular grooves on the heart's exterior indicate the interventricular septum separating the ventricles. The two grooves (the paraconal and subsinuosal grooves) carry similarly-named arteries.

Left side (auricular surface*): the side of the heart where the auricles are seen with the pulmonary trunk in between them.

Right side (atrial surface*): the side of the heart where the vena cavae (cranial and caudal) are seen entering the right atria.

1. Apex: the most caudoventral part of the heart, always formed by the left ventricle (and having a "tip").

2. Base: the hilus of the organ facing dorsocranially. (It is the broad "top" of the heart.) It receives the great veins and sends out the great arteries.

*<u>Sternocostal surface</u> and <u>diaphragmatic surface</u> are terms used to orient the human heart because of the human's ventrodorsally (anterioposteriorly) flattened thorax. The sternocostal surface faces the sternum and the diaphragmatic surface rests on the diaphragm. In domestic animals, with their laterally-flattened thorax, the tendency is to think of the heart from the lateral view, that is right or left sides.

3. Right auricle: seen from the <u>left</u> side of the heart, in front of the pulmonary trunk (c).

4. Left auricle: also seen on the <u>left</u> side of the heart, caudal to the pulmonary trunk.

5. Conus: the expanded outflow from the right ventricle into the pulmonary trunk.

6. Paraconal interventricular groove: the external indication of the interventricular septum separating the ventricles. The groove descends the left side of the heart, adjacent (para-) to the conus of the heart, thus, paraconal.

7. Coronary groove: a depression encircling the heart, except for the conus. The groove externally indicates the separation of the atria and ventricles and contains the coronary vessels.

8. Left atrium: the chamber into which the pulmonary veins empty.

9. Left ventricle: seen best from the left side, caudal to the paraconal groove. On the right side, it is seen caudal to the subsinuosal groove. It forms the caudal boundary of the heart and its apex.

10. Ligamentum arteriosum (arterial ligament): the remnant of the fetal ductus arteriosus (arterial duct) connecting the pulmonary trunk and the aorta.

11. Right atrium (Fig. IX-25): seen from the <u>right</u> side of the heart, with the venae cavae entering it.

12. Right ventricle: makes up most of the heart on the right side, below the coronary groove. It "wraps" around the cranial side of the heart to continue as the pulmonary trunk.

13. Coronary sinus: the termination of the great coronary vein emptying into the right atrium.

14. Subsinuosal interventricular groove: the long depression on the caudal right side of the heart. The groove is below (sub-) the coronary sinus (sinuosal). Like the paraconal interventricular groove, it marks the interventricular septum on the exterior.

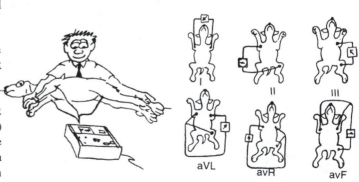

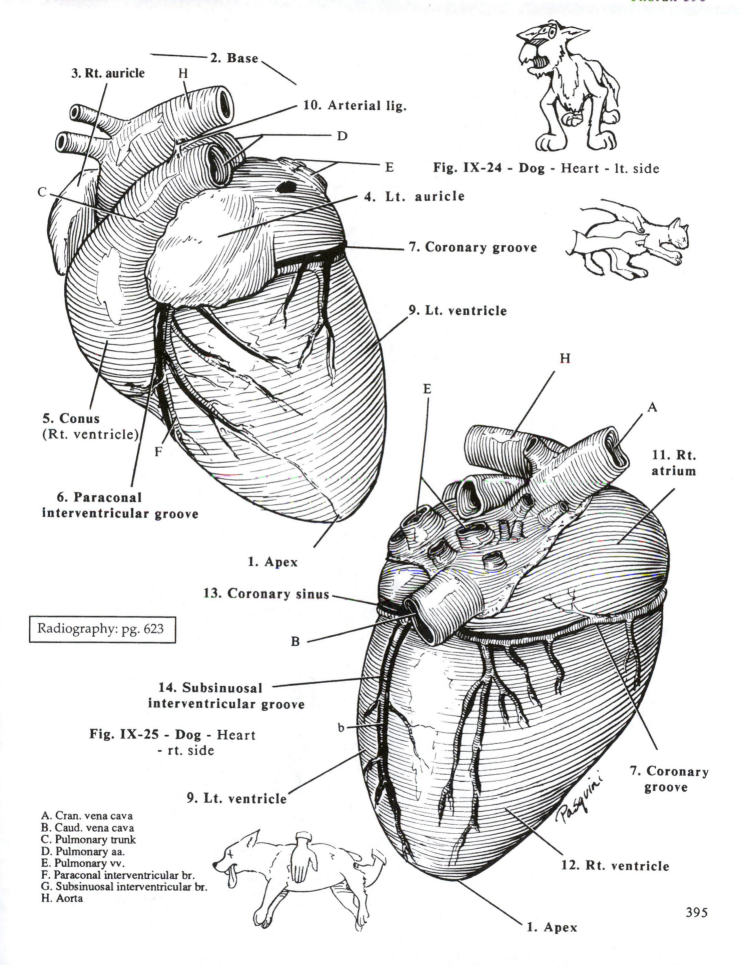

2. Base

3. Rt. auricle

H

10. Arterial lig.

D

E

C

Fig. IX-24 - Dog - Heart - lt. side

4. Lt. auricle

7. Coronary groove

9. Lt. ventricle

H

A

11. Rt. atrium

5. Conus (Rt. ventricle)

F

E

6. Paraconal interventricular groove

1. Apex

13. Coronary sinus

B

Radiography: pg. 623

14. Subsinuosal interventricular groove

Fig. IX-25 - Dog - Heart - rt. side

b

9. Lt. ventricle

7. Coronary groove

A. Cran. vena cava
B. Caud. vena cava
C. Pulmonary trunk
D. Pulmonary aa.
E. Pulmonary vv.
F. Paraconal interventricular br.
G. Subsinuosal interventricular br.
H. Aorta

12. Rt. ventricle

1. Apex

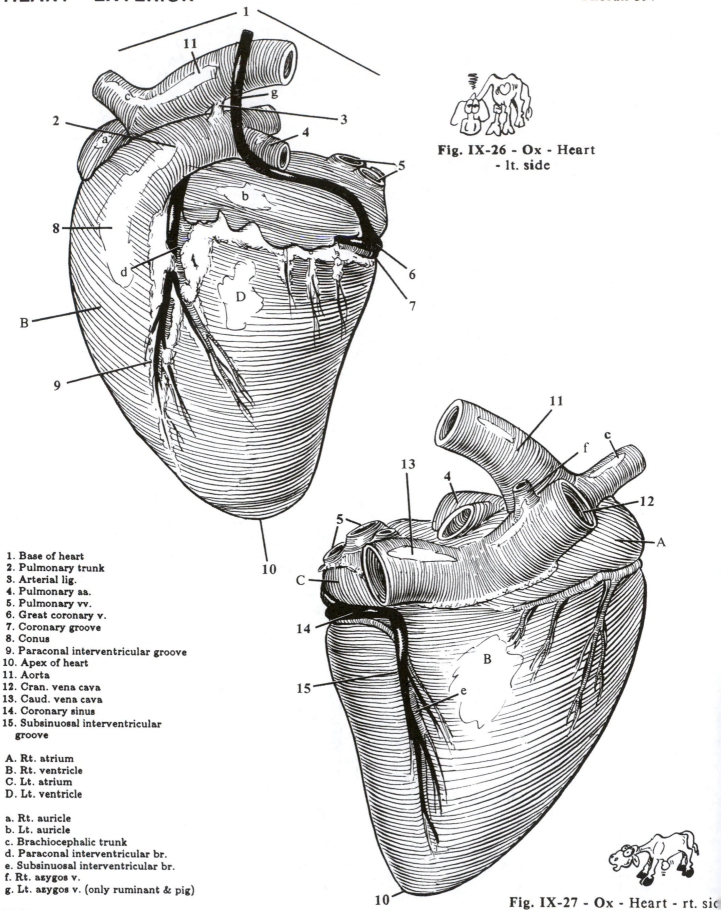

Fig. IX-26 - Ox - Heart - lt. side

Fig. IX-27 - Ox - Heart - rt. side

1. Base of heart
2. Pulmonary trunk
3. Arterial lig.
4. Pulmonary aa.
5. Pulmonary vv.
6. Great coronary v.
7. Coronary groove
8. Conus
9. Paraconal interventricular groove
10. Apex of heart
11. Aorta
12. Cran. vena cava
13. Caud. vena cava
14. Coronary sinus
15. Subsinuosal interventricular groove

A. Rt. atrium
B. Rt. ventricle
C. Lt. atrium
D. Lt. ventricle

a. Rt. auricle
b. Lt. auricle
c. Brachiocephalic trunk
d. Paraconal interventricular br.
e. Subsinuosal interventricular br.
f. Rt. azygos v.
g. Lt. azygos v. (only ruminant & pig)

HEART - EXTERIOR

1. Base

2. Pulmonary trunk

3. Arterial lig.

4. Pulmonary aa.

5. Pulmonary vv.

C

6. Great coronary v.

7. Coronary groove

Fig. IX-28 - Horse - Heart, lt. side

a

8. Conus

B

d

9. Paraconal interventricular groove

10. Apex

D

11. Aorta

12. Cran. vena cava

C

f

c

A

13. Caud. vena cava

14. Coronary sinus

15. Subsinuosal interventricular groove

D   e

B

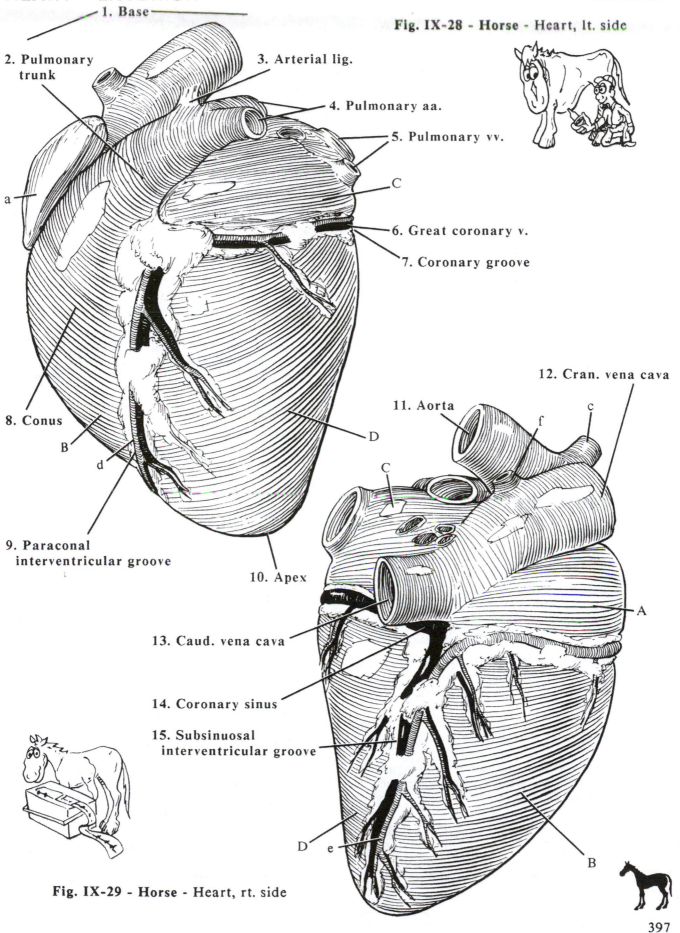

Fig. IX-29 - Horse - Heart, rt. side

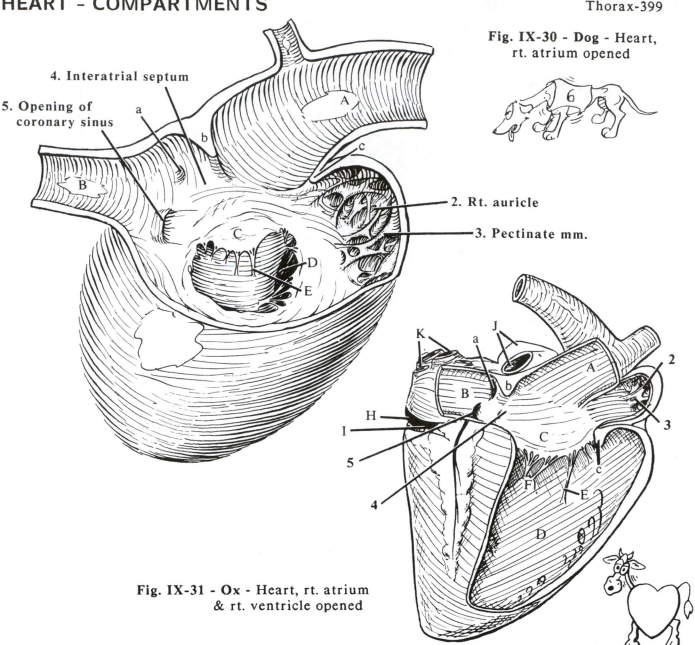

4. Interatrial septum

5. Opening of coronary sinus

A

a

b

B

c

C

D

E

2. Rt. auricle

3. Pectinate mm.

Fig. IX-30 - Dog - Heart, rt. atrium opened

6

K

J

a

b

A

2

B

H

C

3

I

c

5

F

E

4

D

Fig. IX-31 - Ox - Heart, rt. atrium & rt. ventricle opened

COMPARTMENTS of the HEART: the heart has four chambers. The two atria receive blood and pump it down into the respective ventricles, which pump it away from the heart.

1. RIGHT ATRIUM: the compartment receiving deoxygenated blood from the body and most of the heart.

Vena caval sinus (sinus venarum cavarum): the main part of the right atria were the vena cavae and coronary sinus open. This doesn't include the auricle.

2. Right auricle (AW-ri-kl) (L. *auricula*, a little ear): the blind pocket of the atria, characterized by pectinate muscles in its wall.

3. Pectinate muscles: the interdigitating, criss-crossing, muscular bands in the walls of both auricles.

4. Interatrial septum: the wall separating the two atria.

• **Fossa ovale** (oval fossa) (a), a shallow depression in the interatrial septum. It is the vestige of the oval foramen.

5. Coronary sinus: the end of the great cardiac vein which opens into the right atrium.

Intervenous tubercle (b): a projection from the dorsal wall of the right atrium that diverts the flow of both the cranial and caudal vena cava into the right ventricle.

Fossa ovale (a): a remnant of the foramen ovale of the fetus.

Openings into/out of the right atrium: cranial vena cava, caudal vena cava, coronary sinus, and right atrioventricular orifice.

Fig. IX-32 - Horse - Heart, rt. ventricle & rt. atrium opened - rt. side

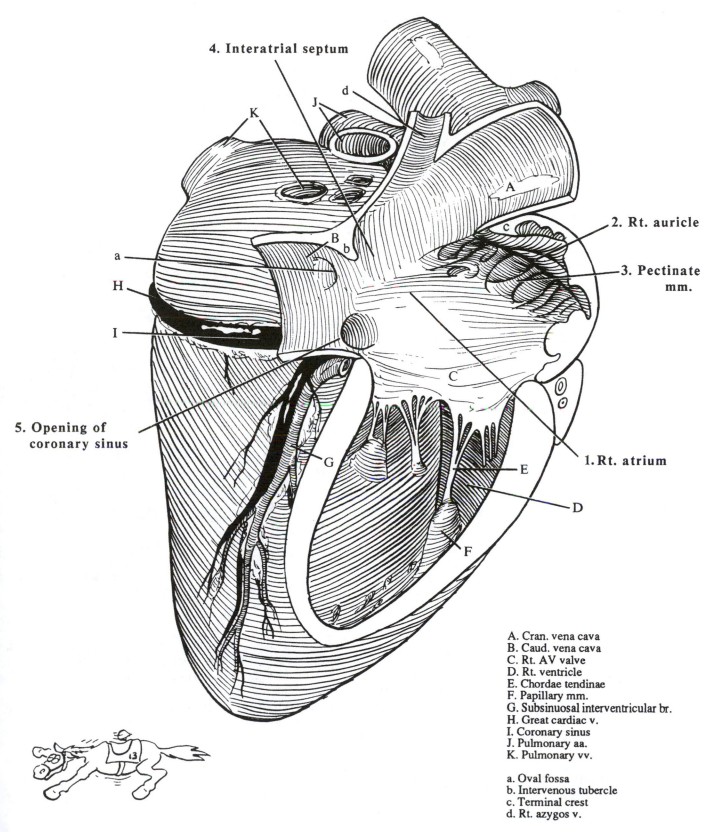

4. Interatrial septum

K

J

d

4. Interatrial septum

A

2. Rt. auricle

c

3. Pectinate mm.

a

H

I

B

b

C

5. Opening of coronary sinus

G

E

1. Rt. atrium

D

F

A. Cran. vena cava
B. Caud. vena cava
C. Rt. AV valve
D. Rt. ventricle
E. Chordae tendinae
F. Papillary mm.
G. Subsinuosal interventricular br.
H. Great cardiac v.
I. Coronary sinus
J. Pulmonary aa.
K. Pulmonary vv.

a. Oval fossa
b. Intervenous tubercle
c. Terminal crest
d. Rt. azygos v.

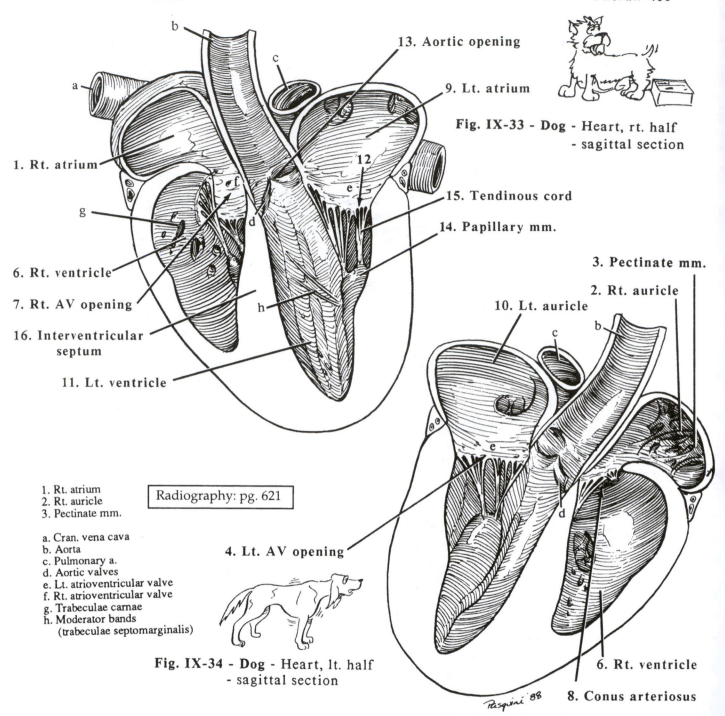

13. Aortic opening

9. Lt. atrium

Fig. IX-33 - Dog - Heart, rt. half
- sagittal section

b

c

a

1. Rt. atrium

g

6. Rt. ventricle

7. Rt. AV opening

16. Interventricular septum

11. Lt. ventricle

12

e

15. Tendinous cord

14. Papillary mm.

3. Pectinate mm.

2. Rt. auricle

10. Lt. auricle

h

d

Radiography: pg. 621

1. Rt. atrium
2. Rt. auricle
3. Pectinate mm.

a. Cran. vena cava
b. Aorta
c. Pulmonary a.
d. Aortic valves
e. Lt. atrioventricular valve
f. Rt. atrioventricular valve
g. Trabeculae carnae
h. Moderator bands
   (trabeculae septomarginalis)

4. Lt. AV opening

b

c

e

d

6. Rt. ventricle

8. Conus arteriosus

Pasquini '88

Fig. IX-34 - Dog - Heart, lt. half
- sagittal section

COMPARTMENTS of the HEART (cont.)

6. RIGHT VENTRICLE: the compartment receiving blood from the right atrium and pumping it, via the pulmonic circulation, through the pulmonary trunk and the pulmonary veins to the lungs. The right ventricular wall is thinner than the left because less pressure is required to move blood through the lungs than through the body.

Openings into/out of the right ventricle: the right AV opening and the pulmonary trunk.

7. Right atrioventricular (AV) opening: the opening between the right atrium and right ventricle, functionally opened and closed by the right **atrioventricular valve.**

8. Conus arteriosus or **conus**: the funnel-shaped outflow of the right ventricle leading to the pulmonary trunk.

Pulmonary opening: the opening in the pulmonary trunk protected by the pulmonary valve.

Moderator band or trabeculae septomarginalis (h): a cord of

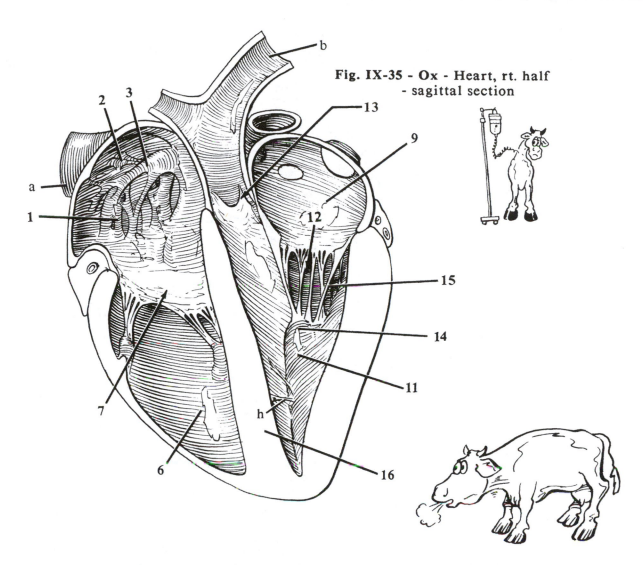

Fig. IX-35 - Ox - Heart, rt. half - sagittal section

myocardium crossing the lumen connecting the outer wall with the interatrial septum. Purkinje fibers travel over these bands to help synchronize contraction and emptying of the ventricle.

9. LEFT ATRIUM: the compartment receiving oxygenated blood from the lungs via the pulmonary veins.

10. Left auricle: a blind pocket with characteristic pectinate muscles as seen in the right auricle.

Openings in/out of the left atrium: the pulmonary veins and the left atrioventricular orifice.

11. LEFT VENTRICLE: the compartment receiving oxygenated blood from the left atrium and sending it out the aorta to the body and the heart (systemic circulation). The left ventricle is thicker walled than the right because of the higher pumping pressure required for systemic circulation.

Openings into/out of the left ventricle: the left AV orifice and the aorta.

12. Left atrioventricular (AV) orifice: the opening between the left atrium and left ventricle; operated by the **left atrioventricular valve.**

13. Aortic opening: the opening from the left ventricle into the aorta. The **aortic valve** prevents backflow from the aorta into the left ventricle.

STRUCTURES COMMON to both VENTRICLES

14. Papillary muscles: the muscular projections serving as attachments for the tendinous cords (chordae tendineae) of the atrioventricular (AV) valves.

15. Chordae tendineae (tendinous cords): the tough strands anchoring the free edges of the atrioventricular (AV) valves to the papillary muscles and preventing eversion of the valve leaflets into the atrium upon ventricular contraction (systole).

16. Interventricular septum: the wall separating the ventricles.

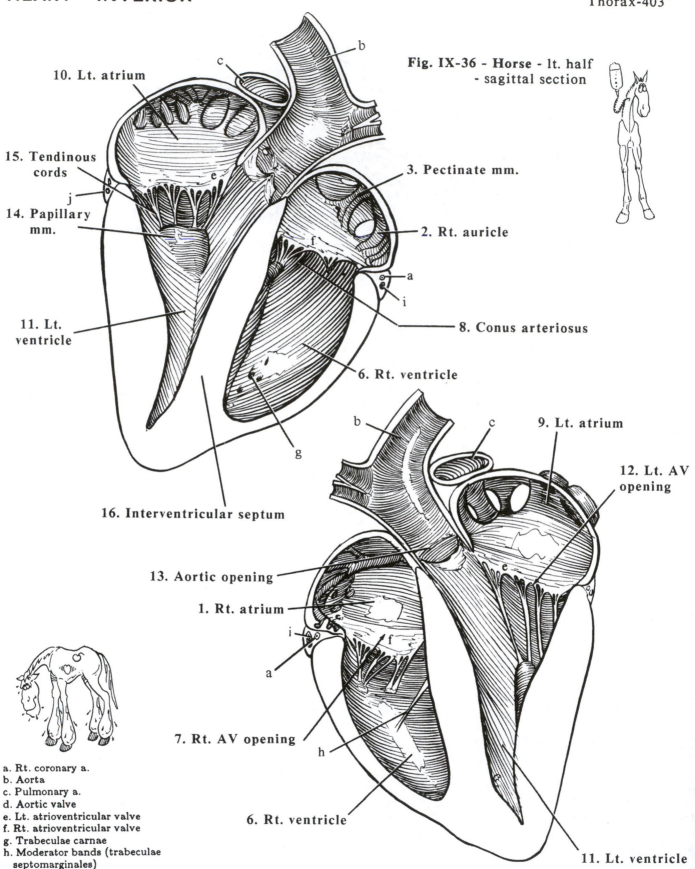

10. Lt. atrium

15. Tendinous cords

14. Papillary mm.

11. Lt. ventricle

16. Interventricular septum

Fig. IX-36 - Horse - lt. half - sagittal section

3. Pectinate mm.

2. Rt. auricle

8. Conus arteriosus

6. Rt. ventricle

9. Lt. atrium

12. Lt. AV opening

13. Aortic opening

1. Rt. atrium

7. Rt. AV opening

6. Rt. ventricle

11. Lt. ventricle

a. Rt. coronary a.
b. Aorta
c. Pulmonary a.
d. Aortic valve
e. Lt. atrioventricular valve
f. Rt. atrioventricular valve
g. Trabeculae carnae
h. Moderator bands (trabeculae septomarginales)
i. Great coronary v.
j. Lt. coronary a. (circumflex br.)

Fig. IX-37 - Horse - Heart, rt. half - sagittal section

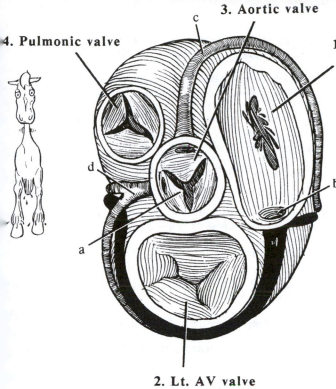

4. Pulmonic valve

3. Aortic valve

c

1. Rt. AV valve

Fig. IX-38 - Horse - Heart,
base of ventricles

d

a

b

2. Lt. AV valve

a. Nodule
b. Opening of coronary sinus
c. Rt. coronary a.
d. Lt. coronary a.
e. Fibrous rings
f. Rt. AV opening
g. Lt. AV opening
h. Aortic opening
i. Pulmonic opening
j. Ossa cordis (ox & older horses)

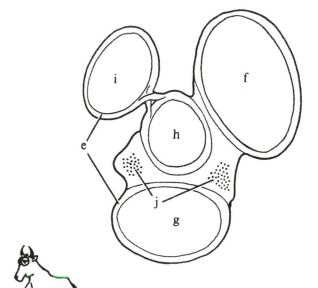

Fig. IX-39 - Ox - Heart skeleton

VALVES OF THE HEART: the fibrous structures guarding the openings between the atria and the ventricles and the ventricles, and the two main heart outflows - the aorta and the pulmonary trunk.

Atrioventricular (ay'tree-oh-ven-TRIK-yoo-lar) **(AV) valves**: prevent backflow into the atria during ventricular (systolic) contractions. The AV valves are anchored in the ventricles by tendinous cords (chordae tendineae) and attach peripherally to the fibrous rings of the cardiac skeleton.

1. Right AV (tricuspid) valve: operates the right AV opening. There are only two major cusps (parietal and septal) in the dog, with intervening secondary cusps. In man and other domestic species, there are three major cusps (angular, parietal and septal), thus "tri-".

2. Left AV (bicuspid, mitral) valve: similar to the right AV valve, but has a heavier construction due to greater pressure of the left ventricle during contraction (systole). (A miter is a two cusp hat worn by bishops in the Catholic church. Someone thought they looked like the left AV valve, hence mitral.)

3. Aortic (semilunar) valve: the three semilunar cusps attached to the aortic fibrous ring in the origin of the aorta.

4. Pulmonary (semilunar) valve: the valve between the conus of the right ventricle and the pulmonary trunk. It is similar to the aortic valve, but of lighter construction.

Memory aid: for the common names of the AV valves: "tri before you bi". This is related to the direction of flow through the heart.

"SKELETON" OF THE HEART: the connective tissue skeleton separating the atria from the ventricles and supplying attachments for the heart valves. It contains cartilage in all the species and two bones (ossa cordis) in the ox and older horses.

403

HEART AUSCULTATION (aws-kul-TAY-shun): listening to heart sounds. Heart sounds are caused by the closing of the different heart valves. Ventricle contraction (systole) causes a rise in ventricular pressure and closure of the AV valves (1st heart sound) and opening of the aortic and pulmonic valves. During ventricular relaxation (diastole), the AV valves open and the aortic and pulmonic (semilunar) valves close (2nd heart sound) due to back pressure in the aorta and pulmonary trunk.

• **Systole**: contraction of the ventricles; occurs between the 1st and 2nd heart sound.

• **Diastole**: relaxation of the ventricles; occurs between the 2nd and 1st heart sounds.

• **1st heart sound** ("lub"): caused by the closure of the AV valves.

• **2nd heart sound** ("dub"): caused by the closure of the semilunar valves (aortic and pulmonic).

LOCATION of the HEART (in most species): from the 2nd or 3rd ICS (intercostal space) to the 5th or 6th ICS and from the sternum about 2/3 of the way up the thorax. The olecranon is located at the 5th ICS in the normal standing animal, therefore, there is very little heart caudal to the arm. To auscultate the heart you need to press up between the triceps brachii muscle and thoracic wall.

• **Tip of the olecranon process**: at the level of the 5th intercostal space when the animal is standing in a normal square position.

POINT OF MAXIMUM INTENSITY (PMI) or puncta maxima: the point on the thoracic wall where a valve sound is loudest. Put the stethoscope at the points listed below and move to find the PMI.

• **Left AV valve**: the left 5th ICS at the level of the olecranon (low).

• **Pulmonic valve**: the left 3rd ICS at the level of the olecranon (low).

• **Aortic valve**: the left 4th ICS at the level of the shoulder (high).

• **Right AV valve**: the right 4th ICS at the level of the olecranon (low).

P^{A}M -3^{4}5: a **memory aid** for the PMI of the valves on the left side of the chest. P, A, M stands for the pulmonic, aortic and mitral valves respectively, and 3, 4, 5 stands for the intercostal spaces where they are found. The staggered positions indicate high or low in each respective spaces.

HEART MURMURS: abnormal sounds caused by bloodflow turbulence, due to valvular or nonvalvular problems.

Valvular murmur: a sound due to a leaky or narrowed valve. To identify murmurs, first determined if the murmur is in systole or diastole. Then, find the PMI of the murmur to determine which valve is affected.

• **Leaky (insufficiency) murmur**: caused by turbulence due to backflow through a valve not fully closed.

• **Narrowing (stenosis) murmur**: a constriction of the opening causing a turbulence past that opening.

• **Systolic murmur**: occurs between the 1st and 2nd heart sounds, when the AV valves should be fully closed and the aortic and pulmonic valves open.

  - **AV leaky (insufficiency)**: systolic murmur (left AV insufficiency is the most common).

  - **Aortic or pulmonic narrowing (stenosis)**: systolic murmur (aortic stenosis is more common, but rare).

• **Diastolic murmur**: occurs between the 2nd and 1st heart sounds, when the aortic and pulmonic valves should be closed and the AV valves opened (AV stenosis or semilunar valve insufficiency).

  - **AV narrowing (stenosis)**: a diastolic murmur (very rare).

  - **Aortic** or **pulmonic leaking (insufficiency)**: a diastolic murmur (rare).

• **Non-valvular murmurs**:

  - **PDA (patent ductus arteriosus)**: a failure of the fetal ductus arteriosus (arterial duct) to close. The resulting murmur sounds like a washing machine. It is continuous, thus, systolic and diastolic.

  - **Interatrial septal defect** (patent foramen ovale): failure of the opening (oval foramen) between the two fetal atria to close.

  - **Interventricular septal defect (ISD)**: failure of the inter ventricular septum to close. It results in a systolic murmur heard loudest on the right side near the sternum.

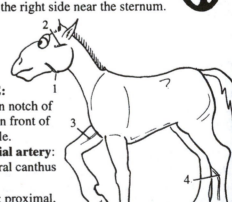

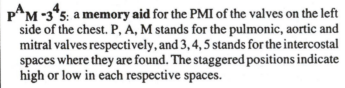

PULSE - HORSE:
1. **Facial artery**: in notch of the mandible just in front of the masseter muscle.
2. **Transverse facial artery**: just caudal to lateral canthus of eye.
3. **Median artery**: proximal, medial side of forearm.
4. **Great metatarsal artery**: between the McIII and Mc IV of the hindlimb.
5. **Digital artery**

CIRCULATION

Fig. IX-40 - Ox
- Rt. thoracic cavity (schematic)

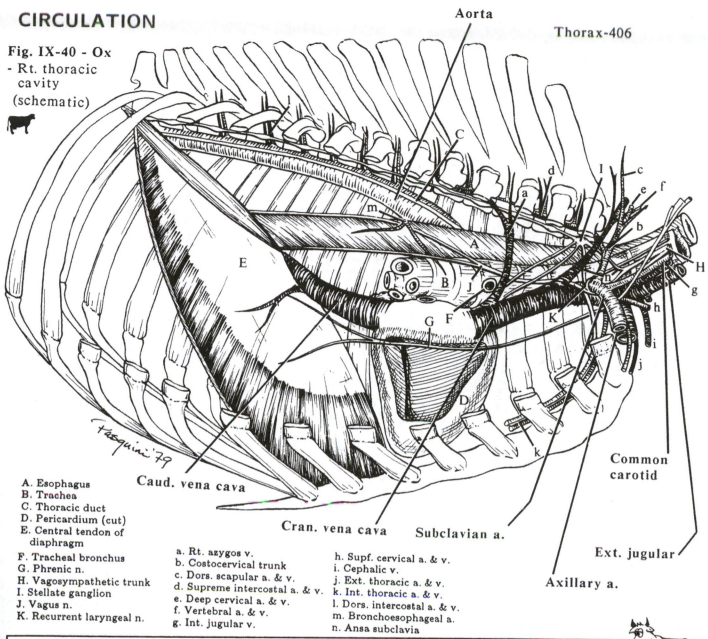

Aorta

Caud. vena cava

Cran. vena cava   Subclavian a.

Common carotid

Ext. jugular

Axillary a.

A. Esophagus
B. Trachea
C. Thoracic duct
D. Pericardium (cut)
E. Central tendon of diaphragm
F. Tracheal bronchus
G. Phrenic n.
H. Vagosympathetic trunk
I. Stellate ganglion
J. Vagus n.
K. Recurrent laryngeal n.

a. Rt. azygos v.
b. Costocervical trunk
c. Dors. scapular a. & v.
d. Supreme intercostal a. & v.
e. Deep cervical a. & v.
f. Vertebral a. & v.
g. Int. jugular v.

h. Supf. cervical a. & v.
i. Cephalic v.
j. Ext. thoracic a. & v.
k. Int. thoracic a. & v.
l. Dors. intercostal a. & v.
m. Bronchoesophageal a.
n. Ansa subclavia

HEART WORMS (dirofilariasis): adult round worms (nematodes - *Dirofilaria immitis*) of the dog live in the right ventricle, causing a great strain on the right side of the heart. This results in enlargement of the right ventricle, pulmonary trunk and pulmonary arteries due to increased pressure required to pump blood through the worm mass, thus, increasing the work load.

Cardiomyopathy
• Primary or idiopathic cardiomyopathies: result in progressive cardiac disease and affect mainly cats and dogs.
  - Hypertrophic cardiomyopathy: an enlarged, thickened heart occuring frequently in cats
  - Dilatative or congestive cardiomyopathy: an enlarged dilated heart causing conjestive heart failure in cats and dogs. Rare, it's the only significant cardiomyopathy in lg. animals.

Myocarditis: inflammation of the heart muscle.

Traumatic reticulopericarditis: uncommon result of hardware disease when a wire from reticulum penetrates the pericardium.

White muscle disease: selenium or vitamin E deficiency affecting cardiac and skeletal muscle mainly in cattle.

High mountain disease: cattle at high altitudes have extra stress on the heart which can lead to heart failure.

Bacterial endocarditis: bacterial vegetative growths on the heart valves.

Atrial fibrillation: in horses and cattle associated with gastrointestinal diseases.

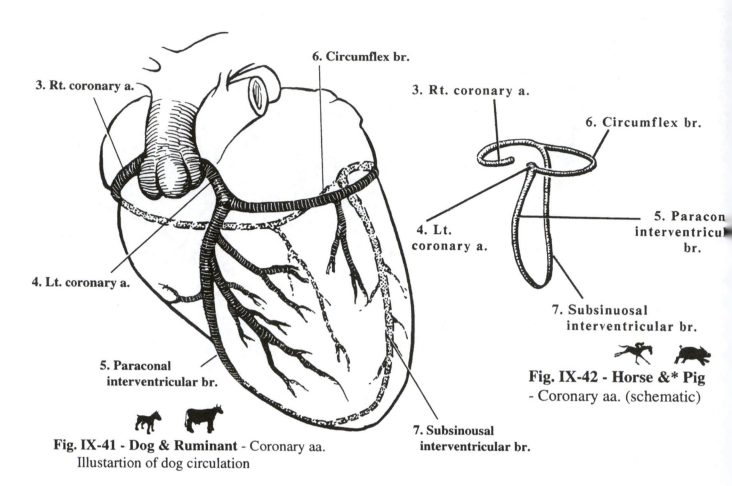

6. Circumflex br.

3. Rt. coronary a.

4. Lt. coronary a.

5. Paraconal interventricular br.

Fig. IX-41 - Dog & Ruminant - Coronary aa.
Illustartion of dog circulation

3. Rt. coronary a.

6. Circumflex br.

4. Lt. coronary a.

5. Paracon interventricul br.

7. Subsinuosal interventricular br.

Fig. IX-42 - Horse &* Pig
- Coronary aa. (schematic)

7. Subsinousal interventricular br.

AORTA: the great artery leaving the left ventricle and arching caudally. It sends oxygenated blood from the left heart to the heart itself and to the rest of the body through its systemic branches. The aorta is divided into the ascending aorta, aortic arch and descending aorta. The descending aorta has thoracic and abdominal segments.

1. ASCENDING AORTA: the initial part of the aorta, originating from the left ventricle at the center of the heart's base.

2. Aortic sinuses: the pockets between the aortic valve's cusps and the vessel wall. Right and left coronary arteries arise from the cranial and left sinuses, respectively.

Coronary (KOR-oh-na-ree) **arteries** (L. *corona*, crown): the arteries encircling the base of the heart like a crown. These are the first branches off the aorta.

3. Right coronary artery: originates from the right aortic sinus. It courses cranially under the right auricle and then to the right in the coronary groove. In some species it continues as the subsinuousal interventricular branch (horse and pig).

4. Left coronary artery: arising from the left aortic sinus, it courses to the left under the left auricle and immediately branches into descending (paraconal) and encircling (circumflex) branches.

In some species, the circumflex branch, after reaching the heart's right side, descends as the subsinuosal interventricular branch.

5. Paraconal interventricular branch: the descending branch of the left coronary artery in the paraconal interventricular groove.

6. Circumflex branch: the branch of the left coronary artery coursing in the coronary groove from the left to the right side of the heart.

7. Subsinuosal interventricular branch: the descending artery in the subsinuosal interventricular groove. This branch is derived from either the right coronary artery or the circumflex branch of the left coronary artery, depending on the species.

SPECIES DIFFERENCES:

Dog and **ruminants**: the left coronary artery gives rise to both the paraconal and subsinuosal interventricular branches.

Horse and **pig**: the rt. coronary artery gives rise to the subsinuosal interventricular branch.

Cat: the subsinuosal interventricular branch can arise from <u>either</u> coronary artery, but usually arises from the circumflex branch of the left coronary artery, as in the dog and ruminants.

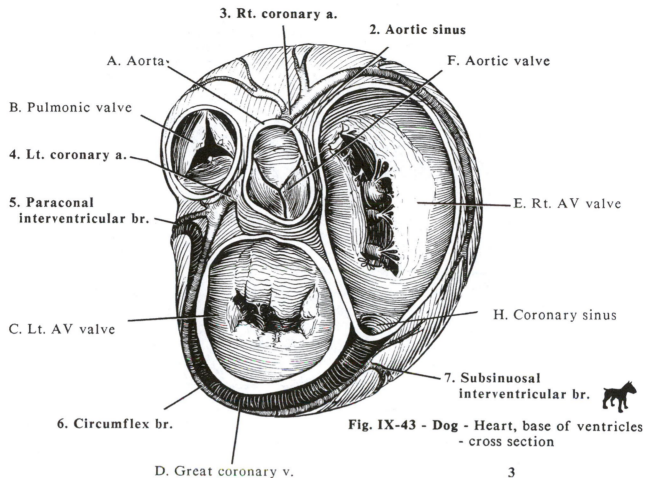

3. Rt. coronary a.

2. Aortic sinus

A. Aorta

F. Aortic valve

B. Pulmonic valve

4. Lt. coronary a.

**5. Paraconal
interventricular br.**

E. Rt. AV valve

C. Lt. AV valve

H. Coronary sinus

**7. Subsinuosal
interventricular br.**

6. Circumflex br.

**Fig. IX-43 - Dog - Heart, base of ventricles
- cross section**

D. Great coronary v.

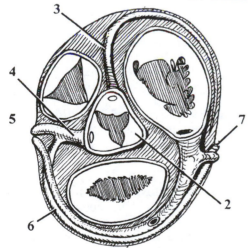

**Fig. IX-44 - Ox - Heart, base of
ventricles - cross section**

A. Aorta   E. Rt. AV valve
B. Pulmonic valve   F. Aortic valve
C. Lt. AV valve   G. Nodule
D. Great coronary v. H. Coronary sinus

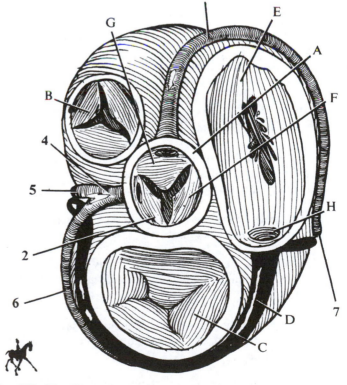

**Fig. IX-45 - Horse - Heart, base of ventricles
- cross section**

407

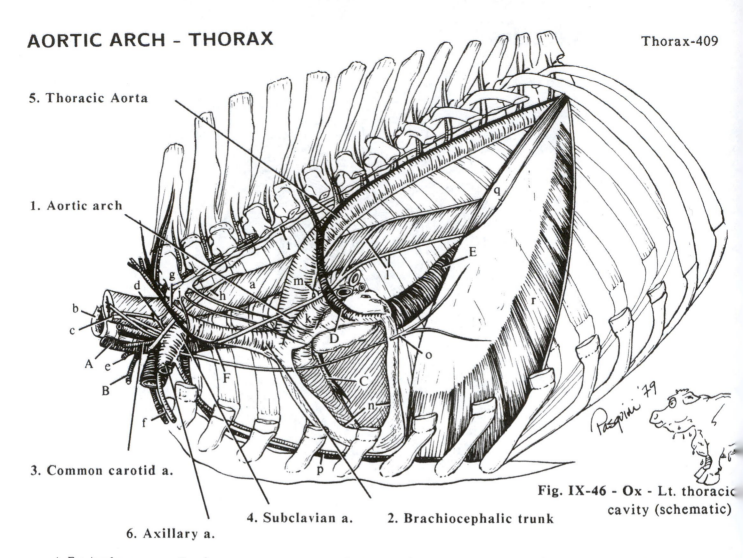

5. Thoracic Aorta

1. Aortic arch

3. Common carotid a.

4. Subclavian a.   **2. Brachiocephalic trunk**

6. Axillary a.

Fig. IX-46 - Ox - Lt. thoracic cavity (schematic)

A. Ext. jugular v.	a. Esophagus	g. Costocervical trunk	m. Recurrent laryngeal n.
B. Cephalic v.	b. Trachea	h. Thoracic duct	n. Pericardium (cut)
C. Paraconal br.	c. Vagosympathetic trunk	i. Sympathetic trunk	o. Phrenic nerve
D. Lt. azygos v.	d. Middle cervical ganglion	j. Cervicothoracic (stellate) ganglion	p. Internal thoracic a. & v.
E. Caud. vena cava	e. Superficial cervical a. & v.	k. Pulmonary trunk	q. Crus of diaphragm
F. Cran. vena cava	f. External thoracic a. & v.	l. Vagus nerve	r. Costal part of diaphragm

1. AORTIC ARCH: the continuation of the ascending aorta, it sends branches to the head, neck, and thoracic limbs.

2. Brachiocephalic trunk: the first branch of the aortic arch, present in all the domestic species. It gives rise to the common carotid artery and the right subclavian artery.

3. Right and **left common carotid arteries:** ascend the neck to supply the head, face, and brain.

4. Right and **left subclavian arteries:** supply the neck, thoracic limb, and the cranial portion of the thoracic wall. Each has many branches:

• Vertebral artery: the first branch off either subclavian artery. It courses cranially to pass through the transverse canal of the cervical vertebrae.

• Costocervical trunk: arises near and lateral to the vertebral artery. Its branches can include the deep cervical, dorsal scapular, supreme intercostal (thoracic vertebral in the dog) and vertebral arteries.

• Superficial cervical artery: arises near the thoracic inlet and runs onto the superficial neck in front of the shoulder.

• Internal thoracic artery: arises opposite the superficial cervical artery and passes on the floor of the thorax.

DESCENDING AORTA: the part of the aorta caudal to the aortic arch, divided into the thoracic aorta and the abdominal aorta by the diaphragm.

5. Thoracic aorta: the division of the descending aorta in the thoracic cavity. It helps supply the thoracic wall via the dorsal intercostal arteries.

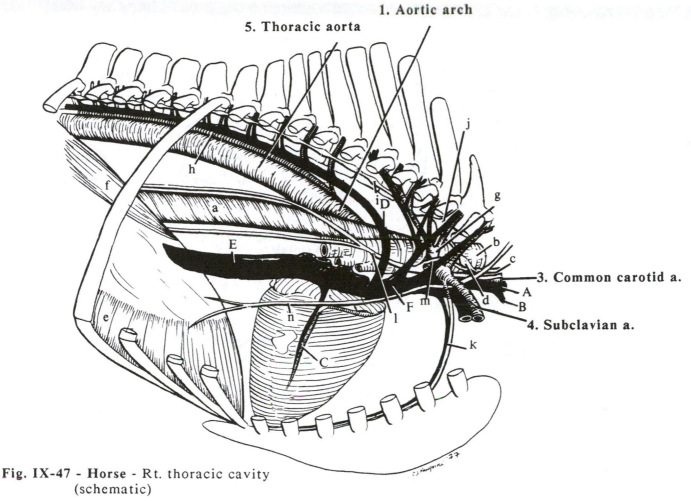

1. Aortic arch

5. Thoracic aorta

3. Common carotid a.

4. Subclavian a.

Fig. IX-47 - Horse - Rt. thoracic cavity (schematic)

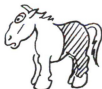

A Ext. jugular v
B Cephalic v.
C. Subsinuosal interventricular
   br. of rt. coronary a. (horse)
D. Azygos v.
E Caud. vena cava
F. Cran. vena cava

a. Esophagus
b. Trachea
c. Vagosymphathetic trunk
d. Middle cervical ganglion
e. Costal part of diaphragm
f. Crus of diaphragm
g. Costocervical trunk

h. Thoracic duct
i. Sympathetic trunk
j. Cervicothoracic (stellate) ganglion
k. Int. thoracic a.
l. Vagus n.
m. Recurrent laryngeal n.
n. Phrenic n.

SPECIES DIFFERENCES

Common carotid arteries: dogs – arise separately; ungulates (hooved animals) – arise by a short, common **bicarotid trunk**.

Branches of the aortic arch:

Carnivores and **pig:** brachiocephalic and left subclavian arteries arise separately from the aortic arch.

Horse and **ruminants:** only the brachiocephalic artery arises from the aortic arch. Both subclavian arteries arise from the brachiocephalic trunk.

Subclavian arteries: branches (vertebral, costocervical, deep cervical, superficial cervical and internal thoracic) vary in their origins between the species:

• **Ruminant:** the vertebral artery arises from the costocervical trunk, thus, the subclavian arteries have only three branches.

• **Carnivores:** the vertebral and costocervical arteries arise separately, thus, the subclavian arteries have four branches.

• **Horse:** the same as the dog on the right - four branches. On the left the deep cervical artery arises from the subclavian, not the costocervical trunk and, thus, the left subclavian has five branches.

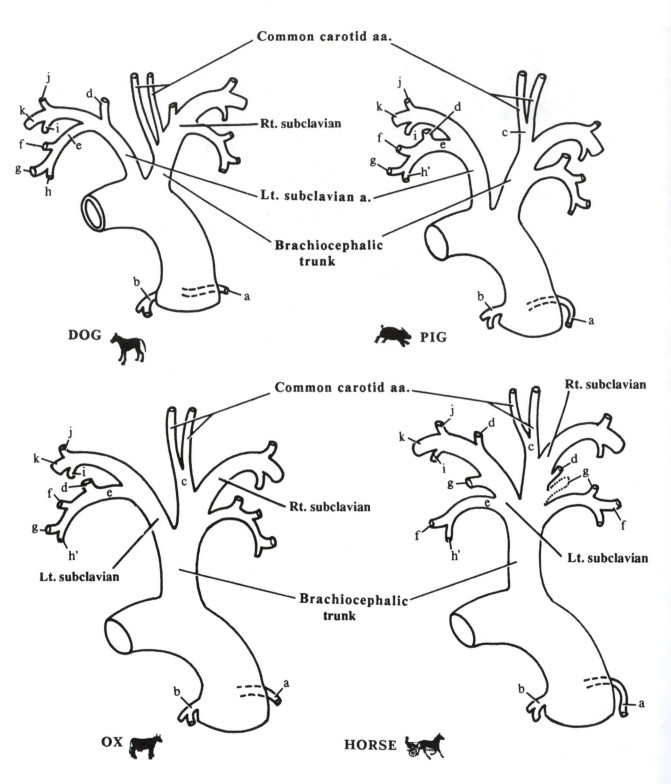

Fig. IX-48-51 - Branches of the Aortic Arch

a. Rt. coronary a.
b. Lt. coronary a.
c. Bicarotid trunk
   (ungulates)
d. Vertebral a.

e. Costocervical trunk
f. Dorsal scapular a.
g. Deep cervical a.
h. Thoracic vertebral a.
   h' Supreme intercostal a.

i. Internal thoracic a.
j. Supf. cervical a.
k. Axillary a.

Fig. IX-52 - Horse - Arteries to neck

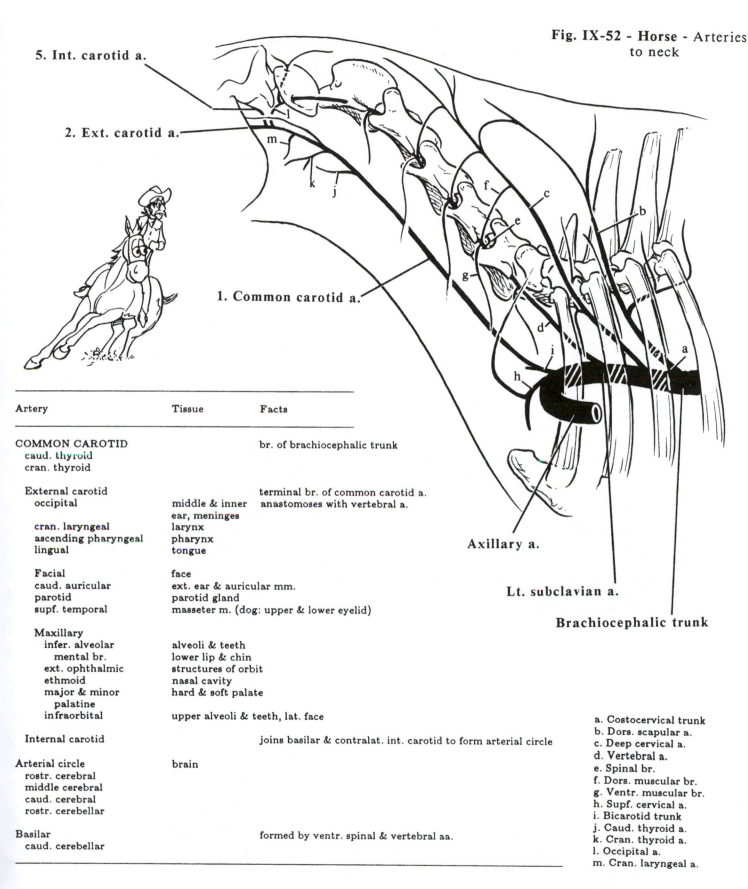

5. Int. carotid a.

2. Ext. carotid a.

1. Common carotid a.

Axillary a.

Lt. subclavian a.

Brachiocephalic trunk

Artery	Tissue	Facts
COMMON CAROTID		br. of brachiocephalic trunk
caud. thyroid		
cran. thyroid		
External carotid		terminal br. of common carotid a.
occipital	middle & inner ear, meninges	anastomoses with vertebral a.
cran. laryngeal	larynx	
ascending pharyngeal	pharynx	
lingual	tongue	
Facial	face	
caud. auricular	ext. ear & auricular mm.	
parotid	parotid gland	
supf. temporal	masseter m. (dog: upper & lower eyelid)	
Maxillary		
infer. alveolar	alveoli & teeth	
mental br.	lower lip & chin	
ext. ophthalmic	structures of orbit	
ethmoid	nasal cavity	
major & minor palatine	hard & soft palate	
infraorbital	upper alveoli & teeth, lat. face	
Internal carotid		joins basilar & contralat. int. carotid to form arterial circle
Arterial circle	brain	
rostr. cerebral		
middle cerebral		
caud. cerebral		
rostr. cerebellar		
Basilar		formed by ventr. spinal & vertebral aa.
caud. cerebellar		

a. Costocervical trunk
b. Dors. scapular a.
c. Deep cervical a.
d. Vertebral a.
e. Spinal br.
f. Dors. muscular br.
g. Ventr. muscular br.
h. Supf. cervical a.
i. Bicarotid trunk
j. Caud. thyroid a.
k. Cran. thyroid a.
l. Occipital a.
m. Cran. laryngeal a.

411

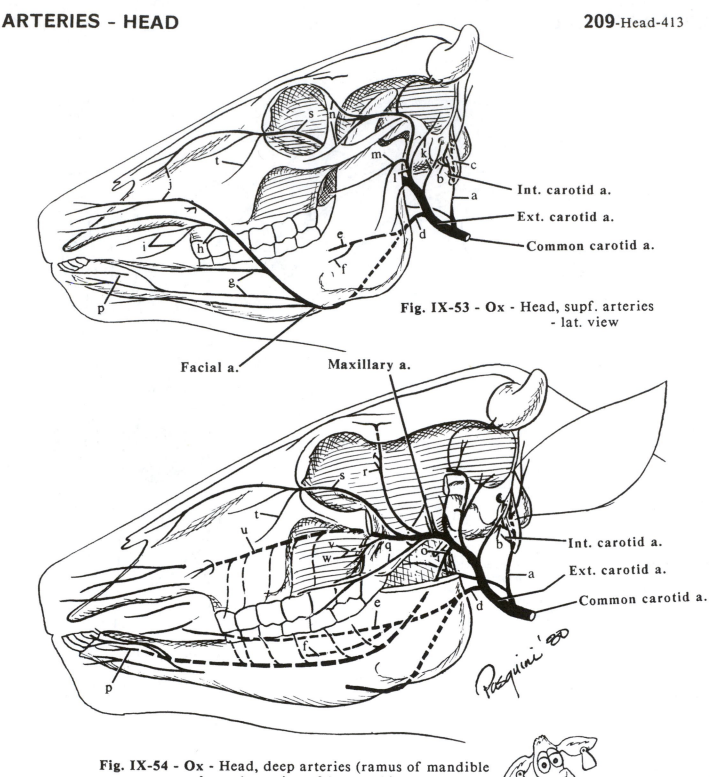

Int. carotid a.

Ext. carotid a.

Common carotid a.

**Fig. IX-53 - Ox - Head, supf. arteries
- lat. view**

Facial a.

Maxillary a.

Int. carotid a.

Ext. carotid a.

Common carotid a.

**Fig. IX-54 - Ox - Head, deep arteries (ramus of mandible
& caud. portion of bony orbit removed)
- lat. view**

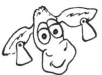

a. Occipital a.
b. Middle meningeal a.
c. Condylar a.
d. Linguofacial trunk
e. Lingual a.
f. Sublingual a.
g. Inferior labial a.
h. Supf. labial a.

i. Angularis oris a.
j. Nasal aa.
k. Auricular aa.
l. Supf. temporal a.
m. Transverse facial a.
n. Palpebral aa.
o. Inferior alveolar a.
p. Mental a.

q. Buccal a.
r. Ext. ophthalmic a.
s. Malar a.
t. Angularis oculi a.
u. Infraorbital a.
v. Sphenopalatine a.
w. Palatine aa.

A. Ventr. spinal aa.
B. Caud. cerebellar a.
C. Rostr. cerebellar a.
D. Caud. cerebral a.
E. Caud. communicating br.
F. Rostr. cerebral a.
G. Middle cerebral a.
H. Olfactory bulb
I. Optic nerve
J. Cerebral hemisphere
K. Pons
L. Cerebellum
M. Medulla oblongata

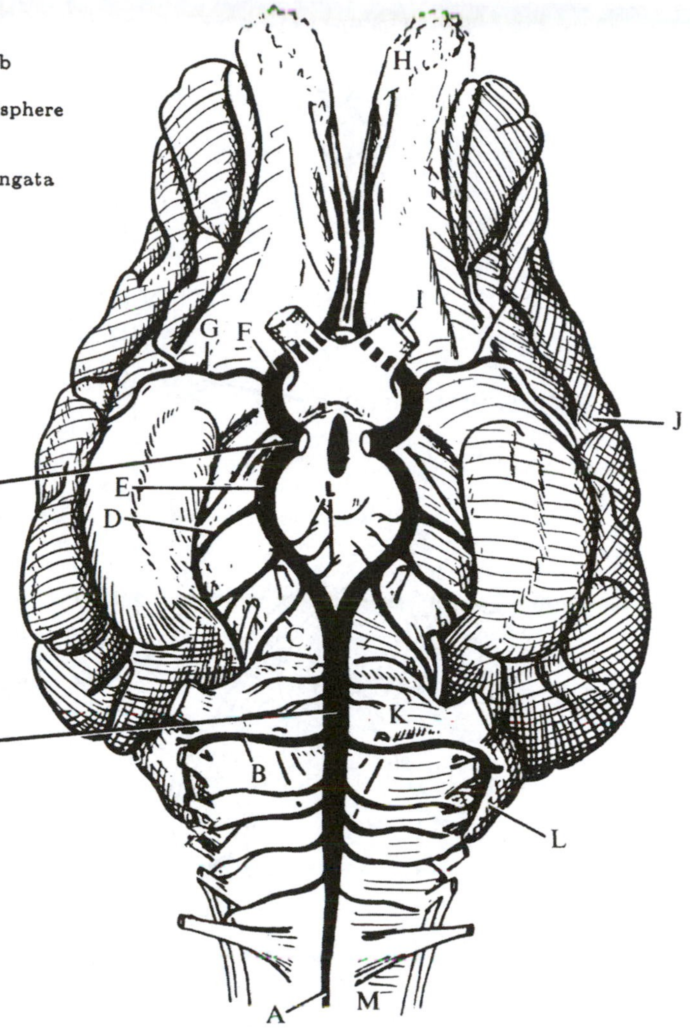

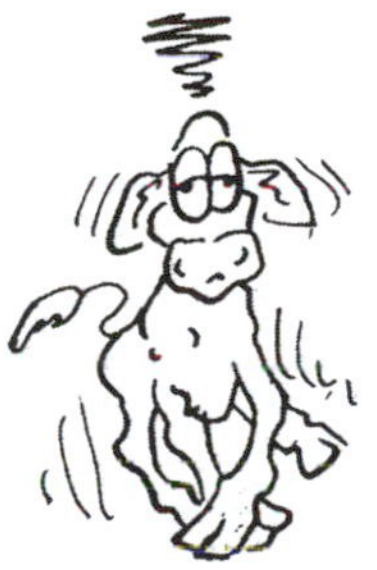

1. COMMON CAROTID ARTERIES (right and left): arise separately or together (bicarotid trunk) from the brachiocephalic trunk. They ascend the neck with the vagosympathetic trunk to terminate in the internal and external carotid arteries supplying the head, face, and brain. The thyroid and laryngeal arteries are the only branches of the common carotid arteries.

2. External carotid artery: the large, direct continuation of the common carotid artery that becomes the maxillary artery. Its first small branch is the occipital artery. It terminates by first giving off a caudal auricular artery and then branching into superficial temporal and maxillary arteries.

3. Linguofacial artery or separate lingual and facial arteries: branch(es) of the external carotid artery. The facial artery winds around the ventral border of the mandible to supply the face.

5. Int. carotid a.

7. Basilar a.

Fig. IX-55 - Ox - Blood supply to brain

4. Maxillary artery: the direct continuation of the external carotid artery to the space below the orbit (the pterygopalatine fossa). Its branches supply the orbit, teeth, chin, nose, nasal cavity and palate.

5. Internal carotid artery: the smaller terminal branch of the common carotid artery. It enters the cranial cavity, joining the basilar artery to form the arterial circle. It has an enlargement, the carotid sinus, near its origin.

6. Arterial circle (circulus arteriosus cerebri, circle of Willis): located ventral to the hypothalamus encircling the infundibular stalk. It is formed by the paired internal carotid arteries and the basilar artery. It supplies the brain.

7. Basilar artery: arises from the vertebral artery and ventral spinal artery.

Blood brain barrier: inability of most substances to cross the capillaries of nervous tissue due to tight connections between the capillary endothelial cells.

VENOUS DRAINAGE OF THE HEAD

Maxillary and **linguofacial veins** join to form the **external jugular vein**. The external jugular veins and **subclavian veins** join to form the brachiocephalic vein in carnivores and pigs. The brachiocephalic veins then join to form the cranial vena cava. In horses and ruminants the external jugular veins and subclavian veins join to form the cranial vena cava.

SPECIES DIFFERENCES

Bicarotid trunk: in ungulates, the common origin of the two common carotid arteries (in carnivores they arise separately).

Internal carotid artery: in **cats** and **ruminants** the part outside the skull degenerates.

Linguofacial trunk: the common origin of the lingual and facial artery in horses and ruminants (in the carnivores and pig they arise separately).

413

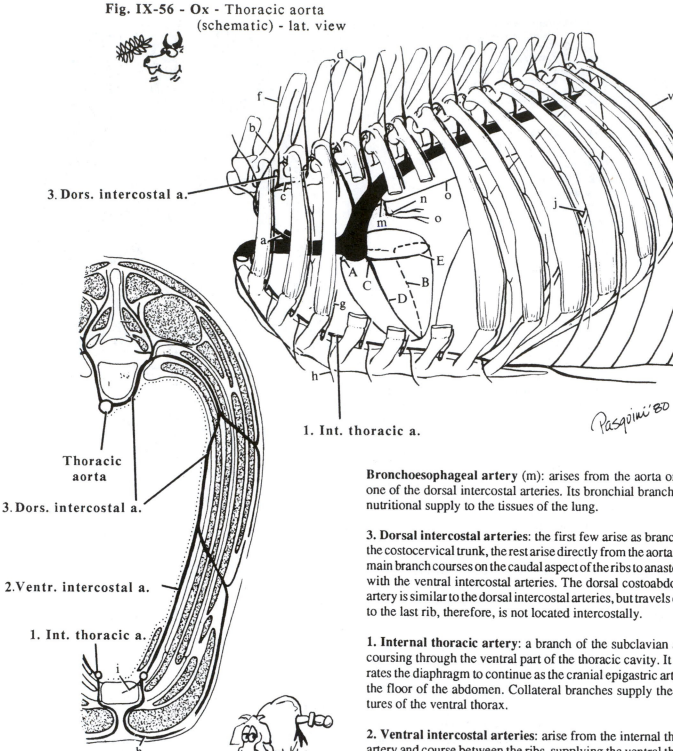

Fig. IX-56 - Ox - Thoracic aorta (schematic) - lat. view

3. Dors. intercostal a.

1. Int. thoracic a.

Pasquini '80

Thoracic aorta

3. Dors. intercostal a.

2. Ventr. intercostal a.

1. Int. thoracic a.

Fig. IX-57 - Ox - cross section (schematic)

Bronchoesophageal artery (m): arises from the aorta or from one of the dorsal intercostal arteries. Its bronchial branch is the nutritional supply to the tissues of the lung.

3. Dorsal intercostal arteries: the first few arise as branches of the costocervical trunk, the rest arise directly from the aorta. Their main branch courses on the caudal aspect of the ribs to anastomose with the ventral intercostal arteries. The dorsal costoabdominal artery is similar to the dorsal intercostal arteries, but travels caudal to the last rib, therefore, is not located intercostally.

1. Internal thoracic artery: a branch of the subclavian artery, coursing through the ventral part of the thoracic cavity. It perforates the diaphragm to continue as the cranial epigastric artery on the floor of the abdomen. Collateral branches supply the structures of the ventral thorax.

2. Ventral intercostal arteries: arise from the internal thoracic artery and course between the ribs, supplying the ventral thoracic wall.

> **CLINICAL**
>
> **Intercostal vessels** and **nerves**: in all species course on the caudal aspects of the ribs. Therefore, an incision to open the thoracic wall (intercostal incision) is made in the middle of the intercostal space.

Fig. IX-58 - Horse - lat. view (schematic)

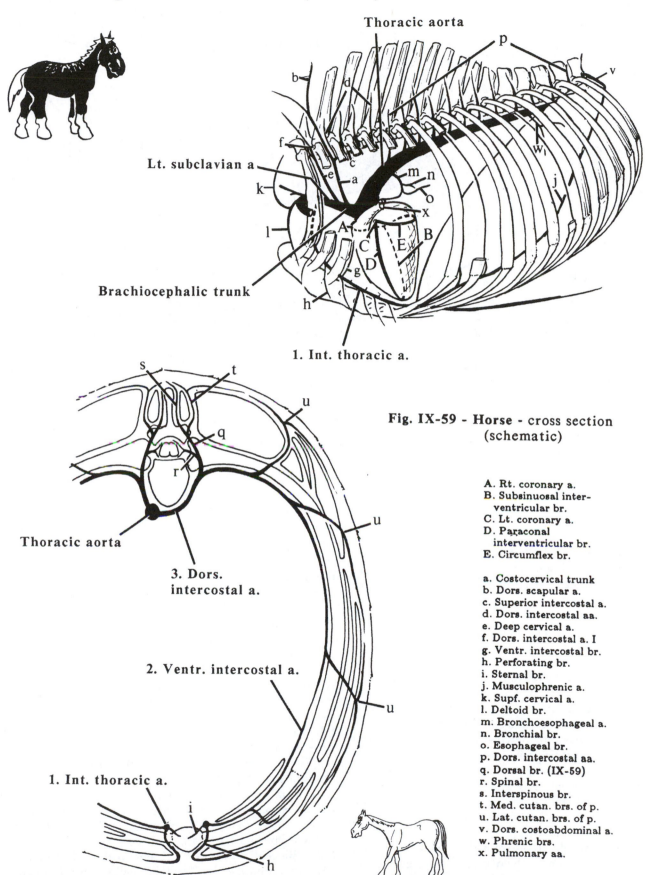

Thoracic aorta

Lt. subclavian a

Brachiocephalic trunk

1. Int. thoracic a.

Thoracic aorta

3. Dors. intercostal a.

2. Ventr. intercostal a.

1. Int. thoracic a.

Fig. IX-59 - Horse - cross section (schematic)

A. Rt. coronary a.
B. Subsinuosal inter-
   ventricular br.
C. Lt. coronary a.
D. Paraconal
   interventricular br.
E. Circumflex br.

a. Costocervical trunk
b. Dors. scapular a.
c. Superior intercostal a.
d. Dors. intercostal aa.
e. Deep cervical a.
f. Dors. intercostal a. I
g. Ventr. intercostal br.
h. Perforating br.
i. Sternal br.
j. Musculophrenic a.
k. Supf. cervical a.
l. Deltoid br.
m. Bronchoesophageal a.
n. Bronchial br.
o. Esophageal br.
p. Dors. intercostal aa.
q. Dorsal br. (IX-59)
r. Spinal br.
s. Interspinous br.
t. Med. cutan. brs. of p.
u. Lat. cutan. brs. of p.
v. Dors. costoabdominal a.
w. Phrenic brs.
x. Pulmonary aa.

AORTIC BRANCHES - 1

I. Dog, **Thoracic arteries**, lateral view, schematic.

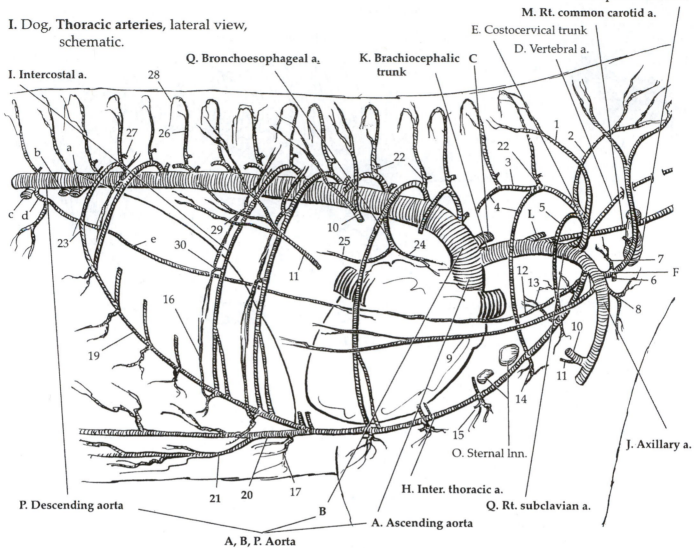

G. Supf. cervical lnn.
M. Rt. common carotid a.
E. Costocervical trunk
D. Vertebral a.
K. Brachiocephalic C
trunk

Q. Bronchoesophageal a.

I. Intercostal a.   28

1 2
22
3
4 L 5
22
10
25 24
12 7
13 6 F
11 8
10
9 11
16
14
19 15
O. Sternal lnn.
J. Axillary a.

27 26
b a
c d
23 e 30
11
29

21 20 17 B H. Inter. thoracic a.
A. Ascending aorta Q. Rt. subclavian a.
P. Descending aorta A, B, P. Aorta

Left side: Aortic branches

A, B, J. Aorta: large unpaired artery coming out of the center of the base of the heart, to the right of the pulmonary trunk.

A. Ascending aorta: the short, first part of the aorta which passes craniodorsally. The right and left coronary arteries arise from the ascending aorta and will be discussed later.

B. Arch of the aorta: the caudal and left bend in the aorta distal to the ascending part.

C. Left subclavian a.: the 2nd branch off the aorta arch, it passes cranially out of the thorax to supply the thoracic limb as the axillary a. It has four branches: vertebral, costocervical trunk, **internal thoracic** and superficial cervical aa.

D. Vertebral a.: a branch of the subclavian a., it arises medially to the costocervical trunk. Travelling with the vertebral n. toward the neck, they enter the transverse canal of the cervical vertebrae. The vertebral a. usually arises before the costocervical trunk.

E. Costocervical trunk: arises from the subclavian a. and extends dorsally to supply the neck, shoulder and cranial costal regions.

F. Superficial cervical a.: arises from the subclavian a., opposite the internal thoracic a., it travels over the superficial area of the neck near the superficial cervical lymph nodes (seen while dissecting the thoracic limb).

G. Superficial cervical lnn.: the large group of lymph nodes located cranially to the shoulder, under the omotransversarius and brachiocephalicus mm.

H. Internal thoracic a.: one of the four branches of the subclavian a. that arises near the first rib and travels inside the ventral thorax.

I. Intercostal a.: are formed by the anastomoses of ventral intercostal a. of the internal thoracic and musculophrenic aa. and the dorsal intercostal a. of the costocervical trunk and aorta. They pass on the caudal border of the ribs in the intercostal spaces with like named veins and nerves.

J. Axillary a.: the direct continuation of the subclavian a. past the first rib to supply the thoracic limb (already cut off with the limb).

K. Brachiocephalic trunk: first branch of the arch of the aorta. As its name implies, it extends cranially to supply the right

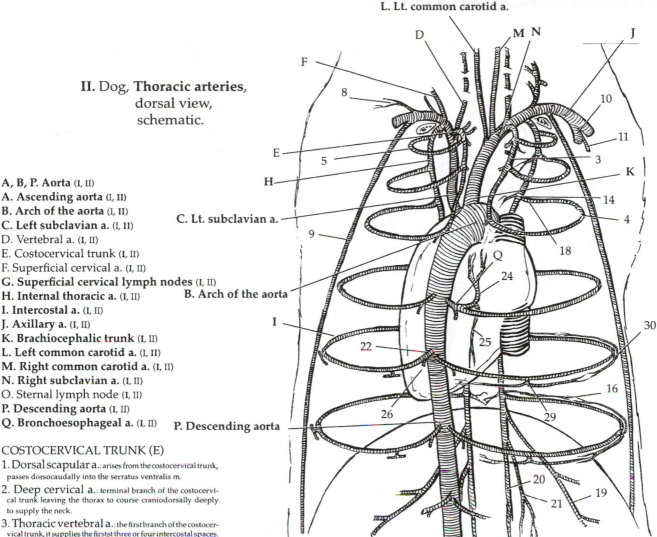

II. Dog, Thoracic arteries, dorsal view, schematic.

L. Lt. common carotid a.

C. Lt. subclavian a.

B. Arch of the aorta

P. Descending aorta

A, B, P. Aorta (I, II)
A. Ascending aorta (I, II)
B. Arch of the aorta (I, II)
C. Left subclavian a. (I, II)
D. Vertebral a. (I, II)
E. Costocervical trunk (I, II)
F. Superficial cervical a. (I, II)
G. Superficial cervical lymph nodes (I, II)
H. Internal thoracic a. (I, II)
I. Intercostal a. (I, II)
J. Axillary a. (I, II)
K. Brachiocephalic trunk (I, II)
L. Left common carotid a. (I, II)
M. Right common carotid a. (I, II)
N. Right subclavian a. (I, II)
O. Sternal lymph node (I, II)
P. Descending aorta (I, II)
Q. Bronchoesophageal a. (I, II)

COSTOCERVICAL TRUNK (E)

1. Dorsal scapular a.: arises from the costocervical trunk, passes dorsocaudally into the serratus ventralis m.

2. Deep cervical a.: terminal branch of the costocervical trunk leaving the thorax to course craniodorsally deeply to supply the neck.

3. Thoracic vertebral a.: the first branch of the costocervical trunk, it supplies the firstst three or four intercostal spaces. It passes above the head of the ribs instead of beneath it.

4. Dorsal intercostal aa. 2-3 or 4: arise from a branch (thoracic vertebral a.) of the costocervical trunk.

5. First intercostal a.: arises from the costocervical trunk.

SUPERFICIAL CERVICAL A. (F)

6. Deltoid branch: a branch of the superficial cervical (occasionally the internal thoracic a.), it passes distally in the groove between the pectoral and brachiocephalicus mm.

7. Suprascapular a.: arises from the superficial cervical a., passes between the supraspinatus and subscapularis mm. with the like named nerve. It supplies the shoulder area.

AXILLARY A. (K)

8. External thoracic a.: first branch of the axillary a. to the superficial pectorals.

9. Lateral thoracic a.: branch of the axillary to the lateral thoracic wall (including axillary lymph node, latissimus dorsi, deep pectoral and cutaneous trunci mm. and cranial and caudal mammary glands).

10. Subscapular a.: arises from the axillary a. and passes dorsocaudally to become superficial near the caudal angle of the scapula.

11. Thoracodorsal a.: arises from the subscapular a. and passes caudally to the latissimus dorsi m. and skin.

INTERNAL THORACIC A. (H)

12. Pericardiophrenic a.: small; it arises from the internal thoracic a. and passes with the phrenic n. to the pericardium and then to the diaphragm. Bronchial branches may arise from the pericardiophrenic a. or internal thoracic a. to the root of the lungs, frequently absent.

13. Thymic branches: pass from the internal thoracic to the thymus.

14. Perforating branches: pass from the internal thoracic a. through interchondral space 2-6 or 7. They give off sternal and ventral cutaneous branches and mammary branches.

15. Sternal branches: pass from the perforating branches to the sternebrae.

16. Ventral cutaneous branches: continuation of the perforating branches of the internal thoracic a.

17. Mammary branches: pass to the mammary gland to developed glands.

18. Ventral intercostal aa.: the first eight arise from the internal thoracic a. and then from the musculophrenic a. They anastomose with the dorsal intercostal a. to form the intercostal a. that pass caudal to the ribs in the intercostal spaces with like named aa. and nn. They may be double in the intercostal spaces 2-10.

19. Musculophrenic a.: a terminal branch of the internal thoracic a., it arises near the eighth rib and passes dorsocaudally in the costodiaphragmatic space between the diaphragm and the costal wall and then pierces the diaphragm to continue along the connection of the diaphragm and the lateral abdominal wall. It gives off ventral intercostal aa. 9-12.

20. Cranial epigastric a.: large terminal branch of the internal thoracic a., arising near the eight intercostal space, perforates the diaphragm to continue on the deep surface of the rectus abdominus m.

21. Superficial cranial epigastric a.: arises in the abdomen from the cranial epigastric a., passes through the rectus abdominus to become superficial supplying the cranial mammary glands and anastomosing with the superficial caudal epigastric a.

AORTA and COSTOCERVICAL TRUNK

22. Dorsal intercostal aa.: the first three or four arise from the costocervical trunk (2nd-3rd or 4th from thoracic vertebral a.) the last eight or nine from the aorta. Those arising from the dorsal surface of the descending aorta start with the fourth or fifth pair. They travel distally on the caudal border of the ribs in the intercostal spaces to anastomose with ventral intercostal aa. of the internal thoracic a. forming the intercostal a.

23. Costoabdominal a.: courses along the caudal border of the last rib, and thus, not in an intercostal space and thus, not an intercostal a.

BRONCHOESOPHAGEAL A.

24. Bronchial branches: arise from the bronchoesophageal a. that supplies the tissue of the lung.

25. Esophageal branches: ascending and descending branches to the interthoracic part of the esophagus.

INTERCOSTAL A. (I)

26. Dorsal branch of the intercostal a.: pass dorsally to the epaxial mm. and end in dorsal cutaneous branches of the skin.

27. Spinal branch: enter the spinal canal through the intervertebral foramen. They divide into dorsal and ventral branches.

28. Dorsal cutaneous branches: supply the skin of the dorsum.

29. Proximal lateral cutaneous branches: branches of the intercostal a.

30. Distal lateral cutaneous branches: branches of the intercostal a., it passes ventral to the latissimus dorsi m. through the cutaneous trunci m. and end in a short dorsal and long ventral branch. They are accompanied by satellite vv. and cutaneous nn.

DESCENDING AORTA (M)

a. Celiac a.
b. Cranial mesenteric a.
c. Renal a.
d. Phrenicoabdominal a.
e. Phrenic a.

AORTIC BRANCHES - 3

Fig III: Branches of the aortic arch, lateral view, schematic

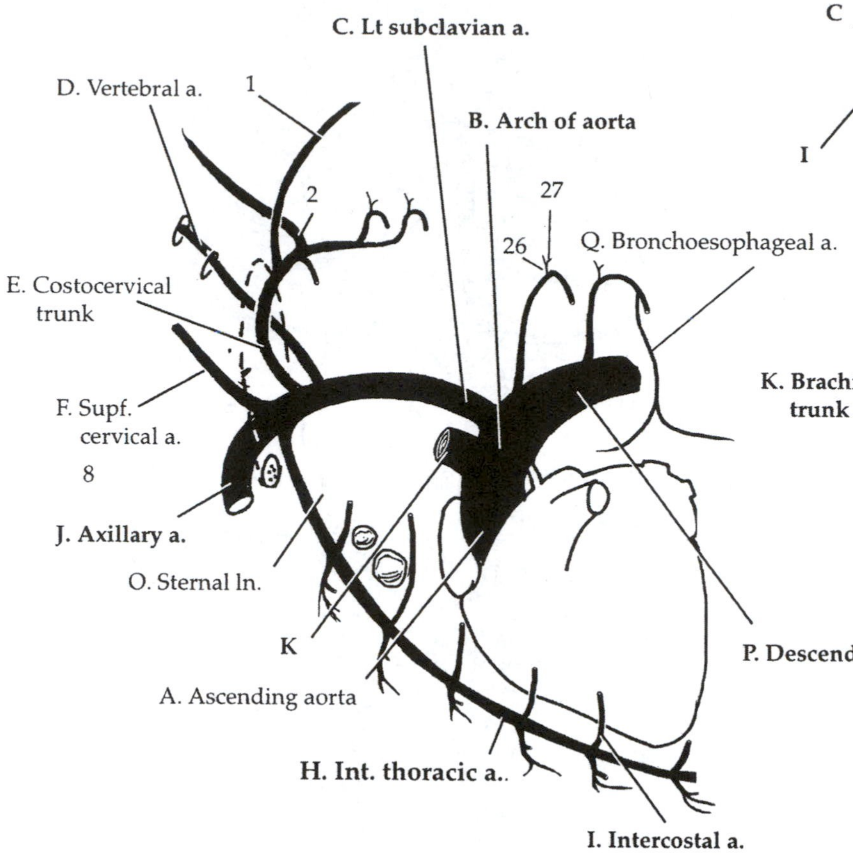

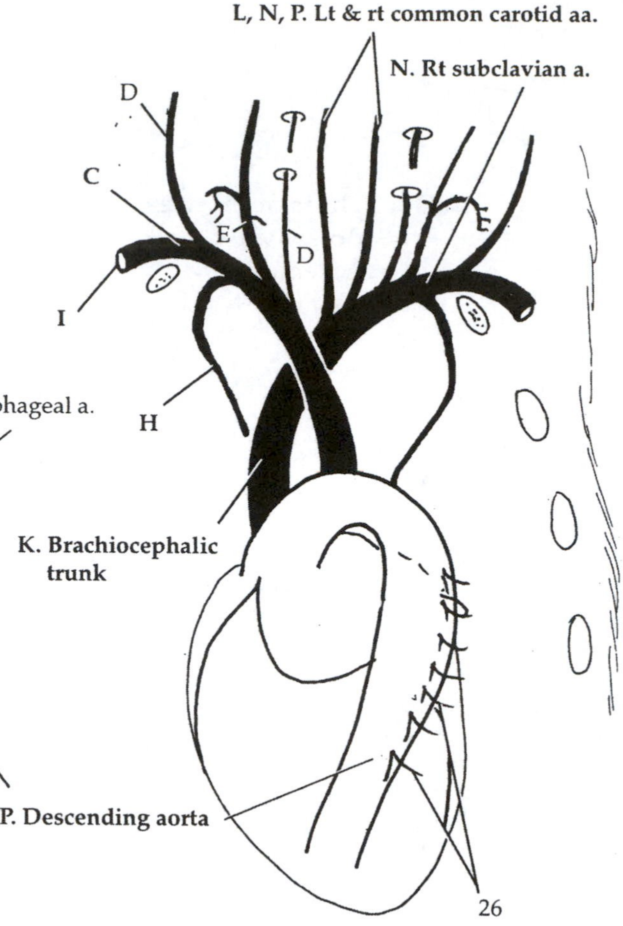

D. Vertebral a.

1

C. Lt subclavian a.

B. Arch of aorta

2

27

E. Costocervical trunk

26

Q. Bronchoesophageal a.

F. Supf. cervical a.

8

J. Axillary a.

O. Sternal ln.

K

A. Ascending aorta

H. Int. thoracic a..

I. Intercostal a.

L, N, P. Lt & rt common carotid aa.

N. Rt subclavian a.

D

C

E

D

I

H

E

K. Brachiocephalic trunk

P. Descending aorta

26

Fig IV: Branches of the aortic arch, dorsal view, schematic

limb, neck and head. The brachiocephalic trunk gives off the left common carotid a., then terminates in the right common carotid and right subclavian aa.

L. Left common carotid a.: extends up the neck with the left vagosympathetic trunk to the head.

M. Right common carotid a.: half of the terminal branch of the brachiocephalic trunk that extends to the head with the right vagosympathetic trunk.

N. Right subclavian a.: the other half of the terminal branch of the brachiocephalic trunk that extends around the first rib to the thoracic limb.

O. Sternal lymph node: located next to the cranial end of the internal thoracic a. before it dives under the transverse thoracis m.

P. Descending aorta: the part of the aorta distal to the arch of the aorta that travels caudally in the dorsal thorax. It is divided into thoracic (M^i) and abdominal (M^{ii}) parts by the diaphragm.

Q. Bronchoesophageal a.: variably arises from the 5th intercostal a. It is the main supply to the tissue of the lung via its bronchial branch. It also gives off a esophageal a. to the esophagus.

R. Cutaneous vessels: emerge with cutaneous nerves from the surface of the thorax and abdomen underneath the skin (if injected, they are red, blue, and white thin strands)

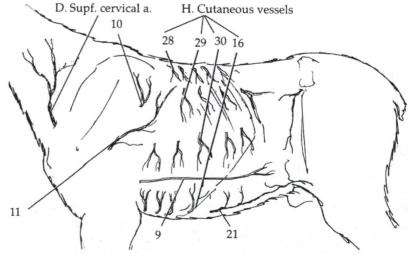

D. Supf. cervical a.

10

H. Cutaneous vessels

28   29 30 16

11

9   21

Fig V: Cutaneous vessels, lateral view

AORTIC BRANCHES - 4

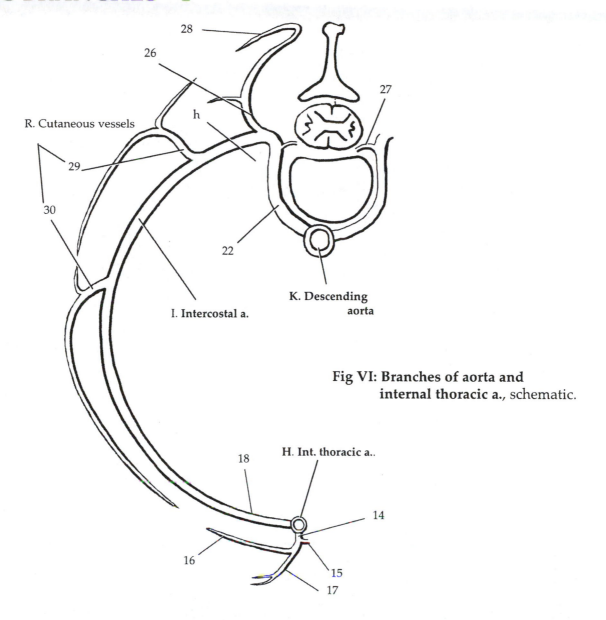

R. Cutaneous vessels

K. Descending aorta

I. Intercostal a.

Fig VI: Branches of aorta and internal thoracic a., schematic.

H. Int. thoracic a..

A, B, P. Aorta
A. Ascending aorta
B. Arch of the aorta
C. Left subclavian a.
D. Vertebral a.
E. Costocervical trunk
F. Superficial cervical a.
G. Superficial cervical lymph nodes
H. Internal thoracic a.
I. Intercostal a.
J. Axillary a.
K. Brachiocephalic trunk
L. Left common carotid a.
M. Right common carotid a.
N. Right subclavian a.
O. Sternal lymph node
P. Descending aorta
<u>**Q. Bronchoesophageal a.**</u>

COSTOCERVICAL TRUNK (B)
1. Dorsal scapular a.
2. Deep cervical a.
3. Thoracic vertebral a.
4. Dorsal intercostal aa. 2-3 or 4
5. First intercostal a.
SUPERFICIAL CERVICAL A.
6. Deltoid branch
7. Suprascapular a.
AXILLARY A. (K)
8. External thoracic a.
9. Lateral thoracia a.
10. Subscapular a.
11. Thoracodorsal a.
INTERNAL THORACIC A.
12. Pericardiophrenic a.
13. Thymic branches
14. Perforating branches
15. Sternal branches
16. Ventral cutaneous branches

17. Mammary branches
18. Ventral intercostal aa.
19. Musculophrenic a.
20. Cranial epigastric a.
21. Superficial cranial epigastric a.
AORTA & COSTOCERVICAL TRUNK
22. Dorsal intercostal aa.
23. Costoabdominal a.
BRONCHOESOPHAGEAL A.
24. Bronchial branches
25. Esophageal branches
INTERCOSTAL A. (I)
26. Dorsal branch of the intercostal a.
27. Spinal branch
28. Dorsal cutaneous branches
29. Proximal lateral cutaneous branches
30. Distal lateral cutaneous branches

VEINS - THORAX

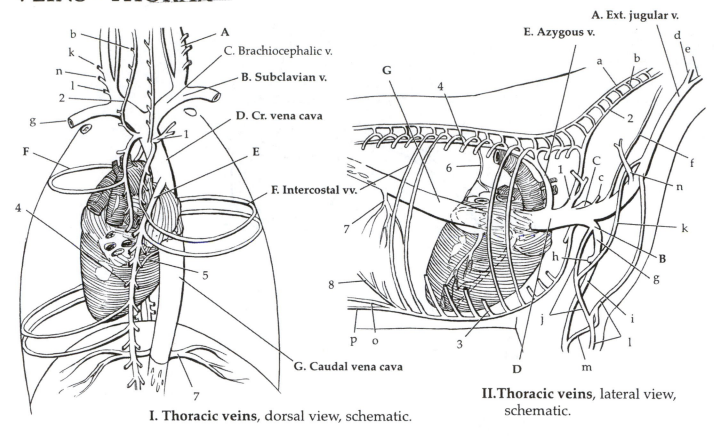

I. Thoracic veins, dorsal view, schematic.

II. Thoracic veins, lateral view, schematic.

1. **Costocervical trunk**: drain several branches - dorsal scapular, dorsal intercostal, deep cervical, supreme intercostal, and vertebral vv.

2. **Vertebral v.**: drains into the costocervical trunk and pass through the transverse vertebral foramens (canal) receiving intervertebral vv.

3. **Ventral intercostal vv.**: pass caudal to the ribs in the intercostal spaces with like named aa. and nn.

4. **Dorsal intercostal vv.**: except for the first three or four cranial ones, empty into the azygous or the hemizygous vv.

5. **Hemizygous v.**: very variable, if present, it lies to the left of the aorta and connects the caudal vena cava and the azygous v.

6. **Bronchoesophageal v.**: variable, passes with like named a. and empties into the azygous v. at the level of the seventh thoracic vertebrae.

7. **Phrenic vv.**: drains the diaphragm.

8. **Musculophrenic v.**

a. **Vertebral plexus**

b. **Intervertebral vv.**: drains the vertebral plexus into the vertebral v.

c. **Caudal thyroid v.**: unpaired v. that empties into where the brachiocephalic vv. merge.

d. **Maxillary v.**

e. **Linguofacial v.**

f. **Internal jugular v.**: tiny vessel in the carotid sheath with the common carotid a. and vagosympathetic trunk. It usually terminates in the terminal end of the external jugular v.

g. **Axillary v.**

h. **Subscapular v.**

i. **Brachial v.**

j. **Axillobrachial v.**

k. **Omobrachial v.**: from the thoracic limb, empties into the caudal end of the external jugular v.

l. **Cephalic v.**: from the thoracic limb, empties into the caudal end of the external jugular v.

m. **Median cubital v.**

n. **Superficial cervical v.**: empties into the external jugular v.

o. **Cranial epigastric v.**

p. **Superficial cranial epigastric v.**

A. External jugular v.: formed by the joining of the linguofacial and maxillary vv. just caudal to the head, it travels down the neck the thoracic inlet.

B. Subclavian v.: continuation of the axillary v. around the first rib. It joins the jugular v. to form the brachiocephalic v.

C. Brachiocephalic v.: formed by the subclavian and external jugular vv. The right and left brachiocephalic vv. join to form the cranial vena cava.

D. Cranial vena cava: the large vessel entering the right side of the heart cranially. It is formed by the joining of the brachiocephalic vv.

E. (Right) azygous v.: arising in the abdomen, it passes through the aortic hiatus and runs in the caudodorsal thorax between the aorta and vertebral bodies. Passing cranially, it arches around the root of the right lung to empty into the cranial vena cava or directly into the right atrium. It drains the dorsal intercostal vv. from both sides as far forward as the third or fourth intercostal spaces (carnivores do not have a left azygous like ruminants).

F. Intercostal vv.: pass caudal to the ribs in the intercostal spaces with like named aa. and nn. They are formed by dorsal and intercostal vv. from the azygous and internal thoracic vv. respectively.

G. Internal thoracic vv.: pass on the floor of the thorax receiving the ventral intercostal vv. Right and left internal thoracic vv. empty by a common trunk into the cranial vena cava.

H. Caudal vena cava: the large vessel entering the right side of the heart caudally returning blood from the abdomen and caudal body.

I. Cat, **Left thoracic limb arteries,**
medium view, schematic.

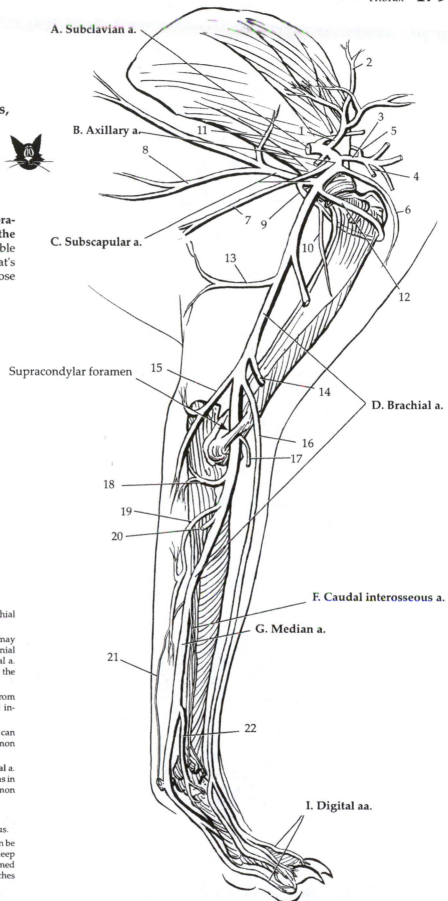

The cat's brachial a. passes through the supracondylar foramen, making it in danger if the
humerus is broken. Besides this and possible
variations of the interosseous vessels, the cat's
thoracic limb aa. are basically similar to those
of the dog.

A. SUBCLAVIAN A.
1. Costocervical trunk
2. Dorsal scapular a.
3. Superficial cervical a.
   4. Deltoid branch
   5. Suprascapular a.
B. AXILLARY
6. External thoracic a.
7. Lateral thoracic a.
C. SUBSCAPULAR A.
8. Thoracodorsal a.
9. Caudal circumflex humeral a.
10. Collateral radial a.
11. Circumflex scapular a.
12. Cranial circumflex humeral a.
D. BRACHIAL A.
13. Deep brachial a.
14. Bicipital a.
15. Collateral ulnar a.
16. Superficial brachial a.
17. Transverse cubital a.
18. Recurrent ulnaris a.
19. Deep antebrachial a.: in the cat arises from the brachial
a.; in the dog from the median a.
E. COMMON INTEROSSEOUS A.: the cat may
not have a common interosseous a. If not present, the cranial
and caudal interosseous aa. arise directly off the brachial a.
with the caudal interosseous a. being the last branch of the
brachial a.
20. Cranial interosseous a.: in the cat arises from
the brachial a. by itself or, like in the dog, with caudal interosseous a.
F. Caudal interosseous a.: very delicate in the cat, it can
arise as the last branch of the brachial a. or from the common
interosseous a. like in the dog.
G. MEDIAN A.: the direct continuation of the brachial a.
in the forearm, just distal to the common interosseous a. (as in
the dog) or from the caudal interosseous a. (but no common
interosseous a. is present).
21. Ulnar a.: usually arises from the median a.
22. Radial a.: runs cranial to the median a. on the radius.
ARTERIES OF THE FOREPAW: as in the dog can be
divided into palmar and dorsal branches and then into deep
and superficial branches. Superficial branches are named
dorsal or palmar common digital aa. and the deep branches
are dorsal or palmar metacarpal aa.
H. DIGITAL AA.

A. Subclavian a.

B. Axillary a.

C. Subscapular a.

Supracondylar foramen

D. Brachial a.

F. Caudal interosseous a.

G. Median a.

I. Digital aa.

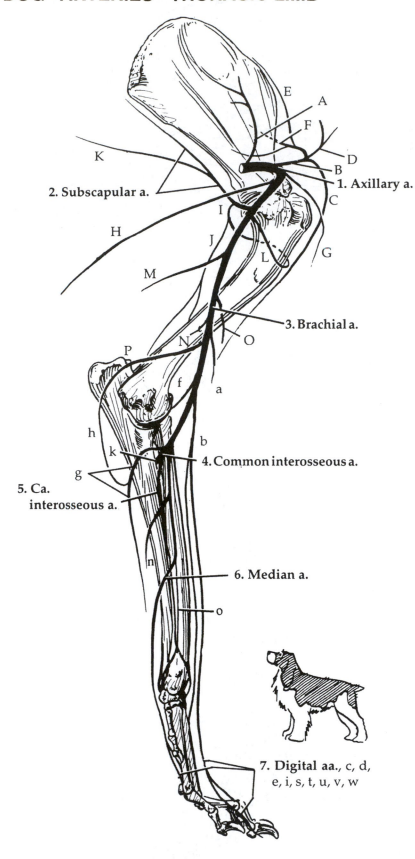

Fig IX-60: Dog - Thoracic limb arteries
- Medial view (schematic)

2. Subscapular a.

K

E
A
F
D
B

1. Axillary a.

C

I

H

J

L

G

M

3. Brachial a.

O

N

P

f

a

h

b

k

4. Common interosseous a.

g

5. Ca.
interosseous a.

6. Median a.

n

o

7. Digital aa., c, d,
e, i, s, t, u, v, w

1. **Axillary artery**: the direct continuation of the subclavian a. around the first rib to the thoracic limb. It supplies the structures of the shoulder and continues as the brachial a. in the arm.
2. **Subscapular artery** (c): passes dorsally along the border of the scapula between the subscapular and teres major muscles.
3. **Brachial artery**: the continuation of the axillary a. on the medial aspect of the arm. It continues as the median a. in the forearm after giving off the common interosseous a.
4. **Common interosseous artery**: the last branch of the brachial a., it dives through the interosseous space between the radius and ulna. It has caudal and cranial interosseous branches in all species.
5. **Caudal interosseous artery**: passes distally between the radius and ulna.
6. **Median artery**: the continuation of the brachial a. past the common interosseous a. It courses distally with the median n. on the medial side of the forearm under the flexor carpi radialis m. Passing through the carpal canal, it joins branches of the common interosseous a. to form the palmar arterial arches. The palmar arches give off palmar metacarpal (from the deep arch) and palmar common digital aa. (from the superficial arch) to supply the palmar aspect of the forepaw. The median a. is the largest artery in the manus in all the domestic species, except the cat (its main supply is the radial a.)
7. **Digital arteries**: the blood vessels of the manus (metacarpus and digits). Their distribution varies between the species. They are numbered from medial to lateral.

Carnivores: arteries of the manus.

- Common digital arteries (dorsal and palmar): the <u>superficial</u> aa. of the metacarpus. They divide into proper digital aa. in the digital region. They are numbered from medial to lateral I-IV depending on location (common digital a. I is between Mc1 and Mc2, common digital a. II is between Mc2 and Mc3, etc.)
- Metacarpal digital arteries (palmar and dorsal): the <u>deep</u> arteries of the metacarpus traveling next to the metacarpal bones. They parallel the larger common digital aa. and usually contribute to the formation of the proper digital aa.
- Proper digital arteries: the distal branches of the common digital aa. in the digits. They extend down the sides of the digits as **axial** and **abaxial** proper digital aa.

Clinical

- **Caudal interosseous a.**: in dogs can't be occluded with a tourniquet in the mid-forearm because it is protected between the radius and ulna. It is also prone to injury if the forearm bones are fractured.

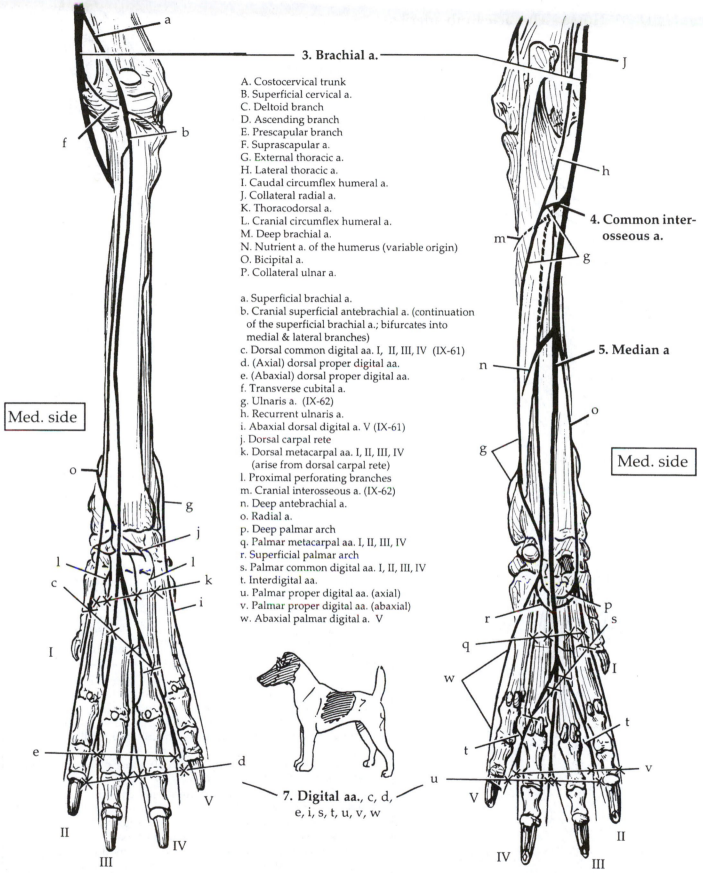

3. Brachial a.

A. Costocervical trunk
B. Superficial cervical a.
C. Deltoid branch
D. Ascending branch
E. Prescapular branch
F. Suprascapular a.
G. External thoracic a.
H. Lateral thoracic a.
I. Caudal circumflex humeral a.
J. Collateral radial a.
K. Thoracodorsal a.
L. Cranial circumflex humeral a.
M. Deep brachial a.
N. Nutrient a. of the humerus (variable origin)
O. Bicipital a.
P. Collateral ulnar a.

a. Superficial brachial a.
b. Cranial superficial antebrachial a. (continuation of the superficial brachial a.; bifurcates into medial & lateral branches)
c. Dorsal common digital aa. I, II, III, IV (IX-61)
d. (Axial) dorsal proper digital aa.
e. (Abaxial) dorsal proper digital aa.
f. Transverse cubital a.
g. Ulnaris a. (IX-62)
h. Recurrent ulnaris a.
i. Abaxial dorsal digital a. V (IX-61)
j. Dorsal carpal rete
k. Dorsal metacarpal aa. I, II, III, IV (arise from dorsal carpal rete)
l. Proximal perforating branches
m. Cranial interosseous a. (IX-62)
n. Deep antebrachial a.
o. Radial a.
p. Deep palmar arch
q. Palmar metacarpal aa. I, II, III, IV
r. Superficial palmar arch
s. Palmar common digital aa. I, II, III, IV
t. Interdigital aa.
u. Palmar proper digital aa. (axial)
v. Palmar proper digital aa. (abaxial)
w. Abaxial palmar digital a. V

4. Common inter-osseous a.

5. Median a

Med. side

Med. side

7. Digital aa., c, d, e, i, s, t, u, v, w

Fig IX-61: Dog - Left forearm & manus
 - Cranial/Dorsal view
 (schematic)

Fig IX-62: Dog - Left forearm & forepaw
 - Caudal/Palmar view
 (schematic)

HORSE - ARTERIES - THORACIC LIMB

Fig IX-63: Horse - Thoracic limb arteries
- Medial view (schematic)

Fig IX-64: Horse - Metacarpal & digital arteries
- Palmar view (schematic)

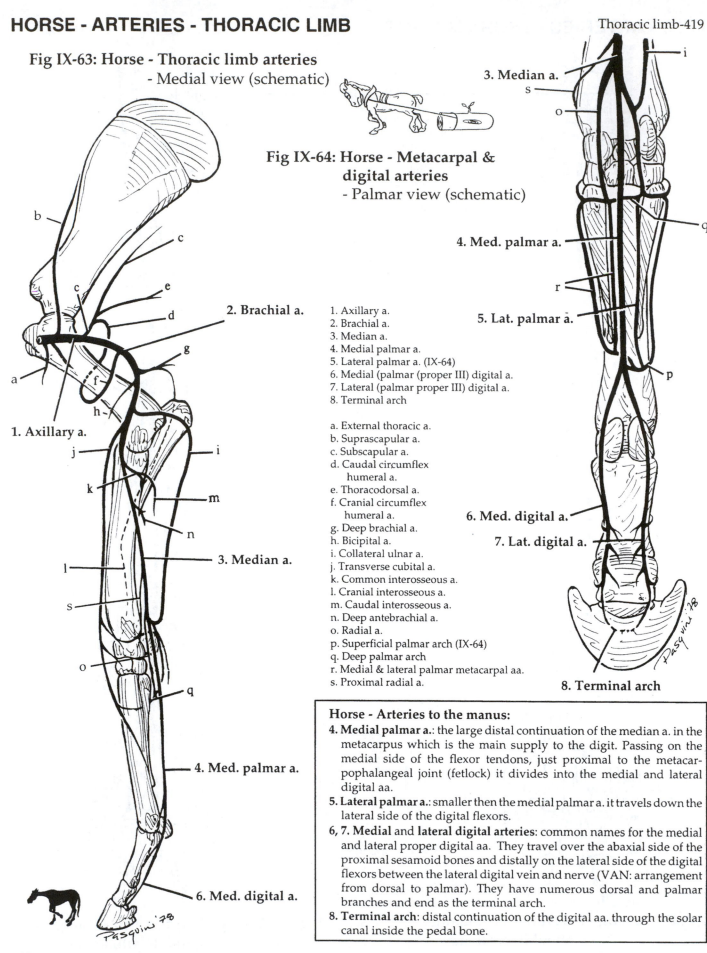

3. Median a.

4. Med. palmar a.

5. Lat. palmar a.

6. Med. digital a.

7. Lat. digital a.

8. Terminal arch

2. Brachial a.

1. Axillary a.

3. Median a.

4. Med. palmar a.

6. Med. digital a.

1. Axillary a.
2. Brachial a.
3. Median a.
4. Medial palmar a.
5. Lateral palmar a. (IX-64)
6. Medial (palmar (proper III) digital a.
7. Lateral (palmar proper III) digital a.
8. Terminal arch

a. External thoracic a.
b. Suprascapular a.
c. Subscapular a.
d. Caudal circumflex humeral a.
e. Thoracodorsal a.
f. Cranial circumflex humeral a.
g. Deep brachial a.
h. Bicipital a.
i. Collateral ulnar a.
j. Transverse cubital a.
k. Common interosseous a.
l. Cranial interosseous a.
m. Caudal interosseous a.
n. Deep antebrachial a.
o. Radial a.
p. Superficial palmar arch (IX-64)
q. Deep palmar arch
r. Medial & lateral palmar metacarpal aa.
s. Proximal radial a.

Horse - Arteries to the manus:
4. **Medial palmar a.:** the large distal continuation of the median a. in the metacarpus which is the main supply to the digit. Passing on the medial side of the flexor tendons, just proximal to the metacarpophalangeal joint (fetlock) it divides into the medial and lateral digital aa.
5. **Lateral palmar a.:** smaller then the medial palmar a. it travels down the lateral side of the digital flexors.
6, 7. **Medial** and **lateral digital arteries:** common names for the medial and lateral proper digital aa. They travel over the abaxial side of the proximal sesamoid bones and distally on the lateral side of the digital flexors between the lateral digital vein and nerve (VAN: arrangement from dorsal to palmar). They have numerous dorsal and palmar branches and end as the terminal arch.
8. **Terminal arch:** distal continuation of the digital aa. through the solar canal inside the pedal bone.

Fig IX-65: Ox - Thoracic limb aa.
- Medial view (schematic)

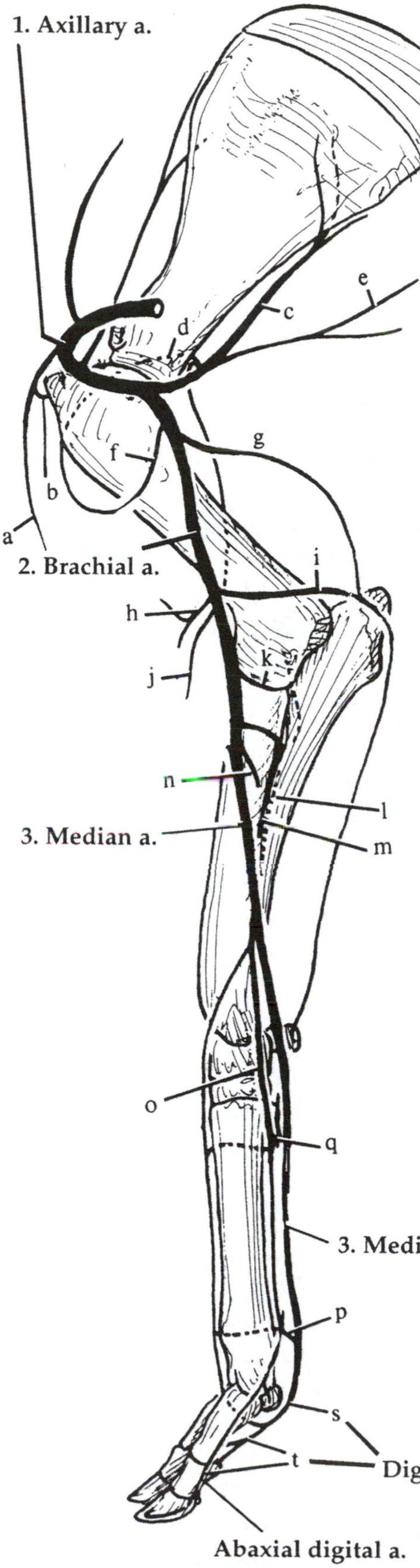

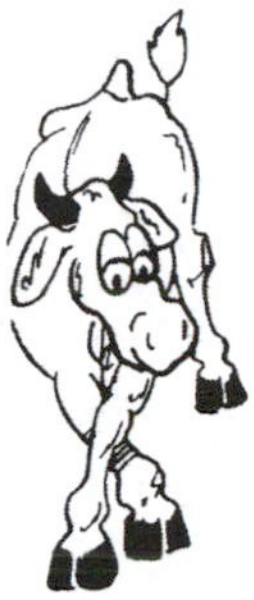

1. Axillary a.

2. Brachial a.

3. Median a.

3. Median a.

o

q

3. Median a.

p

s

t

Digital aa.

Abaxial digital a.

1. Axillary a.
2. Brachial a.
3. Median a.
4. Digital aa.

A. Palmar common
   digital a. III (X-66)
B. Dorsal metacarpal a. III (X-67)

a. External thoracic a.
b. Lateral thoracic a.
c. Subscapular a.
d. Caudal circumflex humeral a.
e. Thoracodorsal a.
f. Cranial circumflex humeral a.
g. Deep brachial a.
h. Bicipital a.
i. Collateral ulnar a.
j. Transverse cubital a.
k. Common interosseous a.
l. Cranial interosseous a.
m. Caudal interosseous a.
n. Deep antebrachial a.
o. Radial a.
p. Superficial palmar arch
q. Deep palmar arch
r. Palmar metacarpal aa. (IX-67)
s. Palmar common digital aa.
t. Palmar proper digital aa.

3. Median a.

l

B

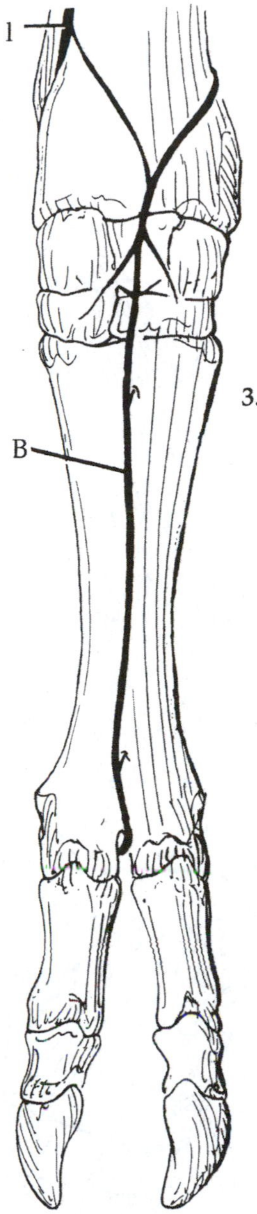

Fig IX-66: Ox - Metacarpal
& digital arteries
- Dorsal view
(schematic)

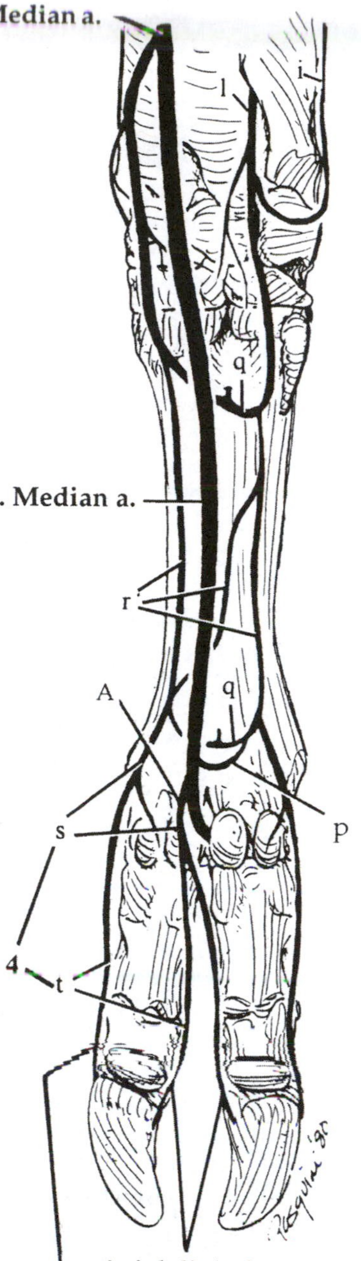

3. Median a.

3. Median a.

r

A

q

s

4

t

P

Axial digital aa.

Abaxial digital a.

Fig IX-67: Ox - Metacarpal
& digital arteries
- Palmar view
(schematic)

3. **Median artery**: in the ox, passes to the distal end of the metacarpus where
   it becomes the palmar common digital artery III which divides into axial
   digital arteries at the fetlock.
- **Axial digital arteries** (palmar proper digital aa. of digits III and IV): supply
   the axial sides of the weight bearing digits.
- **Abaxial digital arteries** (palmar common digital aa. II and IV): pass down
   the abaxial sides of the weight bearing digits.
- Dorsal metacarpal artery III: is the only significant artery of the dorsal side of the manus. It occupies the dorsal
   longitudinal groove of Mc III+IV.

419

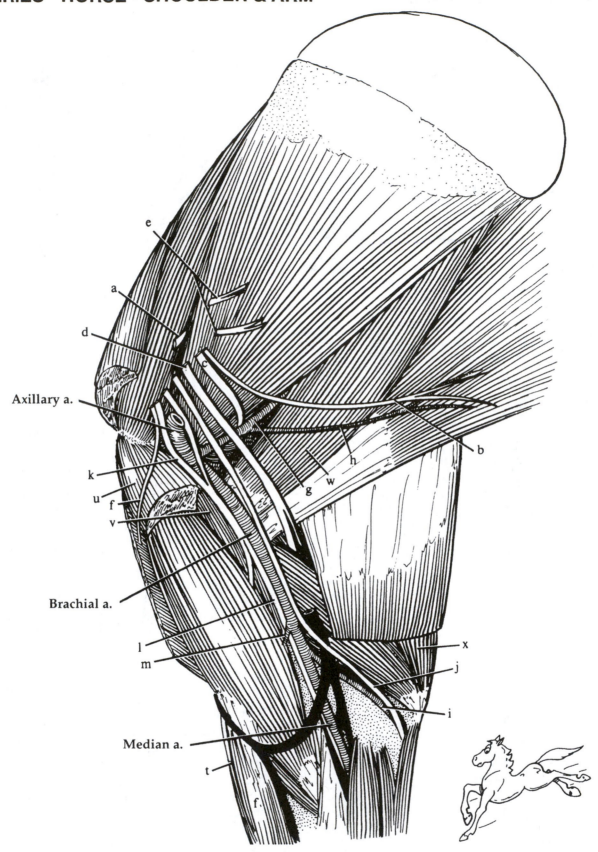

Fig IX-68: Horse - Arteries of the arm
- Medial view

VEINS - THORACIC LIMB

Superficial and deep veins drain the thoracic limb. The deep veins, in the majority, travel with like-named arteries. Superficial veins travel alone just beneath the skin.

- **Accessory cephalic vein**: arises from the dorsal digital arteries. It travels proximally to empty into the cephalic v. on the cranial surface of the forearm above the carpus.

- **Cephalic vein**: arises from the palmar surface of the manus, passes proximally up the forearm and arm, under the brachiocephalic muscle to empty into the external jugular vein. Its branches (omobrachial and axillobrachial vv.) provide other drainage routes.

- **Median cubital vein**: connects the superficially located cephalic vein and the deeply located brachial v. over the flexor surface of the elbow (cubit).

SPECIES DIFFERENCES

Horse: the accessory cephalic v. empties into the cephalic v. near the elbow, not just above the carpus as in the carnivores and ox.

- **"Spur" vein** (eq) or superficial thoracic vein: runs in the superficial fascia at the ventral margin of the cutaneous trunci muscle as it passes towards the axilla.

CLINICAL

- **Venipuncture**: most commonly and easily performed in the dog's cephalic vein. The cephalic and median cubital vv. are held off by finger pressure across the flexor surface of the elbow. A needle is then threaded into the cephalic v. distally on the cranial aspect of the limb.

- **Brachial artery pulse**: palpate on the medial side of the horse's limb through the superficial pectoral muscle just cranial to the medial collateral ligament.

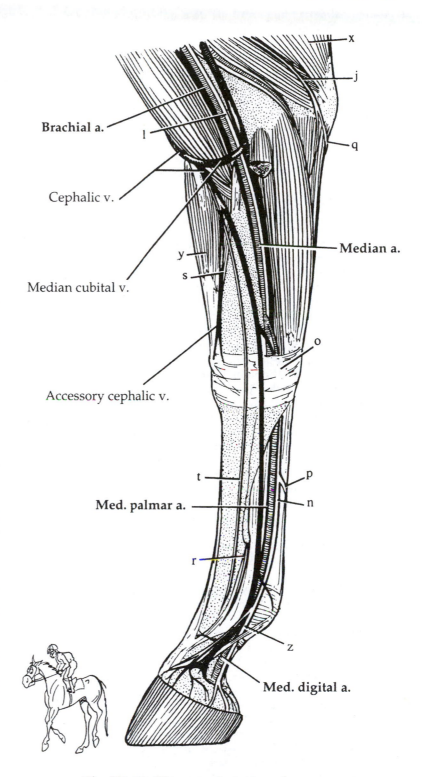

Fig IX-69: Horse - Arteries, forearm
- Medial view

a. Suprascapular n.	i. Collateral ulnar a.	q. Caudal cutaneous antebrachial n. (branch of ulnar n.)	u. Deep pectoral m. (IX-69)
b. Thoracodorsal n.	j. Ulnar n.		v. Coracobrachialis m.
c. Axillary n.	k. Musculocutaneous n.	r. Medial (palmar) metacarpal n.	w. Teres major m.
d. Radial n.	l. Median n.	s. Cranial cutaneous antebrachial n. (branch of axillary n.)	x. Triceps brachii m.
e. Subscapular n.	m. Bicipital a.		y. Extensor carpi radialis
f. Pectoral n.	n. Medial palmar n. (IX-69)	t. Medial cutaneous antebrachial n. (branch of musculocutaneous n.)	z. Medial digital n. (IX-69)
g. Subscapular a.	o. Flexor retinaculum		
h. Thoracodorsal a.	p. Communicating branch		

ABDOMINAL AORTA

1. **Abdominal aorta**: the part of the descending aorta caudal to the diaphragm. It courses along the roof of the abdomen between the caudal vena cava and the psoas muscles. The aorta terminates in the paired external iliac aa. to the pelvic limb, the internal iliac aa. to the pelvis, and the median sacral a. at the level of the last lumbar vertebra. Its main branches to the abdominal viscera are the unpaired celiac, cranial and caudal mesenteric aa., and the paired renal and gonadal aa. Paired parietal (wall) branches are the caudal phrenic a. to the diaphragm, cranial abdomen a. to the abdominal wall, lumbar aa. to the back, and deep circumflex iliac a. (k) to the flank.

Unpaired branches of the abdominal aorta:

2. **Celiac artery**: the first unpaired branch of the aorta arising between the crura of the diaphragm. It branches into splenic, hepatic and left gastric aa. They supply the cranial part of the abdomen (stomach, liver, spleen, and part of the duodenum and pancreas).

3. **Cranial mesentery artery**: the second unpaired branch arises just caudal to the celiac artery. Its branches (i.e., colics, cecal, jejunal) supply most of the intestines.

6. **Caudal mesenteric artery**: the third and last unpaired branch arises from the caudal aorta and passes in the mesocolon to supply the descending colon and rectum.

Paired branches of the abdominal aorta:

4. **Renal arteries**: originating from the aorta caudal to the cranial mesenteric a. and pass to each kidney.

5. **Gonadal arteries and veins (testicular or ovarian)**: the tiny vessels arising from the middle of the abdominal aorta just caudal to the renal aa. supply the gonads.

8. **External iliac arteries**: the large terminal branches of the caudal aorta near the caudal mesenteric artery that pass to the pelvic limbs.

7. **Internal iliac arteries**: the termination of the aorta passing to supply the viscera of the pelvis and part of the hip and thigh.

9. **Median sacral artery**: the unpaired terminal branch of the aorta that passes on midline below the sacrum.

VEINS - ABDOMEN: the paired veins travel with arteries of like name. Those draining areas supplied by unpaired branches of the aorta (celiac, cranial and caudal mesenteric aa.) do not return to the caudal vena cava directly, but join to form the portal vein.

• **Caudal vena cava**: is formed just cranial to the pelvic inlet by the joining of the common iliac vv. Traveling on the roof of the abdomen next to the aorta, it receives veins draining the areas supplied by the paired branches of the aorta. Cranially, it tunnels through the dorsal part of the liver, pierces the diaphragm, passes through a notch in the accessory lobe of the right lung, and empties into the right atrium of the heart.

6. **Portal vein**: the large vein coming from the intestinal mass into the hilus of the liver. It is formed by the joining of the cranial and caudal mesenteric, gastroduodenal, and splenic vv. which drain the areas (GI viscera) supplied by the unpaired branches of the aorta. The portal v. drains into the liver sinusoids of the liver so intestinal blood can be processed and cleaned before entering the general circulation.

• **Liver sinusoids**: spaces in the liver where the portal

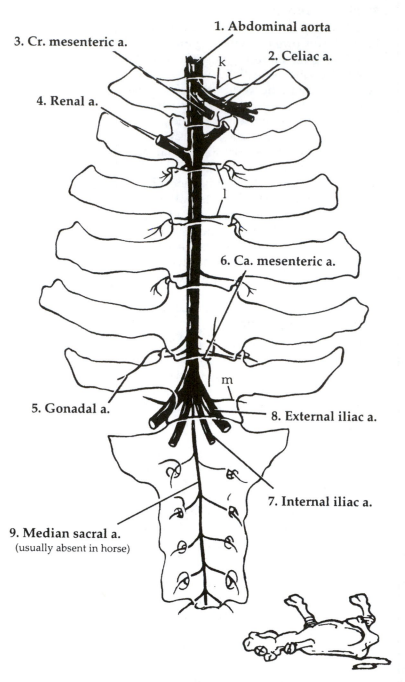

Fig. IX-70: Ox - Abdominal aorta
- Dorsal view
(schematic)

blood is processed.

• **Hepatic veins**: drain the liver (liver sinusoids) directly into the caudal vena cava without leaving the liver. Since the caudal vena cava passes through the edge of the liver and the hepatic veins are in the liver tissue, they can't be seen unless the caudal vena cava is cut open.

5. **Gonadal veins (testicular or ovarian)**: the right gonadal v. enters the caudal vena cava, while the left gonadal v. may enter the left renal v. This is important surgically.

ABDOMINAL AORTA

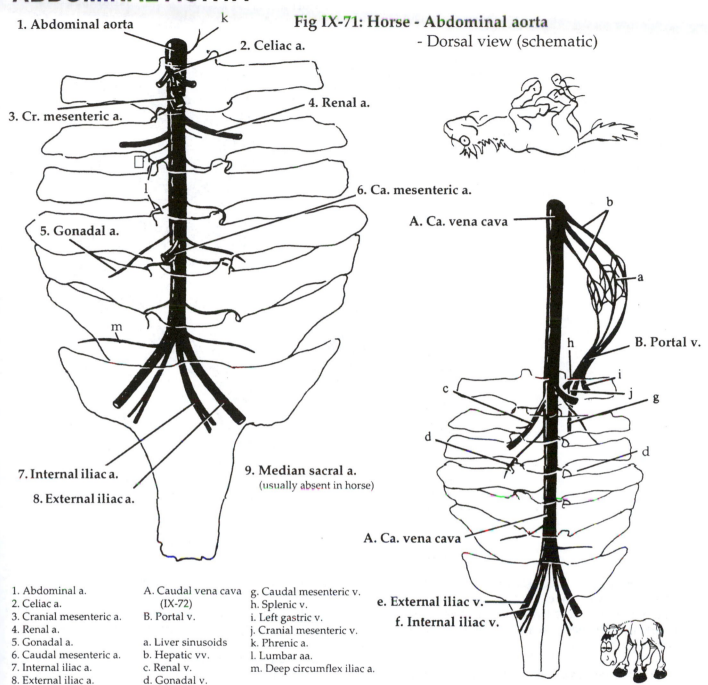

Fig IX-71: Horse - Abdominal aorta
- Dorsal view (schematic)

1. Abdominal aorta
2. Celiac a.
3. Cr. mesenteric a.
4. Renal a.
5. Gonadal a.
6. Ca. mesenteric a.
7. Internal iliac a.
8. External iliac a.
9. Median sacral a.
   (usually absent in horse)

A. Ca. vena cava
B. Portal v.
e. External iliac v.
f. Internal iliac v.

1. Abdominal a.	A. Caudal vena cava	g. Caudal mesenteric v.
2. Celiac a.	(IX-72)	h. Splenic v.
3. Cranial mesenteric a.	B. Portal v.	i. Left gastric v.
4. Renal a.		j. Cranial mesenteric v.
5. Gonadal a.	a. Liver sinusoids	k. Phrenic a.
6. Caudal mesenteric a.	b. Hepatic vv.	l. Lumbar aa.
7. Internal iliac a.	c. Renal v.	m. Deep circumflex iliac a.
8. External iliac a.	d. Gonadal v.	
9. Median sacral a.	e. External iliac v.	
(usually absent in horse)	f. Internal iliac v.	

Fig IX-72: Horse - Caudal vena cava
- Dorsal view (schematic)

SPECIES DIFFERENCES
- **Median sacral artery**: much reduced or absent in the <u>horse</u>. The area it supplies in other species is taken care of by a caudal gluteal a.

CLINICAL
- **Median sacral artery**: used to take blood,"tail bleed", in <u>cattle</u>.
- **Cranial mesenteric artery**: a common site for an aneurysm

(bulging of a blood vessel) in the <u>horse</u>, caused by the parasitic worm, *Strongylus vulgaris*. Parasitic blockage of this artery or its branches may cause colic.
- **Saddle thrombus**: blockage of the termination of the aorta of the cat which results in paralysis of the rear limbs.

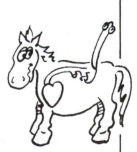

CELIAC ARTERY

Fig. IX-73 - Dog - Viscera supplied by the celiac a. (schematic)

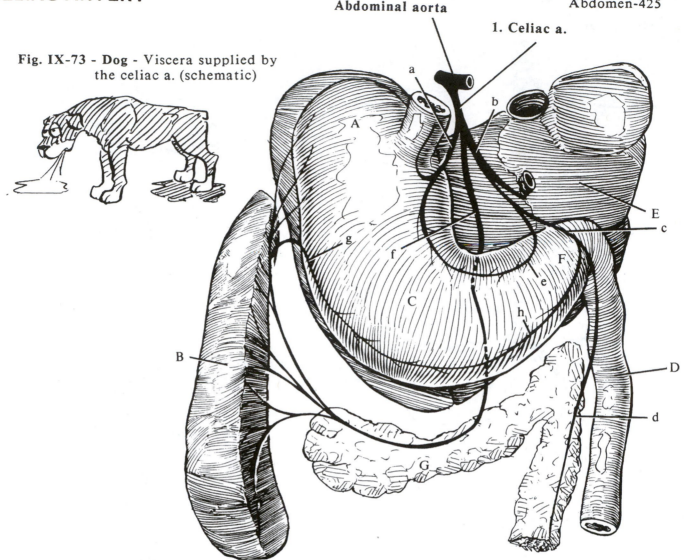

Abdominal aorta

1. Celiac a.

1. Celiac artery: the first visceral branch of the abdominal aorta, arising unpaired between the crura of the diaphragm. It terminates as the hepatic, splenic and left gastric arteries supplying the cranial part of the GI tract (stomach, part of the duodenum, liver and spleen.)

• **Left gastric artery** (a): supplies the left side of the lesser curvature of the stomach.

• **Splenic artery** (f): enters, by many terminal branches, the long hilus of the spleen in the dog. In the ruminant it enters a small hilus.

  • **Left gastroepiloic artery** (g): passes to the greater curvature of the stomach.

  • **Short gastric arteries** (l): arise from the splenic artery and pass to the fundus of the stomach.

• **Hepatic artery** (b): sends hepatic branches to the liver and a cystic branch to the gall bladder. It then continues on to supply

parts of the stomach, duodenum, and pancreas.

• **Right gastric artery** (e): anastomoses with the left gastric artery to supply the lesser curvature of the stomach.

• **Gastroduodenal artery** (c): crosses the stomach to branch into right gastroepiloic and cranial pancreaticoduodenal arteries.

• **Right gastroepiloic artery** (h): supplies the greater curvature along with the left gastroepiloic artery.

• **Cranial pancreaticoduodenal artery** (d): passes distally along the descending duodenum to supply it and the pancreas.

SPECIES DIFFERENCES

Ruminal arteries: travel in the right and left longitudinal grooves of the rumen. Both can arise from the splenic artery.

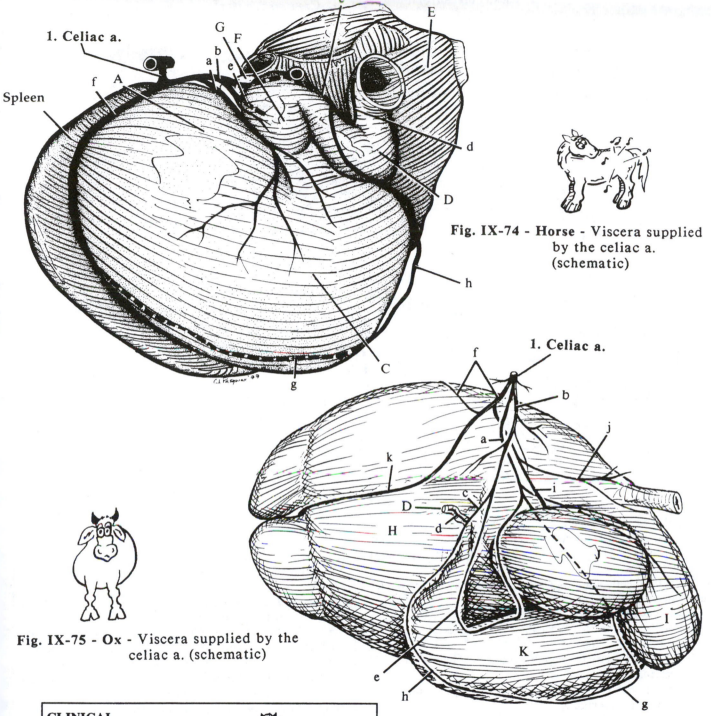

1. Celiac a.

Spleen

Fig. IX-74 - Horse - Viscera supplied by the celiac a. (schematic)

1. Celiac a.

Fig. IX-75 - Ox - Viscera supplied by the celiac a. (schematic)

CLINICAL

Rumenotomy: open the dorsal sac above the longitudinal groove, thereby avoiding its arteries.

Gastrotomy: when opening the stomach in the dog cut between the two curvatures to avoid the major blood vessels.

Splenectomy in the carnivores: the vessels to the spleen must be ligated close to the spleen along the hilus so the short gastric and left gastroepiploic arteries are not compromised.

A. Fundus of stomach	a. Lt. gastric a.
B. Spleen	b. Hepatic a.
C. Stomach	c. Gastroduodenal a.
D. Duodenum	d. Cran. pancreaticoduodenal a.
E. Liver	e. Rt. gastric a.
F. Pylorus	f. Splenic a.
G. Pancreas	g. Lt. gastroepiploic a.
H. Rumen	h. Rt. gastroepiploic a.
I. Reticulum	i. Lt. ruminal a.
J. Omasum	j. Reticular a.
K. Abomasum	k. Rt. ruminal a.

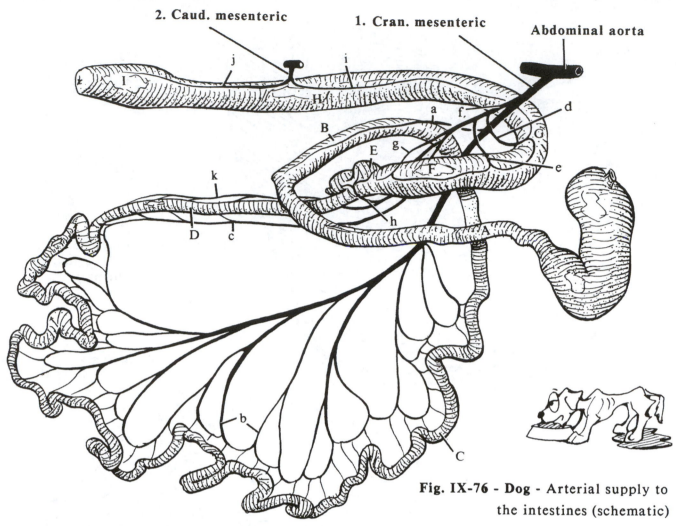

2. Caud. mesenteric   1. Cran. mesenteric

Abdominal aorta

Fig. IX-76 - Dog - Arterial supply to the intestines (schematic)

1. Cranial mesenteric artery: the largest visceral branch of the abdominal aorta, arising just caudal to the origin of the celiac artery. It courses caudoventrally in the mesentery to supply most of the intestines.

• **Caudal pancreaticoduodenal artery**: anastomoses with the cranial pancreaticoduodenal artery.

• **Ileocolic artery**, branches to:
  • **Middle colic artery (d)**: supplies the transverse ("middle") colon.
  • **Right colic artery (e)**: supplies the second half of the ascending colon.
  • **Colic branch of the ileocolic artery (g)**: supplies the first part of the ascending colon.
  • **Antimesenteric ileal artery (k)**: travels on the antimesenteric side of the ileum in the ileocecal fold.

• **Jejunal** and **ileal branches (b)**: come off the continuation of the cranial mesenteric artery. These branches anastomose, making arcades from which short jejunal and ileal arteries extend to reach the organs.

2. Caudal mesenteric artery: the smallest unpaired major branch of the abdominal aorta. It arises near the termination of the abdominal aorta and supplies the descending colon and rectum through its left colic and cranial rectal arteries respectively.

SPECIES DIFFERENCES

Memory aid: consider the ascending colon (AC) to be the "right" colon and divided into two parts. Consider the transverse colon the "middle" colon and the descending colon the "left" colon. Then name the arteries supplying the second part of the right colon, the middle colon and the left colon the right, middle and left colic arteries respectively. This leaves the first part of the AC which is supplied by the colic branch. This simplification works for all the domestic species.

Horse: the first part of the AC is the ventral colons from the cecum to the pelvic flexure (colic branch). The second part is the left and right dorsal colons from the pelvic flexure to the transverse colon (right colic artery).

Ox: the first part of the AC is from the cecum to the central flexure (proximal loop and centripetal coils) (colic branch). The second part is from the central flexure to the transverse colon.

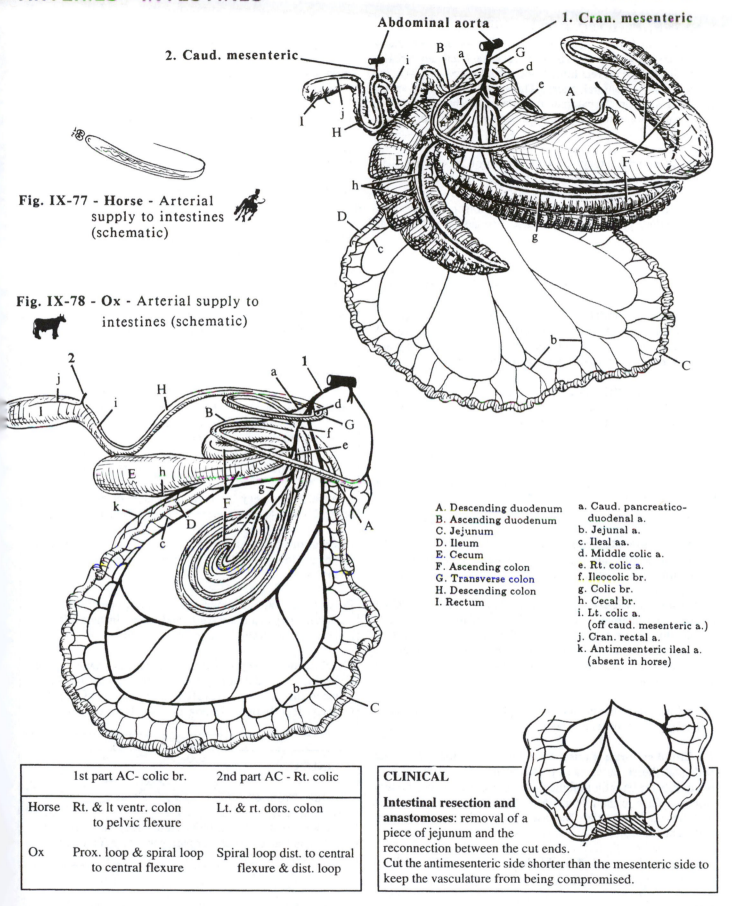

Abdominal aorta

1. Cran. mesenteric

2. Caud. mesenteric

Fig. IX-77 - Horse - Arterial supply to intestines (schematic)

Fig. IX-78 - Ox - Arterial supply to intestines (schematic)

	a. Caud. pancreatico-
A. Descending duodenum	duodenal a.
B. Ascending duodenum	b. Jejunal a.
C. Jejunum	c. Ileal aa.
D. Ileum	d. Middle colic a.
E. Cecum	e. Rt. colic a.
F. Ascending colon	f. Ileocolic br.
G. Transverse colon	g. Colic br.
H. Descending colon	h. Cecal br.
I. Rectum	i. Lt. colic a.
	(off caud. mesenteric a.)
	j. Cran. rectal a.
	k. Antimesenteric ileal a.
	(absent in horse)

	1st part AC- colic br.	2nd part AC - Rt. colic
Horse	Rt. & lt ventr. colon to pelvic flexure	Lt. & rt. dors. colon
Ox	Prox. loop & spiral loop to central flexure	Spiral loop dist. to central flexure & dist. loop

CLINICAL

Intestinal resection and anastomoses: removal of a piece of jejunum and the reconnection between the cut ends. Cut the antimesenteric side shorter than the mesenteric side to keep the vasculature from being compromised.

1. EXTERNAL ILIAC ARTERY: the large branch of the terminal aorta. It gives off the deep femoral artery, then penetrates the abdominal wall through the femoral canal (lacunae) to reach the medial side of the rear limb. Once out of the abdominal cavity it becomes the femoral artery. The caudal abdominal artery usually arises from the external iliac artery after the deep femoral artery and supplies the caudal abdominal wall (carnivores, sheep and cattle).

2. Deep femoral artery: the only branch of the external iliac artery present in all species. It has the following branches:

• **3. Pudendoepigastric trunk**: a short branch off the deep femoral artery giving rise to the caudal epigastric and external pudendal arteries.

　• **4. Caudal epigastric artery**: courses cranially on the deep surface of the straight abdominal muscle (rectus abdominis).

　• **5. External pudendal artery**: passes through the inguinal canal and branches into the superficial caudal epigastric and ventral scrotal or ventral labial arteries (the latter supplying the scrotum or labia of the vulva, respectively).

　　• **6. Superficial caudal epigastric artery**: courses cranially under the skin of the ventral abdominal wall to anastomose with the cranial epigastric artery.

7. INTERNAL ILIAC ARTERIES: the terminal branch of the aorta that enters the pelvic cavity. It branches into caudal gluteal and internal pudendal arteries. This division occurs at different levels, thus, giving rise to either a "long" or "short" internal iliac artery.

8. Internal pudendal artery: can be "short" or "long", depending on where it and the caudal gluteal artery separate. It terminates as the ventral perineal artery and the artery of the penis or clitoris.

9. Prostatic or **vaginal artery**: the branch of either the internal pudendal or internal iliac, depending on which is longer. It supplies the urogenital organs in the pelvic cavity. Its branches are named for the organs they supply: uterine/uterine branch (ductus deferentis artery/branch), urethralis, middle rectal, and caudal vesical arteries.

• **Uterine artery**: the main blood supply to the uterus. It arises differently in the different species.

10. Umbilical artery: arises from the internal iliac or internal pudendal (horse) artery and passes to the apex of the urinary bladder. In the fetus the umbilical arteries were the vascular return from the fetus to the mother. After birth they regress from the umbilicus to the bladder. The last branch of the umbilical artery is the cranial vesical artery.

• **11. Round ligament of the bladder**: the part of the umbilical artery in the edge of the lateral ligament of the bladder. Its lumen is usually obliterated (not patent).

Artery of the penis: the continuation of the internal pudendal artery in the male. It rounds the arch of the ischium and trifurcates:

• **12. Artery of the bulb**: supplies the corpus spongiosum penis.

• **13. Deep artery of the penis**: enters and supplies the corpus cavernosum penis.

• **14. Dorsal artery of the penis**: travels along the dorsal surface of the penis.

Artery of the clitoris: analogous to the artery of the penis. It branches into the artery of the vestibular bulb, the deep artery of the clitoris (except in horses) and dorsal artery of the clitoris (except in horses).

Ventral perineal artery (d): the other terminal branch of the internal pudendal artery. It supplies the perineum.

SPECIES DIFFERENCES

15. Uterine artery: branches off various arteries:
　• Vaginal artery in the <u>carnivores.</u>
　• External iliac artery in the <u>mare.</u>
　• Umbilical artery in the <u>ruminants</u>. The mare and ruminants also have a uterine branch of the vaginal artery.

Internal iliac artery (7): carnivores and horses have short internal iliac arteries; ruminants and pigs have long ones.

Internal pudendal artery (8): carnivores and horses have "long" internal pudendal arteries; ruminants and pigs have "short" ones.

Prostatic or **vaginal artery** (9): arises from the internal pudendal artery in the carnivores and horses. In the ruminants and pig it arises from the internal iliac artery.

16. Obturator artery: usually arising from the cranial gluteal artery in the cat and horse, it travels through the obturator foramen. In the horse it gives off the middle artery of the penis (clitoris). It is absent in the dog and usually absent in the ox.

CLINICAL

"Saddle thrombi": a blood clot at the termination of the aorta seen in cats. This can block the external iliac arteries and result in lameness, paresis or paralysis of the hind limbs.

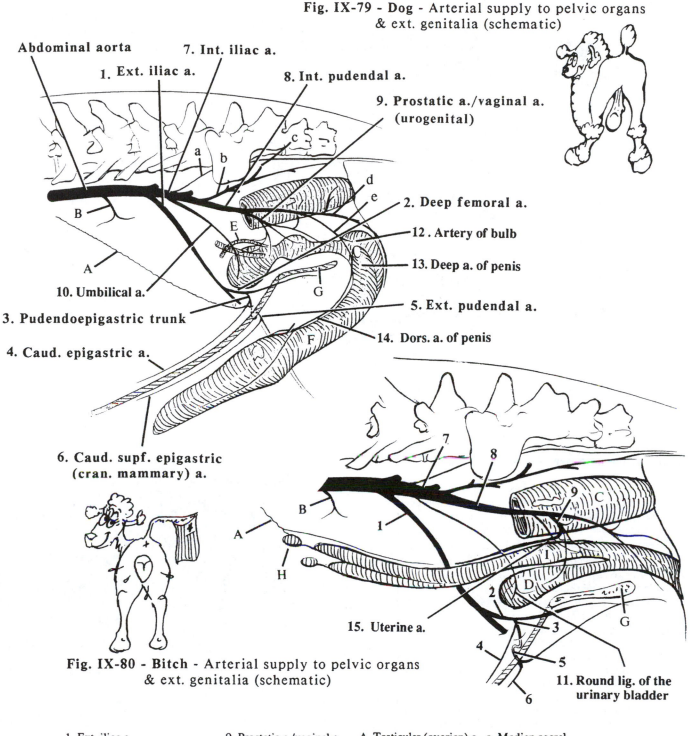

Fig. IX-79 - Dog - Arterial supply to pelvic organs
& ext. genitalia (schematic)

Abdominal aorta

7. Int. iliac a.

1. Ext. iliac a.

8. Int. pudendal a.

9. Prostatic a./vaginal a.
(urogenital)

2. Deep femoral a.

12. Artery of bulb

13. Deep a. of penis

5. Ext. pudendal a.

14. Dors. a. of penis

10. Umbilical a.

3. Pudendoepigastric trunk

4. Caud. epigastric a.

6. Caud. supf. epigastric
(cran. mammary) a.

15. Uterine a.

11. Round lig. of the
urinary bladder

Fig. IX-80 - Bitch - Arterial supply to pelvic organs
& ext. genitalia (schematic)

1. Ext. iliac a.
2. Deep femoral a.
3. Pudendoepigastric trunk
4. Caud. epigastric a.
5. Ext. pudendal a.
6. Caud. supf. epigastric (cran. mammary) a.
7. Int. iliac a.
8. Int. pudendal a.

9. Prostatic a./vaginal a.
10. Umbilical a.
11. Round lig. of bladder
12. Artery of bulb
13. Deep a. of penis
14. Dors. a. of penis
15. Uterine a.

A. Testicular (ovarian) a.
B. Caud. mesenteric a.
C. Rectum
D. Urinary bladder
E. Ductus deferens
F. Body of penis
G. Pelvic symphysis
H. Ovary
I. Uterus

a. Median sacral
b. Caud. gluteal
c. Cran. gluteal
d. Ventral perineal
e. Artery of penis (clitoris)

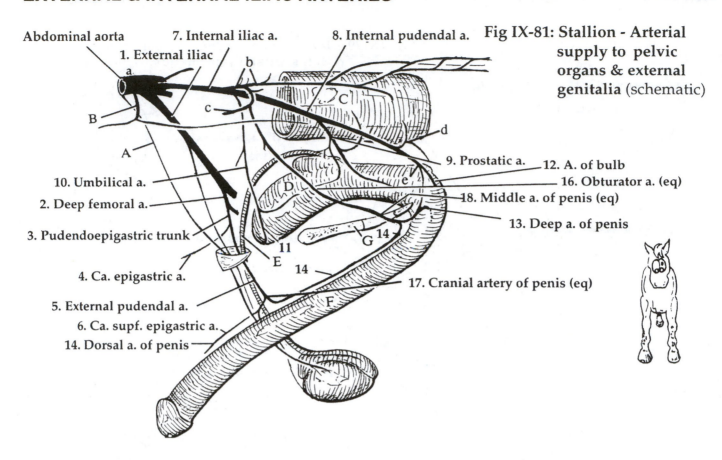

Fig IX-81: Stallion - Arterial supply to pelvic organs & external genitalia (schematic)

Abdominal aorta
7. Internal iliac a.
8. Internal pudendal a.
1. External iliac
10. Umbilical a.
2. Deep femoral a.
3. Pudendoepigastric trunk
4. Ca. epigastric a.
5. External pudendal a.
6. Ca. supf. epigastric a.
14. Dorsal a. of penis
9. Prostatic a.
12. A. of bulb
16. Obturator a. (eq)
18. Middle a. of penis (eq)
13. Deep a. of penis
17. Cranial artery of penis (eq)

Mare: blood supply to uterus: uterine branch of the ovarian a., **uterine a. (from external iliac a.)** and uterine branch of the vaginal a.

15. **Uterine artery**: arises from the external iliac a. near the deep circumflex iliac a. It passes in the mesometrium to the uterus. This artery is not present in the dog and is a branch of the umbilical a. in the ruminant.

Stallion: blood supply to the penis: Artery of the bulb (from internal pudendal a.), deep a. of the penis (from middle a. of penis [from obturator a.]) and cranial a. of the penis (from external pudendal a.)

16. **Obturator artery**: in the horse arises from the cranial gluteal a., a branch of the caudal gluteal a. It passes medial to the shaft of the ilium and through the obturator foramen to continue as the **middle a. of the penis**.

18. **Middle artery of the penis/clitoris**: the continuation of the obturator a. outside the pelvis. It contributes to the dorsal a. of the penis and enters the penis as the deep a. of the penis.

13. **Deep artery of the penis**: the continuation of the middle a. of the penis, entering and supplying the corpus cavernosum.

17. **Cranial artery of the penis**: a unique equine branch of the external pudendal a. passing cranially and caudally on the penis to help supply the dorsal a. of the penis.

12. **Artery of the bulb**: a branch of the termination of the internal pudendal a. (e) passing into the bulb of the penis to supply the corpus spongiosum.

14. **Dorsal artery of the penis**: formed by anastomoses of the middle a., cranial a. of the penis, and a small continuation of the internal pudendal a. (inconsistent).

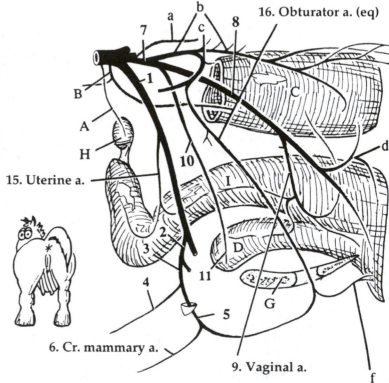

15. Uterine a.
16. Obturator a. (eq)
6. Cr. mammary a.
9. Vaginal a.

Fig IX-82: Mare - Arterial supply to pelvic organs & external genitalia (schematic)

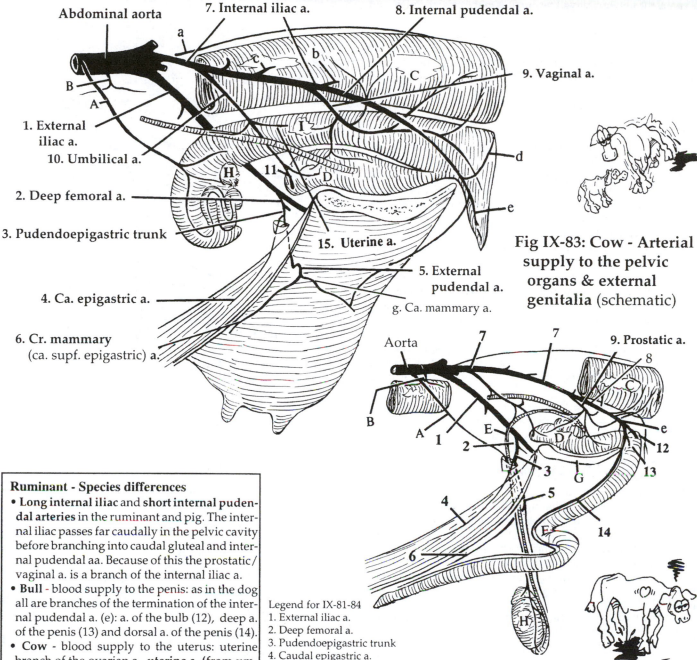

Fig IX-83: Cow - Arterial supply to the pelvic organs & external genitalia (schematic)

Abdominal aorta
7. Internal iliac a.
8. Internal pudendal a.
9. Vaginal a.
a
c
b
C
B
A
1. External iliac a.
10. Umbilical a.
I
d
2. Deep femoral a.
H
11
D
e
3. Pudendoepigastric trunk
15. Uterine a.
5. External pudendal a.
4. Ca. epigastric a.
g. Ca. mammary a.
6. Cr. mammary (ca. supf. epigastric) a.

Aorta
7
7
9. Prostatic a.
8
B
A
1
E
D
e
2
12
3
G
13
4
5
6
F
14
H

Fig IX-84: Bull - Arterial supply to pelvic organs & external genitalia (schematic)

Ruminant - Species differences

• **Long internal iliac** and **short internal pudendal arteries** in the ruminant and pig. The internal iliac passes far caudally in the pelvic cavity before branching into caudal gluteal and internal pudendal aa. Because of this the prostatic/vaginal a. is a branch of the internal iliac a.

• **Bull** - blood supply to the penis: as in the dog all are branches of the termination of the internal pudendal a. (e): a. of the bulb (12), deep a. of the penis (13) and dorsal a. of the penis (14).

• **Cow** - blood supply to the uterus: uterine branch of the ovarian a., **uterine a. (from umbilical a.)** and the uterine branch of the vaginal a. (comparable to the vaginal a. in the dog)

15. Uterine a.: a branch of the umbilical a. in ruminants.

6. "Cranial mammary artery": common name for the superficial caudal epigastric a. in ruminants and the mare.

• **"Caudal mammary artery" (g):** caudal branch of the external pudendal a. (mammary a.) passing around the base of the udder in ruminants.

• **"Milk veins"**, subcutaneous abdominal vein (cranial and caudal superficial epigastric v.): common names for the large satellite veins of the superficial epigastric vv. on the ventral abdomen.

Legend for IX-81-84
1. External iliac a.
2. Deep femoral a.
3. Pudendoepigastric trunk
4. Caudal epigastric a.
5. External pudendal a.
6. Caudal superficial epigastric (cranial mammary) a.
7. Internal iliac a. (long in ruminants)
8. Internal pudendal a.
9. Prostatic a./vaginal a. (genital a.)
10. Umbilical a.
11. Round ligament of the urinary bladder
12. Artery of the bulb
13. Deep artery of the penis
14. Dorsal artery of the penis
15. Uterine a.
    Mare: from external iliac a.
    Cow: from umbilical a.
16. Obturator a. (eq)
17. Cranial artery of the penis (eq)
18. Middle artery of the penis (eq)

A. Testicular (ovarian) a.
B. Caudal mesenteric a.
C. Rectum
D. Urinary bladder
E. Ductus deferens
F. Body of the penis
G. Pelvic symphysis
H. Ovary/testis
I. Uterus

a. Median sacral a.
b. Caudal gluteal a.
c. Cranial gluteal a.
d. Ventral perineal a.
e. Artery of the penis (clitoris)
f. Middle artery of the clitoris (branch of obturator a. in horse)
g. Caudal mammary a.

431

1. **Internal iliac artery**: the terminal branch of the aorta that enters the pelvic cavity. It terminates in the caudal gluteal and internal pudendal aa.
2. **Caudal gluteal artery**: gives off the cranial gluteal a. and then leaves the pelvic cavity with the ischiatic n. to supply the superficial gluteal m. and proximal "hamstring" mm.
3. **Cranial gluteal artery**: arises from the caudal gluteal a. and passes over the greater ischiatic notch to supply the middle gluteal and surrounding muscles.
4. **External iliac artery**: the large terminal branch of the aorta. After giving off the deep femoral a., it penetrates the abdominal wall through the femoral canal (vascular lacunae) as the femoral a. to reach the medial thigh.
5. **Deep femoral artery**: arises from the external iliac a. just inside the abdomen. It gives off the pudendoepigastric trunk and then passes out the femoral canal as the medial circumflex femoral a. (d) which supplies the medial thigh.
6. **Femoral artery**: the continuation of the external iliac a. through the femoral triangle, passing distally to continue as the **popliteal a.** caudal to the stifle joint.
7. **Saphenous artery**: arises from the femoral a. in the femoral triangle. It passes subcutaneously with the medial saphenous v. and saphenous n. on the medial thigh. Past the stifle it divides into cranial and caudal branches in the carnivores and horse.
8. **Caudal femoral artery** (distal caudal femoral a. in carnivores): the last branch of the femoral a. in all species, it passes caudally on the gastrocnemius to supply the caudal thigh ("hamstring") mm.
9. **Popliteal artery**: the continuation of the femoral a. after the caudal femoral a. Passing between the two heads of the gastrocnemius m., it branches into cranial and caudal (small) tibial aa.
10. **Cranial tibial artery**: passes through the interosseous space and then distally on the cranial surface of the crus with the deep branch of the fibular n.
11. **Dorsal pedal artery**: the direct continuation of the cranial tibial a. over the flexor surface of the tarsus.

Perforating tarsal artery: passes between the tarsal or metatarsal bones to reach the plantar aspect of the pes.

• **Metatarsal** and **common digital arteries**: similar to the metacarpal and digital arteries of the forelimb.

SPECIAL
• **Femoral canal** or **vascular lacunae**: the opening between the abdominal cavity and the medial thigh for the passage of the femoral and deep femoral aa.

CLINICAL
• **"Saddle thrombi"**: a blood clot at the termination of the cat's aorta. This can block the external iliac aa. and result in lameness, paresis, or paralysis of the hind limbs.
• **Collateral circulation**: The many different blood vessels supplying the pelvic limb allow ligation (tying off) of the femoral artery without permanent ill effects in a healthy dog.
• **Pulse: palpated in different locations**:
  - Carnivores: femoral a. in the femoral triangle on the medial thigh. During surgeries the dorsal pedal, brachial, lingual or common carotid arteries can also be used.
  - Horse: great metatarsal, facial, and transverse facial arteries can be used.
• **Femoral catheterization**: is used for angiocardiography frequently because of its convenient superficial location.

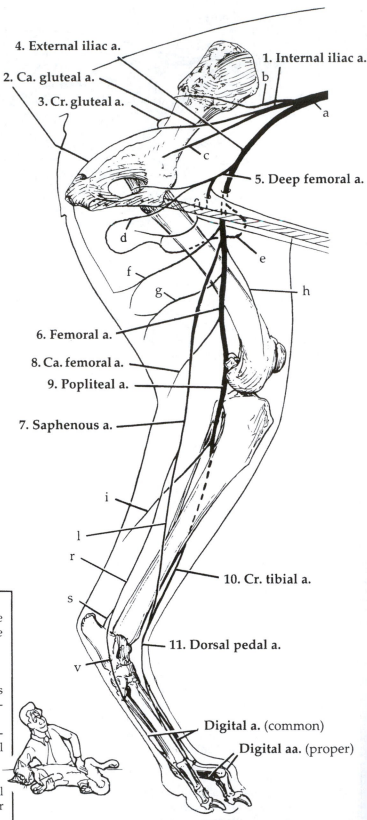

4. External iliac a.
1. Internal iliac a.
2. Ca. gluteal a.
3. Cr. gluteal a.
5. Deep femoral a.
6. Femoral a.
8. Ca. femoral a.
9. Popliteal a.
7. Saphenous a.
10. Cr. tibial a.
11. Dorsal pedal a.
Digital a. (common)
Digital aa. (proper)

Fig IX-85: Dog - Left pelvic limb
- Medial view
(schematic)

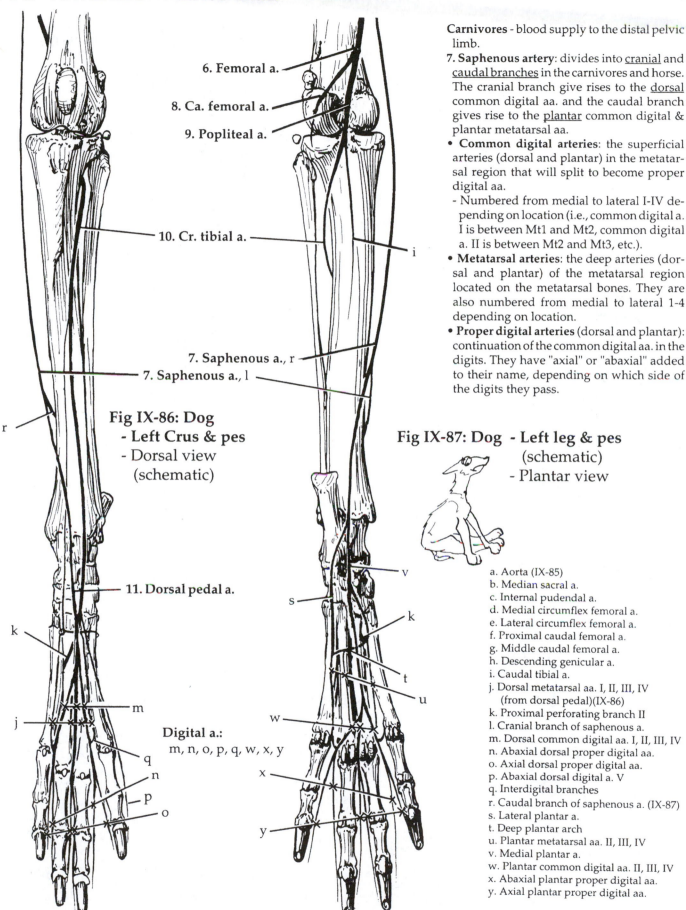

Carnivores - blood supply to the distal pelvic limb.

7. Saphenous artery: divides into <u>cranial</u> and <u>caudal branches</u> in the carnivores and horse. The cranial branch give rises to the <u>dorsal</u> common digital aa. and the caudal branch gives rise to the <u>plantar</u> common digital & plantar metatarsal aa.

- **Common digital arteries**: the superficial arteries (dorsal and plantar) in the metatarsal region that will split to become proper digital aa.
  - Numbered from medial to lateral I-IV depending on location (i.e., common digital a. I is between Mt1 and Mt2, common digital a. II is between Mt2 and Mt3, etc.).
- **Metatarsal arteries**: the deep arteries (dorsal and plantar) of the metatarsal region located on the metatarsal bones. They are also numbered from medial to lateral 1-4 depending on location.
- **Proper digital arteries** (dorsal and plantar): continuation of the common digital aa. in the digits. They have "axial" or "abaxial" added to their name, depending on which side of the digits they pass.

6. Femoral a.

8. Ca. femoral a.

9. Popliteal a.

10. Cr. tibial a.

7. Saphenous a., r

7. Saphenous a., l

**Fig IX-86: Dog
- Left Crus & pes
- Dorsal view
(schematic)**

Fig IX-87: Dog - Left leg & pes
(schematic)
- Plantar view

11. Dorsal pedal a.

Digital a.:
m, n, o, p, q, w, x, y

a. Aorta (IX-85)
b. Median sacral a.
c. Internal pudendal a.
d. Medial circumflex femoral a.
e. Lateral circumflex femoral a.
f. Proximal caudal femoral a.
g. Middle caudal femoral a.
h. Descending genicular a.
i. Caudal tibial a.
j. Dorsal metatarsal aa. I, II, III, IV
   (from dorsal pedal)(IX-86)
k. Proximal perforating branch II
l. Cranial branch of saphenous a.
m. Dorsal common digital aa. I, II, III, IV
n. Abaxial dorsal proper digital aa.
o. Axial dorsal proper digital aa.
p. Abaxial dorsal digital a. V
q. Interdigital branches
r. Caudal branch of saphenous a. (IX-87)
s. Lateral plantar a.
t. Deep plantar arch
u. Plantar metatarsal aa. II, III, IV
v. Medial plantar a.
w. Plantar common digital aa. II, III, IV
x. Abaxial plantar proper digital aa.
y. Axial plantar proper digital aa.

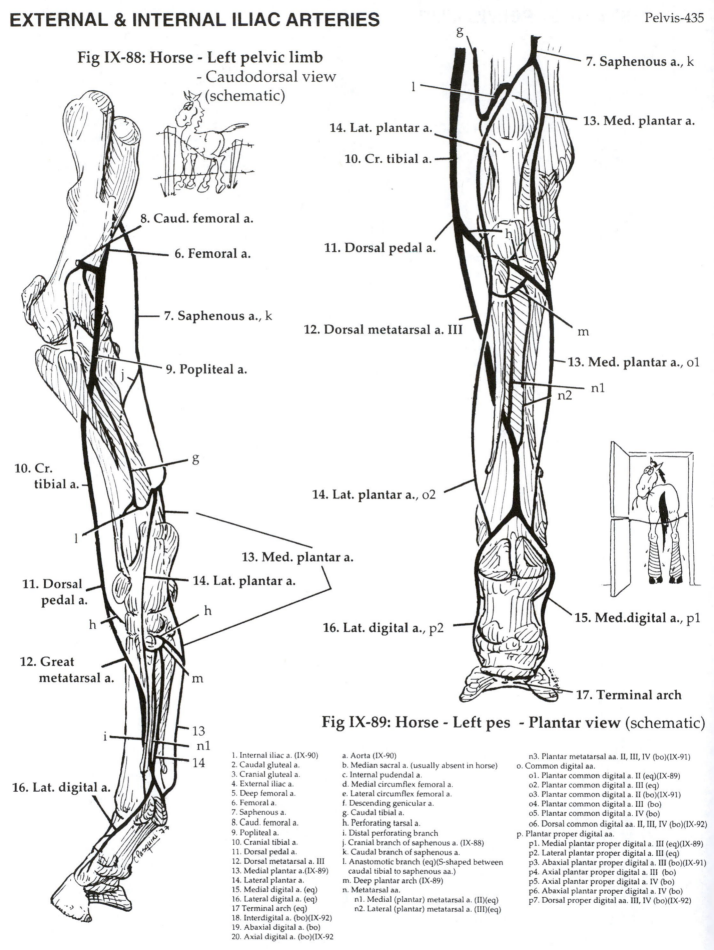

Fig IX-88: Horse - Left pelvic limb
- Caudodorsal view (schematic)

7. Saphenous a., k

14. Lat. plantar a.

13. Med. plantar a.

10. Cr. tibial a.

8. Caud. femoral a.

6. Femoral a.

11. Dorsal pedal a.

7. Saphenous a., k

9. Popliteal a.

12. Dorsal metatarsal a. III

13. Med. plantar a., o1

10. Cr. tibial a.

14. Lat. plantar a., o2

13. Med. plantar a.

14. Lat. plantar a.

11. Dorsal pedal a.

15. Med. digital a., p1

12. Great metatarsal a.

16. Lat. digital a., p2

17. Terminal arch

16. Lat. digital a.

Fig IX-89: Horse - Left pes - Plantar view (schematic)

1. Internal iliac a. (IX-90)
2. Caudal gluteal a.
3. Cranial gluteal a.
4. External iliac a.
5. Deep femoral a.
6. Femoral a.
7. Saphenous a.
8. Caud. femoral a.
9. Popliteal a.
10. Cranial tibial a.
11. Dorsal pedal a.
12. Dorsal metatarsal a. III
13. Medial plantar a.(IX-89)
14. Lateral plantar a.
15. Medial digital a. (eq)
16. Lateral digital a. (eq)
17 Terminal arch (eq)
18. Interdigital a. (bo)(IX-92)
19. Abaxial digital a. (bo)
20. Axial digital a. (bo)(IX-92

a. Aorta (IX-90)
b. Median sacral a. (usually absent in horse)
c. Internal pudendal a.
d. Medial circumflex femoral a.
e. Lateral circumflex femoral a.
f. Descending genicular a.
g. Caudal tibial a.
h. Perforating tarsal a.
i. Distal perforating branch
j. Cranial branch of saphenous a. (IX-88)
k. Caudal branch of saphenous a.
l. Anastomotic branch (eq)(S-shaped between
   caudal tibial to saphenous aa.)
m. Deep plantar arch (IX-89)
n. Metatarsal aa.
   n1. Medial (plantar) metatarsal a. (II)(eq)
   n2. Lateral (plantar) metatarsal a. (III)(eq)

n3. Plantar metatarsal aa. II, III, IV (bo)(IX-91)
o. Common digital aa.
   o1. Plantar common digital a. II (eq)(IX-89)
   o2. Plantar common digital a. III (eq)
   o3. Plantar common digital a. II (bo)(IX-91)
   o4. Plantar common digital a. III (bo)
   o5. Plantar common digital a. IV (bo)
   o6. Dorsal common digital aa. II, III, IV (bo)(IX-92)
p. Plantar proper digital aa.
   p1. Medial plantar proper digital a. III (eq)(IX-89)
   p2. Lateral plantar proper digital a. III (eq)
   p3. Abaxial plantar proper digital a. III (bo)(IX-91)
   p4. Axial plantar proper digital a. III (bo)
   p5. Axial plantar proper digital a. IV (bo)
   p6. Abaxial plantar proper digital a. IV (bo)
   p7. Dorsal proper digital aa. III, IV (bo)(IX-92)

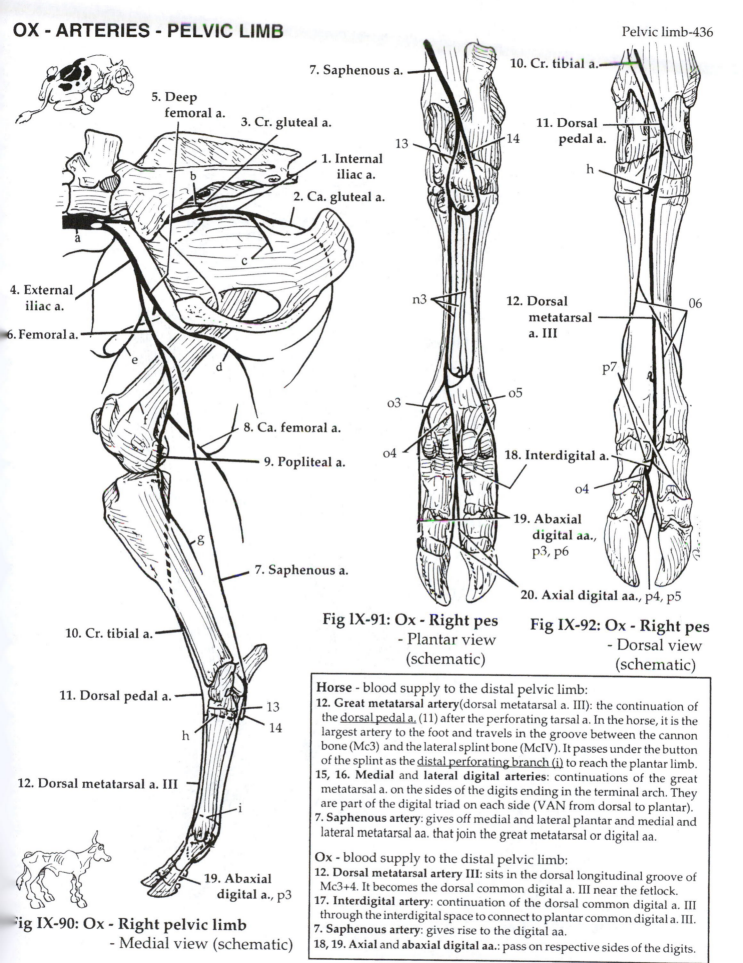

5. Deep femoral a.

3. Cr. gluteal a.

1. Internal iliac a.

2. Ca. gluteal a.

4. External iliac a.

6. Femoral a.

8. Ca. femoral a.

9. Popliteal a.

7. Saphenous a.

10. Cr. tibial a.

11. Dorsal pedal a.

12. Dorsal metatarsal a. III

19. Abaxial digital a., p3

Fig IX-90: Ox - Right pelvic limb
- Medial view (schematic)

7. Saphenous a.

10. Cr. tibial a.

11. Dorsal pedal a.

12. Dorsal metatarsal a. III

18. Interdigital a.

19. Abaxial digital aa., p3, p6

20. Axial digital aa., p4, p5

Fig lX-91: Ox - Right pes
- Plantar view
(schematic)

Fig IX-92: Ox - Right pes
- Dorsal view
(schematic)

Horse - blood supply to the distal pelvic limb:

12. Great metatarsal artery(dorsal metatarsal a. III): the continuation of the <u>dorsal pedal a.</u> (11) after the perforating tarsal a. In the horse, it is the largest artery to the foot and travels in the groove between the cannon bone (Mc3) and the lateral splint bone (McIV). It passes under the button of the splint as the <u>distal perforating branch (i)</u> to reach the plantar limb.

15, 16. Medial and **lateral digital arteries**: continuations of the great metatarsal a. on the sides of the digits ending in the terminal arch. They are part of the digital triad on each side (VAN from dorsal to plantar).

7. Saphenous artery: gives off medial and lateral plantar and medial and lateral metatarsal aa. that join the great metatarsal or digital aa.

Ox - blood supply to the distal pelvic limb:

12. Dorsal metatarsal artery III: sits in the dorsal longitudinal groove of Mc3+4. It becomes the dorsal common digital a. III near the fetlock.

17. Interdigital artery: continuation of the dorsal common digital a. III through the interdigital space to connect to plantar common digital a. III.

7. Saphenous artery: gives rise to the digital aa.

18, 19. Axial and **abaxial digital aa.**: pass on respective sides of the digits.

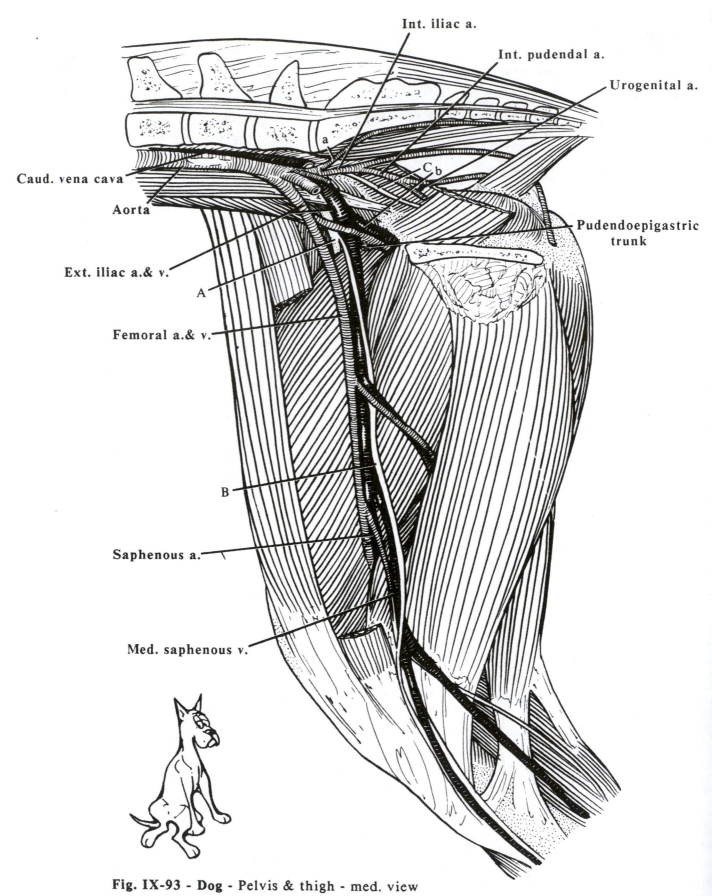

Fig. IX-93 - Dog - Pelvis & thigh - med. view

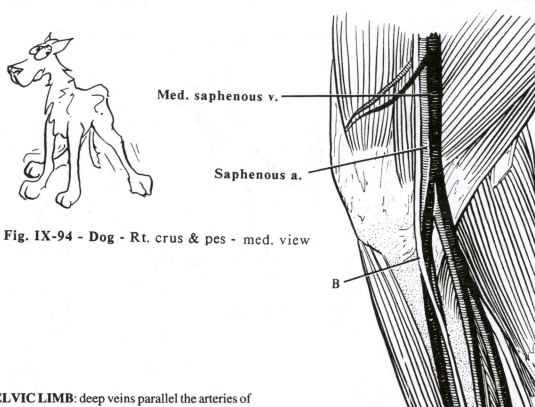

Med. saphenous v.

Saphenous a.

Fig. IX-94 - Dog - Rt. crus & pes - med. view

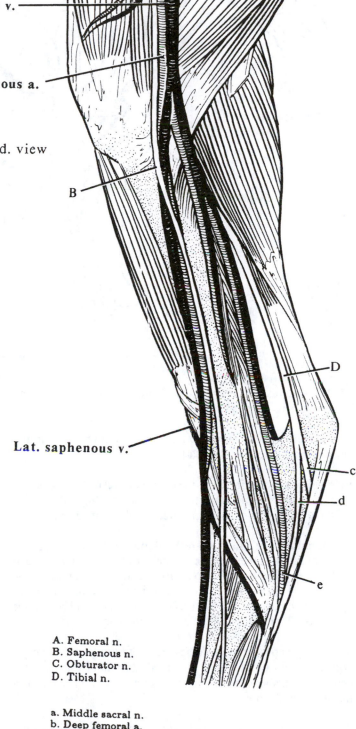

B

D

Lat. saphenous v.

c

d

e

VEINS - PELVIC LIMB: deep veins parallel the arteries of the same name. Superficial drainage occurs via the medial and lateral saphenous veins that do not parallel similarly-named arteries.

Medial saphenous vein: passes on the medial side of the limb with the saphenous artery and vein. It empties into the femoral vein at the apex of the femoral triangle.

Lateral saphenous vein: travels on the lateral side of the limb to enter the caudal popliteal region and empty into the distal caudal femoral vein.

CLINICAL

Lateral saphenous vein: used for venipuncture in the dog when the cephalic vein is unavailable. Injecting where it crosses the lateral side of the leg is difficult because of its mobility. Injecting it more proximally, where it dives into the hamstring muscles, is easier.

Cranial branch of the median saphenous vein: in the horse crosses the dorsomedial aspect of the tarsus. This crosses the "cunean" tendon (medial insertion of the cranial tibial muscle) and the injection site of the dorso-medial pouch of the talocrural joint.

Intravenous local anesthetic of the bovine pes: apply a tourniquet below the tarsus to distend the five superficial veins in the area. Inject any one to anesthetize the distal limb.

A. Femoral n.
B. Saphenous n.
C. Obturator n.
D. Tibial n.

a. Middle sacral n.
b. Deep femoral a.
c. Lat. plantar n. (tibial n.)
d. Med. plantar n. (tibial n.)
e. Med. plantar a.

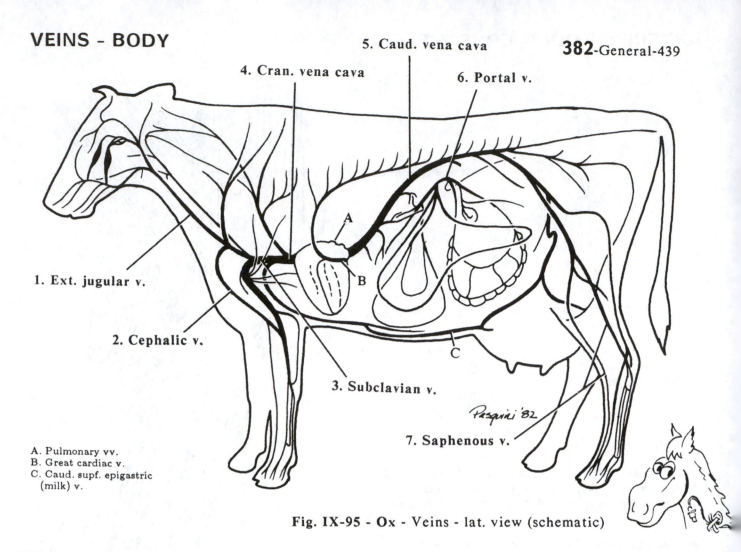

A. Pulmonary vv.
B. Great cardiac v.
C. Caud. supf. epigastric
   (milk) v.

Fig. IX-95 - Ox - Veins - lat. view (schematic)

VEINS: the vessels returning oxygen-depleted blood from the body tissues to the heart.

1. External jugular vein: the large vein in the neck returning blood from the head to the heart.

Veins of the thoracic limb: the deep veins usually parallel the arteries of the limb and take the same names. Superficial veins pass under the skin not accompanied by like-named arteries.

2. Cephalic vein: arises from the digital veins on the palmar aspect of the paw. It extends proximally around the medial side of the forearm just above the carpus to reach the cranial surface of the limb. Here it is joined by the accessory cephalic vein. It continues up the limb crossing the flexor surface of the elbow and lateral side of the arm. It empties into the external jugular vein.

Accessory cephalic vein: arises from the digital veins on the dorsal surface of the paw. It extends proximally to join the cephalic vein above the carpus in the carnivores and ox and near the elbow in the horse.

3. Subclavian vein: the vessel returning blood from the thoracic limb to the heart.

Brachiocephalic vein: found only in the carnivores and pig, formed by the intersection of the external jugular and subclavian veins.

4. Cranial vena cava: the great vessel emptying into the cranial part of the right atrium, returning blood from the head, neck, thoracic limbs and cranial part of the walls of the thoracic cavity.

5. Caudal vena cava: the great vessel emptying into the caudal part of the right atrium, returning blood to the heart from the abdomen, pelvis and pelvic limbs.

6. Portal vein: the large vein carrying essentially all the blood from the abdominal viscera to the liver and its internal sinusoids. Hepatic veins located inside the liver, return to the caudal vena cava.

Veins of the pelvic limb: Deep veins parallel the arteries of the same name. Superficial drainage occurs via the saphenous veins.

7. Medial and **lateral saphenous veins**: the superficial drainage of the pelvic limb. They do not parallel similarly-named arteries. The median saphenous vein travels on the medial side of the limb and empties into the femoral vein in the femoral triangle. The lateral saphenous vein travels on the lateral side of the limb and empties into the caudal femoral vein behind the stifle.

External jugular vein: empties into the brachiocephalic vein in carnivores and pigs; directly into the cranial vena cava in ruminants and horses.

Subclavian vein: empties into the brachiocephalic vein in carnivores and pigs; into the cranial vena cava in ruminants and horses.

Brachiocephalic vein: present only in carnivores and pigs; formed by the convergence of the external jugular and subclavian veins.

Cranial vena cava: formed by the converging of the brachiocephalic vein in carnivores and pigs and by the external jugular and subclavian veins in horses and ruminants.

CLINICAL

Venipuncture: placing a needle into a vein in order to withdraw blood or inject a substance. Sites of venipuncture:

Dog:
- **Cephalic vein**: most common site of venipuncture.
- **Jugular vein**: the second most common site.
- **Lateral saphenous vein**: a third choice, but a poor choice, after the cephalic and external jugular veins.
- **Sublingual vein**: sometimes used during surgery.

Large animals:
- **External jugular vein**: most common site.

Caudal vena caval thrombosis: Cattle, septic thrombi from liver abscesses passing in caudal vena cava to form abscesses in the lungs.

LYMPHATIC SYSTEM: consists of lymphatic tissues and vessels. This system returns protein-rich fluid to the blood circulation that escapes from the blood capillaries into tissue spaces. It is, therefore, part of the circulatory system. The lymphatic system is involved in lymphocyte and antibody production, phagocytosis of particulate matter, and movement of fats from the digestive system to the circulation. Thus, it may be considered part of the hemopoietic (blood forming), immune, reticuloendothelial, and digestive systems. Lymph vessels are not present in the brain, spinal cord, or bone marrow.

The pumping of the heart causes hydrostatic pressure that filters out all components of the blood, except blood cells and platelets, from the capillaries into surrounding tissue. The lymphatic ves-

sels have greater permeability than the capillaries, easily "picking up" proteins and large molecules. Muscle contractions compress the lymphatic vessels, moving the "lymph" along. Lymph nodes are scattered along the course of the lymphatic vessels and contain primitive cells and macrophages. The primitive cells differentiate into lymphocytes and/or plasma cells. Macrophages lining the lymph nodes engulf substances, including metastasizing cancer cells, entering the lymph nodes. Lymphocytes are also produced by the spleen, thymus, and tonsils. The spleen also phagocytoses aged erythrocytes.

Lymph capillaries: blind-ended tubes located throughout the body. More permeable than blood capillaries, they "pick up" the excess interstitial fluid, which is then called "lymph".

Lymphatic vessels: the larger vessels formed by the convergence of lymph capillaries. Similar to veins, the lymphatic vessels differ in having thinner walls, more valves, and lymph nodes along their course.

Lymph nodes (lnn., sin.=ln.): the ovoid or bean-shaped, encapsulated structures located along the course of the medium-sized lymphatic vessels. The lymph nodes function as filters and germinal centers for lymphocytes. Each node has a capsule of fibrous connective tissue. Trabeculae extend from the capsule into the lymph node. The outer cortex and inner medulla make up the parenchyma of the node. Lymph enters the periphery of the lymph node by afferent lymphatic vessels, passes through the parenchymal sinuses, and out the hilus of the lymph node by a single efferent lymphatic vessel. Lymph picks up lymphocytes and is subjected to macrophages as it passes through the node.

Primitive cells: Located in lymph nodes, they differentiate into lymphoctyes and/or plasma cells.

Macrophages: the phagocytic cells lining the walls of the sinuses.

LYMPHOCENTERS: groups of lymph nodes draining the same region of the body in all species. Outlined on the next few pages are the lymphocenters of the body and their major lymph nodes (minor nodes have been ignored). Trunks and ducts drain the lymphocenters back to the general circulation at the so-called "venous angle". The "venous angle" is where the ducts or trunks empty into the large veins in the thoracic inlet.

HEAD and NECK - LYMPHOCENTERS:

1. Parotid lymph node: represents the parotid lymphocenter. It is located under the cranial edge of the parotid gland. It drains the dorsal part of the head, including the orbit and parotid gland, then the lymph continues to the retropharyngeal nodes. It is palpable in the dog and ox.

2. Mandibular lymph nodes: represents the mandibular

lymphocenter and consists of a group of nodes located ventral to the angle of the jaw. They drain that part of the head not drained by the parotid gland to the medial retropharyngeal node. Present in all species, they are palpable in the dog, ox, and horse.

Retropharyngeal lymphocenter: drains the deeper structures of the head and neck, including the pharynx and larynx. They also receive lymph coming from the parotid and mandibular lymph nodes.

• **3. Medial retropharyngeal lymph node**: the largest lymph node of the head and neck, present in all species. It lies between the larynx and the wing of the atlas and is not normally palpable.

• **4. Lateral retropharyngeal lymph node**: usually absent in the dog (palpable if present) and palpable in the ox.

5. Superficial cervical lymph nodes: represent the superficial cervical lymphocenter. They are present in all species and palpable in the dog, ox, and horse. Located in front of the shoulder joint under the superficial neck muscles, they drain the superficial neck and dorsal thorax along with the proximal part of the forelimb.

6. Deep cervical lymphocenter: the chain of deep lymph nodes (cranial, middle and caudal) along the length of the trachea. It drains the deep and ventral structures of the neck into the thoracic duct on the left side or into the lymphatic duct on the right.

A. RIGHT and **LEFT TRACHEAL (JUGULAR) TRUNKS**: traveling along the trachea, draining the lymph nodes of the head and neck . They empty into the thoracic duct on the left side, the right lymphatic duct, or the vessels of the thoracic inlet.

THORACIC LIMB and **THORAX LYMPHOCENTERS**: the thoracic lymphocenters can be divided into parietal (dorsal and ventral thoracic lymphocenters represented by the intercostal and sternal lymph nodes, respectively) and visceral groups (mediastinal and bronchial lymphocenters).

7. Mediastinal lymphocenters: consist of the cranial mediastinal lymph nodes in all species. The carnivores lack the caudal mediastinal lymph nodes that are huge in the ruminants.

8. Bronchial lymphocenters: consist of nodes located around the tracheal bifurcation. All species have left tracheobronchial lymph nodes.

9. Axillary lymph node (part of the axillary lymphocenter): constantly present in all species and palpable in the dog. Located in the axilla, it drains the forelimb and the thoracic wall, including the first three pairs of mammary glands in the dog. The accessory axillary lymph node is present in the cat and inconstant in the dog and ox. The horse has a palpable cubital lymph node.

ABDOMENAL LYMPHOCENTERS:

10. Lumbar lymphocenters: consist of lumbar lymph nodes located along the abdominal aorta. They drain the kidney, loins, adrenal glands, and abdominal portion of the urogenital system, including the testes, into the lumbar trunks or cisterna chyli. The carnivores lack renal lymph nodes.

11. Celiac lymphocenter: consists of splenic, gastric, hepatic, and pancreaticoduodenal lymph nodes that drain associated structures to the cisterna chyli (see below). The ruminants have many nodes associated with the compartments of their stomach.

12. Cranial mesenteric lymphocenter: consists of the jejunal, cecal, and colic lymph nodes. They are located near these organs and drain into the cisterna chyli.

• **13. Cranial mesenteric lymph nodes**: a surprisingly large node located in the root of the mesentery of the dog.

14. Caudal mesenteric lymphocenter: represented by the caudal mesenteric lymph nodes draining the descending colon.

F. VISCERAL TRUNKS: drain the digestive organs to the cisterna chyli or lumbar trunks.

PELVIS and PELVIC LIMB LYMPHOCENTERS

15. Popliteal lymphocenter: represented by the superficial popliteal lymph nodes in the carnivores (palpable in the dog) and the deep popliteal lymph nodes in the other species. They drain the distal limb into the medial iliac center.

16. Ischial lymphocenter: absent in the dog.

17. Deep inguinal lymphocenter: located along the external iliac artery. The horse has deep inguinal lymph nodes.

Superficial inguinal lymphocenter: drains the groin, caudal mammary glands, and scrotum into the iliosacral or deep inguinal lymph nodes.

• **18. Superficial inguinal lymph nodes**: present in all species, they are palpable in the dog, ruminants, and horse. They are also called the mammary or scrotal lymph nodes if they drain the male reproductive organs or the udder (caudal mammae in dogs) as well as the groin.

• **19. Subiliac or "prefemoral" lymph node**: absent in the dog and palpable in the ruminants and horse.

20. Medial iliac and **sacral lymph nodes** (part of iliosacral lymphocenter): located near the termination of the aorta in the abdominal and pelvic cavities. They drain the surrounding region, the pelvic organs, and the hindlimb into the lumbar trunks.

B. LUMBAR TRUNKS: arise from the medial iliac nodes and extend to the cistern chyli. They drain the pelvis, pelvic limb and pelvis, abdominal organs, and abdominal wall.

C. CISTERNA CHYLI: the dilation at the thoracolumbar junc-

Normally Palpable Superficial Lymph Nodes

• Parotid lymph node	- dog, ox
• Mandibular lymph nodes	- dog, ox, horse
• Lateral retropharyngeal lymph node	- ox
• Superficial cervical lymph nodes	- dog, ox, horse
• Axillary lymph node	- dog
• Cubital lymph node	- horse
• Superficial popliteal lymph node	- dog
• Subiliac lymph nodes	- ruminant, horse
• Superficial inguinal lnn.	- dog, ruminant, horse

4. Lat. retropharyngeal ln.

1. Parotid ln.

2. Mandibular lnn.

5. Superficial cervical lnn.

19. Subiliac ln.

18. Superficial inguinal lnn.

Fig IX-96: Ox - Palpable superficial lymph nodes (schematic)

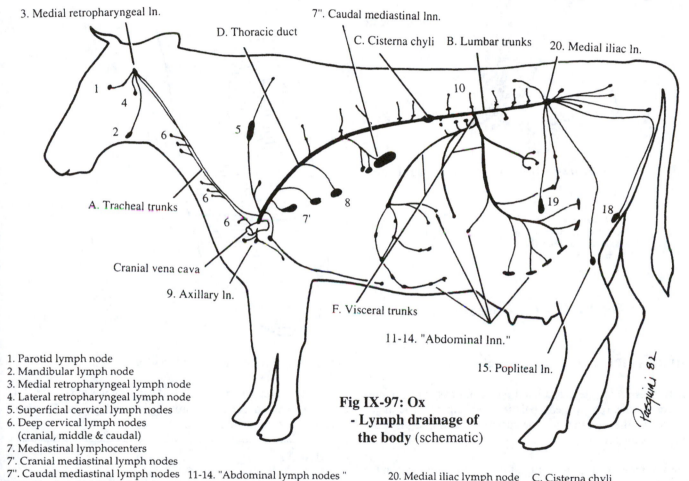

3. Medial retropharyngeal ln.

D. Thoracic duct

7". Caudal mediastinal lnn.

C. Cisterna chyli   B. Lumbar trunks

20. Medial iliac ln.

A. Tracheal trunks

Cranial vena cava

9. Axillary ln.

F. Visceral trunks

11-14. "Abdominal lnn."

15. Popliteal ln.

Fig IX-97: Ox - Lymph drainage of the body (schematic)

1. Parotid lymph node
2. Mandibular lymph node
3. Medial retropharyngeal lymph node
4. Lateral retropharyngeal lymph node
5. Superficial cervical lymph nodes
6. Deep cervical lymph nodes
   (cranial, middle & caudal)
7. Mediastinal lymphocenters
7'. Cranial mediastinal lymph nodes
7". Caudal mediastinal lymph nodes
8. Tracheobronchial lymph nodes
9. Axillary lymph node
10. Lumbar lymph nodes

11-14. "Abdominal lymph nodes"
15. Popliteal lymph node
18. Superficial inguinal lymph nodes
19. Subiliac lymph node (absent in dog)

20. Medial iliac lymph node

A. Tracheal trunks
B. Lumbar trunks

C. Cisterna chyli
D. Thoracic duct
E. Right lymphatic duct (not shown)
F. Visceral trunks

tion receiving lymph from the lumbar and intestinal (visceral) trunks (draining the lymph nodes of the abdomen, pelvis and pelvic limb).

D. THORACIC DUCT: the major lymphatic vessel draining the entire body, except the right thoracic limb, right cranial thorax, and right side of the neck. It begins at the cisterna chyli, passes through the aortic hiatus cranially on the right side between the

azygos vein and the aorta. Passing to the left side of the thorax in the cranial mediastinum, it empties near the thoracic inlet ("venous angle") into the jugular vein or the cranial vena cava.

E. RIGHT LYMPHATIC DUCT: drains the right cranial thorax, right thoracic limb and right side of the neck into the venous system where the cranial vena cava is formed.

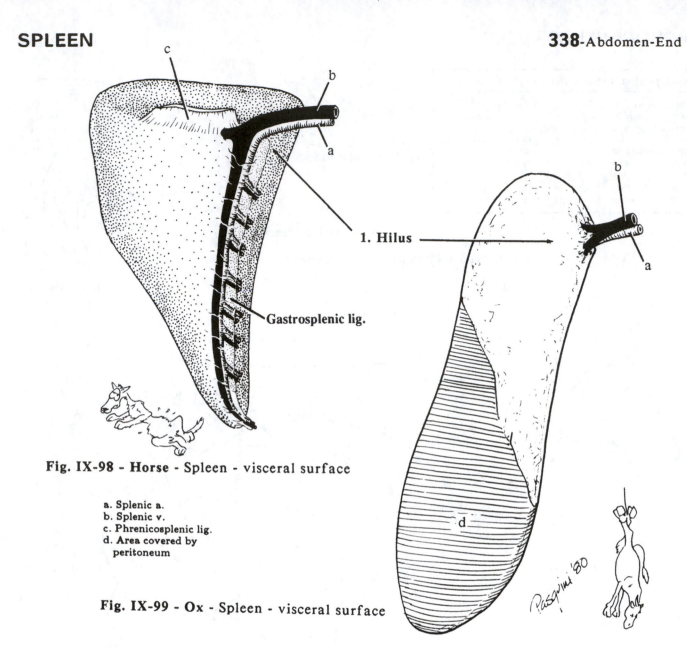

Fig. IX-98 - Horse - Spleen - visceral surface

a. Splenic a.
b. Splenic v.
c. Phrenicosplenic lig.
d. Area covered by
   peritoneum

Fig. IX-99 - Ox - Spleen - visceral surface

1. Hilus

Gastrosplenic lig.

OTHER LYMPHOID STRUCTURES

Tonsils: masses of <u>un</u>encapsulated lymphoid tissue below mucous membranes (pharyngeal, palatine and lingual). The major ones protect the entrance to the larynx and esophagus from incoming pathogens.

Peyer's patches: diffuse accumulation of lymphatic tissue in the wall of the ileum.

Hemal nodes: filter blood instead of lymph found in the ruminants along the aorta. They are easily distinguished from lymph node by their dark, reddish brown color.

SPLEEN: the largest lymphoid organ in the body. It is a flat, elongated structure interposed in the blood stream located next to the left abdominal wall. In the fetus it produces red blood cells. In the adult it stores red blood cells that can be squeezed back into circulation when needed. It also produces lymphocytes, stores iron, and destroys worn out red blood cells.

1. Hilus: the area where vessels and nerves enter the spleen. It is a long groove in the carnivores, horse and pig, and a small indentation in ruminants.

CLINICAL

Splenectomy: removal of the spleen. This is a common procedure in the <u>dog</u>, indicated for tumors in or traumatic rupture of the spleen. Animals do quite well without a spleen.

Superficial lymph nodes: can be an important indicator of an illness because they enlarge and become palpable in response to infection.

Meat inspection and **necropsy:** pathogenic changes in lymph nodes make them important in these disciplines.

Chapter X
Nervous System

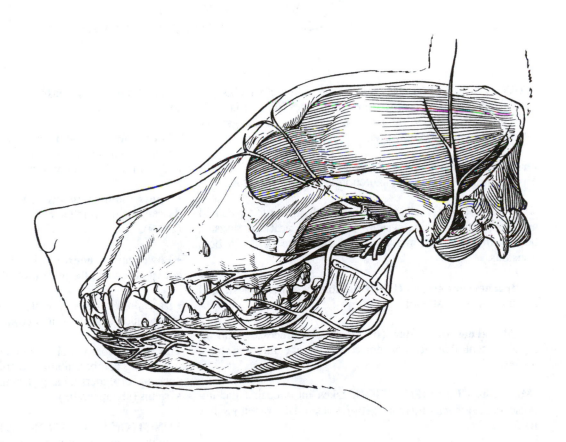

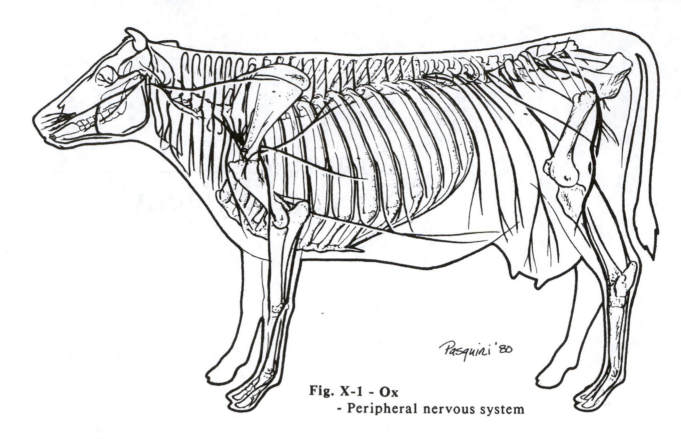

Fig. X-1 - Ox
- Peripheral nervous system

NERVOUS SYSTEM: the control center allowing the body to react to the environment. It stores, integrates, and initiates all appropriate response to information it receives. It is organized into a communication network.

Organization of the Nervous System: Functionally, it can be divided into the somatic and autonomic nervous systems.

STRUCTURAL CLASSIFICATION: divided into the central and peripheral nervous system. This is an artificial division because many of the nerves of the body are partly in both divisions.

Central nervous system (CNS): the control center consisting of the brain and spinal cord.

Peripheral nervous system (PNS): all nerve processes connecting to the central nervous system, consisting of cranial and spinal nerves.

IMPULSE CLASSIFICATION: takes into account the impulses (sensory or motor) carried by nerves and the directions they travel.

Sensory (afferent) system: conducts sensory (afferent) information from the periphery to the central nervous system(CNS). Sensory information travels in ascending tracts from the spinal cord ("lower") to the brain ("higher").

• **Ascending tracts:** sensory fibers in the spinal cord that travel toward the brain.

Motor (efferent) system: consists of motor (efferent) nerves that conduct from higher to lower levels of the central nervous system and from the central nervous system to the periphery.

• **Upper motor neurons (UMN):** extend from the brain down descending tracts in the cord to synapse on lower motor neurons (LMN).

• **Lower motor neurons (LMN):** extend away from the spinal cord and brain to the muscles and glands of the body.

• **Descending tracts:** bundles of upper motor neuron fibers that move caudally in the spinal cord.

This system doesn't hold up under close scrutiny, especially the integrating components in the spinal cord. It is still a valuable concept for understanding damage to the central or peripheral systems (see appendix).

FUNCTIONAL CLASSIFICATION: takes into account the activities that are directed by the nervous system.

Somatic nervous system (soma, body): carries conscious <u>voluntary</u> information from the central nervous system to the skeletal muscles along cranial and spinal nerves. It functions to keep the

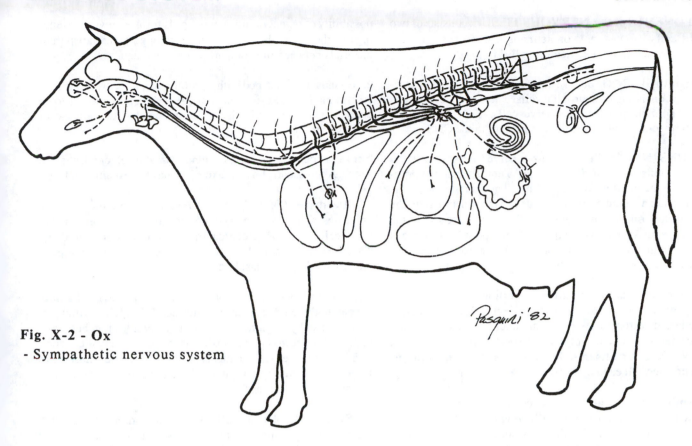

Fig. X-2 - Ox
- Sympathetic nervous system

body in balance with its external environment. This system allows the animal to move and interact with its environment.

Autonomic nervous system (ANS) (*auto*, self; *nomos*, law): carries involuntary information (sensory and motor) to and from smooth muscle, cardiac muscle, and glands of the body along cranial and spinal nerves to the spinal cord and brain. It functions to regulate the balance (homeostasis) of the body's internal environment.

FIBERS - FUNCTIONAL CLASSIFICATION (pg. 560): divides fibers of peripheral nerves according to their function into afferent and efferent nerves which in turn are divided into somatic and visceral divisions, and then subdivided into general and special categories. It also takes into account their embryonic branchial mesoderm origin. Three capital letters (GSA, GSE, SVE, GVA, GVE, SSA, and SSV) are given to each of the subdivisions. Although this may be a convenient shorthand for the neurologists that uses them all the time, it is extremely difficult the student. Not only is it confusing and hard to learn, if not continually used, it is soon forgotten.

FIBERS - SIMPLIFIED FUNCTIONAL CLASSIFICATION: the author proposes a simpler system for teaching purposes. Although it may not hold up to close scrutiny, it reduces the confusion when learning basic neurology.

• **Somatic fibers** (motor and sensory): from nerves of the somatic

nervous system to skeletal muscle; and from skin and deeper somatic structures.

• **Somatic motor (efferent) fibers** (SVE, GSE): supply skeletal (somatic) muscles, no matter what the branchial arch origin.

• **Somatic sensory (afferent) fibers** (GSA): carry sensory information from skin and deeper somatic structures (skeletal muscle, skin, tendons, joint capsules, bones, etc.).

• **ANS fibers:** from nerves of the autonomic nervous system. They innervate smooth muscle, cardiac muscle, and glands. They are subdivided into fibers of the sympathetic and parasympathetic divisions. Sympathetic fibers are carried by branches of all spinal and most cranial nerves. Parasympathetic fibers are restricted to some sacral spinal nerves (pelvic nerve) and only a few cranial nerves (Cn III, VII, IX, and X).

• **ANS motor (efferent) fibers:** these can be further divided into sympathetic and parasympathetic fibers.

• **ANS sensory (afferent) fibers:** carry sensory fibers from blood vessels and viscera throughout the body. Some somatic sensory fibers also affect ANS motor fibers.

• **Special sensory fibers:** carry special sensory information of taste, smell, vision, hearing, and vestibular function to the brain.

NEURON

COMPONENTS of the NERVOUS TISSUE: consists of two types of cells - **nerve cells** or **neurons** and **neuroglial cells**. These are bathed in the **extracellular fluid**.

Neuroglia (nyoo-ROG-lee-ah): the supporting structure of nervous tissue consisting of neuroglial cells. These specialized cells support, nourish and insulate nerve cells. They replace the supporting connective tissue the not present in the CNS.

NEURONS (NYOO-ron) (G. *neuron*, nerve) or **nerve cell**: the functional units of the nervous system. Their specialized properties make the nervous system unique. The largest cells in the body, they are also the most numerous (on the order of 10 to the 12th power, a million million cells). Most of these are in the central nervous system as compared to the peripheral nervous system. A number of characteristics make neurons so specialized that no two cells are identical.

Compartmentalization: the different portions of a neuron have different membrane properties and to a degree different internal organelles, therefore, making them functional and structural compartments. This concept explains how diseases can effect only specific compartments. These specialized compartments communicate with each other by transport systems.

Biochemical specialization: nerves cells are grouped biochemically by their neurotransmitters, allowing each set to carry out specific functions. Clinically, diseases can attack sets of neurons based on their specific neurotransmitters.

Nonreproducible: nerve cells uniquely lack the ability to divide. A neuron dies if it is damaged and its function is lost. Other nerve cells may take over this function.

Complex connections: distinguishes nervous tissue from other tissues and is central to the functioning of nervous tissue. These connections are very precise (e.g., a specific point on the brain is connected to the little finger).

Information: neurons are the information cells of the body. They are specialized to process or integrate information, conduct it to different parts of the body, transfer it from one cell to another, store and/or generate information.

1. Cell body (soma [SOH-ma] or perikaryon): arranged as a nucleus and its neuroplasm (cytoplasm) which contains typical organelles (e.g., mitochondria, RER, and golgi [with the exception of the organelles used in mitosis like the centrioles]). Rough endoplasmic reticulum (RER) is in high concentrations because neurons are the most metabolically-active cells in the body, producing huge amounts of protein. The RER is clumped into large, granular, basophilic inclusions called Nissl (NIS-l) bodies scattered throughout the neuroplasm of the cell body and dendrites, but not in the axon. This feature makes the body the control (trophic) center of the neuron. The cell body sythesizes enzymes and other molecules essential to the normal function and the survival of the other compartments of the neuron (dentrites and axon). If the cell body is damaged, the rest of the cell dies. On the other hand, if an axon in the periphery is damaged, it has the possibility of regenerating. Neurofibrils form a network extending into the nerve fibers, functioning in support and transport of materials between the compartments of the neuron.

2. Nucleus: well-defined with a prominent nucleolus and granular chromatin. After four years of age the nucleus appears to be unable to undergo mitosis, therefore, unable to increase or replace neurons.

Nerve processes: two types extend from the cell dendrites and axons. A cell usually has one axon, but may have many dendrites.

• **3. Dendrites** (DEN-dryt) (G. *dendron*, tree): the multiple processes acting as the receptor portion of the neuron that conduct information (electrical impulses) toward the cell body. They are usually multi-branched processes containing cytoplasmic organelles and Nissl bodies.

• **4. Axon**: carries information (electrical impulses) away from the cell body to other neurons or tissue. It is a long cylindrical process, usually singular, that may have tiny side branches (axon collaterals). Axons have neurofibrils, but no Nissl bodies. Their terminal branches (telodendrites) end in **synaptic knobs** (end feet). The axon usually originates from the axon hillock, a small elevation on the cell body.

• **5. Synaptic knobs** (also called end feet, boutons, or buttons): form the presynaptic side of a synapse (pg. 449) and contain synaptic vesicles that store chemicals for release at the synapse.

CLASSIFICATION of NEURONS: nerves are classified as sensory neurons, motor neurons, or interneurons. 99.997% of the neurons of the CNS are interneurons.

• **Sensory (afferent) neuron**: brings information from receptors in the periphery to the central nervous system. These neurons have their cell bodies located <u>outside</u> the central nervous system.

• **Motor (efferent) neuron**: carries information from the central nervous system to peripheral muscles, glands, or other neurons. The neurons of the motor nervous system have their cell bodies <u>in</u> the central nervous system (brain or spinal cord) and their axons (motor, efferent) extending to the periphery.

• **Interneuron**, association, connecting or internuncial neurons: carry sensory impulses from sensory neurons to motor neurons. The whole interneuron (cell body, dendrites and axon) is located <u>in</u> the CNS (brain or spinal cord).

Classification of neurons based on processes:

• Multipolar: receive many dendrites and has one axon.

• Bipolar: receive one common trunk formed by its dendrites and sends out one axon.

• Unipolar or pseudounipolar: receive one common trunk formed by the axon and dendrite.

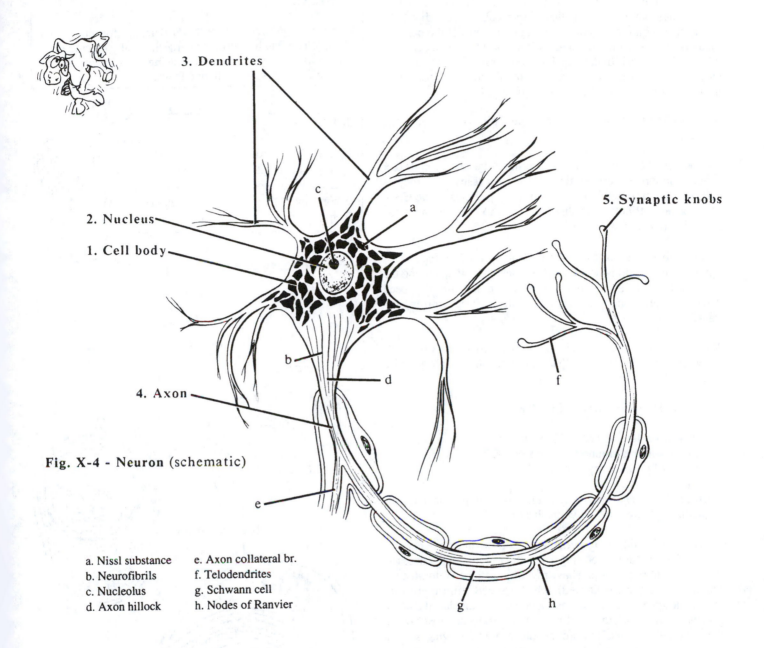

3. Dendrites

5. Synaptic knobs

2. Nucleus

1. Cell body

c

a

4. Axon

b

d

Fig. X-4 - Neuron (schematic)

f

e

g   h

a. Nissl substance	e. Axon collateral br.
b. Neurofibrils	f. Telodendrites
c. Nucleolus	g. Schwann cell
d. Axon hillock	h. Nodes of Ranvier

CLINICAL

Neuritis (noo-RY-tis): inflammation of a nerve.

Compartmentalization: the condition allowing diseases to differentially affect separate parts of the nerve cell.

Neurotransmitters: because neurotransmitters are different for different sets of neurons, disease processes can selectively affect specific sets of neurons.

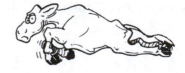

NEUROGLIA

NEUROGLIA (nyoo-ROG-lee-al) (neuro + G. *glia*, glue): the second cellular component of nervous tissue. They are about 10 to 50 times more abundant than nerve cells. Neuroglial cells function as a binding agent to maintain the form of the nervous system. They also provide metabolic support for nerve cells and play a role in repair of damaged nervous tissue. Unlike neurons, they are able to divide, therefore, are the primary source of intrinsic (coming from the tissue itself) tumors.

NEUROGLIA of the CNS: astrocytes, oligodendrocytes and microglia.

Astrocytes (AS-troh-syt) (G. *astron*, star): star-shaped cells that supply support to nervous tissue. The processes of astrocytes extend to form a membrane around the capillaries of the CNS. They bring nutrients from the capillaries to the neurons, thus, providing nutritional support.

Oligodendrocyte (ol'e-goh-DEN-droh-syt) (G. *oligo*, few): Smaller and less branched than astrocytes, they wrap around the axons of nerve cells to form myelin. Myelin increases the speed of conduction along the axon, resulting in faster information transfer.

Microglia (my-KROG-lee-ah) (sin.= microglial cell): the smallest neuroglial cells of the CNS. They migrate and act to phagocytize waste products in nerve tissue.

PERIPHERAL NEUROGLIAL CELLS

1. Schwann cells: the neuroglia of the PNS. They form myelin sheaths by winding around nerve processes. They are the equivalent of the oligodendrocyte of the CNS.

Nodes of Ranvier (rahn-ve-ay)(Fig. X-4,h): unmyelinated gaps between segments of the myelin sheath.

Myelin (MY-e-lin): a lipoprotein (all cell membranes are composed of lipoproteins) forming a sheath around nerve processes. Axons or dendrites can both have myelin sheaths (**myelinated**) or remain naked (**unmyelinated**). Myelin sheaths function to increase the speed of impulse conduction and to insulate the nerve process. In the PNS, the myelin sheath is produced by **Schwann cells** winding themselves around the process, leaving several continuous layers of its cell membrane. The remaining portion of the Schwann cell encircling the sheath is known as the **neurolemma**, which assists in regeneration of injured axons. Schwann cells also enclose unmyelinated fibers, but without the multiple wrappings.

Myelinated fiber: a process having a myelin sheath.

Unmyelinated fiber: a process lacking a myelin sheath, but still having a Schwann cell covering.

CLINICAL

Astrocytes: proliferate after brain damage, forming a scar (gliosis). This can be detrimental, mechanically placing stress on the surrounding brain tissue, causing irritation of adjacent tissue and/or a possible epileptic focus.

CLINICAL

Equine degenerative myelencephalopathy: degenerative demyelination of nerves carrying proprioception (position) sensory fibers. Common cause of ataxia (incoordination) in young horses.

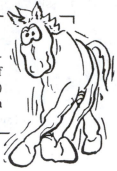

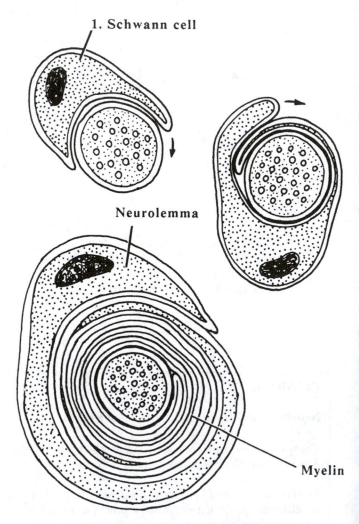

Fig. X-5,6,7 - Schwann cell, wrapping around nerve process

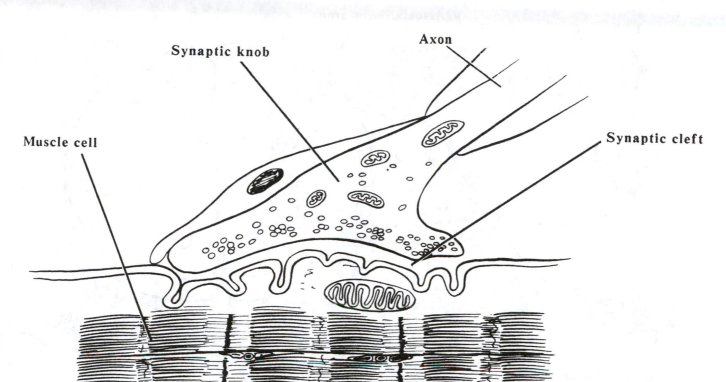

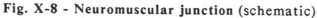

Fig. X-8 - Neuromuscular junction (schematic)

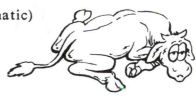

SYNAPSE (SIN-aps) (G. *synapsis,* connection): a specialized site of apposition where information passes from one nerve cell to another cell. The first cell is the presynaptic cell, the second the postsynaptic cell. Between the two cells is a synaptic cleft. The presynaptic cell is always a nerve; the postsynaptic cell can be a nerve, a muscle or a gland.

Nerve action potential (NAP): an electrical event that travels down an axon.

Presynaptic cell: the neuron that is transferring information to the postsynaptic cell.

Synaptic button, bouton, or knob: the terminal end of the presynaptic nerve that is in apposition with the postsynaptic cell. It contains synaptic vesicles.

Synaptic vesicles: membrane-bound organelles containing neurotransmitters located in the synaptic button.

Neurotransmitters: a chemical substance within the synaptic vesicle that mediates information transfer between nerve cells and other cells at synapses. Different sets of neurons use different neurotransmitters.

Postsynaptic cell: the neuron, muscle, or gland receiving infor-

mation from the presynaptic cell.

Receptors: integral proteins inserted in the membrane of the postsynaptic cell. They function to bind with a neurotransmitter, resulting in a change in the membrane of the postsynaptic cell.

Synaptic event: A nerve action potential propagates down the axon to reach the synaptic knob. This causes the synaptic vesicles to release their neurotransmitters into the synaptic cleft. The neurotransmitters diffuse across the cleft to bind to receptors on the postsynaptic membrane. This binding causes a change in the postsynaptic membrane. If the postsynaptic cell is a nerve, it can **initiate** or **inhibit** another nerve action potential in the postsynaptic nerve.

Neuromuscular junction: the synaptic connection between a neuron and muscular tissue where electrical impulses pass from the neuron to the muscle cell. This can result in contraction of the muscle.

CLINICAL

Postparturient paresis/Milk fever: "downer cow" after parturition due to hypocalcemia. Calcium is needed for the release of Ach at the neuromuscular junction. It is treated with IV calcium.

REFLEX ARC

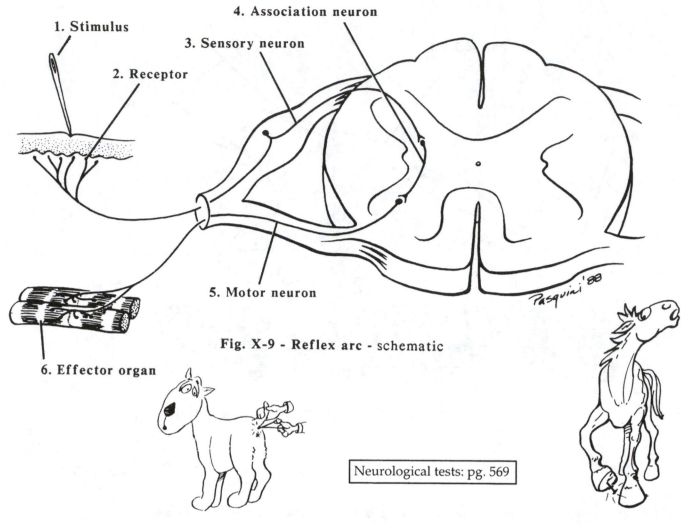

1. Stimulus
2. Receptor
3. Sensory neuron
4. Association neuron
5. Motor neuron
6. Effector organ

Fig. X-9 - Reflex arc - schematic

Neurological tests: pg. 569

REFLEX ARC: the simplest impulse pathway. A reflex is an involuntary response to a sensory stimulus. The reflex arc (the pathway of a reflex) involves a sensory neuron, an interneuron (internuncial neuron), and a motor neuron (the patellar tap lacks an interneuron). Specialized receptors at the end of sensory neurons receive a stimulus, resulting in an impulse. The impulse travels through the dendrite, body, and axon of the sensory neuron into the spinal cord. In the spinal cord, the sensory neuron synapses on an interneuron that carries the impulse to a synapse on a motor neuron. The motor neuron innervates a receptor organ (muscle) to contract (pull away from the stimulus).

• **Stimulus:** a change in the environment (e.g., hot stove).

• **Receptor:** the end of a sensory neuron's dendrite that responds to change (stimulus) by developing a nerve impulse.

• **Sensory (afferent) neuron:** sends sensory impulses to the CNS.

• **Interneuron, association (internucial) neurons:** located in the spinal cord, connect a sensory neuron with a motor neuron. They also can connect with other neurons, thus, send information up to the brain (so when the reflex is over, it can be commented on, "ouch!").

• **Motor (efferent) neuron:** carries an impulse (information) to an effector organ.

• **Effector (target) organ:** the muscle or gland innervated by a motor neuron to react to the stimulus (pull away from the stove).

NUCLEUS: aggregations of nerve cell bodies (perikarya) located in the brain. Their dark color sets the nuclei off from the white nerve fibers.

GANGLION (pl.=ganglia): a group of nerve cell bodies outside the central nervous system, manifested as a swelling of a nerve.

GRAY MATTER: that part of nervous tissue consisting of neuronal cell bodies.

WHITE MATTER: that part of nervous tissue consisting mainly of myelinated nerve fibers.

NERVE: a bundle of nerve processes outside the CNS.

NERVE TRACTS or **FASCICULI** (fah-SIK-yoo ly): nerve fiber bundles of common origin in the brain and spinal cord. They are usually named for their origin and destination.

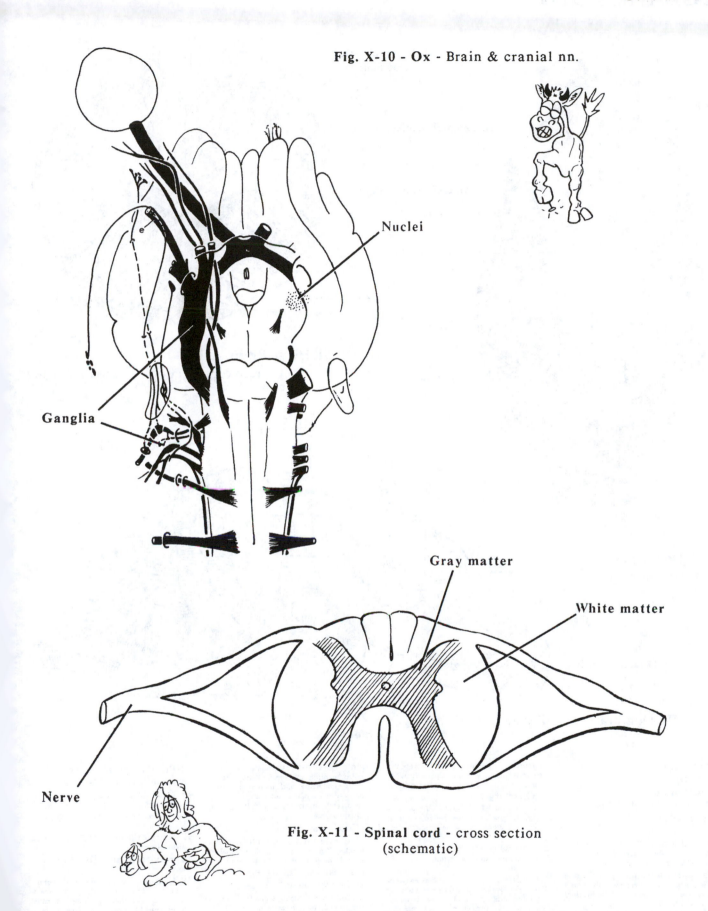

Fig. X-10 - Ox - Brain & cranial nn.

Nuclei

Ganglia

Gray matter

White matter

Nerve

Fig. X-11 - Spinal cord - cross section
(schematic)

CEREBRUM

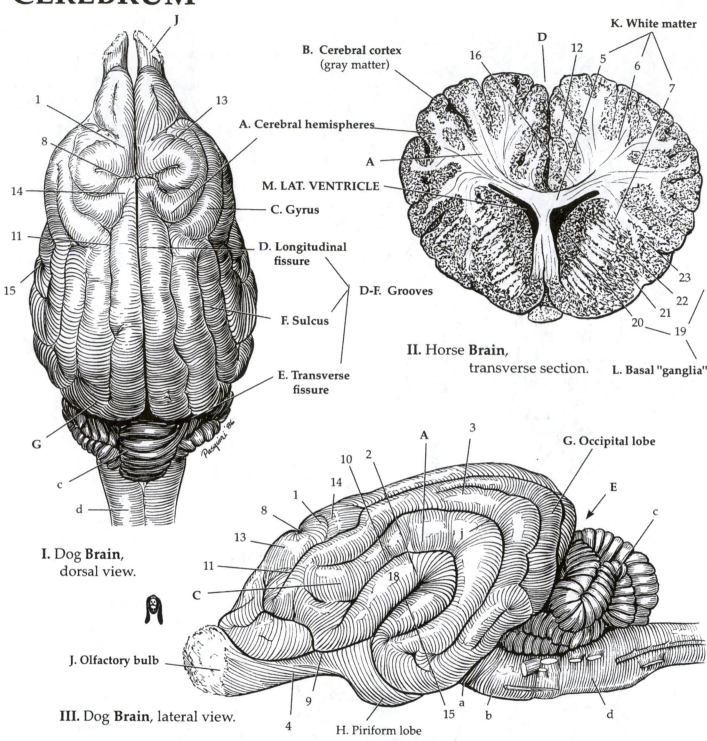

J

1

8

14

11

15

G

c

d

I. Dog Brain, dorsal view.

J. Olfactory bulb

III. Dog Brain, lateral view.

13

B. Cerebral cortex (gray matter)

A. Cerebral hemispheres

M. LAT. VENTRICLE

C. Gyrus

D. Longitudinal fissure

D-F. Grooves

F. Sulcus

E. Transverse fissure

16   D   12   5   6   7   **K. White matter**

A

23   22   21   20   19

II. Horse Brain, transverse section.   **L. Basal "ganglia"**

A   3   **G. Occipital lobe**

10   2

14   E

1   j   c

8

13

11   18

C

9   15   a   b   d

4   **H. Piriform lobe**

a. Midbrain (IV).

b. Pons (IV)

c. Cerebellum (I, II, IV).

d. Medulla oblongata (I, II, IV).

e. Third ventricle (I)

1. **Frontal lobe** (I, III): the rostral part of each cerebral hemisphere. It contains the motor cortex and prefrontal cortex.

2. **Temporal lobe** (III): the lateral side of the cerebrum caudoventral to the lateral fissure. This is the location of the **hearing/auditory** centers.

3. **Parietal lobe** (III): the dorsal part of the cerebrum, it is the somatosensory cortex, that controls conscious proprioception, temperature, pressure, touch and pain sensations.

4. **Olfactory tracts** (III): pass caudally from the bulb to connect to the piriform lobe, amygdala and other parts of the brain. There are lateral and medial olfactory tracts or stria.

5. **Corpus callosum** (II, IV): formed by commissural axons connecting the 2 cerebral hemispheres.

6. **Coronal radiata** (II): wall of axons (white matter) above the corpus callosum radiating into the cortex, formed by commissural, association and projection axons entering or exiting the gyri.

7. **Internal capsule** (II): white matter ventral to the corpus callosum, formed by efferent (projection fibers) and afferent pathways between the cerebral cortex and the brain stem, cerebrum and spinal cord. It continues distally as the corona radiata.

8. **Cruciate sulcus** (I).

9. **Lateral rhinal sulcus** (III): separates the older olfactory cerebrum (rhinencephalon) from the newer cerebrum (neopallium).

10. **Ectosylvian sulcus** (III).

11. **Coronal sulcus** (I, III)

12. **Splenial sulcus** (II): separates the cortex (neopallium) from the archipallium.

13. **Motor area** (I).

14. **Rostral parietal lobe** (I).

15. **Pseudosylvian fissure** (I).

16. **Cingulate gyrus** (II, IV): part of the archipallium (limbic lobe of the cerebral hemispheres) between the corpus callosum and splenial sulcus.

17. **Supracallosal gyri** (IV): part of the archipallium.

18. **Sylvian gyrus** (III): primary auditory cortex.

19. **Corpus striatum** (II): consists of the caudate and lentiform nuclei and the myelinated fibers associated with them. Located at the base of each hemisphere, named for its striated appearance when sectioned.

BRAIN

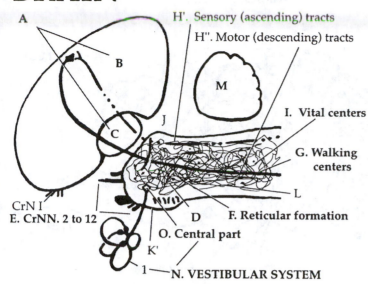

H'. Sensory (ascending) tracts
H". Motor (descending) tracts
I. Vital centers
G. Walking centers
L
F. Reticular formation
O. Central part
N. VESTIBULAR SYSTEM
CrN I
E. CrNN. 2 to 12

I. Brain, schematic, lateral view.

BRAIN: that portion of the central nervous system (CNS) contained within the skull. Functionally, it can be divided into forebrain/proencephalon (cerebrum and diencephalon), brain stem, vestibular system and cerebellum. The brain, like the spinal cord, is also organized into segments, although less distinct.

Encephalon (G. *enkephalos*, brain) is the basis of many medical terms relating to the brain (e.g., encephalitis).

A. FOREBRAIN/PROENCEPHALON (I).

B. **Cerebrum** (I, II, III): forms the bulk of and performs the higher functions of the brain.

C. **Diencephalon** (I, III)*: the rostral brain stem between the cerebrum and the midbrain, surrounding the third ventricle. The diencephalon, a structural component of the brain stem, is functionally related more closely to the cerebrum. The diencephalon is composed primarily of the **thalamus** and the **hypothalamus**.

D. **BRAIN STEM** (I): can be divided into diencephalon, midbrain, pons and medulla. Functionally, it includes the midbrain, pons and medulla oblongata. The brainstem connects the cerebrum, cerebellum and spinal cord; and is also concerned with visceral (internal organs) activities and gives rise to almost all of the cranial nerves. It consists of bundles of nerve fibers and several masses of gray matter (nerve cell bodies) called nuclei.

• **Structures associated with the entire brainstem:**

E. **Cranial nn. 2 to 12** (I): arise from or enter the brainstem. All of the **cranial nn.** except the first (olfactory) are associated with the brain stem.

F. **Reticular formation** (re-TIK-yoo-lar), **reticular activation system** (I): dealing with the level of consciousness, it is housed within the brain stem. It is a network of nerve fibers and islands of gray matter located from the spinal cord to the diencephalon. It is connected to the hypothalamus, basal ganglia, cerebellum and cerebrum. It functions in consciousness and arousal (alertness, depression, stupor and coma). When sensory input comes

into the brain, the reticular formation arouses the cerebral cortex to respond to such input. Without the reticular formation, an animal would remain unconscious or unaware (coma). The reticular information also functions as a filter to all the sensory information coming into the brain, passing on important information to the cerebrum while disregarding others.

G. **Walking centers** (I)(walking motion reflex centers): located in the brain stem. Higher centers initiate and stop the motion through descending motor tracts that cross over in the midbrain. A cat with its cerebrum removed (decerebrate) can be made to walk/run by putting electrodes into the brainstem.

H. Fiber tracts: all ascending and descending nerve tracts must pass through the brainstem.

H'. Sensory (ascending) tracts (I): both proprioceptive fibers and pain, touch and temperature fibers pass through the brainstem.

H". Motor (descending, UMN) tracts (I): pass from the higher brain centers to the rest of the brain and the spinal cord through the brain stem.

I. Vital centers (I): cardiac, vasomotor and respiratory centers are housed in the brainstem.

Parts of the brainstem (excluding the diencephalon which is functionally more closely related to the cerebrum):

J. **Midbrain** (mesencephalon)(III).

K, M. **Metencephalon** (II, III): consists of the pons and the cerebellum.

K. **Pons** (III, IV).

L. **Medulla oblongata** or **medulla** (myelencephalon) (II, III, IV): the caudal portion of the brain stem which continues caudally as the spinal cord.

M. **CEREBELLUM** (I, II, III): the large mass behind the cerebrum, it houses reflex centers coordinating voluntary movements.

N. **VESTIBULAR SYSTEM** (I): controls posture and balance in relationship to gravity and eye movements in relationship to head movements. It is divided into peripheral and central portions.

O. Central vestibular portion (I): includes the vestibular nuclei in the brain stem and centers in the cerebellum.

P. **VENTRICULAR SYSTEM** (III): series of interconnected cavities in the cerebral cortex and brain stem that connect to the subarachnoid space. They are filled with cerebrospinal fluid.

I-XI. Cranial nerves (IV): all but the first (CrN I) arise from or enter the brainstem.

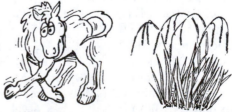

*Roman numerals are used for the cranial nerves and for the figures. When put in parenthesis after a structure's name the Roman numerals indicate which figure they can be found in. Bolding the numeral indicates the best illustration for the structure.

BRAIN

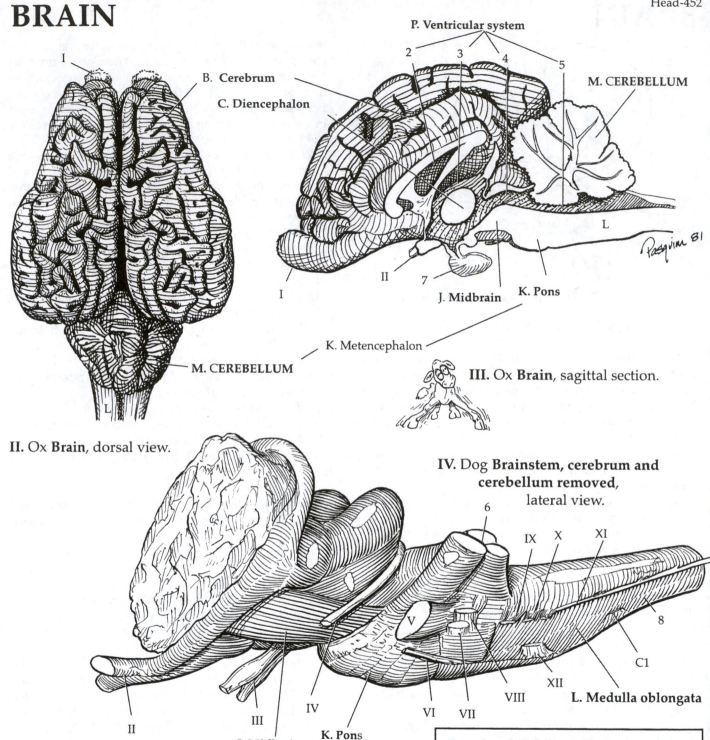

II. Ox Brain, dorsal view.

P. Ventricular system

M. CEREBELLUM

B. Cerebrum

C. Diencephalon

M. CEREBELLUM

J. Midbrain   **K. Pons**

K. Metencephalon

III. Ox Brain, sagittal section.

IV. Dog Brainstem, cerebrum and cerebellum removed, lateral view.

J. Midbrain   **K. Pons**   **L. Medulla oblongata**

I. Olfactory n (CrN 1)(II).
II. Optic n. (CrN 2)(III, IV).
III. Oculomotor n. (CrN 3)(IV).
IV. Trochlear n. (CrN 4)(IV).
V. Trigeminal n. (CrN 5)(IV).
VI. Abducens n. (CrN 6)(IV).
VII. Facial n. (CrN 7)(IV).
VIII. Vestibulocochlear n. (CrN 8)(IV).
IX. Glossopharyngeal n. (CrN 9)(IV).
X. Vagus n. (CrN 10)(IV).
XI. Accessory n. (CrN 11)(IV).
XII. Hypoglossal n. (CrN 12)(IV).
C1. First cervical spinal n. (IV)

1. Peripheral part of the vestibular system (I).
2. Lateral ventricle (III).
3. Third ventricle (III).
4. Mesencephalic aqueduct (III).
5. Fourth ventricle (III).
6. Cerebellar peduncles (IV).
7. Pituitary gland/hypophysis (III).
8. Spinal cord

Functional division of the brain
• Forebrain/prosencephalon (cerebrum and diencephalon)
• Brain stem
• Vestibular system
• Cerebellum

Anatomical divisions of the brain
• Prosencephalon/cerebrum
• Brainstem
  - Diencephalon
  - Midbrain/mesencephalon
  - Metencephalon: pons and cerebellum
  - Myelencephalon (medulla oblongata)

CEREBRUM

CEREBRUM (SER-ee-brum) or telencephalon (L. brain): the largest part of the brain, it carries out the higher brain functions. It receives inputs from sense organs to interpret vision and audition, proprioception and general sensations. It initiates voluntary skeletal muscle movements, stores memory, deals with voluntary motor control, behavior and mental status. Specific areas of the cerebral cortex are interconnected by fiber tracts to coordinate their interactions. Paleopallium ("ancient cortex") is the part of the cortex of the most ancient origin. Including the olfactory bulb, olfactory tracts and piriform lobe, it has retained its association with olfaction, and is separated from the rest of the cortex by the rhinal sulcus. The neopallium constitutes the major part of the cerebrum and is usually what is considered when referring to the cortex or cerebrum. The archipallium, the second oldest part of the cortex, was originally correlated with olfaction, but now has new functions. It is associated with the limbic system. Deep in the cerebral hemispheres (neopallium), it includes the cingulate gyrus and the hippocampus. It is located in the medial wall of the cerebellar hemispheres where it forms a hairpin loop around and over the thalamus. Rhinencephalon ("smell brain"): telencephalon of lower vertebrates that developed for this sense. During evolution, its parts have changed so this term is no longer in favor. When used, it includes the piriform lobe and the hippocampus.

A. Cerebral hemispheres (I, II, III): the two structures created by the dorsally located longitudinal fissure dividing the cerebrum. They are connected deeply by the **corpus callosum**.

B. Cerebral cortex (II): the thin, superficial layer of gray matter made up of neuron cell bodies.

C. Gyri or **convolutions** (I, II, III)(JY-ry) (sin.=gyrus): the numerous folds separated by grooves on the surface of the cerebral hemispheres greatly increasing its surface area.

D-F. Grooves: the depressions between the gyri (convolutions), divided into two groups according to their depth. **Fissures** are deep grooves; **sulci** are shallow.

D. Longitudinal fissure (I, II): the deep groove separating the cerebrum into two cerebral hemispheres.

E. Transverse fissure (I, III): the deep groove separating the cerebellum from the cerebral hemispheres. In the live animal it contains the tentorium cerebelli.

F. Sulci (I, III)(SUL-sy)(sin.=sulcus): the shallow grooves between convolutions (gyri).

Lobes and **functional areas**: the lobes of the cerebral hemispheres named for the bones overlying them. The cortex has been mapped for sensory and motor areas. The motor

area, the caudal part of the frontal lobe, receives axons from motor neurons that cross (decussate) to the opposite side in the brain stem. Therefore, the <u>right</u> hemisphere controls skeletal muscle movements on the body's <u>left</u> side, the left hemisphere controls the body's right side. Specific points in the motor cerebral cortex control specific muscles. Association areas are next to the sensory and motor areas. They analyze sensory input and are concerned with memory, reasoning, judgement and emotional feelings.

G. Occipital lobe (I, III): the caudal part of each cerebral hemisphere housing the centers for **vision**.

H. Piriform lobe (III): the ventral bulge medial to the temporal lobe. It is the oldest part of the cortex (pallium) that initially was purely olfactory (smell).

J. Olfactory bulb (I, III): rostral extremity of the paleopallium that fits in a recess of the ethmoid bone. Fibers of the olfactory nerve pass from the nasal mucosa through the

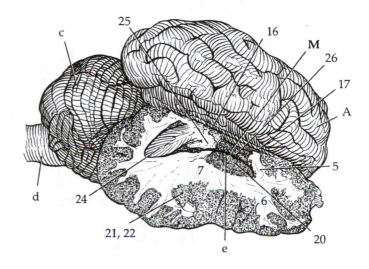

IV. Sheep **Brain**, cut to show basal ganglia, dorsolateral view.

holes of the cribriform plate of the ethmoid bone and enter the olfactory bulb, giving it a shaggy appearance.

K. White matter (II): the myelinated neuronal axons connecting the cortex with other parts of the cortex, brain and spinal cord. **Association fibers** are axons connecting neurons in different parts of the same cerebral hemisphere. **Commissural axons** interconnect both hemispheres, the largest forming the <u>corpus callosum</u>. **Projection fibers** are the efferent and afferent axons connecting the cerebral cortex to other parts of the brain and the spinal cord.

L. Basal nuclei/basal "ganglia" (II): the masses of neuron cell bodies located deep in the white matter of the cerebrum. The basal nuclei are concerned with voluntary and involuntary movements. They include the caudate nucleus, lentiform nucleus (putamen and globus pallidus) and the claustrum. The amygdala is often erroneously included.

M. LATERAL VENTRICLES (II, IV, pg. 473): the two spaces of the ventricular system, each surrounded by a cerebral hemisphere and filled with cerebrospinal fluid (CSF).

20. Caudate nucleus (II): a basal nuclei with a common shape, it has a large head bulging into the lateral ventricle and a slender curving tail following the curve of the lateral ventricles.

21, 22. Lentiform nucleus (II): a basal nuclei located lateral to the caudate nucleus and separated from it by the internal capsule. It is divided by fibers into the globus pallidus and the putamen.

21. Paladium/Globus pallidus (II): lateral part of the lentiform nucleus.

22. Putamen (II): medial part of the lentiform nucleus.

23. Claustrum (II): a basal ganglion located between the lentiform nucleus and the cortex (neopallium).

Amygdala: basal nuclei near the tail of the caudate nucleus (not shown).

24. Hippocampus (IV): a nucleus, it is the ventral curved part of the archipallium beneath the corpus callosum. The fibers of the hippocampus pass cranially as the fornix, lying directly below the corpus callosum. It is important in the learning and storage of long term memories.

25. Fornix (IV): fibers leaving the hippocampus, passing rostrally beneath the corpus callosum and then arching rostrally around the thalamus to enter the hypothalamus and terminate in the mammillary bodies.

26. Choroid plexus in lateral ventricle. (IV).

DIENCEPHALON

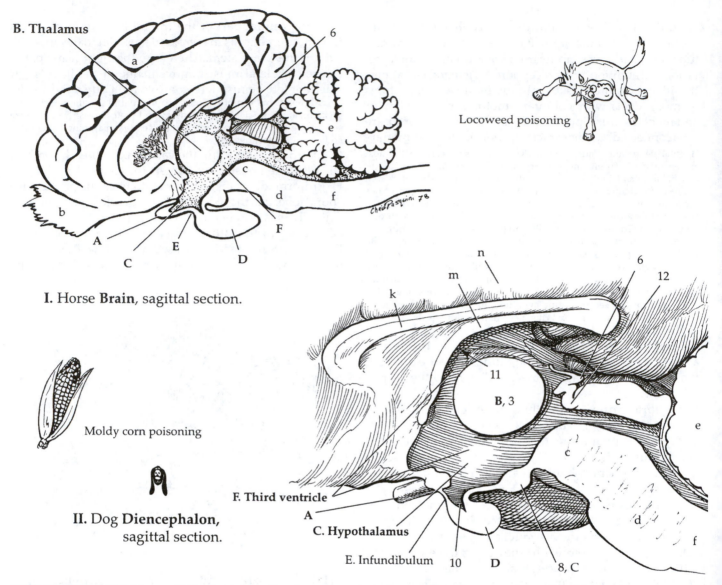

B. Thalamus

6

a

e

b

c

d

f

A

E

F

C

D

I. Horse Brain, sagittal section.

Locoweed poisoning

Moldy corn poisoning

n

m

k

6

12

11

B, 3

c

e

c

f

d

F. Third ventricle

A

C. Hypothalamus

E. Infundibulum   10   **D**   8, C

II. Dog Diencephalon, sagittal section.

DIENCEPHALON (dy-en-SEF-a-lon) (G. *dia*, through + *enkephalos*, brain): the rostral brain stem between the cerebrum and the midbrain, surrounding the third ventricle. Functionally, it can be lumped with the cerebellum into the forebrain. The diencephalon is composed primarily of the **thalamus** and the **hypothalamus***, both having gray matter grouped into nuclei.

A. Optic n. (I, II, III, IV): cranial nerve 2/II enters the brain, crosses as the optic chiasm and continues as the optic tracts through the diencephalon.

B. Thalamus (THAL-a-mus) (G. *thalamos*, inner chamber) (I, II): the deeply located two oval masses, containing many nuclei (gray matter), connected by the **interthalamic adhesion.** The thalamus functions as a <u>central</u> <u>relay</u> <u>center</u> for <u>sensory</u> impulses to the cerebral cortex and contains some motor fibers from the cortex to other brain centers. All senses, except smell, come to the thalamus, which sends them on to their appropriate cerebral cortical areas. The thalamus also interprets an awareness of nonlocalized

pain, touch and temperature. The thalamus is structurally part of the brain stem, but functionally is closely related to the cerebrum, to which it relays information.

C. Hypothalamus (hy-po-THAL-a-mus) (G. *hypo*, under) (I, II): the floor of the diencephalon. Seen in a ventral view of the brain, it is located beneath the thalamus. The hypothalamus communicates with the cortex, thalamus and other parts of the brain, as well as with the pituitary gland via the infundibulum. It is concerned with maintaining hemostasis by regulating visceral activity by its affect on the autonomic nervous system and the endocrine system. The hypothalamus sets appetite, drives of thirst, hunger and sexual desire; and sets emotional states with the limbic system. The hypothalamus regulates the viscera by controlling and integrating the **autonomic nervous system (ANS)**. Through the ANS, it controls heart rate, blood pressure, body temperature and gastrointestinal secretions and motility. Via the pituitary gland, the hypothalamus is the main link between the two regulating systems of the body - the nervous system and the endocrine system. It produces two hormones, antidiuretic hormone (ADH) and

* The diencephalon, besides the thalamus and hypothalamus, consists of the subthalamus, metathalamus and epithalamus.

DIENCEPHALON

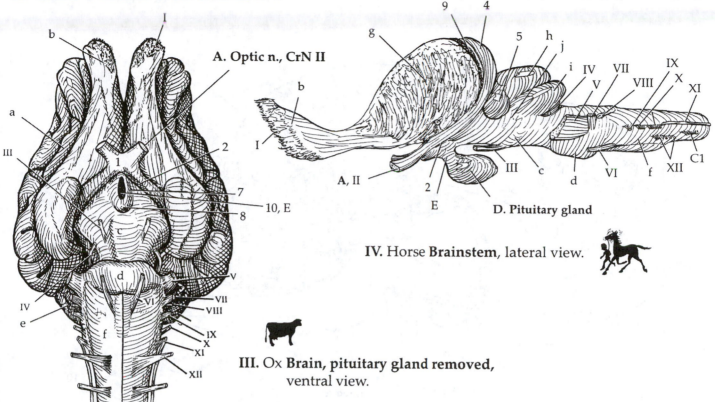

A. Optic n., CrN II

IV. Horse Brainstem, lateral view.

D. Pituitary gland

III. Ox **Brain, pituitary gland removed,** ventral view.

oxytocin, that are sent to the posterior pituitary gland for storage and release. The hypothalamus also serves as an intermediary between the nervous and endocrine systems through production and release of regulating hormones or factors which control hormonal release by the anterior pituitary gland.

- Antidiuretic hormone (ADH): restricts water loss in the kidney. It is produced by the supraoptic nuclei of the hypothalamus.
- Oxytocin (oks-i-TOH-sin): a hormone that stimulates the smooth muscle of the uterus and mammary gland to contract.

D. Pituitary gland (pi-TOO-i-tair'-ee) or **hypophysis** (hy-POF-i-sis) (I, II, IV): the small gland of internal secretion attached to the hypothalamus by the infundibulum. It consists of two main parts: the anterior lobe (adenohypophysis [ad'-i-noh-hy-POF-i-sis) and the posterior lobe (neurohypophysis). Its secretions are important in growth, maturation and reproduction. It usually remains in the skull when the brain is removed due to its location

E. Infundibulum (in'fun-DIB-yoo-lum)(A, **B**, C, D): the stalk attaching the pituitary gland to the hypothalamus. The third ventricle invaginates into the infundibulum, forming an infundibular recess.

F. Third ventricle (I, II, pg. 473): the ventricle enclosed by the diencephalon and encircling the interthalamic adhesion. It communicates with the lateral ventricles through the interventricular foramen and with the mesencephalic aqueduct.

CLINICAL:

Temperature regulation: the hypothalamus of the newborn does not regulate body temperature as efficiently as the hypothalamus of an adult.

1. Optic chiasm (III): the crossing of the medial fibers of the optic nerves.
2. Optic tract (III, IV): that part of the optic pathway between the optic chiasm and the lateral geniculate body.
3. Interthalamic adhesion or intermediate mass (II): that region where the right and left thalamus press together, reducing the third ventricle to an encircling space.
4. Lateral geniculate body (je-NIK-yoo-layt)(IV): a swelling of the thalamus deep to the optic tract which is connected to the ipsilateral rostral colliculi via a brachium (ridge). It receives visual information from the optic tracts and relays it to the cerebral cortex. With the medial geniculate body, it forms the metathalamus (caudolateral part of the thalamus).
5. Medial geniculate body (*genicula*, a little knee)(IV): relays auditory information to the cortex. It is a swelling of the thalamus which is connected to the ipsilateral caudal colliculi via a brachium.
6. Pineal body (II): an endocrine gland located medially in the diencephalic roof (epithalamus). It is believed to help seasonally regulate ovarian activity in relation to changing day lengths. It also produces melatonin, important in circadian rhythms (during a 24 hour period).
7. Tuber cinereum (III): surface feature of the hypothalamus that funnels down to the infundibulum that suspends the hypophysis, it contains nuclei associated with the ANS and hormonal regulation.
8. Mammillary body (corpus mamillare)(II, III): seen caudal to the tuber cinereum, it contains nuclei. It is the part of the limbic system that deals with behavior (controls feeding reflexes [licking, swallowing, etc.]).
9. Choroid plexus of the third ventricle (tela choroidea)(IV): forms the ceiling of the third ventricle.
10. Infundibular recess (recessus neurohypophysialis)(II): the recess of the third ventricle into the infundibulum.
11. Interventricular foramina (II): Monro's foramen: the two connections between the lateral and third ventricles.
12. Caudal commissure (II): part of the diencephalon, its fibers are concerned with the pupillary reflex.

I-XII. Cranial nerves.
C1. Cervical spinal n.

a. Cerebrum (I, III).
b. Olfactory bulb (I, III).
c. Midbrain (I, II, III, IV).
d. Pons (I, II, III, IV).
e. Cerebellum (I, II, III).

f. Medulla (I, II, III, IV).
g. Internal capsule (IV).
h. Rostral colliculus (IV).
i. Caudal colliculus (IV).
j. Brachium of caudal colliculus (IV)
k. Corpus callosum (II)
m. Fornix (II).
n. Cingulate gyrus (II)

MIDBRAIN

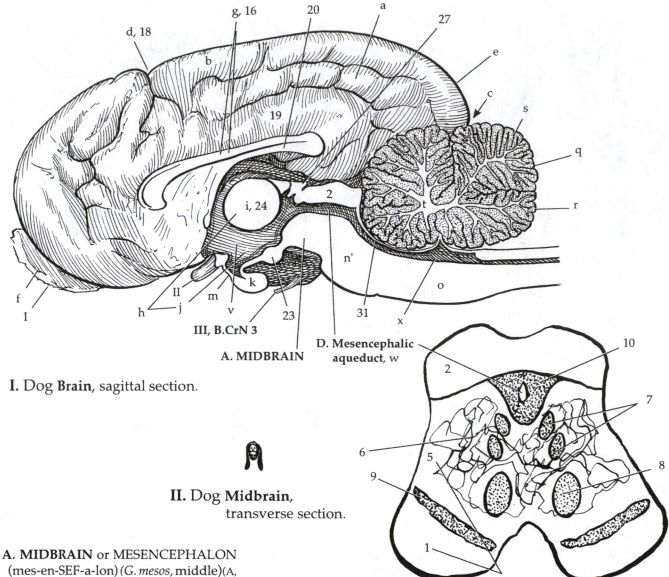

I. Dog Brain, sagittal section.

A. MIDBRAIN

D. Mesencephalic aqueduct, w

III, B.CrN 3

II. Dog Midbrain,
transverse section.

A. MIDBRAIN or MESENCEPHALON
(mes-en-SEF-a-lon) (*G. mesos*, middle) (A,
B, **C**, D): part of the brainstem between the
diencephalon and the pons, it connects
lower brain centers and the spinal cord
with higher brain centers. It consists
of the tectum, tegmentum and crura
cerebri and contains part of the reticular
activation formation. Covered dorsally
by the cerebrum and cerebellum, it is
seen ventrally. It includes the tectum (roof),
rostral and caudal colliculi, red nucleus, and
substantia nigra.

B, C. Cranial nn. 3 and **4** (oculomotor
and trochlear) (**I**, III): have their nerve
cell bodies of origin in and emerge from
the midbrain.

D. Mesencephalic (cerebral) aqueduct
(aqueduct of Sylvius) (**I**, II): the ventricular tube running through the midbrain, connecting the third and fourth
ventricles.

CEREBRUM or telencephalon
a. Cerebral hemispheres (I).
b. Gyri or convolutions (I).
c. Transverse fissure (I).
d. Sulci (I).
e. Occipital lobe (I).
f. Olfactory bulb (I).
g. White matter (I).
h. DIENCEPHALON (I).
i. Thalamus (I).
j. Hypothalamus (I).
k. Pituitary gland (I).
m. Infundibulum (I, III).
n. METENCEPHALON: pons and cerebellum.
n'. Pons (I, III).
o. MEDULLA OBLONGATA or medulla
 (I, II, IV).
p. Pyramids (III).
q. CEREBELLUM (I).
r. Folia (I).
s. Cerebellar cortex (I).
t. Arbor vitae (I).

u. Cerebellar peduncles (IV).
v, x, M. VENTRICLES: lateral ventricle not shown, the
 mesencephalic aqueduct is labeled M.
v. Third ventricle (I).
x. Fourth ventricle (I).

I. Olfactory n (CrN 1) (I).
II. Optic n. (CrN 2) (I).
III. Oculomotor n. (CrN 3) (I).
IV. Trochlear n. (CrN 4) (IV).
V. Trigeminal n. (CrN 5) (III, IV).
VI. Abducens n. (CrN 6) (III).
VII. Facial n. (CrN 7) (III, IV).
VIII. Vestibulocochlear n. (CrN 8) (III, IV).
IX. Glossopharyngeal n. (CrN 9) (III).
X. Vagus n. (CrN 10) (III).
XI. Accessory n. (CrN 11) (III).
XII. Hypoglossal n. (CrN 12) (II).
C1: First cervical n. (III).

MIDBRAIN

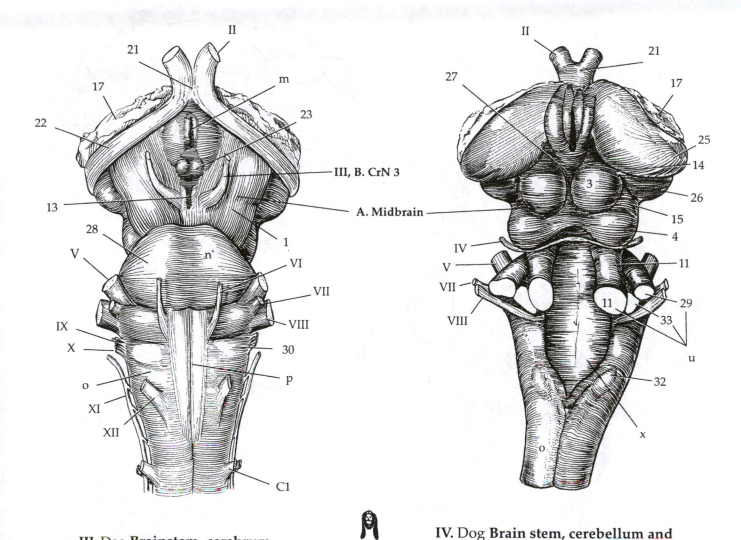

III. Dog Brainstem, cerebrum and cerebellum removed, ventral view.

IV. Dog Brain stem, cerebellum and cerebrum removed, dorsal view.

Midbrain (I, III, IV).

1. **Crus cerebri / cerebral crus** (pl. = crura cerebri)(I, III)*: fiber tracts between the forebrain and the caudal brainstem visible on the ventral surface of the brain. It is the continuation of the internal capsule.

2. **Tectum** (I, II): the roof of the midbrain located dorsal ly to the tegmentum, it is composed of four colliculi (corpora quadrigemina).

3, 4. **Corpora quadrigemina** (IV): the four colliculi making up the tectum of the midbrain.

3. **Rostral colliculi** (ko-Lik-yoo-ly)(sin.= colliculus)(IV): the two rounded eminences containing visual reflex centers and spacial integration centers. They connect to the ipsilateral geniculate body via a ridge (brachium).

4. **Caudal colliculi** (IV): the two rounded eminences behind the rostral colliculi which contain auditory relay and reflex centers. They connect to the ipsilateral medial geniculate body via a prominent ridge (brachium).

5. **Tegmentum** (II): makes up the majority of the midbrain and consists of the reticular formation. It is between the tectum and the substantia nigra. It contains the trigeminal nuclei (rostral sensory nucleus) dealing with proprioception and the trochlear nuclei (CrN IV).

6. **Reticular formation** (II).

7. **Oculomotor nuclei (CrN III)**(II)(principal and parasympathetic [Edinger-Westphal's] nucleus).

8. **Red nuclei** (nucleus ruber) (II): the mass of gray matter that communicates with the cortex, cerebellum and with the spinal cord. Functioning in motor reflexes concerned with maintaining posture, it is associated with the basal ganglia in the control of voluntary movement. They are named for their red color due to their strong blood supply. They are the origins of the rubrospinal tract.

9. **Substantia nigra**(NEYE-grah)(black [Soemmering's] substance)(II): a nucleus containing dark pigmented cells. Belonging to the extrapyramidal system, it plays an important role in regulating the motor output of the cerebrum. It is associated with the basal ganglia in the control of voluntary movement.

10. **Periaqueductal gray / substantia grisea centralis** (II): gray matter surrounding the aqueduct.

11. **Rostral cerebellar peduncle** (IV): connects the midbrain and the cerebellum.

12. **Cerebral peduncle** (pedunculus cerebri)(II): consists of the crus cerebri (ventrally) and the tegmentum (dorsally), separated by the substantia nigra.

13. **Interpeduncular fossa** (II): separates the two crura cerebri caudal to the mammillary bodies.

14. **Brachium of the rostral colliculus** (IV): the arm (ridge) connecting the ipsilateral lateral geniculate body and the rostral colliculi.

15. **Brachium of the caudal colliculus** (IV): the arm (ridge) connecting the ipsilateral medial geniculate body and the caudal colliculi.

16-20. **Telencephalon / cerebrum**

16. **Corpus callosum** (I):

17. **Internal capsule** (III, IV).

18. **Cruciate sulcus** (I).

19. **Cingulate gyrus** (I).

20. **Fornix** (I).

21-27. **Diencephalon** (h, I).

21. **Optic chiasm** (III).

22. **Optic tract** (III).

23. **Mammillary body** (I, III).

24. **Interthalamic adhesion** (I).

25. **Lateral geniculate body** (IV).

26. **Medial geniculate body** (IV).

27. **Pineal body** (I, IV).

Rhombencephalon / hindbrain (pons and medulla)

Pons (n', I, III).

28. **Transverse axons of the pons** (III).

29. **Middle cerebellar peduncle** (IV).

30-33. **Medulla** (o, I, III, IV).

30. **Trapezoid body** (III).

31. **Rostral medullary velum** (I).

32. **Medial cuneate tubercles** (IV).

33. **Caudal cerebellar peduncle** (IV).

*Roman numerals are used for the cranial nerves and for the figures. When put in parenthesis after a structure's name the Roman numerals indicate which figure they can be found in. Bolding the numeral indicates the best illustration for the structure.

PONS - MEDULLA

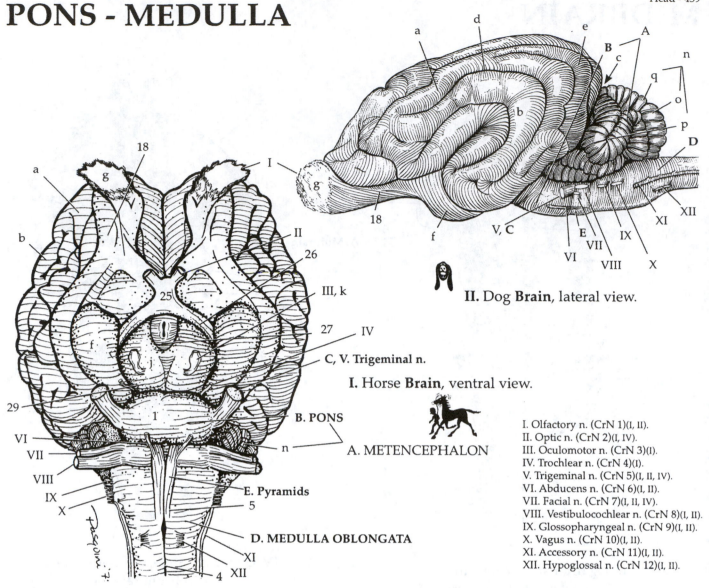

II. Dog Brain, lateral view.

I. Horse Brain, ventral view.

B. PONS

A. METENCEPHALON

E. Pyramids

D. MEDULLA OBLONGATA

C, V. Trigeminal n.

I. Olfactory n. (CrN 1)(I, II).
II. Optic n. (CrN 2)(I, IV).
III. Oculomotor n. (CrN 3)(I).
IV. Trochlear n. (CrN 4)(I).
V. Trigeminal n. (CrN 5)(I, II, IV).
VI. Abducens n. (CrN 6)(I, II).
VII. Facial n. (CrN 7)(I, II, IV).
VIII. Vestibulocochlear n. (CrN 8)(I, II).
IX. Glossopharyngeal n. (CrN 9)(I, II).
X. Vagus n. (CrN 10)(I, II).
XI. Accessory n. (CrN 11)(I, II).
XII. Hypoglossal n. (CrN 12)(I, II).

A. METENCEPHALON(I, II, III): consists of the pons and the cerebellum.

B. PONS (L., bridge)(I, II, IV): the bulge (ventral metencephalon) between the midbrain and the medulla oblongata. Functionally, it bridges the spinal cord and brain, and different parts of the brain. Nuclei within the pons, working with nuclei in the medulla oblongata, regulate breathing.

C. Trigeminal n. (CrN 5/V)(I, II, IV): emerges from the pons. It has its cell bodies (most sensory and all motor) in the pons.

D. MEDULLA OBLONGATA (me-DUL-la ob'long-GAT-a) or **medulla** (I, II, III, IV): the caudal portion of the brain stem which continues caudally as the spinal cord.

E. Pyramids (I, II): the longitudinal swellings formed by motor tracts coming from the cerebral cortex on the ventral surface of the medulla. These tracts cross from one side to the other in the caudal end of the pyramids.

F. Fourth ventricle (III, IV pg. 473): located in the pons and medulla, beneath the cerebellum.

- G. Lateral apertures (foramina of Luschka)(II): openings between the fourth ventricle and the subarachnoid space. They are located directly behind the cerebellar peduncles.

- H. Choroid plexus of 4th ventricle(III): produces cerebrospinal fluid (CSF). It is located only in the caudal half of the ventricle, suspended from the caudal medullary velum.

CRANIAL NERVES: the cell bodies of all or part of several cranial nn. are located in the medulla, including the vestibulocochlear (8/VIII) (cochlear part), glossopharyngeal (9/IX), vagus (10/X), accessory (11/XI) (cranial part), and hypoglossal (12/XII) nerves.

Reticular formation: partially contained in the medulla.

Vital reflex centers: located in the medulla. The cardiac center regulates the rate and strength of heart contractions. The vasomotor center regulates the diameter of the blood vessels, thus, blood pressure. The rhythm of breathing is regulated by the respiratory centers. Because of these vital centers, damage to this part of the brain stem is often fatal. Besides these vital reflex centers, the medulla has "nonvital" reflex centers regulating coughing, sneezing, swallowing and vomiting.

PONS - MEDULLA

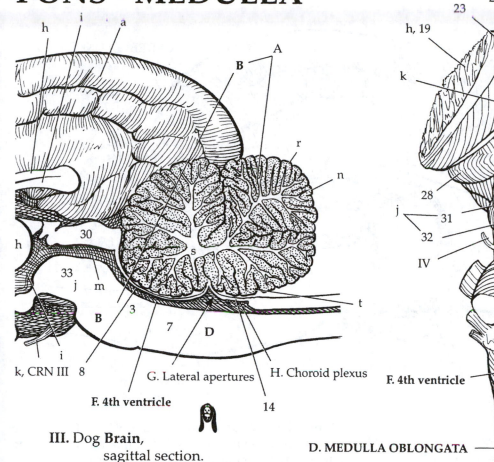

III. Dog Brain, sagittal section.

G. Lateral apertures   H. Choroid plexus

F. 4th ventricle

IV. Horse Brainstem, cerebrum and cerebellum removed, dorsal view.

F. 4th ventricle

D. MEDULLA OBLONGATA

a-g. CEREBRUM
  a. Cerebral hemispheres (I, II).
  b. Gyri or convolutions (I, II).
  c. Transverse fissure (II).
  d. Sulci (II).
  e. Occipital lobe (II).
  f. Piriform lobe (I, II).
  g. Olfactory bulb (I, II).
h, i. DIENCEPHALON
  h. Thalamus (III, IV).
  i. Third ventricle (III, IV).
j. MIDBRAIN or mesencephalon (I, III, IV).
  k. Cranial nn. III (I, III, IV).
  m. Mesencephalic (cerebral) aqueduct (III, IV).
n. CEREBELLUM (I, II, III).
  o. Vermis (II).
  p. Lateral masses (II).
  q. Folia (II).
  r. Cerebellar cortex (III).
  s. Arbor vitae (III).
  t. Flocculonodular lobe (III).

Rhombencephalon/hindbrain: consists of the myelencephalon and metencephalon.
1. Transverse axons of the pons (I): become the middle cerebellar peduncle on each side to the cerebellum.
2. Middle cerebellar peduncle (IV): carry the transverse axons connecting the pons and the cerebellum.

3. Tegmentum (III): dorsal part of the pons.
Medulla
4. Ventral median fissure (I): the longitudinal groove on the ventral surface that continues as the median fissure of the spinal cord.
5. Decussation of the pyramids (I): at the caudal end of the pyramids at the transition of the medulla to the spinal cord.
6. Trapezoid body: the transverse ridge adjacent to the pons area, between the abducens n. and vestibulocochlear n.; the ventral acoustic tract or stria carrying auditory axons from the contralateral cochlear nucleus.
7. Tegmentum of medulla oblongata (III).
8. Rostral medullary velum: covers the rostral part of the fourth ventricle. It contains the decussation of the trochlear n. (CrN4 / IV) coming off the area of the caudal colliculus. The velum is usually removed with the cerebellum.
9, 10. Gracile and medial cuneate tubercles (III, IV): inconspicuous eminences raised by the gracile and cuneate nuclei on the dorsal part of the medulla, flanking the caudal part of the fourth ventricle. They are the terminations of the like named fasciculi of the spinal cord. Second stage nuclei leave the nuclei and immediately decussate to the opposite side to pass rostrally in the ventral medulla as the large tract called the medial lemnicus which ends in the thalamus.
11. Fasciculus cuneatus (IV): the lateral division of the lemniscal system from the cranial trunk, forelimb and neck (sensory - discriminative touch).
12. Fasciculus gracilis (IV): the medial division of the lemniscal system from the hind limb and caudal trunk (sensory - discriminative touch).
13. Caudal cerebellar peduncle (IV): connects the medulla to the cerebellum.
14. Caudal medullary velum (III): ependymal-pia mater

layer forming the roof of the fourth ventricle. It is usually removed when the cerebellum is removed.
15. Median sulcus (IV): marks the floor of the fourth ventricle.
16. Obex (IV): where the dilated fourth ventricle becomes the spinal canal in the spinal cord.
17. Dorsal ventral fissure (IV): the longitudinal groove on the dorsal surface that continues as the dorsal median fissure of the spinal cord.
18-23. Telencephalon
  18. Olfactory tracts (I, II).
  19. Internal capsule (IV).
  20. Corpus callosum (IV).
  21. Caudate nucleus (IV).
  22. Hippocampus (IV).
  23. Fornix (column) (IV).
24-28. Diencephalon
  24. Pineal body (IV).
  25. Optic chiasm (I).
  26. Optic tract (I).
  27. Mammillary body (I).
  28. Lateral geniculate body (IV).
29-34. Midbrain.
  29. Crus cerebri / cerebral crus (I).
  30. Tectum (III).
  31. Rostral colliculi (IV).
  32. Caudal colliculi (IV).
  33. Tegmentum (III).
  34. Rostral cerebellar peduncle (IV).

CEREBELLUM

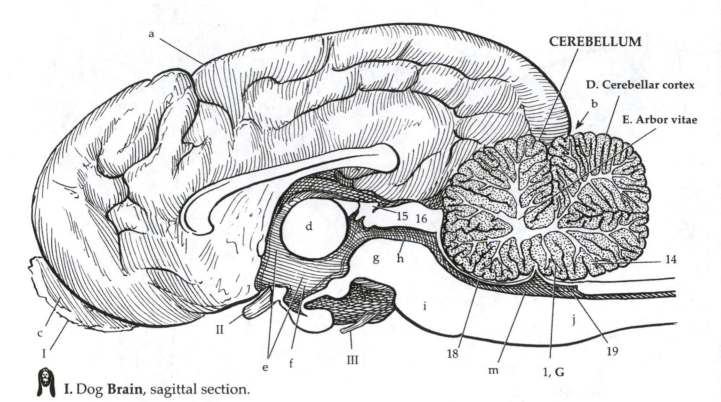

CEREBELLUM

D. Cerebellar cortex

E. Arbor vitae

I. Dog **Brain**, sagittal section.

CEREBELLUM (ser-e-BEL-um): the second largest subdivision of the brain. It is the dorsal metencephalon, located above the pons and medulla, and caudal to the transverse fissure. It is concerned with <u>coordinating</u> movements, but does not initiate them. It also has connections to the vestibular system to help coordinate balance and posture.

Function: a motor reflex center in coordinating subconscious and conscious skeletal muscle movements. Proprioceptors, located in muscles, tendons and joints; sense the relative position of one body part to another. Vestibular receptors of the inner ears and visual receptors of the eyes also provide input related to **proprioception** (sensing position). Information regarding cerebral commands regarding voluntary and involuntary movements are sent to the cerebrum. The cerebellum evaluates these inputs and sends out motor impulses to adjust muscle actions, thus, maintaining posture and balance and coordinating skeletal muscle movements.

A. Vermis (VER-mis) (L. worm)(III): the median part of the cerebellum named for its worm like appearance.

B. Lateral masses/cerebellar hemispheres (hemispherium cerebelli)(III): the parts of the cerebellum on either side of the vermis.

C. **Folia** (folds)(sin:=folium)(folia cerebelli)(IV): parallel ridges on the lateral masses and the vermis that increase the surface area.

D. Cerebellar cortex (I, V): the thin, outer layer of gray matter. Its surface is greatly increased by the folia (folds) on its surface. It consists of three layers; a deep granule cell layer (stratum granulosum), an intermediate Purkinje (pur-KIN-jee) cell layer, and a superficial molecular layer (stratum moleculare). Purkinje (piriform) cells are huge and highly branched and carry the output of the cerebellar cortex.

E. Arbor vitae (AR-bohr VEE-tee; "tree of life")(I): the white matter tracts (medulla of cerebellum) branching into the cerebellum. It is named for its resemblance to a tree and the ancient belief that it was the seat of the soul.

F. Cerebellar peduncles (pe-DUNG-kulz)(II, IV): the bundles of fibers connecting the cerebellum to the brain stem.

G. Flocculonodular lobe (flok-yoo-loh-NOD-yoo-lar)(IV): concerned with balance, it is the oldest lobe of the cerebellum, consisting of a nodule at the ventral vermis and two flocculi lateral to the nodule. It receives information from the vestibular nuclei. .

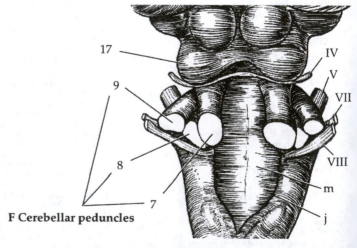

F Cerebellar peduncles

II. Dog **Brainstem**, cerebrum and cerebellum removed, dorsal view.

CEREBELLUM

III, Dog **Brain,** caudal view.

A. Vermis

b

B. Lat. masses

j

5

IV. Dog **Cerebellum,**
ventral view.

12

5

C. Folia

6

4

D

11

13

6

5

12

F. Cerebellar peduncles

1

3

2

10

G. Flocculonodular lobe

V

i

VI

VII

VIII

IX

X

j

XI

k

XII

V. Dog **Cerebellum,**
lateral view.

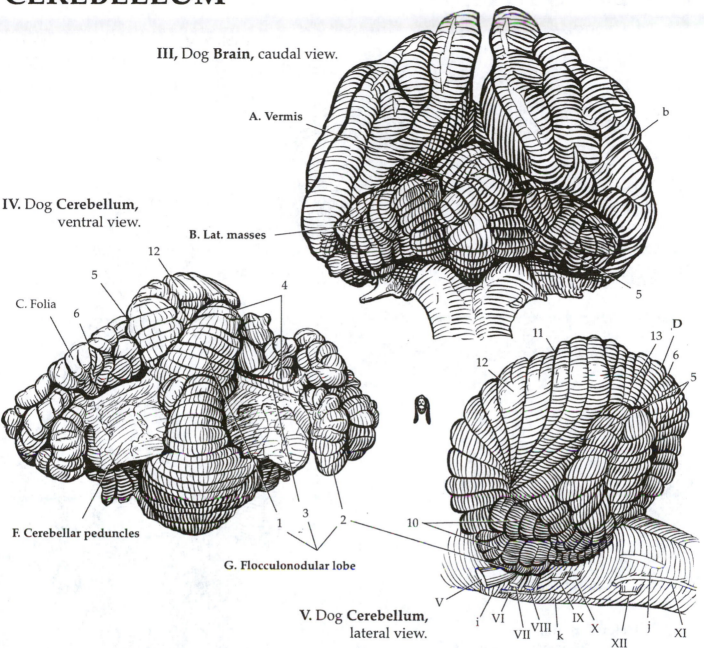

I. Olfactory n. (CrN 1)(I).
II. Optic n. (CrN 2)(I).
III. Oculomotor n. (CrN 3)(I).
IV. Trochlear n. (CrN 4)(II).
V. Trigeminal n. (CrN 5)(II, V).
VI. Abducens n. (CrN 6)(V).
VII. Facial n. (CrN 7)(II, V).
VIII. Vestibulocochlear n. (CrN 8) (II, V).
IX. Glossopharyngeal n. (CrN 9)(V).
X. Vagus n. (CrN 10)(V).
XI. Accessory n. (CrN 11)(V).
XII. Hypoglossal n. (CrN 12)(V).

a-c. CEREBRUM.
  a. Cerebral hemispheres (I).
  b. Transverse fissure (I, II).
  c. Olfactory bulb (I).
d-f. DIENCEPHALON
  d. Thalamus (I).
  e. Third ventricle (I).

f. Hypothalamus (I).
g. MIDBRAIN/mesencephalon (II).
h. Mesencephalic aqueduct (I).
RHOMBENCEPHALON/HINDBRAIN: myel-encephalon and metencephalon.
METENCEPHALON: pons and cerebellum.
  i. Pons (I, IV).
j. MEDULLA OBLONGATA (I, II, III, IV).
  k. Pyramids (V).
  m. Fourth ventricle (I, II).

1. Nodulus/flocculonodular node (I, IV): located at the ventral vermis.
2. Flocculus (plur.=flocculi)(IV, V): located lateral to the flocculonodular node.
3. Flocculonodular tract (IV) (pedunculus flocculi): connects the flocculonodular node and the two flocculi.
4. Uvulonodular fissure (IV): separates the flocculonodular lobe from the rest of the cerebellum.
5. Sulci (sulci cerebelli) (III, IV, V): grooves between the vermis and hemispheres and between parts of the hemispheres.
6. Fissures (fissurae cerebelli)(IV, V): grooves dividing the surface of the cerebellum into folia.

7. Rostral cerebellar peduncle (brachium conjunctivum)(pedunculus cerebellaris rostralis)(II): connects the midbrain and the cerebellum. It consists of motor (efferent) axons going to the red nucleus, reticular formation and thalamus; and sensory (afferent) axons of the rubrospinal and spinocerebellar tract.
8. Middle cerebellar peduncle (brachium pontis)(pedunculus cerebellaris medius)(II): carry the transverse sensory (afferent) axons connecting the pons (pontine nuclei) and the cerebellum.
9. Caudal cerebellar peduncle (pedunculus cerebellaris caudalis)(II): connects the medulla to the cerebellum and consists of sensory (afferent) axons from the spinal cord, vestibular nuclei, olivary nucleus and reticular formation.
10. Paraflocculus (V).
11. Primary fissure (V): divides the cerebellum into a rostral and caudal lobe.
12. Rostral lobe (lobus rostralis)(V).
13. Caudal lobe (lobus caudalis)(V).
14. Uvula (vermis)(I).
15-17. MIDBRAIN.
15. Pineal body (I).
16. Tectum (I).
17. Caudal colliculi (II).
18, 19. MEDULLA.
18. Rostral medullary velum (I).
19. Caudal medullary velum (I).

LIMBIC SYSTEM

Limbic system or the **emotional brain** governs emotional aspects of behavior.

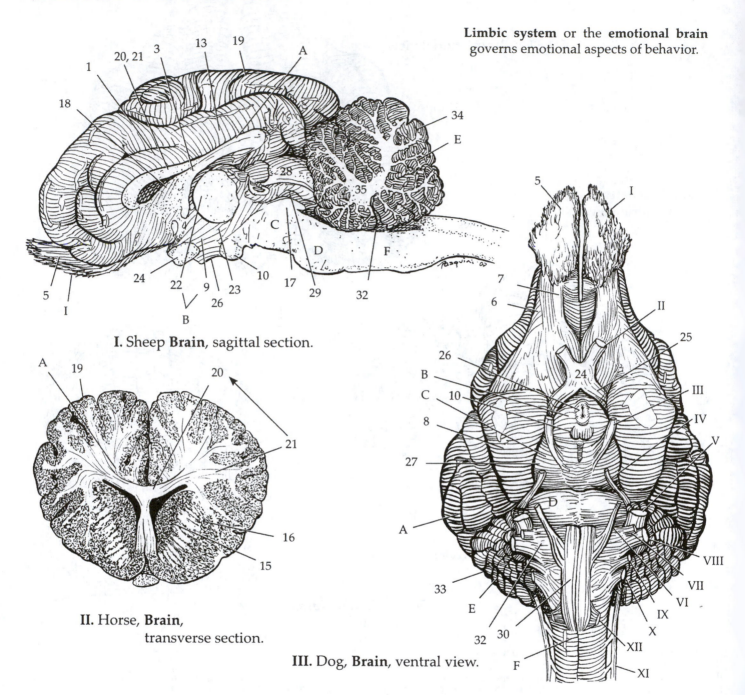

I. Sheep **Brain**, sagittal section.

II. Horse, **Brain**, transverse section.

III. Dog, **Brain**, ventral view.

Limbic system or **emotional brain**: complicated interconnections of the forebrain, hypothalamus and olfactory system. It is often called the "visceral brain" as it deals with visceral motor activity associated with the emotional aspects of behavior, such as fear, anger, pleasure, rage, sexual activity, eating, drinking and sorrow. By causing unpleasant and pleasant feelings about experiences, the limbic system modifies the actions of the animal to help ensure their survival (disliking being hit by a car may lengthen a dog's life). It is divided into a limbic cortex and subcortical nuclei. The cortical part is a ring of tissue deep in the medial side of the cerebral hemispheres, including the hippocampus and fornix, piriform lobe, cingulate gyrus and the fiber tracts connecting them. The subcortical part includes the hypothalamus, thalamic nuclei, caudate nucleus, putamen, amygdala and dorsal part of the midbrain's tegmentum and the fiber tracts connecting them. The amygdaloid body, the almond-shaped nuclei at the tail end of the caudate nucleus in the piriform lobe, appears to act as an interface between the limbic system, the cerebrum and various sensory systems. The hippocampal nuclei in the thalamus and hypothalamus are also components of the limbic system. The limbic system has also been called the "smell brain" (rhinencephalon) because of the erroneous belief that it was concerned primarily with olfaction, although smell is important to this system.

LIMBIC SYSTEM

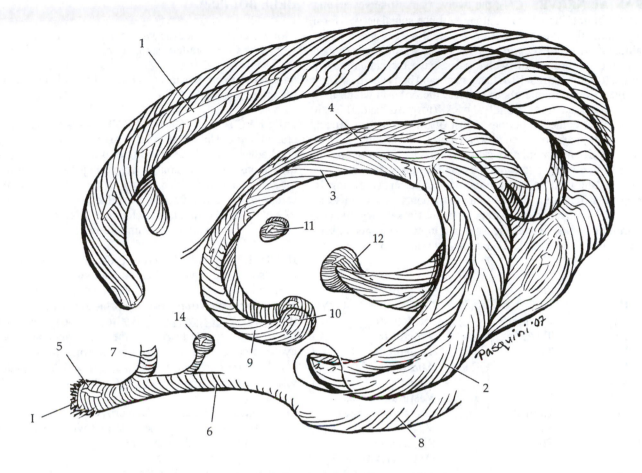

IV. Dog, Lymbic system, three-dimensional schematic (modified from Dyce, Sack, Wensing; Textbook of Veterinary Anatomy)

A. Cerebrum (I, II, III).
B. Diencephalon (I, III)
C. Midbrain (I, III)
D. Pons (I, III)
E. Cerebellum (I, III)
F. Medulla (I, III)

I. Olfactory n. (I, III, IV)
II. Optic n. (III)
III. Oculomotor n. (III)
IV. Trochlear n. (III)
V. Trigeminal n. (III)
VI. Abducens n. (III)
VII. Facial n. (III)
VIII. Vestibulocochlear n. (III)
IX. Glossopharyngeal n. (III)
X. Vagus n. (III)
XI. Accessory n. (III)
XII. Hypoglossal n. (III)

1. **Cingulate gyrus** (I, IV): with the supracallosal gyrus, constitutes the limbic lobe of the cerebral hemispheres. It lies above the corpus callosum.
2. **Hippocampus** (IV): the nucleus beneath the lateral ventricle, part of the limbic system, it is important in learning and storage of long term memories. It is probably the limbic system's control of emotion and behavior by regulating the autonomic, somatic and endocrine systems. It is the ventral curved part of the archipallium beneath the corpus callosum. The fibers of the hippocampus pass cranially as the fornix lying directly below the corpus callosum.
3. **Fornix** (I): fibers leaving the hippocampus, they pass rostrally beneath the corpus callosum and then arching rostrally around the thalamus to enter the hypothalamus and terminate in the mammillary bodies.
4. **Commissure of the fornix or commissure of the hippocampus** (IV): join the right and left hippocampi.
5. **Olfactory bulb** (I, III, IV).
6. **Lateral olfactory tract or stria** (III, IV).
7. **Medial olfactory tract or stria** (III, IV).

8. **Pyriform lobe** (III, IV).
9. **Hypothalamus** (I, IV).
10. **Mammary body** (I, III, IV): part of the limbic system, it also controls feeding reflexes (licking, swallowing, etc.).
11. **Thalamic nuclei** (IV).
12. **Amygdala** (IV): basal nuclei near the tail of the caudate nucleus
13. **Supracallosal gyrus** (I, IV).
14. **Septal nuclei** (IV).
15. **Caudate nucleus** (II).
16. **Putamen** (II).
17. **Dorsal part of the midbrain's tegmentum** (I).
18. **Septum pellucidum** (telencephali)(I): the thin sheet connecting the fornix and callosum after they separate rostrally. It forms the part of the medial wall of the lateral ventricle.
19-21. **TELENCEPHALON.**
19. **Cerebral hemispheres** (I).
20. **Corpus callosum** (I).
21. **White matter** (I).
22-26. **DIENCEPHALON.**
22. **Thalamus, interthalamic adhesion** (I)

23. **Third ventricle** (I).
24. **Optic chiasm** (I, III).
25. **Optic tract** (III).
26. **Infundibulum** (I, III).
27-29. **MIDBRAIN**
27. **Crus cerebri / cerebral crus** (III)
28. **Tectum** (I).
29. **Mesencephalic aqueduct** (I).
METENCEPHALON: pons and cerebellum (D, E).
30-32. **MEDULLA OBLONGATA**
30. **Pyramids** (III).
31. **Trapezoid body** (III).
32. **Fourth ventricle** (I).
33-35. **CEREBELLUM**
33. **Folia** (I, III).
34. **Cerebellar cortex** (I).
35. **Arbor vitae** (I).

CRANIAL NERVES

CRANIAL NERVES (CN): the twelve pairs of nerves arising from the brain. These nerves, along with the spinal nerves, form the peripheral nervous system. All cranial nerves attach to the brain stem, with the exception of Cranial nerve I (olfactory) which enters the cerebrum. All twelve pairs leave the cranial cavity through foramina to reach the head, neck, and body cavities. They are given Roman numerals to indicate the order in which they attach to the brain, from "front" to "back" (rostral to caudal). Their names indicate their functions. Most of the nerves are mixed, meaning they carry both sensory and motor fibers. Some, such as I, II and VIII, are completely sensory, carrying fibers of special senses. Some carry both voluntary and involuntary motor impulses. All these different combinations can be very confusing. In hope of clarification, the different components have been separated into **somatic motor nerves, somatic sensory nerves, autonomic (ANS) nerves** (sensory and motor) and **special sensory nerves.** For a complete functional classification of neurons, see appendix A.

I	On	Olfactory
II	Old	Optic
III	Olympus	Oculomotor
IV	Towering	Trochlear
V	Topps	Trigeminal
VI	A	Abducens
VII	Fat	Facial
VIII	Vested	Vestibulocochlear
IX	German	Glossopharyngeal
X	Viewed	Vagus
XI	Some	Spinal accessory
XII	Hops	Hypoglossal

TYPES OF CRANIAL NERVES:

Mixed nerve: a nerve carrying both **somatic** sensory and motor fibers. They also carry ANS sympathetic motor fibers.

Motor nerve: a nerve carrying primarily **somatic** motor fibers to voluntary (skeletal) mm. These are understood to also carry sensory fibers from muscles innervated by motor fibers. They usually also carry ANS sympathetic motor fibers.

Sensory nerve: a nerve carrying only somatic sensory fibers to the brain.

Special sensory nerve: a nerve carrying special sensory fibers associated with smell, vision, hearing, or taste (special senses).

Autonomic (ANS) fibers: fibers from nerves of the autonomic nervous system. They innervate smooth muscle, cardiac muscle, and glands and are subdivided into fibers of the sympathetic and parasympathetic divisions. Sympathetic fibers are carried by branches of all spinal and most cranial nerves. Parasympathetic fibers are restricted to some sacral spinal nerves (pelvic nerve) and a few cranial nerves (CN III, VII, IX, and X).

CELL BODIES:

Motor neuron: a neuron whose cell body is located in nuclei <u>within</u> the CNS (brain or spinal cord).

Sensory neuron: a neuron whose cell body is located in groups (ganglia) <u>outside</u> the CNS.

1. OLFACTORY (Cn I) NERVE (ol-FAK-toh-ree): the first cranial nerve, entirely **special sensory**, dealing with <u>smell</u>. Its cell bodies, located in the lining of the caudal nasal cavity, send their axons into the cranial cavity through the cribriform plate of the ethmoid bone. The axons join the olfactory bulbs of the cerebrum and travel through the olfactory tracts to the pyriform lobe of the cerebrum. The olfactory nerve is the <u>only</u> cranial nerve not entering or exiting the brain through the brain stem.

II. OPTIC NERVE (Cn II) (OP-tik): the second cranial nerve, it is also <u>special sensory</u>, dealing with **vision**. Its cell bodies are located in the retina of the eye. Their axons combine to form the optic nerve which tranverses the orbit to enter the cranial cavity through the <u>optic foramen</u> (1). Both eyes send axons to both visual cortices. Axons coming from the nasal (medial) sides of the eyeballs cross over in the **optic chiasm**. The visual impulses continue via optic tracts to the thalamus, which relays them to the visual cortex in the <u>occipital lobe</u> of the cerebrum.

Optic chiasm (ky-AZ-um, G. a crossing) (B): the joining of the two optic nerves inside the cranial cavity, just rostral to the hypothalamus. It is the site of crossing of some optic fibers.

Optic tracts (Fig. X-19,i): the paths from the optic chiasm to the thalamus.

Occipital lobe of the cerebrum (Fig. X- 13;1): the location of the visual centers.

III. OCULOMOTOR NERVE (Cn III): The third cranial nerve arises from the midbrain. It is primarily a motor nerve to most of the eye's voluntary (skeletal) extraocular muscles-the dorsal, medial, and ventral rectus muscles, and the ventral oblique muscle. It also is **motor** to the superior palpebral levator, the muscle that raises the upper eyelid.

The oculomotor nerve also has **ANS motor fibers** controlling the involuntary smooth muscles of the eye (ciliary and pupil sphincter muscles). These alter the shape of the lens for focusing (accommodation), and adjust the pupil size. The sensory limb for these visceral reflexes is carried by the <u>optic nerve</u>.

IV. TROCHLEAR (TROK-lee-ar) **NERVE (Cn IV):** the smallest cranial nerve, **motor** to the dorsal oblique muscle of the eyeball.

Fig. X-22 - Ox - Brain (schematic) - ventr.view

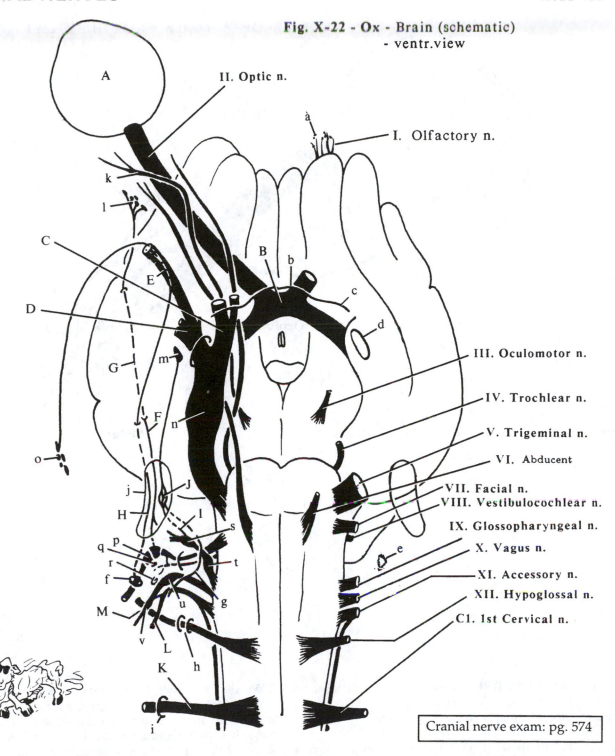

II. Optic n.

I. Olfactory n.

III. Oculomotor n.

IV. Trochlear n.

V. Trigeminal n.

VI. Abducent

VII. Facial n.

VIII. Vestibulocochlear n.

IX. Glossopharyngeal n.

X. Vagus n.

XI. Accessory n.

XII. Hypoglossal n.

C1. 1st Cervical n.

Cranial nerve exam: pg. 574

A. Eyeball
B. Optic chiasm
C. Ophthalmic, maxillary n.(V)
D. Mandibular br. (V)
E. Lingual br. of mandibular n., division of V
F. Major petrosal n.
G. Nerve of pterygoid canal
H. Chorda tympani (VII)
I. Tympanic n.
J. Tympanic plexus
K. First cervical spinal n.

a. Foramina in cribriform lamina
b. Optic foramen
c. Foramen orbitorotundum
d. Oval foramen
e. Int. acoustic meatus
f. Stylomastoid foramen
g. Jugular foramen
h. Hypoglossal canal
i. Lat. foramen of atlas
j. Cavity of middle ear
l. Pterygopalatine ganglion

m. Otic ganglion
n. Trigeminal ganglion (V)
o. Mandibular ganglion
p. Geniculate ganglion (VII)
q. Vestibular ganglion (VIII)
r. Spiral ganglion (VIII)
s. Prox. ganglion (IX)
t. Dist. ganglion (IX)
u. Prox. ganglion (X)
v. Dist. ganglion (X)

Fig. X-23 - Ox - Eyeball & CN II, III, IV & VI

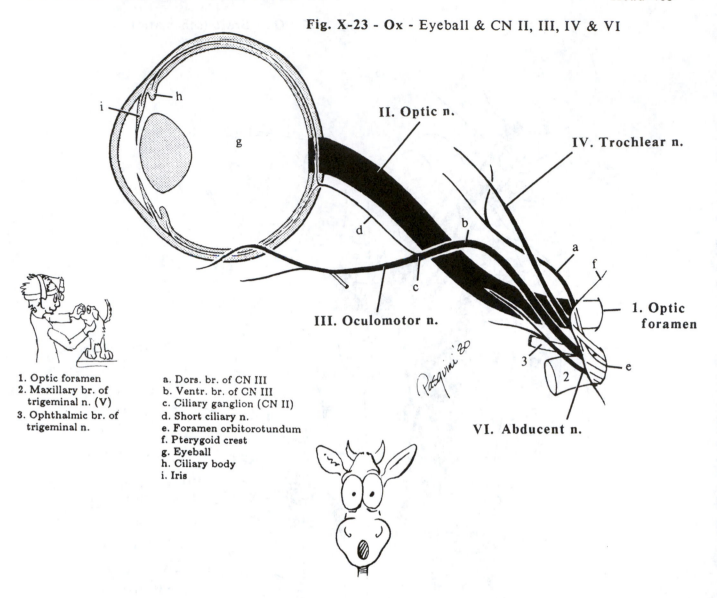

II. Optic n.

IV. Trochlear n.

III. Oculomotor n.

1. Optic foramen

VI. Abducent n.

1. Optic foramen
2. Maxillary br. of trigeminal n. (V)
3. Ophthalmic br. of trigeminal n.

a. Dors. br. of CN III
b. Ventr. br. of CN III
c. Ciliary ganglion (CN II)
d. Short ciliary n.
e. Foramen orbitorotundum
f. Pterygoid crest
g. Eyeball
h. Ciliary body
i. Iris

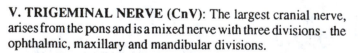

V. TRIGEMINAL NERVE (CnV): The largest cranial nerve, arises from the pons and is a mixed nerve with three divisions - the ophthalmic, maxillary and mandibular divisions.

1. Ophthalmic division (V1) (of-THAL-mik): a **sensory** division to the skin of the forehead, the skin lateral to the eye, most of the nasal cavity and the <u>cornea</u> of the eye. Its cell bodies are located in the trigeminal ganglion within the cranial cavity, but still <u>outside</u> the brain.

• **Infratrochlear nerve** (f): the principal supply to the horn of small ruminants.

• **Long ciliary nerve** (d): supplies sensation to the cornea.

2. Maxillary division (V2): a **sensory** trigeminal subdivision exiting the cranial cavity and traveling rostrally through the infraorbital canal as the infraorbital nerve to innervate the upper teeth. It exits the canal through the infraorbital foramen to innervate the skin of the nose (muzzle) and face, and the oral cavity.

• **Cornual nerve** (j): the major sensory nerve to the horn of the ox.

• **Infraorbital nerve** (n): passes through the infraorbital canal and exits the infraorbital foramen to supply sensory innervation to the middle part of the face.

3. Mandibular division (V3): **mixed nerve** (both **sensory** and

1. Ophthalmic division of CN V

Colored to indicate if
- motor
- sensory
- mixed

Supraorbital n.

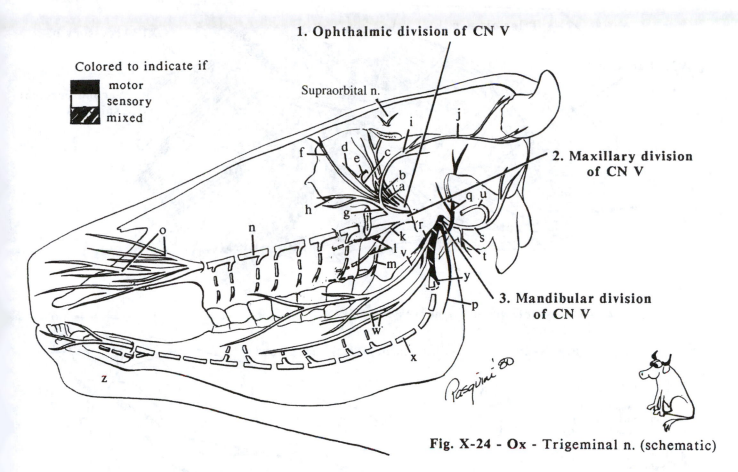

2. Maxillary division of CN V

3. Mandibular division of CN V

Fig. X-24 - Ox - Trigeminal n. (schematic)

a. Lacrimal n.
b. Frontal n.
c. Nasociliary n.
d. Long ciliary n.
e. Ethmoidal n.
f. Infratrochlear n.
g. Zygomatic n.

h. Zygomaticofacial n.
i. Zygomaticotemporal n.
j. Cornual br. of CN V
k. Pterygopalatine n.
l. Major & minor palatine nn.
m. Caud. nasal n.
n. Infraorbital n.

o. Nasal br.
p. Masseteric br. of mandibular div.
q. Deep temporal n.
r. Pterygoid nn.
s. Auriculotemporal n.
t. Parotid brs. of CN V

u. Transverse facial n.
v. Buccal n.
w. Lingual & sublingual nn.
x. Inferior alveolar n.
y. Mylohyoid n.
z. Mental n.

Cranial nerve V exam: pg. 578

motor). It supplies **motor innervation** to the muscles of chewing (mastication). Sensory fibers innervate the lower cheek and jaw, and the rostral two-thirds of the tongue (not taste).

• **Mental nerve** (z): the continuation of the inferior alveolar nerve (x) as it exits the mental foramen. It supplies sensation to the chin.

VI. ABDUCENT (ab-DYOO-sent) or **ABDUCENS** (L., drawing away) **NERVE (Cn VI)**: (Fig. X-23): The sixth cranial nerve, it is the **motor** innervation to two skeletal extraocular muscles of the eye; the lateral rectus and part of the retractor bulbi muscles. It originates from the medulla and exits the cranial cavity to enter the orbit. *Memory Aid*: To remember which muscle it innervates, remember that to abduct (move laterally, as in abducent) the eye requires the lateral rectus.

CLINICAL

Injury to the trigeminal nerve: can result in sensory deficit of the face and drooped jaw due to paralysis of the muscles of mastication.

Infraorbital nerve: can be palpated and anesthetized as it emerges from the infraorbital foramen.

Mental nerve: can be palpated and anesthetized as it emerges from the mental foramen.

Injury to abducens nerve: results in inability to gaze laterally.

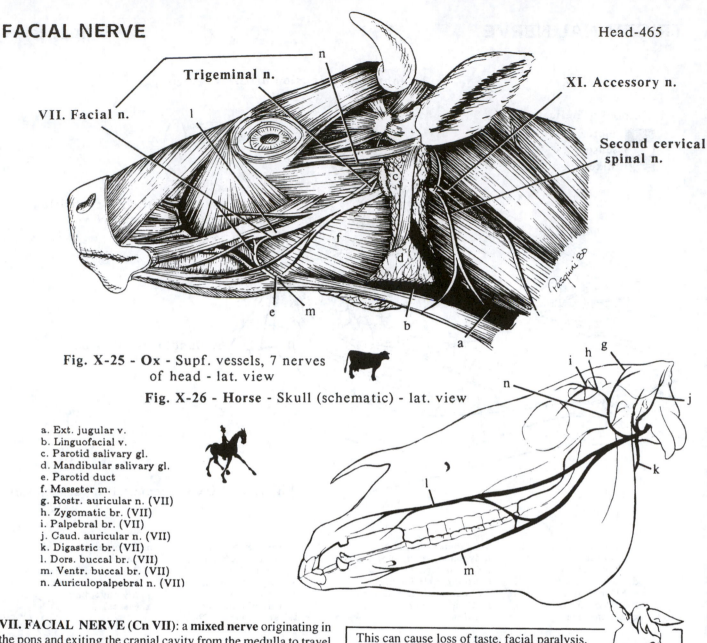

Fig. X-25 - Ox - Supf. vessels, 7 nerves of head - lat. view

Fig. X-26 - Horse - Skull (schematic) - lat. view

a. Ext. jugular v.
b. Linguofacial v.
c. Parotid salivary gl.
d. Mandibular salivary gl.
e. Parotid duct
f. Masseter m.
g. Rostr. auricular n. (VII)
h. Zygomatic br. (VII)
i. Palpebral br. (VII)
j. Caud. auricular n. (VII)
k. Digastric br. (VII)
l. Dors. buccal br. (VII)
m. Ventr. buccal br. (VII)
n. Auriculopalpebral n. (VII)

VII. FACIAL NERVE (Cn VII): a **mixed nerve** originating in the pons and exiting the cranial cavity from the medulla to travel across the face under the skin. It innervates the muscles of facial expression (including the orbicularis oris muscle). **Sensory** branches (chorda tympani nerve) from the rostral two-thirds of the tongue carry the sense of taste to the brain. The facial nerve also carries ANS motor fibers to the **lacrimal gland** (major petrosal), and the sublingual and mandibular salivary glands.

ANS - parasympathetic: innervate the lacrimal glands and salivary glands. **Lacrimalization** is very important because it is only controlled by Cn VII; whereas salivation is also caused by Cn IX.

VIII. VESTIBULOCOCHLEAR NERVE (Cn VIII) (ves-tib'-yoo-loh-KOHK-lee-ar) **(Fig. X1-39, A & B)**: the **special sensory** nerve concerned with hearing and equilibrium. It is divided into two branches; the cochlear and the vestibular. (See pg. 556).

| Cranial n. VII exam: pg. 579 |

CLINICAL

Middle ear infections: can cause paralysis of the facial nerve.

This can cause loss of taste, facial paralysis, and loss of lacrimation. Animals have little vanity about their appearance, the glossopharyngeal nerve also has taste fibers, but without a functioning lacrimal gland or the orbicularis oculi muscle, the eye can seriously dry out.

Auriculopalpebral nerve (n): innervates the eyelids and can be blocked for procedures of the eye.

Buccal branches of the facial nerve: cross the lateral aspect of the masseter muscle. These can be injured, causing facial paralysis (e.g., a horse lying on a harness buckle during surgery [buccal on buckle]).

Facial/trigeminal reflex arc: the facial nerve supplies the motor component to the sensory component of the trigeminal nerve. Pricking the face with a pin checks this arc. If either nerve is paralyzed, then a twitch of the muscles will not be elicited.

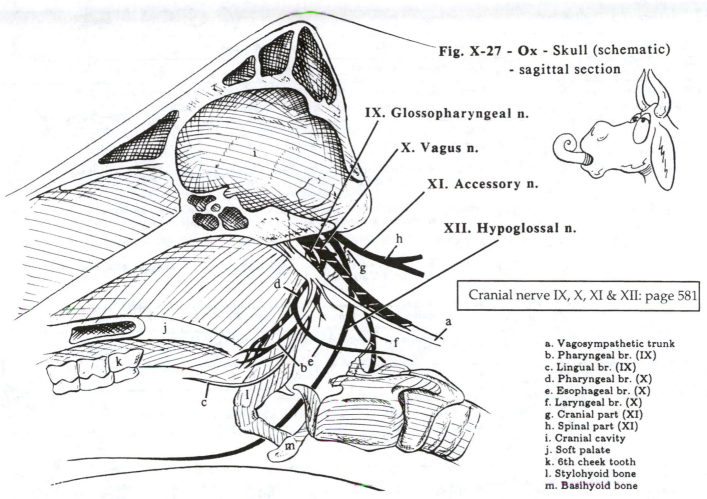

Fig. X-27 - Ox - Skull (schematic) - sagittal section

IX. Glossopharyngeal n.

X. Vagus n.

XI. Accessory n.

XII. Hypoglossal n.

Cranial nerve IX, X, XI & XII: page 581

a. Vagosympathetic trunk
b. Pharyngeal br. (IX)
c. Lingual br. (IX)
d. Pharyngeal br. (X)
e. Esophageal br. (X)
f. Laryngeal br. (X)
g. Cranial part (XI)
h. Spinal part (XI)
i. Cranial cavity
j. Soft palate
k. 6th cheek tooth
l. Stylohyoid bone
m. Basihyoid bone

IX. GLOSSOPHARYNGEAL NERVE (Cn IX) (glos'oh-fa-RIN-jeal): a **mixed** nerve supplying, as its name suggests, the tongue and pharynx. It deals with taste, swallowing and salivation. **Motor fibers** with those of the vagus nerve supply muscles in the pharynx that aid in swallowing. The **special** sense of **taste** from the caudal third of the tongue is carried by the glossopharyngeal nerve. Autonomic (ANS) sensory and motor fibers regulate the secretion of the parotid salivary gland. Sensory (ANS) fibers from the carotid sinus play a major role in sensing and regulating blood pressure.

X. VAGUS NERVE (Cn X) (L. wandering): a **mixed** nerve. Its **motor fibers** innervate the muscles to the pharynx (with the glossopharyngeal nerve) and larynx that control swallowing and vocalization. Its parasympathetic (ANS) fibers to the viscera of the cervical region, the thorax and abdomen regulate these organs' activities (pg. 526). The recurrent laryngeal nerve is part of the vagus that peals off in the thorax and returns up the neck to supply motor innervation to the muscles of the larynx, including the dorsal cricoarytenoideus muscle.

XI. ACCESSORY NERVE (Cn XI): a **motor** nerve to some neck muscles, including the trapezius. It is divided into cranial and spinal portions, with cell bodies located in the medulla and spinal cord, respectively. Both portions leave the cranial cavity together, then branch immediately. The **cranial portion** (g) is the somatic motor innervation to the soft palate, pharynx and larynx dealing with swallowing and vocalization. The **spinal portion** (h) de-

scends into the neck to supply the trapezius muscle and parts of the sternocephalicus, brachiocephalicus and omotransversarius muscles.

XII. HYPOGLOSSAL NERVE (Cn XII): motor nerve supplying the muscles (voluntary) of the tongue, controlling vocalization and swallowing.

CLINICAL:

Damage to the glossopharyngeal or vagus: may cause difficulty in swallowing.

Rabies: of zoonotic importance, causing hydrophobia (fear of water, as in drinking) due to paralysis of the pharynx (IX & X). With pharyngeal paralysis, salivation, or choke first think **rabies**!

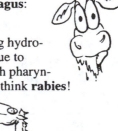

Damage to the recurrent laryngeal nerve: common in race horses, causing paralysis of the muscle that opens the larynx (dorsal cricoarytenoideus), resulting in a condition called "roaring".

Damage to the hypoglossal nerve: causes paralysis to the tongue's muscles and unilateral damage causes deviation of the tongue toward the normal side.

CRANIAL NERVES

CRANIAL NERVE	FUNCTION
I. Olfactory	Special Sense - smell (SVA)
II. Optic	Special Sense - vision (SSA)
III. Oculomotor	Motor - extrinsic eye mm. (dors., med., & ventr. oblique & superior levator) (GSE)
Short ciliary n.	ANS - parasympathetic - ciliary & sphincter pupillae mm. (GVE)
IV. Trochlear	Motor - dors. oblique m. (GSE)
V. Trigeminal	
V_1. Ophthalmic	Sensory - area of forehead (skin of forehead & caud. nose, med. side of eye, eyeball, nasal mucosa) (GSA)
V_2. Maxillary	Sensory - area of upper jaw (skin of lat. eye, nose, upper lip, cheek; mucosa of nasal cavity, soft & hard palate, upper lip; teeth of upper jaw & gums.) (GSA)
V_3. Mandibular	Mixed
	Motor - muscles of mastication (masseter, temporalis, med. & lat. pterygoid, rostr. belly of digastricus & mylohyoid) (SVE)
	Sensory - area of lower jaw (skin of lower chin, lower lips; roots of teeth of lower jaw; mucosa of tongue, oral vestibule, floor of mouth); temporal & zygomatic regions (skin of temporal & zygomatic regions, ext. acoustic meatus, tympanic membrane, parotid salivary gland & guttural pouch in horse) (GSA)
VI. Abducent	Motor - lat. rectus & retractor bulbi mm. (GSE)
VII. Facial	Motor - muscles of facial expression (SVE)
"Intermediate"	Special Sense - taste (rostr. 2/3 of tongue [chorda tympani n.]) (SVA)
	ANS - parasympathetic - lacrimal, nasal & palatine glands; mandibular & sublingual salivary glands. (GVE)
VIII. Vestibulocochlear	
Cochlear	Special Sense - hearing (organ of corti) (SSA)
Vestibular	Special Sense - equilibrium (semicircular canals, utricles & saccule) (SSA)
IX. Glossopharyngeal	Mixed
	Motor - stylopharyngeus caudalis, levator veli palatini, tensor veli palatini mm. (SVE)
	Sensory - pharyngeal region (mucosa of caud. 1/3 of tongue, soft palate, tonsils, pharynx auditory tube & middle ear; carotid sinus & carotid body) (GVA)
	ANS - parasympathetic - parotid & buccal salivary glands (GVE)
	Special Sense - taste (caud. 1/3 of tongue) (SVA)
X. Vagus	Mixed
	Motor - pharyngeal & laryngeal mm. (pharyngeal mm. & skeletal m. of esophagus, caud. cricothyroideus m. [cran. laryngeal n.], intrinsic mm. of larynx except cricothyroid m. [recurrent laryngeal n.]) (SVE)
	Sensory - baroreceptors in aortic arch & chemoreceptors in aortic bodies. (GVA)
	ANS - parasympathetic - pharynx, larynx, trachea, esophagus, thoracic & abdominal organs (GVE)
XI. Accessory	
Ext. br.	Motor - trapezius, sternocephalicus, cleidocephalicus, omotransversarius mm. (SVE)
Int. br.	Motor - intrinsic mm. of larynx via fibers traveling in the recurrent laryngeal n. (CN X) (SVE)
XII. Hypoglossal	Motor - intrinsic & extrinsic mm. of tongue (genioglossus, styloglossus & hyoglossus mm.) (GSE)

Fig. X-28 - Horse - Supf. vessel & nerves of head
- lat. view

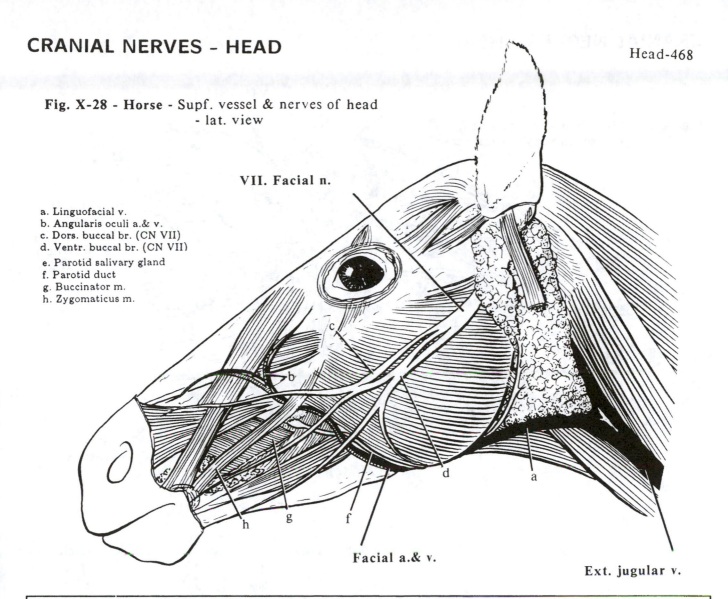

VII. Facial n.

a. Linguofacial v.
b. Angularis oculi a.& v.
c. Dors. buccal br. (CN VII)
d. Ventr. buccal br. (CN VII)
e. Parotid salivary gland
f. Parotid duct
g. Buccinator m.
h. Zygomaticus m.

Facial a.& v.

Ext. jugular v.

HEAD - NERVE BLOCKS: Before general anesthesia allowed animals to be put down and recovered safely, nerve blocks of the head where commonly used. There are several problems of the equine head that require general anesthesia or nerve blocks: teeth removal for abscesses, open tooth roots, sinusitis, draining sinus impactions. Today general anesthesia is used instead, but can be supplemented by specific nerve blocks.

Mental nerve block: anesthetize the mental nerve as it comes out of the mental foramen to anesthetize the lower chin.

Mandibular alveolar nerve block: injection at the mandibular foramen. The foramen is on the medial side of the mandible, opposite the point at which a line across the occlusal surface of the cheek teeth crosses a perpendicular line from the caudal edge of the eye. Insert a 6" needle medial to the mandible straight up to this point and inject anesthetic. This anesthetizes the lower lip, but doesn't get the incisors because those fibers are internal. This block can be used when repairing lacerations of the lower lip.

Infraorbital nerve block: palpate the rostral end of the facial crest. Run your finger dorsally to the infraorbital foramen and palpate the nerve under the levator labii superioris muscle. This block only anesthetizes superficial structures from the point of the foramen to the lip. Remember, nerves do not respect the midline, so do both sides to anesthetize the middle of the upper lip. This can be used when repairing lacerations on the lips or the bridge of the nose. Injecting into the foramen one inch, which is difficult, anesthetizes the face back to the orbit.

Maxillary nerve block: find the caudal angle of the eye and palpate the notch in the lower part of the zygomatic arch, just below the caudal angle of the eye. Pass the needle under the notch and aim rostrally and ventrally to anesthetize the maxillary nerve where it enters into the maxillary foramen. This anesthetizes the upper cheek teeth.

Supraorbital block (a branch of the ophthalmic division): palpate the foramen in the zygomatic process of the frontal bone. Inject a "bleb" of anesthetic over the foramen and rub it in. This anesthetizes the area over the forehead between the eyes. Do not inject into the foramen and thus the eyeball.

467

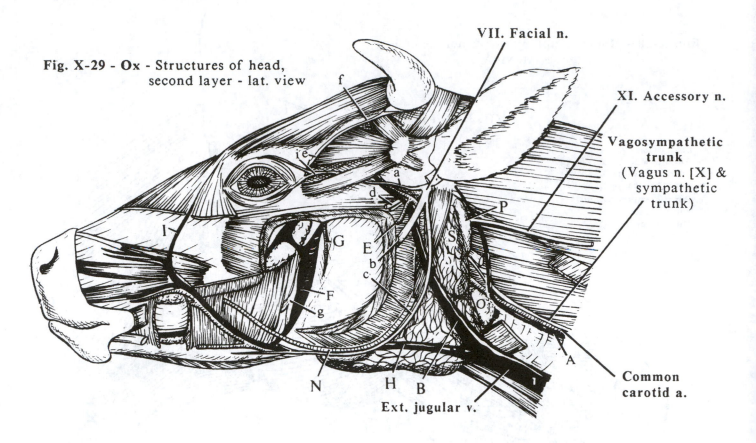

VII. Facial n.

XI. Accessory n.

Vagosympathetic trunk (Vagus n. [X] & sympathetic trunk)

Fig. X-29 - Ox - Structures of head, second layer - lat. view

Common carotid a.

Ext. jugular v.

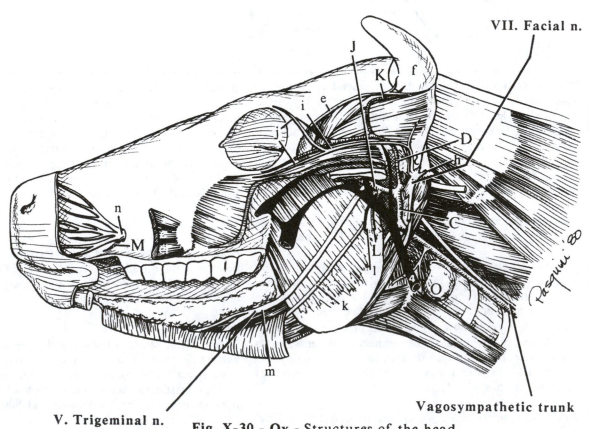

VII. Facial n.

Vagosympathetic trunk

V. Trigeminal n.

Fig. X-30 - Ox - Structures of the head, third layer - lat. view

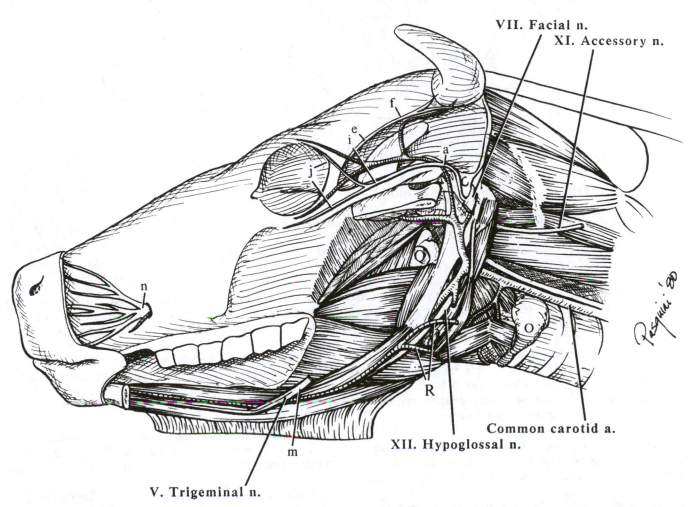

VII. Facial n.
XI. Accessory n.

Common carotid a.

XII. Hypoglossal n.

V. Trigeminal n.

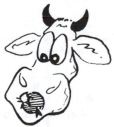

Fig. X-31 - Ox - Structures of the head,
fourth layer - lat. view

A. Int. jugular v. (X-29)
B. Maxillary v.
C. Ext. carotid a. (X-30)
D. Supf. temporal a.& v.
E. Transverse facial a. (X-29)
F. Deep facial v.
G. Buccal a.
H. Linguofacial v.
I. Angularis oculi v.
J. Maxillary a. (X-30)

K. Cornual a.
L. Inferior alveolar a.
M. Infraorbital a.
N. Parotid duct (X-29)
O. Thyroid gland
P. Lat. retropharyngeal lnn.
Q. Med. retropharyngeal lnn. (X-31)
R. Mandibular duct
S. Parotid salivary gland (X-29)

a. Auriculopalpebral n. (VII)(X-29)
b. Dors. buccal br. (VII)
c. Ventr. buccal br. (VII)
d. Auriculotemporal n. (V)
e. Zygomaticotemporal n. (V)
f. Cornual n. (V)
g. Buccal n. (V)
h. Caud. auricular n. (VII)(X-30)
i. Zygomatic br. of auricopalpebral n. (VII)

j. Palpebral br. of
   zygomatic br.(VII)
k. Mylohyoid n. (V)
l. Inferior
   alveolar n. (V)
m. Lingual n. (V)
n. Infraorbital n. (V)

SPINAL CORD

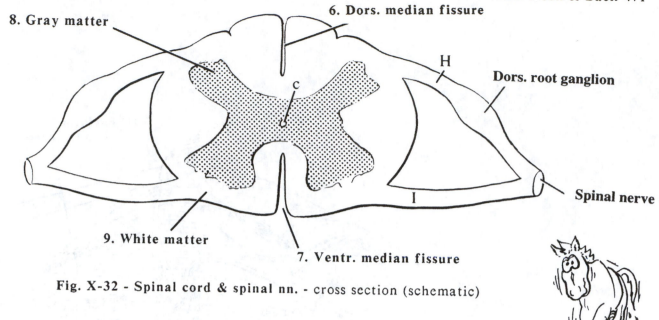

8. Gray matter

6. Dors. median fissure

H

Dors. root ganglion

c

9. White matter

I

Spinal nerve

7. Ventr. median fissure

Fig. X-32 - Spinal cord & spinal nn. - cross section (schematic)

SPINAL CORD: the long column of nervous tissue located within the vertebral (spinal) canal that, along with the brain, makes up the central nervous system (CNS). The spinal cord is the direct continuation of the caudal brain stem (medulla oblongata) beginning at the level of the foramen magnum. It extends only to the lumbosacral region of the spinal canal because the cord grows slower than the spinal column ("back bone"). Because of this the last spinal nerves must pass progressively caudally to reach their exit from corresponding intervertebral foramina.

Divisions of the spinal cord: divided into cervical (C), thoracic (T), lumbar (L), sacral (S) and caudal (coccygeal) regions which give rise to the spinal nerves that exit between the vertebrae.

Spinal segment: a region of the spinal cord from which a pair of spinal nerves arise. The spinal cord stops growing before the spinal column resulting in the spinal cord segments not always lining up with the corresponding vertebrae. The caudal thoracic and cranial lumbar cord segments lie over the vertebrae of the corresponding numbers. The last lumbar, the sacral, the caudal segments and the end of the spinal cord are more cranial to the corresponding vertebrae.

1. Cervical enlargement: the enlargement of the caudal part of the cervical and cranial part of the thoracic spinal cord regions; the spinal nerves serving the thoracic limb (brachial plexus) emerge here.

2. Lumbar enlargement: the enlargement of the spinal cord where nerves to and from the pelvic limb attach.

3. Conus medullaris (KOH-nus med-yoo-LAR-is): the tapered, terminal end of the spinal cord. The location in the vertebral canal varies among the species.

4. Filum terminale (FY-lum ter-min-AL-ee): the fibrous cord derived from the pia mater, extending from the conus to the caudal vertebrae. It helps anchor the spinal cord in the spinal canal.

5. Cauda equina (KAW-da ee-KWY-na) ("Horse's tail"): the structure formed by nerve roots leaving the caudal part of the spinal cord, traveling caudally to reach their exit from the vertebral canal.

6. Dorsal median fissure: the dorsal groove extending the length of the dorsal surface of the spinal cord. Along with the ventral median fissure, it divides the cord into symmetrical lateral halves.

7. Ventral median fissure: the groove extending the length of the ventral surface of the spinal cord.

CROSS SECTIONS of the spinal cord show the fissures mentioned above and a central H-shaped mass of gray matter surrounded by white matter.

• **8. Gray matter**: the nerve cell bodies and synapses organized into the shape of an "H". This is further anatomically divided into horns (columns).

• **9. White matter**: the axons running up and down the cord in specific tracts (fasciculi). These tracts connect the brain and interconnect the various spinal segments of the cord. The myelin around the nerve fibers gives the region its white color.

– **Ascending tracts** are the axons traveling up the spinal cord carrying sensory impulses (information) to the brain.

– **Descending tracts** are the axons of nerve cell bodies in the brain. They travel down the spinal cord carrying motor impulses.

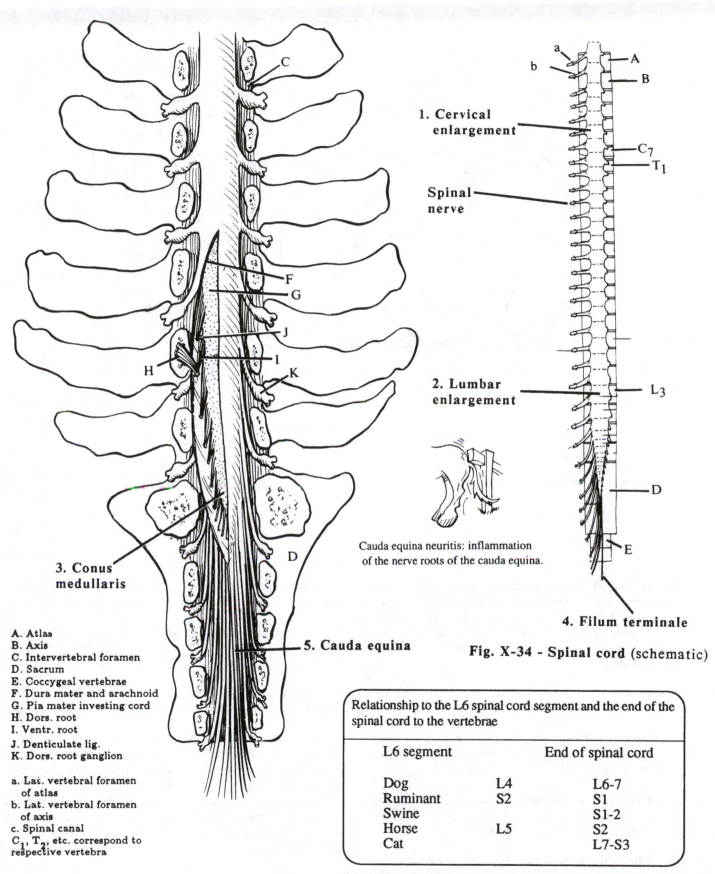

1. Cervical enlargement

Spinal nerve

2. Lumbar enlargement

3. Conus medullaris

5. Cauda equina

4. Filum terminale

Cauda equina neuritis: inflammation of the nerve roots of the cauda equina.

Fig. X-34 - Spinal cord (schematic)

A. Atlas
B. Axis
C. Intervertebral foramen
D. Sacrum
E. Coccygeal vertebrae
F. Dura mater and arachnoid
G. Pia mater investing cord
H. Dors. root
I. Ventr. root
J. Denticulate lig.
K. Dors. root ganglion

a. Lat. vertebral foramen of atlas
b. Lat. vertebral foramen of axis
c. Spinal canal
C_1, T_2, etc. correspond to respective vertebra

Relationship to the L6 spinal cord segment and the end of the spinal cord to the vertebrae		
L6 segment		End of spinal cord
Dog	L4	L6-7
Ruminant	S2	S1
Swine		S1-2
Horse	L5	S2
Cat		L7-S3

Adapted from Applied Veterinary Anatomy, Habel and de Lahunta, 1986

Fig. X-35 - Horse - Spinal cord & meninges
- transverse section (schematic)

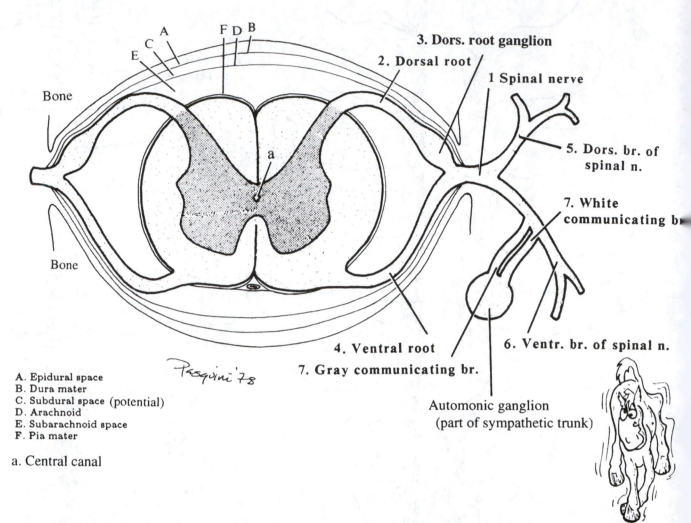

A
C
E
F D B

3. Dors. root ganglion

2. Dorsal root

1 Spinal nerve

Bone

5. Dors. br. of spinal n.

7. White communicating br

Bone

a

Pasquini '78

A. Epidural space
B. Dura mater
C. Subdural space (potential)
D. Arachnoid
E. Subarachnoid space
F. Pia mater

a. Central canal

4. Ventral root

7. Gray communicating br.

6. Ventr. br. of spinal n.

Automonic ganglion
(part of sympathetic trunk)

1. SPINAL NERVES: the joined dorsal and ventral roots arising from the spinal cord. They are mixed nerves carrying sensory impulses toward the spinal cord and motor impulses away from the spinal cord. Just after a spinal nerve emerges through an intervertebral foramen, it splits into dorsal, ventral, and communicating branches.

2. Dorsal (sensory) root: the root bringing sensory fibers to the spinal cord.

3. Dorsal root ganglion: a swelling on the dorsal root containing the cell bodies of the sensory (afferent) neurons (pseudounipolar) making up the dorsal root.

4. Ventral root (motor): the root carrying motor (efferent) nerve fibers from cell bodies in the spinal cord to effector structures (organs, muscles, glands, etc.) of the body.

5. Dorsal branch (rami) of spinal nerves: extend dorsally to

innervate deep muscles and skin above the transverse processes of the vertebrae. It carries sensory and motor fibers.

6. Ventral branch (rami) of spinal nerves: supply the muscles and skin of the limbs and the lateral and ventral areas of the trunk. It also carries motor and sensory fibers.

7. Communicating branches: connect the spinal nerves to the autonomic nervous system (ANS) (sympathetic trunk) (pg. 524).

SPINAL NERVE ORGANIZATION: the endoneurium, a delicate connective tissue that surrounds individual fibers in a spinal nerve. The perineurium, a connective tissue sheath, surrounds bundles of endoneurium-covered nerve fibers (fascicles). A fascicle is a bundle of nerve fibers surrounded by perineurium. The epineurium is the connective tissue covering the entire spinal nerve. It is continuous with the spinal meninges at the intervertebral foramen.

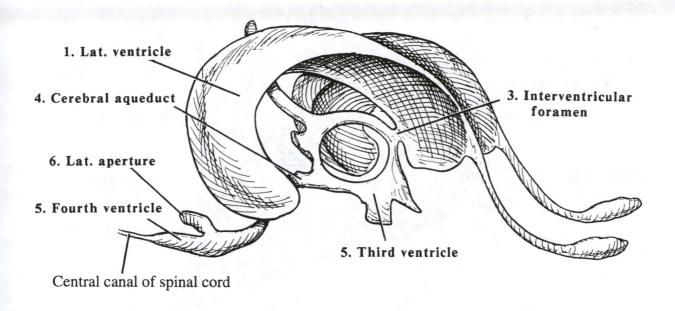

1. Lat. ventricle

4. Cerebral aqueduct

6. Lat. aperture

5. Fourth ventricle

Central canal of spinal cord

3. Interventricular foramen

5. Third ventricle

Fig. X-36 - Ox - Plastic cast of ventricles - craniolat. view

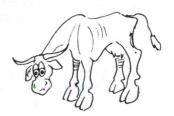

VENTRICLES (VEN-tri-kulz): a series of interconnected cavities in the cerebral hemispheres and brain stem. They are directly continuous with the central canal (Fig. X-32,e) and the subarachnoid space between the meningeal layers (see meninges) surrounding the brain and spinal cord.

1. Lateral ventricles: the largest of the ventricles. There is one located within each cerebral hemisphere.

2. Third ventricle: located in the diencephalon, encircling the interthalamic adhesion.

3. Interventricular foramina: the two channels connecting the third ventricle with the two lateral ventricles.

4. Cerebral (mesencephalic) aqueduct: the small canal running longitudinally through the midbrain to connect the third and fourth ventricles.

5. Fourth ventricle: located between the brain stem and the overlying cerebellum. It is directly continuous with the central canal of the spinal cord.

6. Openings between the fourth ventricle and the subarach-
noid space: two lateral apertures (a).

Choroid (KOH-royd) **plexuses** (G. *choroid* delicate membrane): the capillary network extending into the ventricles from their walls. They secrete cerebrospinal fluid (CSF). The CSF produced in the lateral ventricles circulates through the interventricular foramina to the third ventricle where more fluid is added by the plexuses in its roof. The fluid then passes through the cerebral aqueduct to the fourth ventricle, where its choroid plexus adds more fluid. The fluid then goes to the spinal canal or out through apertures in the roof of the fourth ventricle into the subarachnoid space.

CEREBROSPINAL (se-ree'broh-SPY-nal) **FLUID (CSF):** a clear fluid produced by the choroid plexuses which circulates through the ventricles, central canal and subarachnoid space surrounding both the brain and spinal cord. The brain and spinal cord (CNS) "float" in the cerebrospinal fluid which acts as a protective shock absorber.

Arachnoid villi (granulations): projections of the arachnoid and subarachnoid space into the sagittal dural sinus. They provide escape of the CSF into the general circulation.

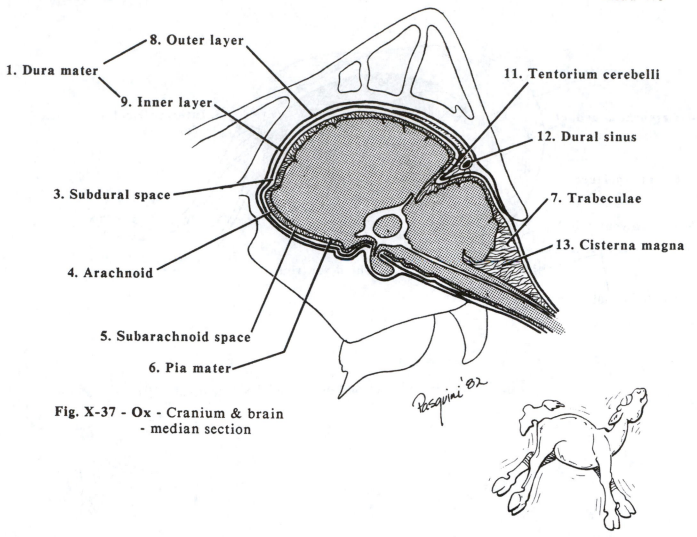

1. Dura mater
8. Outer layer
9. Inner layer
3. Subdural space
4. Arachnoid
5. Subarachnoid space
6. Pia mater

11. Tentorium cerebelli
12. Dural sinus
7. Trabeculae
13. Cisterna magna

Fig. X-37 - Ox - Cranium & brain
- median section

Pasquini '82

MENINGES (me-NIN-jeez) (sin.=meninx) (L. membranes): the three membranes surrounding the brain and spinal cord. The spinal and cranial meninges are continuous at the foramen magnum.

1. Dura mater (DYOO-ra may-ter) (L. *dura* hard + *mater* mother): the outermost meninx made of strong connective tissue. The cranial dura mater has two layers where the spinal dura has one. **Pachymeninx** (G. *pachys* thick + *meninx* membrane) is another name for the dura mater.

2. Epidural space: the cavity between the dura mater and the wall of the vertebral canal. Because the cranial dura mater is fused with the periosteum of the bones of the cranium, there is no epidural space surrounding the brain.

3. Subdural space: a potential space located between the dura mater and the arachnoid.

4. Arachnoid (a-RAK-noyd) (G. *arachne* spider + *eidos* resembles): the delicate middle meninx.

5. Subarachnoid space: the cavity between the arachnoid and the pia mater where cerebrospinal fluid (CSF) circulates.

6. Pia mater (PEE-a-may-ter) (L. *pius* tender + *mater* mother): the innermost meninx, closely investing the spinal cord and brain.

Leptomeninges (G. *leptos* slender + *meninges* membranes): refers to the pia and arachnoid together.

7. Trabeculae (tra-BEK-yoo-lee) (L. beams): connective tissue fibers spanning the subarachnoid space to join the arachnoid and pia.

CRANIAL MENINGES: the three meningeal layers surrounding the brain. The cranial and spinal subarachnoid and pia mater are similar and continuous at the foramen magnum.

Cranial dura mater: the outer membranous covering of the brain, composed of two layers: a tough, outer layer and a thin, inner layer. The two layers of the dura separate over the fissures of the brain; the inner layer extends into the fissures forming partitions and dural sinuses. The cranial dura mater is continuous

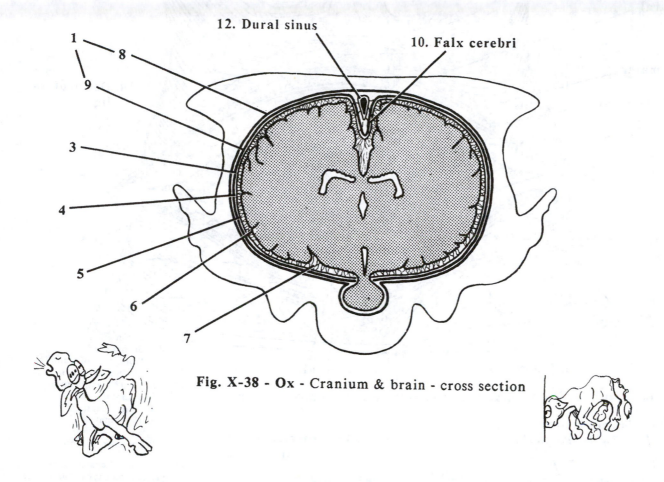

12. Dural sinus

10. Falx cerebri

1
8
9
3
4
5
6
7

Fig. X-38 - Ox - Cranium & brain - cross section

with the spinal dura mater at the foramen magnum.

8. Outer (periosteal) layer: the tough, fibrous layer attached to the bones of the cranium, forming the inner periosteum of the cranial bones.

9. Inner (meningeal) layer: the thinner layer.

Partitions: the folding and protrusion of the inner layer of the dura into the large fissures between parts of the brain.

10. Falx (L."sickle") **cerebri** (falks ser'e-bry): the partition extending into the longitudinal fissure, separating the right and left cerebral hemispheres.

11. Tentorium cerebelli (ten-TOH-ree-um ser'e-BEL-lee): the partition extending into the transverse fissure between the occipital lobes of the cerebral hemispheres and the cerebellum.

12. Dural sinuses: the venous spaces formed where the two dural layers separate from each other. The dural sinuses are filled with venous blood returning to the heart from the brain. The cerebrospinal fluid (CSF) is transferred from the subarachnoid space into these venous sinuses through arachnoid villi and returned to the general circulation. Since secretion and absorption is usually equal, the pressure of the cerebrospinal fluid is relatively constant.

13. Cisterna magna (L. reservoir + large): an expansion of the subarachnoid space located between thecaudal surface of the cerebellum and the dorsal surface of the medulla, just inside the foramen magnum. This is a common site for a CSF "tap" (removal of CSF).

CLINICAL:

Meningitis: inflammation of the meninges.

Internal hydrocephalus (G. *hydro* water + *enkephalos* brain): an accumulation of cerebrospinal fluid in the brain's ventricles due to obstruction of the flow of fluid. The blockage can occur in the cerebral aqueduct or the lateral apertures.

External hydrocephalus: an accumulation of CSF in the subarachnoid space due to interference with absorption into the dural venous sinuses.

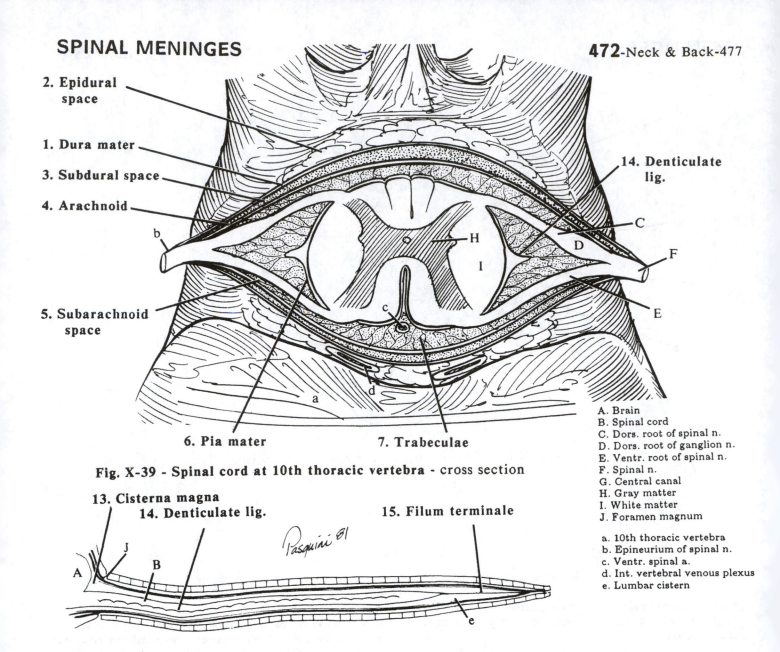

2. Epidural space

1. Dura mater

3. Subdural space

4. Arachnoid

5. Subarachnoid space

14. Denticulate lig.

6. Pia mater

7. Trabeculae

Fig. X-39 - Spinal cord at 10th thoracic vertebra - cross section

13. Cisterna magna
14. Denticulate lig.

15. Filum terminale

Pasquini 81

A. Brain
B. Spinal cord
C. Dors. root of spinal n.
D. Dors. root of ganglion n.
E. Ventr. root of spinal n.
F. Spinal n.
G. Central canal
H. Gray matter
I. White matter
J. Foramen magnum

a. 10th thoracic vertebra
b. Epineurium of spinal n.
c. Ventr. spinal a.
d. Int. vertebral venous plexus
e. Lumbar cistern

Fig. X-40. Ox - Spinal cord & meninges (schematic) - sagittal section

SPINAL MENINGES: the membranes surrounding the spinal cord, continuous with the cranial meninges at the foramen magnum.

14. Denticulate ligaments (L. *dentatus* toothed): the membranous extensions of the pia mater connecting to the dura mater between the spinal nerves; anchoring the spinal cord laterally.

15. Filum terminale: the fibrous strand formed by the meninges attaching the dural tube to the caudal vertebrae.

CLINICAL:

Caudal epidural analgesia: injection of a small volume of analgesic into the epidural space at either the sacrocaudal (S5-Ca1) or first intercaudal space (Ca1-Ca2). This inexpensive, simple procedure is commonly performed on cows, sheep and goats for obstetrical manipulations and surgeries involving the tail, anus, rectum, vulva, perineum and prepuce.

Just enough analgesia to block the sacral and caudal nerves is needed. If the analgesic travels further up the spinal column, it may cause loss of locomotor function of the hindlimbs. Pump the tail up and down while palpating for the first movable space. This may be the sacrocaudal (S5-Ca1) or first intercaudal space (Ca1-Ca2). In older cows the sacrocaudal space ossifies with age. Insert a 1 1/2 to 2" needle on the median plane through disinfected skin between S5-Ca1 or Ca1-Ca2 ventrocranially at an angle of 10° to the vertical. Pass the needle to the floor of the canal, then withdraw needle slightly to be sure you are in the canal. Inject anesthetic. Success causes paralysis of the tail in an animal that remains standing.

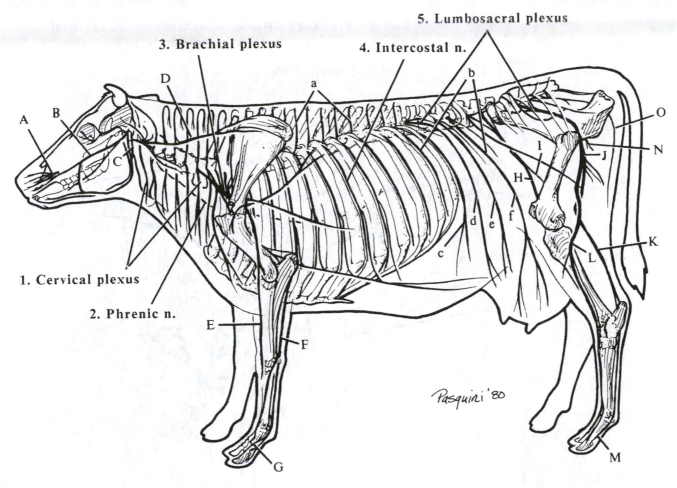

5. Lumbosacral plexus

3. Brachial plexus

4. Intercostal n.

1. Cervical plexus

2. Phrenic n.

Pasquini '80

Fig. X-41 - Ox - Spinal plexuses - lat. view

A. Trigeminal n. (V)	F. Ulnar n.	K. Tibial n.	a. Dors. br. of spinal nn.
B. Facial n. (VII)	G. Digital n.	L. Common fibular n.	b. Ventr. br. of spinal nn.
C. Hypoglossal n. (XII)	H. Femoral n.	M. Digital n.	c. Costoabdominal n.
D. Accessory n. (XI)	I. Saphenous n.	N. Obturator n.	d. Iliohypogastric n.
E. Radial n.	J. Ischiatic n.	O. Pudendal n.	e. Ilioinguinal n.
			f. Genitofemoral n.

SPINAL PLEXUSES (*plexus* braid): the interlacing of the **ventral branches** of spinal nerves adjacent to the vertebreal column in every region except the thorax. The major plexuses so formed are cervical, brachial, and lumbosacral.

1. Cervical plexus (L. *cervix* neck): the joining of many ventral branches of the cervical nerves, supplying structures in the neck.

2. Phrenic nerve: arises from the cervical plexus and supplies motor fibers to the diaphragm. This is why a broken neck can result in respiratory paralysis.

3. Brachial plexus: a network formed by the ventral branches of the last few cervical nerves and the first one or two thoracic nerves. It supplies most of the muscles of the thoracic limb.

4. Lumbosacral plexus: the ventral branches of the lumbar and sacral nerves. It supplies muscles and skin of the abdominal wall, the pelvic limb, external genitalia, rump and perineum.

5. INTERCOSTAL (THORACIC) NERVES: the ventral branches of the thoracic nerves do not form a plexus, but pass in the intercostal spaces as intercostal nerves. They supply the intercostal muscles and the overlying skin. The costoabdominal (last thoracic) nerve runs behind the last rib and helps supply the flank.

DERMATOME (DER-ma-tohm): an area of skin supplied by a single spinal nerve.

Fig. X-42 - Horse - Spinal nerves & brachial
plexus (schematic) - lat. view

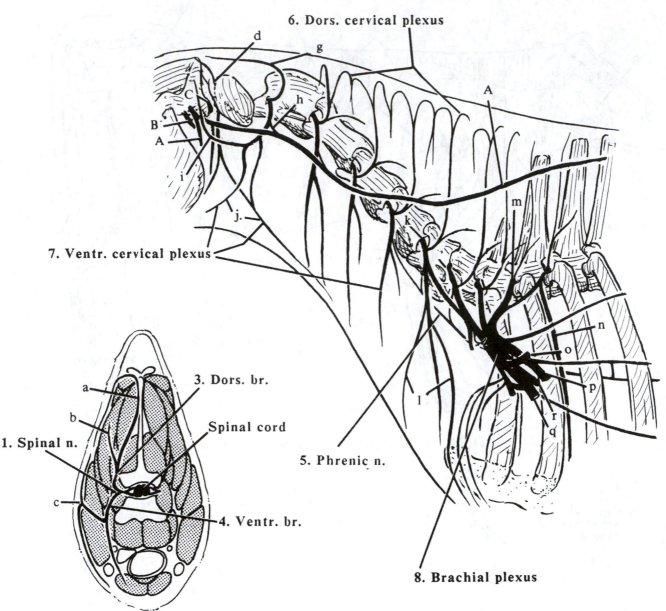

6. Dors. cervical plexus

7. Ventr. cervical plexus

3. Dors. br.

Spinal cord

1. Spinal n.

5. Phrenic n.

4. Ventr. br.

8. Brachial plexus

Fig. X-43 - Horse - Neck - cross section

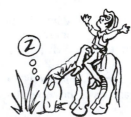

A. Accessory n. (XI)	a. Med. br. of dors. br.	h. Br. to accessory n.	n. Intercostal n.
B. Cran. cervical ganglion	b. Lat. br. of dors. br.	i. Great auricular n.	o. Axillary n.
C. Hypoglossal n. (XII)	c. Cutaneous br.	j. Transverse cervical n.	p. Radial n.
D. Brachial plexus	d. Spinal n. C_1	k. Spinal n. C_6	q. Median n.
	f. Spinal n. C_2	l. Supraclavicular nn.	r. Ulnar n.
	g. Major occipital n.	(cutan. brs. of k)	
	(dors. br.)	m. Spinal n. T_1	

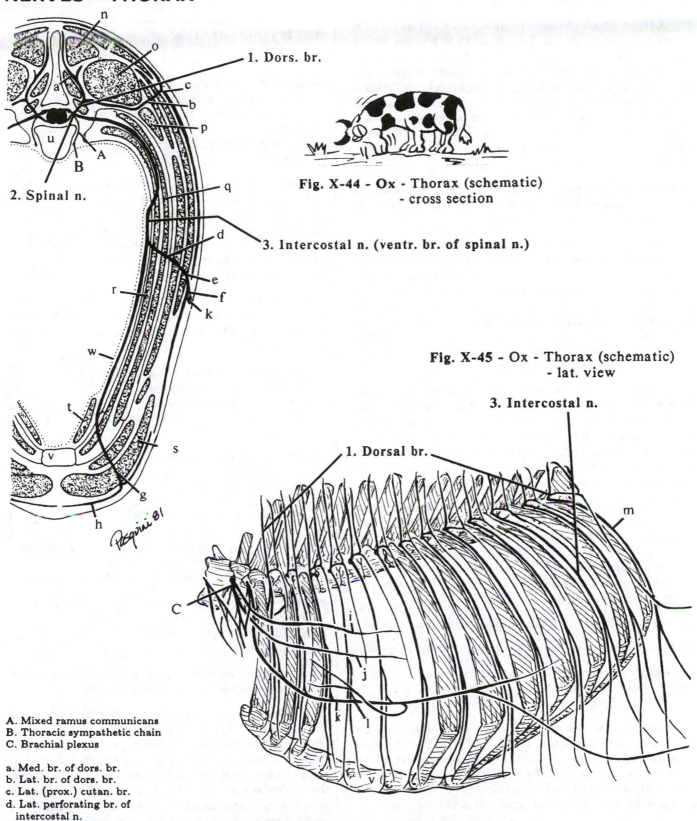

Fig. X-44 - Ox - Thorax (schematic) - cross section

1. Dors. br.

2. Spinal n.

3. Intercostal n. (ventr. br. of spinal n.)

Fig. X-45 - Ox - Thorax (schematic) - lat. view

3. Intercostal n.

1. Dorsal br.

A. Mixed ramus communicans
B. Thoracic sympathetic chain
C. Brachial plexus

a. Med. br. of dors. br.
b. Lat. br. of dors. br.
c. Lat. (prox.) cutan. br.
d. Lat. perforating br. of intercostal n.
e. Lat. (dist.) cutan. br.
f. Connecting br. to lat. thoracic n.
g. Ventr. perforating br. of intercostal n.
h. Ventr. cutan. n.
i. Long thoracic n. (C7-8)

j. Thoracodorsal n. (C7-8)
k. Lat. thoracic n. (C8-T2)
l. Intercostobrachial n.
m. Costoabdominal n. (T13)
n. Spinalis et semispinalis m.
o. Longissimus thoracis m.
p. Iliocostalis thoracis m.

q. Ext. intercostal m.
r. Int. intercostal m.
s. Ascending pectoral m.
t. Transversus thoracis m.
u. 7th thoracic vertebra
v. Sternum
w. Costal pleura

BRACHIAL PLEXUS: the network of nerves formed from the ventral branches of the last few cervical and first one or two thoracic spinal nerves. The nerves arising from this plexus innervate the intrinsic and some of the extrinsic muscles of the thoracic limb and, via the phrenic nerve, the diaphragm. The brachial plexus has roughly the same organization and distribution in all the domestic species, with the exception of the digits. Clinical information can be obtained by knowledge of the muscles innervated, areas of cutaneous sensation, and the spinal cord segments contributing to each nerve.

1. Suprascapular nerve: extends from the brachial plexus around the cranial surface of the neck of the scapula to innervate the infraspinatus and supraspinatus muscles.

2. Radial nerve: supplies the <u>extensors</u> of the elbow, carpus and digits (caudal arm muscles and the craniolateral forearm muscles). Extending from the brachial plexus into the triceps brachii muscle, it then passes around the caudal aspect of the humerus to reach the <u>lateral</u> side of the arm. Continuing distally, it branches into superficial and deep branches to the forearm. The superficial branch of the radial nerve supplies the skin of the craniolateral forearm in all domestic species. It is sensory to the dorsal surface of the manus in all, except the horse.

3. Ulnar nerve: motor to some caudomedial forearm muscles (flexor group) and muscles of the manus. It runs from the brachial plexus on the medial side of the forearm with the median and musculocutaneous nerves. At the elbow, it separates from these nerves to reach the caudal aspect of the forearm. It is sensory to the caudal forearm and palmar manus. In the dog it is the cutaneous innervation to the fifth (most lateral) digit.

4. Median nerve: along with the ulnar nerve, supplies motor innervation to the flexor muscles of the carpus and digits. It, with the ulnar nerve, is sensory to the palmar surface of the manus. The median nerve runs with the brachial vessels and the musculocutaneous and ulnar nerves in the arm. It continues on the medial side of the forearm to divide into medial and lateral palmar nerves, just proximal to the carpus.

5. Long thoracic nerve: innervates the serratus ventralis muscle.

6. Thoracodorsal nerve: innervates the latissimus dorsi muscle.

7. Musculocutaneous nerve: innervates the flexors of the elbow (biceps brachii and brachialis muscles) and the coracobrachialis muscle. It gives off the median cutaneous antebrachial nerve.

8. Axillary nerve: innervates the true flexors of the shoulder (teres major, teres minor and deltoid muscles). It dives between the teres major and subscapular muscles medially to reach the lateral side of the shoulder. Its cutaneous branches supply the lateral surface of the arm and cranial aspect of the forearm (lateral cutaneous brachial and cranial cutaneous antebrachial nerves).

Lateral thoracic nerve (not shown): supplies the cutaneous trunci muscle and cutaneous innervation to the ventrolateral abdominal wall.

SPECIES DIFFERENCES

Horse: the radial nerve doesn't extend past the carpus.

Ungulates: the median and musculocutaneous nerves appear as one nerve in the brachium, except for the musculocutaneous muscular branches. The two nerves are separate in the carnivores.

CLINICAL

"Sweeney" or **"shoulder slip"**: a condition seen in the horse due to injury of the suprascapular nerve. This results in rapid atrophy of the supraspinatus and infraspinatus muscles which produces a prominent scapular spine. Before atrophy, the shoulder is unstable and slips laterally, appearing to be dislocated.

Radial (nerve) paralysis: the most common and clinically significant nerve problem of the forelimb. It is usually due to traumatic injury. Clinical manifestations vary with location of the injury.

"High" radial nerve paralysis: proximal to where the nerve innervates the triceps brachii muscle. This results in an inability to extend the elbow, thus, inability to bear weight on the limb.

"Low" radial nerve paralysis: occurs distal to the triceps innervation, thus, weight can be born on the limb. The extensor muscles of the carpus and digits are affected, manifested clinically in "knuckling over" (dragging the dorsum of the foot on the ground). Most animals compensate by "flipping" the foot forward when moving the limb so the foot lands in the proper position.

Brachial plexus avulsion: results in damage to many nerves of the limb, resulting in a flaccid limb that is dragged.

Ulnar or medial nerve damage: little clinical manifestation due to the overlap of their motor innervations.

Panniculus (cutaneous trunci) response: contraction of the cutaneous trunci muscle in response to a pin prick. The sensory component of the reflex passes over the spinal nerves to the spinal cord at the level of the pin prick. The information passes up the spinal cord to the motor nerves of the lateral thoracic nerve in the caudal cervical region. This test is done systematically from caudal to cranial along the thorax. A positive panniculus response indicates the spinal cord is intact from roughly the level of the stimulus to the cervical area. A negative panniculus response may indicate the level of spinal cord damage (see Appendix - pg. 566).

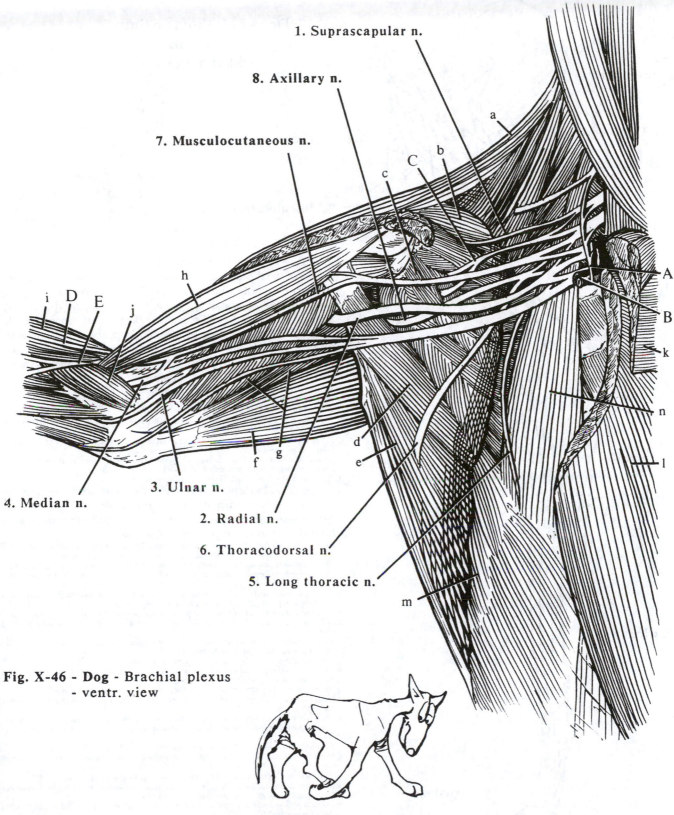

1. Suprascapular n.

8. Axillary n.

7. Musculocutaneous n.

4. Median n.

3. Ulnar n.

2. Radial n.

6. Thoracodorsal n.

5. Long thoracic n.

Fig. X-46 - Dog - Brachial plexus
- ventr. view

A. Phrenic n.
B. Axillary a.& v.
C. Subscapular n.
D. Supf. radial n., med. br.
E. Med. cutan. antebrachial n.

a. Brachiocephalicus m.
b. Supraspinatus m.
c. Subscapular m.
d. Teres major m.
e. Latissimus dorsi m.

f. Tensor fasciae antebrachii m.
g. Triceps brachii m.
h. Biceps brachii m.
i. Extensor carpi radialis m.
j. Pronator teres m.

k. Supf. pectoral m.
l. Deep pectoral m.
m. Serratus ventralis m.
n. Scalenus m.

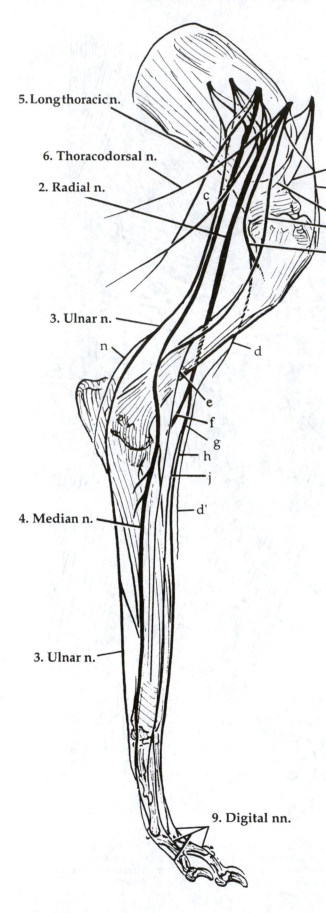

5. Long thoracic n.

6. Thoracodorsal n.

2. Radial n.

3. Ulnar n.

4. Median n.

3. Ulnar n.

9. Digital nn.

Fig X-47: Dog - Left thoracic limb
(schematic)
- Medial view

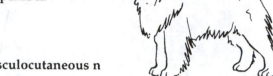

1. Suprascapular n.

7. Musculocutaneous n

8. Axillary n.

DOG: Nerves of the forearm and manus: except for the radial n., nerves of the thoracic limb, including their cutaneous branches (sensory), are not significant clinically. This is because they are rarely damaged, and if they are, the gait is not appreciably affected. Even in brachial plexus avulsion, using sensory loss to determine the exact nerves affected is probably of academic interest only and will have little effect on treatment. Having said this, the names of most of the less clinically significant nerves and cutaneous branches are listed below.

a. Subscapular nerves (C6-8): are motor to the subscapular m.

b. Pectoral nerves (cranial and caudal): are motor to the pectoral muscles.

c. Lateral thoracic nerve: is motor to the serratus ventralis m.

d. Cranial lateral cutaneous brachial nerve: a branch of axillary n., it is sensory to the lateral side of the arm.

d'. Cranial cutaneous antebrachial nerve: a branch of the axillary n., it is sensory to the cranial aspect of the antebrachium with the radial and musculocutaneous nn.

e. Medial cutaneous antebrachial nerve: the sensory branch of the musculocutaneous n. to the medial antebrachium. Unlike the horse it doesn't reach the carpus.

f. Deep branch of radial n. (motor): dives into the extensor muscles of the digit .

g. **Superficial branch of radial nerve: sensory to the skin of the craniolateral forearm and dorsal surface of the manus. Sensation can be tested to support a diagnosis of radial nerve damage if knuckling over or dropped elbow is noted.**

h. Medial branch of superficial radial n.: travels with the cephalic v.; at the manus it gives off a dorsal digital n. I to the dewclaw and continues on as the abaxial dorsal digital n. II.

i. Abaxial dorsal digital n. II.: passes on the dorsomedial side of the most medial main digit (II).

j. Lateral branch of superficial radial n.: travels with the cephalic v., and distal to the carpus, branches into common digital nn.

k. Dorsal common digital nn. II, III, IV: travel distally in the dorsal junction of the metacarpal bones to split into proper digital nn. at the metacarpophalangeal joints.

l. Axial dorsal proper digital nn. II, III, IV, V: pass on the dorsoaxial side of the corresponding digits.

m. Abaxial dorsal proper digital nn. III, IV: pass on the dorsoabaxial side of the corresponding digits.

n. Caudal cutaneous antebrachial nerve: arises from the ulnar n. in the arm and passes to supply sensation to the caudal aspect of the forearm.

o. Dorsal branch of the ulnar n.: is sensory to the lateral side of the paw.

p. Abaxial dorsal digital n. V: continuation of the dorsal branch of the ulnar nerve on the dorsolateral (abaxial) aspect of the most lateral digit.

q. Palmar branch of the ulnar nerve: passes through the carpal canal and continues in the manus to supply (motor) the interosseous muscle and, with the median n., sensation to the palmar manus.

r. Superficial branch of the palmar branch of the ulnar n.: splits into the common palmar digital n. IV and the abaxial palmar digital n. V to the palmarolateral/abaxial side of the most lateral digit (V).

s. Common palmar digital n. IV: sensory to digits IV and V.

t. Abaxial palmar digital n. V: sensory to the palmarolateral/abaxial side of the most lateral digit (V).

u. Deep branch of palmar branch of the ulnar n.: forms palmar metacarpal nn.

v. Palmar metacarpal nn. I, II, III, IV: pass in palmar grooves between metacarpal bones to reinforce the common digital nn. at the metacarpophalangeal joints.

w. Abaxial palmar digital n. I: branch of the median n., it passes on the medial side of the most medial main digit (II).

x. Common palmar digital nn. I, II, III: branches of the median n., they pass distally above the metacarpal bone junctions. After being reinforced by the metacarpal nn., they, along with the common palmar digital n. IV, branch into proper digital nn.

y. Axial palmar proper digital nn. II, III, IV, V: branches of common palmar digital nn., they pass on the palmaroaxial side of the corresponding digits.

z. Abaxial palmar proper digital nn. III, IV: branches of the common palmar digital nn., they pass on the palmaroabaxial side of the corresponding digits.

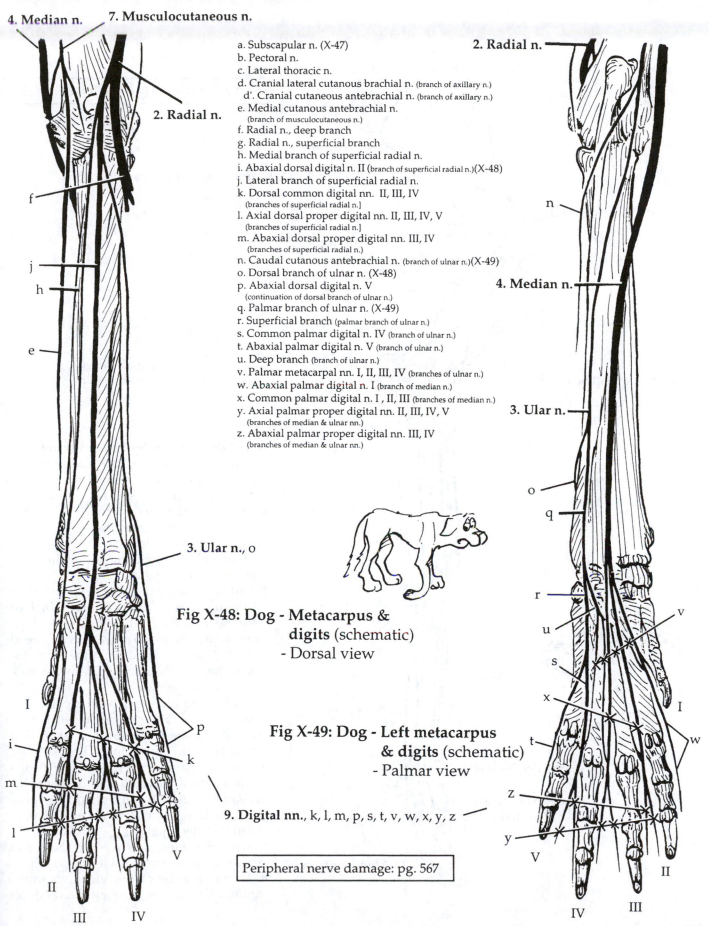

4. Median n.   7. Musculocutaneous n.

2. Radial n.

2. Radial n.

a. Subscapular n. (X-47)
b. Pectoral n.
c. Lateral thoracic n.
d. Cranial lateral cutanous brachial n. (branch of axillary n.)
d'. Cranial cutaneous antebrachial n. (branch of axillary n.)
e. Medial cutanous antebrachial n.
   (branch of musculocutaneous n.)
f. Radial n., deep branch
g. Radial n., superficial branch
h. Medial branch of superficial radial n.
i. Abaxial dorsal digital n. II (branch of superficial radial n.)(X-48)
j. Lateral branch of superficial radial n.
k. Dorsal common digital nn. II, III, IV
   (branches of superficial radial n.]
l. Axial dorsal proper digital nn. II, III, IV, V
   (branches of superficial radial n.]
m. Abaxial dorsal proper digital nn. III, IV
   (branches of superficial radial n.)
n. Caudal cutaneous antebrachial n. (branch of ulnar n.)(X-49)
o. Dorsal branch of ulnar n. (X-48)
p. Abaxial dorsal digital n. V
   (continuation of dorsal branch of ulnar n.)
q. Palmar branch of ulnar n. (X-49)
r. Superficial branch (palmar branch of ulnar n.)
s. Common palmar digital n. IV (branch of ulnar n.)
t. Abaxial palmar digital n. V (branch of ulnar n.)
u. Deep branch (branch of ulnar n.)
v. Palmar metacarpal nn. I, II, III, IV (branches of ulnar n.)
w. Abaxial palmar digital n. I (branch of median n.)
x. Common palmar digital n. I , II, III (branches of median n.)
y. Axial palmar proper digital nn. II, III, IV, V
   (branches of median & ulnar nn.)
z. Abaxial palmar proper digital nn. III, IV
   (branches of median & ulnar nn.)

n

4. Median n.

3. Ular n.

o

q

3. Ular n., o

r

v

u

s

Fig X-48: Dog - Metacarpus &
digits (schematic)
- Dorsal view

Fig X-49: Dog - Left metacarpus
& digits (schematic)
- Palmar view

I

x

w

I

p

t

i

k

z

m

l

y

V

V

II

II

III

IV

9. Digital nn., k, l, m, p, s, t, v, w, x, y, z

IV

III

Peripheral nerve damage: pg. 567

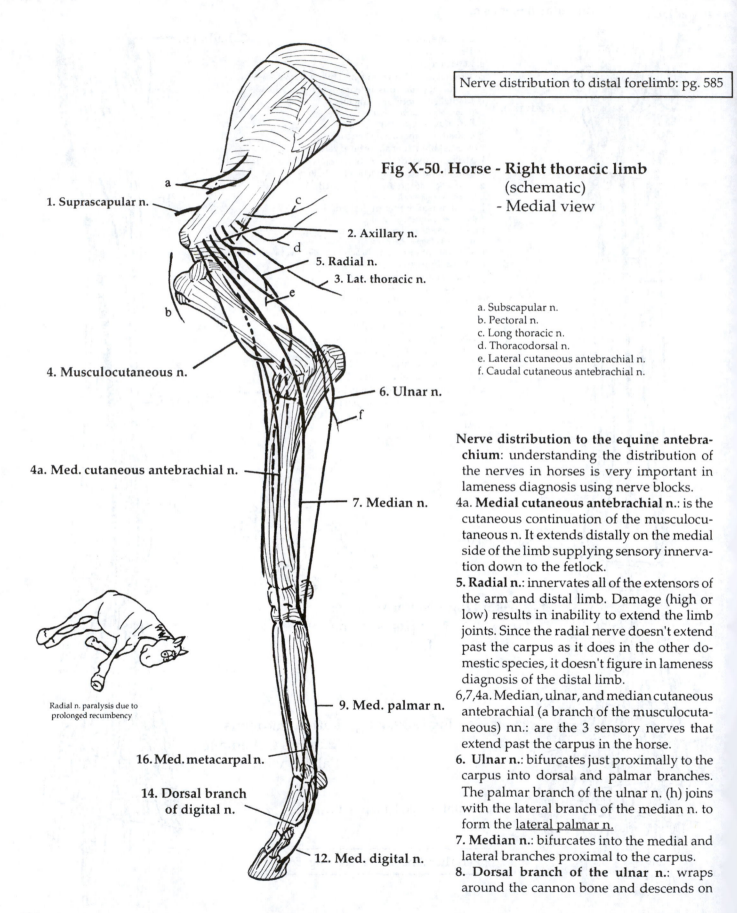

1. Suprascapular n.

a

1. Suprascapular n.

c

2. Axillary n.

d

5. Radial n.

3. Lat. thoracic n.

e

b

4. Musculocutaneous n.

6. Ulnar n.

f

4a. Med. cutaneous antebrachial n.

7. Median n.

9. Med. palmar n.

16. Med. metacarpal n.

14. Dorsal branch
of digital n.

12. Med. digital n.

Radial n. paralysis due to
prolonged recumbency

Nerve distribution to distal forelimb: pg. 585

Fig X-50. Horse - Right thoracic limb
(schematic)
- Medial view

a. Subscapular n.
b. Pectoral n.
c. Long thoracic n.
d. Thoracodorsal n.
e. Lateral cutaneous antebrachial n.
f. Caudal cutaneous antebrachial n.

Nerve distribution to the equine antebra-chium: understanding the distribution of the nerves in horses is very important in lameness diagnosis using nerve blocks.

4a. **Medial cutaneous antebrachial n.**: is the cutaneous continuation of the musculocu-taneous n. It extends distally on the medial side of the limb supplying sensory innerva-tion down to the fetlock.

5. **Radial n.**: innervates all of the extensors of the arm and distal limb. Damage (high or low) results in inability to extend the limb joints. Since the radial nerve doesn't extend past the carpus as it does in the other do-mestic species, it doesn't figure in lameness diagnosis of the distal limb.

6,7,4a. Median, ulnar, and median cutaneous antebrachial (a branch of the musculocuta-neous) nn.: are the 3 sensory nerves that extend past the carpus in the horse.

6. **Ulnar n.**: bifurcates just proximally to the carpus into dorsal and palmar branches. The palmar branch of the ulnar n. (h) joins with the lateral branch of the median n. to form the underlined lateral palmar n.

7. **Median n.**: bifurcates into the medial and lateral branches proximal to the carpus.

8. **Dorsal branch of the ulnar n.**: wraps around the cannon bone and descends on

the dorsolateral side of the cannon region to supply sensory innervation down to the lateral fetlock.

9. **Medial** and 10. **lateral palmar nn.**: travel down either side of the flexor tendons. At the level of the fetlock they continue as the palmar digital nn.

- 9. **Medial palmar n.**: is the direct continuation of the median palmar n. (all median n. fibers).
- 10. **Lateral palmar n.**: is formed by a branch of the median and the palmar branch of the ulnar nn. (median and ulnar nn. fibers).

11. **Communicating branch**: carries fibers from the medial palmar n. (median n. fibers) to the lateral palmar n. (ulnar and median nn. fibers).

12. **Medial** and 13. **lateral digital nn.**: the direct continuation of the medial and lateral palmar nn. past the level of the fetlock. They continue distally with the similarly-named arteries abaxial to the sesamoid bones, then distally on the palmar digit. They pass on the sides of the flexor tendons under the ligament of the ergot to innervate the heel region of the foot. (*NAV: medial and lateral palmar digital nn.)

- Digital triad: the digital vein, artery and nerve on each side of the digit. These triads are arranged vein, artery, nerve (VAN) from dorsal to palmar/plantar.

14. **Dorsal branches of the digital nn.**: passes distally to provide sensory innervation to the toe region of the foot. They arise on each side from the digital nn. near the fetlock. Crossing the abaxial surface of the proximal palmar sesamoid bones with a digital nn., the dorsal branch diverges dorsally from the digital n. and extends distally to the toe.

15. **Deep branch of the lateral palmar n.** or **deep branch of the ulnar n.**: arises at the level of the carpus. It dives deep to the suspensory ligament to which it supplies. It then branches into lateral and medial metacarpal nn.

16, 17. **Medial** and **lateral metacarpal nn.**: are extensions of the deep branch of the lateral palmar n. They course distally, deep against the junctions of the splint bones and the cannon bone. At the buttons of the splints they become superficial and continue to the fetlock joint. (*NAV: medial and lateral palmar metacarpal nn.)

*Palmar is removed from the labels of the digital and metacarpal nerves' names to reflect common clinical jargon. NAV = Nomina anatomica veterinaria

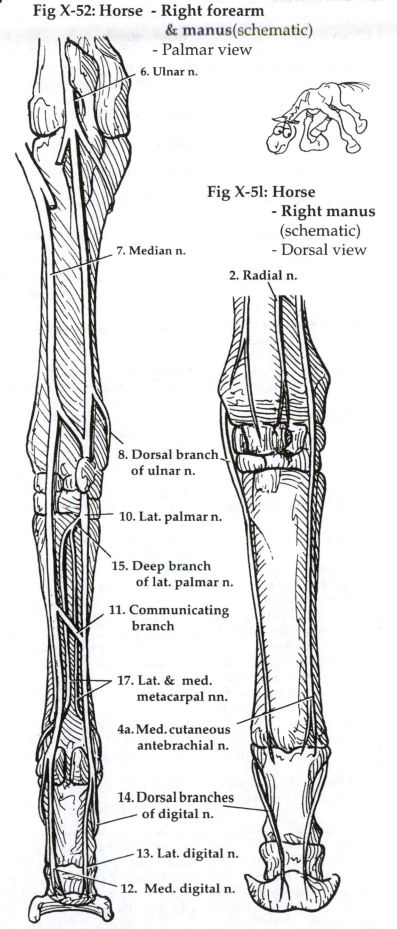

Fig X-52: Horse - Right forearm & manus (schematic) - Palmar view

6. Ulnar n.

7. Median n.

8. Dorsal branch of ulnar n.

10. Lat. palmar n.

15. Deep branch of lat. palmar n.

11. Communicating branch

17. Lat. & med. metacarpal nn.

13. Lat. digital n.

12. Med. digital n.

Fig X-5l: Horse - Right manus (schematic) - Dorsal view

2. Radial n.

4a. Med. cutaneous antebrachial n.

14. Dorsal branches of digital n.

BRACHIAL PLEXUS

Nerve	Motor: muscles	Sensory: region
Suprascapular n.	Motor: **supraspinatus & infraspinatus mm.**	
Subscapular n.	Motor: subscapular m.	
Pectoral nn.	Motor: pectoral m.	
Long thoracic n.	Motor: serratus ventralis m.	
Thoracodorsal n.	Motor: latissimus dorsi m.	
Lateral thoracic n.	Motor: **cutaneous trunci m.**	Sensory: ventral thoracic & abdominal walls
Musculocutaneous n.	Motor: flexors of elbow (coracobrachialis, biceps brachii & brachialis mm.)	
- Medial cutaneous antebrachial n.	....	Sensory: medial forearm (Eq: down to fetlock)
Axillary n.	Motor: flexors of shoulder .... (teres major, teres minor & deltoid mm.)	Sensory: cranial arm & forearm
Radial n.	Motor: **extensors of elbow, carpus & digits** (triceps brachii, anconeus, tensor fasciae antebrachii, extensor carpi radialis, common digital extensor, lateral digital extensor, lateral ulnar, oblique carpal extensor & supinator mm.)	
- Cutaneous branch(es)		Sensory: craniolateral forearm in all species & dorsal manus in all, except the horse
Ulnar n.	Motor: some flexors of forearm & muscles of manus	Sensory: caudal forearm, lateral side of metacarpus & digits
- Caudal cutaneous antebrachial n.		Sensory: caudal forearm
- Dorsal branch		Sensory: dorsolateral metacarpus, down to fetlock (Eq)
- Palmar branch (Eq)		
. Lateral palmar n. (Eq)		Sensory: w/ medial palmar to metacarpus & digits (Eq)
.. Deep branch (Eq)		Sensory: proximal suspensory area
... Medial & lateral metacarpal nn. (Eq)		Sensory: fetlock (Eq)
. Lateral digital n. (Eq)		Sensory: w/ medial digital n. to heel (Eq)
.. Dorsal branch (Eq)		Sensory: toe (eq)
Median n.	Motor: most of flexors of forearm	Sensory: w/ ulnar to manus
. Medial palmar n. (Eq)		Sensory: w/ lateral palmar to metacarpus & digits
. Medial digital n. (Eq)		Sensory: w/ lateral digital n. to heel (Eq)
.. Dorsal branch (Eq)		Sensory: toe (Eq)

* **Bold type** is used to highlight nerves that have "common" clinical significance.

• Besides radial nerve paralysis (and maybe the lateral thoracic n. in the panniculus response) most individual nerves do not have common clinical significance except in the horse.

• Horse (Eq): besides Sweeney (suprascapular n.) and radial nerve paralysis, the rest of the highlighted nerves are important for nerve blocks to diagnose lameness.

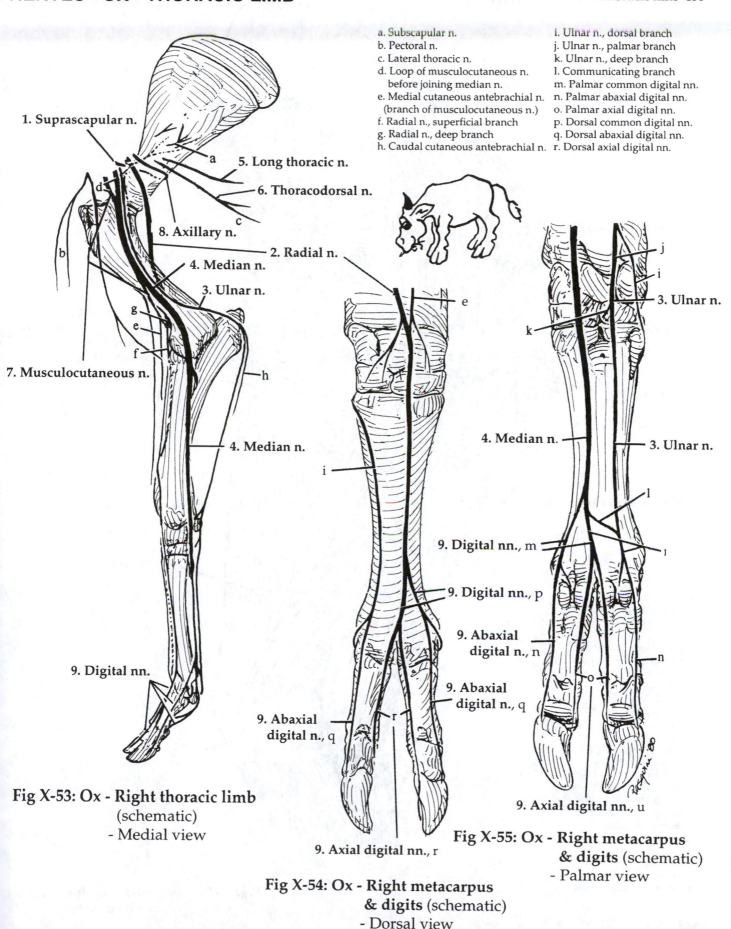

a. Subscapular n.
b. Pectoral n.
c. Lateral thoracic n.
d. Loop of musculocutaneous n. before joining median n.
e. Medial cutaneous antebrachial n. (branch of musculocutaneous n.)
f. Radial n., superficial branch
g. Radial n., deep branch
h. Caudal cutaneous antebrachial n.

i. Ulnar n., dorsal branch
j. Ulnar n., palmar branch
k. Ulnar n., deep branch
l. Communicating branch
m. Palmar common digital nn.
n. Palmar abaxial digital nn.
o. Palmar axial digital nn.
p. Dorsal common digital nn.
q. Dorsal abaxial digital nn.
r. Dorsal axial digital nn.

1. Suprascapular n.
5. Long thoracic n.
6. Thoracodorsal n.
8. Axillary n.
2. Radial n.
4. Median n.
3. Ulnar n.
7. Musculocutaneous n.
4. Median n.
9. Digital nn.

3. Ulnar n.
4. Median n.
3. Ulnar n.

e

9. Digital nn., m
9. Digital nn., p
9. Abaxial digital n., n
9. Abaxial digital n., q

i

9. Abaxial digital n., q
9. Axial digital nn., r

o

n

9. Axial digital nn., u

Fig X-53: Ox - Right thoracic limb
(schematic)
- Medial view

Fig X-54: Ox - Right metacarpus & digits (schematic)
- Dorsal view

Fig X-55: Ox - Right metacarpus & digits (schematic)
- Palmar view

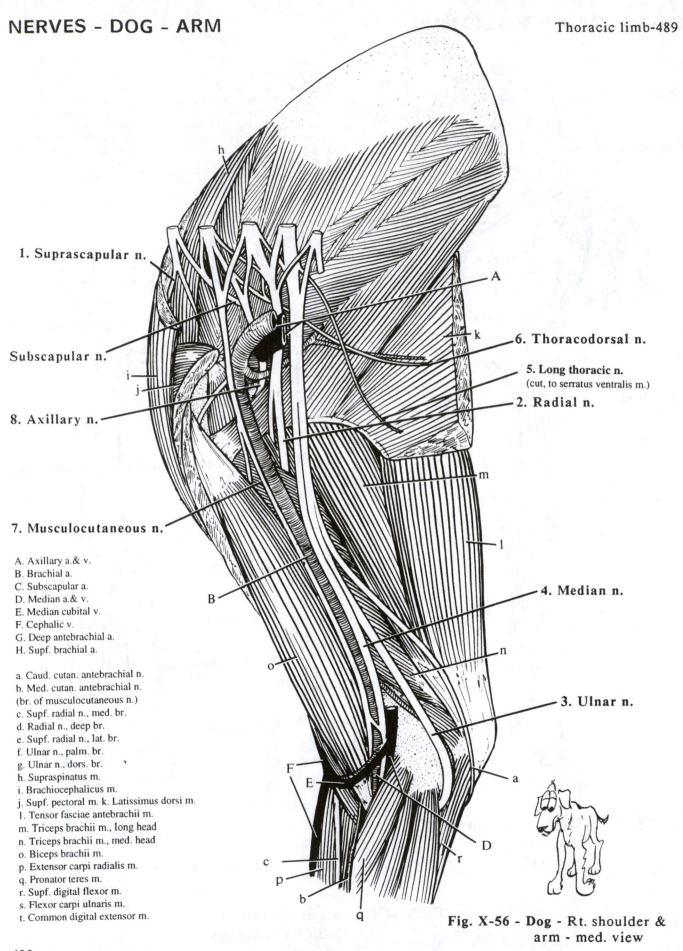

1. Suprascapular n.

Subscapular n.

8. Axillary n.

7. Musculocutaneous n.

A. Axillary a.& v.
B. Brachial a.
C. Subscapular a.
D. Median a.& v.
E. Median cubital v.
F. Cephalic v.
G. Deep antebrachial a.
H. Supf. brachial a.

a. Caud. cutan. antebrachial n.
b. Med. cutan. antebrachial n.
(br. of musculocutaneous n.)
c. Supf. radial n., med. br.
d. Radial n., deep br.
e. Supf. radial n., lat. br.
f. Ulnar n., palm. br.
g. Ulnar n., dors. br.
h. Supraspinatus m.
i. Brachiocephalicus m.
j. Supf. pectoral m. k. Latissimus dorsi m.
l. Tensor fasciae antebrachii m.
m. Triceps brachii m., long head
n. Triceps brachii m., med. head
o. Biceps brachii m.
p. Extensor carpi radialis m.
q. Pronator teres m.
r. Supf. digital flexor m.
s. Flexor carpi ulnaris m.
t. Common digital extensor m.

6. Thoracodorsal n.

5. Long thoracic n.
(cut, to serratus ventralis m.)

2. Radial n.

4. Median n.

3. Ulnar n.

Fig. X-56 - Dog - Rt. shoulder & arm - med. view

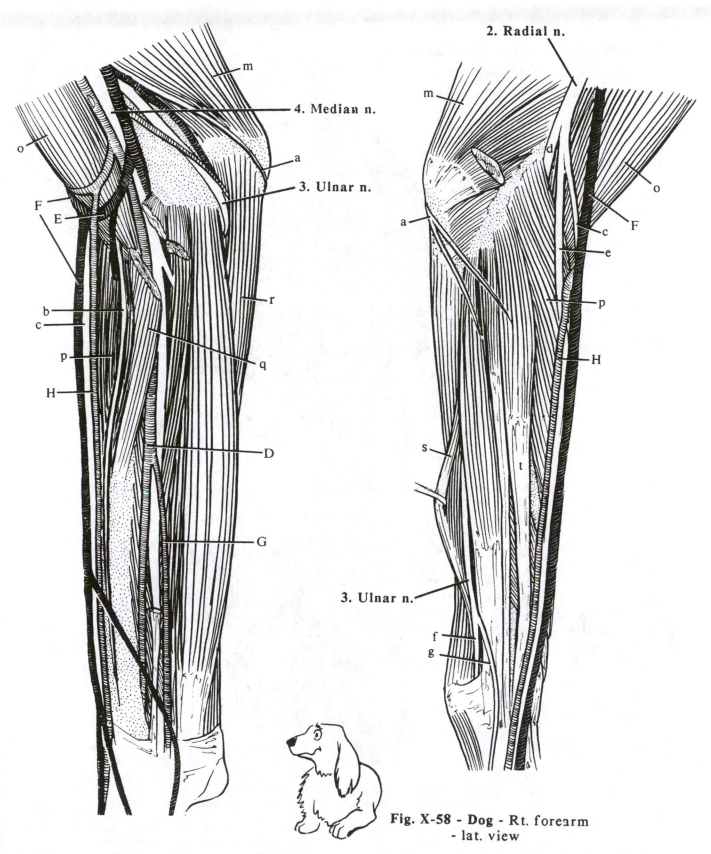

2. Radial n.

m

d

a

o

F

c

e

p

H

s

t

3. Ulnar n.

f

g

**Fig. X-58 - Dog - Rt. forearm
- lat. view**

m

4. Median n.

a

3. Ulnar n.

o

F

E

r

b

c

p

H

q

D

G

**Fig. X-57 - Dog - Rt. forearm
- med. view**

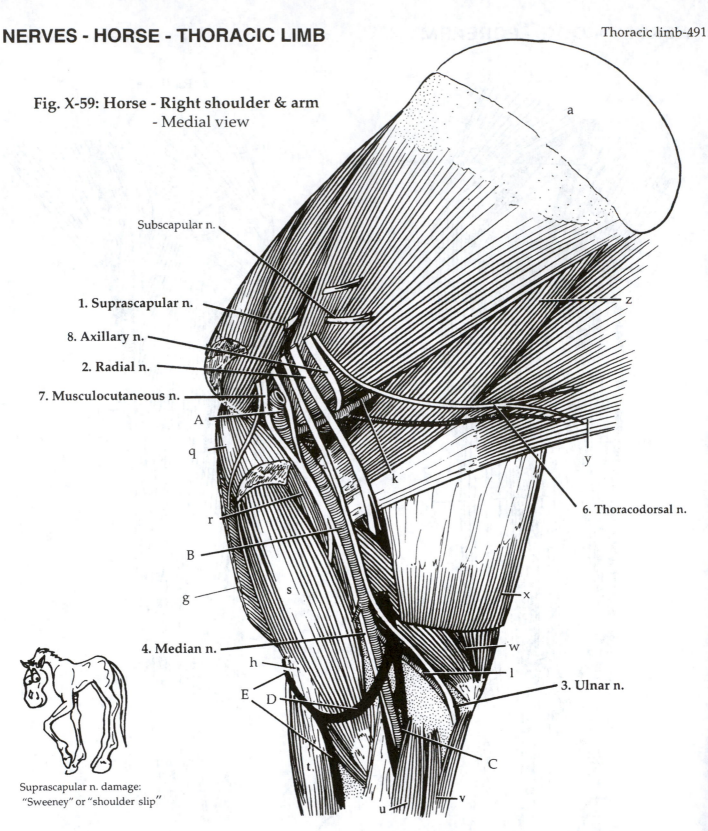

Fig. X-59: Horse - Right shoulder & arm
- Medial view

Subscapular n.

1. Suprascapular n.

8. Axillary n.

2. Radial n.

7. Musculocutaneous n.

A

q

r

B

g

4. Median n.

h

E   D

t.

6. Thoracodorsal n.

3. Ulnar n.

C

z

y

k

s

x

w

l

u   v

Suprascapular n. damage:
"Sweeney" or "shoulder slip"

A. Axillary a.
B. Brachial a.
C. Median a.& v.
D. Median cubital v.
E. Cephalic v.
F. Medial palmar a. & v. (X-60)
G. Medial digital a. & v.

a. Scapular cartilage
b. Caudal cutanous antebrachial n.
   [branch of ulnar n.]
c. Lateral cutanous antebrachial n.
   [branch of radial n.]
d. Radial n., deep branch
e. Subclavius m.
f. Subscapular m.
g. Superficial pectoral m.
h. Lacertus fibrosis

i. Ulnaris lateralis m. (X-61)
j. Common digital extensor m.
k. Subscapular a.
l. Collateral ulnar a.& v. (X-59)
m. Accessory cephalic v. (X-60)
n. Radial a.& v.
o. Button of splint
p. Flexor tendons (SDF, DDF)
q. Deep pectoral m. (X-59)
r. Coracobrachialis m.

s. Biceps brachii m.
t. Extensor carpi radialis m.
u. Flexor carpi radialis m.
v. Flexor carpi ulnaris m.
w. Triceps brachii m.
x. Tensor fasciae antebrachii m.
y. Latissimus dorsi m.
z. Teres major m.

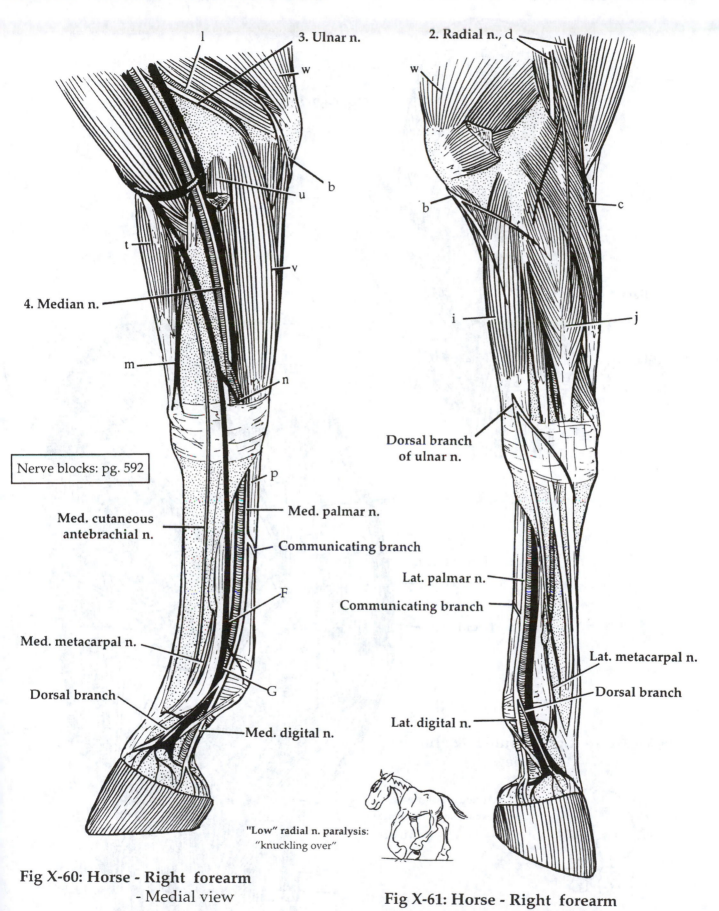

l

3. Ulnar n.

w

2. Radial n., d

w

b

u

b

c

t

v

4. Median n.

i

j

m

n

Nerve blocks: pg. 592

Dorsal branch
of ulnar n.

p

Med. palmar n.

Med. cutaneous
antebrachial n.

Communicating branch

Lat. palmar n.

Communicating branch

F

Med. metacarpal n.

Lat. metacarpal n.

Dorsal branch

Dorsal branch

G

Lat. digital n.

Med. digital n.

"Low" radial n. paralysis:
"knuckling over"

Fig X-60: Horse - Right forearm
- Medial view

Fig X-61: Horse - Right forearm
- Lateral view

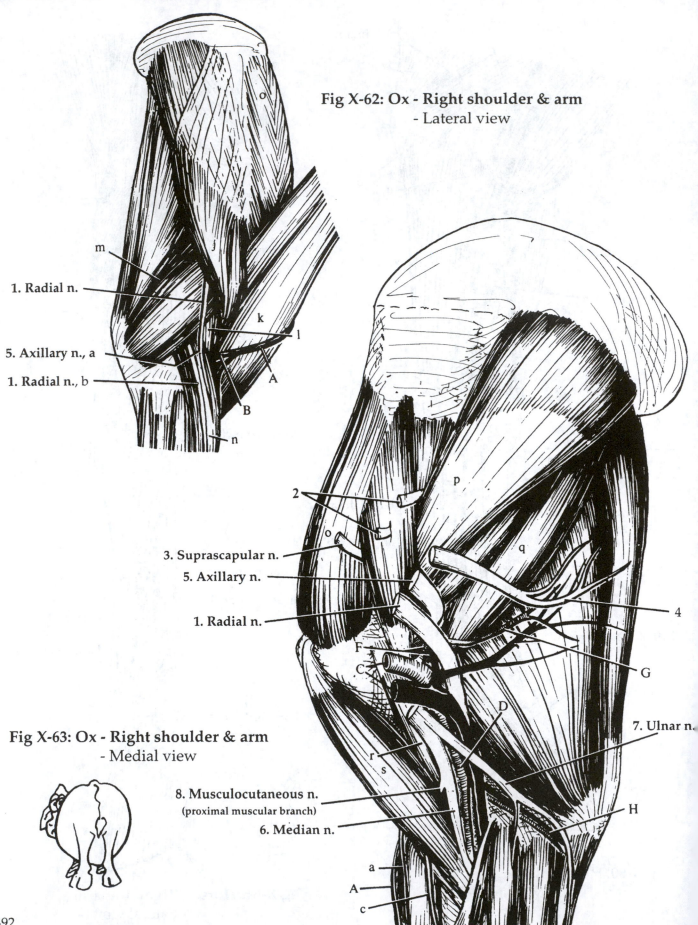

Fig X-62: Ox - Right shoulder & arm
- Lateral view

m

1. Radial n.

5. Axillary n., a

1. Radial n., b

k

l

A

B

n

o

2

o

3. Suprascapular n.

5. Axillary n.

1. Radial n.

p

q

4

F

C

G

D

r

s

7. Ulnar n.

Fig X-63: Ox - Right shoulder & arm
- Medial view

8. Musculocutaneous n.
(proximal muscular branch)

6. Median n.

H

a

A

c

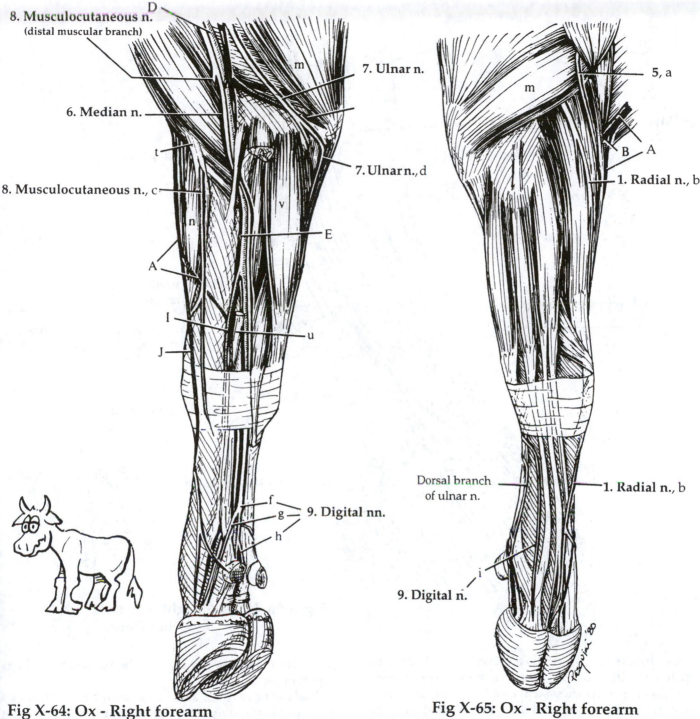

8. Musculocutaneous n.
(distal muscular branch)

D

m

7. Ulnar n.

6. Median n.

t

7. Ulnar n., d

8. Musculocutaneous n., c

v

n

E

A

I

u

J

f

g — 9. Digital nn.

h

5, a

m

B   A

1. Radial n., b

Dorsal branch
of ulnar n.

1. Radial n., b

i

9. Digital n.

Fig X-64: Ox - Right forearm
- Medial view

Fig X-65: Ox - Right forearm
- Lateral view

1. Radial n.
2. Subscapular n.
3. Suprascapular n.
4. Thoracodorsal n.
5. Axillary n.
6. Median n.
7. Ulnar n.
8. Musculocutaneous n.
9. Digital nn.

A. Cephalic v. (X-62)
B. Median cubital v.
C. Axillary a.& v. (X-63)
D. Brachial a.& v.
E. Median a.& v. (X-64)
F. Subscapular a.& v. (X-63)
G. Thoracodorsal a.& v.
H. Collateral ulnar a.& v.
L. Radial a.& v. (X-64)
J. Accessory cephalic v.

a. Cranial cutaneous antebrachial n.
   (branch of axillary n.) (X-62)
b. Radial n., superficial branch
c. Medial cutaneous antebrachial n.
   (branch of musculocutaneous n.) (X-63)
d. Caudal cutaneous antebrachial n.
   (branch of ulnar n.) (X-64)
e. Superficial branch of palmar branch
   (of ulnar n.) (X-65)
f. Palmar common digital nn.
   (branches of lat. & med. plamar) (X-64)
g. Palmar abaxial digital nn.
h. Palmar axial digital nn.
i. Dorsal common digital nn. (X-65)

j. Deltoid m. (X-62)
k. Brachiocephalicus m.
l. Brachialis m.
m. Triceps brachii m.
n. Extensor carpi radialis m.
o. Supraspinatus m.
p. Subscapularis m. (X-63)
q. Teres major m.
r. Coracobrachialis m.
s. Biceps brachii m.
t. Lacertus fibrosus (X-64)
u. Flexor carpi radialis m.
v. Flexor carpi ulnaris m.

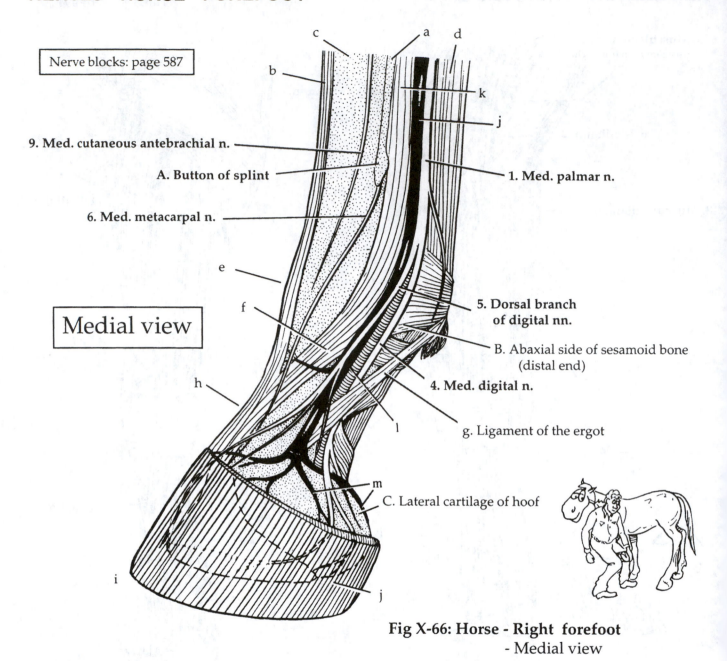

Nerve blocks: page 587

9. Med. cutaneous antebrachial n.

A. Button of splint

6. Med. metacarpal n.

Medial view

1. Med. palmar n.

5. Dorsal branch of digital nn.

B. Abaxial side of sesamoid bone (distal end)

4. Med. digital n.

g. Ligament of the ergot

C. Lateral cartilage of hoof

Fig X-66: Horse - Right forefoot
- Medial view

Nerve blocks (see page 587) are used to locate the site of pain when diagnosing lameness in horses (see appendix). Blocks are performed systematically starting **distally** and **moving proximally**. Block bilaterally because pain doesn't know where the midline is. Blocking a nerve carrying pain will cause the animal to "go sound" (eliminating lameness) on that limb. If the animal does not "go sound" with a block, then block higher. If two or more blocks are needed for the animal to go sound, the problem is located between the last two blocks.

- Since 90% of all lamenesses are in the foot, most will be isolated with just three different nerve blocks: the palmar digital, abaxial sesamoidean, and low palmar).

A. "Heel" or **palmar digital (PD) nerve block**: anesthetizes the heel area of the foot. Block the medial and lateral digital nn. above the lateral cartilages of the hoof on the palmar aspect of the digit.

B. "Toe and pastern" or **abaxial sesamoid block**: anesthetizes the toe and the pastern. Block the medial and lateral digital nn. and their dorsal branches as they cross the distal end of the abaxial side of the sesamoid bones.

C. "Fetlock", low palmar or **four point block**: anesthetizes the fetlock and distally. Block 6 nerves a hand's breadth (4") above the fetlock:

- Medial and lateral palmar nn. on the sides of the flexor tendons.
- Medial and lateral metacarpal nn. as they emerge from under the buttons of the splints.
- Medial cutaneous antebrachial n. and dorsal branch of the ulnar n. dorsal to the buttons of the splints.

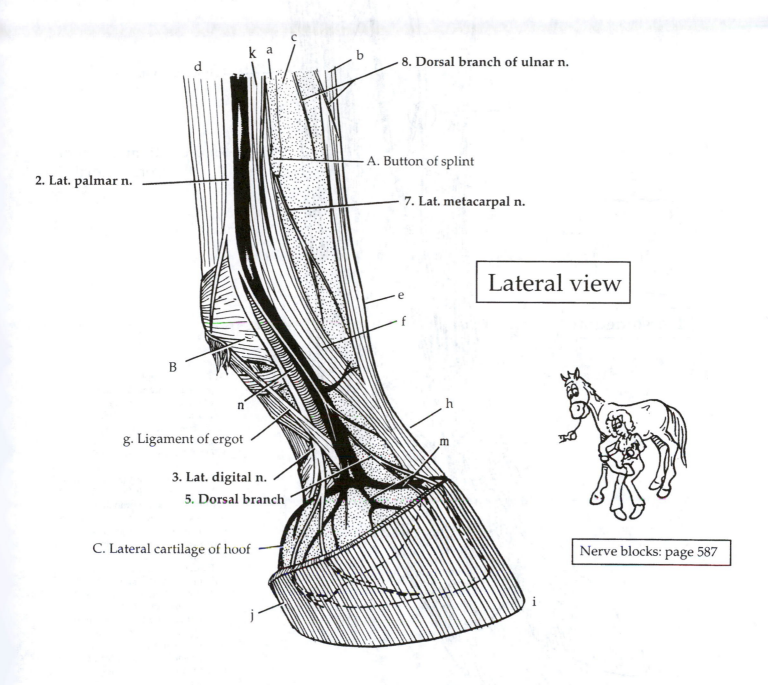

8. Dorsal branch of ulnar n.

A. Button of splint

7. Lat. metacarpal n.

2. Lat. palmar n.

Lateral view

e

f

B

h

n

m

g. Ligament of ergot

3. Lat. digital n.

5. Dorsal branch

C. Lateral cartilage of hoof

Nerve blocks: page 587

j

i

d k a c b

Fig X-67: Horse - Forefoot
- Lateral view

1. Medial palmar n.
2. Lateral palmar n.
3. Lateral (palmar) digital n.
4. Medial (palmar) digital n.
5. Dorsal branch of digital nn.
   (medial & lateral)
6. Deep branch of lateral palmar n.
   7. Medial (palmar) metacarpal n.
   8. Lateral (palmar) metacarpal n.
9. Dorsal branch of ulnar n.
10. Medial cutaneous antebrachial n.
    (branch of musculocutaneous n.)

A. Button of splint (hand's breadth/4"
   above fetlock)
B. Abaxial side of sesamoid bone
C. Lateral cartilage of hoof

a. Splint bone (Mc2)
b. Extensor tendon
c. Cannon bone (Mc3)
d. Flexor tensons (SDF & DDF)
e. Level of fetlock
f. Extensor branch of suspensory
   ligament
g. Ligament of ergot

h. Level of pastern
i. Toe area
j. Heel area
k. Suspensory ligament
l. Medial digital a. & v.
m. Coronary venous plexus
n. Lateral digital a.

495

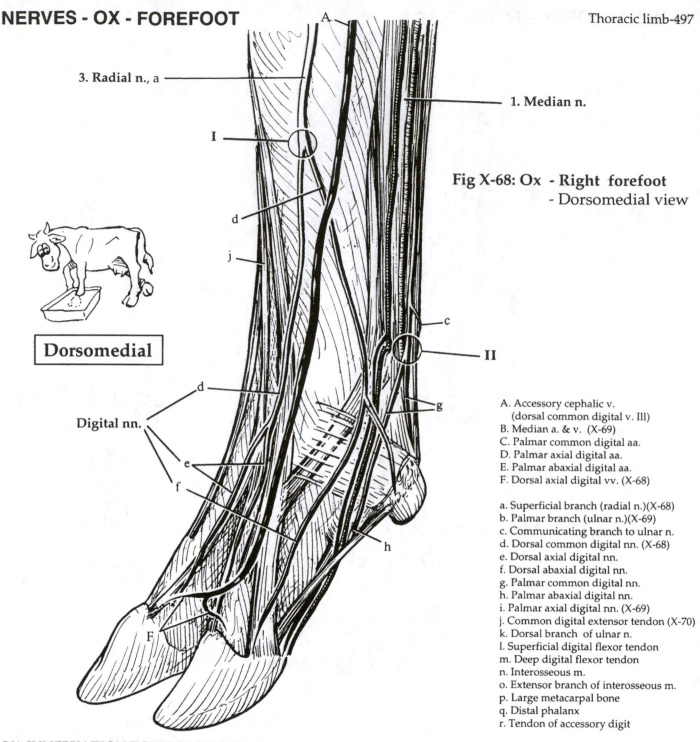

3. Radial n., a

1. Median n.

I

d

j

Dorsomedial

d

Digital nn.

e

f

c

II

g

h

F

Fig X-68: Ox - Right forefoot
- Dorsomedial view

A. Accessory cephalic v.
   (dorsal common digital v. Ill)
B. Median a. & v. (X-69)
C. Palmar common digital aa.
D. Palmar axial digital aa.
E. Palmar abaxial digital aa.
F. Dorsal axial digital vv. (X-68)

a. Superficial branch (radial n.)(X-68)
b. Palmar branch (ulnar n.)(X-69)
c. Communicating branch to ulnar n.
d. Dorsal common digital nn. (X-68)
e. Dorsal axial digital nn.
f. Dorsal abaxial digital nn.
g. Palmar common digital nn.
h. Palmar abaxial digital nn.
i. Palmar axial digital nn. (X-69)
j. Common digital extensor tendon (X-70)
k. Dorsal branch of ulnar n.
l. Superficial digital flexor tendon
m. Deep digital flexor tendon
n. Interosseous m.
o. Extensor branch of interosseous m.
p. Large metacarpal bone
q. Distal phalanx
r. Tendon of accessory digit

OX: INNERVATION TO THE FOREFOOT

1. **Median nerve**: supplies sensory innervation to 3 of the 4 palmar surfaces of the digits (axial and abaxial of medial digit and axial of lateral digit), all but the abaxial side of the lateral digit, which is supplied by the ulnar n.
2. **Ulnar nerve**: has palmar and dorsal branches.
 - **Palmar branch of the ulnar nerve**: supplies the interosseous muscle and, with the median n., the palmar abaxial side of the lateral digit.
 - **Dorsal branch of the ulnar nerve**: supplies the dorsal abaxial surface of the lateral digit (4).
3. **Superficial branch of the radial nerve**: supplies sensory inner- vation to 3 of 4 surfaces of the dorsal digits; the lateral side of digit

CLINICAL:

Blocking out the distal limb of the ox can be done with nerve blocks, a ring block, or intravenous regional anesthesia.
- **Nerve blocks of the thoracic limb - ox:**
 - **I. Superficial radial nerve block**: palpate the nerve in the mid- metacarpus, medial to the common digital extensor tendon. Inject anesthetic at this point.
 - **II. Median nerve block**: inject on the medial side in the groove between the interosseous m. and the flexor tendons.
 - Blocking the ulnar nerve can be done in two ways. Inject the ulnar n. 1 hand's breadth (4") above the accessory carpal bone where it emerges between the flexor carpi ulnaris and ulnaris lateralis mm. OR block its palmar and dorsal branches sepa-

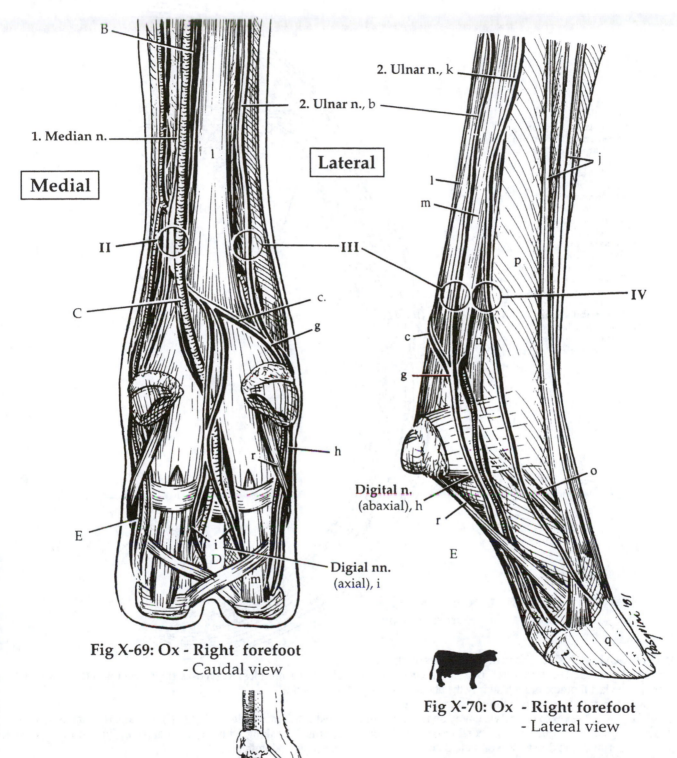

B

1. Median n.

2. Ulnar n., b

2. Ulnar n., k

Medial

Lateral

l

II

III

IV

C

c.

g

j

l

m

p

c

n

g

E

h

r

i

D

m

Digial nn.
(axial), i

Digital n.
(abaxial), h

r

E

o

q

Fig X-69: Ox - Right forefoot
- Caudal view

Fig X-70: Ox - Right forefoot
- Lateral view

rately:

. **III. Dorsal branch of the ulnar nerve
block**: inject the groove between the
cannon bone and the interosseous m.

. **VI. Palmar branch of ulnar nerve
block**: redirect the needle used for the dorsal ulnar n. and inject
the groove between the interosseous m. and the flexor tendons.

• **Ring block**: another way to desensitize the distal limb is to
encircling the metacarpus with a local anesthetic agent.

• **Intravenous technique**: the simplest way to block out the distal
limb it to use a tourniquet to raise the
large veins of the foot. Then inject an
anesthetic agent in one of them to
anesthetize the lower limb in a
retrograde fashion This has similar
results to nerve blocks, is more
reliable, requires no special
knowledge of anatomy, and only
1 injection ia needed.

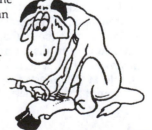

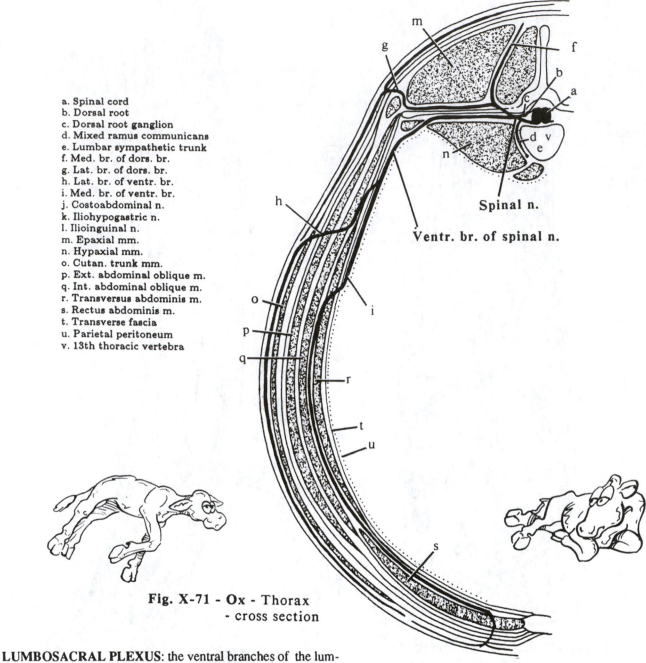

a. Spinal cord
b. Dorsal root
c. Dorsal root ganglion
d. Mixed ramus communicans
e. Lumbar sympathetic trunk
f. Med. br. of dors. br.
g. Lat. br. of dors. br.
h. Lat. br. of ventr. br.
i. Med. br. of ventr. br.
j. Costoabdominal n.
k. Iliohypogastric n.
l. Ilioinguinal n.
m. Epaxial mm.
n. Hypaxial mm.
o. Cutan. trunk mm.
p. Ext. abdominal oblique m.
q. Int. abdominal oblique m.
r. Transversus abdominis m.
s. Rectus abdominis m.
t. Transverse fascia
u. Parietal peritoneum
v. 13th thoracic vertebra

Spinal n.

Ventr. br. of spinal n.

**Fig. X-71 - Ox - Thorax
- cross section**

LUMBOSACRAL PLEXUS: the ventral branches of the lumbar and sacral nerves. The first three or four lumbar ventral branches and the last thoracic branch supply the abdominal wall. The lumbosacral plexus to the pelvic limb is formed by the ventral branches of L_4 to S_2. Nerves to the pelvic cavity and the genitalia arise from the ventral branches of the sacral nerves (pudendal, caudal rectal, perineal and dorsal nerve to the penis).

Abdominal nerves: The first three or four ventral lumbar branches are distributed to the abdominal wall (iliohypogastric, ilioinguinal, genitofemoral, and lateral cutaneous femoral nerves) along with the last thoracic (costoabdominal) nerve. These are important in flank surgery in the ox and horse. These branches travel in a caudoventral direction. They pierce the transverse abdominis muscle at the transverse processes and travel caudoventrally between it and the internal abdominal oblique. They supply the

abdominal muscles and send lateral and ventral cutaneous branches to the skin.

Costoabdominal nerve (T13) (j): not a part of the lumbosacral plexus, but, along with the first couple of lumbar nerves, innervates the abdominal wall.

Iliohypogastric nerve (L_1 or Ll &2) (k): in animals with six lumbar vertebrae (ox and horse), it is formed by the ventral branches of L_1. In animals with seven lumbar vertebrae (carnivores) there are cranial (L_1) and caudal (L_2) iliohypogastric nerves.

Ilioinguinal nerve (L_2 or L_3) (l): in animals with six lumbar vertebrae, formed by L_2; with seven lumbar vertebrae, L_3.

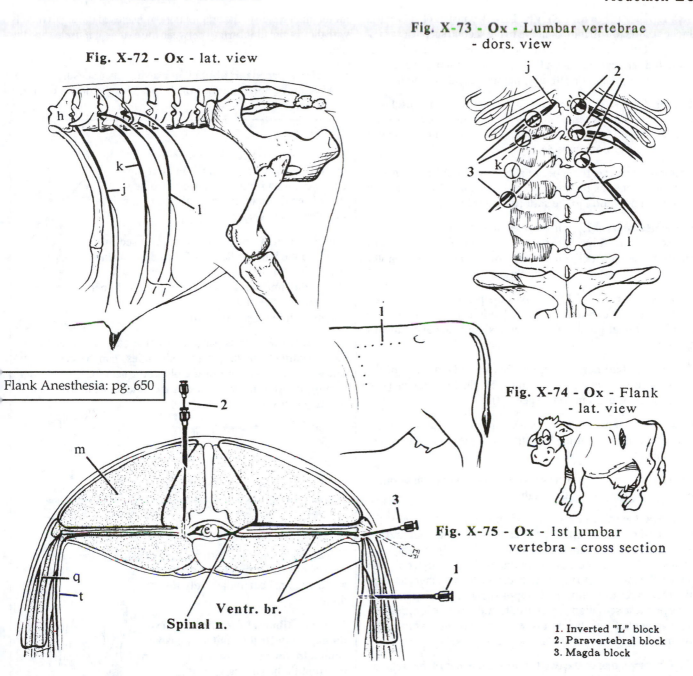

Fig. X-72 - Ox - lat. view

Fig. X-73 - Ox - Lumbar vertebrae - dors. view

Flank Anesthesia: pg. 650

Fig. X-74 - Ox - Flank - lat. view

Fig. X-75 - Ox - 1st lumbar vertebra - cross section

Ventr. br.
Spinal n.

1. Inverted "L" block
2. Paravertebral block
3. Magda block

Genitofemoral nerve (L3 & 4): divides into a genital branch supplying the external genital organs and the inguinal region (cranial part of the udder in the cow) and a femoral branch supplying the skin over the medial thigh.

CLINICAL (see Appendix for more) (pg. 650)

Standing flank surgery in the ox: opening the paralumbar fossa to deal with such problems as "hardware disease", dystocia, displaced abomasum, etc. The first three or four ventral lumbar nerves and the last thoracic nerve are anesthetized in flank surgery of the ox and horse.

Local anesthesia for a flank surgery: concerned with T13, L1 and L2 nerves and can be done in a number of ways:

1. Inverted "L" block: injections are done in the abdominal wall, from the subcutaneous area to the peritoneum, in the pattern shown.

2. Paravertebral block: blocks all branches of the spinal nerves.

3. Distal paralumbar analgesia or **Magda block**: blocks only the ventral and lateral dorsal branches of the spinal nerves.

NERVE SUPPLY to the PELVIC LIMB: consists of the ventral branches of the fourth lumbar nerve to the second sacral nerve (L_4 - S_2) of the lumbosacral plexus (caudal cutaneous femoral, femoral, cranial gluteal, caudal gluteal, caudal clunial, obturator, ischiatic, tibial, common (fibular) peroneal, and pudendal).

1. Femoral nerve (L_{4-6}): innervation of the extensor muscles of the stifle (quadriceps femoris). It passes through the psoas muscles, out of the abdominal cavity and through the femoral canal to the quadriceps femoris muscle.

2. Saphenous nerve: the superficial branch of the femoral nerve, supplying cutaneous innervation to the medial side of the limb and motor innervation to the sartorius muscle.

3. Obturator nerve (L_{4-6}): innervates most of the medial adductor muscles of the thigh. It extends from the lumbosacral plexus through the pelvic cavity on the body of the ilium and obturator foramen to the medial side of the thigh.

Lumbosacral trunk: (L_7-S_2): leaves the pelvis over the greater ischiatic notch to continue as the ischiatic nerve. It gives three branches - cranial gluteal, caudal gluteal and caudal cutaneous femoral nerves.

7. Cranial gluteal nerve: supplies flexors and extensors of the hip (tensor fasciae latae, middle and deep gluteal muscles [also the superficial gluteal in some species]).

8. Caudal gluteal nerve: supplies the superficial gluteal muscles and the proximal part of the hamstring muscles, thus, the extensors of the hip.

Caudal cutaneous femoral nerve: supplies cutaneous innervation over the caudal aspect of the thigh.

4. Ischiatic (sciatic) nerve ($L_{6\ or\ 7}$-S_2): the largest nerve of the lumbosacral plexus, supplying the caudal thigh muscles and, by its terminal branches (tibial and common fibular [peroneal]), the muscles of the crus and pes. It continues the lumbosacral trunk caudal to the hip joint, to run distally caudal to the femur and deep to the biceps femoris muscle. It supplies the hamstring muscles and the pelvic association (internal obturator [except in ruminants and pigs], gemelli and quadratus femoris). It branches mid-thigh into tibial and common (fibular) peroneal nerves.

5. Tibial nerve: one of the two terminal branches of the ischiatic nerve. It runs between the two heads of the gastrocnemius muscle to reach and supply the caudal muscles of the crus. It splits at the level of the point of the hock into medial and lateral plantar nerves. The plantar nerves continue down the plantar aspect of the pes mainly supplying sensation.

Caudal cutaneous sural nerve: cutaneous branch of the tibial nerve arising above the stifle.

6. Common peroneal (fibular*) nerve: the other terminal branch of the ischiatic nerve, coursing around the lateral side of the crus (over fibula). It supplies the craniolateral muscles of the crus (deep peroneal branch) and the skin of the craniolateral crus and dorsal foot (superficial peroneal branch).

Deep peroneal (fibular*) nerve (n. peroneus profundus): supplies motor innervation to the craniolateral muscles of the leg. It travels with the cranial tibial artery between the extensor muscles and the tibia.

Superficial peroneal (fibular) nerve: mainly a sensory nerve. It divides on the dorsal surface of the pes into the dorsal common digital nerves.

CLINICAL

Femoral nerve deficiency: inability to extend the stifle results in the inability to bear weight on limb. There may also be a loss of sensation on the medial side of the limb (saphenous nerve).

Obturator nerve paralysis: can becaused by injury to the intrapelvic par of the nerve during parturition (birth). This results in inability to adduct the limb and is most noticable on slippery floors where the limbs slip sideways. This is common in foaling and calving.

"Downer cow": a postpartum cow that cannot rise to stand. This syndrome, having many etiologies, can be caused by injury to the pelvic part of the obturator nerve due to trauma during parturition. The animal cannot adduct its limb to stand, but may recover.

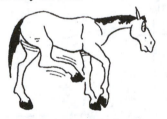

Tibial n. paralysis

Tibial nerve damage: affects theextensors of the tarsus and flexors of the digits. The tarsus drops and the animal cannot actively flex the digits.

Common fibular* (peroneal) nerve damage: affects the digital extensors similar to low radial nerve paralysis in the front limb. This can result in "knuckling over".

Spastic paresis/Elso heel: hereditary condition where calves ' hock and stifle are extended at all times when standing. This has been treated by cutting the tibial nerve to the gastrocnemius muscle

Stretching/spastic syndrome: episodes of spasms and extendion of hindlimbs of adult cattle

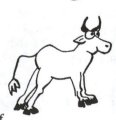

* **Fibular nerve may be** used instead **of peroneal** to avoid confusion with the perineal branches of the pudendal nerve of the pelvis. It also helps distinguish it from the tibia because it passes over the fibula (lateral side of limb. This option is allowed by the N. A . V.

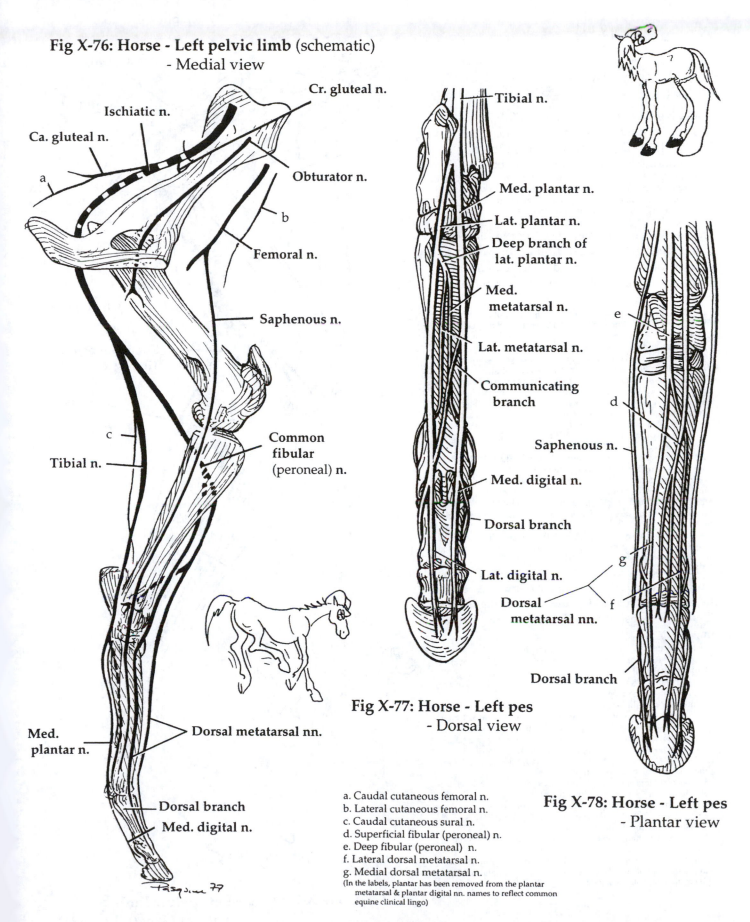

Fig X-76: Horse - Left pelvic limb (schematic)
- Medial view

Cr. gluteal n.

Ischiatic n.

Ca. gluteal n.

a

Obturator n.

b

Femoral n.

Saphenous n.

c

Tibial n.

Common
fibular
(peroneal) n.

Med.
plantar n.

Dorsal metatarsal nn.

Dorsal branch

Med. digital n.

Tibial n.

Med. plantar n.

Lat. plantar n.

Deep branch of
lat. plantar n.

Med.
metatarsal n.

Lat. metatarsal n.

Communicating
branch

Saphenous n.

Med. digital n.

Dorsal branch

Lat. digital n.

Dorsal
metatarsal nn.

e

d

g

f

Dorsal branch

Fig X-77: Horse - Left pes
- Dorsal view

Fig X-78: Horse - Left pes
- Plantar view

a. Caudal cutaneous femoral n.
b. Lateral cutaneous femoral n.
c. Caudal cutaneous sural n.
d. Superficial fibular (peroneal) n.
e. Deep fibular (peroneal) n.
f. Lateral dorsal metatarsal n.
g. Medial dorsal metatarsal n.
(In the labels, plantar has been removed from the plantar
   metatarsal & plantar digital nn. names to reflect common
   equine clinical lingo)

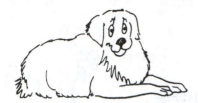

DOG - Nerves of the LEG and PES:

Axis of the paw: passes between the third and fourth digits. Digital nerves facing the axis are axial and those that face away are abaxial.

• According to NAV (Nomina Anatomica Veterinaria) superficial nn. of the metapodium (metacarpus and metatarsus) are common digital nn. and the deep nn. are metacarpal/metatarsal nn. Nerves in the digits arising from the bifurcation of common digital nn. are proper digital nn. Those originating from other sources are just digital nn.

6. Common fibular (peroneal) nerve: branches into superficial and deep fibular nn. which extend distally to divide into dorsal metatarsal and digital nn. that supply the dorsal surface of the pes.

• **Superficial peroneal (fibular) nerve (e):** supplies motor innervation to the peroneus brevis and lateral digital extensor, and then continues as a sensory n. It divides on the dorsal surface of the paw into the dorsal common digital nn.
- Abaxial dorsal digital nerves II and V (h): extend on the abaxial (medial and lateral) sides of the metatarsus and digits.
- Dorsal common digital nerves II, III, and IV (g): extend distally above the dorsal junctions of the metatarsal bones to be joined by the dorsal metatarsal nn. proximal the metatarsophalangeal joint. Upon reaching the digits, the dorsal common digital nn. branch into axial and abaxial dorsal proper digital nn.
  . Axial dorsal proper digital nerves II, III, IV, and V (j): pass down the axial side of corresponding digits.
  . Abaxial dorsal proper digital nerves III and IV (k): pass down the abaxial side of the corresponding digits.
• **Deep fibular (peroneal) nerve (f):** supplies motor innervation to the craniolateral muscles of the leg. It passes deep between the muscles to reach the cranial surface of the tibia and then passes distally with the cranial tibial a. At the tarsus, it divides into dorsal metatarsal nn. II, III, and IV.
- Dorsal metatarsal nerves II, III, and IV (i): pass distally in the junctions between the metatarsal bones to join the dorsal common digital nn. above the metatarsophalangeal joint.

5. Tibial nerve: supplies all the muscles of the caudal leg and is sensory to the plantar aspect of the pes. Just proximal to the talocrural joint the tibial n. divides into medial and lateral plantar nn.

- Medial plantar nerve (l): the smaller branch of the tibial n. that branches to form the plantar common digital nn. and the abaxial plantar digital n. II.
  . Abaxial plantar digital n. II (m): passes down the medial aspect of the metatarsus and medial digit.
  . Plantar common digital nerves II, III, and IV (n): extend distally in the plantar junction of the metatarsal bones to be joined by the plantar metatarsal nn. Upon reaching the digits (near the level of the metatarsophalangeal joints) the plantar common digital nn. branch into axial and abaxial plantar proper digital nn.
  . Axial plantar proper digital nerves II, III, IV, and V (r): pass down the axial side of the corresponding digits.
  . Abaxial plantar proper digital nerves III and IV (s): pass down the abaxial side of the corresponding digits.
- Lateral plantar nerve (o): larger and deeper than the medial plantar nerve, it divides into plantar metatarsal nn. I, II, III and IV which join the plantar common digital nn.
  . Abaxial plantar digital nerve V (p): passes down the lateral side of the pes.
  . Plantar metatarsal nerves II, III, and IV (q): pass in the junctions of the metatarsal bones and join the plantar common digital nn. above the metatarsophalangeal joints.

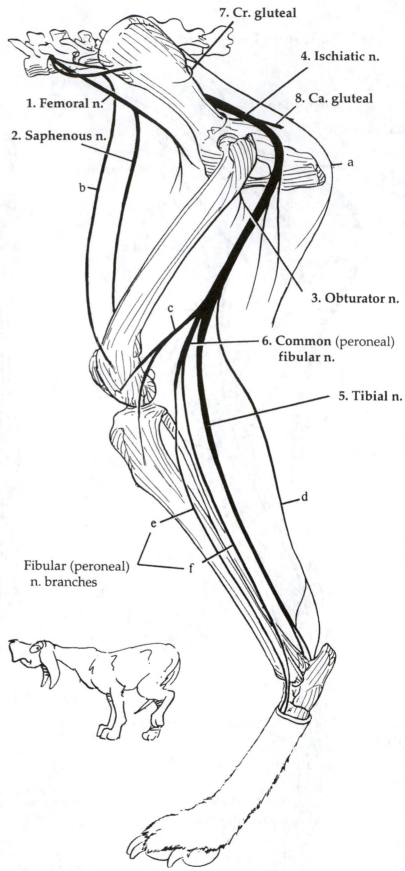

7. Cr. gluteal

4. Ischiatic n.

8. Ca. gluteal

1. Femoral n.

2. Saphenous n.

a

b

3. Obturator n.

6. Common (peroneal) fibular n.

5. Tibial n.

c

d

e

f

Fibular (peroneal) n. branches

Fig X-79: Dog - Left pelvic limb
- Lateral view (schematic)

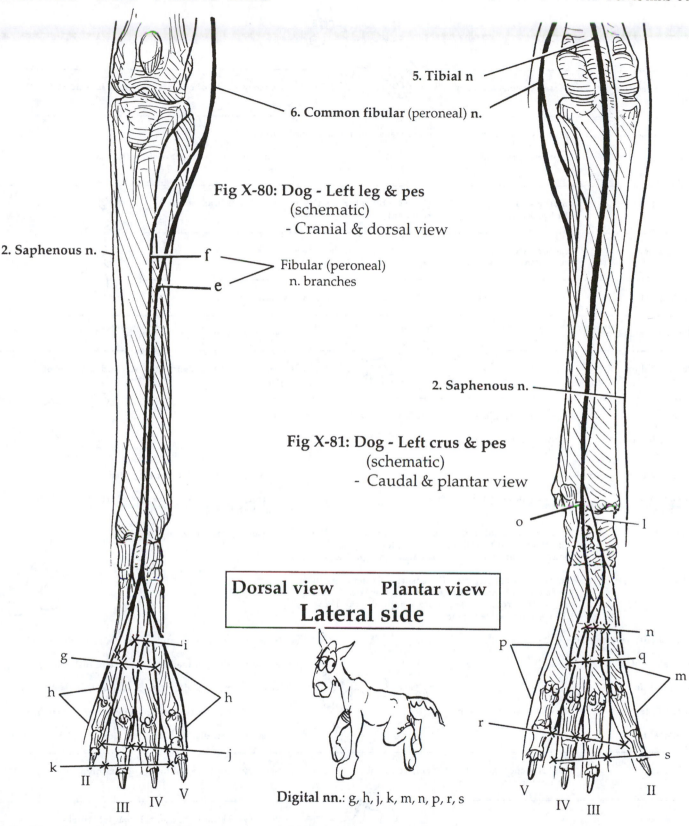

5. Tibial n

6. Common fibular (peroneal) n.

Fig X-80: Dog - Left leg & pes
(schematic)
- Cranial & dorsal view

2. Saphenous n.

f

e

Fibular (peroneal)
n. branches

2. Saphenous n.

Fig X-81: Dog - Left crus & pes
(schematic)
- Caudal & plantar view

o

l

Dorsal view	Plantar view
Lateral side	

g

h

i

h

j

k

II

III

IV

V

P

n

q

m

r

s

V

II

IV

III

Digital nn.: g, h, j, k, m, n, p, r, s

a. Caudal cutaneous femoral n.
b. Lateral cutaneous femoral n.
c. Lateral cutaneous sural n.
d. Caudal cutaneous sural n.
e. Superficial fibular n.
f. Deep fibular n.

g. Dorsal common digital nn. II, III, IV
h. Abaxial dorsal digital nn. II, IV
i. Dorsal metatasal nn. II, III, IV
j. Axial dorsal proper digital nn. II, III, IV, V

k. Abaxial dorsal proper digital nn. III, IV
l. Medial plantar n.
m. Abaxial plantar digital n. II
n. Plantar common digital nn. II, III, IV
o. Lateral plantar n.

p. Abaxial plantar digital n. V
q. Plantar metatarsal nn. II, III, IV
r. Axial plantar proper digital nn. II, III, IV, V
s. Abaxial plantar proper digital nn. III, IV

NERVES	MOTOR	SENSORY
Lateral cutaneous femoral	motor - psoas major m.	sensory - skin of craniomed. thigh & cran. stifle
Femoral (L4-6)	motor - extensors of stifle (quadriceps femoris) & iliopsoas mm.	
Saphenous	motor - sartorius m.	sensory - med. aspect of limb from stifle to metatarsus
Obturator (L4-6)	motor - to adductors of thigh (ext. obturator, pectineus, adductor & gracilis mm.) (int. obturator m. in pig & ruminants)	
Cranial gluteal	motor - extensors & flexors of hip (supf., middle & deep gluteal mm., & tensor fascia lata m.) (some species - supf. gluteal m.)	
Caudal gluteal	motor - extensors of hip (supf. gluteal, biceps femoris & semitendinosus mm.	
Caudal cutaneous femoral		sensory - caud. aspect of thigh
Caudal clunial nn.		sensory - skin of caudomed. & caudolat. face of thigh
Ischiatic	motor - deep gluteal, int. obturator, gemelli mm.	
Common fibular (peroneal)	motor - biceps femoris m.	
Lateral cutaneous sural		sensory - skin on lat. aspect of leg
Superficial fibular	motor - lat. digital extensor m.	sensory - skin on dors. aspect of crus & pes (horse just to fetlock)
Deep fibular	motor - dorsolat. flexors of hock & extensors of digits (cranial tibial, third fibular, long digital extensor, lat. digital extensor & short digital extensor mm.)	sensory - structures of foot
Tibial	motor - hamstring mm. (biceps femoris, semitendinosus & semimembranosus) to extensors of hock & flexors of digits (gastrocnemius, popliteal, supf. digital flexor & deep digital flexor mm.)	
Caudal cutaneous sural		sensory - to skin of caud. aspect of leg (crus).
Medial plantar		sensory - skin on medioplant. face of metatarsus
Digital nn.		sensory - med. digits or med. side of horse's digit
Lateral plantar	motor - interosseus m.	sensory - skin of lateroplant. surface of metatarsus
Digital nn.		sensory - lat. digits (horse, lat. side of digit)
Caudal rectal	motor - coccygeus, levator ani, ext. anal sphincter mm.	sensory - ischiorectal fossa (not carnivores)
Cranial clunial		sensory - skin of craniolat. hip & lat. thigh.
Middle clunial		sensory - skin of dorsolat. hip & thigh.

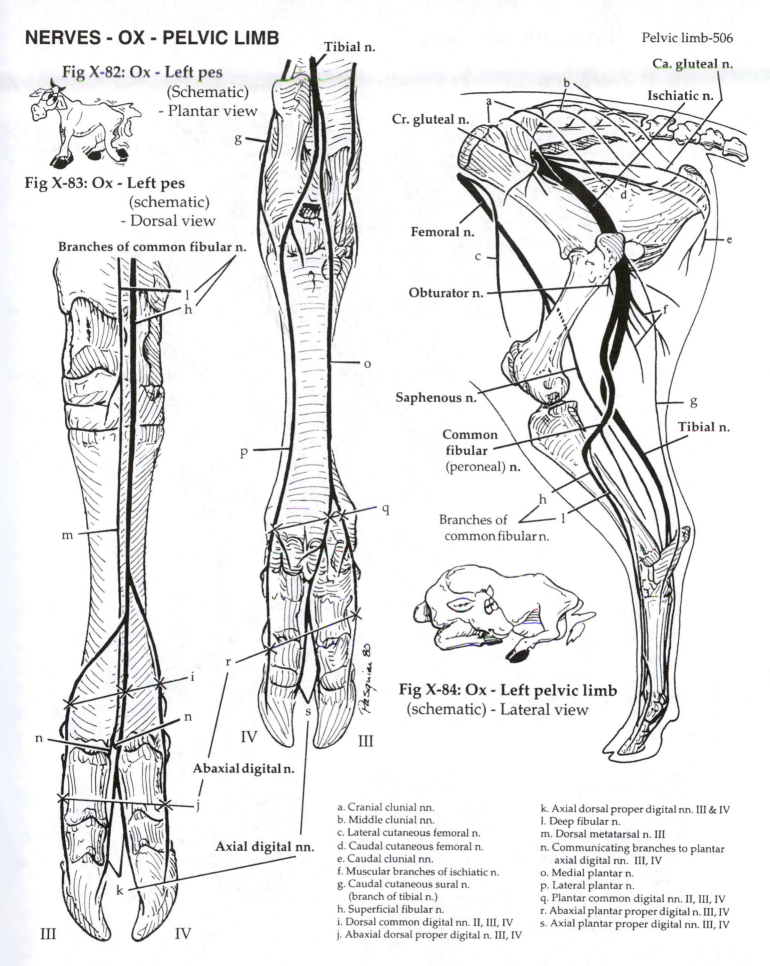

NERVES - OX - PELVIC LIMB

Fig X-82: Ox - Left pes
(Schematic)
- Plantar view

Fig X-83: Ox - Left pes
(schematic)
- Dorsal view

Branches of common fibular n.

Tibial n.

g

l
h

o

p

q

r

s

IV

III

Abaxial digital n.

Axial digital nn.

m

i

n

n

j

k

III

IV

PASquini 80

Ca. gluteal n.

Cr. gluteal n.

Ischiatic n.

b

a

d

Femoral n.

c

e

Obturator n.

f

Saphenous n.

g

Common fibular (peroneal) n.

Tibial n.

h

Branches of common fibular n.

l

Fig X-84: Ox - Left pelvic limb
(schematic) - Lateral view

a. Cranial clunial nn.
b. Middle clunial nn.
c. Lateral cutaneous femoral n.
d. Caudal cutaneous femoral n.
e. Caudal clunial nn.
f. Muscular branches of ischiatic n.
g. Caudal cutaneous sural n.
 (branch of tibial n.)
h. Superficial fibular n.
i. Dorsal common digital nn. II, III, IV
j. Abaxial dorsal proper digital n. III, IV

k. Axial dorsal proper digital nn. III & IV
l. Deep fibular n.
m. Dorsal metatarsal n. III
n. Communicating branches to plantar
 axial digital nn. III, IV
o. Medial plantar n.
p. Lateral plantar n.
q. Plantar common digital nn. II, III, IV
r. Abaxial plantar proper digital n. III, IV
s. Axial plantar proper digital nn. III, IV

505

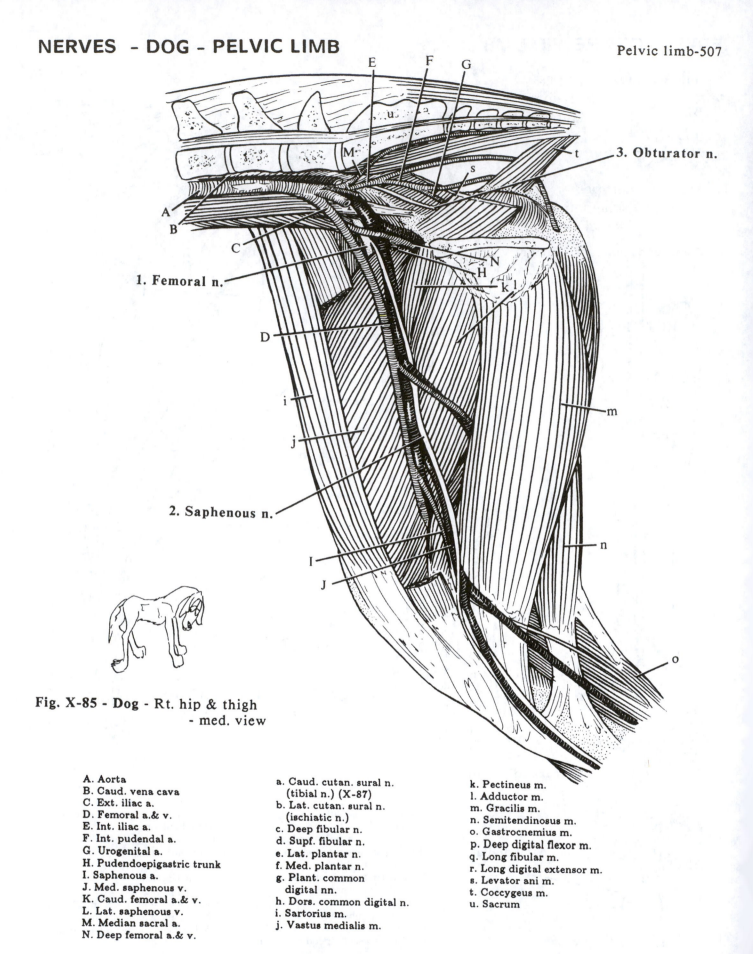

Fig. X-85 – Dog - Rt. hip & thigh
- med. view

A. Aorta
B. Caud. vena cava
C. Ext. iliac a.
D. Femoral a.& v.
E. Int. iliac a.
F. Int. pudendal a.
G. Urogenital a.
H. Pudendoepigastric trunk
I. Saphenous a.
J. Med. saphenous v.
K. Caud. femoral a.& v.
L. Lat. saphenous v.
M. Median sacral a.
N. Deep femoral a.& v.

a. Caud. cutan. sural n.
   (tibial n.) (X-87)
b. Lat. cutan. sural n.
   (ischiatic n.)
c. Deep fibular n.
d. Supf. fibular n.
e. Lat. plantar n.
f. Med. plantar n.
g. Plant. common
   digital nn.
h. Dors. common digital n.
i. Sartorius m.
j. Vastus medialis m.

k. Pectineus m.
l. Adductor m.
m. Gracilis m.
n. Semitendinosus m.
o. Gastrocnemius m.
p. Deep digital flexor m.
q. Long fibular m.
r. Long digital extensor m.
s. Levator ani m.
t. Coccygeus m.
u. Sacrum

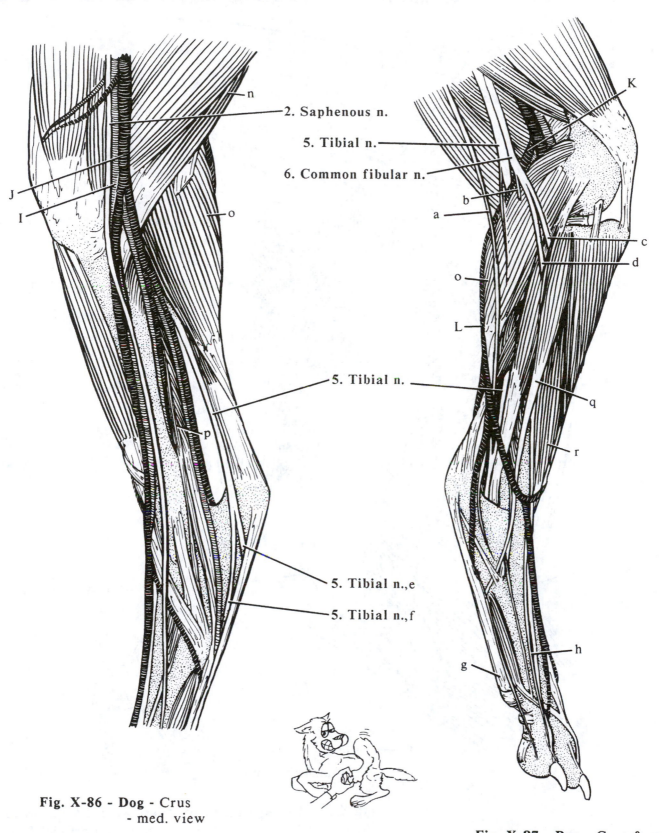

2. Saphenous n.

5. Tibial n.

6. Common fibular n.

5. Tibial n.

5. Tibial n.,e

5. Tibial n.,f

Fig. X-86 – Dog - Crus
- med. view

Fig. X-87 – Dog - Crus & pes
- lat. view

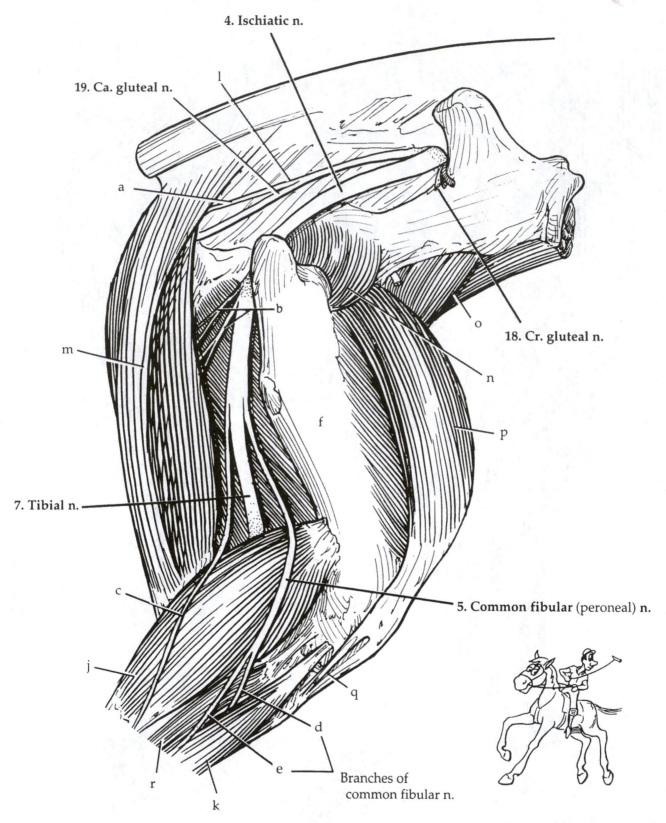

4. Ischiatic n.

19. Ca. gluteal n.

l

a

18. Cr. gluteal n.

b

o

m

n

7. Tibial n.

f

p

c

5. Common fibular (peroneal) n.

j

q

d

r

e

Branches of
common fibular n.

k

Fig X-88: Horse - Right hip, deep layer (biceps femoris,
tensor fascia latae, superficial &
middle gluteal muscles removed)
- Lateral view

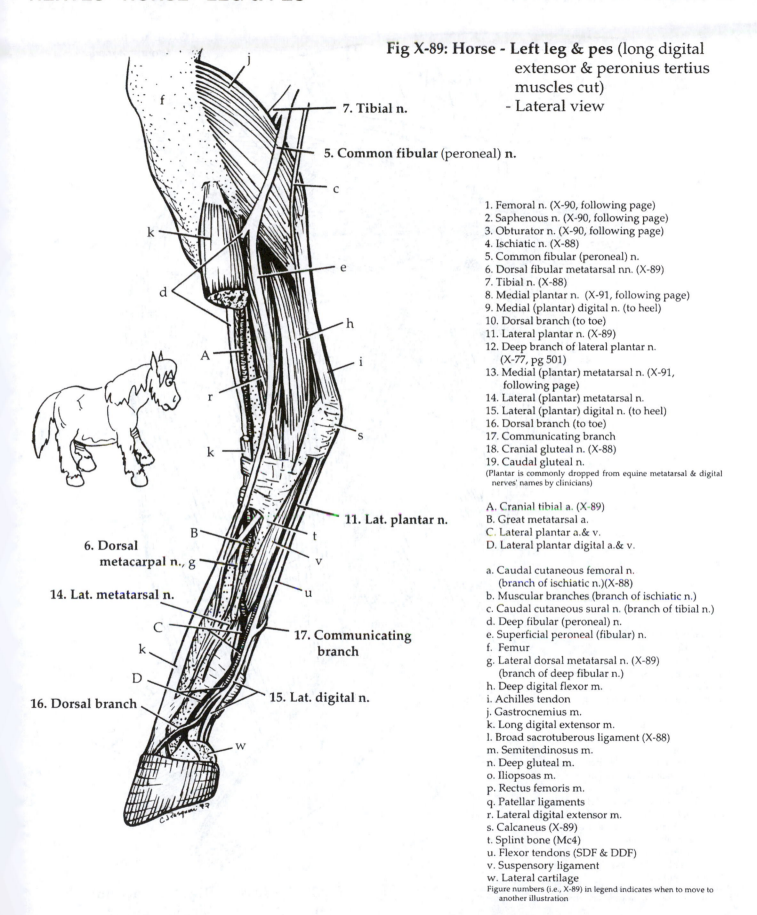

Fig X-89: Horse - Left leg & pes (long digital extensor & peronius tertius muscles cut) - Lateral view

7. Tibial n.

5. Common fibular (peroneal) n.

11. Lat. plantar n.

6. Dorsal metacarpal n., g

14. Lat. metatarsal n.

17. Communicating branch

15. Lat. digital n.

16. Dorsal branch

1. Femoral n. (X-90, following page)
2. Saphenous n. (X-90, following page)
3. Obturator n. (X-90, following page)
4. Ischiatic n. (X-88)
5. Common fibular (peroneal) n.
6. Dorsal fibular metatarsal nn. (X-89)
7. Tibial n. (X-88)
8. Medial plantar n. (X-91, following page)
9. Medial (plantar) digital n. (to heel)
10. Dorsal branch (to toe)
11. Lateral plantar n. (X-89)
12. Deep branch of lateral plantar n.
    (X-77, pg 501)
13. Medial (plantar) metatarsal n. (X-91,
    following page)
14. Lateral (plantar) metatarsal n.
15. Lateral (plantar) digital n. (to heel)
16. Dorsal branch (to toe)
17. Communicating branch
18. Cranial gluteal n. (X-88)
19. Caudal gluteal n.
(Plantar is commonly dropped from equine metatarsal & digital
  nerves' names by clinicians)

A. Cranial tibial a. (X-89)
B. Great metatarsal a.
C. Lateral plantar a.& v.
D. Lateral plantar digital a.& v.

a. Caudal cutaneous femoral n.
   (branch of ischiatic n.)(X-88)
b. Muscular branches (branch of ischiatic n.)
c. Caudal cutaneous sural n. (branch of tibial n.)
d. Deep fibular (peroneal) n.
e. Superficial peroneal (fibular) n.
f. Femur
g. Lateral dorsal metatarsal n. (X-89)
   (branch of deep fibular n.)
h. Deep digital flexor m.
i. Achilles tendon
j. Gastrocnemius m.
k. Long digital extensor m.
l. Broad sacrotuberous ligament (X-88)
m. Semitendinosus m.
n. Deep gluteal m.
o. Iliopsoas m.
p. Rectus femoris m.
q. Patellar ligaments
r. Lateral digital extensor m.
s. Calcaneus (X-89)
t. Splint bone (Mc4)
u. Flexor tendons (SDF & DDF)
v. Suspensory ligament
w. Lateral cartilage
Figure numbers (i.e., X-89) in legend indicates when to move to
  another illustration

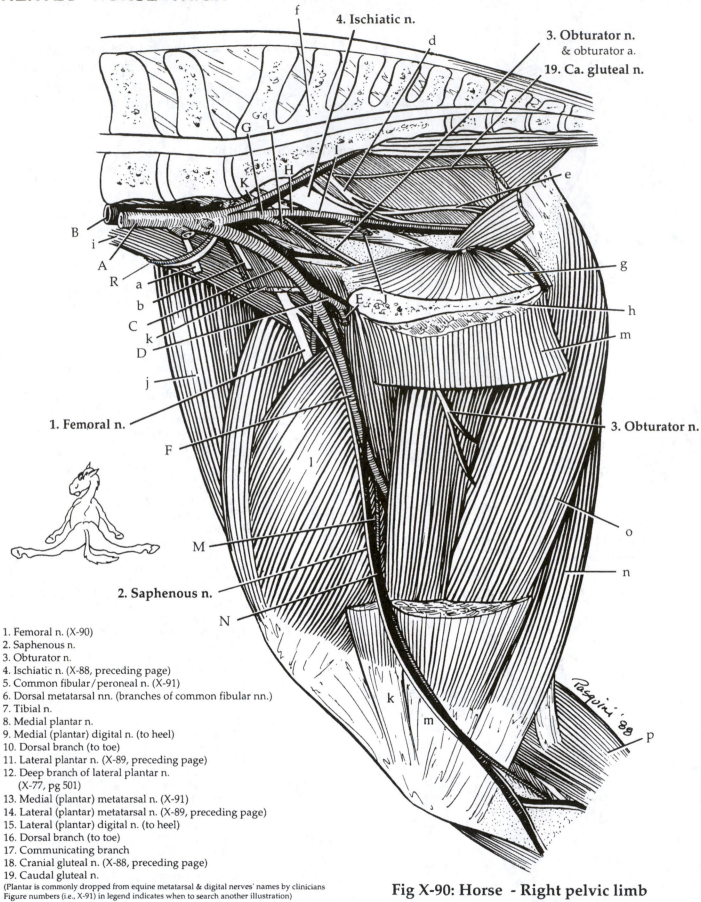

Fig X-90: Horse - Right pelvic limb
- Medial view

1. Femoral n. (X-90)
2. Saphenous n.
3. Obturator n.
4. Ischiatic n. (X-88, preceding page)
5. Common fibular/peroneal n. (X-91)
6. Dorsal metatarsal nn. (branches of common fibular nn.)
7. Tibial n.
8. Medial plantar n.
9. Medial (plantar) digital n. (to heel)
10. Dorsal branch (to toe)
11. Lateral plantar n. (X-89, preceding page)
12. Deep branch of lateral plantar n.
    (X-77, pg 501)
13. Medial (plantar) metatarsal n. (X-91)
14. Lateral (plantar) metatarsal n. (X-89, preceding page)
15. Lateral (plantar) digital n. (to heel)
16. Dorsal branch (to toe)
17. Communicating branch
18. Cranial gluteal n. (X-88, preceding page)
19. Caudal gluteal n.

(Plantar is commonly dropped from equine metatarsal & digital nerves' names by clinicians
Figure numbers (i.e., X-91) in legend indicates when to search another illustration)

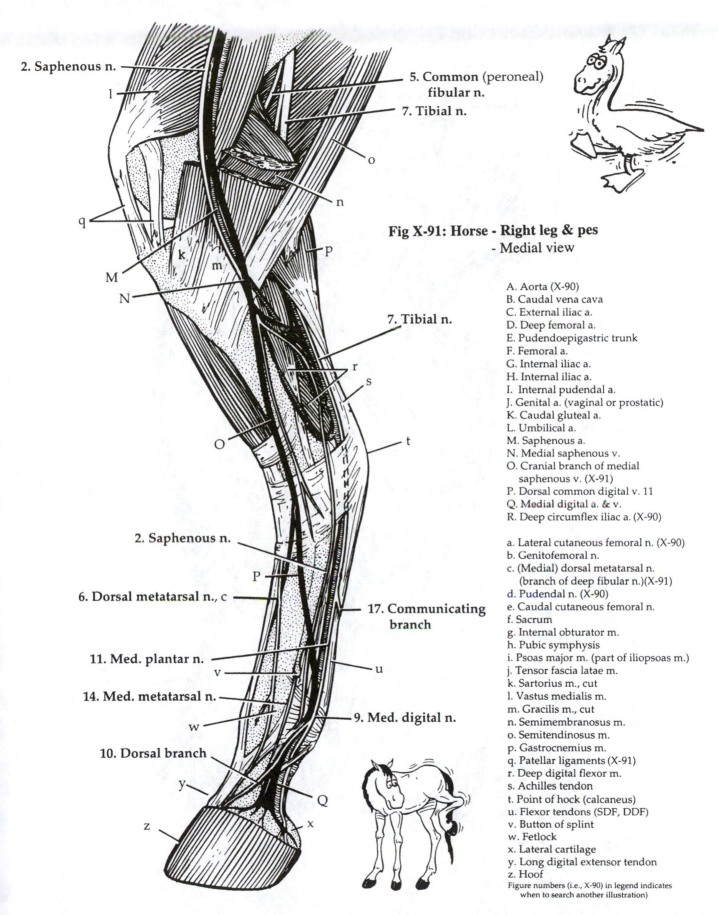

2. Saphenous n.

l

5. Common (peroneal) fibular n.

7. Tibial n.

o

n

q

p

k

m

M

N

Fig X-91: Horse - Right leg & pes
- Medial view

7. Tibial n.

r

s

O

t

2. Saphenous n.

P

6. Dorsal metatarsal n., c

17. Communicating branch

11. Med. plantar n.

v

u

14. Med. metatarsal n.

w

9. Med. digital n.

10. Dorsal branch

y

Q

z

x

A. Aorta (X-90)
B. Caudal vena cava
C. External iliac a.
D. Deep femoral a.
E. Pudendoepigastric trunk
F. Femoral a.
G. Internal iliac a.
H. Internal iliac a.
I. Internal pudendal a.
J. Genital a. (vaginal or prostatic)
K. Caudal gluteal a.
L. Umbilical a.
M. Saphenous a.
N. Medial saphenous v.
O. Cranial branch of medial saphenous v. (X-91)
P. Dorsal common digital v. 11
Q. Medial digital a. & v.
R. Deep circumflex iliac a. (X-90)

a. Lateral cutaneous femoral n. (X-90)
b. Genitofemoral n.
c. (Medial) dorsal metatarsal n. (branch of deep fibular n.)(X-91)
d. Pudendal n. (X-90)
e. Caudal cutaneous femoral n.
f. Sacrum
g. Internal obturator m.
h. Pubic symphysis
i. Psoas major m. (part of iliopsoas m.)
j. Tensor fascia latae m.
k. Sartorius m., cut
l. Vastus medialis m.
m. Gracilis m., cut
n. Semimembranosus m.
o. Semitendinosus m.
p. Gastrocnemius m.
q. Patellar ligaments (X-91)
r. Deep digital flexor m.
s. Achilles tendon
t. Point of hock (calcaneus)
u. Flexor tendons (SDF, DDF)
v. Button of splint
w. Fetlock
x. Lateral cartilage
y. Long digital extensor tendon
z. Hoof
Figure numbers (i.e., X-90) in legend indicates when to search another illustration)

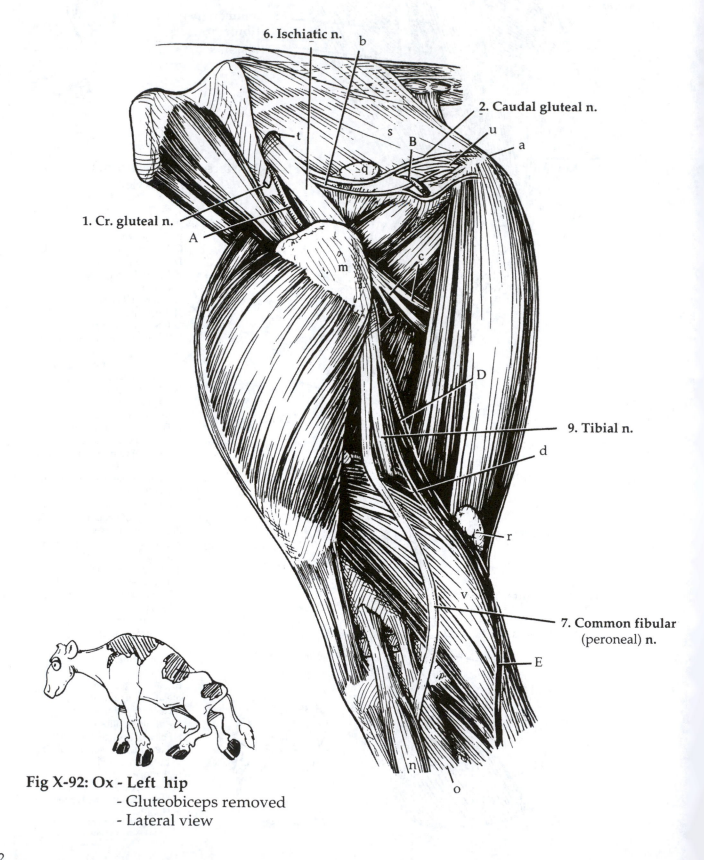

6. Ischiatic n.

2. Caudal gluteal n.

1. Cr. gluteal n.

9. Tibial n.

7. Common fibular
(peroneal) **n.**

Fig X-92: Ox - Left hip
- Gluteobiceps removed
- Lateral view

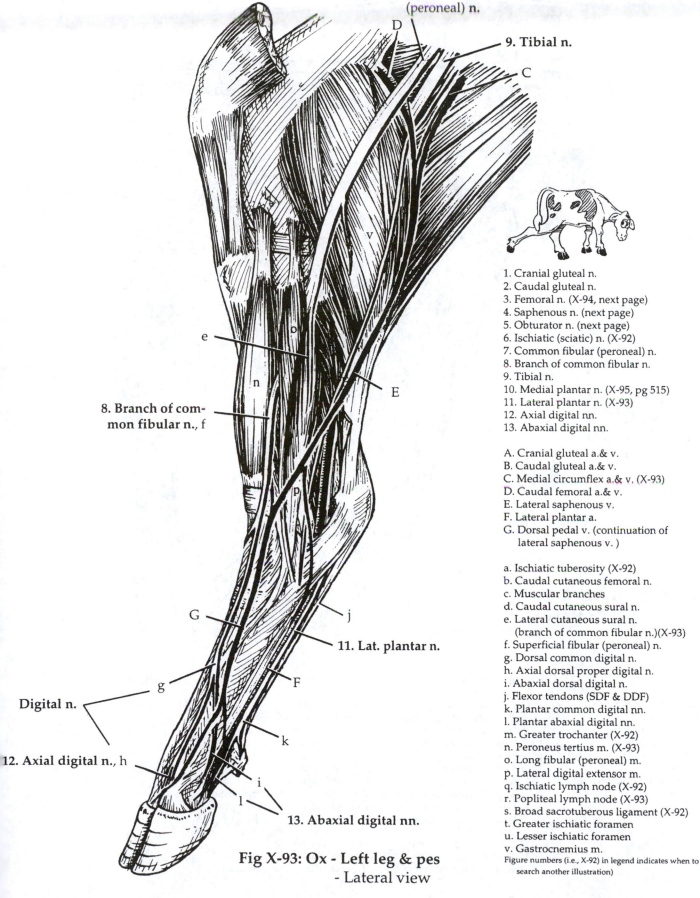

7. Common fibular (peroneal) n.

9. Tibial n.

D

C

8. Branch of common fibular n., f

e

n

o

v

E

p

G

j

g

F

11. Lat. plantar n.

Digital n.

k

12. Axial digital n., h

i

l

13. Abaxial digital nn.

Fig X-93: Ox - Left leg & pes
- Lateral view

1. Cranial gluteal n.
2. Caudal gluteal n.
3. Femoral n. (X-94, next page)
4. Saphenous n. (next page)
5. Obturator n. (next page)
6. Ischiatic (sciatic) n. (X-92)
7. Common fibular (peroneal) n.
8. Branch of common fibular n.
9. Tibial n.
10. Medial plantar n. (X-95, pg 515)
11. Lateral plantar n. (X-93)
12. Axial digital nn.
13. Abaxial digital nn.

A. Cranial gluteal a.& v.
B. Caudal gluteal a.& v.
C. Medial circumflex a.& v. (X-93)
D. Caudal femoral a.& v.
E. Lateral saphenous v.
F. Lateral plantar a.
G. Dorsal pedal v. (continuation of
   lateral saphenous v.)

a. Ischiatic tuberosity (X-92)
b. Caudal cutaneous femoral n.
c. Muscular branches
d. Caudal cutaneous sural n.
e. Lateral cutaneous sural n.
   (branch of common fibular n.)(X-93)
f. Superficial fibular (peroneal) n.
g. Dorsal common digital n.
h. Axial dorsal proper digital n.
i. Abaxial dorsal digital n.
j. Flexor tendons (SDF & DDF)
k. Plantar common digital nn.
l. Plantar abaxial digital nn.
m. Greater trochanter (X-92)
n. Peroneus tertius m. (X-93)
o. Long fibular (peroneal) m.
p. Lateral digital extensor m.
q. Ischiatic lymph node (X-92)
r. Popliteal lymph node (X-93)
s. Broad sacrotuberous ligament (X-92)
t. Greater ischiatic foramen
u. Lesser ischiatic foramen
v. Gastrocnemius m.
Figure numbers (i.e., X-92) in legend indicates when to
   search another illustration

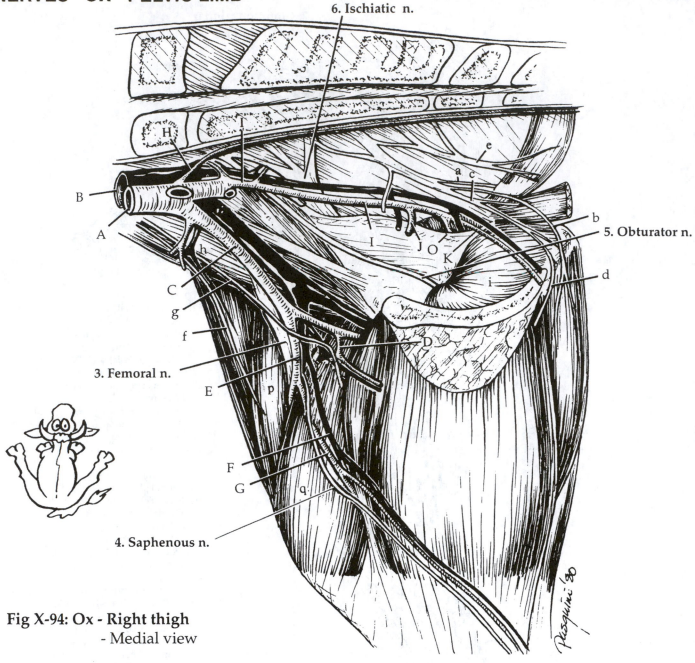

Fig X-94: Ox - Right thigh
- Medial view

Labels on figure: 6. Ischiatic n., H, B, A, C, g, f, 3. Femoral n., E, F, G, 4. Saphenous n., p, q, e, a, c, I, J, O, K, i, D, b, 5. Obturator n., d, h

1. Cranial gluteal n. (X-92, pg 512)
2. Caudal gluteal n.
3. Femoral n. (X-94)
4. Saphenous n.
5. Obturator n.
6. Ischiatic (sciatic) n.
7. Common fibular (peroneal) n. (X-96)
8. Branches of common fibular n.
9. Tibial n. (X-95)
10. Medial plantar n.
11. Lateral plantar n. (X-93, pg 513)
12. Axial digital nn. (X-96)
13. Abaxial digital nn.

A. Aorta (X-94)
B. Caudal vena cava
C. External iliac a.
D. Pudendoepigastric trunk
E. Femoral a. & v.
F. Medial saphenous v.
G. Saphenous a.
H. Median sacral a.
I. Internal iliac a.
J. Genital a. (prostatic or vaginal)
K. Internal pudendal a.
L. Medial plantar a. (superficial branch) (X-95)
M. Dorsal pedal a. (X-96)
N. Digital a.
O. Caudal gluteal a. (X-94)

a. Proximal cutaneous branch of pudendal n. (X-94)
b. Distal cutaneous branch of pudendal n.
c. Deep perineal n.
d. Superficial perineal n.
e. Caudal rectal n.
f. Lateral cutaneous femoral n.
g. Genitofemoral n.
h. Psoas major m.
i. Intrapelvic part of external obturator m.
j. Plantar common digital n. (X-95)
k. Plantar abaxial digital n.
l. Dorsal common digital n.
m. Dorsal axial digital n.
n. Deep fibular (peroneal) n.
o. Superficial fibular (peroneal) n.

p. Rectus femoris m. (X-94)
q. Vastus medialis m.
r. Gastrocnemius m.
s. Peroneus tertius m. (X-95)
t. Long digital extensor m. (X-96)

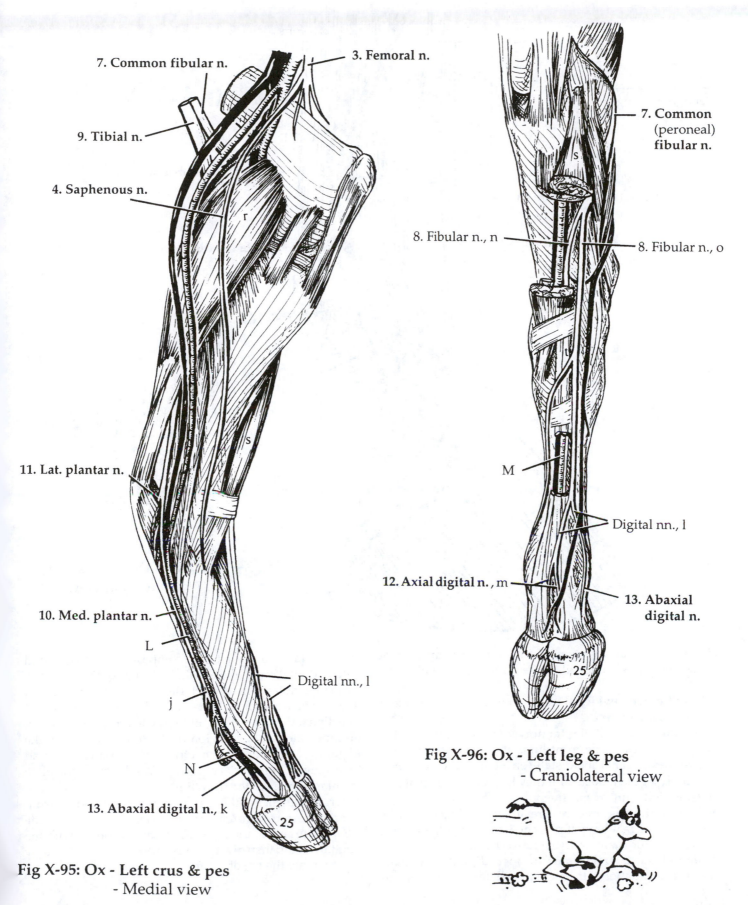

7. Common fibular n.

3. Femoral n.

9. Tibial n.

4. Saphenous n.

r

7. Common (peroneal) fibular n.

s

8. Fibular n., n

8. Fibular n., o

s

11. Lat. plantar n.

M

Digital nn., l

12. Axial digital n., m

13. Abaxial digital n.

10. Med. plantar n.

L

j

Digital nn., l

N

13. Abaxial digital n., k

25

25

Fig X-95: Ox - Left crus & pes
- Medial view

Fig X-96: Ox - Left leg & pes
- Craniolateral view

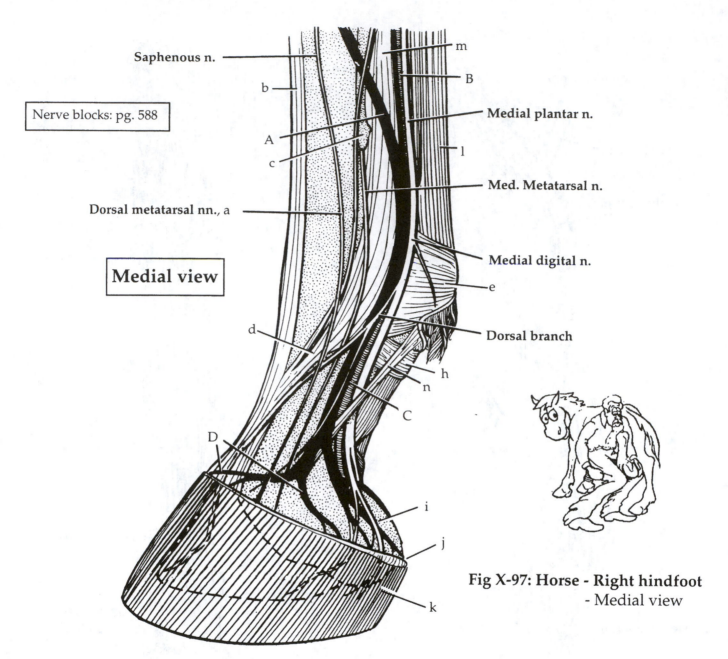

Saphenous n.

b

Nerve blocks: pg. 588

A

c

Dorsal metatarsal nn., a

Medial view

d

D

m

B

Medial plantar n.

l

Med. Metatarsal n.

Medial digital n.

e

Dorsal branch

h

n

C

i

j

k

Fig X-97: Horse - Right hindfoot
- Medial view

Horse - Nerve supply to pes: is similar to the manus, except that there are also dorsal nerves to the distal end of the limb.

• **Tibial nerve**: divides above the tarsus into medial and lateral plantar nerves.

• **Medial** and **lateral plantar nerves** (c): correspond to the palmar nerves of the front limb; they pass through the tarsal (flexor) canal and distally on either side of the flexor tendons. At the fetlock joint they become the medial and lateral digital nn., respectively.

• **Communicating branch**: is relatively slight and may be absent in the rear limb. If present, it may be palpated as it passes laterodistally over the flexor tendons.

• **Medial** and **lateral** (plantar proper) **digital nerves**: the direct continuation of the medial and lateral plantar nerves

past the level of the fetlock (comparable to medial and lateral digital nn. of the forelimb). They continue distally with the similarly-named arteries over the abaxial sides of the proximal sesamoid bones, then distally on the sides of the digital flexor tendons under the ligament of the ergot to innervate the heel region of the foot. Along with the digital v. and a., they form a triad on each side. The triad is arranged vein, artery, nerve (VAN) from dorsal to plantar, similar to the front limb.

• **Dorsal branches** of the digital nerves: similar to the front limb, arise from the digital nn. at the fetlock. They cross the abaxial surface of the proximal sesamoid bones with the digital nn. and then diverge to extend dorsally and distally to innervate the <u>toe</u> of the foot.

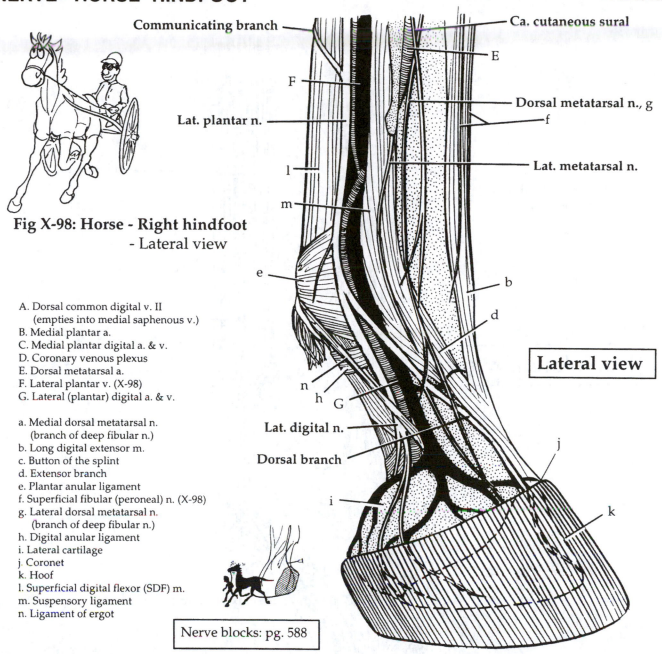

Fig X-98: Horse - Right hindfoot
- Lateral view

Labels on figure: Communicating branch, Ca. cutaneous sural, F, E, Lat. plantar n., Dorsal metatarsal n., g, f, l, Lat. metatarsal n., m, e, b, d, n, h, G, Lat. digital n., Dorsal branch, i, j, k, **Lateral view**

A. Dorsal common digital v. II
   (empties into medial saphenous v.)
B. Medial plantar a.
C. Medial plantar digital a. & v.
D. Coronary venous plexus
E. Dorsal metatarsal a.
F. Lateral plantar v. (X-98)
G. Lateral (plantar) digital a. & v.

a. Medial dorsal metatarsal n.
   (branch of deep fibular n.)
b. Long digital extensor m.
c. Button of the splint
d. Extensor branch
e. Plantar anular ligament
f. Superficial fibular (peroneal) n. (X-98)
g. Lateral dorsal metatarsal n.
   (branch of deep fibular n.)
h. Digital anular ligament
i. Lateral cartilage
j. Coronet
k. Hoof
l. Superficial digital flexor (SDF) m.
m. Suspensory ligament
n. Ligament of ergot

Nerve blocks: pg. 588

• **Deep branch of the lateral plantar nerve**: arises in the proximal cannon bone region and supplies the suspensory ligament, then continues as the metatarsal nn. (comparable to the deep branch of the lateral palmar n. in the front limb).

• **Medial** and **lateral (plantar) metatarsal nerves**: are extensions of the deep branch of the lateral plantar n. They course distally, deep in the junctions of the splint and cannon bone. At the buttons of the splints they become superficial and continue to the fetlock joint (comparable to the metacarpal nn. of the frontlimb).

• **Saphenous nerve**: is sensory to the dorsomedial side of the pes down to the fetlock. It corresponds to the medial cutaneous antebrachial n. in the forelimb.

• **Caudal cutaneous sural nerve**: corresponds to the dorsal branch of the ulnar nerve in the forelimb as it is sensory to the dorsolateral side of the pes down to the fetlock.

• **Dorsal metatarsal nerves**: are the main difference between the fore- and rear limb, as there are no corresponding branches in the thoracic limb. They are why a ring block is added to the four point or fetlock block to completely block out the fetlock area. Medial and lateral dorsal metatarsal nn. are the continuation of the deep peroneal n. They pass down the dorsal surface of the cannon bone to supply sensation to the fetlock and continue as dorsal digital nerves to the digits and dorsal hoof. The superficial fibular (peroneal) n. also passes down the dorsal surface of the metatarsus to the level of the fetlock. There are no corresponding branches in the thoracic limb.

See page 492 for specific nerve blocks.

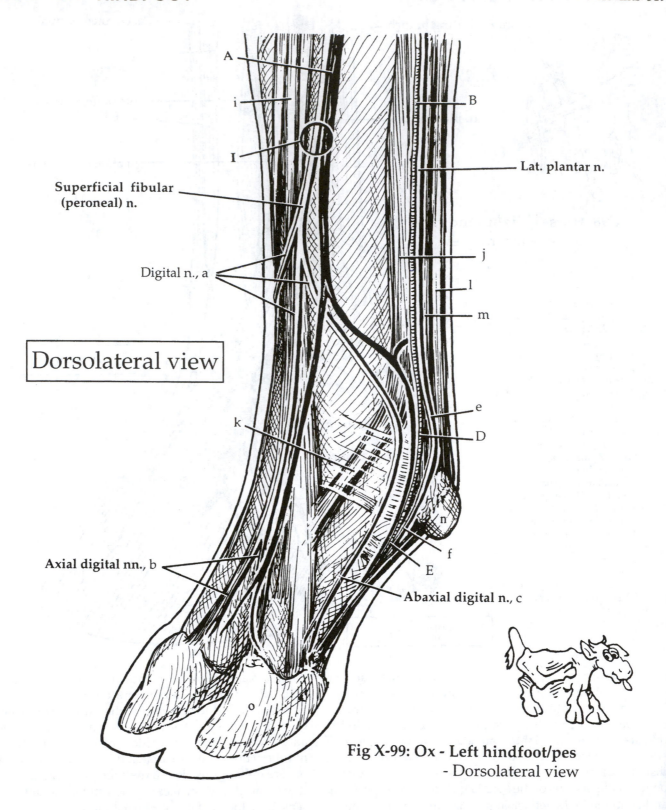

A

i

I

Superficial fibular
(peroneal) n.

Digital n., a

Dorsolateral view

B

Lat. plantar n.

j

l

m

e

D

k

n

f

E

Axial digital nn., b

Abaxial digital n., c

o

Fig X-99: Ox - Left hindfoot/pes
- Dorsolateral view

I-III. Digital n. blocks (pg 519)

A. Lateral saphenous v. (cranial branch)
B. Lateral plantar a. (superficial branch)
C. Medial plantar a. (superficial branch)
D. Plantar common digital a.
E. Plantar abaxial digital a.
F. Plantar axial digital a.

a. Dorsal common digital nn. II, III, IV (X-99)
b. Axial dorsal proper digital nn. III & IV
c. Abaxial dorsal proper digital n. III (not shown), IV
d. Lateral plantar n. (X-96)
e. Plantar common digital nn. II, III, IV
f. Abaxial plantar proper digital n. III, IV
g. Axial plantar proper digital nn. III, IV (X-100)
h. Medial plantar n. (X-100)

i. Tendon of long digital extensor m. (X-101)
j. Interosseous m. (X-99)
k. Extensor branch of interosseous m.
l. Tendon of superficial digital flexor m.
m. Tendon of deep digital flexor m.

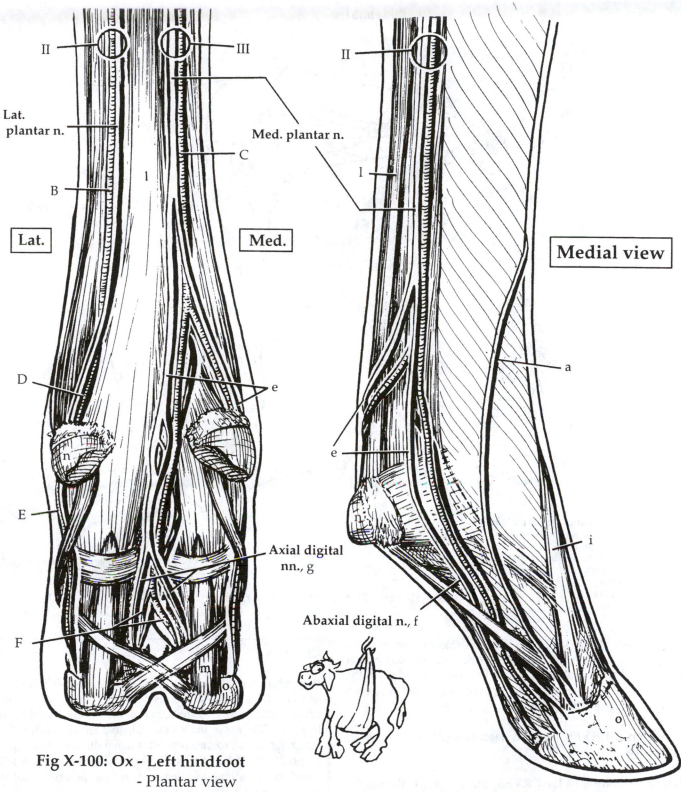

Lat.
plantar n.

Med. plantar n.

Lat.

Med.

Medial view

Axial digital
nn., g

Abaxial digital n., f

Fig X-100: Ox - Left hindfoot
- Plantar view

Fig X-101: Ox - Lt. hindfoot
- Medial view

Nerve Blocks - Ox

I. Fibular (peroneal) nerve blocks: block the superficial fibular (peroneal) nerve by injecting on either side of the dorsal branch of the lateral saphenous vein at the level of the mid-metatarsus. Block the deep fibular (peroneal) n. through the same site by going deep to the extensor tendons.

II. Plantar nerve blocks: inject the medial and lateral plantar nn. by injecting next to the flexor tendons on both sides.

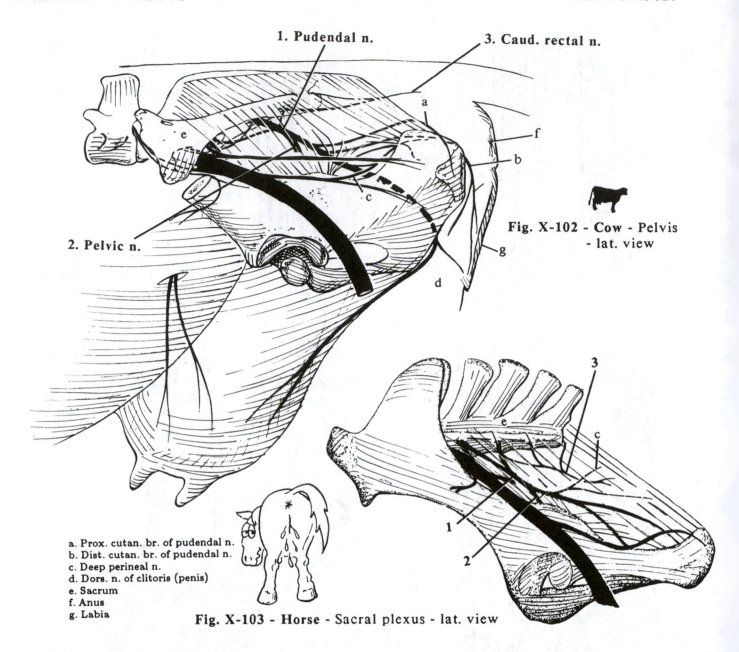

1. Pudendal n.

3. Caud. rectal n.

2. Pelvic n.

Fig. X-102 - Cow - Pelvis - lat. view

a. Prox. cutan. br. of pudendal n.
b. Dist. cutan. br. of pudendal n.
c. Deep perineal n.
d. Dors. n. of clitoris (penis)
e. Sacrum
f. Anus
g. Labia

Fig. X-103 - Horse - Sacral plexus - lat. view

1. PUDENDAL NERVE: supplies the internal and external genitalia, rectum and perineal area. Arising from the ventral branches of the sacral nerves, it travels obliquely through the pelvic cavity. Its main branches are the superficial and deep perineal nerves and the dorsal nerve of the penis.

2. PELVIC NERVES: the parasympathetic (ANS) nerve supply to the pelvic area.

3. CAUDAL RECTAL NERVES: nerve supply to the anus.

CLINICAL

Pudendal nerve block: will block the anal and perineal region and in bulls will cause protrusion of the penis. Palpate the nerves rectally on the medial aspect of the broad sacrotuberous ligament. The nerve leaves the palpable lesser ischiatic foramen just dorsal to the palpable internal iliac artery. Insert a 5" needle medial to the sacrotuberous ligament and inject anesthetic. Continue to inject as you pull the needle out to anesthetize the caudal rectal nerves.

Caudal rectal nerves: can be damaged during anal sac removal resulting in paresis or paralysis of the external anal sphincter muscle.

Fig. X-105 - Ox - Needle placement (schematic) - dors. view

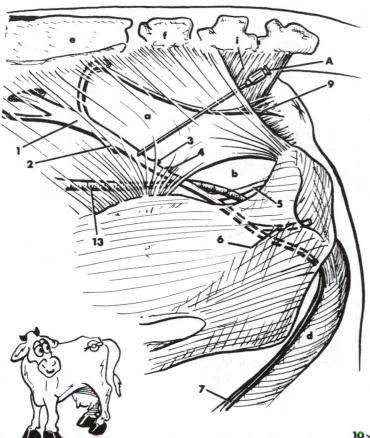

Fig. X-104 - Ox - Needle placement (schematic) - lat. view

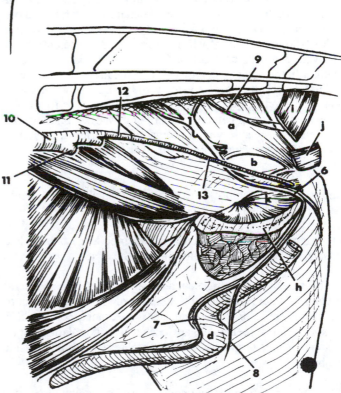

1. Pudendal n. (S2-4)
2. Pelvic n.
3. Proximal cutaneous branch of 1 (cut)
4. Distal cutaneous branch of 1 (cut)
5. Deep perineal n.
6. Superficial perineal n.
7. Dorsal n. of penis
8. Scrotal branch
9. Caudal rectal n.
10. Aorta
11. External iliac a. (cut)
12. Internal iliac a.
13. Internal pudendal a. (on medial aspect of broad sacrotuberous ligament)

A. Needle (18 g, 3.5") in deepest part of ischiorectal fossa
B. Gloved hand in rectum

Internal iliac artery is palpated rectally an inch cranial to the craniodorsal end of the lesser ischiatic foramen. The pudendal n. is dorsal to this point. The internal iliac a. branches into caudal gluteal and internal pudendal arteries in the region of the lesser ischiatic foramen.

a. Broad sacrotuberous ligament
b. Lesser ischiatic foramen
c. Rectum (opened dorsally)
d. Penis
e. Sacrum
f. First caudal vertebra
g. Ischium
h. Pubic symphysis
i. Coccygeus m.
j. Levator ani m.
k. Intrapelvic part of external obturator m.

Fig. X-106 - Ox - Needle placement (schematic) - med. view

AUTONOMIC NERVOUS SYSTEM

AUTONOMIC (aw'-toh-NOM-ik) **NERVOUS SYSTEM (ANS)**: that portion of the nervous system operating involuntarily or automatically to keep the animal's body stable. Without conscious effort, it regulates smooth muscle, cardiac muscle and glands (visceral structures) in the maintenance of normal internal stability (homeostasis) of the organism, and, when needed, deals with emergency situations. It regulates heart rate, intestinal motility, body temperature and blood pressure, among other visceral activities. The ANS, although said to be involuntary, is still controlled by higher centers in the brain, such as the cerebral cortex, hypothalamus and medulla oblongata. These centers interconnect and connect directly to the two divisions of the ANS.

TWO DIVISIONS of the ANS: the ANS is divided into two divisions, the sympathetic and parasympathetic. The visceral structures (smooth muscle, cardiac muscle and glands) usually have a dual innervation (sympathetic and parasympathetic). The action of the two divisions usually have opposite effects, as in the heart where the parasympathetic slows the rate and the sympathetic speeds it up. This allows a finer control of such activities.

Reflex arcs: Autonomic functions are mainly controlled by reflex arcs. Sensory (visceral afferent) fibers enter the spinal cord or brain stem via spinal or cranial nerves. These fibers carry sensory impulses from smooth muscle, cardiac muscle and glands (visceral effectors structures), as well as from specialized visceral receptors throughout the body. In the spinal cord or brain stem, they synapse with ANS motor neurons whose fibers (visceral efferent fibers) innervate the visceral structure (smooth or cardiac muscles or glands). In the somatic nervous system (dealing with voluntary skeletal muscles), there is usually only **one** motor (efferent) neuron; the autonomic nervous system has **two**. The first is the preganglionic motor neuron whose fiber leaves the spinal cord or brain stem to synapse with a postganglionic efferent neuron in ganglia. The postganglionic motor fiber innervates the visceral structure.

Ganglion (pl.=ganglia): collection of nerve cell bodies outside the central nervous system.

1. Visceral [effector] structures: the smooth muscle, cardiac muscle, and glands being controlled by the ANS.

2. ANS sensory (afferent) neurons: carry stimuli from a visceral effector or other receptor to the spinal cord via the dorsal root of the spinal nerve or to the brainstem via cranial nerves. ANS sensory (afferent) cell bodies are located in the dorsal root ganglia of spinal nerves or ganglia of the cranial nerves, located outside the brain.

ANS motor (efferent) neurons: carry motor impulses to a visceral effector by **two** motor (efferent) neurons. This is different from the somatic system, where reflex arcs have only one motor (efferent) neuron.

3. Preganglionic (pree'-gang-lee-ON-ik) **neuron**: an ANS motor neuron whose fiber extends from the CNS to synapse in an autonomic (motor) ganglion with a postganglionic neuron.

4. Postganglionic neuron: also an ANS motor (efferent) neuron whose fiber extends from a ganglion to the visceral structure (visceral effector) innervated.

The motor (efferent) outflow of the sympathetic division comes from the thoracolumbar segments of the spinal cord. Preganglionic motor (efferent) cell bodies are located in the lateral gray column (a) of the spinal cord. The motor fibers leave the spinal cord by the ventral root (D), pass through the spinal nerves and the white communicating branch (E) to reach the ganglia of the sympathetic trunk (G). In the ganglion the fiber has three possible pathways:

I. Synapse with postganglionic neurons in the sympathetic trunk ganglion. Postganglionic fibers then return to the spinal nerves by the communicating branch to be distributed to the periphery.

II. Ascend or descend within the sympathetic trunk to other ganglia where they will have the same three choices.

III. Pass through the ganglion to a peripherally located collateral ganglion to synapse on postganglionic neurons (e.g., splanchnic nerves [I])(4).

Ventral and dorsal branches of the spinal nerves: (not roots) carry visceral and somatic sensory (afferent) fibers.

A. Spinal nerve: the nerve carrying both somatic and autonomic sensory and motor fibers between the periphery and the spinal cord. These fibers include visceral sensory (afferent) fibers towards the spinal cord, and visceral motor (efferent) fibers back to effector organs.

B. Dorsal root: carries somatic and visceral sensory (afferent) fibers entering the spinal cord.

C. Dorsal root ganglion: the location of cell bodies of sensory neurons.

D. Lateral gray column: area where the preganglionic nerve cells are located.

E. Ventral root: carries somatic and visceral motor fibers leaving the spinal cord.

F-G. Communicating branches*: connect the spinal nerves with the sympathetic trunk.

G. Sympathetic trunk: the series of connected ganglia (H) lying

---

* There are two types of communicating branches, white and gray, which are indistinct from each other in most domestic animals. Thoracic and cranial lumbar nerves have both white and gray communicating branches. The other spinal nerves only have gray branches. White communicating branches are formed by myelinated preganglionic fibers, connecting thoracic and lumbar spinal nerves with the ganglia of the sympathetic trunk. The myelin of the fibers gives the branch its white color. Gray communicating branches connect the sympathetic trunk to all spinal nerves. They carry unmyelinated (thus, a gray color) postganglionic fibers from the chain ganglion to the spinal nerves to innervate vessels and skin glands.

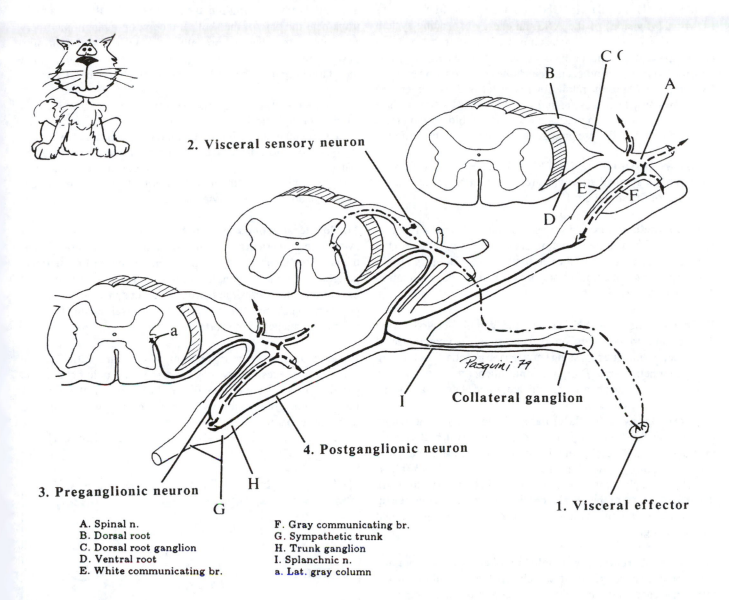

2. Visceral sensory neuron

Collateral ganglion

I

4. Postganglionic neuron

3. Preganglionic neuron

G

H

1. Visceral effector

A. Spinal n.
B. Dorsal root
C. Dorsal root ganglion
D. Ventral root
E. White communicating br.

F. Gray communicating br.
G. Sympathetic trunk
H. Trunk ganglion
I. Splanchnic n.
a. Lat. gray column

Fig. X-107 - Sympathetic supply (schematic)

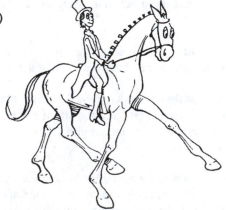

on either side of the vertebral column. It extends from the base of the skull to the sacral region of the vertebral column. The ganglion only receive preganglionic fibers from the sympathetic (thoracolumbar) division of the ANS. Preganglionic fibers that pass through the sympathetic trunk form the splanchnic nerves (I) that pass to collateral ganglia around the unpaired branches of the aorta.

ANS - SYMPATHETIC DIVISION

SYMPATHETIC DIVISION (thoracolumbar [thoh-ra-koh-LUM-bar] division) of the ANS: an energy-expending system that counterbalances the parasympathetic system to maintain homeostasis when the body is at rest. In an emergency, this division overrides the other and spends the body's energy reserves. Its activation dilates the pupils, increases the heart rate, opens the lung's airways, decreases gut motility, dilates the blood vessels in the skeletal muscles, increases glucose in the blood, and erects hair on the back. All these prepare the animal for "fight or flight".

THORACOLUMBAR OUTFLOW: The motor (efferent) outflow of the sympathetic division comes from the thoracolumbar segments of the spinal cord.

1. Sympathetic trunk: the series of connected ganglia lying on either side of the vertebral column. It extends from the base of the skull to the sacral region of the vertebral column. The ganglia only receive preganglionic fibers from the sympathetic (thoracolumbar) division of the ANS.

2. Trunk ganglia (GANG-lee-a): the ganglia located in the thoracolumbar region of the sympathetic trunk. They are connected by preganglionic fibers passing between the ganglia, thus forming the sympathetic trunk. Postganglionic fibers arising from these ganglia innervate the heart, bronchi, lungs and abdominal organs.

3. Cervicothoracic (stellate) ganglion: the largest autonomic ganglion in the body. It is located near the vertebral column medial to the first rib. Preganglionic fibers reaching this ganglion can synapse on postganglionic nerves to the heart and neck (blood vessels, sweat glands, etc.) or pass through it. If they pass through, they can synapse in the middle cervical ganglion or continue up the cervical part of the sympathetic trunk to synapse in the cranial cervical ganglion.

4. Vertebral nerve: postganglionic fibers arising from the cervicothoracic ganglion. It travels up the neck through the transverse canal and sends fibers (gray communicating branches) to the cervical spinal nerves to supply vessels and skin glands.

5. Ansa subclavia: two cord-like structures that connect the cervicothoracic ganglion and the middle cervical ganglion. They pass around the subclavian artery and are made of preganglionic fibers.

6. Middle cervical ganglion: a group of sympathetic postganglionic cell bodies located at the thoracic inlet.

7. Sympathetic trunk (cervical portion): the preganglionic fibers passing from the middle cervical ganglion up the neck to synapse in the cranial cervical ganglion. These fibers travels with the vagus nerve.

8. Vagosympathetic trunk: the combined vagus and sympathetic trunk in the neck. These are fused together. Fibers of the vagus pass down the trunk while sympathetic fibers pass up the trunk. The vagus leaves the sympathetic trunk at the thoracic inlet.

9. Cranial cervical ganglion: the terminal end of the sympathetic trunk near the base of the skull. It receives preganglionic fibers from the sympathetic thoracolumbar outflow and transmits postganglionic fibers to the head which follow arteries to reach their target organs. These fibers pass through the middle ear.

10. Splanchnic (SPLANK-nik) **nerves**: the preganglionic fibers passing through the sympathetic trunk without synapsing. They leave the sympathetic trunk at the caudal thoracic and the lumbar regions to pass to **collateral ganglia** or the **adrenal gland**. They synapse in these ganglia with postganglionic neurons. The postganglionic fibers travel with arteries to reach their target organs (abdominal and pelvic viscera.)

11. Collateral ganglia (prevertebral): the large ganglia located away from the vertebral column around the unpaired branches of the aorta (**celiacomesenteric ganglion** and **caudal mesenteric ganglion**). Collateral ganglia receive preganglionic fibers that pass through the sympathetic trunk without synapsing, and send postganglionic fibers to the viscera along vessels arising from the unpaired branches of the aorta.

12. Hypogastric nerves: the sympathetic innervation to the pelvic region. Presumably they carry preganglionic fibers to the ganglia of the pelvic plexus on the sides of the rectum. Postganglionic fibers presumably leave the ganglion and extend to the target organs.

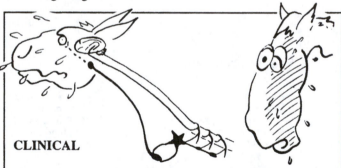

CLINICAL

Horner's syndrome: a group of signs due to loss of sympathetic innervation to the head. The problem can be anywhere along the path of sympathetic fibers (from the hypothalamus down the spinal cord to the cranial thoracic limb segments, up the neck, through the middle ear, to the orbit (thoracic roots avulsion, abscesses in neck, middle ear infections, orbital abscesses, etc.)

Clinical signs of Horner's syndrome:
• Retraction of the eyeball (enophthalmos) resulting in:
• Protrusion of the third eyelid
• Drooping of the upper eyelid (ptosis)
• Constriction of the pupil (miosis)

• Horse: sweating on ipsilateral (same) side of neck and face.

• Ox: loss of sweating on ipsilateral (same) side of planum nasale

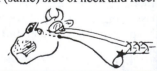

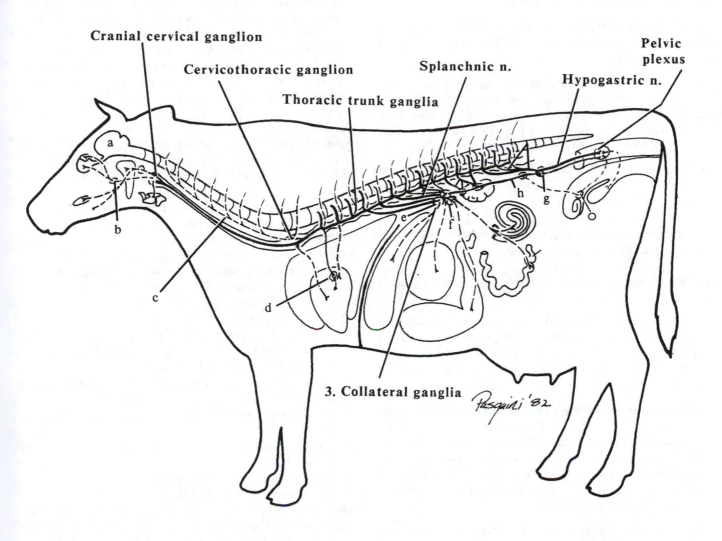

Fig. X-108 - Ox - Sympathetic division (schematic)

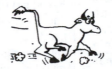

a. Brain
b. Otic ganglion
c. Vertebral n.
d. Cardiac ganglion
e. Cran. mesenteric ganglion
f. Celiac ganglia
g. Caud. mesenteric ganglion
h. Intermesenteric plexus

PARASYMPATHETIC DIVISION (craniosacral division) of the ANS: the energy-conserving system. It is mainly concerned with homeostasis ("day-to-day living"). It slows the heart rate and increases the motility of the GI tract so food can be absorbed and utilized or stored. It also brings the body back to rest after an emergency sympathetic stimulus is over.

CRANIOSACRAL OUTFLOW: the parasympathetic division has its outflow through certain cranial and sacral nerves. Thus, it has a "pair a" outflows.

Terminal (intramural) ganglia: the ganglia of the parasympathetic division located close to or in the wall of the organ they innervate. They receive long preganglionic fibers from the parasympathetic division of the ANS and send short postganglionic fibers to the effector organs.

Cranial outflow: the parasympathetic fibers carried by cranial nerves III, VII, IX and X (oculomotor, facial, glossopharyngeal and <u>vagus</u>). The brain stem contains motor nuclei of the cell bodies of the <u>pre</u>ganglionic parasympathetic fibers. The fibers leave the brain stem via the above cranial nerves to synapse with <u>post</u>ganglionic fibers in terminal ganglia.

Cranial nerves carrying parasympathetic preganglionic motor fibers:

1. Oculomotor nerve (Cn III): carries preganglionic fibers to the ciliary ganglion to synapse on postganglionic fibers to the smooth muscles that constrict the pupil and "accommodate" (adjust the shape of) the lens of the eye. A mixed nerve, it also carries somatic fibers to the extrinsic eye muscles.

2. Facial nerve (Cn VII): carries preganglionic fibers to the pterygopalatine (ter'i-goh-PAL-a- tin) (B) and the mandibular ganglia (C). Postganglionic fibers extend to the lacrimal gland, the glands of the nasal mucosa, palate, pharynx and the mandibular and sublingual salivary glands. A mixed nerve, it also carries somatic fibers to the muscles of facial expression and special sensory fibers of taste.

3. Glossopharyngeal nerve (Cn IX): transmits preganglionic fibers to the otic ganglion (E). Postganglionic fibers extend to the parotid salivary gland and zygomatic salivary gland in carnivores. A mixed nerve, it also carries somatic fibers and special sensory fibers of taste.

4. Vagus nerve (Cn X): the majority of the cranial parasympathetic outflow, it also carries somatic innervation to skeletal muscles. It carries long <u>pre</u>ganglionic fibers to synapse in the terminal ganglia of the organs of the thorax and abdomen. At least part of the vagus passes through the celiacomesenteric plexus without synapsing on their way to the abdominal organs. Short <u>post</u>ganglionic fibers innervate the organs such as the heart, lungs, liver, stomach, pancreas, small intestine, kidneys and part of the colon.

• Recurrent laryngeal nerve: branches off the vagus in the thorax and returns up the neck to innervates most of the intrinsic muscle of the larynx. Small twigs branch off to cardiac plexus and to the esophagus and trachea

526

Sacral parasympathetic outflow: has its motor cell bodies in the sacral spinal cord. The fibers leave the spinal canal by the ventral roots to unite as the pelvic nerve.

5. Pelvic nerve: formed by parasympathetic preganglionic fibers from the sacral spinal cord. They branch into the pelvic plexus on either side of the rectum. The pelvic plexus also contains ganglia (presumably sympathetic, receiving preganglionic fibers over the hypogastric nerves.) Postganglionic sympathetic and parasympathetic fibers extend to the terminal colon, rectum, ureters, urinary bladder and reproductive organs.

Neurotransmitters

• **Acetylcholine** (a-see-til-KOHL-leen) is the neurotransmitter of the parasympathetic division's nerve fibers and the sympathetic postganglionic fibbers called cholinergic fibers

• **Norepinephrine** (nor'-ep-ee-NEF-rin) (noradrenalin): neurotransmitter of postganglionic sympathetic fibers, called adrenergic (ad'- ren-ER-jik) fibers

• Parasympathetic division: cholinergic (koh'-lin-ER-jik) parasympathetic fibers result in more specific action than those of the sympathetic division, because:

a. Parasympathetic preganglionic fibers synapse on fewer postganglionic fibers

b. Parasympathetic postganglionic parasympathetic fibers are less widespread in their distribution to effector organs

c. Acetylcholine is deactivated quickly.

• Sympathetic division: has a more widespread and longer lasting action than the parasympathetic division because:

a. Preganglionic fibers synapse on many postganglionic fibers

b. Postganglionic fibers have widespread distribution to effector organs

c. Norepinephrine is degraded slowly

d. Norepinephrine enters the blood.

• These effects help the parasympathetic division go about its day-to-day specific chores, while the sympathetic division, when called upon, can charge the entire body for "fight or flight".

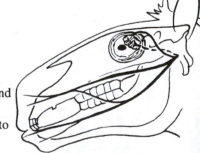

Clinical

Facial nerve paralysis: due to ear infections can paralyze the lacrimal gland and the orbicularis oculi muscles causing the eye to dry severely.

Oculomotor dysfunction: will affect the pupils of the eye (see Appendix - pg. 574)

Vagal dysfunction: usually not a clinical problem, except in the ruminant where it can cause vagal indigestion and bloat.

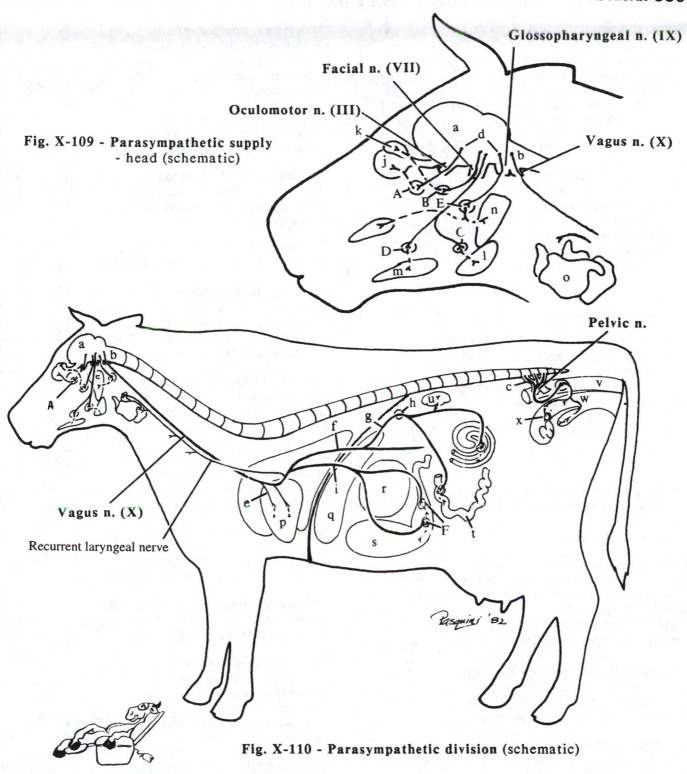

Glossopharyngeal n. (IX)

Facial n. (VII)

Oculomotor n. (III)

Vagus n. (X)

**Fig. X-109 - Parasympathetic supply
- head (schematic)**

Pelvic n.

Vagus n. (X)

Recurrent laryngeal nerve

Pasquini '82

Fig. X-110 - Parasympathetic division (schematic)

A-F. Terminal ganglia	a. Brain	h. Celiac plexus	q. Liver
A. Ciliary ganglion	b. Brainstem	i. Ventr. vagal trunk	r. Omasum
B. Pterygopalatine ganglion	c. Ventr. root of	j. Eye	s. Abomasum
C. Mandibular ganglion	sacral spinal n.	k. Lacrimal gland	t. Intestines
D. Sublingual ganglion	d. Parasympathetic	l. Mandibular salivary gland	u. Kidney
E. Otic ganglion	nuclei	m. Sublingual salivary gland	v. Rectum
F. Terminal ganglion	e. Vagal cardiac n.	n. Parotid salivary gland	w. Uterus
	f. Dors. vagal trunk	o. Larynx	x. Ovary
	g. Br. to celiac plexus	p. Heart	

CLINICAL - NERVOUS SYSTEM

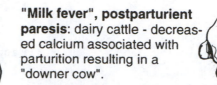

Spinal dysfunction: focal or diffuse
- Focal dysfunction: due to trauma, infection, inflammation, degeneration, malformations, verminous, tumors, etc.
- Diffuse/multifocal dysfunction: due to rabies, tetanus, botulism, meningomyelitis, toxicity, infection, verminous, etc.

UMN (upper motor nerve) dysfunction: occurs in cord above level of nerves reaching limbs and results in loss of inhibition of UMNs on lower motor neurons
- Clinical signs = "thumbs up" signs
  - Spastic paresis or paralysis
  - Increased to normal tone
  - Increased to normal reflexes
  - Extended limbs
  - Slow atrophy of muscles

LMN (lower motor neuron) dysfunction: lesion in peripheral nerves or in spinal cord where LMNs originate and results in loss of motor innervation to periphery.
- Clinical signs = "thumbs down"
  - Flaccid paresis or paralysis
  - Decreased or absent tone
  - Decreased or absent reflexes
  - Fast atrophy of muscles

Equine protozoal myeloencephalitis (EPM): protozoa migrate through spinal cord and brain #1 cause of multifocal, asymmetric neurologic disease in horses.

Cattle grubs, verminous myelitis: organophosphate killing of heel fly larvae after they have reached the spinal cord resulting in spinal cord dysfunction. This condition is less significant economically than meat and hide damage due to migrating larvae.

"Star gazing", polioencephalomalacia (PEM): cattle - thiamine deficiency (required for carbohydrate metabolism) resulting in decreased glucose to brain.

Thromboembolic meningoencephalitis (TEME): cattle, Haemophilus bacterial, systemic infection affecting brain, lungs, joints and reproduction.

Circling disease, Listeriosis: cattle - #1 bacterial infection of the brain stem associated with silage feeding. Microabscesses in the brain stem result in head tilt and circling (vestibular signs).

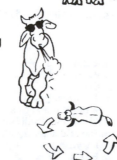

"Milk fever", postparturient paresis: dairy cattle - decreased calcium associated with parturition resulting in a "downer cow".

Lead toxicity: cattle - #1 inorganic poisoning resulting in CNS and gastrointestinal clinical signs.

"Bovine bonkers", Urea toxicity: cattle - feeding excessive urea as a nonprotein nitrogen source, the resulting ammonium is toxic to the CNS.

Tick paralysis: induced ascending, symmetrical flaccid paralysis due to tick.

Botulism, "forage poisoning", "shaker foals": relatively rare in cattle and horses, higher in wild waterfowl and chickens. *Clostridium botulinum* bacteria cause a rapidly fatal motor paralysis.

Tetanus, "lockjaw": all animals susceptible with horse most sensitive. *Clostridium tetani* bacteria multiply in deep puncture wounds producing a neurotoxin that results in a sawhorse stance and lockjaw due to extensor rigidity, and possible respiratory paralysis. Always keep horse's tetanus immunization current and booster for any wounds.

Locoweed poisoning: toxicity of Oxytropis and Atragalus plants to cattle, sheep and horses; resulting in various clinical signs including CNS.

Equine encephalomyelitis (EEE, WEE): horses - toga virus transmitted by mosquito resulting in CNS dysfunctional signs.

Yellow star thistle poisoning, nigrapallidal encephalomalacia: Horse - plant poising that causes liquifaction of brain nuclei, resulting in dysfunction and death due to starvation/dehydration.

"Dummies", neonatal maladjustment syndrome: horses- etiology unknown, day old aimless wandering, "barking", weakness and ataxia.

Rabies: virus causing progressive fatal neurological disease. Clinical signs are highly variable (furious, dumb and paralytic forms).

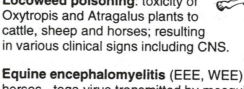
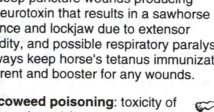
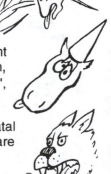

Chapter XI
Common Integument
Eye - Ear

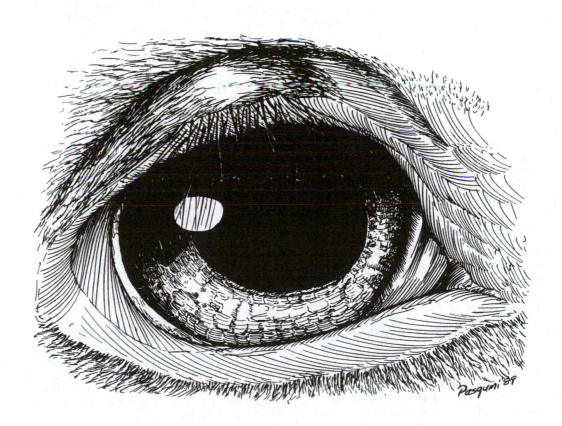

COMMON INTEGUMENT

COMMON INTEGUMENT (in'TEG-yoo-ment): consists of the skin, hair, skin glands (including the mammary glands), claws, hooves, and horns.

Skin or **cutis**: the thin organ covering the body, protecting underlying tissues from injury, drying, and bacterial invasion. It helps regulate body temperature, excretes water and salts through sweat glands, senses the environment and synthesizes Vitamin D3.

STRUCTURE of the SKIN: consists of two layers, a superficial epithelium (ep'i-THEE-lee-um) (epidermis) upon a deeper, fibrous layer (dermis or corium), which lies on a layer of loose connective tissue (subcutis).

1. Epidermis: superficial layers of the skin, consisting of continually renewed stratified squamous epithelium. The epidermis is divided into five layers. Cells divide in the deepest layer and push outward to form the more superficial layers. As they grow outward they die, become keratinized, and are finally shed from the outermost layer. The basal layer (stratum basale) is the deepest layer and consists of a single sheet of cuboidal to columnar cells capable of cell division. These cells multiply, pushing out to form the more superficial layers. The layer above the stratum basale is the spiny layer (stratum spinosum), composed of polyhedral cells. When prepared for microscopic examination, the cells may take on a "prickly" or "spiny" appearance. This layer varies in thickness from one region of the body to another. Often the stratum spinosum and stratum basale are collectively called the germinal layer (stratum germinativum). The granular layer (stratum granulosum), the third layer, is composed of squamous cells in different stages of degeneration, and contain keratohyalin granules involved in forming keratin. The clear layer (stratum lucidum), an inconsistently-present fourth layer, is made of flat, dead squamous cells containing translucent droplets of eleidin, which give this layer its name (lucidum = clear). Eleidin comes from keratohyalin and becomes keratin. The outermost layer, the horny layer (stratum corneum), consists of flat, dead, cornified cells completely filled with keratin, a waterproofing protein.

2. Dermis (DER-mis) or **corium**: the layer of skin directly below and separated from the epidermis by a basement membrane. It consists of collagenous and elastic connective tissue containing blood vessels, nerve fibers, glands and hair follicles. The papillary region or layer is the dermis immediately beneath the epidermis. Small finger-like projections, dermal papillae, project up into the epidermis, greatly increasing the surface area between the two layers, thus, holding them together. The deepest layer of the dermis, the reticular region or layer, is responsible for variations in skin thickness. It is named for the arrangement of collagenous fibers into a network (reticulum).

3. SUBCUTANEOUS LAYER or **superficial fascia** (sub'kyoo-TAY-nee-us), hypodermis or subcutis: the layer of areolar connective tissue and interspersed fat connecting the skin to underlying structures, such as bones and muscles. This layer is often called subcutaneous tissue or superficial fascia.

APPENDAGES OF THE SKIN: the hair, hooves, claws, sebaceous glands, and sweat glands associated with the skin.

4. Sweat glands or **sudoriferous glands** (syoo'doh-RIF-er-us): simple, coiled, tubular glands of the skin that open independently of hair follicles. Merocrine (MER-oh-krin) (eccrine) sweat glands, the predominant type of sweat glands in man, are restricted to the footpads of carnivores, the frog of the horse, the nasolabial region of ruminants and swine, and the pig carpus. Apocrine (AP-oh-krin) sweat glands predominate in the domestic species and are distributed throughout the skin. Sweat glands

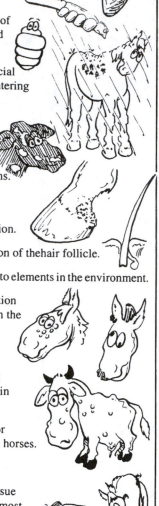

CLINICAL

Blister: a fluid-filled separation between the epidermis and dermis.

Skin parasites: fleas, lice, mites, chiggers, onchocerciasis, Habronema spp., flies

Cattle grubs (hypodermiasis): larvae of Heel fly that migrate through meat and skin causing large economic losses.

Rain scald (dermatophilosis): superficial bacterial infection (*Dermatophilus*) entering through damaged skin.

Ringworm (dermatophytosis): fungal infection of skin.

Wounds: one of most common conditions encountered by veterinarians.

Grease heel (pastern dermatitis): crusting and seborrheic dermatitis common in skin of horse's pastern region.

Folliculitis/furunculoses: inflammation of the hair follicle.

Contact dermatitis: allergic reactions to elements in the environment.

Hives (uticaria): hypersensitivity reaction resulting in wheals (localized edema in the dermis) most common in horses.

Sarcoids: #1 neoplasia of horses.

Squamous cell carcinoma: malignant neoplasia, usually of nonpigmented skin at mucocutaneous junctions.

Melanoma: benign or malignant tumor which is most significant in older gray horses.

Warts (papilloma): caused by a virus.

Proud flesh: exuberant granulation tissue in wound healing by second intention most common in the distal limbs of horses.

Photodermatitis: sunburn caused by photosensitizing or hepatotoxic substances.

help maintain body temperature of the domestic species. The horse sweats the most ("lathering up") of the domestic species, the cat and dog the least.

5. Sebaceous glands or **oil glands** (se-BAY-shus): simple alveolar holocrine glands usually connected to hair follicles. The cells lining the glands disintegrate to form the secretion **sebum** (SEE-bum). Sebum is an oily substance consisting of a mixture of cholesterol, protein, and inorganic salts, which is released into the hair follicle to lubricate the skin and prevent excessive evaporation. Sebum of the fleece of sheep is called lanolin.

HAIR: the long, slender, filamentous appendage of the skin composed of keratinized (dead) epithelial cells. Each hair consists of a shaft and a root. The root is contained in a depression (hair follicle). Associated with hair follicles are sebaceous glands and a bundle of smooth muscle, the

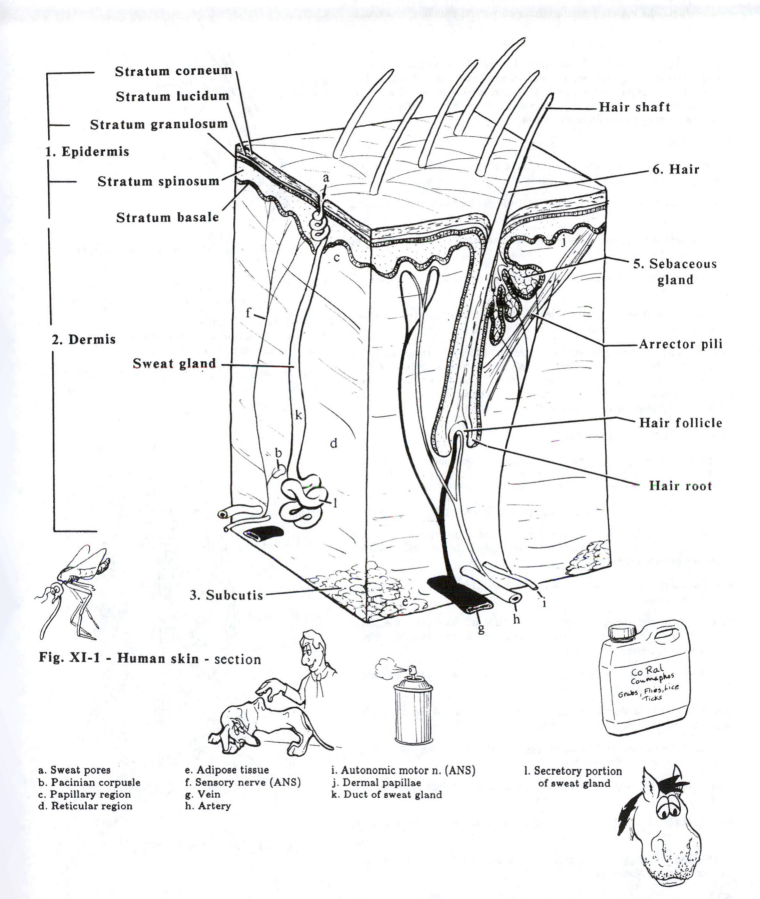

Stratum corneum

Stratum lucidum

Stratum granulosum

1. Epidermis

Stratum spinosum

Stratum basale

2. Dermis

Sweat gland

3. Subcutis

Hair shaft

6. Hair

5. Sebaceous gland

Arrector pili

Hair follicle

Hair root

Fig. XI-1 - Human skin - section

a. Sweat pores
b. Pacinian corpusle
c. Papillary region
d. Reticular region

e. Adipose tissue
f. Sensory nerve (ANS)
g. Vein
h. Artery

i. Autonomic motor n. (ANS)
j. Dermal papillae
k. Duct of sweat gland

l. Secretory portion of sweat gland

Co Ral
Coumaphos
Grubs, Flies, Lice
Ticks

SKIN

arrector pili muscle, connecting the side of the hair to the dermis. During stress, cold or fright the muscle pulls the hair into vertical positions, resulting in "goosebumps" in humans. In domestic species, this produces a trap for insulating air or making the animal appear more intimidating.

Hair follicles: horses and cattle have single hair follicles. Dogs have compound hair follicles with a single primary hair and a group of smaller secondary hairs. Pigs have single follicles grouped in clusters. Cats have a single follicle with a primary guard hair surrounded by clusters of compound follicles. The compound follicles have three primary hairs with many secondary hairs.

Types of hair:

• **Bristles**: the hair coat of the pig; the cilia (eyelashes), vibrissae (hairs of the nostril), and "beard" (hair of the submandibular region) of the goat.

• **Guard hairs**: the outer coat ("topcoat") of the domestic species, except the sheep and pig.

• **Wool hair**: the wavy, fine, short, inner coat ("undercoat"). This is the hair type of the fleece of sheep.

• **Long (horse) hair**: the long hair of the horse - forelock, mane, tail, and "feathers" (behind the fetlock).

• **Tactile hair**: stiff, sensory hair in some of the domestic species on the upper and lower lip, chin, cheek, around the eye, and the carpus.

Color of hair: determined by complicated genetic factors governing the amount of pigment (melanin) in the hair. There are only three hair pigments: black, brown, and yellow. The great variation in color is due to combinations or absence of these three pigments. Gray hairs of aging result from loss of pigment; white hair is due to absence of pigment and presence of air in the hair shaft.

SPECIALIZED GLANDS of the SKIN:

Carpal glands: in pigs just proximal to the carpus on the caudomedial side of the leg. They produce pheromones to sexually stimulate the mating partner. They also mark the sow during mating as the boar's "property".

Caudal (coccygeal) **glands**: in carnivores on the dorsum of the root of the tail.

Ceruminous glands: in all domestic species, found in the wall of the external auditory canal. They produce "ear wax" which protects the tympanic membrane from foreign bodies (pg. 551).

Circumanal glands: in carnivores around the anus. They can become neoplastic (perianal adenoma).

Circumoral or **perioral glands**: only in cats, located in the skin around the mouth, especially the lower lip. Their functional significance, although called the "cleaning glands", is probably for marking.

Glands of the anal sac: in carnivores, in the walls of the anal sacs, they secrete into the anal sacs for storage.

Glands of the inguinal sinus: in sheep on either side of the udder or scrotum. The odor may help the lamb locate the udder.

Glands of the infraorbital sinus: in sheep found in the infraorbital sinus just rostral to the eye, used for marking.

Glands of the interdigital sinus: in sheep between the digits, used as "trail markers".

Glands of the nasal skin: in artiodactyls (even-toed animals) in the skin of the nose.

Horn glands: in goats and some sheep just caudal to the base of the horn (similar location in hornless animals).

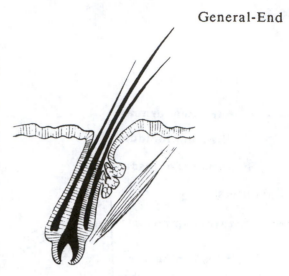

Fig. XI-2 - Dog - Section of skin (schematic)

Mental (chin) glands: in pigs a wart-like skin eminence on the chin. It has both tactile and secretory (marking) functions.

Preputial glands: located in the prepuce, their secretions mix with degenerated cells to form a substance called smegma, which is significant in the horse.

Subcaudal gland: in goats, the two glands below the tail that are said to be responsible for the buck's characteristic smell.

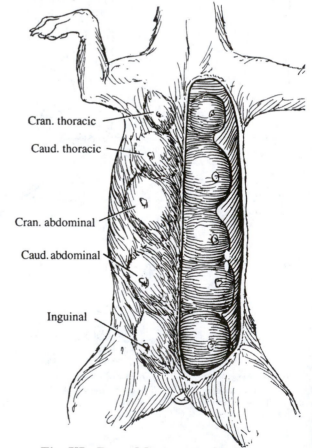

Cran. thoracic

Caud. thoracic

Cran. abdominal

Caud. abdominal

Inguinal

Fig. XI - Dog - Mammary glands

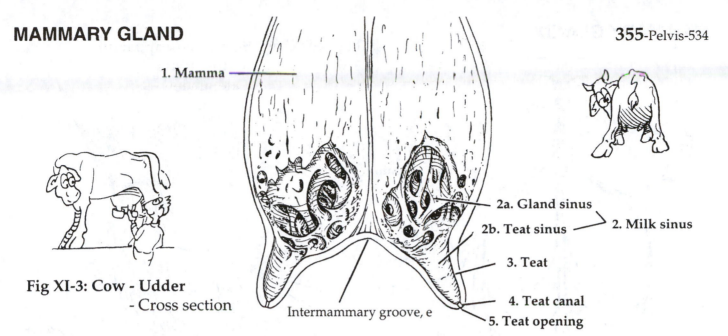

1. Mamma

2a. Gland sinus

2b. Teat sinus — 2. Milk sinus

3. Teat

4. Teat canal

5. Teat opening

Fig XI-3: Cow - Udder
- Cross section

Intermammary groove, e

Mammary gland: (mammae): a modified sweat gland that nourishes the young. It consists of the mamma and the teat. Undeveloped in both the male and female at birth, the female mammary gland begins to develop as a secondary sex characteristic at puberty. With the birth of the first young and the first lactation, the mammary gland attains its full size and function. When suckling by the young stops, milk production ceases and the gland regresses. Shortly before the next and subsequent parturitions, the gland is stimulated by hormonal changes to produce milk.

- **Mamma** (pl. = mammae): the glandular structure associated with a teat.
  - Lobes: the internal compartments of the mamma, separated by adipose tissue (fat). The lobes are divided into lobules. Lobules consist of connective tissue containing alveoli, the grapelike clusters of milk-secreting cells of the mammary gland.
  - **Milk (lactiferous) ducts**: large ducts conveying milk from the alveoli to the milk sinus. The openings of the lactiferous ducts convey milk formed in the alveolus to the gland sinus.
- **Milk (lactiferous) sinus**: the large milk storage cavity within the teat and the glandular body.
  - 2a. Gland sinus: part of the milk sinus within the glandular body.
  - 2b. Teat sinus: part of the milk sinus within the teat.
- **3. Teat** or **papilla**: the projecting part of the mammary gland containing part of the milk sinus.
- **4. Teat canal, papillary duct** or "streak canal": the canal leading from the teat sinus to the teat opening. It is lined with stratified squamous epithelium thrown into longitudinal folds. The cells of the canal produce a sebaceous plug in the teat canal.
- **5. Teat opening**: the opening of the teat canal. The exit point for milk or the entrance point for bacteria into the mammae.
- **Sphincter muscle**: the muscular fibers around the teat opening that prevent milk flow except during sucking or milking.

Cow: the mammary gland of the cow takes on added significance due to the importance of milk as a human food source.
- **Udder**: the term designating all the mammae in the ruminant and the mare (sometimes used for the sow also). In the cow it hangs from the caudal abdomen and pelvis, thus, is partly covered laterally by the thigh.
- **Quarters**: the 4 parts of the bovine udder, each associated with one teat. All 4 quarters are completely separated from each other.

The intermammary groove (e) is the sagittal external indication of the separation of the 2 halves of the udder.
- **3 layers of the teat wall**: Skin: the naked, sensitive skin; **middle layer**: connective tissue, smooth muscles, and many veins (erectile tissue), and the **mucosal layer**. These layers should be approximated when repairing a teat laceration.
- **Furstenberg's rosette**: relatively inconspicuous radiation of the longitudinal ridges of teat canal mucosa into the teat sinus.
- **Annular fold**: a constriction between the glandular and the teat parts of the milk sinus. It consists of muscular fibers, connective tissue, and circular venous channels ("Furstenburg's venous ring").

Clinical:
- **Mastitis**: inflammation of the mammary gland / udder. It is the most costly disease in adult dairy cows. As the quarters are separate from each other, an infection in only 1 quarter is possible. Infections can still spread directly between the quarters on the same side. Medicine injected into 1 quarter will not reach the other quarters, but IV injection of antibiotics will reach all quarters.
- **Low spider**: overdeveloped **Furstenberg's rosette** that may block the opening of the teat canal.
- **High spider**: stenosis near the annular fold at the base of the teat. Occasionally it has to be cut to allow milk into the teat sinus. The instrument should be directed by palpation to the center of the constriction so the peripheral venous ring is avoided.
- **"Milking out"**: the complete emptying of a quarter.
- **Dry period**: cows are "dried up" by stopping "milking out" about 2 months before birth. This ensures that milk production will be high after birth.
- **Udder and teat conditions**: bovine herpes mammillitis, udder acne, pseudocowpox, teat chapping and cracking, and warts.
- **"Milk knots"**: superficial dilations of the lactiferous ducts that are filled with milk. These are palpable and will disappear as they are emptied during milking.

MAMMARY GLAND

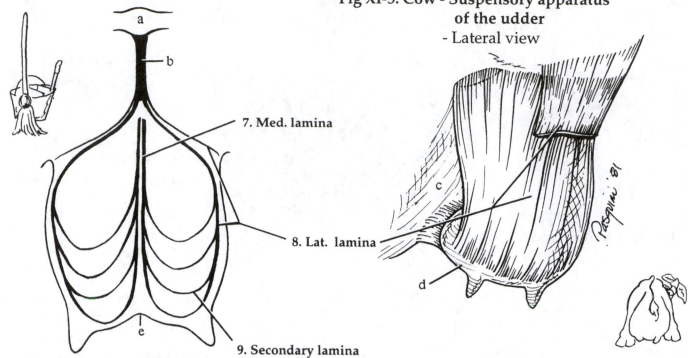

7. Med. lamina

8. Lat. lamina

9. Secondary lamina

**Fig XI-4: Cow - Suspensory apparatus
of the udder** (schematic)

**Fig XI-5: Cow - Suspensory apparatus
of the udder**
- Lateral view

a. Pelvic symphysis   d. Udder
b. Symphyseal tendon   e. Intermammary groove
c. Body Wall

- **Suspensory apparatus**: the specialized attachment of the udder, best developed in the cow. In the cow it attaches to the symphyseal tendon (below the pelvic symphysis) and the ventral abdominal wall. It consists of **4 primary laminae** (medial and lateral sheets of connective tissue) applied to the lateral and medial side of each half of the udder and meeting at the teats. They form the capsule of the udder.
  - **Medial lamina of the suspensory apparatus**: the 2 elastic sheets arising mainly from the ventral abdominal wall near the linea alba and extending ventrally between the 2 halves of the udder. Due to its elastic fibers, as the udder fills, it stretches more than the lateral laminae and the teats angle laterally (helping to prevent the teats from dragging).
  - **Lateral laminae of the suspensory apparatus**: the sheet of dense connective tissue passing from the subpelvic tendon caudally and the abdominal wall cranially over the lateral side of the udder.
  - **Secondary laminae**: seven to ten sheets connecting the medial and lateral primary laminae that divide the mammary gland into lobes.
  - **Subpelvic tendon or symphyseal tendon**: arises from the pelvic symphysis and gives rise to the medial thigh muscles.
- **Blood supply (cow)**: the external pudendal (mammary) aa. are the main blood supply to the cow's udder with a small contribution from the internal pudendal aa. The mammary aa. have a sigmoid flexure to allow stretching when the udder fills with milk. They bifurcate into cranial and caudal mammary branches, forming a circle around the base of the udder. The ventral perineal aa. (branches of the internal pudendal aa.) enter the caudal part of the circle. In small ruminants the blood supply to the udder is entirely from the mammary (external pudendal) aa.
- **Venous drainage**:
  - **Venous circle of the udder in the cow**: encircles above the base of the udder. Blood enters it from 1 or 2 perineal vv. and from superficial and deep vv. draining the udder. Drainage from the udder is through the external pudendal (mammary) vv., or milk veins (superficial epigastric vv.), not the ventral perineal vv. (which

only drains towards the udder).
- Superficial udder vv. pass <u>craniodorsal</u> from the teats ("Furstenburg's venous ring") to empty into the venous circle. They can be distinguished visually by their direction from the <u>dorsocaudally</u> directed udder's subcutaneous lymphatics.
- **"Furstenburg's venous ring"**: the venous circle at the junction of the teat and gland sinuses.
- **Mammary branch of the ventral perineal vv.**: drain into the caudal part of the venous circle of the udder. They have valves preventing dorsocaudal flow away from the udder.
- **"Milk veins", subcutaneous abdominal (cr. and ca. superficial epigastric) vv.**: the large, tortuous veins on the ventral abdomen draining the udder with the external pudendal vv. The "milk vv." form during the cow's first pregnancy by anastomoses of the cr. and ca. superficial epigastric vv. They have incompetent valves allowing blood to flow in both directions. The milk vv. can pass though the abdominal wall to join the cranial epigastric or the internal thoracic vv. or, rarely, pass forward to join the external thoracic v., resulting in a milk v. all the way to the axilla.
- **"Milk well"**: where a "milk vein" travels through the abdominal wall caudal to the costal arch and joins the internal thoracic v.
- **External pudendal (mammary) vv.**: drain though the inguinal canal. It has a sigmoid flexure to allow stretching when the udder fills.

Clinical:
- **Rupture of the suspensory apparatus in the cow**: disastrous and on the rise due to the demand for ever-greater production.
- **Amputation of half of the udder**: either right or left halves can be removed because of the double medial suspensory ligaments.
- **Milk veins**: are conveniently used for IV injection and collecting blood even though there is a high chance of hematoma formation. Having incompetent valves, they disappear when the animal is put in dorsal recumbency so mark them first.

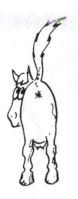

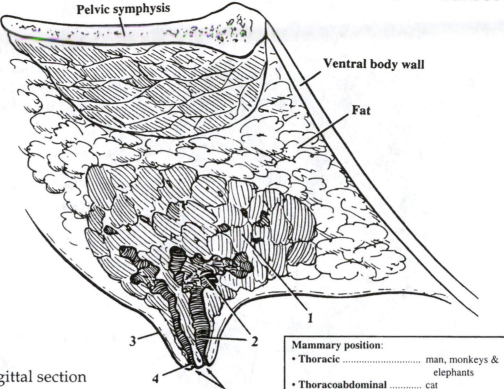

1. Mamma
2. Milk sinus
3. Teat
4. Teat canal
5. Teat openings

Fig XI-6: Horse - Udder
- Parasagittal section

Mammary position:	
• **Thoracic**	man, monkeys & elephants
• **Thoracoabdominal**	cat
• **Thoracoabdominoinguinal**.	dog & pig
• **Inguinal**	horse & ruminants

- **Nerve supply to the udder in ruminants**:
- Ventral branches of L1 and L2 (iliohypogastric and ilioinguinal) nerves: supply the skin of the cranial forequarters.
- Genitofemoral nerve: supply the skin over the middle udder, the gland substance, and deep part of the teat wall.
- Mammary branches of the pudendal nerve: supply the caudal aspect of the udder (hindquarters).
- **Lymphatic drainage cow:**
- **Afferent lymphatic ducts** of the udder: pass <u>dorsocaudal</u> to reach the mammary lymph nodes. They may be apparent under the skin.
- **Mammary (superficial inguinal) lymph nodes**: two nodes at the dorsocaudal side of the udder. There is usually a palpable large, kidney-shaped node between the caudal side of the base of the udder and thigh and a smaller node that is too deep to be palpated.
- **Efferent vessels**: pass into the abdomen through the inguinal canal to empty into the deep inguinal node.

Species differences:
- **Bitch**: usually have 10 mammae, 5 (4 - 6) on each side separated by an intermammary groove. Teats of an animal that has been pregnant are always larger than those of an animal that has never been pregnant.
- **Queen**: 8 mammae, 4 on each side.
- **Sow**: 14 (10 - 18) mammae, seven on each side, usually.
- **Cow**: 4 mammae, 2 (quarters) on each side, bound into an udder.
- **Goat** and **sheep**: 2 mammae in a pendulous udder.
- **Mare**: 2 mammae in a small udder.
- **Male - teats**: usually have the same number and position as females. Ruminants have teats on the cranial surface of the scrotum. They are often absent in the horse and, if present, are located beside the prepuce.

Accessory teats or **supernumerary teats (polythelia)**: extra teats that may or may not be connected to primary mammary gland tissue in both females and males. These extra teats can be associated with extra glandular complexes (polymastia: extra mammae). These are often removed in the cow and goat (doe) as they may interfere with milking.

- **Cow**: often caudal to the other 4, but can be between or cranial to them.
- **Sheep**: usually cranial to normal ones.
- **Bulls, rams** and **bucks**: if found, are usually cranial to the scrotum.
- **Lymph drainage in the bitch**: the cranial 2-3 pairs drain through the axillary, accessory axillary, and sternal lymph nodes; the caudal 2-3 pairs through the superficial inguinal lymph nodes.

Clinical:
- Cow: anaesthetizing the teat and udder.
  - Teat anaesthesia: ring block at the base of the teat, including the skin and muscular tissue; or an inverted V line block.
  - Forequarter: paravertebral anesthesia of L1, L2, and L3 spinal nn. or segmental lumbar epidural anesthesia of L1, L2 and L3 spinal nn.
  - Caudal teat and escutcheon areas of the udder: block the perineal n. in the standing cow; or high caudal epidural or lumbosacral epidural anesthesia in recumbent ruminants.
- Dog: mammary tumors comprise 50% of all canine tumors and 50% are malignant. There is no proof that lumpectomy (removal of only the tumor) or radical mastectomy is any better for survival time.
- Cat: mammary tumors comprise 20% of all tumors, but 85% are malignant. Radical mastectomy is the treatment of choice (TOC) in cats due to the high percentage of malignancy.
- **Colostrum**: the mammary secretion in the first few days after parturition. It has a different composition than normal milk, with essential nutrients and immunoglobulins (antibodies). It also has a laxative effect to stimulate the expulsion of the neonate's first stool (meconium).
- **Horse, ruminant** and **pig**: <u>colostrum</u> is especially important in these species because their placentae do not allow transfer of antibodies between the mother and fetus.

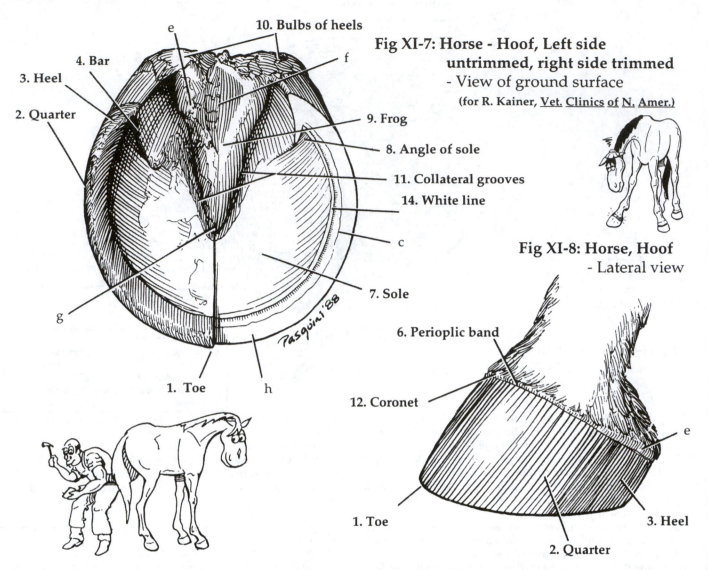

Fig XI-7: Horse - Hoof, Left side untrimmed, right side trimmed
- View of ground surface
(for R. Kainer, Vet. Clinics of N. Amer.)

e
10. Bulbs of heels
4. Bar
3. Heel
2. Quarter
f
9. Frog
8. Angle of sole
11. Collateral grooves
14. White line
c
7. Sole
g
Pasquini '88
1. Toe
h

Fig XI-8: Horse, Hoof
- Lateral view

6. Perioplic band
12. Coronet
e
1. Toe
2. Quarter
3. Heel

Foot of horse: the hoof and the structures within it. The foot skeleton consists of the middle and distal phalanges (pastern and coffin [pedal] bones), the coffin joint, the navicular bone, and the lateral cartilages of the distal phalanx. Many ligaments and tendons of the common/long digital extensor and deep digital flexor muscles insert on the bones of the foot.

• **Hoof** (ungula): the horny epidermis covering the digit's distal end; divided into the wall, sole, and frog.

• **Wall** (paries): the visible part of the standing horse's hoof. It is thickest at the toe and gradually thins toward the heels. The medial wall is steeper than the lateral side. The wall grows at roughly 1/3" per month.

1. **Toe**: the dorsal part of the wall. It is usually about 60° to the ground.

2. **Quarters**: the medial and lateral wall parts.

3. **Heels** (or angles): the palmar or plantar aspect of the wall.

4. **Bars**: the extension of the wall from the back (palmar/plantar side) of the foot towards the toe. They are seen on either side of the frog from the ground surface.

5. **Periople**: the outer, thin, shiny layer of the hoof.

6. **Perioplic band**: soft horn, a few millimeters thick, adjacent to the coronet. It widens out over the heels.

7. **Sole**: the concave surface between the frog and wall that faces the ground.

8. **Angles of the sole**: medial and lateral, located between where the bars and the wall meet at the heels.

9. **Frog** (cuneus ungulae): the wedge-shaped structure between the sole, bars, and bulbs. Its apex points towards the toe. The central sulcus is a depression in the center of the frog between its two crura. The frog is often called the "heart of the horse's foot" because its compression forces blood out of the foot back toward the body. It is homologous with the digital pads of other species.

10. **Bulbs of the heels**: the expanded part of the frog on the palmar aspect of the foot which are covered by periople. With the frog, they form the pad (torus ungula) of the horse.

11. **Collateral (paracuneal) grooves** (sulci): the sulci separating the frog from the bars and sole. These should be

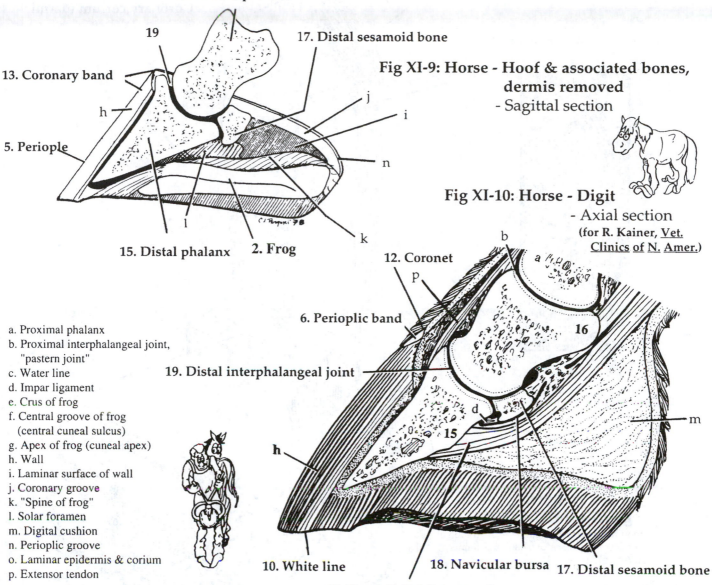

16. Middle phalanx

19

17. Distal sesamoid bone

13. Coronary band

h

5. Periople

j

i

n

Fig XI-9: Horse - Hoof & associated bones, dermis removed
- Sagittal section

Fig XI-10: Horse - Digit
- Axial section
(for R. Kainer, <u>Vet. Clinics of N. Amer.</u>)

15. Distal phalanx   **2. Frog**

k

a. Proximal phalanx
b. Proximal interphalangeal joint, "pastern joint"
c. Water line
d. Impar ligament
e. Crus of frog
f. Central groove of frog (central cuneal sulcus)
g. Apex of frog (cuneal apex)
h. Wall
i. Laminar surface of wall
j. Coronary groove
k. "Spine of frog"
l. Solar foramen
m. Digital cushion
n. Perioplic groove
o. Laminar epidermis & corium
p. Extensor tendon

12. Coronet

p

b

6. Perioplic band

19. Distal interphalangeal joint

16

d

h

15

m

10. White line   **18. Navicular bursa**   **17. Distal sesamoid bone**

20. Deep digital flexor tendon

periodically cleaned or "thrush" may develop.

12. Coronet: the junction of the hoof (periople) and the skin.

13. Coronary band: the proximal part of the hoof overlying the coronary corium.

14. White line or **white zone:** the junction between the wall and sole on the ground surface of the foot. It is the external indication of the sensitive internal structures. Therefore, a nail driven up the white line would reach sensitive tissue. (The NAV uses white zone to avoid confusion with the linea alba of the abdomen. In practice, most horsemen wouldn't be confused, having never heard of the linea alba, and couldn't translate it if they had.)

15. Distal phalanx or **coffin/pedal bone:** embedded in the hoof (coffin).

16. Middle phalanx or **short pastern:** forms the coffin joint with the distal phalanx.

17. Distal sesamoid bone or **navicular bone:** redirects the deep digital flexor tendon.

18. Navicular bursa: situated between the deep digital flexor tendon and the distal sesamoid (navicular) bone to reduce friction between the two.

19. Distal interphalangeal joint (DIP/coffin joint): the articulation between the middle and distal phalanges embedded in the hoof.

20 Deep digital flexor tendon: crosses the navicular bursa to attach to the distal phalanx.

21. Common/long digital extensor tendon: attaches to the extensor process of the distal phalanx in the fore and hind limbs, respectively.

• **Hoof** (collateral, ungual) **cartilages:** two sagittal cartilage plates attach to the wings of the distal phalanx. They project slightly above the hoof where they can be palpated.

1. Perioplic corium (dermis)

2. Coronary corium (dermis)

2. Coronary corium (dermis)

a

c   b

2. Coronary epidermis

11. subcutis

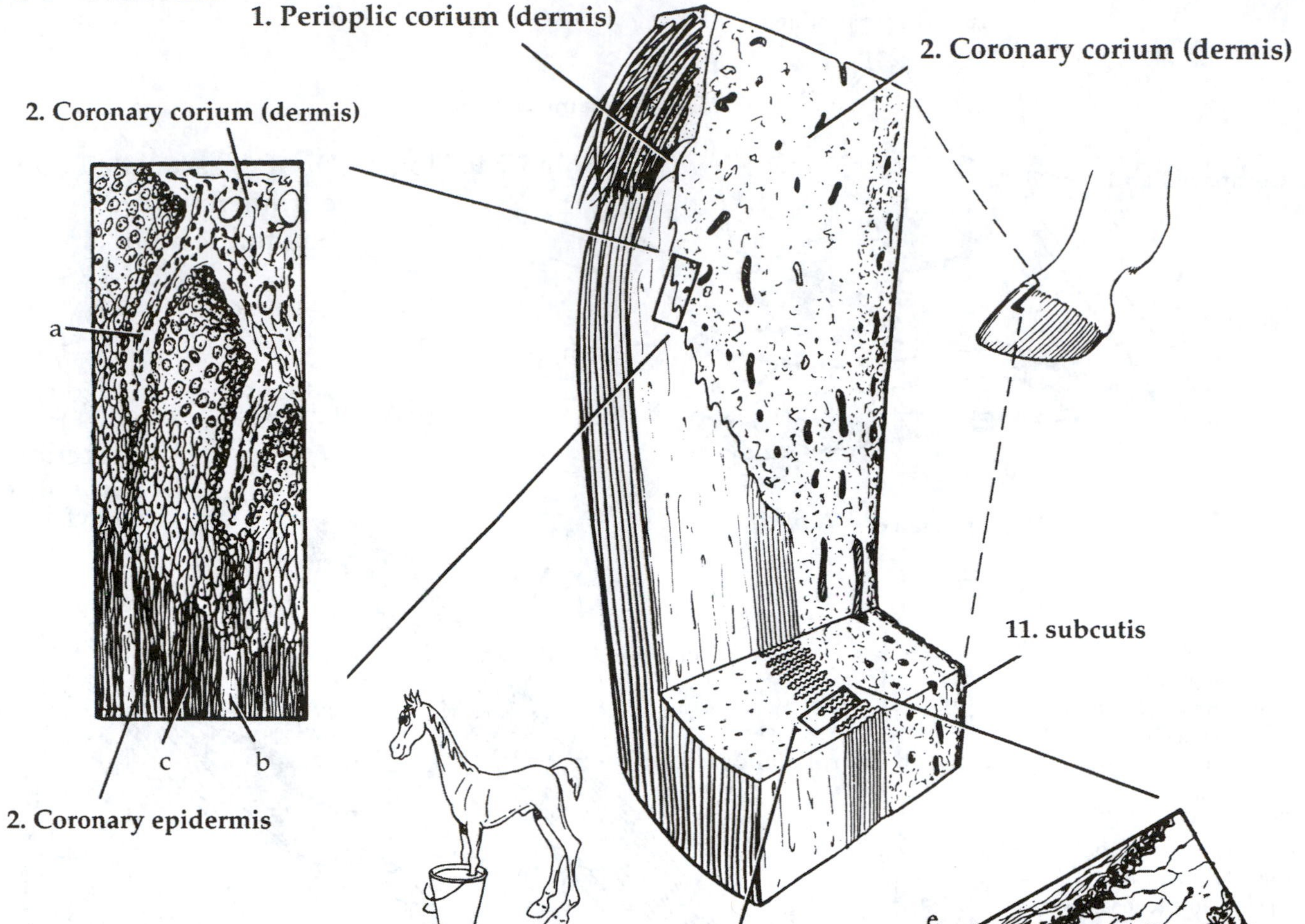

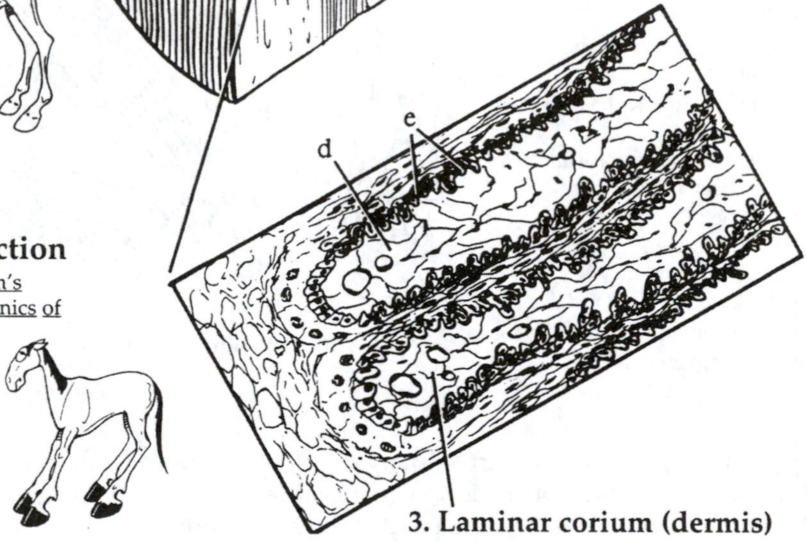

Fig XI: Horse - Hoof wall, coronary region - three dimensional dissection

(modified from J. Daugherty's illustration in <u>Adam's Lameness in Horses</u>, Stashak for R.Kainer, <u>Vet. Clinics of N. Amer.</u>)

a. Papilla
b. Tubular horn
c. Non-tubular horn
d. Primary lamina
e. Secondary laminae

d   e

3. Laminar corium (dermis)

Structure of foot: the covering of the foot is modified skin (integument) and, <u>like the skin</u>, consists of an outer epidermis (the hoof) and an underlying dermis (corium). The subcutis connects the dermis to the internal structures of the foot.

• **Corium** or **dermis**/pododerm (KO-ree-um) (pl. = coria): the highly vascular part of the integument of the foot providing nourishment for the overlying epidermis (hoof). Nerves are located in the corium (dermis), but not in the horny hoof (epidermis), making the corium the sensitive part ("quick") of the foot. By attachments to the deep structures of the foot, the corium holds the hoof in place. The corium is divided into 5 parts: periople, coronary, laminar, sole, and frog. Each coria, except the laminar, has

pegs (papillae) extending into the horny epidermis. Around these pegs (dermal papillae), the germinal epidermis builds tubular and non-tubular horn. The tubular horn develops from the epidermis around the papillae as it grows away from the papillae. The nontubular horn develops from the germinal epithelium between the papillae. The vascular subcutis attaches the corium (dermis) to the periosteum of the distal phalanx.

1. **Perioplic corium** (corium [dermis] limbi): the thin band of dermis that is continuous proximally with the dermis of the skin. It widens out over the bulb of the heel, and produces the thin, shiny, external layer (perioplic epidermis [stratum externum]) of the wall.

2. **Coronary corium** (corium [dermis] coronae): the thick

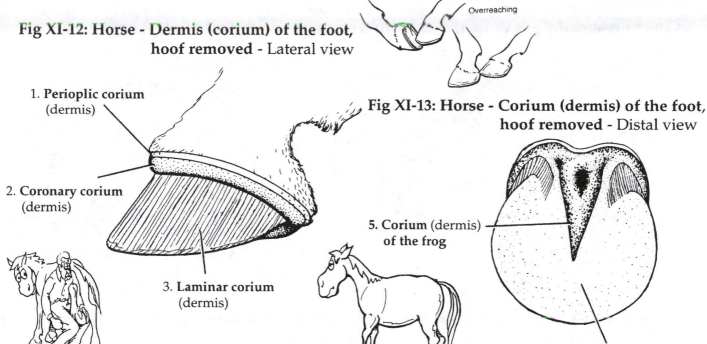

Fig XI-12: Horse - Dermis (corium) of the foot, hoof removed - Lateral view

1. **Perioplic corium** (dermis)

2. **Coronary corium** (dermis)

3. **Laminar corium** (dermis)

Fig XI-13: Horse - Corium (dermis) of the foot, hoof removed - Distal view

5. **Corium** (dermis) **of the frog**

4. **Corium** (dermis) **of the sole**

band of dermis (coronary band) just distal to the perioplic corium. Located in the coronary groove of the hoof (Fig XI-9, j), its papillae provide the template for tubular and non-tubular horn of the wall's bulk. The corium's deep surface connects to the ligaments and cartilages of the distal phalanx by a very vascular connective tissue subcutis called the coronary cushion.

3. **Laminar corium (sensitive laminae)** (corium [dermis] parietis): the nonpigmented dermis suspending the distal phalanx's lateral and dorsal sides (parietal surface) to the hoof wall. Its papillae are modified into elongated primary laminae (sheets) oriented perpendicular to the parietal surface of the distal phalanx. Secondary laminae extend off the primary laminae at acute angles. The laminae interdigitate with the laminae of the laminar epidermis of the hoof, tightly binding hoof (epidermis) to corium (dermis). The deep surface of the laminar dermis is attached by the subcutis to the periosteum of the distal phalanx.

4. **Corium of the sole** (corium [dermis] soleae): the dermis underlying and nourishing the horny sole.

5. **Corium of the frog** (corium [dermis] cunei): the pigmented dermis underlying and nourishing the horny frog. The deep surface of the dermis blends with the digital cushion (Fig XI-10, m).

Epidermis or **hoof**: the part of the integument overlying the dermis (corium). The epidermal layer next to the corium is the germinal layer as would be expected in a skin structure. Here cells divide and push away from the dermis, hardening as they move away to form the hard hoof.

6. **Perioplic epidermis**: the light band marking the junction between the hoof and skin (its proximal edge is the coronet). It arises around the papillae of the perioplic corium.

Growing down toward the ground as a shiny, thin, external layer of the hoof wall (stratum externum) in young animals, it usually is worn away in older horses.

7. **Coronary epidermis (stratum medium)**: the middle, highly keratinized hoof wall layer extending distally from the coronary corium that nourishes it. This layer forms the bulk of the wall of the hoof.

- **Coronary groove**: the sulcus that cups the coronary corium (Fig XI-9, j).

8. **Laminar epidermis**: the inside layer of the hoof (stratum internum) that interdigitates with the laminae of the corium, connecting the hoof to the parietal surface of the distal phalanx. Overlying the laminar corium's primary and secondary laminae, the germinal layer of the laminar epidermis multiplies, pushing the cells perpendicularly away to join the coronary epidermis. The arrangement of interdigitating laminar corium and epidermis greatly increases the surface area and strength of the bond between the hoof and underlying structures. As the laminar corium (sensitive) rounds the toe of the distal phalanx it becomes the sole dermis. The non-pigmented laminar epithelium (insensitive) continues from this turning point to the ground surface of the hoof, forming the **white line**.

9. **Sole epidermis**: similar to the coronary epidermis, consisting of pigmented tubular and non-tubular horn.

10. **Frog epidermis**: similar to the coronary epidermis, but more elastic and not fully keratinized. Its tubular horns are slightly wavy, thus, softer.

- **Central spine (spinae cunei)**, "spine of the frog" or "frog stay" (Fig XI-9, k): the projection on the inner side of the frog epidermis that attaches to the frog corium.

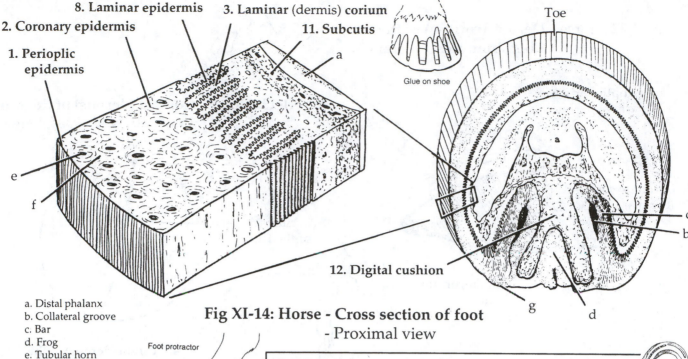

8. Laminar epidermis

2. Coronary epidermis

1. Perioplic epidermis

3. Laminar (dermis) corium

11. Subcutis

Glue on shoe

Toe

a

e

f

c

b

12. Digital cushion

g

d

Fig XI-14: Horse - Cross section of foot
- Proximal view

a. Distal phalanx
b. Collateral groove
c. Bar
d. Frog
e. Tubular horn
f. Intertubular (nontubular) horn
g. Bulb of heel

Foot protractor

11. Subcutis: the layer of connective tissue joining the corium to the coffin bone, cartilages of the hoof, and tendons of the foot.

12. Digital cushion: the wedge-shaped mass of relatively avascular, white elastic fibers, and fat overlying the frog and attaching to the cartilages of the hoof. It absorbs concussive forces.

• Coronary cushion: the subcutaneous tissue just deep to the coronary corium. It contains a large coronary venous plexus.

CLINICAL
13. White line: the junction between the wall and sole on the ground surface of the foot. It is formed by the insensitive laminae reaching the ground surface. An important landmark in horse shoeing, used to ensure the sensitive laminar corium is not invaded, a nail is driven into the hoof on the outside of this line. With experience, a nail can be driven inside and angled across the line without entering the sensitive laminae. "Nail prick" is when a nail is driven into the sensitive laminae.

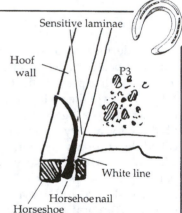

Sensitive laminae

Hoof wall

P3

White line

Horseshoe nail

Horseshoe

Fig: Schematic longitudinal section of hoof wall showing horseshoe nail entering the sensitive laminae

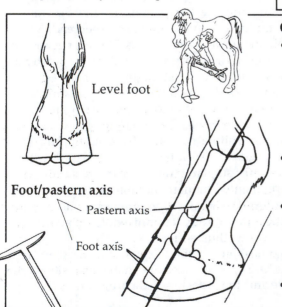

Level foot

Foot/pastern axis

Pastern axis

Foot axis

Conformation of the horse's foot

• Foot (hoof) axis: the angle of the foot in relation to the ground surface. When viewed from the front, all legs should be perpendicular to the ground. From the side, it is the angle the dorsal surface of the hoof makes with the ground. An ideal angle from the side is unimportant compared to a correct foot/pastern axis. A rough estimate of the ideal foot axis when the pastern foot axis is correct is 60° for the front and hind feet (45-50° for the front foot, 50-55° for the hindfoot.)

• Pastern axis: the angle of the proximal phalanx (long pastern) with relation to the ground. This axis should be in the same plane as the foot axis.

• **Foot/pastern axis**: should be equal and form a continuous line. If the angles of the foot and pastern axes are not equal, then the horse has a broken foot-pastern axis. This is more important then the foot axis. The foot axis can be manipulated by horseshoers to make a straight foot-pastern axis, even if this deviates from the ideal foot axis.

• **Level foot**: a foot with equal length to the medial and lateral quarters and heels.

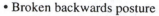

Broken foot pastern axis: when the foot and pastern axis are not equal and continuous from the lateral view.

- Broken backwards posture
  - **"Club foot":** dorsal angle to the ground of greater than 60° due to a flexural deformity.
  - **Coon foot:** the foot axis is steeper than the pastern axis.
- **Run under heel, Low heel-long toe:** a foot with an angle of less than 45°.

Off-level foot: a foot with a lower quarter than the opposite quarter which can result in problems.

- **Sheared heels:** hoof imbalance with break down between the bulbs of the heels.

Flat foot: a foot with little concavity to the sole.

Thin wall and sole: inheritable condition predisposing to sole bruising.

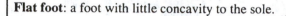

Contracted heels: narrower than normal foot in it's palmar/plantar aspect due to nonweight bearing on the heels.

- **Hoof bound:** a lameness due to chronic contracted heels.

Laminitis or **founder:** inflammation of the laminae of the foot (feet) which can result in rings on the hoof and pedal rotation.

- **Dropped foot:** uncoupling of the laminar epidermis and dermis due to laminitis; allowing the pull of the deep digital flexor to rotate the toe of the distal phalanx downward, pushing on the sole, thus causing a "dropped foot/sole".

"Seedy toe": separation at the white line from the ground surface as a result of laminitis. This can develop into "gravel".

- **Subsolar abscess:** a common condition in horses.

- **Puncture wounds of sole:** can result in abscesses. Their severity may differ if they are outside of or into the frog. Those into thefrog can disasterously effect deeper structures (navicular bursa, coffin joint or synovial sheath of digital flexors.)

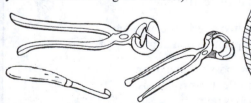

"Gravel": a drainage tract up the sensitive laminae and out the skin above the coronet, resulting from an abscess of a crack in the white line.

- **Bruise: common condition in horses.**
  - **"Corn":** a bruise (contusion) of the medial angle of the sole.

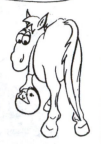

Navicular syndrome: chronic progressive intermittent lameness due to problems of the navicular bone, navicular bursa, coffin joint, deep digital flexor tendon and/or associated structures. Estimated to cause 1/3 of all forelimb lamenesses.

Pedal osteitis: demineralization of the distal phalanx due to inflammation.

Pedal fractures: fractures of the distal phalanx.
- Extensor process fractures of the coffin bone

Navicular disease

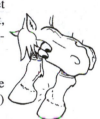

Buttress foot: swelling of the dorsal coronet due to tears of the extensor tendon's attachment, fractures of the extensor process or distal phalanx, or to low ringbone.

Low ringbone: osteoarthritis or degenerative joint disease of the DIP (distal interphalangeal) joint.

Thrush: a degenerative condition of the frog associated with filth, resulting in black necrotic material.

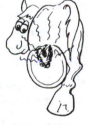
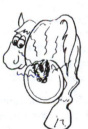

Sidebones: calcification of the lateral cartilages, usually an incidental finding with age, but can lead to lameness if they fracture.

- **Quittor:** chronic inflammation of the lateral cartilages of the hoof characterized by draining tracts just proximal to the hoof.

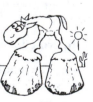

Brittle feet: dry feet with cracks in the hoof wall.

- **Toe crack, quarter crack** and **heel crack** (sand cracks): breaks in the hoof wall starting from the ground surface or the coronary border. Toe, quarter, or heel indicates the location of the crack on the hoof.

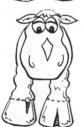

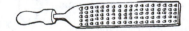

FOOT - OX

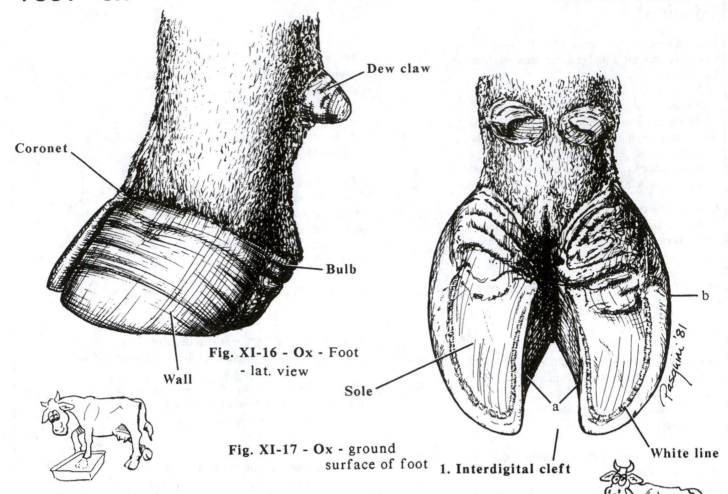

Fig. XI-16 - Ox - Foot
- lat. view

Fig. XI-17 - Ox - ground
surface of foot **1. Interdigital cleft**

FOOT of the OX and PIG: the ox and pig have two weight bearing digits, the horse one. Otherwise, they are basically anatomically the same. The foot skeleton is formed by the middle and distal phalanges, the distal interphalangeal joints (coffin joints) and the distal sesamoid bones. Many ligaments and the tendons of the common/long digital extensor and deep digital flexor muscles attach to these two phalanges.

Hooves: the epidermis of the wall, sole and heels; similar to the horse, except they have no frog, bars or secondary laminae.

Corium (dermis): the sensitive vascular layer underlying the hoof consisting of perioplic, coronary, laminar, sole, and bulb dermis.

1. Interdigital cleft: the space between the two hooves.

Hoof pads or **bulbs** (tori ungulae): highly keratinized cushions on the palmar/plantar aspect of the foot.

CLINICAL

Ulceration of sole: at junction of sole and heel due to trauma of solar corium.

Bruised sole: common condition due to trauma.

Subsolar abscess: due to puncture of the sole.

Foot rot: inflammation of the interdigital subcutaneous tissue of foot.

Corkscrew claw: an inherited condition of lateral hindlimb abaxial horn growth underneath the sole.

Claw (hoof) cracks: separations in the hoof wall.

Laminitis (founder): inflammation of laminae, not as dramatic as in the horse (no rotation, usually subclinical).

Interdigital dermatitis: a wet inflammation of the interdigital cleft.

Corns (interdigital fibroma): proliferation of the tissue in the interdigital cleft due to chronic irritation.

Septic pedal arthritis: a serious condition often treated by amputation of a digit.

Removal of a digit: possible and often done in the ox because it has two, thus, can still stand if one is removed.

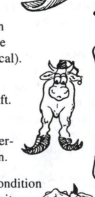
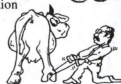

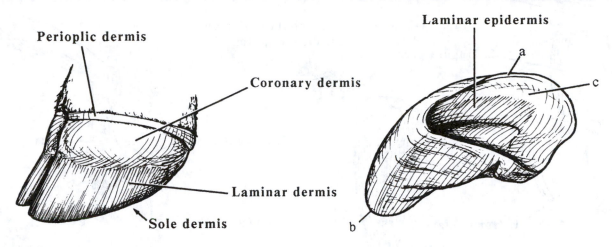

Perioplic dermis

Coronary dermis

Laminar dermis

Sole dermis

Fig. XI-18 - Ox - Foot, hoof removed
showing dermis - lat. view

Laminar epidermis

a

c

b

Fig. XI-19 - Ox - Hoof
- dorsomed. view

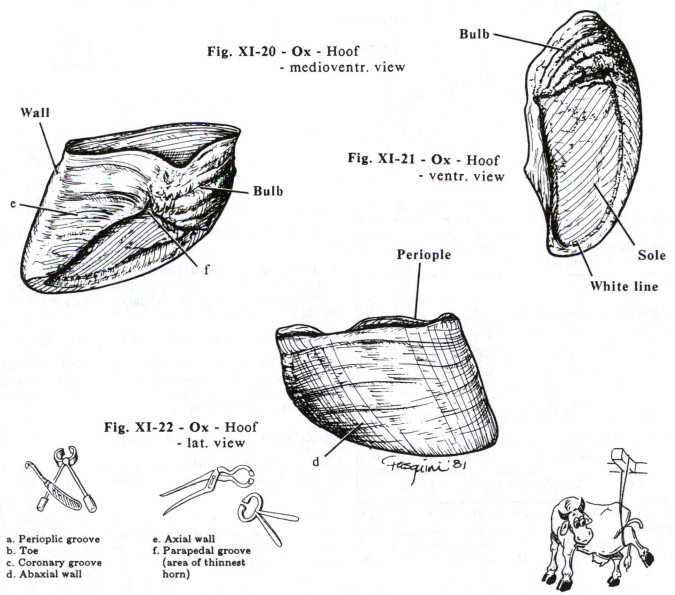

Fig. XI-20 - Ox - Hoof
- medioventr. view

Bulb

Fig. XI-21 - Ox - Hoof
- ventr. view

Sole

White line

Wall

e

f

Bulb

Periople

Fig. XI-22 - Ox - Hoof
- lat. view

d

Pasquini '81

a. Perioplic groove
b. Toe
c. Coronary groove
d. Abaxial wall

e. Axial wall
f. Parapedal groove
(area of thinnest
horn)

CLAW - ERGOT - CHESTNUT

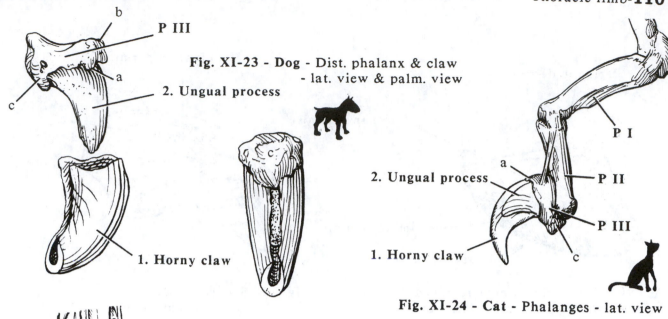

Fig. XI-23 - Dog - Dist. phalanx & claw
- lat. view & palm. view

2. Ungual process

1. Horny claw

3. Metacarpal pad

4. Digital pad

Fig. XI-24 - Cat - Phalanges - lat. view

2. Ungual process

1. Horny claw

a. Ungual crest
b. Extensor process
c. Flexor process

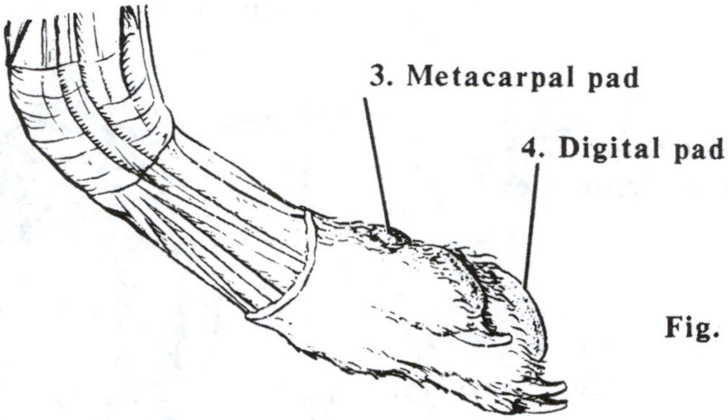

Fig. XI-25 - Dog - dist. forelimb

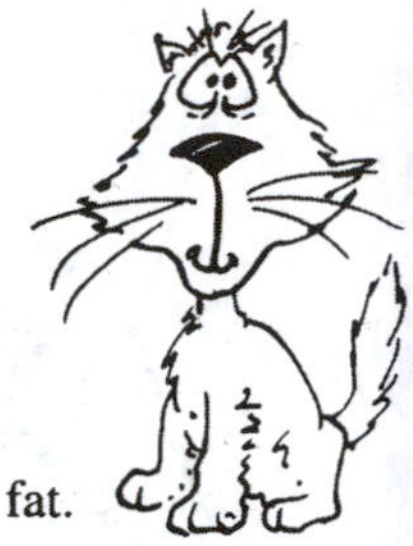

1. CLAW: a modification of the epidermis in the carnivores, conforming to and enclosing the **ungual process** (2) of the distal phalanx (P III). The claw consists of a wall and a sole growing away from the underlying dermis. The dermis nourishes the wall and connects it to the ungual process.

CLINICAL

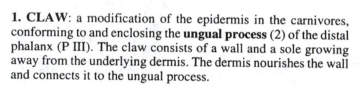

Nail trimming: claws grow very fast and must be trimmed or worn down or they can curve around and enter the paw, especially the dew claw which normally gets little wear. If they are cut too short the dermis may be exposed (**"quicked"**) causing pain and bleeding.

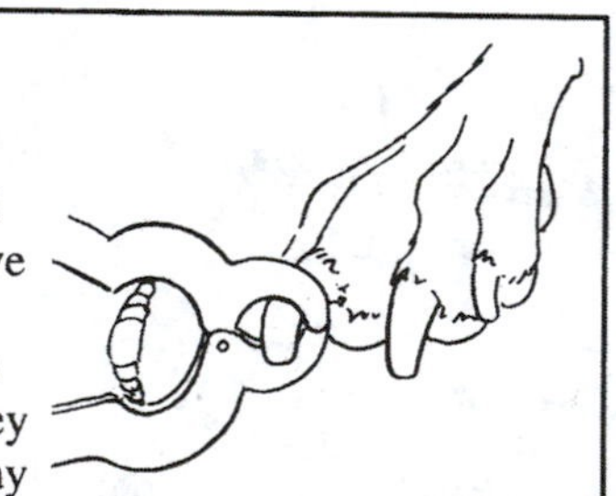

Declaw (onychectomy): removal of the claws of cats. To prevent regrowth, the dorsal aspect of the ungual crest must be removed. This is usually done by removing the entire distal phalanx by cutting through the distal phalangeal joint.

PADS - CARNIVORES (tori): the hairless, cushion-like pads on the palmar/plantar side of the limbs. The toughest skin on the dog, the epidermis is thick and highly keratinized with a rough surface due to many papillae. The underlying dermis contains

sweat glands along with fibroelastic tissue and fat.

Carpal pad: located palmar to the carpus. The carnivores lack tarsal pads.

3. Metacarpal (metatarsal) pad: the heart-shaped pad on the palmar/plantar surface at the level of the proximal metacarpophalangeal (metatarsophalangeal) joints. These joints rest on the pad when the dog is standing.

4. Digital pads: the small pad over the distal end of each digit.

Ruminant – the hoof pads or bulbs are comparable to the digital pads of carnivores. The metacarpal, metatarsal, carpal and tarsal pads are missing in all the domestic species, except the carnivore and the horse (chestnuts and ergots).

ERGOT and CHESTNUT of the HORSE

Ergot: a small mass of horny material on the palmar/plantar surface of the fetlock. They are buried in the "feathers" (long hair behind the fetlock).

Chestnut or "night eyes": a small horny mass on the forearm's medial surface above the carpus and on the medial surface of the tarsus. The tarsal chestnut is usually absent in donkeys and occasionally absent in horses.

Fig. XI-26 - Ox - Horn
- longitudinal section

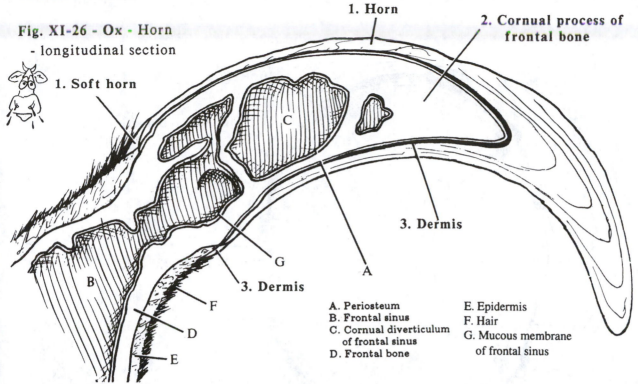

1. **Horn**

2. **Cornual process of frontal bone**

1. **Soft horn**

3. **Dermis**

3. **Dermis**

A
G
B
F
D
E
C

A. Periosteum
B. Frontal sinus
C. Cornual diverticulum of frontal sinus
D. Frontal bone

E. Epidermis
F. Hair
G. Mucous membrane of frontal sinus

1. HORN (cornu): the covering of the cornual process of the frontal bone (2) in all three domestic ruminants. They are present in both sexes. The cornual process starts from a horn bud and grows out as a solid structure that becomes hollowed out (pneumatized) by about 6 months of age. The horn is epidermal tissue formed similarly to the hoof wall. The underlying dermis has papillae providing the template for the germinal layer of the epidermis (horn) to form tubular and nontubular horn. The epikeras is the ring of soft horn marking the transition between skin and horn. Like the periople of the hoof, it grows out and covers the horn with a thin shiny layer. Horns are permanent and grow throughout life. The soft horn at the base is similar to the periople of the hoof.

SPECIES DIFFERENCES

Cattle: the horns are located at the caudolateral end of the head.

Sheep and goats: the horns are located behind the orbits.

Polled: ruminants not having horns.

Pregnancy grooves - cow: the grooves (cornual rings) on the external surface of the horns, caused by slowing of growth near the end of gestation and during lactation. A rough estimate of a cow's age can be made by assuming an annual pregnancy; count the number of rings and add to the age of first pregnancy.

Cornual rings - sheep and goats: circumferential grooves on the horn. More distinct than in the cow, 9-12 are produced per year.

CLINICAL

Dehorning: removal of horns. This is best done by removing the horn bud when a calf or kid is between 5 to 10 days of age.

Dehorning of calves: can be done as soon as the horn bud is palpable, by chemical means, cauterization or surgical excision of the horn bud and surrounding skin.

Dehorning young cattle: once the horn has broken through the skin for at least one inch, the above methods for calves will not work. A Barnes dehorner or a small saw can be used.

Dehorning adult cattle: remove the horn close to the skull proximal to the epikeras so no horn can be produced later. This also insures that the branches of the cornual artery will be cut before they enter the horn or hemorrhage can't be controlled.

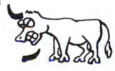

Saws, horn shears and dehorning wires are all used.

Dehorning of young goats: may best be done under general anesthesia because of hemorrhage, and the cranium under the horn buds is thin and easily opened to the brain.

Cornual nerve block - cattle: inject the cornual nerve (a branch of the trigeminal nerve) midway between the eye and the base of the horn just below the temporal line. This will anesthetize most cattle, if it doesn't, do a ring block around the base of the horn.

Cornual and infratrochlear nerve blocks in goats: inject the cornual nerve at the caudal ridge of the root of the zygomatic process of the frontal bone to a depth of 1/2 inch; inject the infratrochlear nerve dorsomedial to the eye close to the edge of the bony orbit.

Sinusitis: common sequel to dehorning because in animals over 7 months old the cornual sinus is opened.

EYE

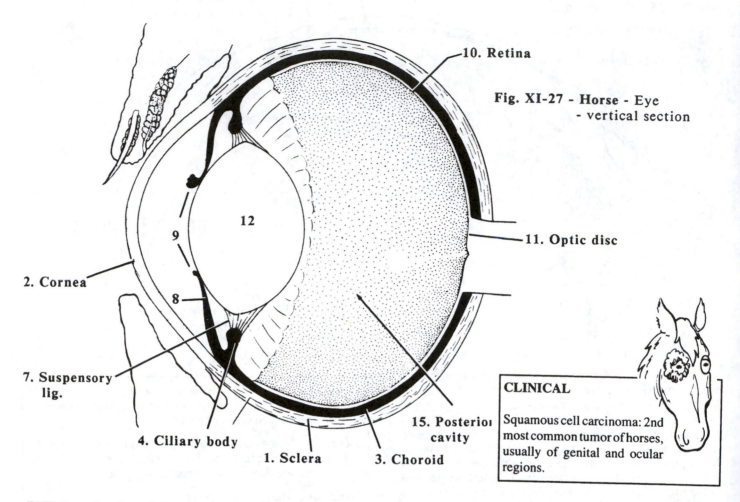

10. Retina

Fig. XI-27 - Horse - Eye
- vertical section

11. Optic disc

2. Cornea

7. Suspensory lig.

4. Ciliary body

1. Sclera

3. Choroid

15. Posterior cavity

CLINICAL

Squamous cell carcinoma: 2nd most common tumor of horses, usually of genital and ocular regions.

EYE (L. *oculus*, G. *opthalmos*): the organ of sight, consisting of the eyeball and its accessory structures. Light passes through the transparent structures of the eye (cornea, aqueous humor, pupil, lens and vitreous humor) to reach the receptor organs (rods and cones) of the retina. The resulting nerve impulses are then conducted by the optic nerve to the visual center of the brain.

Descriptive terms: the eye is one of the few areas where the human nomenclature is used - anterior, posterior, superior and inferior.

EYEBALL (L. *bulbus oculi*): the eyeball can be divided into three layers - fibrous tunic, vascular tunic and nervous tunic (retina).

Fibrous tunic: the outer coat of the eyeball. It is divided into the sclera and the cornea.

• **1. Sclera** (SKLE-ra)(G. *scleros* hard) or "the white of the eye": the caudal part of the fibrous coat consisting of fibrous tissue. It gives shape and protects the inner structures of the eye.

• **2. Cornea** (KOR-nee-a): the transparent anterior part of the fibrous coat that lets light into the eyeball. Its collagenous fibers

are organized in a series of layers that don't interfere with the passage of light - anterior epithelium, anterior limiting ("Bowman's") membrane, substantia propria, posterior limiting ("Descemet's") membrane, and posterior epithelium.

• Limbus (Fig. XI-29,e): the junction of the sclera and cornea.

Vascular tunic or **uvea** (YOO-vee-a): the middle layer of the eyeball (choroid, ciliary body and iris) consisting mainly of blood vessels and smooth muscle that supply nutrition to the eyeball, and control the shape of the lens and the size of the pupil.

• **3. Choroid** (KOH-royd): the posterior part of the vascular tunic. It is a thin, dark, highly vascular membrane inside the sclera. It supplies the retina and serves to absorb light not reflected out of the eyeball.

– **Tapetum lucidum**: specialized reflective area of the choroid. It is the reason animal's eyes glow when light is shined in them at night; not present in man and pigs.

• **4. Ciliary body** (SIL-ee-ar'ee): the thickest portion of the vascular tunic between the choroid and the iris. It consists of the ciliary muscle and the ciliary processes.

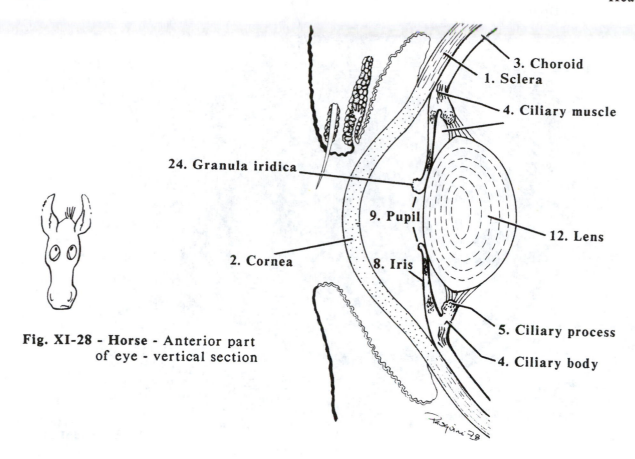

Fig. XI-28 - Horse - Anterior part
of eye - vertical section

3. Choroid
1. Sclera
4. Ciliary muscle
24. Granula iridica
9. Pupil
12. Lens
2. Cornea
8. Iris
5. Ciliary process
4. Ciliary body

–6. Ciliary processes: folds on the inner surface of the ciliary body that anchor the zonular fibers.

7. Suspensory ligaments or **zonular fibers**: attach the lens to the ciliary body, hold the lens in position, and allow the shape of the lens to change due to actions of the ciliary muscles. Contraction of the muscles causes the ciliary ring to shrink towards the lens taking tension off the fibers. This allows the lens to take on a round appearance when focusing on close objects. Relaxing the muscles, as when gazing at the horizon, puts tension on the fibers which stretches the lens thin.

8. Iris: the colored, doughnut-shaped part of the eye surrounding the pupil. It has two layers of muscle reacting to light to increase or decrease the size of the pupil, regulating the amount of light entering the eyeball. The circular, smooth pupillary constrictor muscles constrict the pupil when stimulated by the parasympathetic fibers. The radiating, smooth pupillary dilator muscles dilate the pupil when stimulated by the sympathetic fibers. The color of the iris is determined by the number of pigment cells in it. A high number gives a brown color, a very low number a blue color.

9. Pupil: the central opening of the iris that lets light into the eye.

10. Retina (RET-i-na) ("nervous" coat): the inner coat of the eye, functioning in image formation. The retina contains three layers

of neurons: photoreceptors, bipolar neurons, and ganglion neurons.

• **Photoreceptors**: the light sensitive, first layer of the retina. Dendrites of photoreceptors are the cones and rods.

–**Rods**: dendrites sensitive to dim light (night vision) and shapes.

– **Cones**: dendrites sensitive to color and sharpness of vision.

• **Bipolar neurons**: the intermediate layer of the retina receives impulses from the rods and cones and passes them to the neuronal ganglia.

• **Ganglion neurons**: the inner layer of the retina which pass the impulse in their axons to the optic nerve.

• **11. Optic disc**: the area on the retina where the axons from the ganglion neurons leave the eye as the optic nerve. Having no rods or cones, this area is called the "blind spot".

12. LENS: the transparent, biconvex body of the eye suspended behind (posterior) the iris by the suspensory ligaments. It constitutes part of the refractive mechanism of the eye. The lens has a dense capsule and is arranged in layers of transparent dead cells, like an onion.

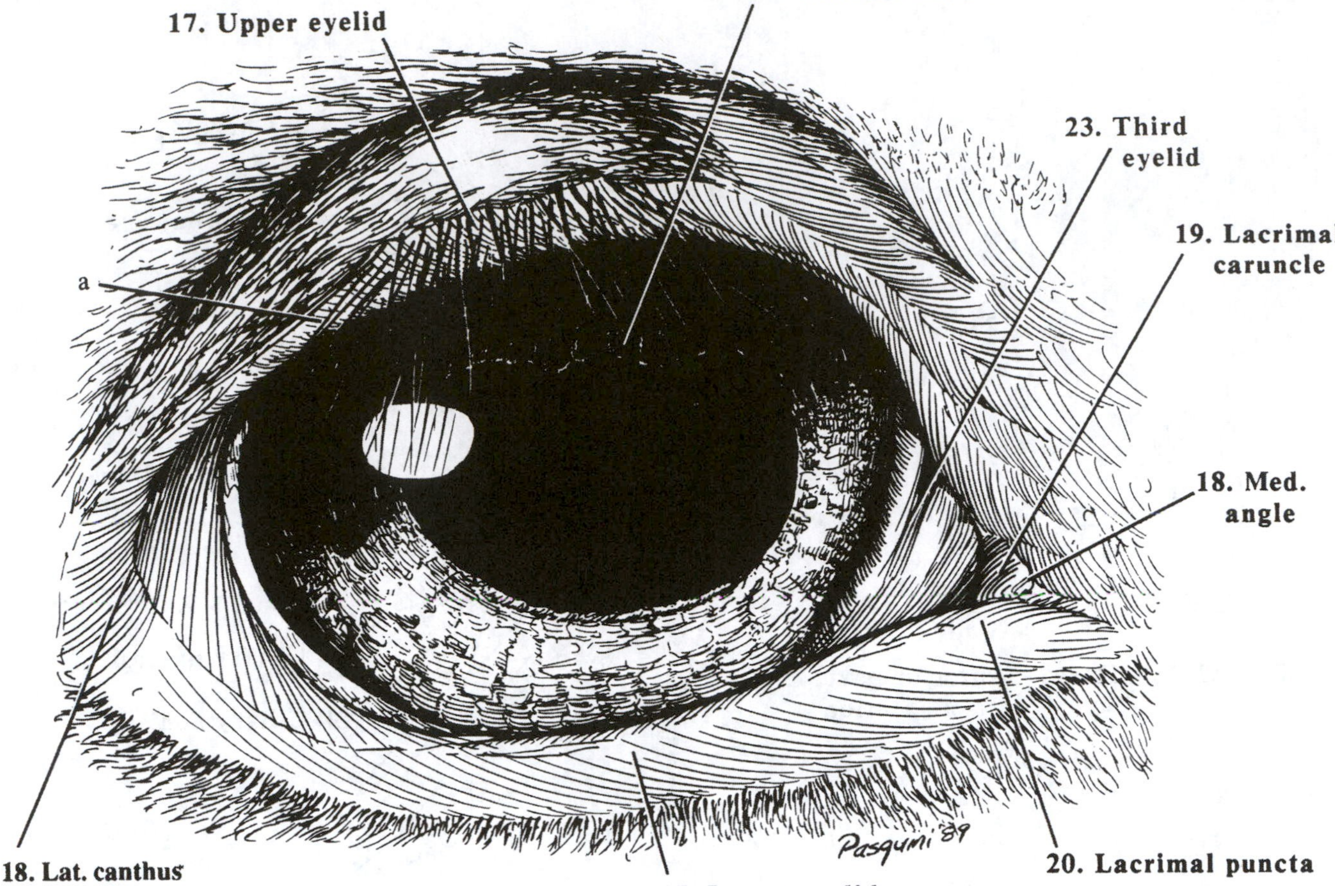

17. Upper eyelid

24. Granula iridica

23. Third eyelid

19. Lacrimal caruncle

18. Med. angle

a

18. Lat. canthus

20. Lacrimal puncta

17. Lower eyelid

Pasquini '89

Fig. XI-29 - Horse - Rt. eye

INTERIOR of the EYE: the cavity of the eye, divided by the lens and iris into three chambers.

13. Anterior chamber: the space between the cornea and the iris.

14. Posterior chamber: the space between the iris and lens.

• **Aqueous humor**: watery fluid, similar to cerebrospinal fluid, filling the posterior and anterior chambers. Aqueous humor is secreted by the ciliary processes into the posterior chamber, flows through the pupil into the anterior chamber, and drains at the periphery into the scleral venous plexus which leads to the veins of the eye. It functions to maintain the intraocular pressure and as a nutrient and waste transport medium.

15. Vitreous chamber: the larger space lying between the lens and retina. It is filled with vitreous humor.

Vitreous body: the jelly-like substance that fills the vitreous chamber, maintains the shape of the eye and holds the retina in place.

ACCESSORY STRUCTURES of the EYE

17. Upper and **lower eyelids** or **superior** and **inferior palpebrae**: the two movable folds protecting the rostral surface of the eyeball. The tarsus is a fibrous plate supporting the margin of the eyelid. Tarsal ("Meibomian") glands open in series onto the

margin of the lid.

Cilia or eyelashes: hairs coming out of the eyelids. There are sebaceous and ciliary glands associated with the cilia.

18. Lateral and **medial commissures** or **canthi** (sin. = **canthus**): the point where eyelids meet.

19. Lacrimal caruncle: a triangular prominence in the medial angle.

20. Lacrimal puncta: openings into lacrimal canals on upper and lower eyelids near the medial angles (pg. 558).

Conjunctiva: the special mucous membrane lining the eyelid and the eyeball.

• **21. Palpebral conjunctiva**: lines the inner surface of the eyelid.

• **22. Bulbar conjunctiva**: the reflection of the palpebral conjunctiva onto the eyeball.

23. Third eyelid (palpebra tertia) or "nictitating membrane": the fold of conjunctiva, reinforced by cartilage, located between the eyelid's medial angle and the eyeball. Retraction of the eyeball causes the third eyelid to move across and protect the eyeball. The gland of the third eyelid is a lacrimal gland.

EYE

21. **Palpebral conjunctiva**

17. **Upper eyelid**

13. **Anterior chamber**

Fig. XI-30 - Ox - Anterior part of eye - vertical section

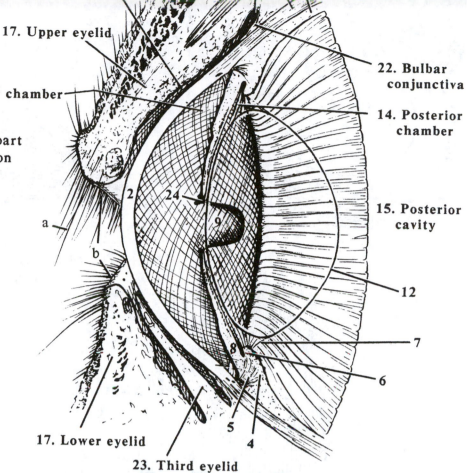

22. **Bulbar conjunctiva**

14. **Posterior chamber**

15. **Posterior cavity**

1. Sclera
2. Cornea
3. Choroid
4. Ciliary body
5. Ciliary m.
6. Ciliary process
7. Suspensory lig.
8. Iris
9. Pupil
10. Retina
11. Optic disc
12. Lens

a. Cilia
b. Palpebral fissure
c. Fornix of the conjunctiva
d. Tarsal glands

17. **Lower eyelid**

23. **Third eyelid**

SPECIES DIFFERENCES

24. **Corpora nigra** (L. black body) or **granula iridica**: several black masses at the upper and lower edges of the iris in the horse and ruminants.

CLINICAL

Cherry eye: hypertrophy and prolapse of the gland of the third eyelid is common in young dogs.

Keratitis: inflammation of the cornea.

Conjunctivitis: inflammation of the conjunctiva.

Cataract: the loss of lens transparency. The most common cause is aging.

Glaucoma: a group of eye diseases characterized by an increase in intra-ocular pressure which causes physiological changes in the optic disk and typical defects in the field of vision.

Stye or **hordeolum**: inflammation of the glands associated with the cilia.

Entropion: the inversion of the margins of the eyelids.

Ectropion: the eversion of the margins of the eyelids.

Moon blindness (equine recurrent uveitis, periodic-ophthalmia): inflammation of the iris, ciliary body and choroid.

Pinkeye (infectious bovine keratitis): a common condition of cattle leading to economic loss, caused by *Moraxella bovis* (bacteria).

Cancer eye: #1 neoplasm of cattle, multifactorial etiology (trauma, white faced, hereditary).

Enucleation (removal) of the eyeball: common in cattle as a treatment for cancer eye.

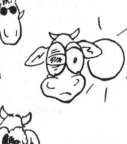
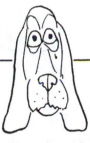

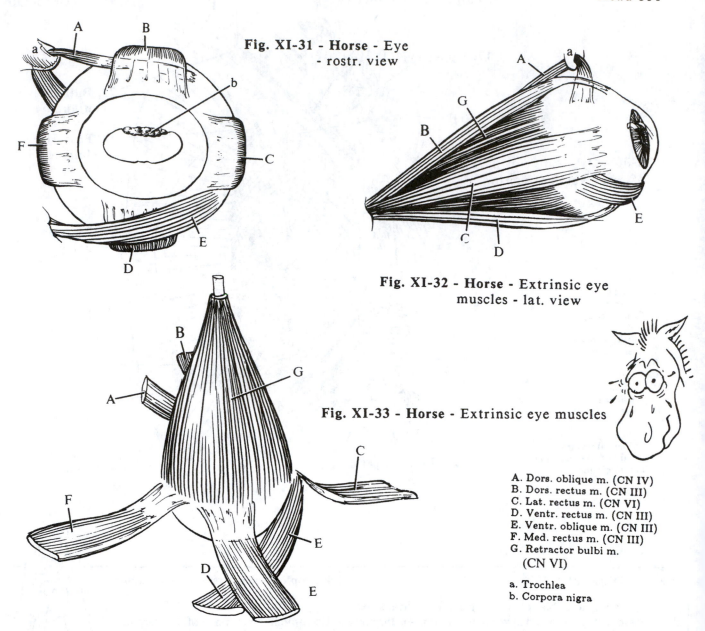

Fig. XI-31 - Horse - Eye - rostr. view

Fig. XI-32 - Horse - Extrinsic eye muscles - lat. view

Fig. XI-33 - Horse - Extrinsic eye muscles

A. Dors. oblique m. (CN IV)
B. Dors. rectus m. (CN III)
C. Lat. rectus m. (CN VI)
D. Ventr. rectus m. (CN III)
E. Ventr. oblique m. (CN III)
F. Med. rectus m. (CN III)
G. Retractor bulbi m.
 (CN VI)

a. Trochlea
b. Corpora nigra

MUSCLES of the EYE: divided into intrinsic and extrinsic groups. Intrinsic muscles consist of the pupillary sphincter, pupillary dilator and ciliary muscles which deal with size of the pupil and lens shape (accommodation). Extrinsic muscles move the eyeball and are located behind it. They are the four rectus muscles (dorsal, ventral, medial, and lateral), two oblique muscles (dorsal and ventral) and the retractor bulbi muscles. Humans lack a retractor bulbi muscle. The muscles in the legend are followed by the nerves innervating them.

Memory aid: for the innervation of the extrinsic muscle of the eye: $Do_4(LrRb)_6Rest_3$. The trochlear (CnIV) innervates the muscle that passes around the trochlea (a) - dorsal oblique. The abducens (CnVI) innervates the muscle that abducts the eye - lateral rectus, and the retractor bulbi. The oculomotor (CnIII) innervates all the rest.

Levator palpebrae superioris muscle: does not attach to the eye, but to the upper eyelid. It elevates the upper eyelid and is innervated by the oculomotor nerve (CNIII).

Orbicularis oculi muscle: surrounds the eye and functions to close it. It is innervated by the palpebral branch of the facial nerve (CNII).

CLINICAL

Facial nerve paralysis: caused by damage to the facial nerve (CnVII). This distorts the face which bothers the owner, not the animal. It becomes a clinically significant problem if the orbicularis oculi muscle is affected and the animal can't shut its eye, and the lacrimal gland losses its facial innervation leading to serious drying of the eye.

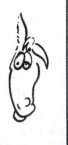

EAR

1. Auricular cartilage

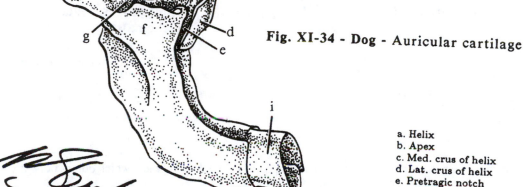

Fig. XI-34 - Dog - Auricular cartilage

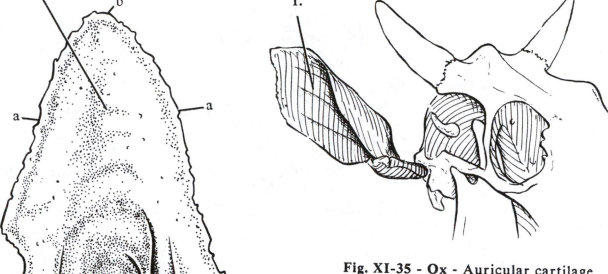

Fig. XI-35 - Ox - Auricular cartilage & skull

a. Helix
b. Apex
c. Med. crus of helix
d. Lat. crus of helix
e. Pretragic notch
f. Tragus
g. Intertragic notch
h. Antitragus
i. Anular cartilage

EAR (L. *auris*; G. *ous*): the organ of hearing and balance. It is divided into three portions - the outer, middle, and inner.

OUTER EAR: the pinna and the external auditory meatus.

Pinna (L. a feather, wing, or fin) or **auricle**: the fleshy appendage attached to the side of the skull by muscles and ligaments, making it very mobile. It functions to catch and direct sound waves toward the middle ear (ear drum).

1. Auricular cartilage: the elastic framework of the pinna and external auditory meatus, covered on both sides with skin.

External auditory meatus: the passageway from the pinna to the ear drum.

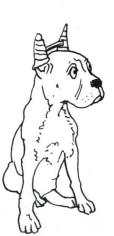

CLINICAL

Auricular hematoma: occurs in dogs, cats and pigs due to trauma (scratching, head shaking) that rupture blood vessels of the ear.

Necrotic ear syndrome of swine: necrosis of the pinna in weaned and growing pigs probably due to fighting followed by infection.

Otitis externa: inflammation of the external ear canal, it is the most common disease of the external ear canal in dogs and cats, but uncommon in large animals.

Cerumen (se-ROO-min)(L. *cera* wax) or earwax: brown, waxy material secreted by glands in the ext. auditory meatus.

EAR

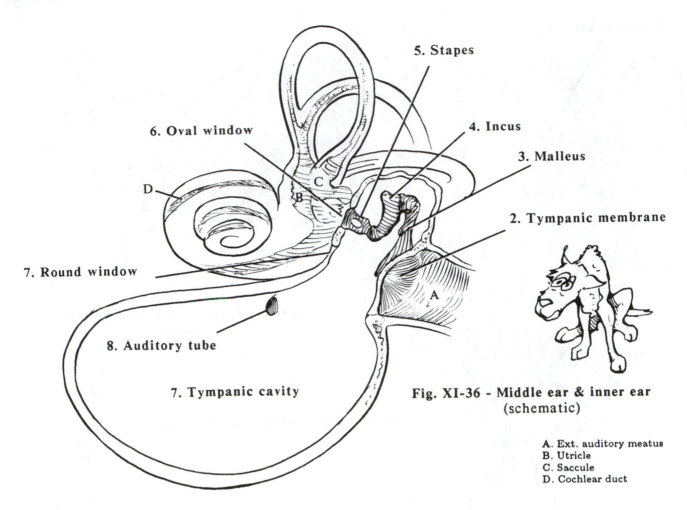

5. Stapes

6. Oval window

4. Incus

3. Malleus

D

C

B

2. Tympanic membrane

7. Round window

A

8. Auditory tube

7. Tympanic cavity

Fig. XI-36 - Middle ear & inner ear
(schematic)

A. Ext. auditory meatus
B. Utricle
C. Saccule
D. Cochlear duct

1. MIDDLE EAR or tympanic cavity: the part of the ear inside of and including the tympanic membrane. It contains the auditory ossicles and the opening to the auditory tube.

2. Tympanic membrane (tim-PAN-ik) or **ear drum**: the thin, semitransparent partition between the external auditory meatus and the middle ear. The ear drum is vibrated by sound waves.

Auditory ossicles (ear bones): the three bones extending across the middle ear from the ear drum to the oval window of the cochlea. They transmit and amplify vibrations of the ear drum to the oval window, setting up vibrations in the fluid of the cochlea.

• 3. Malleus (the "hammer"): the small bone connecting the inner surface of the tympanic membrane and the incus.

• 4. Incus ("anvil"): the ossicle between the malleus and stapes.

• 5. Stapes ("stirrup"): the smallest bone in the body. Its base fits into the oval window.

6. Oval (vestibular) window: one of two openings between the middle and inner ear. It is filled by the base of the stapes, which pushes inward.

7. Round (cochlear) window: the other opening between the middle and inner ear, located below the oval window and covered by a secondary tympanic membrane, which bulges outward with fluid movement.

8. Auditory tube (eustachian tube): the passageway between the middle ear and nasopharynx. It functions to equalize pressure on both sides of the ear drum, protecting it from rupture. Swallowing or yawning opens the auditory tube, allowing air into the middle ear.

CLINICAL

Auditory tube (8): a potential path for spread of infection from the nasopharynx to the middle ear. The pharyngeal opening of the auditory tube allows air into the middle ear to aid in equalizing pressure differences on either side of the tympanic membrane (why chewing gum on airplanes is done).

Otitis media: inflammation of the middle ear usually due to spread of infection from the external ear canal through the tympanic membrane. Spread from the pharynx up the external auditory tube is also possible. This can effect the facial and sympathetic nerves passing through the middle ear and result in facial palsy and/or Horner's syndrome (see page 524).

GUTTURAL POUCHES

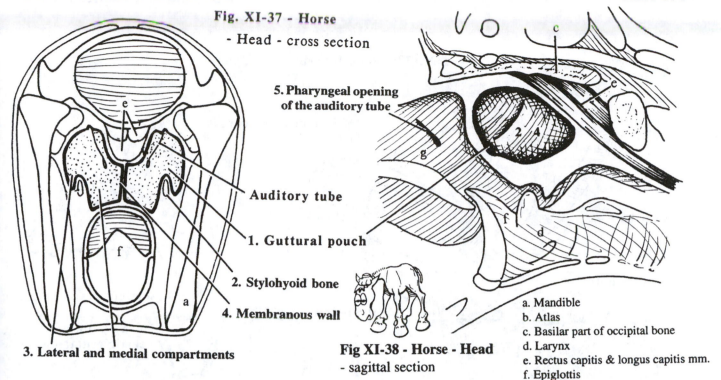

Fig. XI-37 - Horse
- Head - cross section

5. **Pharyngeal opening of the auditory tube**

Auditory tube

1. **Guttural pouch**

2. **Stylohyoid bone**

4. **Membranous wall**

3. **Lateral and medial compartments**

Fig XI-38 - Horse - Head
- sagittal section

a. Mandible
b. Atlas
c. Basilar part of occipital bone
d. Larynx
e. Rectus capitis & longus capitis mm.
f. Epiglottis

1. GUTTURAL POUCH (GUT-ur-al): large, air filled, ventral diverticulae of the auditory tubes in the **horse**. They are located between the cranium, wing of atlas and the pharynx.

2. Stylohyoid bone: partially separates the pouch into compartments

3. Lateral and medial compartments of the guttural pouch.

4. Median membranous wall: made of the mucous membrane of each guttural pouch meeting on the midline.

5. Pharyngeal opening of the auditory tube: small slits in the lateral nasopharyngeal wall that open into the auditory tubes, thus, into the guttural pouches.

Structures crossing the dorsocaudal aspect of the medial pouch:
• Cranial nerves VII, IX, XI & XII
• Cranial sympathetic trunk
• Internal carotid artery

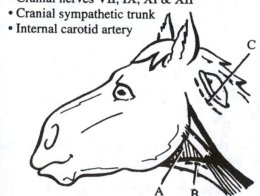

CLINICAL

Guttural pouch tympani: filling of the pouch with air in foals when can't escape through the pharyngeal opening of auditory tube. If unilateral, the median membranous wall can be surgically opened to allow air to enter other pouch and out its opening.

Guttural pouch infections: respiratory diseases can extend into the guttural pouches from the pharynx.

Guttural pouch empyema: purulent material in the pouch, which can become chondroid (hard concretions of inspissated pus). Pus is seen as a fluid line in a standing lateral radiograph of the guttural pouches. Chondroids are removed by surgery.

Guttural pouch mycosis: fungal infection typically affecting the dorsocaudal medial compartment over the internal carotid artery. Erosion of the pouch can result in inflammation of the cranial nerves and rupture of the internal carotid artery resulting in dysphagia (difficult eating) and epistaxis (nose bleeding).

Endoscopy of the guttural pouch: performed by passing a endoscopic tube through the ventral nasal meatus into the pharyngeal opening of the auditory tube, thus, into the guttural pouch. Drainage can be performed with a catheter along the same route.

Surgical approaches to the guttural pouch:
A. Viborg's triangle: incision between tendon of the sterno-cephalicus muscle, linguofacial vein and ramus of the mandible
B. Modified Whitehouse: skin incision ventral to the linguofacial vein and blunt dissection along the larynx to the guttural pouch.
C. Hyovertebrotomy: incision ventral to the wing of the atlas.

Fig. XI-39 - Bony labyrinth

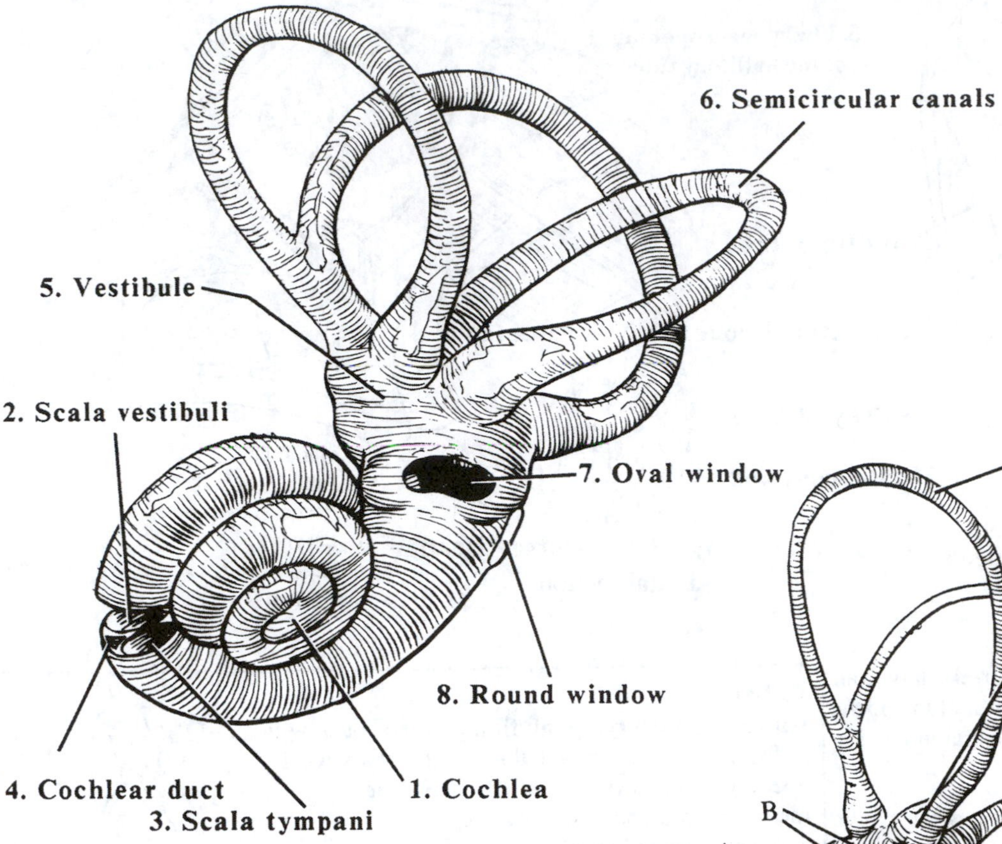

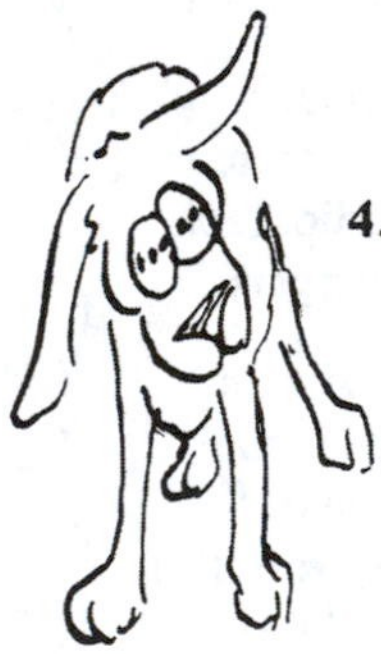

6. Semicircular canals

5. Vestibule

2. Scala vestibuli

7. Oval window

8. Round window

4. Cochlear duct

3. Scala tympani

1. Cochlea

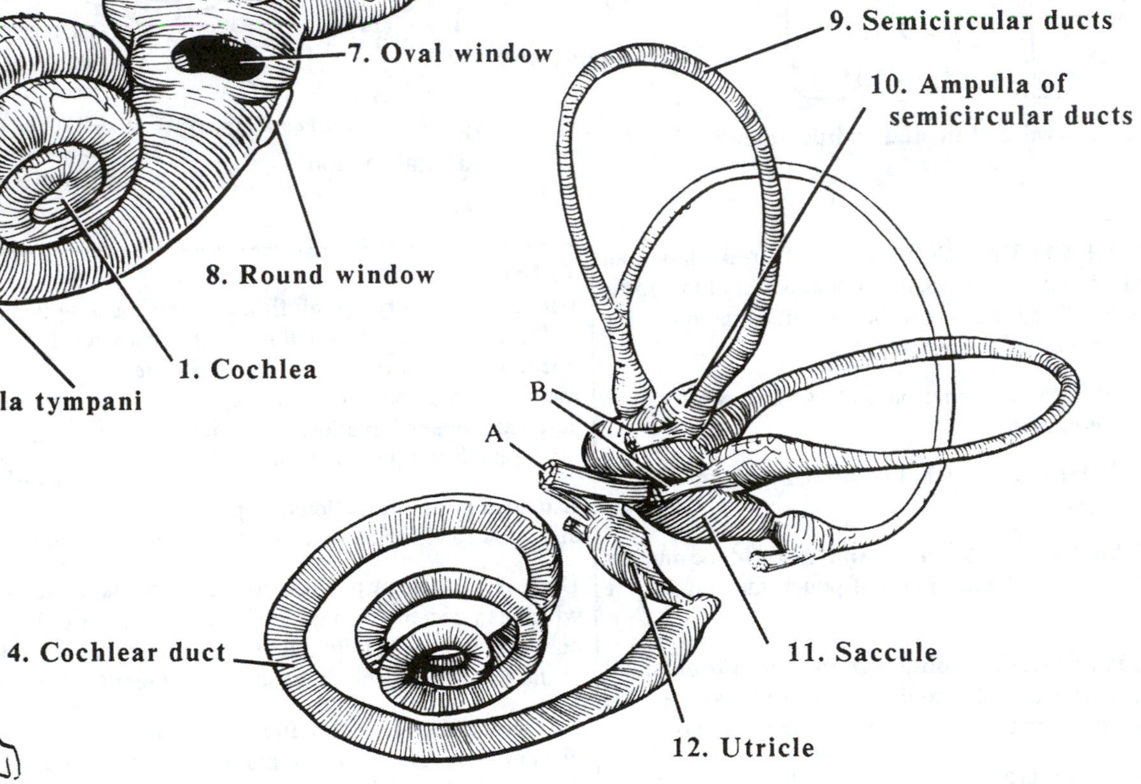

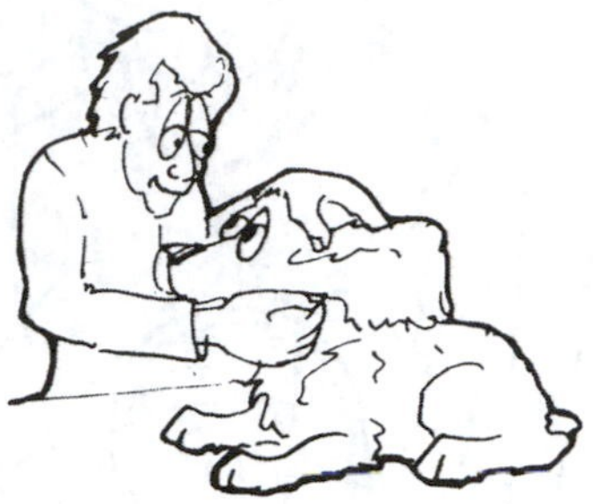

9. Semicircular ducts

10. Ampulla of semicircular ducts

B

A

11. Saccule

12. Utricle

4. Cochlear duct

Fig. XI-40 - Membranous labyrinth

INNER EAR: consists of the bony (osseous) and membranous labyrinth.

Bony (osseous) labyrinth (Fig. XI-39): a series of cavities in the temporal bone; lined with periosteum and divided into the vestibule, cochlea, and semicircular canals.

• **Perilymph:** fluid within the bony labyrinth, surrounding the membranous labyrinth.

Membranous labyrinth (Fig. XI-40): a series of tubes and sac within the bony labyrinth.

• **Endolymph:** fluid within the membranous labyrinth.

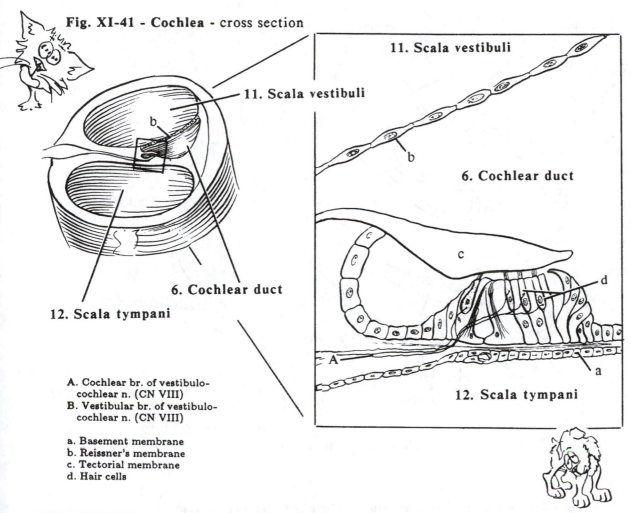

Fig. XI-41 - Cochlea - cross section

11. Scala vestibuli

11. Scala vestibuli

b

6. Cochlear duct

c

d

A

a

6. Cochlear duct

12. Scala tympani

12. Scala tympani

A. Cochlear br. of vestibulocochlear n. (CN VIII)
B. Vestibular br. of vestibulocochlear n. (CN VIII)

a. Basement membrane
b. Reissner's membrane
c. Tectorial membrane
d. Hair cells

1. COCHLEA (KOHK-lee-a) (L. snail shell): the snail shell-like part of the inner ear associated with hearing. The cochlea consists of an outer bony coil and an inner membranous cochlear duct.

Bony labyrinth – cochlea (Fig. XI-30): a bony, spiral canal making a number of turns around a central bony core, the modiolus (moh-DY-oh-lus). The membranous cochlear duct divides the bony spiral labyrinth into two channels – the scala vestibuli and the scala tympani.

• **2. Scala vestibuli**: the canal of the bony labyrinth communicating with the vestibule, the middle ear at the oval window, and the scala tympani at the apex of the cochlea.

• **3. Scala tympani**: the continuation of the scala vestibuli from the apex of the cochlea to the round window.

Membranous labyrinth: a membranous tube separating the two canals of the bony labyrinth and forming the cochlear duct.

• **4. Cochlear duct** or **scala media**: the spiral canal extending from the base to the apex of the cochlea, between the canals of the

bony labyrinth. It is filled with endolymph and contains the spiral organ.

• **Spiral organ** or **organ of Corti** (Fig. XI-33): the organ of hearing consisting of a series of hair cells on the inner surface of the membranous labyrinth. Bending of the free ends of hair cells by vibrating endolymph generates a mechanical signal transmitted by the cochlear branch of the vestibulocochlear nerve (CN VIII) to the brain where it is perceived as sound.

Clinical

Otitis interna: inflammation of the inner ear which can affect balance resulting in vestibular signs (head tilt and circling to effected side), ataxia (general incoordination) and nystagmus (involuntary eye movement) with the fast phase away from the effected side.

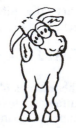

• Infection rarely ascends the vestibulochochlear and facial nerves to the brainstem, resulting in brainstem abscesses, meningitis and possible death.

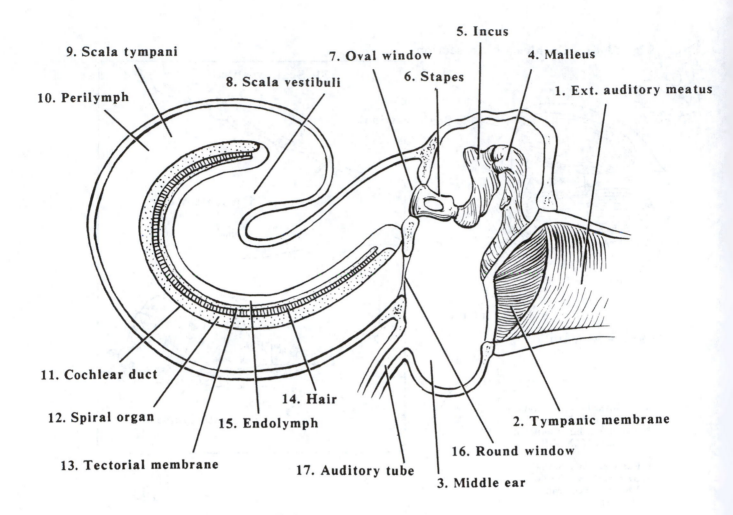

9. Scala tympani

10. Perilymph

8. Scala vestibuli

7. Oval window

5. Incus

6. Stapes

4. Malleus

1. Ext. auditory meatus

11. Cochlear duct

12. Spiral organ

13. Tectorial membrane

14. Hair

15. Endolymph

17. Auditory tube

2. Tympanic membrane

16. Round window

3. Middle ear

Fig. XI-42 – Ext. auditory meatus, middle & inner ear (schematic)

PHYSIOLOGY of HEARING

Sound waves reaching the ear are directed by the **pinna** to the **external auditory meatus** (1) and then to the tympanic membrane (2).

The **tympanic membrane** (2) is vibrated by the sound waves.

The **malleus** (4), connected to the tympanic membrane's inner surface, passes on and amplifies vibrations via the **incus** (5) and **stapes** (6) to the oval window (7).

Vibrations of the **oval window** by the stapes sets the **perilymph** (10) into a wave motion that travels through the **scala vestibuli** (8) and **scala tympani** (9) to the round window (16).

The **round window** (16) bulges into the middle ear and then back into the scala tympani, reversing the fluid wave movement.

Vibrations of the scala vestibuli and scala tympani generate wave motion of the **endolymph** (15) within the **cochlear duct** (11), displacing the hair cells of the spiral organ (12).

The movement of the **hair cells** (14) **of the spiral organ** develops a nerve impulse.

The nerve impulse passes through the **cochlear branch** of the **vestibulocochlear nerve (CNVIII)** to the hearing centers in the brain.

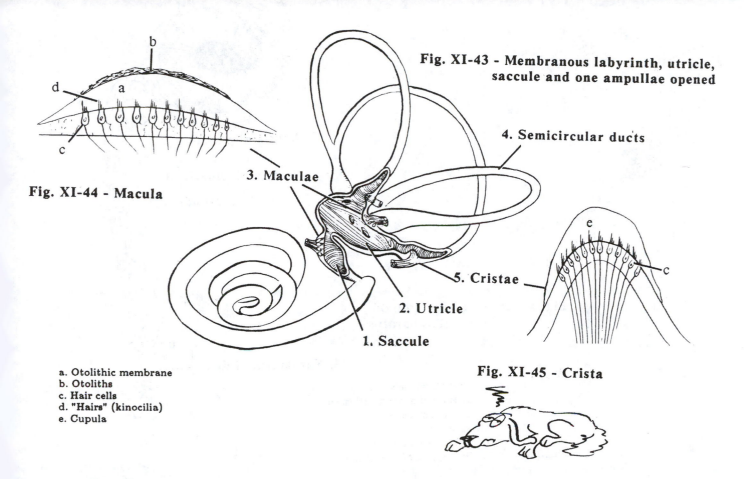

Fig. XI-43 - Membranous labyrinth, utricle, saccule and one ampullae opened

4. Semicircular ducts

3. Maculae

5. Cristae

2. Utricle

1. Saccule

Fig. XI-44 - Macula

a. Otolithic membrane
b. Otoliths
c. Hair cells
d. "Hairs" (kinocilia)
e. Cupula

Fig. XI-45 - Crista

VESTIBULE (Fig.XI-39): the central, expanded portion of the inner ear.

Membranous labyrinth of the vestibule (1,2): consists of two sacs called the utricle and the saccule.

1. Saccule: a sac of the membranous labyrinth.

2. Utricle: connected to the saccule by a small duct.

3. Maculae (MAK-yoo-lee) (sin. = macula): static equilibrium receptors located perpendicular to each other in the utricle and saccule.

Hair (receptor) cells (c): the receptor cells of maculae carrying impulses to the vestibular branch of the vestibulocochlear nerve (CNVIII). The otolithic (oh-toh-LITH-ik) membrane (a) is a gelatinous layer over the hair cells in which the "hairs" (kinocilia) (d) are embedded. The otoliths (b) are calcium carbonate crystals forming a layer over the otolithic membrane.

PHYSIOLOGY of STATIC EQUILIBRIUM: The otolithic membrane (a) is moved by the weight of the otoliths (b) under the pull of gravity. Thus, static equilibrium is concerned with "body (head) position" relative to gravity. This bends the hair cells (c) embedded in the otolithic membrane, generating a nerve action

potential. The impulse is carried by the vestibular branch of the vestibulocochlear nerve to the brain.

SEMICIRCULAR CANALS: the three bony canals arising from the vestibule, arranged at approximately right angles to each other.

Ampulla: an enlarged swelling at the end of each semicircular canal.

Membranous labyrinth (fig. XI-35): lines the bony labyrinth.

4. Semicircular ducts: the membranous labyrinth of the semicircular canals communicating with the utricle.

5. Crista: the receptor organ found in the ampulla of each semicircular duct. Composed of hair (receptor) cells and supporting cells, it senses <u>motion</u> of the head. The cupula (e) is a gelatinous mass covering the crista.

PHYSIOLOGY of DYNAMIC EQUILIBRIUM: When the head moves, endolymph pushes the cupula (e) bending the hair cells (c) which send impulses via the vestibular branch of the vestibulocochlear nerve (CNVIII) to the brain, thus, detecting angular (rotational) acceleration or deceleration of the head.

LACRIMAL APPARATUS

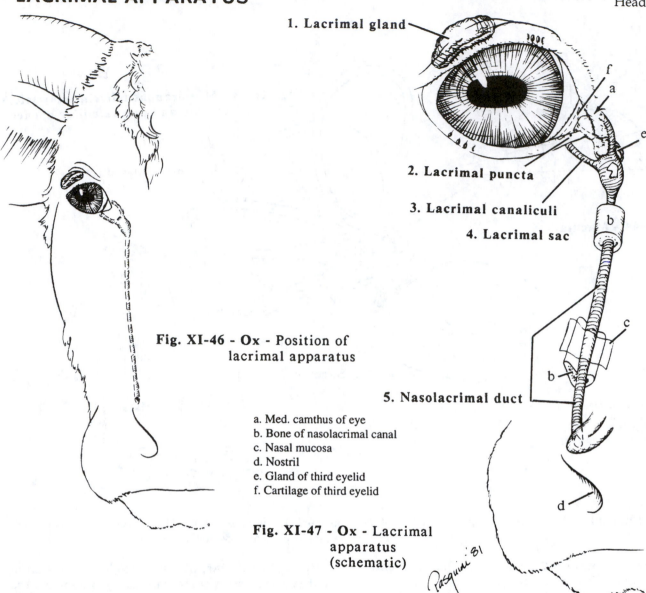

1. Lacrimal gland

2. Lacrimal puncta

3. Lacrimal canaliculi

4. Lacrimal sac

Fig. XI-46 - Ox - Position of
lacrimal apparatus

5. Nasolacrimal duct

a. Med. camthus of eye
b. Bone of nasolacrimal canal
c. Nasal mucosa
d. Nostril
e. Gland of third eyelid
f. Cartilage of third eyelid

Fig. XI-47 - Ox - Lacrimal
apparatus
(schematic)

LACRIMAL APPARATUS: the group of structures that manufacture and drain away tears.

1. Lacrimal gland: the pink gland lying on the dorsolateral aspect of the eyeball. It releases its seromucous secretions via a number of ducts onto the surface of the eyeball.

2. Lacrimal puncta: the openings of the lacrimal canaliculi on the upper and lower eyelids near the medial angle (canthus).

3. Lacrimal canaliculi: the small canals from the lacrimal puncta to the lacrimal sac.

Lacrimal sac: located in a fossa in the lacrimal bone's orbital surface, it marks the beginning of the nasolacrimal duct.

5. Nasolacrimal duct: the duct extending from the lacrimal sac to the rostral part of the nasal cavity, first traveling in a bony canal in the lacrimal and maxillary bones and then deep to the nasal

mucosa before opening into the rostral nasal cavity.

Innervation: parasympathetic innervation by the facial nerve (CnVII). These fibers are in the area of the middle ear along with the sympathetic innervation.

CLINICAL

Middle ear infection: can affect the parasympathetic fibers of the facial nerve to the lacrimal gland and cause decreased secretion of the lacrimal gland, resulting in keratoconjunctivitis sicca.

Keratoconjunctivitis sicca: drying of the cornea and conjunctiva due to malfunction of the lacrimal gland. This can be treated by transposing the parotid duct to the inside of the upper eyelid. When the dog sees food it will salivate ("spit") onto its cornea.

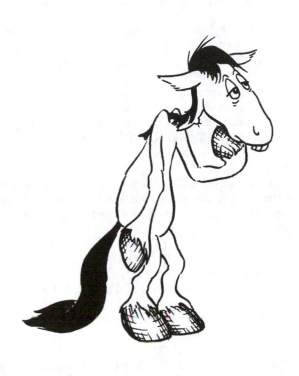

Appendix

TYPES OF NERVES

SIMPLIFIED FUNCTIONAL CLASSIFICATION of NERVE FIBERS. The functional classification of nerve fibers is confusing (complicated); with the words special, general, visceral, and somatic meaning different things for different neurons. Students have difficulty learning the complicated method and soon forget it if not constantly used. For learning purposes, this text simplifies this classification by dividing the nerves consisting of certain fibers into three groups: 1. Motor and sensory fibers, 2. ANS fibers, and 3. Special sensory fibers. The simplified and old "complicated" functional classifications are compared as a reference for books that use the complicated method.

1. Motor and **sensory fibers: somatic** motor fibers to skeletal muscle and somatic sensory fibers from skin and deeper somatic structures (skeletal muscle, skin, tendons, bones, etc.).

2. ANS fibers (motor and sensory): fibers to and from smooth muscle, cardiac muscle, and glands. These fibers, both motor and sensory fibers, are part of the autonomic nervous system (ANS). They are subdivided into fibers of the sympathetic and parasympathetic divisions. Sympathetic fibers are carried by branches of all spinal and most cranial nerves. Parasympathetic fibers are restricted to some sacral spinal roots (pelvic nerve) and only a few cranial nerves (Cnn III, VII, IX and X):

3. Special sensory fibers: fibers carrying taste, smell, vision, hearing & vestibular function over a few cranial nerves (Cnn I, II, VII, VIII, and IX.

NERVE FIBERS: nerves can have any combination of these fibers. Nerves that innervate skeletal muscle carry sensory information from the muscle. The sensory component is understood, but ignored in naming motor nerves. All spinal nerves and most cranial nerves possessing ANS sympathetic motor fibers are ignored in this classification. The initials indicate the complicated functional classification of fibers carried by each type of nerve.

• **Mixed nerve:** consist of both somatic sensory and motor fibers (e.g., radial nerve).

• **Motor nerve:** motor innervation to skeletal muscle, no somatic sensory fibers (e.g., facial nerve)

• **Sensory nerve:** carries only sensory fibers (e.g., ophthalmic and maxillary division of the trigeminal nerve)

• **Special sensory nerve:** carry special sensory fibers of smell, taste, vision, hearing and balance (e.g., optic, vestibulocochlear).

• **Nerves carrying ANS fibers:** all spinal nerves and some cranial nerves.

Outlined below is the relationship of the "simplified" functional classification to the actual "complicated" functional classification.

MOTOR (SVE, GSE) and **SENSORY FIBERS** (GSA): the somatic motor fibers (SVE and GSE) supply striated skeletal muscle. The difference between SVE and GSE is the type of embryonic tissue the muscles from which they innervate are derived. GSA fibers carry sensory information from SVE & GSE supplied muscles. GSA fibers also carry sensory information from skin and other deep structures other than muscles and are called sensory fibers. The simplified method groups all these (SVE, GSE & GSA) into motor and sensory fibers.

• **Special visceral efferent (SVE):** motor fibers supplying striated skeletal muscle derived from embryonic branchial arch mesoderm. These are found in only a few <u>cranial nerves</u>:

> viz. - Muscles of mastication (Cn V)
> - Muscles of facial expression (Cn VII)
> - Muscles of palate, pharynx, esophagus, & larynx (Cnn IX, X & XI)
> - Trapezius muscle (Cn XI)

• **General somatic efferent (GSE):** motor fibers supplying striated skeletal muscle with the exception of those derived from branchial arch mesoderm. Such fibers are found in branches of all spinal and some cranial nerves:

> viz. - Extraocular muscles (Cnn III, IV, & VI);
> - Muscles of the tongue (Cn XII)
> - Striated muscles of the neck, trunk, tail, diaphragm, thoracic and pelvic limbs (spinal nerves)
> - Striated sphincters of the urinary and gastrointestinal tracts (pudendal n.)

• **General somatic afferent (GSA):** sensory fibers supplying the body surface (skin and subcutaneous tissue) as well as deeper structures (bones, skeletal muscles, tendons, etc.) derived from embryonic somatic mesoderm. Fibers are found in branches of all spinal nerves, but only a few cranial nerves.

> viz. - Skin of head and face, and lining of the nasal and oral cavities (Cn V)
> - Skin of the rest of body, tendons, ligaments, joint capsules and skeletal muscles throughout the body.

ANS FIBERS, motor (GVE) and **sensory** (GVA): carry motor (GVE) and sensory (GVA) fibers to and from smooth muscle, cardiac muscle, and glands, respectively.

• **General visceral efferents (GVE):** motor fibers supplying smooth muscle, cardiac muscle, and glands throughout the body. This fiber classification may be subdivided into sympathetic and parasympathetic components, which are part of all spinal nerves and most cranial nerves (sympathetic GVE). Some may be restricted to sacral spinal roots forming the pelvic nerve and a few cranial nerves (parasympathetic GVE):

560

TYPES OF NERVES

viz.· Parasympathetic GVE:
- Smooth muscle of the ciliary body and iris (Cn III)
- Salivary, nasal, and lacrimal glands (Cnn VII & IX)
- Smooth muscle of cervical, thoracic & abdominal viscera & cardiac muscle (heart)(Cn X)
- Smooth muscle of the pelvic viscera (pelvic nerve)

Sympathetic GVE (cranial nerves & spinal nerves):
- Smooth muscle, glands, and blood vessels of the skin of head, trunk & limbs
- Smooth muscle of cranial, cervical, thoracic & pelvic blood vessels and viscera
- Cardiac muscle of the heart

• General visceral afferent (GVA): sensory fibers supplying blood vessels and viscera throughout the head and body, and the endodermally-derived mucosa of the respiratory and gastrointestinal tracts caudal to the nasal and oral cavities. Such fibers are carried in branches of every spinal nerve and probably most cranial nerves:

viz. - Chemoreceptors and baroreceptors associated with the internal carotid artery & aortic arch (Cnn IX & X)
- Mucosa of the nasopharynx, oropharynx & laryngopharynx (Cnn XI & X)

- Blood vessels, glands, & viscera of cranial cervical, thoracic, abdominal & pelvic regions
- Blood vessels & glands of the limbs

SPECIAL SENSORY FIBERS (SVA & SSA): carry special sensory information of taste, smell, vision, hearing & vestibular function.

• Special visceral afferents (SVA): sensory fibers responsible for carrying to the brain information related to taste and smell. All such fibers are associated with cranial nerves:

viz. - Taste receptors ("taste buds") in the tongue, palate & epiglottis (Cnn VII, XI & X)
- Olfactory receptors on the nasal epithelium (Cn I)

• Special somatic afferent (SSA): sensory fibers responsible for carrying to the brain information related to vision, hearing and vestibular function (balance, body position, etc.). All such fibers are associated with cranial nerves:

viz. - Photoreceptors in retina (Cn II)
- Auditory receptors of the cochlea in the inner ear (Cn VIII - cochlear part)
- Receptors in the vestibular apparatus in the inner ear (Cn VIII - vestibular part)

Classification - functional fiber	Somatic NS		ANS		Special senses	
Simplified	Motor	Sensory	Motor	Sensory	Special sensory Taste, smell	Vision, hearing, balance
Detailed	SVE, GSE	GSA	GVE	GVA	SVA	SSA

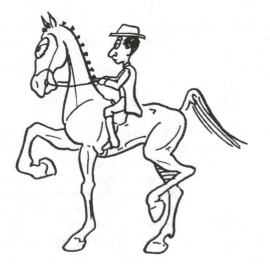

NEUROANATOMY

Neuroanatomy and neurology, historically, have been portrayed as requiring an elite knowledge to master. This section attempts to simplify neuroanatomy for the future practicing veterinarian, not the future neurologist. A basic understanding of the "skeleton" of neuroanatomy will help the "country" veterinarian to localize neurological lesions without fancy equipment. This is an introduction to build on, thus, touches only on a limited number of structures. Once these are learned, the more advanced literature will hopefully be less daunting to the student. Localizing lesions in the nervous system requires a basic understanding of how the nervous system is organized, its structures, and connections. The nervous system can be divided into a central nervous system (CNS) which includes the brain and spinal cord; and a peripheral nervous system consisting of the cranial and spinal nerves and ganglia. The nervous system is also organized in a segmental fashion consisting of peripheral spinal and cranial nerves and the part of the central nervous system from which they arise.

SPINAL CORD: can be divided into segments.

1. Spinal cord segment and its pair of spinal nerves: A spinal cord segment is demarcated by the pair of spinal nerves that arise from it. Spinal nerves consist of sensory and motor fibers that pass over the dorsal (sensory) and ventral (motor) roots, respectively.

2. Reflex arcs: the functional units of the nervous system. They are programmed motor actions. A reflex arc consists of a receptor, a sensory neuron, usually one or more interneurons, a motor neuron, and an effector.

3. Lower motor neuron (LMN): the efferent neuron of a reflex arc that connects the spinal cord to the muscles and glands of the body. The lower motor neuron can be spontaneously active. Modification of the reflex arc by higher centers produces specific actions.

4. Upper motor neurons (UMN): pass in <u>descending motor tracts</u> that connect higher centers (the brain and brain stem) with the lower motor neurons of the reflex arcs. They usually act to inhibit the spontaneous activity of the lower motor neuron until an action is desired. They then stimulate the lower motor neuron to produce a programmed action.

5. Ascending sensory tracts: carry sensory (afferent) information up the spinal cord to higher centers in the spinal cord and brain. Sensory (afferent) neurons carry such information as pain, temperature, touch, and proprioception from the periphery up the spinal cord to the brain. The main information used clinically is superficial pain, deep pain, and proprioception.

• 6. Proprioceptive fibers: sense the position of different body parts in relationship to each other and to the environment. This sense is carried from receptors in the skin, fascia, muscles, and joints up peripheral nerves to the spinal cord. Proprioceptive fibers then travel up the spinal cord to pass through the brain stem to reach the cerebellum and cerebral cortex. The cerebral cortex interprets this information and sends motor information down descending tracts to reflex arcs to make adjustments in <u>posture</u>.

The cerebellum uses proprioceptive information to coordinate posture and movement. Loss of proprioception can indicate a lesion anywhere along this path: in a peripheral nerve, the spinal cord, brain stem, cerebrum, or cerebellum. Postural reactions are used to evaluate proprioception.

• 7. Superficial and deep pain sensory fibers: travel up the peripheral nerves, spinal cord, and brain stem to the cerebrum to be perceived.

Myotome: the muscles or muscle groups innervated by a spinal nerve (LMN).

Dermatome: the area of skin innervated by one spinal nerve (sensory). Knowing the spinal segments innervating myotomes and dermatomes can be used to localize lesions.

BRAIN: also organized into segments, although less distinct. Functionally, it can be divided into cerebrum, thalamus, brain stem, vestibular system, and cerebellum.

8. Cerebrum: includes the cerebral hemispheres and basal nuclei. It deals with voluntary motor control, behavior, and mental status. It interprets vision and audition, proprioception, and general sensations.

9. Thalamus: a part of the brain stem. Functionally, it is closely related to the cerebrum to which it relays information. It also controls the autonomic nervous system (ANS) and the endocrine system.

10. Brainstem: functionally includes the midbrain, pons, and medulla oblongata.

• Walking motion reflex centers: located caudal to the midbrain. Higher centers initiate and stop the motion through descending motor tracts that <u>cross over</u> in the midbrain. A cat with its cerebrum removed (decerebrate) can be made to walk/run by putting electrodes into the brainstem.

• Reticular activating system: Housed in the brain stem, it is concerned with the conscious level (alertness, depression, stupor, and coma).

• Cranial nerves II to XII: associated with the brainstem.

11. Vestibular system: controls posture and balance in relationship to gravity; and eye movements in relationship to head movements. It is divided into peripheral and central portions.

• Peripheral vestibular centers: located in the inner ear, they consist of the labyrinth, receptors, and the vestibular nerve.

• Central vestibular portion: includes the vestibular nuclei in the brain stem and centers in the cerebellum.

12. Cerebellum: concerned with coordinating movements, but does not initiate them. It also has connections to the vestibular

NERVOUS SYSTEM

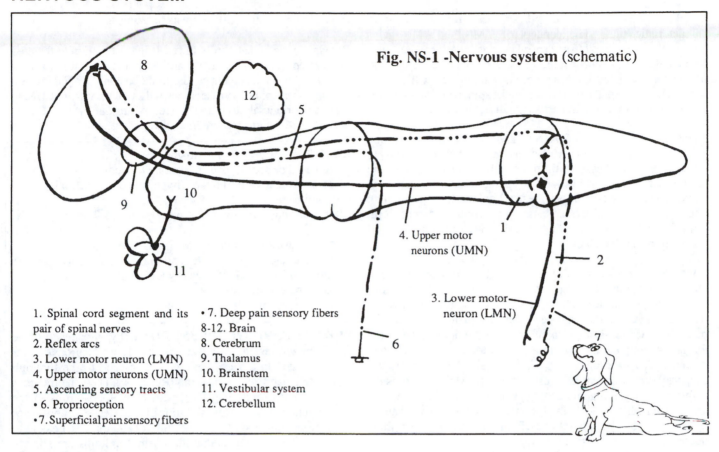

Fig. NS-1 -Nervous system (schematic)

1. Spinal cord segment and its pair of spinal nerves
2. Reflex arcs
3. Lower motor neuron (LMN)
4. Upper motor neurons (UMN)
5. Ascending sensory tracts
• 6. Proprioception
• 7. Superficial pain sensory fibers
• 7. Deep pain sensory fibers
8-12. Brain
8. Cerebrum
9. Thalamus
10. Brainstem
11. Vestibular system
12. Cerebellum

4. Upper motor neurons (UMN)

3. Lower motor neuron (LMN)

system to help coordinate balance and posture.

DEFINITIONS: Once the organization and functions of the different parts of the central nervous system are understood, lesions affecting each part can be discerned. First, some terms need to be understood:

Analgesia: the absence of pain perception.

Depression: an awake animal that is relatively unresponsive to its environment.

Stupor: an animal that sleeps unless aroused by a strong stimulus.

Coma: an unconscious animal that can't be aroused. Complete disconnection of the reticular activation system from the cerebral cortex causes coma and is usually due to a severe brain stem lesion.

Paralysis: the complete loss of motor activity.

Paresis (weakness): the partial loss of voluntary motor activity. Paresis and paralysis are due to partial or complete loss, respectively, of voluntary motor stimulation due to damage of either UMNs or LMNs. The suffix -paresis and -plegia are used to describe paresis and paralysis, respectively:
• Monoparesis or monoplegia: one limb is involved.
• Hemiparesis or hemiplegia: both limbs on one side.
• Tetraparesis/quadraparesis or tetraplegia/ quadriaplegia: all four limbs are involved.

• Paraparesis or paraplegia: only the pelvic limbs.

Flaccid paresis or **paralysis:** decreased or no tone with paresis or paralysis due to lesions of LMNs.

Spastic paresis or **paralysis:** extra tone (hypertonicity) with paresis or paralysis due to lesions of UMNs.

Hypertonicity: excessive muscle tone (not tetany which is rigid, fixed muscle contraction).

Ataxia: a lack of coordinated movements with or without spasticity or paresis. Lesions of the entire nervous system neuroaxis may cause ataxia. Although not specific, it shows up frequently and is indicative of the nervous system.

Tremor: small, rapid, alternating movements at rest.

• **Intention tremor:** a tremor that becomes worse with initiation of a movement and disappears at rest. It indicates cerebellar disease.

Myoclonus (flexor spasm): coarse jerking moments of muscle groups at rest.

Dysmetria (Gr. *dys*, abnormal + *metron*, measure): improper measuring of distance in muscular activity, either too short or too long a range of motion (e.g., goose stepping). Cerebellar disease causes dysmetria (especially hypermetria).

LMN / UMN

UMN or LMN: spinal cord and peripheral injuries will have characteristic signs. The concept of UMN and LMN helps differentiate peripheral from central lesions; and, if central, helps localize the level of the lesion. The central nervous system will not regenerate. If the cord is severed, function below the lesion will not be restored. Partial damage to the spinal cord may recover in time, but after a certain period it will not improve.

LOWER MOTOR NEURON (LMN): the final common pathway from the central nervous system (brain or spinal cord) to a muscle or gland. These are the motor parts of the reflex arcs. The somatic nervous system has one LMN per reflex arc, the autonomic nervous system has two LMNs (preganglionic and postganglionic). The cell bodies of a LMNs are located in the brain and spinal cord. They leave the CNS over the ventral roots, spinal nerves, and cranial nerves to reach the periphery.

LMN damage: can affect the nerve in the periphery or its cell body in the spinal cord segment or brain stem, causing loss of activity of the muscle or gland innervated, resulting in paresis or paralysis. This is a flaccid type ("limp as a dish rag") paresis or paralysis due to loss of the spontaneous stimulation of the LMN. Partial or complete damage to a lower motor neuron results in decreased (hypotonia) to no tone (atonia) and decreased reflexes (hyporeflexia) to absent reflexes (areflexia). LMN damage results in fast atrophy (neurogenic atrophy) within one week. These signs are very valuable in localizing lesions. (With lower motor neuron dysfunction point your thumb to the floor to indicate that everything decreases or disappears).

UPPER MOTOR NEURON (UMN): a central nervous system neuron that effects lower motor neurons. UMNs are responsible for initiating and maintaining conscious movements and for tone in the extensor muscles to maintain posture. Located totally in the central nervous system, they project down descending motor tracts onto lower motor neurons, either directly or through interneurons. The ultimate UMNs are in the cerebral cortex (voluntary center, the seat of true consciousness). There are two populations of UMNs - excitatory and inhibitory. The excitatory UMNs, under normal conditions, are kept inactive, thus, the descending tracts usually inhibit LMN activity. LMNs are spontaneously active without the input of UMN. If the UMNs are damaged, the LMNs increase their activity.

UMN damage causes loss of the ability to initiate voluntary motor activity, and possibly uncontrolled hyperactivity due to decrease of inhibition on LMNs. (Therefore, point your thumb up with UMN damage to indicate that activity goes up). In UMN diseases the tone will be normal to increased. Reflexes will tend to be normal or increased (normoreflexia or hyperreflexia). They will show a spastic paresis or paralysis. The atrophy is a disuse type (not neurogenic), because the LMNs are intact. These LMNs still stimulate the muscles through reflexes, thus, the atrophy will have a slow onset. An animal with a minimal UMN loss and the ability to walk may not develop significant atrophy. To compensate for posture, the extensors have more tone than the flexors. So with loss of upper motor neuron input on lower motor neurons the extensors are facilitated more than the flexors, resulting in an extended limb with spastic paresis or paralysis.

Damage to the spinal cord will result in dysfunction to the area innervated (LMN damage), and hyperactivity to muscles innervated from segments caudal to the lesion (UMN damage). Damage to a spinal cord segment will show LMN, not UMN, signs to peripheral structures its reflex arc innervates. This is because UMN signs require intact LMNs.

LMN disease signs (thumb down)
- Decreased or absent tone (hypotonia to atonia)
- Decreased to absent reflexes (hyporeflexia to areflexia)
- Flaccid paralysis
- Rapid atrophy (neurogenic atrophy) within 5-7 days

UMN disease signs (thumb up)
- Normal to increased muscle tone (normotonia to hypertonia)
- Normal to increased reflexes (hyperflexia)
- Spastic paresis to paralysis
- Slow (disuse) atrophy

SHIFF-SHERRINGTON SYNDROME: hyperextension of the forelimbs with lesions to the thoracic spinal cord. Neurons (border cells), located in the L_{1-4} spinal cord, ascend to the forelimb centers to synapse on interneurons (Renshaw). These interneurons synapse on and inhibit extensor lower motor neurons in the cervical enlargement. This inhibition of the extensors coordinates walking movements between the limbs of quadrupeds. Lesions to this pathway remove inhibition, so the forelimbs are slightly hyperextended. Lower and upper motor neurons are still intact to the thoracic limb, therefore, this is neither an upper or lower motor neuron sign. This is the only time a spinal cord injury will show signs cranial to the point of the injury. It is usually a bad sign prognostically, indicating a serious lesion of the spinal cord. The hind limb would show UMN signs (activity goes up) when Shiff-Sherington signs are seen in the forelimb. This often causes confusion in localization.

UMN/ LMN - localization of lesions: Knowing the difference between LMN and UMN signs can be used to localize a spinal cord lesion. LMN signs always take preference to UMN signs clinically. If both are affected, the signs will be LMN because UMN signs require intact LMNs.

Example 1:
- Signs: flaccid paralysis, absent reflexes, decreased (↓) tone, rapid atrophy and loss of proprioception to the pelvic limbs with normal thoracic limbs.

- Indicates a L_4-S_1 spinal cord lesion (Area 4) (LMN signs to pelvic limbs).

Example 2:
- Signs: spastic paresis, increased (↑) reflexes and tone to the left pelvic limb and flaccid paralysis, decreased (↓) reflexes and tone to the left thoracic limb and loss of proprioception to all limbs.

LMN / UMN

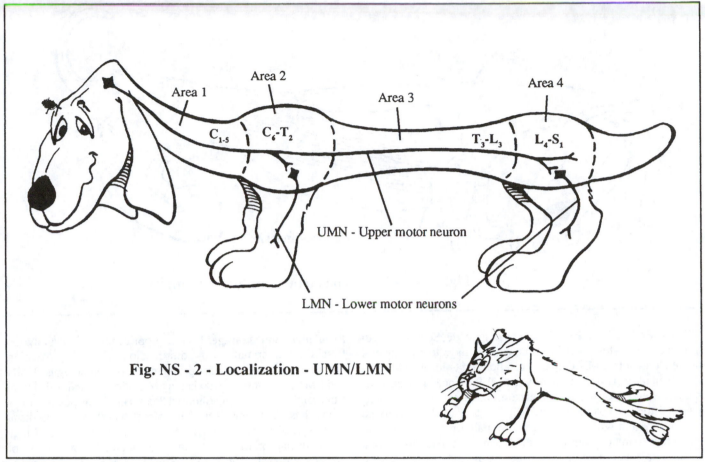

Fig. NS - 2 - Localization - UMN/LMN

Labels in figure:
Area 1, Area 2, Area 3, Area 4
C_{1-5}, C_6-T_2, T_3-L_3, L_4-S_1
UMN - Upper motor neuron
LMN - Lower motor neurons

• Indicates a unilateral C_6-T_1 spinal cord lesion (Area 2) on the left (LMN signs to the left thoracic limb and UMN signs to left pelvic limb).

Example 3:
• Signs: spastic paresis, increased (↑) reflexes and tone and loss of proprioception in the pelvic limbs with normal thoracic limbs.

• Indicates: a T_3-L_3 spinal cord lesion (Area 3)(UMN signs in pelvic limbs - note absence of a Shiff-Sherrington sign in the thoracic limbs).

Example 4:
• Signs: spastic paresis, increased (↑) reflexes and tone and loss of proprioception to all limbs.

• Indicates a C_{1-5} spinal cord lesion (Area 1) or brain lesion (UMN signs to all limbs).

Example 5:
• Signs: spastic paresis, increased (↑) reflexes and tone and loss of proprioception to the left pelvic limb, and normal thoracic limbs.

• Indicates a unilateral T_3-L_3 spinal cord lesion (Area 3) on the left (UMN signs to left pelvic limb).

Example 6:
• Signs: hyperextended thoracic limb, increased (↑) reflexes and tone and loss of proprioception in the pelvic limbs.

• Indicates: a T_3-L_3 spinal cord lesion (Area 3)(UMN signs in pelvic limbs and a Shiff-Sherrington sign in the thoracic limbs).

Table 1 LESION - LMN/UMN - LOCALIZATION
Lesion 1 – transect spinal cord from C_{1-5}: • No LMN signs to either limb • UMN signs & proprioceptive deficits to all limbs
Lesion 2 – in cervical enlargement, C_6-T_2: • LMN to thoracic limb • UMN signs & proprioceptive deficits to pelvic limbs
Lesion 3 – damage in T_3-L_3: • No effect on thoracic limb (+/- Shiff-Sherington) • UMN signs & proprioceptive deficits to pelvic limb
Lesion 4 – damage to L_4 - S_1 • No effect on thoracic limb • LMN to pelvic limb, even if UMN are also damaged

565

SENSORY

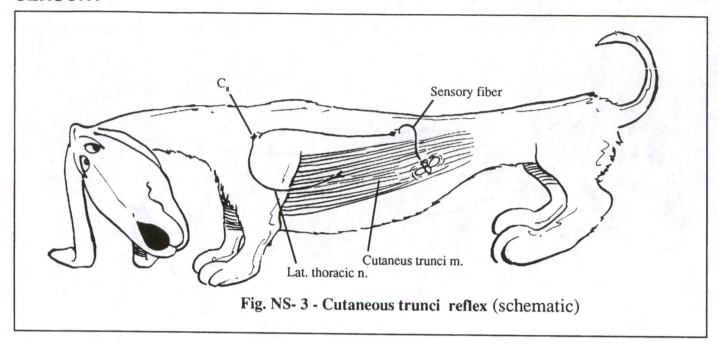

Fig. NS- 3 - Cutaneous trunci reflex (schematic)

OBSERVATION of PAIN: may be diagnostic. Sensory loss to a dermatome (which would occur with damage to a peripheral nerve along with LMN damage) can be used to localize lesions. Assessment of pain is in three parts: (1) Presence or location of pain, (2) Perception of superficial pain, and (3) Perception of deep pain. History and palpation will help locate pain. Lesions to the nervous system will cause decrease in pain distal to the lesion. Therefore, palpate from distal to proximal. Palpate just strong enough to elicit pain. Palpate the limbs and the trunk in a systematic manner.
- Limbs - palpate from distal to proximal.
- Trunk - palpate.
- Vertebral pain - palpate.
  - Lumbosacral region - press over the lumbosacral junction, or extend the hip to stretch the ischiatic nerve.
- Neck - flex and extend the neck carefully.

Ascending sensory tracts: carry sensation up the spinal cord to higher centers. Clinically, the loss of these sensations (superficial pain, deep pain and proprioception) can help localize lesions in spinal cord compression and provide prognostic indicators.

Superficial pain sensory fibers: These are lost about the same time as motor functions. **Superficial pain perception** is evaluated by using a gentle pinch of a pair of hemostats to the skin. If superficial pain is perceived, deep pain will also be perceived. Perception causes a behavioral change such as looking toward the stimulus or attempts to bite. A withdrawal of the structure (limb) from the stimulus is a reflex, it DOES NOT require perception.

Deep pain: the first sensory fibers to show signs and the last to disappear (**first to show, last to go**). Loss of deep pain is a bad prognostic sign. Deep pain is evaluated when superficial pain is absent. Increase the pressure of the superficial pain pinch and watch for a behavioral change (attempt to bite).

Proprioception damage: loss of proprioception is usually the first sign in spinal cord compression. Therefore, testing proprioception will indicate problems before other signs (UMN and LMN) are present. Ataxia may be noticed which is different from cerebellar ataxia. The animal doesn't know the position of its limbs, thus, can't adjust them. The animal may stand with its distal limbs spread (base wide stance), may knuckle over, and may delay initiation of movement. For localization, losses of proprioception are interpreted the same as LMN/UMN signs (i.e., loss of proprioception in the thoracic limb indicates a lesion in the spinal cord segment C_5-T_1 or cranial to C_5).

Cutaneous trunci reflex or panniculus reflex: a normal reflex where a stimulus (e.g., a fly) to the lateral trunk causes the cutaneus trunci muscle to twitch. Sensory fibers extend from their dermatomes (bands of skin sensation) obliquely craniodorsally to synapse in the thoracolumbar spinal cord segments. Ascending sensory tracts extend up the spinal cord to the cell body of the lateral thoracic nerve in spinal cord segment C_8. The <u>lateral thoracic nerve</u> supplies motor innervation to the cutaneous trunci muscle. The dermatomes are one or two vertebrae caudal to the point of origin of the sensory nerves. If a panniculus response is absent caudally and then appears cranial to a specific point (e.g., transverse plane through L_1) the lesion is in the spinal cord up to two vertebrae cranially (at T_{12}-T_{13}). This response is not found over the sacral or cervical areas.

Hyperesthesia: abnormal increase in sensitivity. Lesions to a spinal cord segment will cause a focal hyperesthesia to the dermatome supplied.

Diffuse or **multifocal pain**: often due to inflammation.

Focal pain: often due to compression of the spinal cord or nerve root.

PERIPHERAL NERVES

PERIPHERAL NERVE LESIONS: problems localized to only one limb (monoparesis) by LMN signs. The problem is in the specific nerve roots, nerve or group of nerves or muscles they innervate. These can be evaluated by knowing the motor and the cutaneous innervation of the limbs, then mapping the deficits. Damage to individual nerves will result in little gait abnormalities, except in the case of the radial, femoral, ischiatic, or peroneal nerves. All peripheral nerve damage will show loss of cutaneous sensation (analgesia) to the dermatomes they innervate.

BRACHIAL PLEXUS

Suprascapular nerve damage (C_{6-7}): causes marked atrophy to the supraspinatus and infraspinatus muscles. This is called "sweeney" in horses. Before atrophy, this will cause lateral slipping of the shoulder in the horse.

Musculocutaneous nerve damage (C_{6-8}): analgesia to medial surface of the forelimb and inability to flex the elbow.

Radial nerve damage (C_6-T_2): depending on the level of damage, will show different muscular deficits. If above the innervation of the triceps brachii muscle, the animal will not be able to bear weight on the limb because it can't extend the elbow, and the paw will knuckle over. Damage distal to the triceps brachii will result in knuckling over because the paw can't be extended. Analgesia will be to the dorsal surface of the paw and forelimb in the dog. In horses, the radial nerve only reaches the carpus.

Median nerve damage (C_8-T_2): will have little gait abnormalities, maybe a little sinking of the carpus and metacarpophalangeal joints. There will be partial loss of analgesia to the palmar surface of the paw.

Ulnar nerve damage (C_8-T_2): analgesia to the lateral digit (V) of the paw.

Sympathetic nerve damage: although not part of the brachial plexus, their preganglionic fibers travel over the roots of the brachial plexus and can be damaged with the brachial plexus nerves. Signs are miosis, ptosis, and enophthalmia (Horner's syndrome).

Avulsions of the roots of the brachial plexus: the pulling off of the spinal roots from the spinal cord due to trauma (hit by car). Signs exhibited will depend on the number of roots involved. If all roots of C_6-T_1 are involved, the limb will be paralyzed and drag on the ground, along with loss of sensation distal to the elbow.

LUMBOSACRAL PLEXUS:

Obturator nerve damage (L_{4-6}): will cause lateral slipping on a slick surface due to loss of adductor muscle control.

Femoral nerve damage (L_{3-6}): will result in severe gait deficits; the animal can't bear weight on the pelvic limb because it can't extend the stifle. Analgesia occurs on the medial surface of the limb.

Ischiatic nerve damage (L_5-S_2): results in knuckling over (peroneal nerve), but has the ability to bear weight (intact femoral nerve). There will be loss of sensation below the stifle, except on the medial side (saphenous nerve).

Peroneal damage (L_5-S_2): results in knuckling over due to inability to extend the digits. Cutaneous sensation is lost to the dorsal surface of the leg and pes.

Tibial nerve damage (L_5-S_2): results in dropping of the hock and analgesia to the plantar side of the paw.

SYSTEMIC or MULTIFOCAL NERVOUS SYSTEM DISEASE: do not have signs consistent with a single focal lesion; have diffuse or multifocal signs (e.g., inflammation, nutritional, toxic, or metabolic diseases). Inflammation usually causes diffuse or multifocal pain.

Table 2 - Peripheral nerves - thoracic limb		
Nerve & spinal cord segment		**Clinical sign of damage**
Suprascapular	C_{6-7}	Motor - atrophy of supraspinatus and infraspinatus muscles
Musculocutaneous	C_{6-8}	Sensory loss - med. side of limb Motor - inability to flex elbow

Radial	C_6-T_2	Motor -
		  High - inability to bear weight
		  Low - knuckling over
		Sensory loss - dors. forelimb (only to carpus in horse)

Median	C_8-T_3	Motor - little effect Sensory loss, partial - palmar paw
Ulnar	C_8-T_3	Motor - little affect Sensory - analgesia fifth digit
Sympathetic	C_8-T_3	Miosis, ptosis & enophthalmia

Table 3 - Peripheral nerves - pelvic limb		
Nerve & spinal cord segment		**Clinical sign of damage**
Obturator	L_{3-6}	Motor - lateral slipping
Femoral	L_{3-6}	Motor - inability to bear weight Sensory loss - med. limb (saphenous)
Sciatic	L_5-S_2	Motor - nuckling over Sensory loss - all leg and pes, except med. surface
Peroneal	L_5-S_2	Motor - knuckling over Sensory loss - dorsal leg & pes
Tibial	L_5-S_2	Motor - little affect Sensory loss - plantar leg and pes

BRAIN

Lesions of the brain stem (midbrain, pons and medulla oblongata): by affecting the reticular activation system, will decrease degrees of consciousness from depression to stupor to coma. Deficits in cranial nerves III to XII, arising from the brain stem may indicate brain stem lesions. Walking motion reflexes are generated in centers caudal to the midbrain. Higher centers initiate the motion through descending motor tracts that <u>cross over</u> in the midbrain. Therefore, the midbrain is a clinical localization point for most motor tract systems. Lesions rostral to the midbrain (cerebro-diencephalic disorders) affect the contralateral (opposite) side of the body with proprioceptive deficits, but a normal gait. Lesions caudal to the midbrain (brain stem and spinal cord) cause ipsilateral (same side) proprioceptive deficits with an abnormal gait. An animal with a normal gait and proprioceptive deficits on both sides has a lesion in the midbrain.

Lesion to the vestibular system: affects the ability to control posture in relationship to gravity; and eye movements in relationship to head movements. Head tilt, nystagmus, ataxia, possibly circling, and strabismus are all signs of vestibular disease. Central vestibular disease will also affect other motor and sensory centers in the brain stem, resulting in postural deficits (proprioception) and <u>paresis</u> (UMN). Depression is also seen with central lesions. Peripheral vestibular disease will not produce UMN signs (paresis). Peripheral lesions also don't affect proprioceptive fibers, but the postural reactions appear abnormal (ataxic) because of loss of balance.

Cerebellar lesions: cause incoordination of movements (ataxia), intention tremors, and abnormal movements of the head and body. Lesions can also cause signs of vestibular disease, including head tilt and nystagmus.

Cerebral lesions to the cerebral hemispheres or basal nuclei: may produce alterations in behavior and seizures. A normal gait (the walking centers are caudal to the midbrain) with abnormal postural reactions may be seen because proprioceptive fibers pass to the cerebral cortex. Damage to the occipital (vision) lobe will result in loss of vision, with normal pupillary responses.

Lesions to the thalamus: functionally related to the cerebrum, showing similar signs. Autonomic and endocrine abnormalities (polyuria, polydypsia, altered sleep patterns) are also possible.

Table 4 - Lesions of brain - signs

Brain stem:
Proprioceptive deficits with a normal gait indicate a lesion in or rostral to the midbrain
Proprioceptive deficits with abnormal gait indicate a lesion caudal to the midbrain
- Proprioceptive deficits (unilateral) and normal gait, a lesion rostral to midbrain on contralateral side
- Proprioceptive deficits (bilateral) and normal gait, a lesion probably in the midbrain
- Proprioceptive deficits (unilateral) and abnormal gait, a lesion caud. to the midbrain on ipsilateral side
- Decreased levels of consciousness (depression, stupor, coma)
- Deficits in cranial nerves III - XII

Vestibular system:
- Head tilt, nystagmus, asymmetric ataxia with possibly circling, and strabismus
Central vestibular disease
- Postural deficits (proprioception)
- Paresis (UMN)
- Depression
Peripheral disease
- No paresis
- Postural deficits (balance)
- No depression

Cerebellum:
- Incoordination of movements (ataxia), tremors, abnormal movements of the head
- Vestibular disease signs, including head tilt and nystagmus

Cerebrum:
- Alterations in behavior
- Seizures
- Normal gait with abnormal postural reactions (proprioception loss)
- Loss of vision (occipital lobe) with normal pupillary responses

Diencephalon:
- Cerebral signs
- Autonomic and endocrine abnormalities (polyuria, polydypsia, altered sleep patterns)

NEUROLOGIC TESTS

We discussed the segmental organization of the nervous system, the general functions of each segment, and the signs that lesions produce at each segment. Now we will discuss ways to evaluate different clinical signs.

POSTURAL REACTIONS: although not very specific, they are very sensitive indicators of abnormalities. If an animal doesn't have a profound gait deficit or obvious paralysis or paresis, postural reactions can establish the presence of slight paresis (weakness) or a proprioceptive deficit. They do not localize the problem. All postural reactions should be done on carpet or grass to keep the animal from slipping. Some of these reactions don't belong together physiologically speaking, but are convenient to do at the same time.

Screening postural reactions: hopping and proprioceptive positioning are more sensitive than other postural reactions. If they are normal, all other postural reactions will be normal. If they are abnormal, checking other reactions may be helpful.

Proprioceptive positioning: tests proprioceptive (sensory) information passing up the spinal cord to the cerebral cortex. Place the foot knuckled over (the dorsal surface of the paw down) on the floor. The animal should immediately reposition the foot to the normal position. To avoid touching the limb of small animals, the animal's paw can be placed on a folded piece of paper. Hold the animal's head up so they can't see its foot, and slide the paper laterally. The animal should immediately replace the limb properly. Proprioception tests are extremely sensitive tests, especially to evaluate the integrity of CNS proprioceptive tracts. If there is a consistent deficit with this test, there is a nervous system problem.
• A normal gait and proprioceptive loss indicates a lesion rostral to the midbrain; it can be in the sensory cortex.
• Proprioception is the first thing lost in spinal cord compression.

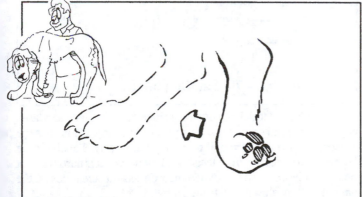

Fig. NA- 4 - Proprioceptive positioning

Hopping reaction: evaluates motor function, proprioception (both conscious and unconscious), and cerebellar function. Thus, although very sensitive, it doesn't localize a lesion. Suspend the dog (arm under belly) and allow one limb to touch the ground. Force weight on the supporting limb to check for weakness, while supporting the chin. Hop the animal forward and laterally. Do this

to all four limbs, looking for asymmetry between any limb and the other three limbs. With a large animal, lift one limb and push so the animal has to hop on the other limb, or push it laterally while standing and walking so it has to step laterally. Pulling the tail laterally can also be used to test the rear limb. This provides information about motor, sensory or cerebellar circuitry.
• Weakness may result in collapse after just standing or after one or two hops.
• Proprioceptive lesion: results in extremely delayed initiation of the hop.
• Cerebellar lesion: results in an exaggerated step when they hop. This is because the main cerebellar output is inhibitory.

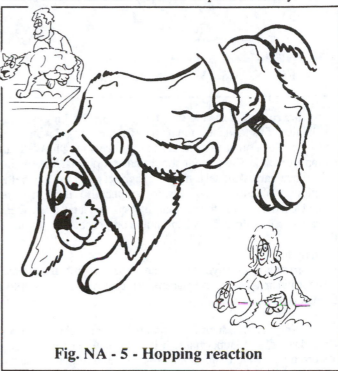

Fig. NA - 5 - Hopping reaction

If the animal has a normal gait and proprioceptive loss is indicated by the hopping reflex, the lesion is rostral to the midbrain. If there is an abnormal gait and proprioceptive loss, then the lesion is in or caudal to the midbrain. An animal that shows deficits in the right forelimb hopping reaction may have a lesion on the left side, rostral to the midbrain; or a lesion on the right side, caudal to the midbrain.

These two screening postural reactions, hopping and proprioceptions, are the most sensitive tests. If normal, the other postural reactions will be normal. If abnormal, then the following postural tests can be performed.

Extensor postural thrust: holding the animal up by its armpits, lower the hindlimbs to the floor. Normal animals will extend the rearlimbs and move them caudally. Pressing down may cause collapse in mild hindlimb paresis (paraparesis).
• Weakness, may result in collapse.
• Proprioceptive lesions - result in extremely delayed initiation of the caudal movement.

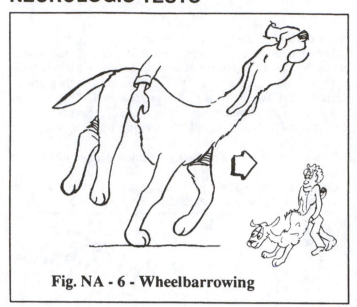

Fig. NA - 6 - Wheelbarrowing

Wheelbarrowing: tests the integration of the forelimb walking mechanism. Suspend the animal on its forelimbs by elevating the abdomen. Push on each shoulder to evaluate strength. Walk the animal forward. The animal should have a normal, alternating gait. Wheelbarrowing tests motor, proprioception and cerebellar functions. Problems may be central or peripheral. Wheelbarrowing should be done with the animal sighted and unsighted (head elevated or blindfolded). Vision may compensate for placing a limb.
• Strength
• Incoordination with hypermetric steps seen in cerebellar disease.
• Abnormal or delayed limb placement is typical of proprioceptive problems.

   • **Wobbler syndrome:** common in Thoroughbred horses, Great Danes, and Dobermans. It is a cervical vertebral column abnormality, which ultimately results in minimal to severe compression on the spinal cord. If minimal, there may be a partial loss of sensory and motor function. Severe deficits in the hindlimb, but nothing obvious in the forelimb, may be seen even though the white matter tracts to the forelimb are also effected. If a young Great Dane comes in with rear limb deficits, the first rule out is "wobbler" due to breed predilection. Wheelbarrowing an animal blindfolded will bring out subtle deficits (forelimb) that sighted wheelbarrowing doesn't. If a dog with hind limb deficits stumbles on its thoracic limbs when blind folded, it is tetraplegic, not paraplegic. To block vision, some people elevate the head, but never elevate the head if a neck lesion is suspected. Two human eye patches, a surgical mask, or even your hand will do nicely.

Hemistanding - hemiwalking: done if weakness on one side (hemiparesis) is found with other postural tests. Support one side of the body and both limbs on that side, while the animal stands and walks on the opposite limbs. Then alternate to test both sides of the body. A normal dog should be able to stand this way for 3 minutes (but they usually get bored in 20 seconds). Have an assistant press down on the hind limb and then the forelimb to assess strength. Then move it forward to see an alternating

hopping gait (the foreleg jumps forward and takes position and then the rear limb jumps forward and takes position).
• Delays or improper placement may indicate a proprioceptive lesions.
• Stumbling or collapse may indicate a motor lesion.
• A cerebellar lesion may be indicated by a hyperexaggerated gait.

PLACING REACTIONS: Placing reactions and postural reactions test for different things. They are placed together because they are convenient to perform together. Placing reactions are <u>highly specific</u> tests, unlike postural reactions. The two types of placing reactions are tactile and visual.

Visual placing reactions: sensitive evaluations of visual deficits, not proprioception. A sighted dog moved toward a table will anticipate it by reaching out. A dog held in a vulnerable position, not cuddled, will be more likely try to reach for the table. Do this on all four limbs.
• Tests the vision pathway

Tactile placing: belongs in <u>spinal cord evaluation</u> because it specifically tests for sensation. Hold the dog's head up so it can't

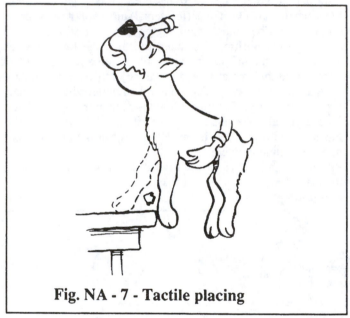

Fig. NA - 7 - Tactile placing

see the table, and touch the dorsal surface of its forepaw to a table edge. The animal should place its paw on the table. This tests the sensory branch of the radial nerve (specific test). Touching the lateral side of the fifth digit tests the ulnar nerve. It is harder to test on the hindlimbs, because when their dorsal surface touches, the animal will reach with its front limbs.
• Tests specific sensory nerves

RIGHTING REFLEX: tests the vestibular apparatus. Normal connections between the **vestibular apparatus** by way of the eighth cranial nerve (vestibulocochlear) to the spinal cord are required. An animal placed on its side will usually try to maintain at least sternal recumbency. This is a specific test for the eighth cranial nerve, not proprioception.
• Tests vestibular pathway

NEUROLOGIC TESTS

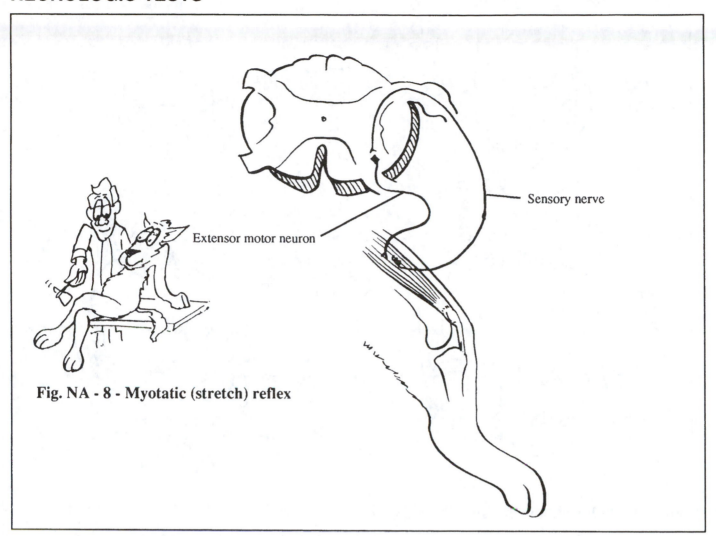

Extensor motor neuron

Sensory nerve

Fig. NA - 8 - Myotatic (stretch) reflex

SPINAL REFLEXES: controlled by reflex arcs, consisting of a sensory neuron, usually at least one interneuron, and a motor neuron (LMN). They receive input from higher centers by way of UMNs and send sensory information up the spinal cord to higher centers. They <u>do not</u> require higher center input and will be present even if the spinal cord has been severed cranial to the reflex. The animal is put in lateral recumbency to evaluate the spinal reflexes.

Myotatic or **stretch reflex**

•**Patellar, quadriceps** or **knee jerk reflex**: A stretch reflex that tests the femoral nerve, its nerve roots, and spinal cord segment L_{4-6}. With the dog in lateral recumbency, the stifle is supported with the tarsus slightly flexed. The patellar ligament is struck with an instrument (plexor). There should be a brisk contraction of the quadriceps muscle, causing extension of the stifle. Taping the patellar ligament stretches the muscle spindle. The sensory nerve passes to the spinal cord and synapses directly on a motor nerve (without an interneuron) which causes the muscle to contract.
• Exaggerated with or without clonus - UMN disease cranial to L_4
• Absent or depressed - LMN disease, can be due to disruption anywhere in the reflex arch, sensory fiber, motor fiber, spinal cord segment or whole peripheral nerve.
• Normal - intact reflex arc, including its spinal cord segment. This doesn't say that the spinal cord (UMNs) is intact cranial to this segment.

• **Extensor carpi radialis reflex**: a stretch reflex that tests the radial nerve, its roots, and spinal cord segments C_7-T_2. With the animal in lateral recumbency, the elbow is supported with the elbow and carpus flexed. Tap the extensor muscles just distal to the elbow. This will result in extension of the carpus. Less reliable than the quadriceps reflex, it is the most reliable myotatic reflex of the frontlimb.
• Exaggerated - UMN disease cranial to C_7
• Absent or depressed - LMN disease, can be due to disruption anywhere in the reflex arch, sensory fiber, motor fiber, spinal cord segment or whole peripheral nerve.
• Normal - intact reflex arc, including its spinal cord segment. There may still be UMN disease cranial to C_7.

Other stretch reflexes are the cranial tibial, gastrocnemius, triceps and biceps reflexes. The books say these are harder to elicit and more difficult to assess. The withdrawal (flexor) reflexes that follow are easier to evaluate than these.

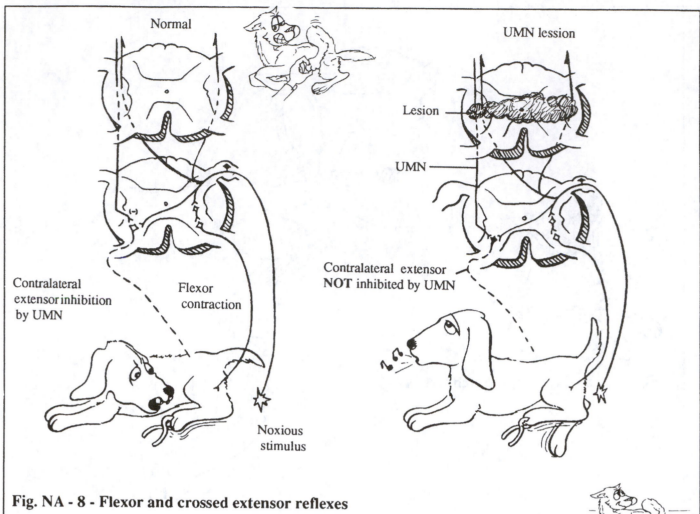

Fig. NA - 8 - Flexor and crossed extensor reflexes

Modified from Kip Carter's illustration in *Veterinary Neurology*, Oliver, Horlein, Mayhew; W.B. Saunders Co., 1987

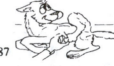

Withdrawal (flexor, pedal) reflex and pain perception: with the animal in lateral recumbency and the limb extended, pinch a toe of the hindlimb first and then the forelimb. A normal response is flexion of the joints, with withdrawal of the toe from the stimulus. This works by reflex arcs. The stimulus is cutaneous or deep pain, depending on the force of the pinch. Use the minimum amount of force to elicit the reflex. Sensory fibers synapse on interneurons in the spinal cord segments. These synapse on motor neurons to the flexor muscle to cause contraction, thus, flexion of the joints of the limb. Simultaneously assess if the pain reaches the cerebrum by noting behavioral changes (biting, looking towards stimulus). This assesses:

• Normal withdrawal - intact peripheral nerve and spinal cord
   segment
   Hindlimb: L_6-S_2
   Forelimb: C_7-T_2
• Depressed or absent - disruption of the reflex arc
   Unilateral: peripheral nerve lesion
   Bilateral: spinal cord lesion, total loss of pain perception

implies a large lesion, since pain pathways are bilateral
• Normal with perception: normal spinal cord segments and spinal cord between stimulus input and brain.
• Withdrawal reflexes don't require the animal to feel the stimulus, they will be elicited with UMN disease and may even be exaggerated. They are decreased in LMN disease or with a sensory nerve lesion.

Crossed extensor reflex: normal in the walking animals; but abnormal in the recumbent animal. During walking, when one limb is picked up (flexed) the other limb extends to bear the added weight. In the recumbent animal, this reflex is not needed and is inhibited by higher centers through UMNs. Pinch a paw to elicit a withdrawal (flexor) reflex. Extension of any other limb is abnormal and indicates blocking of descending, inhibitory pathways. A positive result:
• Indicates a chronic, potentially severe spinal cord injury
   Unilateral crossed extensor reflex, lateralizing the lesion
   to the same side.

NEUROLOGICAL TESTS

Extensor thrust reflex: gently spread the digits with your finger. Normally this will cause extension of the limb. This is hard to assess, but may be exaggerated in UMN disease.

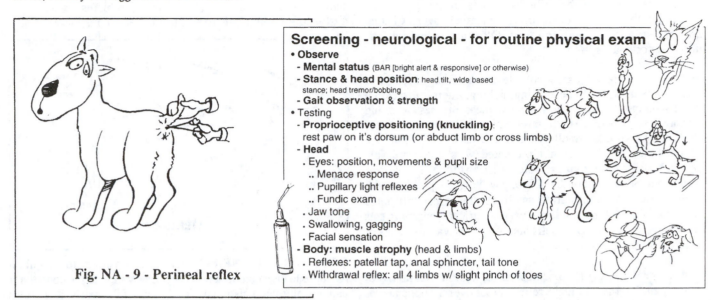

Screening - neurological - for routine physical exam
- **Observe**
  - **Mental status** (BAR [bright alert & responsive] or otherwise)
  - **Stance & head position**: head tilt, wide based stance; head tremor/bobbing
  - **Gait observation & strength**
- **Testing**
  - **Proprioceptive positioning (knuckling)**: rest paw on it's dorsum (or abduct limb or cross limbs)
  - **Head**
    - . Eyes: position, movements & pupil size
      - .. Menace response
      - .. Pupillary light reflexes
      - .. Fundic exam
    - . Jaw tone
    - . Swallowing, gagging
    - . Facial sensation
  - **Body: muscle atrophy** (head & limbs)
    - . Reflexes: patellar tap, anal sphincter, tail tone
    - . Withdrawal reflex: all 4 limbs w/ slight pinch of toes

Fig. NA - 9 - Perineal reflex

Perineal reflex: pain stimulus to the perineal region will cause contraction of the anal sphincter and flexion of the tail. The perineal region and anal sphincter are innervated by the sacral spinal cord segments and the pudendal nerve, the same segments innervating the urinary bladder. The tail is innervated by the caudal nerves. Assesses:
• Sacral spinal cord and cauda equina. Good for bladder and sphincter problems.

Extensor toe (Babinski) sign (pes sign): an abnormal reflex of the pes (hindpaw). Scratch, with a blunt instrument, the plantar aspect of the pes from hock to toe. No reaction or withdrawal are normal reactions. Fanning the toes or extending the limb is abnormal. This reflex can also be obtained on the manus. Evaluation:
• Indicates a chronic and potentially severe spinal cord lesion.

Cutaneus trunci reflex or panniculus reflex (see pg. 566): is a normal reflex to twitch the skin. Sensory fibers extend from their dermatomes (bands of skin sensation) obliquely craniodorsally to synapse in spinal cord segments T_8-L_4. Ascending sensory tracts extend up the cord to the cell body of the lateral thoracic nerve in spinal cord segment C_8. The thoracic nerve supplies motor innervation to the cutaneus trunci muscle. The dermatomes are one or two vertebrae caudal to the point of origin of the sensory nerves. If a panniculus response is present caudally and then disappears cranial to a specific point the lesion is in the spinal cord two vertebrae cranially.

Neuro Exam - Problems - Summary
- **Identify that a neuro problem exists**
  - **General observations**
    - . Mental attitude, consciousness, behavior, seizures
    - . Stance & head position
  - **Gait & strength**
  - **Postural reactions** if still unsure
    - . Proprioceptive positioning reaction
    - . Hemistands & Hemiwalks
    - . Hopping
    - . Wheelbarrowing
- **Localize once identified**
- **Localize to brain**
  - **Cranial nerve exam**
    - . CrN 2 Menace reflex ± obstacle course
    - . CrN 3 Pupillary light reflex (also CrN1)
    - . ANS: Pupillary symmetry
    - . CrN 4 Eye position
    - . CrN 5 Palpebral reflex
    - . CrN 6 Eye position
    - . CrN 7 Menace, corneal & palpebral reflexes
    - . CrN 8 Loud noise
    - . CrN 8 Nystagmus, head tilt (unilateral)
      - .. DDx: Central vestibular: depression & weakness
    - . CrN 9,10: Gag Reflex, Cough Reflex
    - . CrN 12: Pull on tongue
  - **"Head signs"**: mentation, consciousness, seizures, behavior, head tilt, tremors, circling, cranial nerves, etc.
  - **"Head signs" + gait**: localize part of brain
- **Specific signs of part of brain**

- **Localize in spinal cord** or brain
  - **UMN/LMN signs**
    - **Spinal reflexes**
      - .. Patellar reflex
      - .. Withdrawal reflex of rear limb
      - .. Cutaneous trunci reflex
      - .. Withdrawal reflex of forelimb
      - .. Anal reflex
    - **Muscle tone**: palpation
      - .. ↓Tone/flaccidity = LMN
      - .. Normal tone
      - .. ↑Tone: UMN
  - **Sensation:**
    - . Proprioception
    - . Superficial pain
    - . Deep pain
    - . Map superficial sensation: if LMN signs

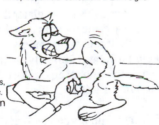

From Pasquini & Pasquini. *Tschauner's Guide to Small Animal Clinics.*, Sudz Publishing

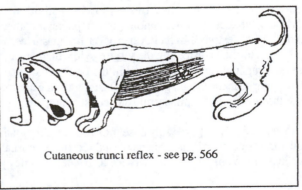

Cutaneous trunci reflex - see pg. 566

CLASP-KNIFE RESPONSE - UMN: a delayed, abrupt collapse of a hyperextended limb. An animal with upper motor nerve (UMN) problems will have an extended limb due to release of the LMNs. Pressing on the limb will slightly increase the tone in the limb due to the pad pressure reflex. After a moment of continual pressure, the limb collapses abruptly. This is a indication of upper motor neuron syndrome.

CRANIAL NERVE EXAM

OLFACTORY NERVE, Cn I: carries the special sense of smell. Olfactory receptors, located in the neuroepithelium of the nasal mucosa, pass through the cribriform plate to synapse in the olfactory bulb. Second order neurons then travel down the lateral olfactory stria to the pyriform lobe. Olfaction is tied into the limbic (emotional) system.

To evoke a response use a volatile non-irritating substance. Proper responses would be sniffing, licking, interest if pleasant smell; wincing, backing away from unpleasant ones. Irritating substances (e.g. alcohol) to the nasal cavity will evoke a response which may look like smelling. Food is excellent if not in a recognizable container or not presented with a recognizable approach. Bring food from a remote source on a tongue derpessor. Destruction of any part of the pathway will cause a problem with smell. Nasal tumors may affect smell, but this is insignificant to the tumor. Clinically smell is not very significant, except in cats which depend heavily on smells and will show various bouts of anorexia if they can't smell.

OPTIC NERVE, Cn II: special sense of sight. It has no motor component. Light striking the retina passes over the optic nerves to the optic chiasm, then on to the optic tracts to synapse in the lateral geniculate nuclei. Neurons then pass over the optic radiations to the occipital lobe for visual interpretation.

Damage can affect any part of the pathway. Loss of vision can be due to ocular diseases, nervous system diseases, or both. Corneal diseases will affect vision by clouding the lens. Diseases of the lens, e.g., cataracts, affect vision. The retina can undergo atrophy. More than Cn II is necessary for proper vision (accommodation, pupil size (CNIII), blinking the eye, tear film (CN VII), conjugation of eye movement (CN III, IV, VI). However, if an image can't be formed (CN II), the animal is blind.

In the dog, 75% of the optic fibers of one optic nerve cross over to the opposite (contralateral) optic tract and 25% stay in the ipsilateral optic tract. In cats there is a 65% cross over. Therefore, the optic tracts carry mainly vision from the opposite eye to the occipital lobe. Clinically, animals behave as if all fibers cross over. If the right occipital lobe is damaged, the animal will appear blind in the left eye.

History: animals can be fairly blind before many owners realize it. Stumbling on stair cases or poor night vision is often the first sign of visual degeneration. **Visually observe,** from a distance, the animal at rest and moving while taking the history. **Obstacle courses:** using objects from your clinic. A dimer switch may be helpful to evaluate day and night visions.

Visual placing reaction: evaluate vision although it is placed with postural reactions for convenience (see placing reactions).

Menace response (Cn II - Cn VII): blinking in response to potentially harmful objects advancing toward the eye. Make a threatening gesture toward the eye without windpuffs or noise. A positive response is blinking. For unknown reasons, absence of connection from the cerebellum abolishes the response. Since the

visual pathway, facial nerve (Cn VII), and cerebellum are all involved, this response doesn't localize the lesion. It is another sign for visual dysfunction, facial nerve problems, or cerebellar dysfunction. If blind, there will be no menace response.

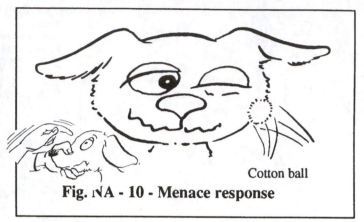
Fig. NA - 10 - Menace response
Cotton ball

OCULOMOTOR NERVE, Cn III: constricts the pupil in response to elevated light levels by innervation to the constrictor papillae muscle. It also innervates some of the extrinsic muscles of the eye.

Cn II and Cn III are tied together and can be evaluated together by checking the menace response, size of the resting pupil and the palpebral light reflexes. First check for vision in each eye by the menace response or visual placing reaction. Then look at the resting pupils (without shining a light in them). Finally, check the pupillary light reflex. Practice drawing quick schematics by incorporating the visual pathways and pupillary light reflex pathways as done on the following pages. Draw an X through the structure affected. Using the schematic and Chart 5 (pg. 576) will help to characterize the lesion.

• **Pupillary light reflex:** used to monitor patients with head trauma, to determine the degree of trauma, to localize the lesion, and to monitor degradation or improvement of an animal. A rapid change from one format to another may warn of deleterious changes that require immediate intervention to reverse. The pupillary light reflex involves the central visual light pathway before the thalamus. Therefore, cerebral diencephalic disease will not abolish the reflex, but may alter it.

Shine a light onto the retina. Impulses pass over the optic nerve, the optic chiasm and optic tracts. Collaterals of the optic tract peel off at the rostral end of the midbrain to synapse on midbrain nuclei (pretectal nucleus). These neurons synapse ipsilateral or contralateral in the accessory oculomotor nuclei (parasympathetic nucleus, Edinger-Westphal). Whichever cross at the chiasm recross in the midbrain to end up affecting the same eye in which the light was shone. Preganglionic fibers travel in the oculomotor nerve (Cn III) to synapse in the ciliary ganglion. Postganglionic neurons innervate the constrictor pupillary muscle, constricting the pupil.

Light shone in a dog's left eye will cause more constriction in the left pupil (direct side) than in the right pupil (indirect or consensual), because 75% of the optic fibers cross twice to affect the same eye

PUPILLARY LIGHT REFLEX

Cranial nerves: pg. 460

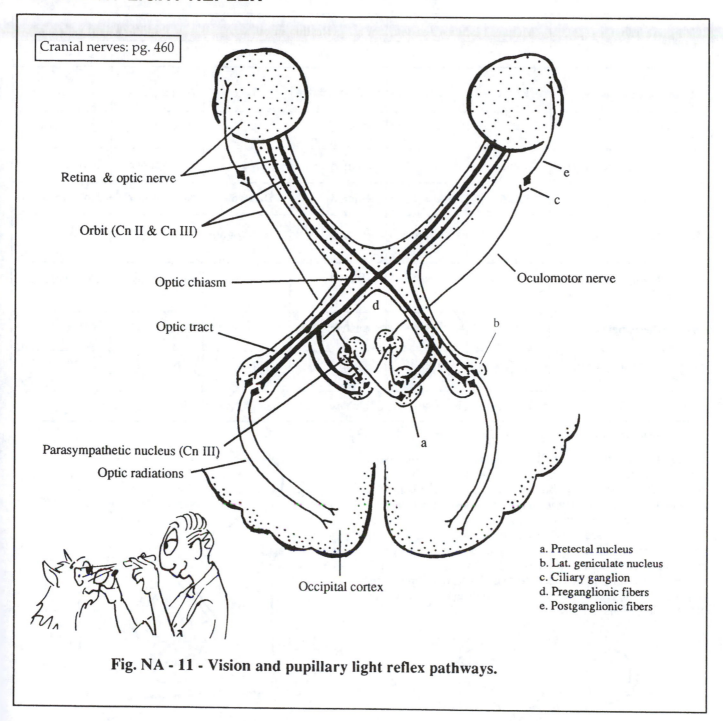

Retina & optic nerve

Orbit (Cn II & Cn III)

Optic chiasm

Optic tract

Parasympathetic nucleus (Cn III)

Optic radiations

Occipital cortex

Oculomotor nerve

e
c
d
b
a

a. Pretectal nucleus
b. Lat. geniculate nucleus
c. Ciliary ganglion
d. Preganglionic fibers
e. Postganglionic fibers

Fig. NA - 11 - Vision and pupillary light reflex pathways.

and 25% end up in the other eye. Therefore, the left pupil should constrict quicker, more efficiently, and to a greater degree than the right (dynamic contraction anisocoria). This is normal in dogs and cats. Direct and indirect pupillary reflexes are named for the eye in which the light is shone, not for the eye that responds. The **direct pupillary light reflex** constricts the pupil in which a light is shown. The **indirect pupillary light reflex** constricts the pupil in the opposite eye in which the light is shone.

Sympathetic innervation to the iris: arises from the hypothalamus and travels down the cervical spinal cord. The preganglionic fibers arise from the first three thoracic spinal cord segments. They travel through the sympathetic trunk and then the vagosympathetic trunk up the neck to synapse in the cranial cervical ganglion. Postganglionic fibers pass through the middle ear and then into the orbit to reach the pupil. These innervate the pupillary dilator muscle to dilate the pupil. Injury anywhere along this pathway will cause the pupil to be more constricted.

PUPILLARY LIGHT REFLEX

Complete lesion LEFT side	Menace response / vision		Resting pupil		Pupillary light reflexes	
	Lt. eye	Rt. eye	Lt. eye	Rt. eye	Light in lt. eye	Light in rt. eye
Retina or optic nerve	Blind	N	Slightly dilated	N	No response	N*
Oculomotor	N	N	Dilated	N	Constrict rt.	Constrict rt.
Orbit (both CnII & CnIII)	Blind	N	Dilated	N	No response	Constrict rt.
Optic chiasm	Blind	Blind	Dilated	Dilated	No response	No response
Optic tract	N	Blind	N	N or Slightly dilated	N*	N*
Parasympathetic nucleus (bliateral)	N	N	Dilated	Dilated	No response	No response
Sympathetic nerves	N	N	Constricted	N	N*	N*
Optic pathway past optic tract	N	Blind	N	N	N*	N*

* N (normal) for the pupillary light reflexes is constriction of both eyes when the light is shone in the eye.

Modifies from Oliver JE Jr and Lorenz MD: *Veterinary Neurology*. Phildelphia, W. B. Saunders co., 1987

Damage to the left retina or left optic nerve (prechiasmatic damage): Clinically, although not the same diseases, they have the same effect to the visual and pupillary pathways. When light is shone in the left eye, neither pupil will constrict because its pathway is blocked. Light in the right eye will cause both to constrict because crossover at the optic chiasm is not blocked. The menace response will be absent in the blind, left eye. The right eye will have sight and show a menace response. At rest, the left pupil will only be partially dilated because it is still getting indirect tone from light coming into the right eye. If the right eye is covered the dilation will become total.

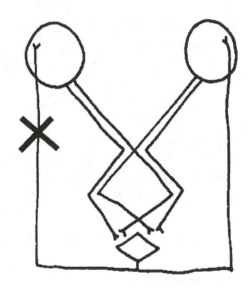

Fig. NA - 13 - Left oculomotor nerve (Cn III) damage

Left oculomotor nerve (Cn III) damage: light can get to accessory parasympathetic (ANS) nuclei and cross over can occur. Thus, the right pupil will constrict with light shone in either eye (direct and indirect response). Parasympathetic innervation is lost to the left eye so it will be unresponsive to light shone in either eye. The resting pupil will be totally dilated due to the loss all parasympathetic innervation. Both eyes have normal vision, thus, menace responses.

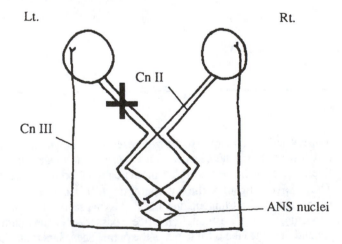

Fig. NA - 12 - Lt. retina or optic n. damage

PUPILLARY LIGHT REFLEX

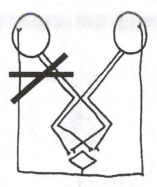

Fig. NA - 14 - Left postorbital problem (abscess)

Left postorbital problem (abscess): affects both the optic and oculomotor nerves on that side. The right eye will be normal, except it will have no indirect pupillary response (light in the left eye). The left eye is blind (no menace response) with no oculomotor innervation (no pupillary response), therefore totally dilated. The only response will be the direct pupillary (on the right-normal-side).

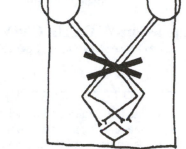

Fig. NA - 15 - Total chiasmatic lesions

Total chiasmatic lesions: less common in animals than in humans. Vision and crossover are blocked so the eyes will not see (no menace response) and there will be no parasympathetic innervation (both pupils totally dilated). With subtotal lesions there will be progressive degrees of these signs.

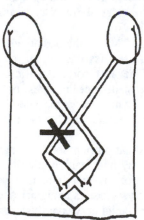

Fig. NA - 16 - Left optic tract (postchiasmatic) lesions

Left optic tract (postchiasmatic) lesions: 75% of the fibers in the optic tract originate from the opposite side, animals with lesions postchiasmatically tend to act contralaterally (opposite side) blind although precise and careful evaluation may show vision

intact in the contralateral nasal field (temporal retina). Pupils will still constrict with light shown in either eye because the minor pathways are still present. The resting right pupil will be partially dilated (still has minor crossover) and covering the eye will not have an effect. The menace response will be absent in the blind right eye.

Midbrain lesion effecting the parasympathetic nucleus: rarely unilateral. It will not effect the visual pathway, thus, the animal can see. It will eliminate all parasympathetic innervation to both eyes, thus, the pupils will be dilated and have no pupillary responses.

Fig. NA - 17 - Midbrain lesion effecting parasympathetic nucleus

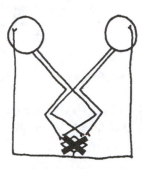

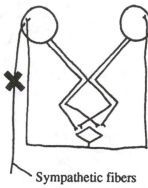

Sympathetic fibers

Fig. NA - 18 - Lesions of left sympathetic pathway

Parasympathetic nucleus

Lesions of the left sympathetic pathway: result in constriction of the resting pupil on the side affected. They will have no affect on vision or the pupils. The lesion can be anywhere along the sympathetic pathway, from the hypothalamus down the cervical spinal cord to segment T_2, over the sympathetic and vagosympathetic trunks from the thorax to the cranial neck, or in the sympathetic postganglionic fibers passing through the middle ear and orbit.

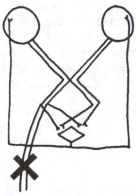

Fig. NA - 19 - Left lesion to the visual pathway past the optic tracts

Left lesion to the visual pathway past the optic tracts (lateral geniculate nucleus, optic radiations and primary visual [occipital] cortex): the animal acts contralaterally blind (blind in right eye). There will be no effect on the pupillary light reflexes because the lesion is past this pathway. It may cause some pupillary constriction because of loss of occipital inhibition (UMN) to the parasympathetic nucleus.

CRANIAL NERVES

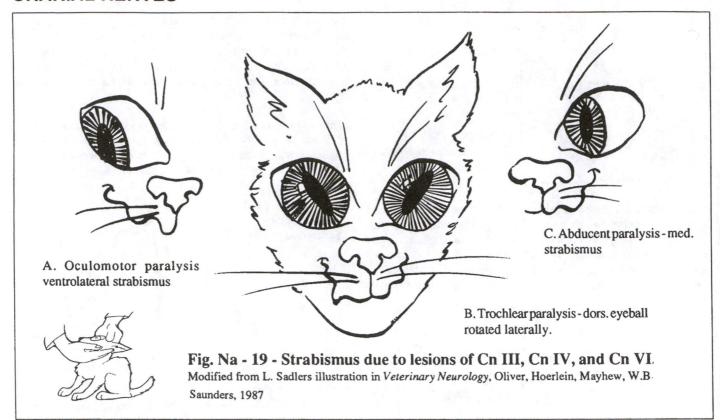

A. Oculomotor paralysis ventrolateral strabismus

C. Abducent paralysis - med. strabismus

B. Trochlear paralysis - dors. eyeball rotated laterally.

Fig. Na - 19 - Strabismus due to lesions of Cn III, Cn IV, and Cn VI.
Modified from L. Sadlers illustration in *Veterinary Neurology*, Oliver, Hoerlein, Mayhew, W.B. Saunders, 1987

OCULOMOTOR, TROCHLEAR and ABDUCENT, Cn III, IV and VI: evaluated together because they all function to move the eye. The parasympathetic innervation of the oculomotor nerve (Cn III) was considered previously. To evaluate, observe the resting position of the eyes, test the ability to move the eyes by following something (throw a cotton ball across the animal's field of vision). Vestibular eye movements are evaluated by moving the head up or down and from side to side.

The oculomotor (Cn III) and trochlear (Cn IV) nerves originate from the midbrain; the abducent nerve (Cn VI) from the pons. All three leave the orbital cavity through the orbital fissure. The vestibular nuclei in the medulla connect to the nuclei of these nerves and voluntary motor centers by the medial longitudinal fasciculus (MLF) located in the center of the brain stem. Movement of the head stimulates the vestibular receptors of the inner ear which pass to the vestibular nuclei and through the MLF to the cells bodies of these three eye muscle nerves. This causes a normal nystagmus with the fast phase in the direction of the head movement.

Strabismus: abnormal position of the eyeball. Lesions to Cn III, IV and VI will cause strabismus.
- Oculomotor lesion - ventrolateral strabismus
- Abducent lesion - medial strabismus
- Trochlear paralysis - not detectable in round pupils. Dorsal side of the eyeball is rotated laterally.

Voluntary following: determine if an animal can see or not, visual placing is a better test. Throw a cotton ball across the visual field and note if the animal follows it with his eyes. A cotton ball is easy to see and doesn't make noise when it lands. An object which makes noise could cause an auditory following, thus, a false positive visual following.

Nystagmus at rest is always abnormal and is usually due to a vestibular system problem.

TRIGEMINAL NERVE, Cn V: three main divisions – the ophthalmic, maxillary, and mandibular –which are all sensory. The mandibular division is also motor to the muscles of mastication.

Pinching or touching the face with a hemostat will test for sensation. Look for a reaction. Use a tissue forceps if you can't get a reaction from a light touch. The last resort is scarification of the nasal mucosa (very painful). Test all three branches - ophthalmic, the medial canthus of the eye; maxillary, the lateral canthus, maxillary region or nasal mucosa; and mandibular, the chin.

Palpating the muscles of mastication (temporalis, masseter and digastricus muscles) for atrophy and manipulating the jaw for tone tests the motor division of the mandibular nerve. These muscles are massive and paralysis results in significant atrophy and loss of mass. Whereas, in facial nerve paralysis, there is no loss of mass in the thin muscles of facial expression, just facial deviation.

The sensory neurons are located in the trigeminal ganglion in the cranial cavity. Their fibers enter the pons. The motor nucleus of Cn V is located in the pons. Motor fibers project down to the spine

CRANIAL NERVES

and up to the facial nucleus for the corneal and palpebral reflexes.

Corneal and palpebral reflexes: used clinically to evaluate the depth of anesthesia.

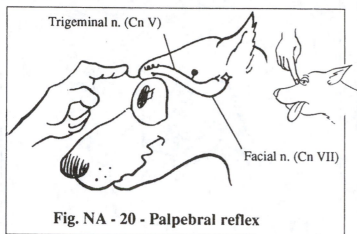

Fig. NA - 20 - Palpebral reflex

Palpebral reflex: a Cn V-VII reflex (trigeminal - facial nerves). Touching the eyelid sends sensory information over the trigeminal nerve (ophthalmic nerve of the maxillary division) to synapse with the facial nerve in the brain stem. Motor fibers of the facial (auriculopalpebral) nerve cause the obicularis oculi muscle to contract (blink). Blinking before the eyelids are touched is a menace response, therefore, repeat a number of times for a positive response. This reflex is used to evaluate depth of anesthesia; especially when an animal is becoming too light.

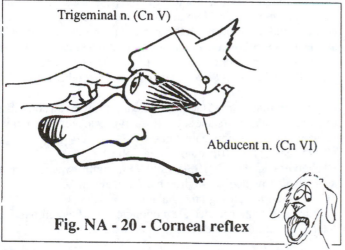

Fig. NA - 20 - Corneal reflex

Corneal reflex: Cn V - VI reflex (trigeminal - abducent): touch only the cornea to stimulate the maxillary nerve (long ciliary nerve of the ophthalmic division). Retraction of the globe is due to connections to Cn VI (abducent) which innervates the retractor bulbi muscle. Blinking will also occur and is partly due to a menace response. Look for retraction of the globe. A corneal reflex is abolished at a deeper stage of anesthesia than the palpebral reflex. Therefore, it a danger signal for an animal getting too deep in anesthesia.

"Dropped jaw" (idiopathic trigeminal neuropathy): a common, acute problem caused by bilateral disease of the mandibular division. This happens without any other deficiencies and is usually self limiting; most animals return to normal in 21 days. The client usually thinks the animal has a broken jaw. The main concern is hydration since the animal has difficulty swallowing with its mouth open.

• Damage to one of the divisions past their separation into three branches will cause sensory loss to the area innervated.
• Damage proximal to the separation will cause loss of sensation to the face and loss of the palpebral and corneal reflexes.
• Unilateral disease of the mandibular division will initially result in deviation of the jaw to the side of the lesion. With atrophy (chronic) of the pterygoid muscle, it will deviate away from the side of the lesion.
• Brain stem nuclear damage can happen to either or both of the sensory or motor nuclei, resulting in sensory or motor loss or both. There should be signs of other brain stem damage.

FACIAL NERVE, Cn VII: has many different functions, motor to the muscles of facial expression, taste, lacrimal and salivary innervation. Taste has little clinical significance. Atrophy of the muscles of facial expression isn't noticeable, but results in deviations and deficits of facial reflexes.

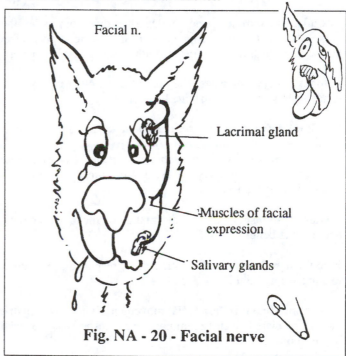

Fig. NA - 20 - Facial nerve

The facial and vestibulocochlear nerves (Cnn VII & Cn VIII) travel from the brain together through the internal acoustic meatus. Then Cn VII leaves Cn VIII and crosses the middle ear cavity. Therefore, an ear infection can cause severe facial nerve problems. The facial nerve leaves the skull through the stylomastoid foramen. The branches of the facial nerve innervate the muscles of facial expression. The auriculopalpebral branch innervates the obicularis oculi muscle to close the eyelids. The ventral and dorsal buccal branches cross the masseter muscle superficially. Autonomic fibers leave the facial nerve internally and come out the orbital fissure to innervate the lacrimal gland.

CRANIAL NERVES

• Peripheral lesions distal to the stylomastoid foramen result in paralysis to the area supplied. They do not affect lacrimation.

   – Paralysis of the auriculopalpebral branch, thus, the obicularis oculi muscle, causes widening of the palpebral fissure in small animals and ptosis (bulging eye) in large animals and some dogs (Pekinese).

   – Buccal branches: paralysis would result in deviations of the face (drooping lip or ear and pulling of the nose to the normal side. Chronically, it will result in deviation towards the lesion from fibrous atrophy).

• Inner ear infections can damage all the branches, resulting in facial deviations, loss of lacrimation and salivary function, and taste. This is often accompanied by vestibular signs (close proximity of Cn VIII) and Horner's syndrome (if the sympathetic nerves are affected).

• A lesion in the cranial cavity between the brain and the internal acoustic meatus will affect all branches of the facial nerve. This is usually accompanied by vestibular signs (CnVIII), but not Horner's syndrome.

• Brain stem damage to the facial nerve affects all or some of the components, depending on the size of the lesion. It is accompanied by other brain stem signs (paresis, proprioceptive deficits, alteration of level of consciousness, and other cranial nerve deficits).

Buccal nerve damage (peripheral) is common in horses when the horse's head is left on an unpadded surface during surgery. (The buccal nerve in the horse is located under the buckle of the halter.)

Palpebral nerve damage: the animal can't close the eyelids, resulting in secondary exposure keratitis.

Lacrimal deficiency: very serious due to drying of the cornea.

Salivation problems: compensation from glands on the opposite side and by the glands on both side innervated by the glossopharyngeal nerve.

Menace response: gives you information on the facial and optic nerves. It is better for Cn II .

Palpebral reflexes: Cn V - VII reflex, response to palpebral touch, causing blinking.

Trigeminal facial reflex: facial movements when touching the face are mediated by the trigeminal nerve (sensory) and the facial nerve (motor).

Shirmer tear test: filter paper put in the corner of eye for a period of time to wick tears. The amount of wick is compared to a standard scale to measure relative amount of lacrimation.

VESTIBULOCOCHLEAR NERVE: has two divisions, the cochlear dealing with hearing (audition) and the vestibular dealing with movement of the head in relation to gravity and movement.

Cochlear division: deafness must be bilateral in an alert animal to evaluate completely without electrophysiologic instruments. Test by making a loud noise out of the animals vision and note

behavioral changes (looking towards noise). A central lesion usually doesn't cause extreme deficits in audition in a conscious animal. Therefore, look for the problem in a deaf dog's ears.

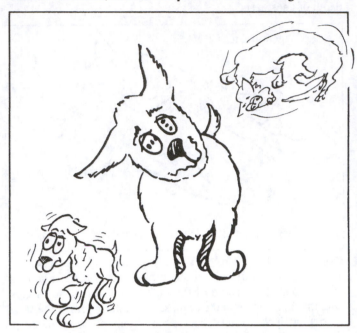

Vestibular proprioception: perceiving position of the head in relationship to gravity and motion. The vestibular apparatus has five components, the three semicircular canals, the utricle and the saccula. The saccula and utricle are responsible for static position and linear motion. The semicircular canals are responsible for angular motion. From the receptors in the semicircular canals, utricle and saccula of the inner ear, most of the nerve fibers pass to the four vestibular nuclei in the medulla oblongata and cerebellum. Fibers for these nuclei pass to many other structures:

• Down the spinal cord to facilitate extensor muscles on both sides and inhibit ipsilateral (same side) flexor muscles. This is important in maintaining posture against gravity.
• To the cerebellum (flocculonodular lobes)
• To motor nuclei of Cn III, IV, and VI to control vestibular eye movements (by medial longitudinal fasciculus (MLF).
• Cerebral cortex through the thalamus
• Reticular formation to mediate motion sickness. Overall, animals seldom vomit in the face of vestibular disease.

Signs

• Head tilt is a classic sign of vestibular disease. The tilt is usually toward the side of the problem.
• Leaning toward the affected side: due to loss of ispsilateral extensor tone in limbs and vertigo.
• Circling and falling to the affected side. Dogs and cats will lean and walk against a wall.
• Reluctance to lie on the good side because it worsens the vertigo and they do not like it.
• Ataxic gait due to cerebellar connections.
• Brain stem lesion - Altered proprioception and motor pathways

CRANIAL NERVES

resulting in abnormal gait and abnormal postural reactions.
• Inability to right themselves, alter their posture.
• Nystagmus due to connections to the nerves of the extrinsic eye muscles.

Nystagmus: at rest is always abnormal and usually indicates vestibular dysfunction. It is repeated, involuntary, rapid movement of the eyeball, which may be horizontal, vertical, rotary or mixed, i.e., of two varieties. Both eyes are effected and usually move together (conjugate). The eyes will move to the same side as the lesion and snap back. Nystagmus is named for its fast (snap) component. If the animal's eyes move to the left and snap back to the right it is a right horizontal nystagmus, even though the lesion is on the left. In vertical nystagmus the eyes move up and down. Rotary nystagmus is deviation around the central axis.

Peripheral vs central lesion: differentiated by the type of nystagmus. A **vertical nystagmus** indicates a central lesion (99% of time). Horizontal and rotary nystagmus can be peripheral or central. **Disconjugate nystagmus,** different nystagmus in the eyes (e.g., horizontal in one and rotary in the other) is caused by a central lesion. Nystagmus that changes from one form to another (e.g., horizontal to rotary) with changing head position is due to a central lesion.

Positional nystagmus: inducing nystagmus in an animal without spontaneous nystagmus by changing head position. This can be due to a peripheral lesion as long as the nystagmus is not vertical, is conjugate and doesn't change to a different type with various head positional changes.

Unilateral otitis (ear infection): affecting the inner ear gives classical vestibular signs: head tilt, circling, leaning, falling, and possible nystagmus. These may be accompanied by Horner's syndrome (sympathetic nerves) and facial paralysis because these nerves also pass through the middle ear. Facial paralysis is critical because of lacrimal problems (dry eye) and inability to close the eye, not because of the distortion of facial features (dogs aren't vain). The loss of lacrimation requires constant artificial tears or surgical relocation of the parotid duct.

Idiopathic vestibular disease: an acute disease of unknown cause in animals. The presenting signs are severe unilateral vestibular signs indistinguishable from vestibular disease due to trauma or inner ear disease. The animal may not be able to stand, lies on the floor paddling its legs, with nystagmus and total disorientation. A self limiting disease, it resolves spontaneously without treatment in a few weeks with the only residual sign a possible slight head tilt. Many of these old dogs are probable needlessly put to sleep.

GLOSSOPHARYNGEAL and VAGUS NERVES IX & X:
Cnn IX & X arise together from a motor nucleus in the medulla (nucleus ambigus). They leave the skull together and do not diverge until they are some distance from the skull. It is almost impossible to have a lesion in one without the other. Therefore, when an animal has pharyngeal paralysis it indicates cranial nerve IX and X. With pharyngeal paralysis first think **RABIES!** The glossopharyngeal nerve also innervates the parotid and zygomatic salivary glands, but salivation isn't a clinical problem because other salivary glands compensate and there is dual innervation on both sides. Taste to the root of the tongue also is not a clinical problem.

Pathway: IX, X & XI leave the cranial vault through the jugular foramen and exit the skull by the temporooccipital fissure.

Gag reflex test: stick a tongue depressor or a laryngeal scope paddle down the throat. Do not use a wooden swab or something the animal can bite in half.

VAGUS, Cn X: since it supplies innervation to the pharynx, larynx and esophagus, clinically look for pharyngeal, laryngeal and esophageal problems. Megaesophagus is a prime sign of Cn X paralysis. This results in regurgitation of formed esophageal masses (tube of food).

Left recurrent laryngeal nerve: peals off from the vagus nerve in the thorax and passes around the arch of the aorta. It then travels up the neck to innervate most of the laryngeal muscles, most notably the cricoarytenoideus dorsalis. The cricoarytenoideus dorsalis is the only muscle that opens the glottic cleft. Paralysis of the recurrent laryngeal nerve results in "roarers", laryngeal hemiplegia in horses. The primary complaint is lack of exercise tolerance. (The roaring is sounds irritating but running out of gas near the finish line costs money.)

Parasympathetic motor: rarely do true cardiovascular or gastrointestinal signs point directly to vagal nerve lesions except in the ruminants. Vagal indigestion in ruminants causes eructation failure and bloat. Such animals are often culled for slaughter.

SPINAL ACCESSORY, Cn XI: arises from a nucleus (nucleus ambiguus) in spinal cord segments C_1 to C_5. Its fibers leave the spinal cord and travels up to enter the cranial vault through the foramen magnum; and then join the vagus. Cervical roots from XI innervate neck muscles, omotransversarius, brachiocephalic, trapezius and sternocephalicus (muscles that move the head). With accessory nerve damage:
• Cervical muscle atrophy. If chronic, you may get fibrous atrophy and torticollis. Observe and palpate for symmetry of muscles on both sides of the neck.

HYPOGLOSSAL NERVE, Cn XII: motor to the muscles of the tongue. Prehension of food and water is done with the tongue. If the tongue is paralyzed the animal can't lap correctly.
• Unilateral paralysis will cause deviate to the side of the lesion at first and then over time away from the lesion as muscles atrophy.

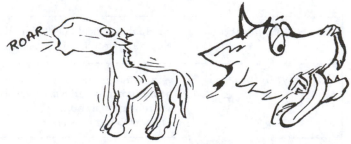

CRANIAL NERVE EXAM	Test & positive response (+)	Lesion localization
I Olfactory	• Odor stimulus	• Usually nasal cavity
II Optic nerve 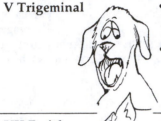	• Obstacle courses: vision • Placing reactions • Menace response • Fundascope	• See Pupillary light reflex chart on page 576
II & III	• Pupillary light reflex	• See Pupillary light reflex chart page 576
III, IV and VI, oculomotor, trochlear & abducens nerves	• Strabismus	• Oculomotor lesion: ventrolateral strabismus • Abducens lesion: medial strabismus • Trochlear paralysis: dorsal side rotated laterally (not detected in round pupils)

V Trigeminal 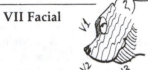	• Muscles of mastication
	  - Palpate muscles of mastication
	  - Open jaw, check tone
	• Sensory
	  - Light touch
	  - Palpebral reflex: V-VII reflex
	  - Corneal reflex: V-VI reflex
		• Past where 3 divisions separate: sensory loss to area innervated (V1: forehead, V2: maxillary region, V3: mandibular region)
		• Proximal to separation: loss of sensation to entire face & loss of the palpebral & corneal reflexes
		• Brain stem nuclear - sensory or motor loss or both plus other brain stem signs

VII Facial 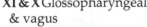	• Schirmer tear test - lacrimation
	• Palpebral reflex (Cr.nn. V-VII)
	• Trigeminal/facial nn. reflex (Cr.nn. V-VII)
	• Check symmetry of face
	• Menace response (Cr.nn. II-VII)
		• Peripheral damage: facial paralysis, no effect on lacrimation
		  - Auriculopalpebral branch - widening of palpebral fissure: small animals & ptosis: large animals.
		  - Buccal branches - deviations of face
		• Middle ear infections - all branches (eyelids, loss of lacrimation) ± vestibular signs, ± Horners
		• Damage in cranial cavity between brain & internal acoustic meatus: affect all branches of facial n., + vestibular signs but no Horner's
		• Brain stem - variable facial branch signs, accompanied by other brain stem signs

VIII Vestibulocochlear
Cochlear division
 	
Vestibular proprioception 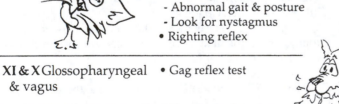
	• Deafness bilateral in alert animal
	
	• Observation of signs
	  - Head tilt
	  - Leaning towards the affected side
	  - Circling & falling to affected side
	  - Ataxic gait
	  - Abnormal gait & posture
	  - Look for nystagmus
	• Righting reflex
		• Nystagmus
		  - Vertical: central lesion (99% of time).
		  - Horizontal & rotary: peripheral or central lesions
		  - Disconjugate nystagmus: central lesions
		• Unilateral otitis: classical vestibular signs + Horner's syndrome & facial paralysis (in middle ear disease)

XI & X Glossopharyngeal & vagus	• Gag reflex test	• Pharyngeal paralysis - think Rabies 1st
X Vagus	• Evaluate clinical signs • Laryngoscope • Esophgoscope	• Parasympathetic - ruminant vagal indigestion - eructation failure & bloat • Recurrent laryngeal nerve: laryngeal hemiplegia in horses & Bouvier de Flandres dogs
XI - Spinal accessory 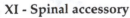	• Palpate cervical muscle for atrophy, • Chronic problem: fibrous atrophy & torticollis.	
XII - Hypoglossal 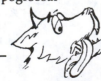	• Pull on tongue • Observe tongue deviates toward lesion initially, in time chronic fibrosis causes tongue to deviate away from the lesion	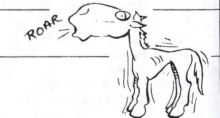

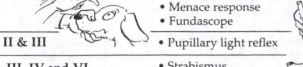

Equine - Nerve & Joint Blocks

NAMES used in this text	OTHER NAMES

NERVE BLOCKS — PERINEURAL BLOCKS

Heel block — **Palmar digitalblock***
PD Block

Pastern/foot block — **Abaxial sesamoid nerve block**
ASNB
High palmar digital block

Fetlock block — **Low palmar** (volar) **block**
Low 4 point block

Metacarpal block — **High (palmar) 4 point block**
• Hight palmar n. block
• High metacarpal n. block

Proximal metacarpal block — **Deep branch of lateral palmar nerve block**
Infiltration of suspensory ligament

Carpus & distal nerve block — **Median & ulnar nerve block**

Tarsus & distal nerve block — **Tibial & peroneal nerve block**

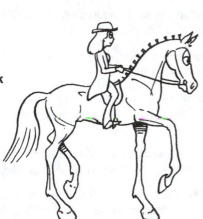

JOINT BLOCKS

Navicular bursa block — Podotrochlear bursa block

Dorsal approach to fetlock, pastern & coffin joints — Dorsal approaches to the metacarpophalangeal, prox. and distal interphalangeal joints

Palmar approach to fetlock joint — Palmar approach to metacarpo/metatarsophalangeal joint

Palmar approach to pastern — Palmar approach to proximal interphalangeal joint

Carpal joint injection — Antebrachiocarpal & middle intercarpal joints
• **Dorsal approach**
• **Palmar approach** to antebrachiocarpal joint

Elbow joint block — Cubital joint block
Caudolateral approach to elbow

Shoulder joint block — Scapulohumeral joint block

Bicipital bursa block — Intertubercular bursa block

Tibiotarsal block — Talocrural block

DIP joint block — **Distal intertarsal joint block**

TMt block — **Tarsometatarsal joint block**

Stifle blocks
• **Medial femorotibial pouch block**
• **Lateral femorotibial pouch block**
• **Femoropatellar pouch block**
  - **Lateral approach**

Hip block — Coxofemoral joint block

Trochanteric block

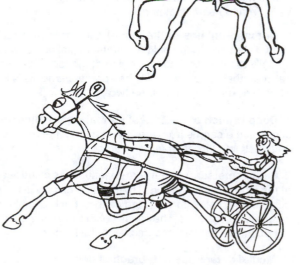

* Most commonly used term
for blocks in **bold**

583

Nerves - Distal Forelimb - Horse

NERVES - EQUINE ANTEBRACHIUM: understanding the distribution of the nerves is important in lameness diagnosis using nerve blocks. Draw a simple line schematic of the nerves to the distal thoracic limb. Once this can be quickly done, placing the nerve blocks & knowing which structures they block will be easier to understand.

Radial nerve: does <u>not</u> extend past the carpus as it does in the other domestic species.

Median, ulnar & medial cutaneous antebrachial (a branch of the musculocutaneous) **nerves:** the 3 nerves passing the carpus in the horse.

1. Median nerve: bifurcates into the medial & lateral branches proximal to the carpus.

2. Ulnar nerve: bifurcates just proximal to the carpus into dorsal & palmar branches.

3. Dorsal branch of the ulnar nerve: wraps around the cannon bone & descends on the dorsolateral side of the cannon region to the fetlock.

4. Palmar branch of the ulnar nerve: joins with the lateral branch of the median nerve to form the <u>lateral palmar nerve</u>.

5, 6. Medial & lateral palmar nerves: travel down either side of the flexor tendons. At the level of the fetlock, they give off a dorsal branch & continue as the palmar digital nerves. The median palmar nerve consists of only median fibers. The lateral palmar nerve has both ulnar & median nerve fibers.

7. Communicating branch: crosses over the palmar aspect of the flexor tendons about halfway down the metacarpus, where it is palpable. It carries fibers from the medial palmar nerve (median nerve fibers) to the lateral palmar nerve (ulnar & median nerve).

8, 9. Medial & lateral palmar digital nerves: pass distally on the palmar aspect of the digit to innervate the <u>heel</u> of the foot. They form a triad along with the digital vein & artery on each side. These triads are arranged vein, artery and nerve (*memory aid:* VAN) from dorsal to palmar/plantar.

10. Dorsal branches of the digital nerves: pass distally for a short distance with the palmar/plantar digital nerves & then pass dorsally to innervate the <u>toe</u> region of the foot. The relationship between the digital nerves & their dorsal branches is important when blocking only one of the two.

11. Deep branch of the lateral palmar nerve (ulnar nerve): arises at the carpus from the lateral palmar nerve, dives deep & branches into the palmar metacarpal nerves.

12. Palmar metacarpal nerves: continuations of the deep branch of the lateral palmar nerve. They course distally in the junctions between the splint bones & the cannon bone deep to the suspensory ligament. They pass under the buttons of the splints to become superficial & continue to the fetlock.

13. Medial cutaneous antebrachial nerve: the cutaneous continuation of the musculocutaneous nerve. It extends distally to the fetlock.

NERVE BLOCKS

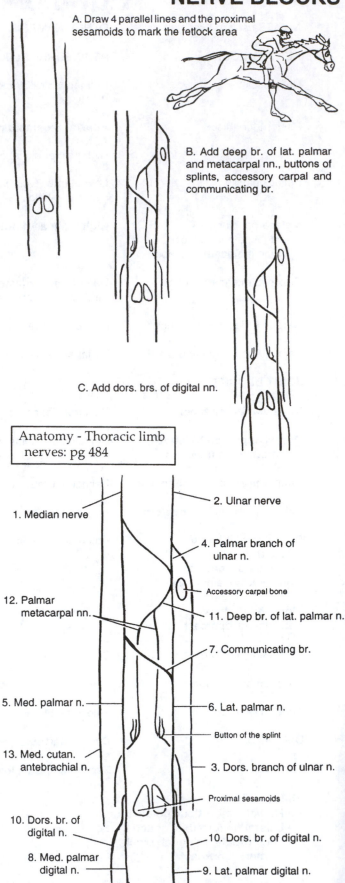

A. Draw 4 parallel lines and the proximal sesamoids to mark the fetlock area

B. Add deep br. of lat. palmar and metacarpal nn., buttons of splints, accessory carpal and communicating br.

C. Add dors. brs. of digital nn.

Anatomy - Thoracic limb nerves: pg 484

1. Median nerve
2. Ulnar nerve
4. Palmar branch of ulnar n.
Accessory carpal bone
12. Palmar metacarpal nn.
11. Deep br. of lat. palmar n.
7. Communicating br.
5. Med. palmar n.
6. Lat. palmar n.
Button of the splint
13. Med. cutan. antebrachial n.
3. Dors. branch of ulnar n.
Proximal sesamoids
10. Dors. br. of digital n.
10. Dors. br. of digital n.
8. Med. palmar digital n.
9. Lat. palmar digital n.

Figure: Simple line schematic to nerves of the distal thoracic limb

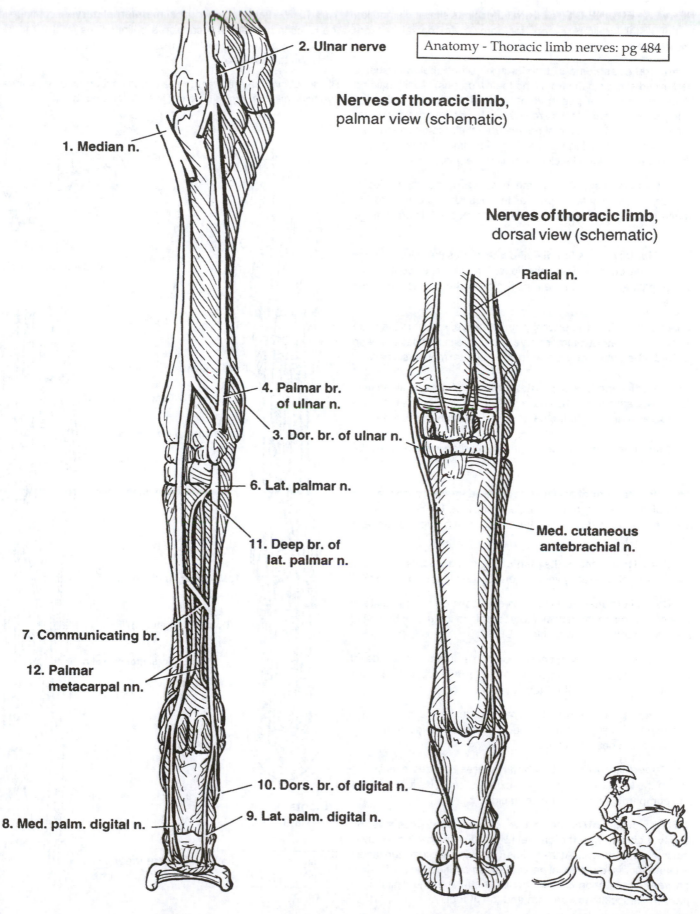

2. Ulnar nerve

Anatomy - Thoracic limb nerves: pg 484

Nerves of thoracic limb,
palmar view (schematic)

1. Median n.

Nerves of thoracic limb,
dorsal view (schematic)

Radial n.

4. Palmar br.
   of ulnar n.

3. Dor. br. of ulnar n.

6. Lat. palmar n.

11. Deep br. of
    lat. palmar n.

Med. cutaneous
antebrachial n.

7. Communicating br.

12. Palmar
    metacarpal nn.

10. Dors. br. of digital n.

8. Med. palm. digital n.

9. Lat. palm. digital n.

NERVES - EQUINE DISTAL HINDLIMB: has similar distribution to the distal forelimb, except for some extra dorsal sensory branches.

Perineural anesthesia of the distal hindlimb (below tarsus) is performed similar to the front limb (below carpus). Additional ring blocks dorsal to the pastern/foot (abaxial sesamoid), fetlock (4 point) & metatarsus blocks are advised to get the added innervation of the dorsal metatarsal nerves from the peroneal nerve that have no corresponding nerves in the forelimb. Extreme caution should be used when blocking hindlimb nerves.

1. Tibial nerve: supplies all the muscles of the caudal leg & sensory to the plantar aspect of the pes. Just proximal to the talocrural joint the tibial nerve divides into medial & lateral plantar nerves.

2 & 3. Plantar nerves (medial and lateral): as the palmar nerves pass distally on the sides of the flexor tendons. They continue as do the palmar nerves to the heel region of the foot as the digital nerves.

4. Deep branch of the lateral plantar nerve: similar to the deep branch of the lateral palmar nerve in the forelimb. It passes deep and branches into the medial and lateral plantar metatarsal nerves.

5 & 6. Medial and lateral plantar metatarsal nerves: lie against the metatarsal bones. They pass further distally then the metacarpal nerves to innervate the pastern and possibly the coronet.

7. Communicating branch: connects medial and lateral plantar nerves, it may be absent.

8 & 9. Plantar digital nerves (medial and lateral): continuations of the plantar nerve to the heel region of the foot. The neurovascular bundle is arranged as the in the thoracic limb - vein, artery and nerve (VAN).

10. Dorsal branches of the plantar digital nerves: as in the front limb arise at the fetlock joint & extend to the toe region of the foot.

11. Caudal cutaneous sural nerve: passes on the dorsolateral side of the limb to the fetlock (comparable to the dorsal branch of the ulnar nerve in the thoracic limb).

12. Saphenous nerve: passes on the dorsomedially side of metatarsus to the fetlock (comparable to the medial cutaneous anterbrachial nerve in the thoracic limb).

• **Common peroneal nerve:** a branch of the ischiatic nerve, it branches into superficial and deep peroneal nerves at the proximal leg near the stifle.

13. Superficial peroneal (fibular) nerve: passes distally between the long and lateral digital extensor muscles to the fetlock (no comparable nerve in the thoracic limb).

14. Deep peroneal (fibular) nerve: passes deep to reach the tibia & travel distally with the cranial tibial artery below the extensor muscles and tendons. At the tarsus it divides to become the medial & lateral dorsal metatarsal nerves, which continue in the junction between the cannon & splint bones (MtII-IV) to the digits. They pass the fetlock to the pastern and toe of foot.

15 & 16. Medial & lateral dorsal metatarsal nerves: continue in the junction between the cannon & splint bones (MtII-IV) to the digits. They pass the fetlock to the pastern and toe (no comparable nerves in the forelimb).

Blocks above the metatarsus are usually accomplished by intra-synovial injection of the different joints & cunean bursa.

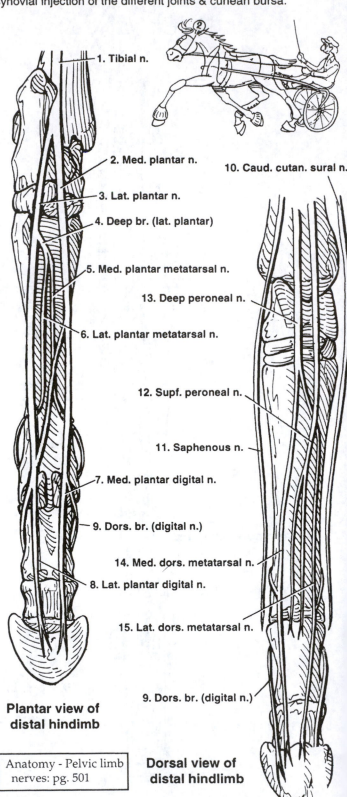

1. Tibial n.
2. Med. plantar n.
3. Lat. plantar n.
4. Deep br. (lat. plantar)
5. Med. plantar metatarsal n.
6. Lat. plantar metatarsal n.
7. Med. plantar digital n.
9. Dors. br. (digital n.)
8. Lat. plantar digital n.

10. Caud. cutan. sural n.
13. Deep peroneal n.
12. Supf. peroneal n.
11. Saphenous n.
14. Med. dors. metatarsal n.
15. Lat. dors. metatarsal n.
9. Dors. br. (digital n.)

Plantar view of distal hindimb

Dorsal view of distal hindlimb

Anatomy - Pelvic limb nerves: pg. 501

Lameness - Nerve Blocks

BLOCKS - LAMENESS DIAGNOSIS: lameness is the consequence of pain or mechanical interference (rare). Nerve blocks & intrasynovial anesthesia stop pain perception, thus, lameness (horse "goes sound"), helping to localize the problem.

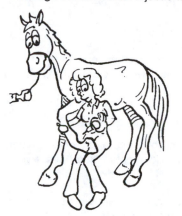

- First identify the lame limb by palpation & observing the animal at rest & in motion. Once the limb has been identified, nerve blocks may be performed to localize the problem area of the limb.
- **Start distally** (lower) & **move proximally** (higher) to localize the problem.
- Block nerves above the area to be anesthetized because the nerve branches spread out as they move distally.
- Block bilaterally (pain doesn't know where the midline is).
- If a limb is blocked sound (no lameness) & the opposite limb is also affected, that limb will then appear lame.
- Look for changes in degree of lameness, not 100% soundness with a block.
- Block higher if the animal doesn't "go sound" with a block.
- Problem is distal to last block performed to achieve soundness.
- Problem is between last 2 blocks used to achieve soundness.
- Blocking to soundness is not a definitive diagnosis, but localizes the source of lameness.
- Thorough radiographic, ultrasound or scintigraphic examination of localized area must follow.

Procedure for nerve blocks:

- Restrain the horse with the handler & the veterinarian standing on the <u>same</u> side of the animal.
  - <u>Do not</u> tranquilize the horse as this will mask the effects of the blocks.
  - A twitch may be helpful in some horses during insertion of the needle.
  - Blocks can be performed with the horse weight bearing or nonweight bearing, depending on the performer's preference.
  - Lifting & flexing the leg gives better control for most blocks.

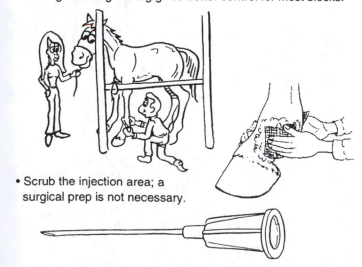

- Scrub the injection area; a surgical prep is not necessary.

- **Use a small needle** (22 gauge 5/8th inch) to minimize pain.
  - Insert the needle <u>quickly</u> upward so if the horse moves, the needle won't be jabbed into the limb.

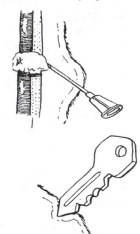

- Let the animal calm down
  - Then attach the syringe using both hands
  - Inject a little anesthetic subcutaneously
  - Then move the needle to the area of the nerve
  - Inject the anesthetic solution at a moderate rate
  - Infuse the anesthetic as closely as possible to the desired nerves in order to produce a limited field of anesthesia

- Aspirate before injecting to avoid injecting into a vessel.
- Injection should not be difficult. If it is, then the needle may be interdermal or in a tendon, redirect the needle & try again.

- Massage the area after injection.

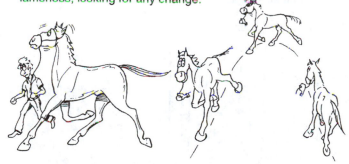

- **Check success of block**: by pushing a blunt object (ball-point pen or key) into area of skin that is desensitized by block

- **Exercise**: once the block has been performed & checked, **exercise the horse** in the same manner that showed the original lameness, looking for any change.

Nerve blocks (perineural block), depending on the article or veterinarian, vary in minor ways, especially for the metacarpal region. Distal to the carpus & tarsus nerve blocks are performed in roughly the same manner except that ring blocks are added to for the dorsal metatarsal nerves that have no comparable nerves in the thoracic limb.

Types of Nerve Blocks: point, line, & ring blocks

- **Point block** (perineural anesthesia): blocking a specific nerve directly at one site. This blocks the nerve & its branches distal to the site of injection.

- **Line block**: produced by infiltrating the anesthetic along a line. This numbs the nerve branches crossing the line.

- **Ring block or field block**: achieved by injecting anesthetic in a complete or partial circle around the limb.

Heel Block (Palmar Digital Block)

"Heel block" or Palmar digital (volar) nerve block (PD): anesthetizes the palmar/plantar digital nerves innervating the palmar/plantar (heel) aspect of the foot.

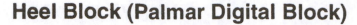

Anatomy - Nerves: pg. 494

Dist. thoracic limb, lat. view

- **Procedure** (same in front & hindlimbs):
  - Put horse in stocks & do block while weight bearing if cooperative. A nose twitch may be necessary. If the horse is fractious lifting the foot & placing the hoof between your knees will give more control.

  - Location: palpate the neurovascular bundle (pulse in digital artery) along the dorsal border of the flexor tendons in the pastern region. Palpate the lateral cartilages.
    . Neurovascular bundle is arranged VAN (vein, artery & nerve) from dorsal to palmar/plantar.

  - **Needle:** Insert the needle just proximal to the ungual cartilage at the level of the pastern joint.
    . Aspirate & inject 1-2 ml of local anesthetic SQ (5/8" 22 gauge) across the vascular bundle.
    . Use a small amount of anesthetic so it doesn't diffuse to the dorsal branch.

An alternative is to push up the ergot & locate its tensed ligament. Inject through the middle of this ligament to block the nerve passing under it.

- **Check:** 3-5 minutes after injecting with a ball point pen or key into the skin over the **bulbs of the heel**. Also test the coronet over the toe to check that the dorsal branches have <u>not</u> been blocked. Hoof testers are also good for testing to see if deep structures (navicular bone) are anesthetized.

Boundaries of injection site
- Palmar/plantar - Flexor tendons
- Distal - Ungual cartilage
- Dorsal - Digital artery

Schematic, nerves

Heel block — Dors. br. — Digital n.

1. Metacarpal n.
2. Digital n.
3. Dorsal branch of digital n.
4. Ligament of ergot
5. Digital v. & a.
6. Palmar digital n.

a. Flexor tendons
b. Lateral cartilage
c. Possible abberant branch

Heel block

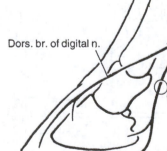

Conditions blocked:
- Shoeing problems
- Bruising of palmar/plantar sole
- Thrush
- Navicular diz
- Navicular fxs
- Palmar fxs of P3
- Digital cushion & bulb lesions

Partially blocked
- Coffin joint problems (synovitis, arthritis)
- Laminitis

Dorsal portion (toe) of the foot is unaffected

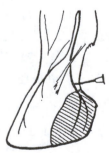

Area desensitized by heel block

Dors. br. of digital n.

Digital n.

Heel block

Schematic, lat view

Pastern/Foot Block - ASNB

"Pastern/Foot" nerve block,
Abaxial sesamoidean nerve block (ASNB), High digital block

- **Blocks:** pastern & entire foot

- **Procedure**: (same in front & hindlimbs)
  - Do in stock with horse weight bearing or outside stock in nonweight bearing if fractious animal.

- **Location**: abaxial sides at distal end of proximal sesamoids
  - Palpate the palmar digital nerve & its dorsal branch over the sides of the proximal sesamoid bones ("pop" them under your fingers). Move distally & locate the base of the sesamoids.

- **Inject** 3 to 5 ml (5/8" 22 gauge needle) of local anesthetic SQ.
  - Blocking distally from where the nerves can be palpated prevents the anesthetic from going too far proximally, possibly anesthetizing the fetlock area.

- **Check**: with a blunt object over the whole coronet

- **Comment: intrasynovial blocks - further localization**
  - If horse goes sound with a pastern/foot block, the coffin & pastern joints can be blocked after the perineural blocks have worn off (pg 597).

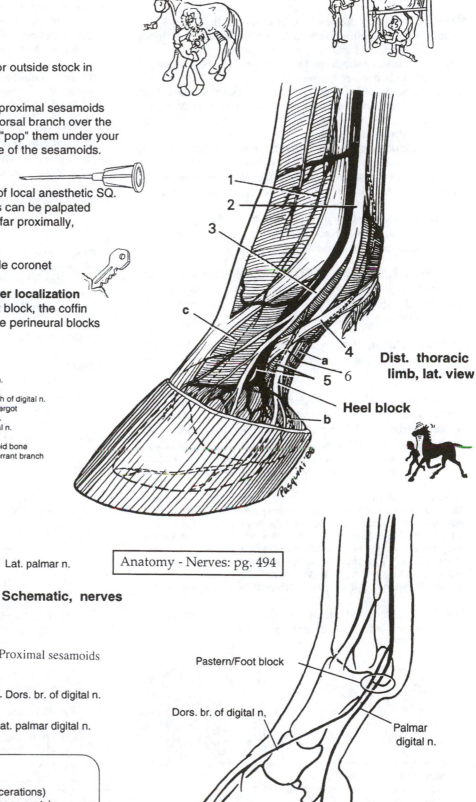

1. Metacarpal n.
2. Palmar n.
3. Dorsal branch of digital n.
4. Ligament of ergot
5. Digital v. & a.
6. Palmar digital n.

a. Dist. sesamoid bone
b. Possible aberrant branch

Dist. thoracic limb, lat. view

Heel block

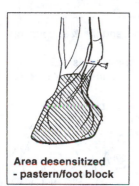

Area desensitized - pastern/foot block

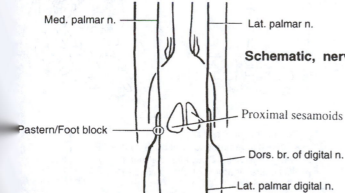

Med. palmar n.

Lat. palmar n.

Schematic, nerves

Anatomy - Nerves: pg. 494

Pastern/Foot block

Proximal sesamoids

Dors. br. of digital n.

Lat. palmar digital n.

Pastern/Foot block

Dors. br. of digital n.

Palmar digital n.

Schematic, lat view

Conditions blocked:
- Pastern joint (synovitis, DJD)
- Pastern area (dist. sesamoidean strain, lacerations)
- Coffin joint (Synovitis, DJD, Subchondral bone cysts)
- Toe of foot (bruises, abscesses, canker, laminitis, seedy toe, shoeing problems, fxs of P3)
- Heel (already ruled out with the heel block)

Fetlock block, Low palmar (volar) block, or 4-point block

- **Nerves blocked to desensitize the fetlock distally:**
  - **Medial & lateral palmar nerves:** located on each side, between the flexor tendons & the suspensory ligament.
  - **Medial & lateral palmar metacarpal nerves:** found emerging beneath the buttons of the splint bones.
  - **Cutaneous sensation** (many references ignore these branches)
    . **Dorsal branch of the ulnar nerve:** crosses just dorsal to where the lateral metacarpal nerve emerges from beneath the button of the lateral splint.
    . **Musculocutaneous nerve branch** (medial cutaneous antebrachial nerve): traveling on the medial surface of the antebrachium near where the medial metacarpal nerve becomes subcutaneous near the button of the medial splint.

- **Procedure:** hold the limb up & flex the fetlock, taking tension off the flexor tendons. Block about 4" above the fetlock (where the epiphysis narrows down to the diaphysis).

  - **Palmar nerves:** inject 3 ml SQ (5/8" 22-g) of local anesthetic between the flexor tendons & the suspensory ligament on each side. It is <u>critical</u> to stay in the subcutis to avoid injecting into the tendon sheath.

  - **Palmar metacarpal nerves:** pass a needle (5/8" 22-gauge) under the buttons of the splints & infuse the area with 3 ml of anesthetic.

  - **Dorsal branch of the ulnar & the medial cutaneous antebrachial nerves:** block by leaving a "bleb" subcutaneously as the needle is withdrawn after performing the metacarpal nerve blocks. Many references don't block these, if not blocked realize it may result in only partial blocking of the cutaneous sensation over the fetlock.

  > Anatomy - Nerves: pg. 494

- Alternate procedure
  - Direct the needle (3" 22-gauge) from the palmar aspect of the limb dorsally to the palmar nerve between the flexor tendons & the suspensory ligament. Inject the palmar nerve (3 ml). Without removing the needle, push the flexor tendons to the side & direct the needle dorsally under the button of the splint (3 ml). Inject the metacarpal nerve. As you withdraw the needle leave a "bleb" of anesthetic under the skin to get the cutaneous nerve. Repeat this on the other side.

- **Check** after 3 to 5 minutes by pressing a blunt object (ball point pen, key) into the skin around the fetlock.

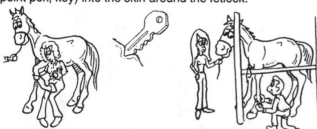

Boundaries of injection site:
- Palmar nerves between the flexor tendon & suspensory ligament
- Metacarpal nerves under the buttons of the splints
- Cutaneous nerves as you withdraw from the buttons of the splints

Low plantar block - hindlimb

- **Similar to the low palmar block of the forelimb, except:**
  - **Ring block of dorsal metatarsus:** desensitizes the 2 additional nerves (dorsal metatarsal nerves) that have no comparable nerves in the thoracic limb.

- **Nerves to hindlimb fetlock** (comparable nerves in the thoracic limb are in parentheses).
  - Medial & lateral plantar nerves (medial & lateral palmar)
  - Medial & lateral plantar metatarsal nerves (medial & lateral metacarpal)
  - **Medial & lateral dorsal metatarsal nerves** from deep peroneal (no comparable nerves in the thoracic limb) pass between the dorsal surfaces of the splint bones & cannon bone.
- Caudal cutaneous sural nerve (found laterally on the tibia) (dorsal branch of ulnar)
- Saphenous nerve (on medial side) (medial cutaneous antebrachial)

- **Procedure:**
  - Block plantar nerves as in forelimb (metatarsal nerves - block under the buttons of splint)
  - **Dorsal ring (field) block instead of bleb** to desensitize dorsal metatarsal nerves & caudal cutaneous sural & saphenous nerves to desensitize the entire dorsal surface of the fetlock distally

  > Anatomy - Nerves: pg. 516

- **Inject:**
  - Plantar nerves between the flexor tendons & suspensory ligament
  - Metatarsal nerves under the buttons of the splints
  - Cutaneous nerves with a ring block of the dorsal surface of the cannon bone

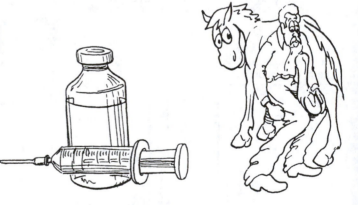

Conditions blocked:
- Fetlock joint (subchondral bone cysts of P1, McIII. Synovitis, DJD, septic arthritis)
- Collateral ligament strain/sprain
- Sesamoiditis
- Prox. sesamoid fractures
- P1 fractures
- Condylar fractures - McIII (cannon bone)

Since 90% of all lameness is in the foot,

most lameness will be isolated with these blocks (Heel, Pastern/ foot & Fetlock). If the horse is still lame, continue up the limb.

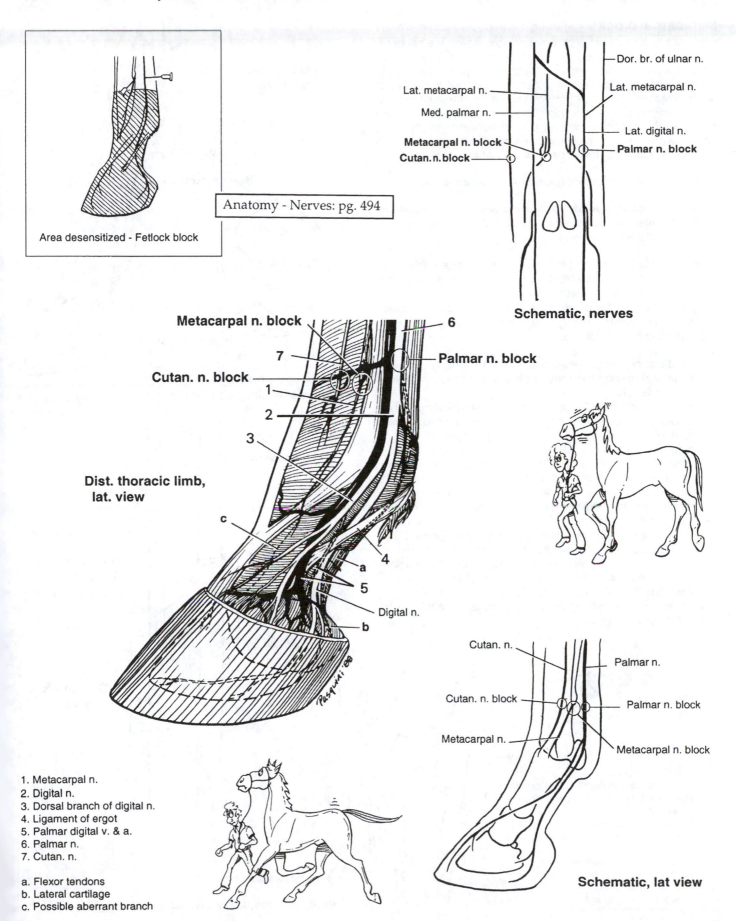

Area desensitized - Fetlock block

Anatomy - Nerves: pg. 494

Schematic, nerves

Dor. br. of ulnar n.

Lat. metacarpal n.

Lat. metacarpal n.

Med. palmar n.

Lat. digital n.

Metacarpal n. block

Cutan. n. block

Palmar n. block

Metacarpal n. block

Palmar n. block

Cutan. n. block

6

7

1

2

3

Dist. thoracic limb, lat. view

c

4

a

5

Digital n.

b

Cutan. n.

Palmar n.

Cutan. n. block

Palmar n. block

Metacarpal n.

Metacarpal n. block

Schematic, lat view

1. Metacarpal n.
2. Digital n.
3. Dorsal branch of digital n.
4. Ligament of ergot
5. Palmar digital v. & a.
6. Palmar n.
7. Cutan. n.

a. Flexor tendons
b. Lateral cartilage
c. Possible aberrant branch

Metacarpal block, High 4 point block NERVE BLOCKS

Metacarpal blocks: confusing & varied. Different people use different block locations & different combinations. The palmar & metatcarpal nerves supply most of the metacarpus. They may be blocked separately to desensitize the deep or superficial structures of the metacarpus. Blocked together they desensitize all or most of the metacarpus depending on how proximally they are performed. All metacarpal blocks are done above the mid-cannon region because of the communicating branch between the medial & lateral palmar nerves. The communicating branches can be felt on the palmar surface of the superficial digital flexor tendon.

High palmar 4 point block (palmar & metacarpal nerves)

- **Blocks**: metacarpal region, except the origin of the suspensory ligament, inferior check ligament of deep digital flexor & the proximal splints and cannon.

- **High palmar block**: used to anesthetize the superficial metacarpal structures by blocking the medial and lateral palmar nerves at the proximal metacarpus.
- **High metacarpal block**: anesthetizes the metacarpal nerves, thus, most of the suspensory ligament and the interosseous ligaments of metacarpal bones

- **Procedure**: nonweight bearing or weight bearing
  - **Palmar nerves: on the sides of the flexor tendons, below the deep fascia**
    . Insert a needle (5/8" 22 gauge) above communicating branch, through the deep fascia to the palmar nerve located between the deep digital flexor and the suspensory ligament.
    . Inject 5 ml of local anesthetic & repeat on the other side.
    - This anesthetizes the superficial metacarpal region, but will <u>not</u> desensitize all of the deep structures of the metacarpus.
    - If a SQ bleb is seen while injecting you are too superficial since the nerves are deep to the deep fascia.
  - **Metacarpal nerves: in the junction between the cannon bone & the splints, deep to the suspensory ligament**
    . Insert a needle (1" 22-gauge) distal to the carpus, between the splints (metacarpal II & IV) & the suspensory ligament down to the cannon bone (metacarpal III) on both sides.
    . Inject 3 to 5 ml of local anesthetic.
    . Blocks: Deep structures of the metacarpus, except proximal metacarpus

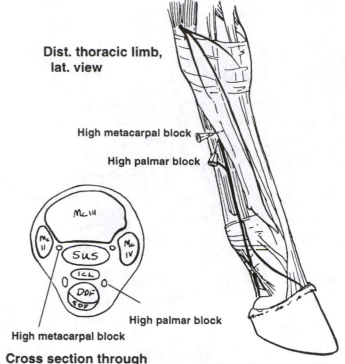

Dist. thoracic limb, lat. view

High metacarpal block

High palmar block

Mc III

Mc II

Mc IV

SUS

ICL

DDF

SDF

High palmar block

High metacarpal block

Cross section through metacarpal region, schematic

Anatomy: pgs. 484, 491

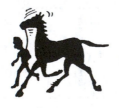

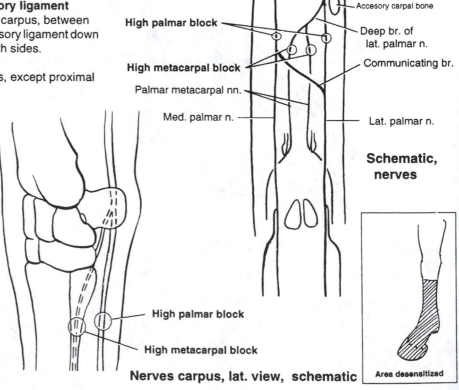

Median nerve

Ulnar nerve

Accesory carpal bone

High palmar block

Deep br. of lat. palmar n.

High metacarpal block

Communicating br.

Palmar metacarpal nn.

Med. palmar n.

Lat. palmar n.

Schematic, nerves

- Conditions blocked:
  - Bowed tendon (tendonitis) & tenosynovitis
  - Stress fractures of cannon bone (McIII)
  - Bucked shins
  - Splint bone fractures
  - Middle & low desmitis of suspensory lig.
- Not blocked:
  - High suspensory desmitis
  - Splints
  - High splint fractures
  - Inferior check ligament

High palmar block

High metacarpal block

Nerves carpus, lat. view, schematic

Area desensitized

Proximal metacarpal block

Metacarpal nerves from deep branch of lat. palmar n.
- The lateral palmar nerve passes in the carpal canal before it gives off its deep branch at the level of the heads of the splints. The deep branch bifurcates into the metacarpal nerves that pass against the palmar surface of the metacarpal bones.
- Blocking the deep innervation to the proximal metacarpus can be performed in 2 ways. If either of these block cause soundness after a negative high 4 point block, the problem is pinpointed to the proximal metacarpus.

Deep branch of the lateral palmar nerve ("Deep ulnar" nerve) block

- Blocking the deep branch of the lateral palmar nerve & its deep branch in the carpal canal

- **Procedure**:
  From the lateral side, insert a needle (1" 20 gauge) midway between the accessory carpal bone & the head of the lateral splint (McIV). Penetrate the flexor retinaculum to the carpal bones. Aspirate & redirect if synovial fluid appears in hub of needle. Inject 5 ml of local anesthetic.

Local infiltration of the suspensory ligament:

- Blocking the branches (metacarpal nerves) of the deep branch of the lateral palmar nerve just distal to the carpus.

- An alternate procedure which has a higher incidence of infiltrating the palmarodistal pouching of the carpometacarpal joint. Confusion with carpal lesions can be avoided by blocking the carpal joints (p 598) first and then infiltrating the suspensory ligament if horse remains lame.

- **Procedure**:
  - Flex the carpus
  - Insert the needle (1" 22 gauge) between the check ligament of DDF & the origin of suspensory ligament at the level of the head of the splint bones (Mc II & IV).
  - Inject 6 ml of local anesthesia both medially & laterally.

Blocks: Same as deep branch of lateral palmar nerve (above)

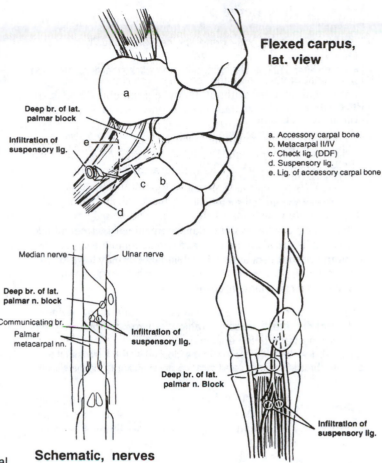

Flexed carpus, lat. view

Deep br. of lat. palmar block

Infiltration of suspensory lig.

a. Accessory carpal bone
b. Metacarpal II/IV
c. Check lig. (DDF)
d. Suspensory lig.
e. Lig. of accessory carpal bone

Median nerve — Ulnar nerve

Deep br. of lat. palmar n. block

Communicating br.
Palmar metacarpal nn.

Infiltration of suspensory lig.

Deep br. of lat. palmar n. Block

Infiltration of suspensory lig.

Schematic, nerves

Nerves carpus, palmar view, schematic

Anatomy: pgs. 484, 491

Nerves carpus, lat. view, schematic

Deep br. of lat. palmar n. block

Infiltration of suspensory lig.

Injections, schematic, palmar view

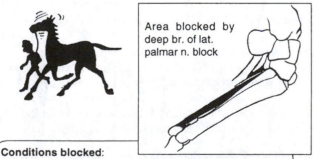

Area blocked by deep br. of lat. palmar n. block

Conditions blocked:
- Deep seated osseous lesions of cannon & splint bones
- Proximal fracture
- Avulsion of the suspensory ligament, or exostoses
- Splints (periostitis between the splints & the cannon bone)
- Desmitis of check ligament of DDF
- Structures also blocked by high metacarpal nerve block

Combining a high metacarpal & deep branch of lateral palmar nerve blocks or suspensory ligament infiltration: blocks: all the structures of the metacarpus
- Tendinitis & tenosynovitis
- Bucked shins
- Stress fractures of cannon bone (McIII)
- Splint bone fractures
- Suspensory desmitis
- **Splints**
- Desmitis of check ligament of DDF

Median & Ulnar Nerve Block

Median & ulnar nerve block
• Desensitizes the entire lower limb from the carpus distally.
• This block is infrequently done, the carpus is usually blocked with intra-synovial blocks (p 598).
• Best done after other nerve blocks have worn off, so that desensitization can be checked.

• **Procedure**
  - **Ulnar nerve block:**
    . Palpate groove (between the flexor carpi ulnaris & ulnaris lateralis muscles) 4" above the accessory carpal bone on the palmar aspect of the forearm.
    . Inject 10 ml of local anesthetic SQ (1", 21 guage)
    .. Nerve is deep to the deep fascia, so a SQ bleb upon injection indicates you are too superficial.
  - **Median nerve:**
    . Palpate the caudal border of flexor carpi radialis on medial side of distal forearm a hand's breadth proximal to the chestnut.
    . Insert needle (21guage, 1.5") obliquely cranially towards the caudal radius. Aspirate, if blood is in the hub, slightly withdraw & inject 10 ml of local anesthetic.

• Check if distal blocks have worn off, or not performed previously
  - Ulnar nerve: blunt probe of craniolateral metacarpus
  - Median nerve: craniomedial side of pastern
• The musculocutaneous nerve may be blocked where it crosses the lacertus fibrosis to eliminate all cutaneous sensation to the distal limb

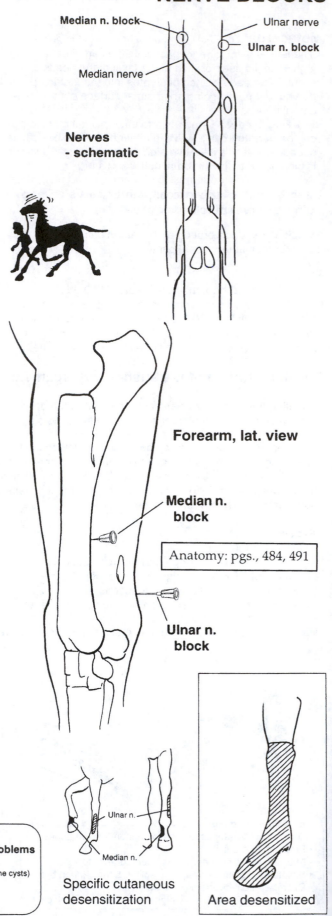

Nerves - schematic

Forearm, lat. view

Median n. block

Anatomy: pgs., 484, 491

Ulnar n. block

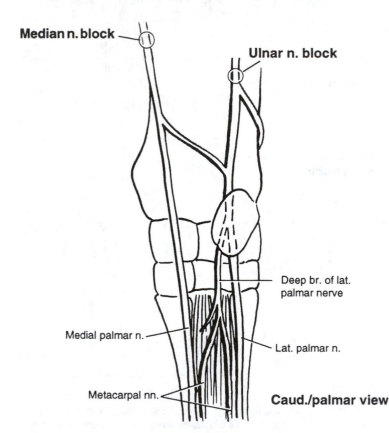

Median n. block

Ulnar n. block

Deep br. of lat. palmar nerve

Medial palmar n.

Lat. palmar n.

Metacarpal nn.

Caud./palmar view

Ulnar n.

Median n.

Specific cutaneous desensitization

Area desensitized

Structures blocked (carpus distally)
• **Eliminate distal limb if upper arm (forearm, elbow, arm or shoulder) problems suspected**
  • Intercarpal joint problem (synovitis, DJD, intercarpal ligament strain, carpal fractures, subchondral bone cysts)
  • Carpal tunnel syndrome
  • Intercarpal problems are better checked with intra-articular anesthesia
  • Can replace deep branch of the lateral palmar nerve block or suspensory ligament infiltration

Tibial & Fibular (peroneal) Nerve block

Hindlimb: lat. view

- Infrequently done to desensitize tarsus and distal limb
- **Procedure**
  - **Tibial block:**
    . From the medial side of the limb, palpate the tibial n. 4" above the point of the hock between the Achilles' tendon & the deep digital flexor tendon on the medial side. The tibial nerve lies on the back of the deep digital flexor muscle.
    . Desensitize the skin with 1 ml of anesthetic (25 gauge).
    . Insert needle (18 gauge 1.5") to the area of nerve & inject 15-25 ml of local anesthetic
  - **Deep & superficial peroneal nerves**
    . Palpate the septum between the long & lateral digital extensor muscles 4" above the tarsus where the muscle bellies taper.
    . Desensitize the skin over the nerves (25 gauge needle).
    . Insert needle (2" 22 gauge) between the long & lateral digital extensors 4" above the point of tarsus. Penetrate down to the tibia. Aspirate & inject 10-15 ml of local anesthetic to anesthetize the deep peroneal nerve.
    . Retract needle & inject 10-15 ml of local anesthetic superficially to desensitize the superficial peroneal nerve.

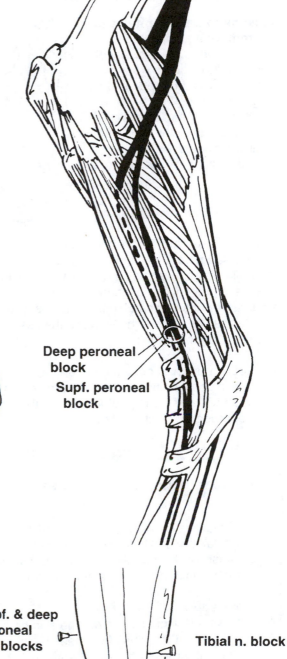

Deep peroneal block

Supf. peroneal block

Structures blocked:
- Blocks out entire distal limb (eliminates distal limb if stifle or higher problem is suspected).

Tibial n. block

Anatomy: pgs. 501, 509, 511

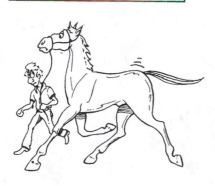

Supf. & deep peroneal nn. blocks

Tibial n. block

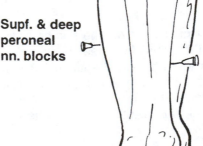

Hindlimb: medial view

Hindlimb: caud. view

Joint Blocks

Arthrocentesis (ar'thro-sen-TEE-sis): the puncturing & aspiration of a joint

Reasons to arthrocentes a joint:

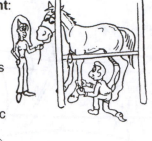

- To remove a sample for visualization (e.g., viscosity of synovial fluid) or lab work
- To administer therapeutic drugs (e.g., antibiotics)
- To administer a diagnostic substance (dye) for radiographic contrast studies
- To administer an anesthetic

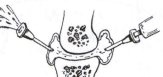

Joints & bursae are blocked to localize pain to a specific blocked structure. The higher risk in these injections over nerve blocks necessitates the observation of total surgical asepsis to prevent contamination. There is also the danger of damaging articular cartilage, thus, causing degenerative joint disease or acute arthritis. Nevertheless, they are very valuable diagnostic tools.

An injection of an anesthetic into a joint of a lame horse which then goes sound localizes the problem to that joint. If the horse remains lame, that joint is not the problem; or it was not properly anesthetized.

Surgical access to a joint: arthroscopic surgery is becoming popular & requires knowing where to access joints. More than one entrance is often necessary for such surgeries.

Joint pouches: focal points where the joint capsule protrudes between osseous & soft tissue structures. The pouches may or may not be swollen, thus, may or may not be palpable. The joint is accessible through these pouches. Avoiding the articular cartilage is desirable, but not always possible. Protrusion of the joint capsule (pouches) sometimes allows a needle to enter the joint cavity away from the articular cartilages. If it becomes necessary to enter between the articular cartilages, use a small needle & restrain the animal to minimize movement & possible scarification of the cartilage.

To locate the injection site:
1. Locate the level of the joint by palpating the regional structures
2. Locate the injection sites by palpating their boundaries
3. Insert the needle & aspirate synovial fluid
   - If you are injecting a large quantity of local anesthetic, remove the same amount of synovial fluid before injection.

Navicular (podotrochlear) bursa block

Anatomy - Joints: pg. 117

Anesthetizes the navicular bursa and, by diffusion, the navicular bone. This block is difficult & rarely done because of the probability of deep infection. If performed, it is done after the heel block has worn off.

- **Procedure:**
  - Make a SQ injection under the skin on midline, just above the bulbs of the heel
  - Direct the needle (2 inch, 20-gauge) through this point, dorsally & parallel to the ground until it hits bone (navicular bone)
  - Back off slightly & inject 5 ml of anesthetic into the bursa

Proximal approach, alternate procedure:
- Procedure
  - Insert the needle above the lateral cartilage of P3
  - Angle the needle towards the opposite heel between the middle phalanx & DDF tendon
  - Use radiographic control

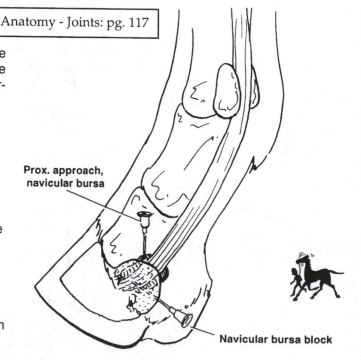

Prox. approach, navicular bursa

Navicular bursa block

Dorsal approach to the fetlock, pastern & coffin joints:

- **Procedure:** same for all 3 joints
  - Insert the needle (1 1/2" 20-gauge) proximal to the joint, under the common/long digital extensor tendon laterally, & pass obliquely into the dorsal pouch
  - Inject 5 ml of local anesthetic

- Coffin joint is within the hoof wall, therefore it cannot be palpated, but only mentally visualized. Insert the needle above the coronet, lateral to & under the extensor tendons into the dorsal pouch.

Palmar approach to coffin joint
- Procedure:
  - Spinal needle placed slightly above deepest indentation of the fossa above the bulbs of the heel
  - Direct needle dorsally & distally toward midpoint between the coronet & toe of the foot

Anatomy - Joints: pg. 117

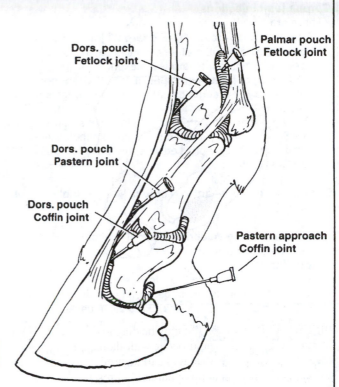

Digit - lat. view

Palmar approach to the fetlock:
- An easier alternative to the dorsal approach
- **Procedure**:
  - Flex the fetlock
  - Palpate the boundaries of the palmar pouch (suspensory lig & cannon bone just proximal to the joint)
  - Insert the needle (1" 18-gauge) dorsal to the suspensory ligament & palmar to the cannon bone
  - Inject 5 ml of local anesthetic

Boundaries:
- Dorsal pouches
  - Proximal to the joint
  - Obliquely under the extensor tendon
- Palmar pouch of fetlock
  - Proximal - button of splint bone
  - Dorsal - cannon bone
  - Distal - proximal sesamoid bone
  - Palmar - suspensory ligament

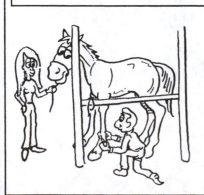

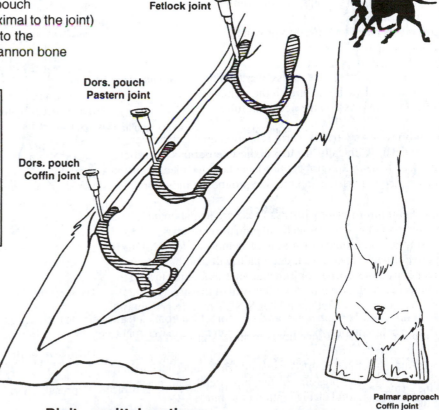

Digit - sagittal section   **Digit, palmar view**

Carpal Joint Blocks

Carpus joint injections
- There are 3 main joints in the carpus
  - **Antebrachiocarpal** or **"Radiocarpal" joint**: doesn't communicate with the other carpal joints. Dorsally it opens wide when the carpus is flexed.
  - **Middle carpal joint**/intercarpal joint: also opens dorsally on flexion & communicates with the carpometacarpal joint.
  - **Carpometacarpal joint**: too small to access with a needle. Fortunately it communicates with the middle carpal joint, thus, is blocked when the middle carpal joint is anesthetized.

Dorsal approaches - antebrachiocarpal & middle carpal joints:

- **Blocks:** either the antebrachiocarpal joint or the middle & carpometacarpal joints
- **Procedure:**
  - Flex the carpus to open the joints
  - Palpate the depressions of both joints on either side of the tendon of the extensor carpi radialis muscle
  - Insert a needle (1" 20-gauge) medially or laterally to the tendon & into the depressions
  - Put a syringe on the needle, aspirate 10 ml of synovial fluid & inject 10 ml of local anesthetic
- **Location:** depression on either side of the extensor carpi radialis

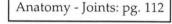

Anatomy - Joints: pg. 112

Carpus - dors. flexed view

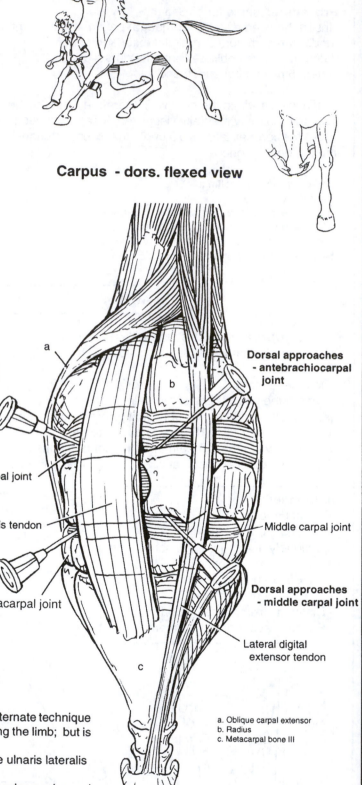

Dorsal approaches - antebrachiocarpal joint

Antebrachiocarpal joint

Extensor carpi radialis tendon

Carpometacarpal joint

Middle carpal joint

Dorsal approaches - middle carpal joint

Lateral digital extensor tendon

a. Oblique carpal extensor
b. Radius
c. Metacarpal bone III

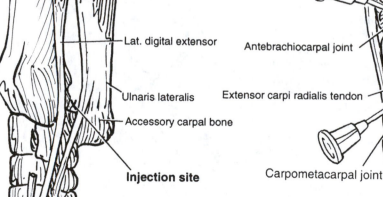

Lat. digital extensor

Ulnaris lateralis

Accessory carpal bone

Injection site

Carpus, lat. view

Palmarolateral pouch approach - antebrachiocarpal joint: an alternate technique that is safer for the articular cartilage, can be done without flexing the limb; but is more difficult to perform.
- Locate the depression between the accessory carpal bone, the ulnaris lateralis muscle & lat. digital extensor muscle
- Insert the needle (1.5" 20-gauge) perpendicular to the limb into the depression and into joint space
- Remove synovial fluid & inject 10 ml of anesthetic.

Elbow (Cubital) Joint

- Difficult to anesthetize; fortunately seldom needed as elbow problems are quite rare.

Lateral approach to the elbow:
- Procedure:
  - Locate the lat. collateral lig. between the palpable lat. epicondyle proximally & the origin of the lat. digital extensor distally
  - Feel the space cranial or caudal to the lat. collateral lig.
  - Slide needle (2 1/2" 18-gauge) into either of these spaces
  - Aspirate & inject 10 ml of local anesthetic
- Boundaries: cranial or caudal to the lateral collateral ligament at the level of the elbow joint

Caudolateral approach to the elbow
- Alternate approach to the elbow joint
- Procedure
  - 18 g 3.5" needle inserted from the caudolat. side, proximal to the elbow joint
  - Direct the needle between the olecranon process of the ulna and the lateral epicondyle of the humerus into the caudal pouch over the olecranon fossa

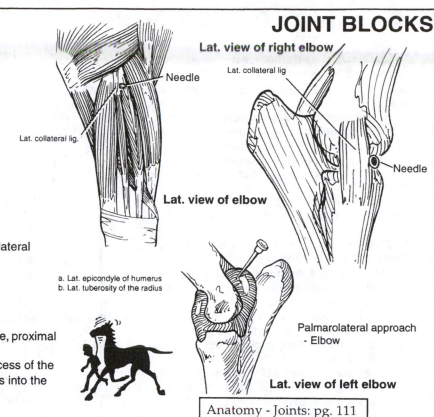

JOINT BLOCKS

Lat. view of right elbow

Lat. collateral lig

Needle

Lat. collateral lig.

Lat. view of elbow

Needle

a. Lat. epicondyle of humerus
b. Lat. tuberosity of the radius

Palmarolateral approach - Elbow

Lat. view of left elbow

Anatomy - Joints: pg. 111

Shoulder Joint Block:

- **Procedure:**
  - Palpate the notch betwee the cran. & caud. prominences (greater tubercle - humerus)
  - Insert the needle (3 1/2" 18 gauge spinal) through the notch at an angle caudal, distal, & medial in order to get into the joint space (greater tubercle extends proximally & cranially above the level of the joint)
  - Aspirate a liberal amount of synovial fluid & inject 10 to 20 mls of local anesthetic
- Injection site: notch in greater tubercle

Intertubercular (bicipital) bursa block:
- The shoulder joint & the intertubercular bursa in the horse are separate structures that do not communicate. Access to the bursa is blocked from the lateral side by the greater tubercle
- **Procedure**:
  - Insert the needle (2 1/2-6" 18-gauge) at the level of the deltoid tuberosity
  - Slide the needle up the cranial surface of the humerus, deep to the biceps brachii & into the intertubercular groove and bursa
  - If the needle goes past the bursa, resistance will be met as it enters the biceps tendon
    . Back off & aspirate synovial fluid
  - Inject 10 ml of anesthetic solution
  - In a large horse this procedure may require a six inch needle

Infraspinatus bursa block: rarely done

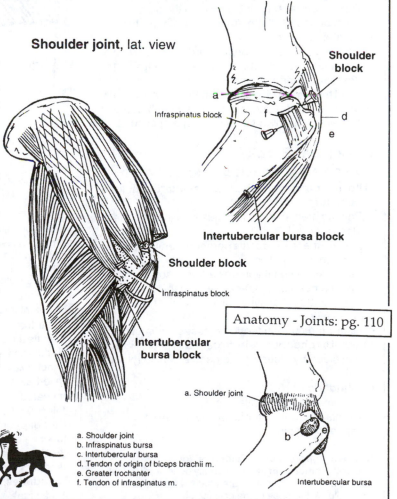

Shoulder joint, lat. view

Shoulder block

a

Infraspinatus block

f

d

e

Intertubercular bursa block

Shoulder block

Infraspinatus block

Intertubercular bursa block

Anatomy - Joints: pg. 110

a. Shoulder joint

b

e

a. Shoulder joint
b. Infraspinatus bursa
c. Intertubercular bursa
d. Tendon of origin of biceps brachii m.
e. Greater trochanter
f. Tendon of infraspinatus m.

Intertubercular bursa

TARSUS/HOCK - anatomy: has 4 distinct joints
- **Tarsocrural, talocrural or "tibiotarsal" joint**: articulation between the tibia & the trochlea of the talus
  - Communicates with the prox. intertarsal joint
  - 3 pouches in which the joint capsule protrudes subcutaneously: dorsal, medioplantar & lateroplantar. These are all connected, therefore, injection in any one anesthetizes all 3 & the prox. intertarsal joint
- **Proximal intertarsal joint**: articulation between the talus & calcaneus proximally & the central & 4th tarsal bones distally
  - Direct communication with the tarsocrural joint, therefore <u>never</u> injected directly
- **Distal intertarsal & tarsometatarsal joints**: plane joints with little motion, thus, the joint spaces are very narrow & difficult to place a needle in. They are, however, most often affected by bone spavin & injected for diagnosis more often than the easier to inject talocural joint. They interconnect in roughly one third of horses.
  - **Distal intertarsal joint, DIT**: between the central, 3rd & fused 1st & 2nd tarsal bones. It does not communicate with any other joint so has to be injected specifically. It is extremely narrow & hard to consistently inject.
  - **Tarsometatarsal joint**: between the distal row of tarsal bones (3rd, 4th, fused 1st & 2nd, & the metatarsal bones)
- **Cunean tendon**: the medial tendon of insertion of the cranial tibial muscle. It inserts on the fused 1st & 2nd tarsal bone. It crosses the dorsomedial surface of the tarsus where bone spavin usually occurs.
  - **Cunean bursa**: under cunean tendon & dorsomedial tarsus (over the site of bone spavin)

Talocrural Blocks
Dorsomedial pouch block:
- **Blocks**: tarsocrural & proximal intertarsal joint
- **Procedure**:
  - Palpate med. malleolus cranially to the calcanean tuberosity
  - Palpate the tendon of the peroneus tertius cranially to the medial malleolus
  - Move distally until you feel a large, soft spot
  - Insert a needle (1" 20-gauge) into this soft spot
  - Aspirate 20 ml of synovial fluid & inject 20 ml of anesthetic
- Distally the cunean tendon crosses the tarsus
- **Medial saphenous vein** crosses this pouch & must be avoided by inserting the needle behind (plantar to) it.
- **Boundaries**:
  - Proximal: medial malleolus
  - Cranial: peroneus tertius muscle or med. saphenous vein

Alternate approaches to Talocrural joint
- **Lateral plantar approach (a)**: rarely done. Inject into the soft spot in the "V" shaped area between the lateral malleolus & the body of the calcaneus

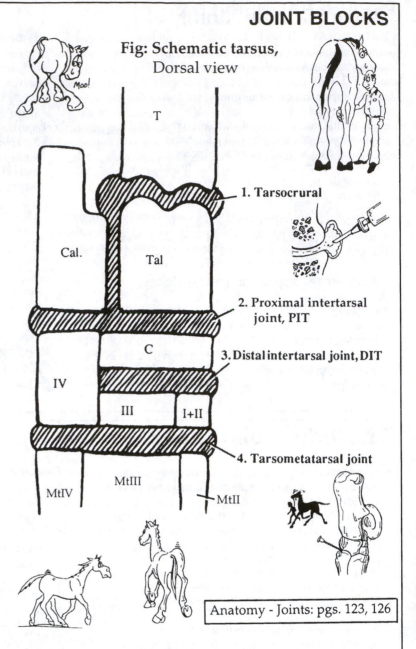

Fig: Schematic tarsus, Dorsal view

T

Cal.

Tal

1. Tarsocrural

2. Proximal intertarsal joint, PIT

C

3. Distal intertarsal joint, DIT

IV

III

I+II

4. Tarsometatarsal joint

MtIV

MtIII

MtII

Anatomy - Joints: pgs. 123, 126

- **Medial plantar approach (b)**: hard to palpate, it also is rarely done. Palpate the deep digital flexor tendon between the medial malleolus & the calcanean tuberosity. Pass the needle between the caudal edge of the tibia & the tendon of the deep digital flexor muscle at the level of the medial malleolus. Avoid the synovial sheath of the deep digital flexor tendon by going dorsal to it.

DIT (distal intertarsal) **joint injection**
- **Procedure**:
  - Palpate the gap between the fused 1st & 2nd, 3rd, & central tarsal bone on the <u>medial</u> side of the hock with a fingernail
  - Inject a little anesthetic SQ at this site
  - Insert a needle (1" 22-gauge) into this junction. This may require repeated redirection of the needle
  - Inject 5 ml of anesthetic
  - If the gap can't be palpated, draw a straight line from the palpable distal tubercle of the talus to the palpable space between the heads of the 3rd & 2nd metatarsal bones. Palpate the proximal border of the cunean tendon & inject where it crosses this line.
- **Boundaries**: junction of central, 3rd & fused 1st & 2nd tarsal bones (med. side)

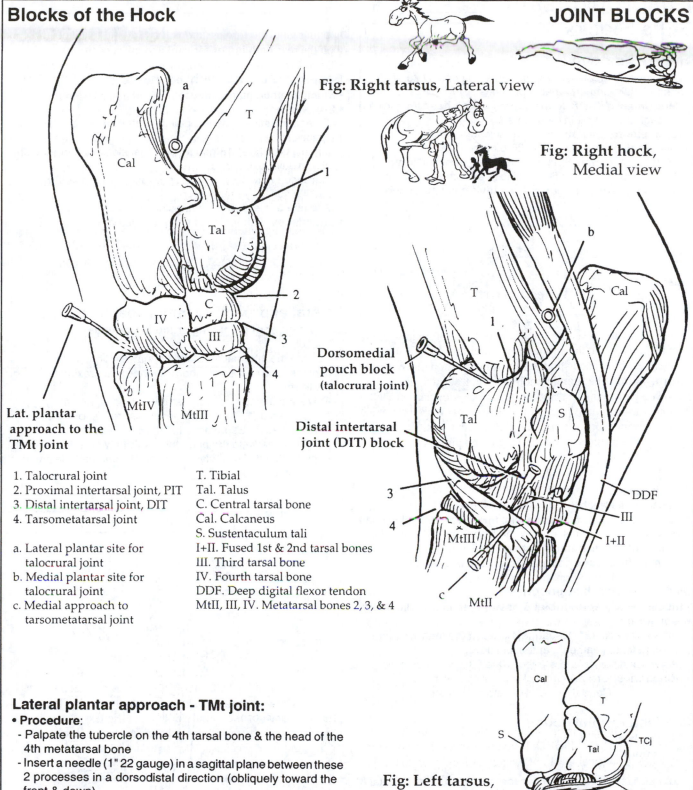

Fig: Right tarsus, Lateral view

Fig: Right hock, Medial view

Lat. plantar approach to the TMt joint

Dorsomedial pouch block (talocrural joint)

Distal intertarsal joint (DIT) block

1. Talocrural joint
2. Proximal intertarsal joint, PIT
3. Distal intertarsal joint, DIT
4. Tarsometatarsal joint

a. Lateral plantar site for talocrural joint
b. Medial plantar site for talocrural joint
c. Medial approach to tarsometatarsal joint

T. Tibial
Tal. Talus
C. Central tarsal bone
Cal. Calcaneus
S. Sustentaculum tali
I+II. Fused 1st & 2nd tarsal bones
III. Third tarsal bone
IV. Fourth tarsal bone
DDF. Deep digital flexor tendon
MtII, III, IV. Metatarsal bones 2, 3, & 4

Fig: Left tarsus, Medial view

Lateral plantar approach - TMt joint:
- **Procedure:**
  - Palpate the tubercle on the 4th tarsal bone & the head of the 4th metatarsal bone
  - Insert a needle (1" 22 gauge) in a sagittal plane between these 2 processes in a dorsodistal direction (obliquely toward the front & down)
  - Inject 5 ml of anesthetic
- **Boundaries:** 4th tarsal bone
  4th metatarsal bone

Medial approach to the tarsometatarsal joint (c): alternate, more difficult approach to the TMt joint. Inject distal to the site for the distal intertarsal joint (DIT) where the 3rd, fused 1st and 2nd tarsal bones and the metatarsal bone all meet. Their site is so small that it is difficult to hit. Put a bleb of anesthetic under the skin and repeatedly redirect the needle to find the site.

Cunean bursa injection:
- **Procedure**:
  - Slide a needle (1" 22-gauge) under the palpable distal border of the cunean tendon on the <u>dorsomedial</u> side of the hock
  - Inject 10 ml of anesthetic
- Differentiate cunean bursitis from bone spavin. If a lame horse improves within 20 minutes, it is a bursitis problem.

Stifle Blocks

Stifle - Anatomy

- Stifle joint: 3 separate compartments - medial & lateral femorotibial & femoropatellar pouches
  - **Med. femorotibial & femoropatellar pouches** communicate through a small slit in most horses
  - **Lat. femorotibial pouch** communicates with the **femoropatellar pouch** only 25% of the time
  - **Med. & lat. femorotibial** pouches <u>never</u> communicate
  - Inflammation of the stifle may close all communications, therefore, **each joint has to be individually assessed**

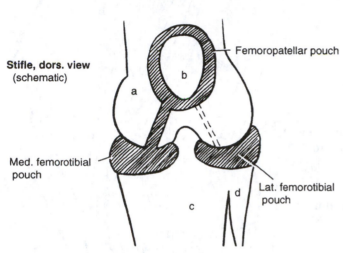

Stifle, dors. view (schematic)

Femoropatellar pouch

Med. femorotibial pouch

Lat. femorotibial pouch

Stifle blocks

- Procedure for each:
  - Identify the level of the stifle joint (med. trochlear ridge often mistaken for the patella). Flex the limb & move the patella which is more distal than first thought
  - Identify the specific boundaries of each pouch

Medial femorotibial pouch:

- **Blocks: med. femorotibial** & possibly femoropatellar pouch
- **Procedure:**
  - Insert a needle (3", 18-gauge) between the med. collateral & med. patellar ligaments at the joint level
  - Aspirate synovial fluid & inject 10 to 20 ml of anesthetic
- **Boundaries:** Cranial - medial patellar ligament
  Caudal - medial collateral ligament

Lat. femorotibial pouch:

- **Blocks**: lateral femorotibial pouch
- **Procedure**:
  - Palpate the 2 prominences of the extensor groove of the tibia to visualize where the 2 extensor muscles run (long digital & peroneus tertius)
  - Palpate the lat. collateral lig. between the lat. epicondyle of the femur & the origin of the lat. digital extensor
  - Insert a needle (3" 18-gauge) caudal to the tendons, pointing proximally
  - Aspirate synovial fluid & inject 10 to 20 ml of anesthetic
- **Boundaries**:
  - Cranial - combined tendon of peroneus tertius & long digital extensor
  - Caudal - lateral collateral ligament

Femoropatellar pouch: easy to access

- **Blocks**: femoropatellar pouch
- **Procedure**:
  - Extend the stifle, grasp & pull the patella to widen the joint space
  - Insert a needle (2" 18-gauge) on either side of the intermediate (middle) patellar lig.
  - Advance the needle 2 inches between the patella & the patellar surface of the femur
  - Aspirate & inject 20 ml of anesthetic
- **Boundaries**: Either side of intermediate patellar ligament

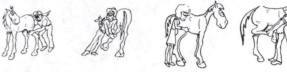

Lateral approach to femoropatellar joint

- **Less danger of damaging articular cartilage**
- Procedure
  - Palpate the intermediate (middle) patellar lig. (find the depression on the tibial tuberosity then feel proximally along the ligament)
  - Move laterally to locate the lateral patellar ligament
  - Direct needle (1.5" 18 g) perpendicular to the long axis of the femur about 2" proximal to lat. condyle of the tibia
  - Advance needle to the bone then withdraw slightly (1-2 mm)
  - Aspirate 20 ml of synovial fluid & inject a comparable amount of local anesthetic

a. Femur
b. Patella
c. Tibia
d. Fibula
e. Miniscus
f. Biceps femoris m.
g. Lat. femoropatllar lig.

Anatomy - Joints: pgs. 120, 122

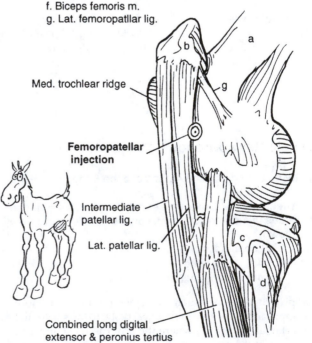

Med. trochlear ridge

Femoropatellar injection

Intermediate patellar lig.

Lat. patellar lig.

Combined long digital extensor & peronius tertius

Lat. approach, lat. view

STIFLE

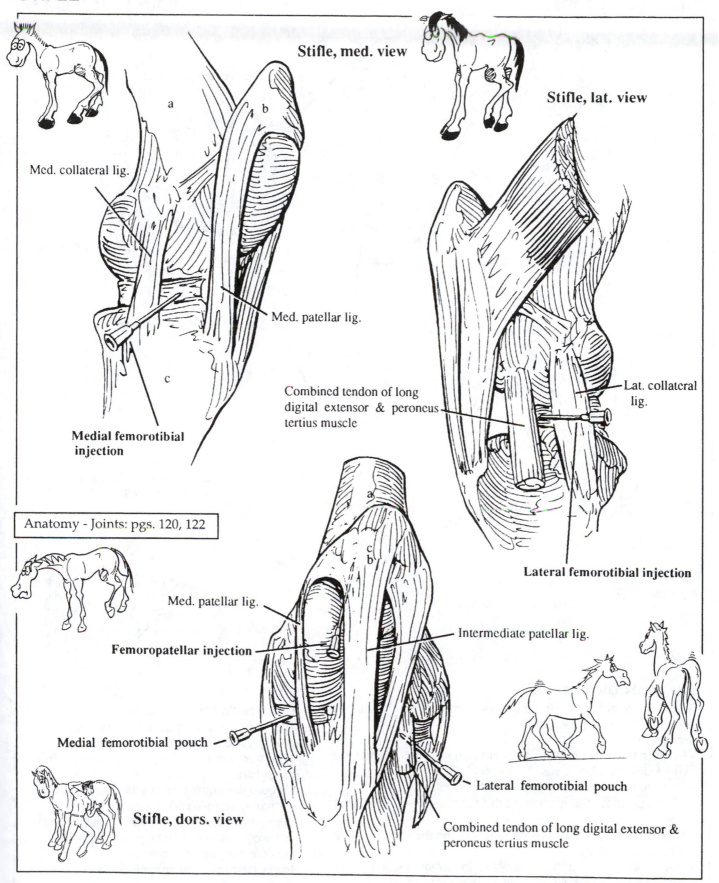

Stifle, med. view

Stifle, lat. view

Med. collateral lig.

a

b

Med. patellar lig.

c

Combined tendon of long digital extensor & peroneus tertius muscle

Medial femorotibial injection

Lat. collateral lig.

Lateral femorotibial injection

Anatomy - Joints: pgs. 120, 122

Med. patellar lig.

a

c
b

Femoropatellar injection

Intermediate patellar lig.

Medial femorotibial pouch

Lateral femorotibial pouch

Stifle, dors. view

Combined tendon of long digital extensor & peroneus tertius muscle

602a

Hip Joint Block

Anatomy - Joints: pg. 118

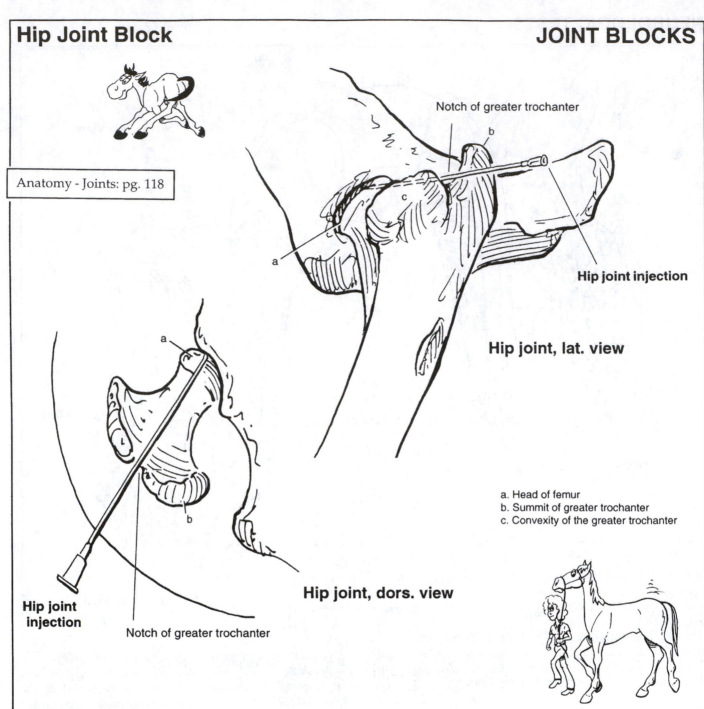

Notch of greater trochanter

Hip joint injection

Hip joint, lat. view

a. Head of femur
b. Summit of greater trochanter
c. Convexity of the greater trochanter

Hip joint, dors. view

Hip joint injection

Notch of greater trochanter

Hip joint block:
- Very hard to achieve, especially in well muscled horses & may require redirecting the needle
- **Procedure**:
  - Palpate the summit of the greater trochanter two thirds of the way from the tuber coxae to the ischiatic tuberosity
  - Palpate or estimate the location of the convexity
  . Then estimate the location of the notch between the 2 (not palpable)
  - Insert a 6 inch needle (16-gauge) through the notch distally & slightly cranially
  - Walk the needle up the neck of the femur into the joint
  - Aspirate synovial fluid and inject 10 to 15 ml of anesthetic
- **Boundaries**: Notch of greater trochanter

Trochanteric bursa injection:
- Trochanteric bursa is between the accessory gluteal muscle (of the middle gluteal) & the greater trochanter
- **Procedure**:
  - Palpate the cranial part of the greater trochanter (convexity)
  - Insert a needle (3" 18-gauge) 2 inches distal to the convexity & direct it proximomedially over the convexity into the bursa
  - Inject 10 ml of local anesthetic

RADIOGRAPHY - INTRODUCTION

Radiology: the branch of medical science which deals with the use of radiant energy in the diagnosis and treatment of disease. This section is to help students start to understand radiology. It is not meant to be an in-depth presentation, but an introduction. Radiology, as a diagnostic modality, is selected when the history and physical exam suggests a possible benefit. Radiology seldom yields a final diagnosis, but contributes in the creation of an adequate differential diagnoses list.

Radiography: The study of the physics, photochemistry and electronic technologies used to form a high quality radiographic image.

Radiograph: a visible image formed by passage of ionizing radiation (energy) through the body, interaction of the escaped radiation with intensifying screens, the action of subsequent emitted light with film and the effect of developing chemicals.

X-ray machine: An X-ray beam is generated by passing an electron beam through a vacuum between a cathode and an anode. The positively charged anode attracts the electrons (opposite charges attract). A few percent of the electrons will pass close to the nuculi of the anode, interact with the electrostatic charge and convert their kinetic energy in to X-rays (photons) while the rest just create heat. The tube enclosure is shielded and a series of lead shutters allows the diagnostic beam to exit.

Cassettes: hold the radiograph film sandwiched between intensifying screens. They come in a number of sizes: 8"x10", 10"x12" 12"x14" and 14"x 17" (or metric equivalents). The object to be radiographed is placed on the cassette, between it and the tube head.

Collimator (misnomer for Beam Limiting Device): the part of the x-ray machine allowing restriction of the size of the beam leaving the machine.

X-ray film: a piece of plastic with a bilayer of silver halide emulsion. When exposed to light or x-rays, the silver halide is activated, which makes it reactive with the weak reducing solution of the developer. Silver halide which is reduced becomes microscopic crystals of silver metal, which appear black. The reduced silver metal is insoluble in the weak solvent of the fixer so it remains. The unreacted silver halide is soluble in fixer and will be removed (cleared). A film may be seen in several states:

• **Exposed; undeveloped; unfixed:** a film removed from the box in daylight (looks the same unexposed, but YOU cannot see it in the dark). It will be opaque with a greyish-green cast due to the emulsion (silver halide) covering it.

• **Exposed; developed; fixed:** film that has been subjected to light or x-rays and developed (i.e. a typical radiograph, exposed areas are black, unexposed regions clear).

• **Unexposed; developed; fixed:** a film removed from the box and developed in the dark room without being subjected to light or x-rays. All the inactivated silver halide is washed away in the

fixer, leaving only the transparent bluish piece of plastic. It is called "white" because films are looked at on a white viewer.

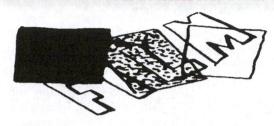

• **Exposed; undeveloped; fixed:** a film that had a virtual image from exposure to light or x-rays, but was not developed, no silver was precipitated so it all was removed by the fixer, resulting in a clear sheet.

• **Exposed; developed; unfixed:** a film with an image that was made visible by the developer, but because the unreacted silver halide was not removed by the fixer, the image is black and green instead of black and white.

• The radiograph is basically a negative, therefore, the whiter the film, the more underexposed it is. The darker a film, the more overexposed.

Viewer: a fluorescent light source for viewing radiographs.

Spotlight or hot light: a strong source of light placed behind the film to view over-exposed areas (darker than desired). A spotlight can make these areas still readable in some cases.

FLASHLIGHT ANALOGY: You can learn a lot about radiography using a flashlight. Radiant (x-rays) energy is a form of energy having many of the same properties as visible light. Both are generated from a source and transmitted as a primary beam. The primary beam is propagated until it strikes an object, where three things can happen: reflection (scatter), further transmission (penetration) or absorption.

• **Reflection or Compton scatter:** the redirection of a percentage of the primary beam striking an object's surface. Scatter radiation is a hazard to the operator as it is not limited to the region between the tube head and the cassette. In Compton Scatter the original photon interacts with an orbital electron which is accelerated and ejected from the atom. A secondary photon of x-ray is produced with less energy than the original and at a different direction of travel.

• **Penetration or transmittance:** the passing of part of the primary beam through the object. Light can be seen through a piece of paper. If more paper is added to the first, a smaller percentage will be transmitted. On the other hand the same thickness of tinfoil will transmit much less than paper (density). Therefore, transmittance is influenced by both thickness and density (atomic weight).

• **Absorption or Photoelectric effect:** the third possibility for the x-ray. This can be felt when the paper held in front of a light

RADIOGRAPHY - INTRODUCTION

source gets warmer. The x-ray photon ceases to exist and its energy is converted to kinetic energy of an orbital electron which is ejected from the atom (i.e., heat).

Inverse square law: Intensity varies with the square of the distance. With visible light or x-rays, doubling the distance quarters the effective power. Therefore, any change of the distance between the x-ray emitter and the cassette film will greatly change the exposure. The use of standard distances for different techniques eliminates distance as a variable.

Divergence: the spreading of the primary beam as it moves away from the source. Scatter also diverges. Therefore, the closer the object is to the cassette, the less divergence, thus, the smaller and sharper its image. The farther from the cassette the larger (magnification effect) and fuzzier (geometric blurring) will be the image. Shine a light on your hand next to a wall. The closer to the wall, the smaller and sharper the shadow; the further from the wall the larger and fuzzier the shadow. Parts placed on the cassette will be sharp and almost actual size; parts away from the cassette will be abnormally enlarged and fuzzy. Always place the side of the animal you are interested in against the cassette so it will be sharp and close to actual size.

Radiographic density: the actual penetrative ability of x-rays to pass through a object and reach the film. Radiographic density of a part is determined by its thickness and its atomic weight. A piece of tin foil is denser (higher atomic weight) than a sheet of paper, thus, will stop more transmittance of light or x-rays. But paper can be stacked (thicker) sufficiently to stop as much transmittance as the piece of tin foil. Therefore, atomic weight and thickness go hand in hand. Although fat feels and looks more dense than water, it is not (fat floats). Air and fat have little reflection, little absorption, and a high degree of transmission to the film, thus, their images on the film will be black. Bone and metal have little transmission allowing less x-rays to reach the film, making their images white. Water densities fall between these in transmission, appearing as shades of gray. Water densities are the soft tissue densities of the body (viscera, muscles and fluids). Soft tissue radiographs are differences between very close densities, therefore, shades of grey. If a water density is thick enough (liver), it can appear as white or whiter than bone. Thickness plays a part in the appearance of overlapping densities also. Two bones that cross will appear whiter where they cross due to the greater thickness.

Markers: lead "R"s and "L"s placed on the cassette are used to tell which side of the animal has been placed on the film (down). These also designate which limb is radiographed if only one limb is shown. In addition to these markers, the film should have a label identifying the client, animal, date and facility performing the study, and if a time study, the time elapsed after the procedure was started.

Patient preparation: radiographs must be taken with a minimal amount of movement. For some animals this may be minimal restraint, whereas others will have to be sedated or anesthetized. For some procedures (e.g., radiographs of the spine) the animal must be anesthetized. Sand bags can be used to properly place the animal in relation to the beam direction. Some studies, such as abdominal radiographs, are compromised by food and fecal material in the GI tract. These patients are prepared by withholding food 12 hours prior to radiography and perhaps using an enema.

Artifacts: (definition: made by human hand) things seen on a radiograph that are not part of the animal. These can be due to a number of causes. Dirt, wet hair, ointments or iodine (radiopaque material) can cause artifacts on radiographs. Therefore, clean the animal first. Artifacts are also caused by static discharge, processing mistakes and physical damage to screens or films.

SAFETY: should be foremost in your mind whenever radiographing. Although invisible, X-rays are very dangerous and additive over time. Never place any part of your body or a helper's body in the primary beam. Wear lead aprons, gloves and stand behind a lead shield when ever possible to block secondary (scatter) radiation. A common misconception is that lead aprons and gloves protect you from the primary beam. This is not true. They only protect from scatter radiation. The beam should always be collimated to no larger than the size of the cassette or region being studied.

ALARA: As Low As Reasonably Achievable. The USNRC regulation concerning radiation exposure to human beings. Any use of ionizing radiation MUST be controlled by the operator to limit human exposure to be As Low As Reasonably Achievable.

BASIC SCHEME OF RADIOGRAPHIC DENSITIES
Commit this to memory!!

- AIR: Less radiodens than fat - black
- FAT: less radio-dense than water - black
- WATER: less radio-dense than bone - gray
- BONE: less radiodense than metal - white
- METAL: most dense - white

A<F<W<B<M or M>B>W>F>A

Memory Aid for radiographic densities mnemonic Bubbles, Blubber, Blood, Bones and Bullets, corresponding to the densities Gas; Fat; Water; Bones (Mineral); Metal.

RADIOGRAPHY - INTRODUCTION

BEAM DIRECTION: named for where the beam first passes into the body or part of body followed by where it exits the body or part to reach the film. Films shot from opposite direction are difficult to differentiate without markers on the film. A caudal/cranial and a cranial/caudal view will look identical in small animals because radiographs have no depth. <u>Do not</u> try to read or see depth in a radiograph.

•**Lateromedial, LM,** or **lateral view:** the beam enters the lateral side and leaves the medial side of a limb. Small animal extremities are usually exposed as mediolateral projections.

• **Craniocaudal** or anteroposterior (AP) **view:** the beam enters the front side of a limb and exits the back surface above the carpus/tarsus.

• **Caudocranial view:** the beam enters the back of the limb and exits the front. It is difficult to differentiate this view from a craniocaudal view.

• **Dorsopalmar/dorsoplantar, DP** or anteroposterior (AP) **view:** shot from the front to the back of a limb below the proximal end of the carpus/tarsus.

• **Palmodorsal/plantodorsal** or **PD view:** the beam passes from the back to the front of a limb below the proximal end of the carpus/tarsus.

•**Lateral projection of a major body cavity** (abdomen, thorax): named by the beams exit surface or the surface closes to the cassette. An animal in left lateral recumbency (left side down) when radiographed produces a left lateral view.

ANATOMICAL LANDMARKS: certain organs or structures with specific locations are used to ascertain the side of the body or limbs in a film. Anatomical landmarks should always be used to check if the markers are correct. (Nature put on the landmarks, people put on the markers, who do <u>you</u> trust?) Use radiographic landmarks to get your bearings. A few of the common radiographic landmarks are:

Anatomical Landmarks
• Apex of the heart - left
• Gas bubble in the fundus of the stomach - left
• Descending colon - left
• Cranial kidney - right; Caudal kidney - left
• Anticlinal vertebra - vertical vertebrae, usually T_{11} in dogs.
• Head of humerus - caudal
• Radius - cranial
• Olecranon - caudal
• Distal end of ulna - lateral and caudal
• Accessory carpal bone - lateral and palmar
• Dew claw - medial
• Patella - cranial
• Fibula - lateral
• Calcaneus lateral and plantar

READING FILMS:

Survival Law!: Read in a systematic manner. Extract maximum information from the entire film. Do not miss something important by jumping at the most obvious. Determine what region is radiographed (shoulder or thorax etc.). Knowing the anatomy is necessary for reading films. Anatomical landmarks help you orient the views and indicate the direction of the beam. If lateral and medial structures are silhouetted (on the edges of structure), then the beam was directed craniocaudal, dorsopalmar or dorsoventral depending on what was radiographed (i.e., a view showing the outline of the radial [lateral structure] and ulnar carpal bone [medial structure] or the lateral edges of the ribs [lateral structures]). Silhouetted caudal and cranial structures indicate beam was directed lateromedial or mediolateral (i.e., accessory carpal bone silhouetted or chest with spines of vertebrae and sternum on the edges of the film).

CHECKLIST: Do not look at the lines, grays and shadows of a radiograph and try to identify what anatomic structure they represent. Instead work from a list of the structures that you expect to see and locate each in a specific order. The first approach will 'miss' agenesis (absence) of an organ, because there is nothing to see.

Two-dimensional / three-dimensional: A radiograph is a two dimensional representation of a three dimensional object. To extrapolate the third dimension at least two radiographs must be taken at 90° to each other. A dorsoventral view of the abdomen will have the medial to lateral and cranial to caudal dimensions, but will lack the dimension in the plane of the beam, dorsal to ventral. The lateral view will have the cranial to caudal and the dorsal to ventral dimensions, but lack the lateral to medial dimension. With both views (lateral and DV) all three dimensions are present and three dimensional information can be extrapolated. If, in the DV view, a buckshot shows up superimposed on the kidney, it could be anywhere in the plane of the beam (subcutaneous, below, in, or above the kidney). Another view is needed to place the buckshot in three dimensions. A lateral view showing the buckshot overlapping the kidney would now place it in the kidney.

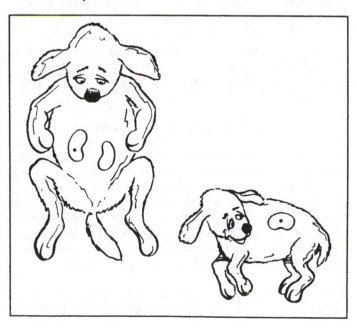

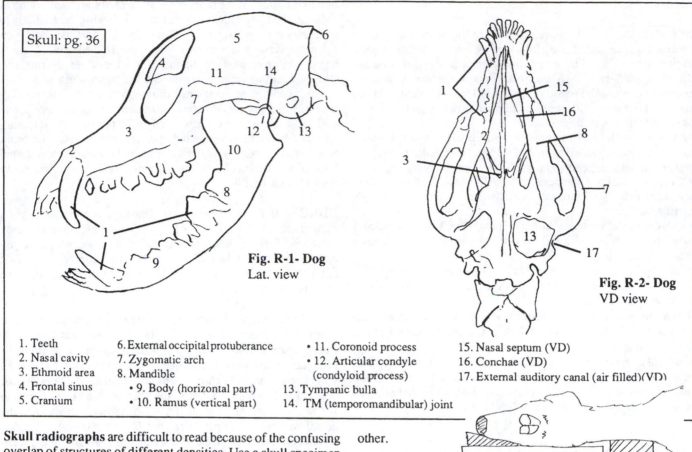

Skull: pg. 36

Fig. R-1- Dog
Lat. view

Fig. R-2- Dog
VD view

1. Teeth	6. External occipital protuberance	• 11. Coronoid process
2. Nasal cavity	7. Zygomatic arch	• 12. Articular condyle
3. Ethmoid area	8. Mandible	(condyloid process)
4. Frontal sinus	• 9. Body (horizontal part)	13. Tympanic bulla
5. Cranium	• 10. Ramus (vertical part)	14. TM (temporomandibular) joint

15. Nasal septum (VD)
16. Conchae (VD)
17. External auditory canal (air filled)(VD)

Skull radiographs are difficult to read because of the confusing overlap of structures of different densities. Use a skull specimen to help read skull radiographs and position shots. All skull radiographs should be done under anesthesia because they need to be perfectly positioned. There are 3 types of skulls in dogs relative to the proportions of the facial bones and the cranial vault. This variation must be taken into account when viewing normal skull films - doliocephalic, larger facial component (i.e. long nosed breeds, such as the collie) - mesaticephalic: (i.e. beagle) - brachiocephalic: shorter facial component (i.e. Boston Terrier). Some indications for the skull radiographs are neurological problems (hydrocephalus), nasal or mandibular problems (fractures), maxilla (rhinitis, neoplasm), primary tumors of skull (soft tissue swelling), mass behind the eye, teeth diseases, and middle ear problems.

Many different positions are used in skull radiography to look at the different structures. The dorsoventral and lateral are standard views. Open mouth, lateral oblique of the mandible or upper jaw views are shot at 45° angle to separate the teeth of the opposite jaws. Occlusal views are shot by placing the cassette in the mouth and directing the beam in a DV or VD direction. This isolates the upper or lower jaw respectively from the other jaw. The lateral oblique (to see the TM joint), frontal or fronto-occipital (for the frontal sinuses), opened mouth VD or DV and foramen magnum are all different views to highlight specific structures.

Be able to identify the structures listed after the different views. Look for symmetry on the DV view by comparing one side to the other.

Cat differences: The cat's skull is constructed differently than the dog and these differences need to be known. Cats have greater doming of the frontal and nasal bones, smaller frontal sinuses (may be absent in Persians), more complete bony orbits and wider skull because the zygomatic arches are wider

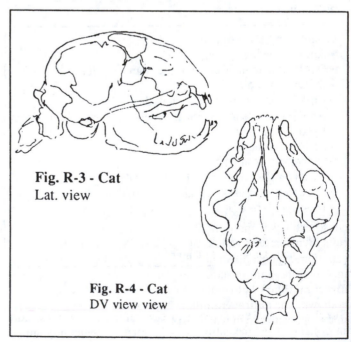

Fig. R-3 - Cat
Lat. view

Fig. R-4 - Cat
DV view view

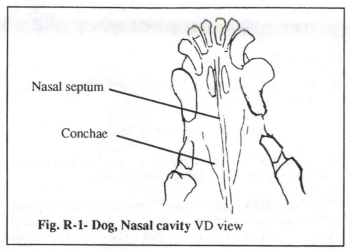

Fig. R-1- Dog, Nasal cavity VD view

Nasal cavity: in the DV view, compare each side for opacity or lucency. Increased soft tissue caused by inflammation or a mass may increase the opacity. When there is a difference in the density of one half of the nasal cavity (heminasum) compared with the other, look for the fine detail of the nasal conchae. If conchal detail is present on both sides then the densest side is diseased (exudate, blood, tumor). If conchal detail is missing from one side then it is the diseased side regardless of whether it is dense (exudate, blood, tumor) or lucent (usually fungal rhinitis).

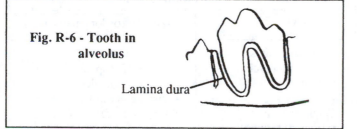

Fig. R-6 - Tooth in alveolus

Lamina dura

Teeth: locate the crown, root and pulp cavity. Note the presence or absence of the lamina dura. It is the side of the alveoli the beam passes through. This makes it appear as a white line separated by a space (periodontal space) from the tooth root. If this is eroded or missing, it indicates a problem with the tooth. The periodontal space is between the lamina dura and the tooth root and is occupied by the periodontal membrane.

Pharynx: Radiographically, its soft structures are contrasted against the air opacity. The pharynx is located ventral to vertebrae C_1-C_2 and is best visualized on a lateral projection. Structures of the pharynx:

A. Soft plate: separates the oropharynx from the nasopharynx and can be seen radiographically.

B. Nasopharynx: air-illed area above the soft palate

C. Oropharynx: air-filled continuation of the oral cavity below the soft palate.

D. Laryngopharynx: the common part of the pharynx filled by the larynx in the lateral projection.

E. Hyoid bones: suspend the larynx from the skull - stylohyoid, epihyoid, ceratohyoid, basihyoid, and thyrohyoid. As bones, they are visible radiographically. The most common clinical radiographic findings are fractures.

• **G. Basihyoid**: seen end on in the lateral projection; making it appear very white (dense).

H. Laryngeal cartilages: make up the skeleton of the larynx - epiglottis, thyroid, cricoid and arytenoid. With age the cartilages can mineralize, especially in large or chondrodystrophic breeds. The cricoid cartilage is the first to become calcified.

• **I. Cricoid cartilage**: the easiest to see.

• **J. Epiglottis**: also easy to see at the rostral end of the larynx. In the horse the normal position of the tip of the epiglottis is dorsal to the soft palate.

The pharynx is evaluated for decreased or increased contrast and displacement. Decreased contrast can be due to inflammation, masses, or a normal finding in brachiocephalic breeds. Increased contrast is due to air around the pharynx (retropharyngeal air) (e.g., penetrating wounds or rupture of the structures of the pharynx or esophagus). Ventral displacement can be due to retropharyngeal masses. Laryngeal, tonsillar or thyroid masses can displace the pharynx laterally. With fractures of the hyoid apparatus the pharynx can be displaced caudally. The pharynges of brachiocephalic dogs are difficult to interpret because there is less air, therefore, less contrast in the pharyngeal region.

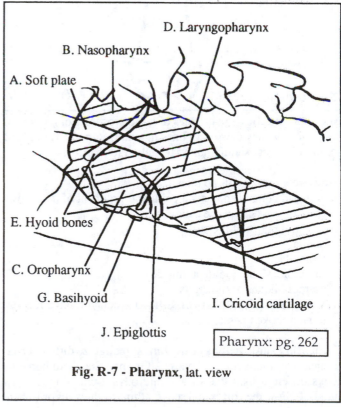

Fig. R-7 - Pharynx, lat. view

Pharynx: pg. 262

LIMBS

Endochondral ossification: the formation of long bones by transforming a cartilaginous model into bone. Bone replacement takes place in three primary ossification centers - the diaphysis and the two epiphyses. This results in a bone capped with articular cartilage and two cartilage discs (metaphyseal growth plates or physes) between the diaphysis and the two epiphyses. Lengthening of bone occurs at the epiphyseal side of the metaphyseal plate. Lengthening stops when the epiphyseal plates are completely replaced by bone. During growth, radiographically, the epiphysial cartilage appears as a radiolucent line (dark line), called the physis by radiologists, separating the diaphysis from the two epiphyses.

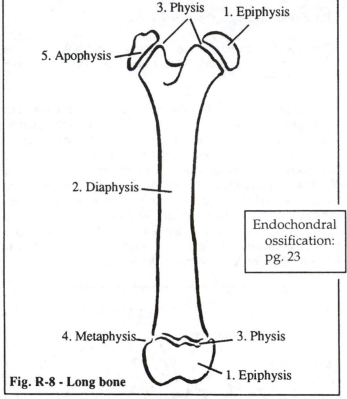

3. Physis
1. Epiphysis
5. Apophysis
2. Diaphysis

Endochondral ossification: pg. 23

4. Metaphysis
3. Physis
1. Epiphysis

Fig. R-8 - Long bone

Accessory ossification centers of large processes of individual bones also display these dark lines in young animals. These (and sesamoid bones) should not be mistaken for fractures.

• Anconeal process of the ulna
• Sesamoid bone of the lateral collateral ligament of the elbow
• Accessory ossicle of the caudal scapula
• Sesamoid bones of the stifle
  Patella
  2 Fabellae
  Sesamoid of the popliteal muscle
• Sesamoid bones of the digits
• Os penis: sometimes has two ossification centers and can appear to be a broken penis.

Evaluating radiographs of the limbs: recognize different anatomical variations for the bones. A German Shepherd humerus looks different than that of a chondrodystrophic dog (Dachshund). Follow the cortex and see if it thins or thickens or if there

are breaks in it. Know the locations of the nutrient foramina so they are not mistake for lytic (dissolved) areas.

Radiographing limbs:

• Long bones of the limbs: include the proximal and distal joints in the film.

• Joints of the limbs: center the joint in film.

• Comparison films: take the opposite limb if there is a question as to what you are seeing and compare the two.

VIEWS OF THE LIMBS: the most common are the lateral view and the craniocaudal or dorsopalmar/plantar. The different views silhouette different sides of the bones and can be identified by what is in silhouette.

Lateral view of limb bones and joints: place the affected limb on the cassette. Pull the affected limb forward and the unaffected limb backwards. The lateral view silhouettes the cranial and caudal surfaces of the bones.

Craniocaudal or anterior-posterior (AP) or dorsopalmar view: silhouettes the medial and lateral structures of the limb.

Structures silhouetted - thoracic limb	
Lat. view	Cranocaud or dorsopalm. view
Cran. structures: • Greater tubercle • Radius Caud. structures: • Head of humerus • Ulna • Accessory carpal bone	Lat. structures: • Spine of scapula • Greater tubercle • Distal end of ulna • Accessory carpal bone Med. structures: • Radial carpal bone • Dew claw

JOINTS - synovial (diarthrodial): consist of the following components:

1. Joint space: in a radiograph, is actually the joint space <u>and</u> the articular cartilage, since the cartilage is invisible in radiographs.

2. Articular cartilage: caps the ends of the bones making up the joint. It can't be seen on the radiograph, only inferred.

3. Joint capsule: surrounds the joint space and attaches at the edge of the articular cartilage. It can't be seen on radiographs unless calcified.

Degenerative joint disease (DJD): a disease affecting synovial joints due to mechanical problems and degrading changes in the articular cartilage. It can be caused by congenital or acquired deformities of the bones and joints, infection or trauma. Some important terms relating to DJD follow:

SHOULDER JOINT

- **Osteophyte** (OS-tee-oh-fyt): an osseous (bony) outgrowth.

- **Sclerosis** (Slee-ROH-sis) (Gr. *sklerosis* hardness): hardening, in bone, referring to the increase in density of a bone.

- **Ankylosis** (ang'ki-LOH-sis): immobility and consolidation of a joint due to disease, injury or surgical procedure.

- **Lysis** (LY-sis) (Gr. *lysis* dissolution): destruction or decomposition, seen as reduced density in bones (blacker).

Radiographic possibilities in DJD (degenerative joint disease):
- Narrowing or disappearance of the joint space.
- Osteophyte formation, most often at the articular margins
- Subchondral bone sclerosis
- Joint deformities
- Lytic and proliferative changes where the joint capsule and ligaments attach around the joint.
- Ankylosis (complete or partial)

SHOULDER JOINT or scapulohumeral joint: the synovial joint between the head of the humerus and the glenoid cavity of the scapula. The lateral and craniocaudal views are standard for the shoulder. Take the lateral view by placing the dog in lateral recumbency with the affected leg down on the cassette. Push the affected limb dorsally and pull the unaffected limb ventrally and caudally to separate the limbs. To take a craniocaudal (AP) view of the shoulder, rotate the limb medially to pull the scapula away from the thorax.

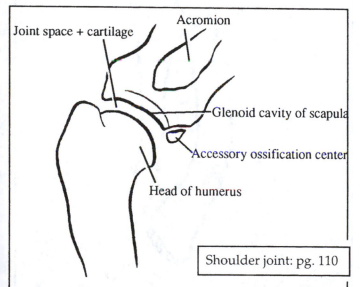

Joint space + cartilage

Acromion

Glenoid cavity of scapula

Accessory ossification center

Head of humerus

Shoulder joint: pg. 110

Fig. R-9 - Shoulder joint radiograph (schematic)

When viewing shoulder films the joint space should be of equal width all around the head of the humerus. The head of the humerus should be smooth and round, with no flattening. Check for fractures of the spine of the scapula in the craniocaudal view. Do not confuse the accessory ossification center of the caudal aspect of the scapula with OCD (osteochondrosis dissecans) which occurs on the caudal aspect of the head of the humerus

(covered below). Remember to look at all the film, noticing structures other than the shoulder joint - neck, cervical vertebrae, air-filled trachea, ribs, and lung fields (air-filled).

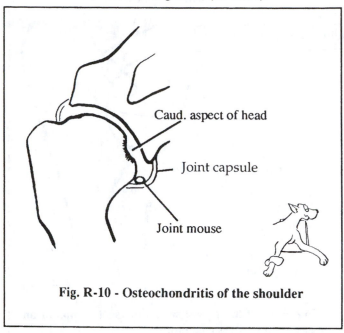

Caud. aspect of head

Joint capsule

Joint mouse

Fig. R-10 - Osteochondritis of the shoulder

Osteochondrosis: a defect in endochondral ossification which causes the deeper layers of the articular cartilage to die. If something goes wrong in osteochondral ossification, the cartilage continues to grow and thicken. Beyond a certain thickness, diffusion from the synovial fluid can't reach the deeper layer, which dies. The etiology is unknown. Excessive nutrition and stress may have something to do with it. It tends to be bilateral. It is seen in 4 to 10 month old, rapidly growing, large breeds. It may occur as a subchondral bone cyst, which is a misnomer because it isn't a secreting membrane, rather a wad of necrotic cartilage with a sclerotic layer around it. Osteochondrosis tends to happen in predictable anatomical sites.

Sites - osteochondrosis
- Shoulder - caudal aspect of the head of the humerus
- Medial humeral condyle - bears more weight
- Medial or lateral femoral condyle
- Trochlea of talus

The caudal aspect of the head of the humerus is the primary site for osteochondrosis. Radiographically, cartilage is not seen so the subchondral bone is checked to see if it indicates that the cartilage is damaged. This may appear as flattening or cratering of the caudal aspect of the head of the humerus with subchondral bone sclerosis (thickening). The lateral radiograph shows this best.

Osteochondrosis dissecans: a form of osteochondrosis that has a dissected flap of cartilage. The cartilage above the dead cartilage fractures and forms a flap. Dissecans means a dissecting flap. The fragment can calcify and/or break off and float around in the synovium and is then called a " joint mouse".

609

ELBOW JOINT: a complicated joint between the humerus, radius and ulna. Three important radiographic structures are listed below:

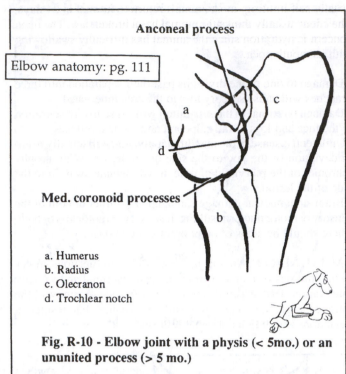

Anconeal process

Elbow anatomy: pg. 111

Med. coronoid processes

a. Humerus
b. Radius
c. Olecranon
d. Trochlear notch

Fig. R-10 - Elbow joint with a physis (< 5mo.) or an ununited process (> 5 mo.)

• **Anconeal process of the ulna**: the proximal projection of trochlear notch. It is an accessory ossification center in most dogs.

• **Coronoid processes of the ulna**: medial and lateral processes of the distal end of the trochlear notch. The **medial** coronoid process is larger and is not an accessory ossification center.

• Sesamoid bone in the lateral collateral ligament of the elbow: present in some dogs, do not mistake it for a fracture. Radiograph the other limb if there is doubt.

Ununited anconeal process: failure of the anconeal process to unite with the ulna. It should unite at about 5 to 6 months of age. It tends to occur in large breed dogs (German Shepherds) and tends to be bilateral. This disease is now felt to be related to OCD. If it has not united after 5 months of age it is considered ununited. You see a straight or ragged radiolucent line. The process may or may not be displaced. There may be degenerative changes in the elbow (DJD). The best view is the flexed lateral elbow which pulls the anconeal process out of the olecranon fossa of the humerus.

Osteochondrosis of the elbow: failure of endochondral ossification on the medial condyle of the humerus. The craniocaudal view is taken to try to see a subchondral lucency. This often accompanies ununited anconeal process.

Fragmented medial coronoid process: believed to be a syndrome of osteochondrosis. It is incorrectly called an ununited coronoid process because it is not a separate ossification center. The cartilaginous precursor undergoes improper development and fragments. It is cartilage so it can't be seen. Rounding off of the medial coronoid process may be seen. Rarely is the cartilage joint mouse seen, unless it calcifies. Most of the time you only see secondary degenerative joint disease (DJD). The earliest site of DJD is bone proliferation on the cranial aspect of the olecranon process. Bone build up (sclerosis) can also occur where the joint capsule attaches. Often it is a diagnosis of inference - a young dog with some kind of elbow dysplasia (developing DJD) with no evidence of other osteochondroses or ununited anconeal process. OFA will now certify elbows. A flexed lateral film is sent in for evaluation.

Premature closure of the physis: usually due to trauma. This is most common in the distal physis of the ulna or radius. Compare the opposite limb's physis on radiographs. Closure of either the physis of the ulna or the radius will cause deformities in the other bone and subluxation and/or degenerative joint disease of the joints on either end of these bones. Look for loss of the radiolucent physeal line on radiographs.

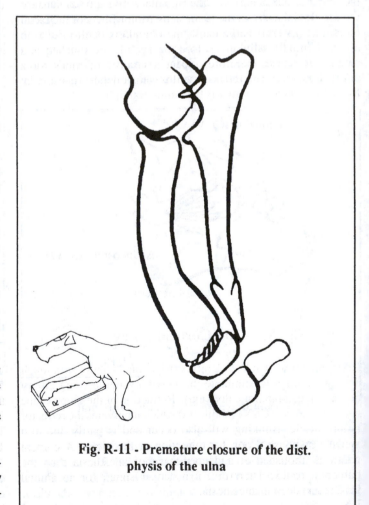

Fig. R-11 - Premature closure of the dist. physis of the ulna

610

PELVIC LIMB - HIP JOINT

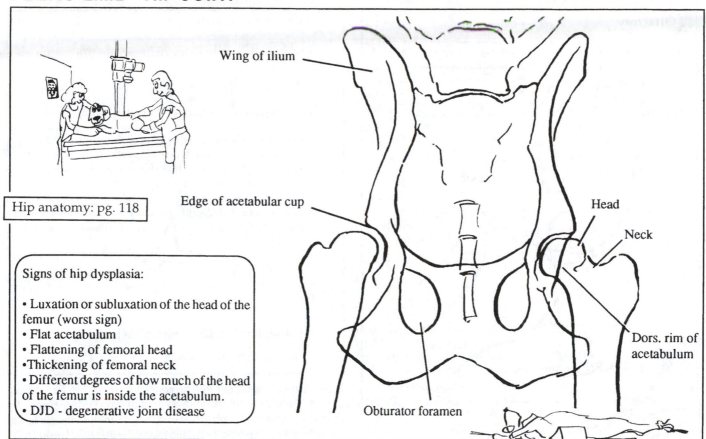

Wing of ilium

Hip anatomy: pg. 118

Edge of acetabular cup

Head

Neck

Dors. rim of acetabulum

Obturator foramen

Signs of hip dysplasia:

• Luxation or subluxation of the head of the femur (worst sign)
• Flat acetabulum
• Flattening of femoral head
•Thickening of femoral neck
• Different degrees of how much of the head of the femur is inside the acetabulum.
• DJD - degenerative joint disease

HIP JOINT: a ball-and-socket joint allowing great range of motion, but sacrificing stability.

Acetabular rim: the craniodorsal ridge is an accessory ossification area. This can be mistaken for a chip fracture.

Physeal scar: normal remnant of the closed physis.

Fovea capitis: an indention on the head of the femur where the round ligament of the head of the femur attaches. This appears as a normal flattening of the femoral head on radiographs. Rotation of the limb medially will hide it in VD films.

Hip dysplasia view: Place the dog in dorsal recumbency with the limbs pulled caudally and rotated slightly medially to place the femurs parallel to each other, the patellas (or patelae) centered in the trochlea of the femur. Superimpose the femur and the ischiatic tuberosity similarly on both sides. The film should include views from below the stifle to just above the hip bones. The pelvis must be level (no rotation). Rotation will make one acetabulum look very deep and one very shallow, therefore, one joint will appear better. Rotation can be checked by looking at the symmetry of obturator foramen. Rotation will cause the "up" foramen to appear rounder and larger, and the "down" side smaller and more elliptical. Rotation also causes the width of the wings of the ilium to be different. The OFA will not certify a dog until it reaches two years of age.

50%-60% of the head of the femur should be inside the dorsal rim

of the acetabulum. Look for congruency (parallel lines) between the head of the femur and the acetabular cup, especially in the cranial third. A tangential line drawn from the edge of the cranial acetabular cup should be as close to perpendicular to the axis of the skeleton as possible. A non-perpendicular line would infer a shallow acetabular cup. Degenerative change (DJD, osteoarthrosis, osteoarthritis) first shows up as osteophyte proliferation along the neck of the femur. This may look like a thickened neck of the femur. Osteophyte proliferation tends to occur where the joint capsule attaches. Lastly, you can see some spurring (proliferation along the edges of the cup of the acetabulum). Any signs of DJD indicates problems. There are a number of treatments for hip dysplasia, ranging from aspirin, cutting off the head of the femur, to hip replacement.

Pelvic fracture: "rule of thumb" - if one fracture is seen, look for two more (one may be a luxation of the hip). The pelvis is a box, if it breaks in one part, it has to break in two more locations in order to displace.

Legg perthes: avascular aseptic necrosis of the femoral head and neck. Loss of blood supply to the head or neck causes the head to become irregular (dissolve away). Over time it will collapse and become flattened and deformed. Treatment is to remove the head and neck, which small dogs tolerate very well. Etiology is unknown. It occurs from 3 to 11 months of age and is usually unilateral, but can be bilateral. This disease occurs in small breeds (Poodle).

STIFLE

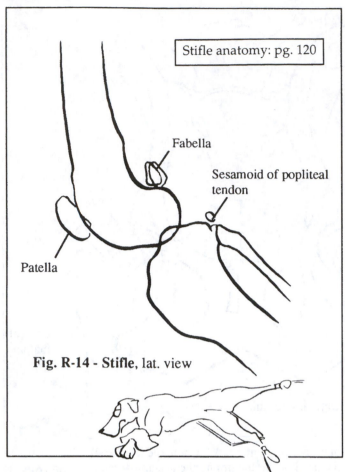

Stifle anatomy: pg. 120

Fabella

Sesamoid of popliteal tendon

Patella

Fig. R-14 - Stifle, lat. view

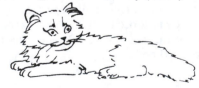

STIFLE: a composite joint between the femur, patella, tibia and fibula.

Sesamoid bones of the stifle: the patella, two fabellae and the sesamoid bone in the popliteal tendon.

Tibial tuberosity: in young dogs, has a growth plate which looks like a fracture.

Skyline view: place the animal in sternal recumbency. Flex the stifle and place the animal on its knees. This view shows the depth of the trochlear groove, the patella and the femoropatellar joint space. The groove is shallow in dogs that have patellar luxation. This can be repaired by deepening the groove surgically.

Subpatellar Fat Pad: On the mediolateral projection of the stifle there is a radiolucent (fat) density seen in the triangle formed by the femur, tibia and distal patellar ligament. A small gray area is seen in the stifle joint apex, which represents the synovial fluid of the stifle. Intra-articular diseases, most common: Cruciate ligament rupture, will cause effusion of the joint and this is seen as the water density (gray) encroaching on the fat density (black).

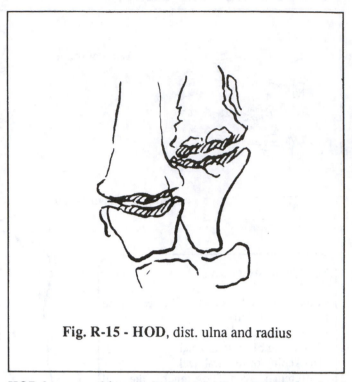

Fig. R-15 - HOD, dist. ulna and radius

HOD, hypertrophic osteodystrophy: occurs in 3 to 7 month old dogs. It tends to occur in the distal end of long bones, especially the ulna, radius and tibia. The etiology is unknown, but felt to involve an excessive plane of nutrition. The animals present with swelling around the metaphyseal region of the long bones of the limbs, fever and lameness. The classical radiographic signs are bone cuffing around the metaphyseal region and double physes. This is a self limiting disease that resolves with time. The animal is treated for pain.

HO, hypertrophic osteopathy: lamellar periosteal proliferation on the long bones of the extremities, causing lameness and pain. The etiology is unknown, but it is associated with space occupying lesions of the thorax - tumor or chronic pneumonia. Radiographically there is periosteal proliferation around the diaphyses of affected bones. It usually starts in the metacarpal and metatarsal bones and then progresses to involve the long bones of all four limbs and the carpus and tarsus. Treatment of the associated thoracic lesion usually results in regression of the bony lesions.

PANOSTEITIS: occurs in 5 month to 2 year old dogs (German Shepherd). They present with shifting leg lameness. It tends to occur in more than one bone at more than one time. It can be almost anywhere, but it tends to occur in the humerus, ulna and femur. Classically what is seen are nodular opacities to complete opacification of the medullary cavities. With time there may be smooth periosteal and endosteal reactions. Reactions are most prominent near the nutrient foramen. When it goes away it tends to leave a vacant look to the medullary cavity (dark) with a course trabecular pattern. You may find any stage of this on different bones. The etiology is unknown. This is also a self limiting disease.

SPINAL RADIOGRAPHS

It is critical to have quality radiographs taken of an anesthetized animal to evaluate spinal problems. It is essential that the spine is aligned straight without rotation. Rotation of a VD/DV film is evaluated by seeing the sternum superimposed over the spine.

TRIADS: Look at general aspects and compare each vertebra with others. Look at them in triads (3's), comparing each vertebra to the one in front and to the one behind. Compare the size, shape and opacity of adjacent vertebrae. Check the alignment of the vertebrae by tracing the dorsal and ventral edges of the vertebral canal. It should be smooth and continuous. A step defect occurs when one of the vertebrae is out of alignment, causing a "step" in one of the edges of the spinal canal.

INTERVERTEBRAL DISC SPACES: evaluated to get an indication of the state of the intervertebral discs. The radiolucent intervertebral discs themselves cannot be visualized. Narrowing of the space may indicate a protruded disc. The intervertebral space between T_{10} and T_{11} is normally narrower than the other spaces. Cervical intervertebral spaces are normally wider than other spaces. A space further from the center of the film, due to divergence of the beam will be viewed obliquely, thus, appear narrower than it is. Thus, only the 6 to 8 vertebrae in the center of the film can be evaluated for joint space differences. Do not take long films of the entire spinal column to save time and money.

INTERVERTEBRAL FORAMINA: Called the "windows" to the spinal cord", (look like Snoopy's little bird buddy, Woodstock, in profile), should not abruptly change size from one to another. The radiolucent spinal cord can't be viewed. A calcified nuclei or disc is a major finding and is a radiopacity found in a intervertebral disc space or spinal canal seen through the intervertebral foramen.

Cats - lumbar vertebrae are relatively longer and narrower than in the dog.

DENS: the cranial projection of the axis that articulates with the ventral arch of the atlas. The dens may not develop (agenesis) or it may be fractured. It may be imaged with a lateral, a DV, or an open mouth radiograph.

" SLEDS" or **transverse process of C$_6$:** in three parts, making it a landmark for cervical films.

ANTICLINAL VERTEBRA: the upright vertebra, usually T_{11}, where the incline of the spinous processes change from caudal to cranial.

MYELOGRAM: the injection of a positive contrast medium into the spaces around the spinal cord (subarachnoid space). This will make the subarachnoid space visible as two white lines separated by a space (the invisible spinal cord). These contrast lines should be smooth, reflecting the smoothness of the spinal canal. Remember the spinal cord has a cervical and a lumbar enlargement that are normal. Look for any deviations in the contrast lines, therefore, in the cord. A break or thinning in the subarachnoid space that looks as if it is pushed outward indicates

a swelling of the spinal cord. A break appearing to be pushed inward could be due to a mass outside the meninges (herniation of a disc). A thinner dorsal column can be normal if balanced with a thicker ventral column. Contrast medium is heavier than CSF, so gravity can be used to move it up or down the subarachnoid space.

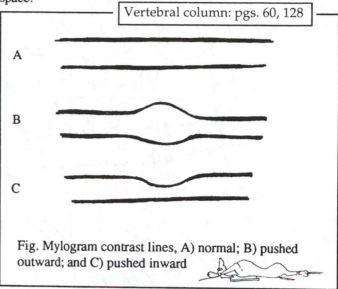

Vertebral column: pgs. 60, 128

A

B

C

Fig. Mylogram contrast lines, A) normal; B) pushed outward; and C) pushed inward

THORACOLUMBAR MYELOGRAM: direct the needle between the spinous processes of L_5 and L_6. The spine of vertebrae L6 is palpated in front of the line drawn between the tuber coxae. Pass it through the ligamentum flavum into the spinal canal. Staying on the midline is critical. The needle is then advanced through the canal until it contacts the dorsal surface of the vertebral body. This usually goes through the conus medullaris, but causes few neurological problems. Withdraw the needle a little into the ventral subarachnoid space. Remove the stylette and hopefully CSF will flow out the needle. If unsure of the needle's position, inject a small amount and then take a film. The most common error is placement of the needle in the epidural space (epiduralgram).

CERVICAL MYELOGRAM: The cisterna magnum is entered to do a cervical myelogam. This is a relatively large space where a CSF sample can be taken and contrast medium can be placed. Flex the head and palpate the wings of the atlas, spine of the axis, and the occipital protuberance. Draw a line between the wings and a line from the occipital protuberance to the spine of the axis. Place the needle on the midline 1/2 inch in front of the line between the wings. Go roughly parallel to the caudal wall of the skull and feel for the "pop" of resistance as the needle passes through the dorsal atlantooccipital ligament. Stop when through the ligament. Do not pith (needle through the brain stem) the dog. Pull out the stylette and look for CSF flow to tell if you are in the right place. Pull the stylette out any time resistance is felt or you are unsure if you are in or not, and look for CSF fluid. If you hit bone, either pull out and start again or walk the needle off the bone. Collect CSF for analysis and then inject the contrast medium. Never aspirate CSF so the spinal cord is not "sucked" into the needle or change pressure in the subarachnoid space resulting in herniation of the brain stem.

THORACIC RADIOLOGY

Anatomy: pgs. 70, 224, 225, 318, 405

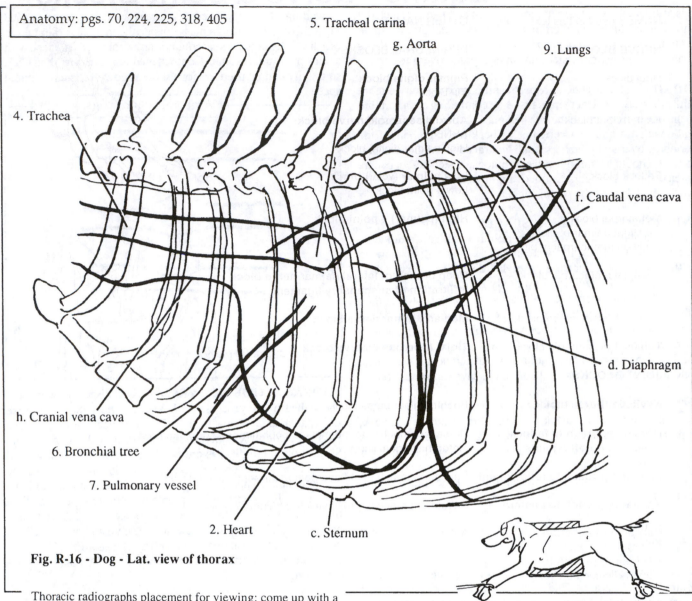

5. Tracheal carina

g. Aorta

9. Lungs

4. Trachea

f. Caudal vena cava

d. Diaphragm

h. Cranial vena cava

6. Bronchial tree

7. Pulmonary vessel

2. Heart

c. Sternum

Fig. R-16 - Dog - Lat. view of thorax

Thoracic radiographs placement for viewing: come up with a placement system that works for you. Then always follow it for standard views to eliminate an unnecessary variable. The 1st rule of thoracic radiography is to have all of the thorax in the film, including part of the neck, part of the abdomen, the vertebral bodies and the sternum. Thoracic films are shot at the peak of full inspiration. The cavity is bigger during inspiration, resulting in less contact between the diaphragm and the heart. In expiratory films the lungs are deflated, thus, more opaque and easy to confuse with pathologic change. Among the problems requiring thoracic radiographs are a cough, heart problems, dyspnea, and abnormal lung sounds.

VD and DV (as the beam sees it): place the film so that the right side of the animal is to your left for both VD and DV views. (Minority opinion: Some radiologists place the images in the position they were taken so the VD has the patient's right to the viewer's left [face-to-face] and the DV has the patient's right to the viewer's right. This forces the viewer to remember the gravitational and projection differences in the two views.)

Lateral views: place on the viewer so that the cranial side of the animal is to the left. (Minority opinion: Some radiologists prefer to place the images on the viewer in the manner they were obtained. A left lateral would be viewed with the head to the viewer's right, a right lateral, with the head to the viewer's left. This encourages the viewer to consider gravitational effects.)

"R" or "L" marker: on a lateral film of the trunk indicates the side the animal was lying on when the film was taken (right or left lateral recumbency). In VD/DV films, these markers orient the right and left sides of the animal. A quick check of the markers is the apex of the heart, located to the left in the VD or DV views.

Cat thorax: similar to the dog, but more triangular and more lucent than the dog's. The heart is also a bit more upright on the lateral view.

THORACIC RADIOLOGY

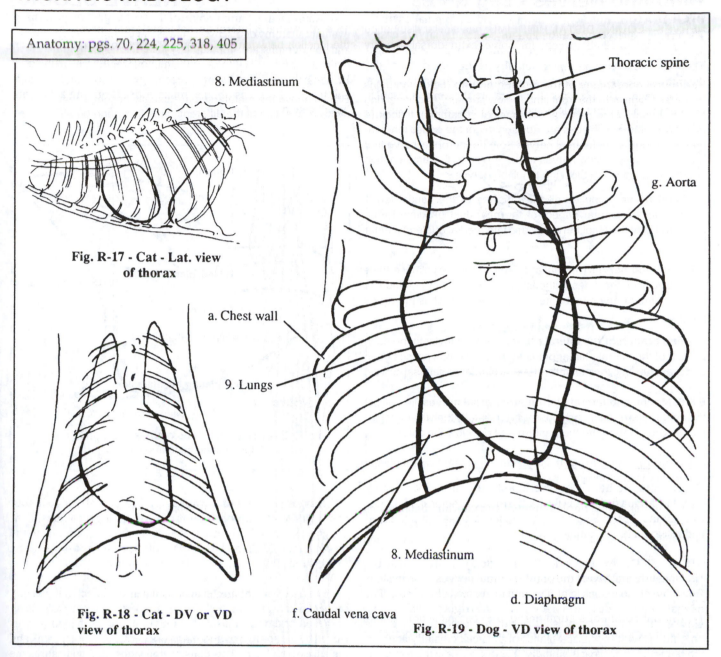

Anatomy: pgs. 70, 224, 225, 318, 405

8. Mediastinum

Fig. R-17 - Cat - Lat. view of thorax

Thoracic spine

g. Aorta

a. Chest wall

9. Lungs

8. Mediastinum

d. Diaphragm

f. Caudal vena cava

Fig. R-18 - Cat - DV or VD view of thorax

Fig. R-19 - Dog - VD view of thorax

Evaluating and reading thoracic films: can be done by an area, organ or a combination of the two. The area approach can be done diagonally from the upper caudal to lower cranial or starting at the center and moving outward, or from the outside to the inside. The organ approach looks at individual organs and organ systems systematically. A list of the organs looked at and a brief hint of for what follows:

1. Borders of thorax:
• a. Chest wall
• b. Thoracic spine
• c. Sternum
• d. Diaphragm
• e. Any of the thoracic limbs in the film.

2. Heart: shape, size, position and opacity.
3. Great vessels: shape, size, position and opacity.
• f. Caudal vena cava
• g. Aorta
• h. Cranial vena cava
4. Trachea: for position and diameter.
5. Tracheal carina
6. Bronchial tree
7. Pulmonary vessel: shape, size, position and opacity.
8. Mediastinum: for shifts, width and any abnormal density or masses.
9. Lungs: for increased or decreased opacities.
10. Pleural cavities: for fluid or air.

DIAPHRAGM - MEDIASTINUM

DIAPHRAGM: divides the thoracic and abdominal cavities. The cranial surface of the diaphragm (water density) is easily visualized by its contrast to the adjacent air density of the lungs. The liver and stomach project cranially against the dome of the diaphragm. Being water dense, they are hard to distinguish from the diaphragm. The right and left crura are the dorsal muscular parts of the diaphragm attaching to the ribs and ventral bodies of the lumbar vertebrae.

– Esophogram: barium study of the esophagus and pharynx to evaluate anatomy or disease. Contrast medium is given by mouth and radiographs are immediately taken. The radiographs will delineate longitudinal folds of the mucous membrane in the dog. In the cat the proximal 3/4 of the esophagus has longitudinal folds and the last 1/4th has oblique mucosal folds, giving a "herring bone" pattern.

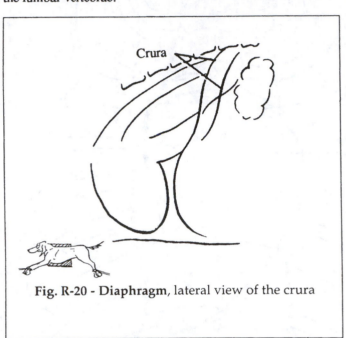

Fig. R-20 - **Diaphragm**, lateral view of the crura

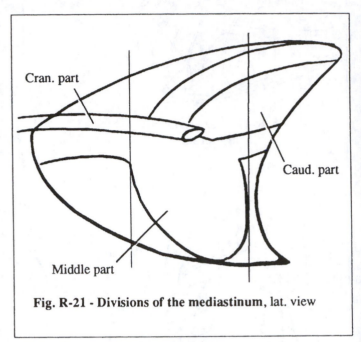

Fig. R-21 - **Divisions of the mediastinum**, lat. view

Diaphragmatic hernia: a severe problem with a 50% fatality rate. The hernia may allow the liver, stomach and/or small bowel to enter the thorax. The herniated organs often are strangulated and release a large volume of fluid.

MEDIASTINUM: the space (or imaginary wall) formed between the serosal layers of the two pleural cavities. The space is filled by all the organs of the thorax, except the lungs. The mediastinum divides the thoracic cavity into right and left halves. Unlike the pleural cavities, it is not a closed cavity, but is continuous with the fascial planes of the neck cranially and into the retroperitoneal space caudally. Therefore, air in the mediastinum can travel up the neck or into the retroperitoneal space. The dorsal mediastinum between the lungs is straight. The ventral mediastinum is very irregular in contour, due to the thymus, heart, and vena cavae. The mediastinum is divided into parts:

1. Cranial part of the mediastinum: the portion in front of the heart. It is contains the esophagus, trachea, thymus (if present), vessels in front of the heart, etc.

• Esophagus: usually not visible on a radiograph unless it contains swallowed air (aerophagia), because it is surrounded by the similar water densities of the mediastinum. Air around it, as in pneumomediastinum, will make it visible. Chest survey films of the esophagus should include the cervical and thoracic portions, including the caudal pharynx and cranial abdomen.

– Esophageal and pharyngeal foreign bodies: lodge in four common sites due to constriction of surrounding structures: 1. At the pharyngeal side of the esophageal opening, 2. Cranial to the thoracic inlet, 3. Cranial to the base of the heart, and 4. At cardia of the stomach.

– Persistent right aortic arch: congenital defect in the development of the aortic arches. This results in the esophagus passing to the left of the aorta instead of the right. The esophagus is thus ringed by the aorta, ligamentum arteriosum, pulmonary trunk and the base of the heart. This constriction stops food and causes the esophagus to balloon cranial to the base of the heart (or the ring).

– Megaesophagus: acquired or congenital dilatation of caudal cervical and thoracic esophagus. This results in ventral displacement of the trachea and heart.

– Tracheal-esophageal stripe: a line caused by the air in a megaesophagus and air in the trachea contrasting the adjacent walls of the two structures.

– Esophageal cone: the VD appearance of a megaesophagus as it passes caudally to the diaphragm.

• Sail sign: an oblique soft tissue opacity due to the thymus in the ventral part of the cranial mediastinum seen in VD or DV views.

MEDIASTINUM

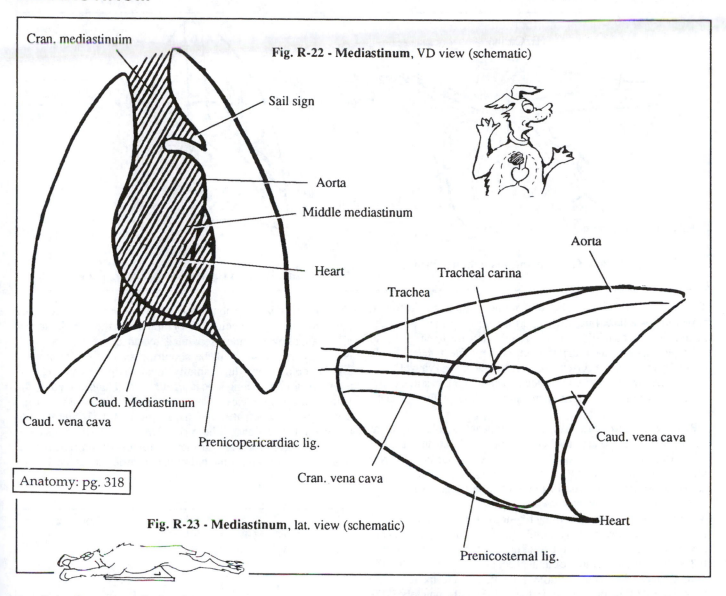

Fig. R-22 - **Mediastinum**, VD view (schematic)

Cran. mediastinuim

Sail sign

Aorta

Middle mediastinum

Heart

Caud. Mediastinum

Caud. vena cava

Prenicopericardiac lig.

Anatomy: pg. 318

Aorta

Tracheal carina

Trachea

Caud. vena cava

Cran. vena cava

Heart

Fig. R-23 - **Mediastinum**, lat. view (schematic)

Prenicosternal lig.

A sail sign is a normal finding in cats and young dogs.

• **Mediastinal lymph node**: located in the cranial mediastinum dorsal to sternebrae two. These are not seen unless enlarged (e.g., lymphosarcoma, common in cats).

2. Middle part of the mediastinum: the portion containing the heart and its pericardial sac, esophagus, bifurcation of the trachea, etc.

3. Caudal part of the mediastinum: the portion caudal to the heart; containing the aorta, esophagus, caudal vena cava, and vagal trunks.

• **Phrenicopericardiac ligament**: seen on the left side extending from the apex of the heart to the diaphragm. It forms the left side of the caudal mediastinum.

4, 5. Dorsal and ventral portions of the mediastinum: divided

by the trachea and the esophagus.

Visible structures of the mediastinum: most structures are not seen, except the air-filled trachea and tracheal bifurcation, the heart and the aorta.

Pneumomediastinum: air in the mediastinum. This causes an increased radiolucency of the mediastinum contrasting the water densities (esophagus and vessels), making them visible. This air can pass up the fascial planes of the neck or into the retroperitoneal space.

Mediastinal shift: moving of the mediastinum to the right or left. Know the normal position of the mediastinum in the VD or DV view so shifts can be detected (i.e. unilateral pneumothorax, pleural effusion, diaphragmatic hernia).

Mediastinal masses: change the shape and density of the mediastinum.

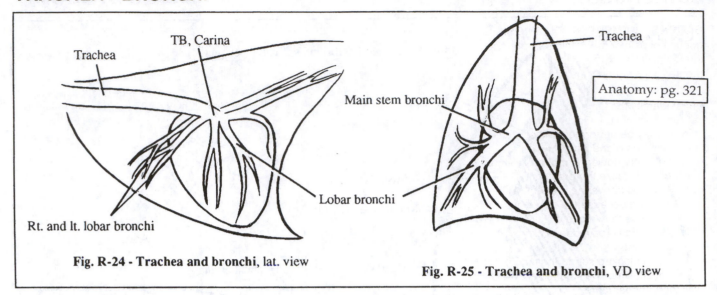

Fig. R-24 - **Trachea and bronchi**, lat. view

Fig. R-25 - **Trachea and bronchi**, VD view

Anatomy: pg. 321

Trachea: an air filled tube within the cranial mediastinum, appearing as a dark line (air). It terminates over the base of the heart at the tracheal bifurcation. In a DV view the trachea should be superimposed over the thoracic spine. The tracheal angle normally is 15° to the vertebral column in the lateral view. Dorsal deviation of the trachea can be due to a cranial mediastinal mass, excess fat, right heart enlargement or an expiratory film (artifact).

TB, Tracheal bifurcation or carina: appears as a black, circular density above the base of the heart. It appears darker than the rest of the trachea because of its greater cross sectional area. (This is incorrectly referred to as the carina by radiologists. The carina is actually a ridge at the base of the tracheal bifurcation.)

Mainstem bronchi or primary bronchi: the two continuations of the trachea into the lungs. Only the air in the major bronchi normally show up. Due to the thickness of the caudal lobe (more tissue density), the air in the caudal bronchi shows better than the cranial ones. The right middle bronchus is the most ventral (dependent) of the bronchi, thus, the right middle lung lobe is the primary site for aspiration pneumonia. The second most common site is the cranial right lung lobe. A light, inhaled foreign body (grass awn), which moves by air flow and not gravity, will tend to take a straight shot to the right caudal lobe.

"Cowboy legs": bowing of the principal bronchi due to enlargement of the left atria or the tracheobronchial lymph nodes in a DV/VD view.

Separation of principal bronchi in the lateral view: due to an enlargement of the left atrium. This causes the left principal bronchus to be elevated and both bronchi to be seen as a "V" on its side, extending caudally from the tracheal bifurcation in a lateral view. Normally they are superimposed.

Bronchogram: air in bronchi showing up because of fluid in the lung tissue causing a contrast between the tissue and bronchi. They will appear as a black tubes (air) in white (water) surroundings.

Pulmonary triad: a lobar bronchus with its associated lobar pulmonary artery and vein. Radiographically, the vessels appear as a pair of water lines separated by an air line (bronchus). Normally the vessels will be about the same size. Pulmonary arteries come from the cranially located right ventricle. The artery to the cranial lung lobe is located dorsal (and cranial) to the vein in the lateral view. The pulmonary veins flow into the caudally-located left atrium, thus, are more ventral (lateral view) and central (VD view). These positions allow a straight shot to their respective heart compartments without crossing each other. In the DV or VD views the pulmonary arteries are at the 4 and 8 o'clock positions.

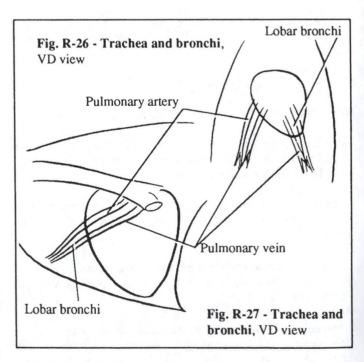

Fig. R-26 - **Trachea and bronchi,** VD view

Fig. R-27 - **Trachea and bronchi,** VD view

Memory Aid: Pulmonary veins are always ventral and central (medial).

LUNGS

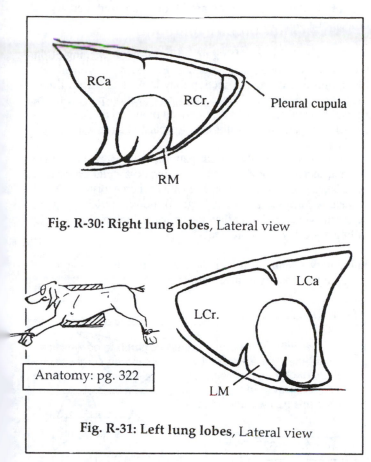

Fig. R-30: Right lung lobes, Lateral view

Anatomy: pg. 322

Fig. R-31: Left lung lobes, Lateral view

Pleural effusions: fluid in the pleural space (i.e., water, [hydrothorax], air [pneumothorax], chyle [chylothorax] and pus [pyothorax]).

Scalloped appearance or leafing: to the lung borders due to pleural effusions pushing the lungs away from the body wall and filling the lung fissures. Fluid lines will be seen in the fissures between the lobes or pseudolobes of the lungs. There will be loss of detail, obscuring the heart and diaphragm

Pneumothorax: air in the pleural space.

Skin folds: may be mistaken for fluid lines. They usually can be traced past the boundaries of the thorax. Skin folds can also be mistaken for the borders of the lungs, causing a false diagnosis of pneumothorax.

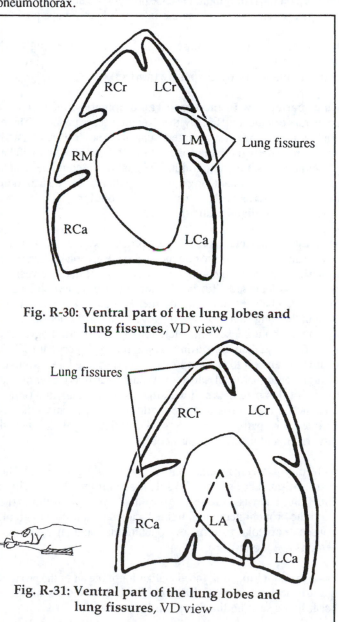

Fig. R-30: Ventral part of the lung lobes and lung fissures, VD view

Fig. R-31: Ventral part of the lung lobes and lung fissures, VD view

LUNGS: should not be seen on radiographs because they are air densities (black). The left lung anatomically has two lung lobes - cranial and caudal. The cranial lobe, divided into cranial and caudal parts, is considered one lobe by anatomists. Radiologists often speak of 3 left lung lobes (cranial, middle and caudal), the caudal part of the cranial lobe being the radiologist's middle lobe. The right lung has 4 lung lobes -cranial, middle, caudal and accessory both anatomically and radiographically. The cranial lobe of the right lung is seen in front of the cranial lobe of the left lung in a lateral view. This shows up as a separate, round, air filled structure that can be confusing. (Note: the Radiologist's scheme of 7 lung lobes holds in all species, where in the horse the anatomist's nomenclature must consider only 2 lobes to exist.)

Lobular pattern of lungs and the lung fissures: normally don't appear unless there is fluid or air in the pleural cavity (as opposed to fluid in the lungs), a collapsed lung or pleural thickenings.

PLEURAL CAVITIES: potential not real spaces, because serous tension holds the visceral pleura of the lungs to the parietal pleura of the thoracic wall. Thus, they are normally not visible radiographically. Fluid (pleural effusion) or air (pneumothorax) in the pleural space causes the lungs to separate from the chest wall.

Cupula of pleural cavity: the cranial extent of the pleural cavity, normally extending past the first rib.

LUNG FIELDS

Basically, lungs are evaluated for fluid and air. Radiographically, air is black. A normal lung field has a black background with fluid (soft tissue) structures (vessels) passing through it. Evaluate lungs for an increase (more radiopaque) or decrease (more radiolucent) in density of their parenchyma. These changes can be generalized or localized, solitary or multiple. Compare the two sides of the thorax in the DV view. They should both be of equal opacity.

If an animal is dyspneic (difficult or labored breathing) do not compromise it by taking a VD view, instead take a DV.

Interstitium or parenchyma: the framework of the lungs, consisting of muscle tissue, cells making up the alveolar spaces, lymphatics, connective tissue, vessels and nerves. Normally this is a very dark air-filled network because the fine structures do not show up on the radiograph. Disease processes can cause them to enlarge and show up, making the interstitium more opaque.

Hyperlucent chest: increased radiolucency to the lung field which can be due to emphysema, hyperventilation, undercirculation or overexposure (artifact).

Lung patterns with increased radio-opacities: the different appearance of the lung field with different disease patterns. There are four basic lung patterns: interstitial, alveolar, bronchiolar and vascular. Usually more than one pattern and often all four will be present on the same radiograph. The goal is to determine which is the most predominant lung pattern or patterns. The distribution of the lung patterns can be lobar, isolated to one lobe; diffuse, over whole lung or hilar, around the hilus.

• **Interstitial pattern**: some disease processes cause the interstitial tissue to become more opaque due to the alveolar: interstitial ratio shifting toward the interstitial. As this continues the vessels become harder to see - "fuzzy". In the normal lung, the pulmonary vessels can be seen to the third order branches. Air can still be seen in the lung field because the alveoli are still filled with air. The number one cause of an interstitial pattern on a radiograph is an incorrectly taken film during expiration (expiratory film). This causes the alveoli to be compressed and thus, the interstitium is a larger component of the lung volume (artifact). Pathologic causes of this pattern are - interstitial fibrosis, interstitial (viral) pneumonia, atelectasis, allergic conditions, lung worms. A nodular interstitial pattern has masses differentiated by their size and dispersion and usually means neoplasia.

• **Alveolar pattern**: results from the alveoli filling with fluid. The vessels disappear because the soft tissue around them is filled with fluid. There is no air seen in the lung (alveoli) resulting in the air in the bronchi being highlighted, called an air bronchogram. Causes of alveolar pattern are - pneumonia, pulmonary edema, hemorrhage (contusion).

– **Air bronchiogram**: the visualization of the air of the bronchi due to the lung being filled with fluid. The vessels disapear because the surrounding lung is filled with fluid.

• **Bronchiolar pattern**: enlarged or increased density of bronchiolar walls.

– **Peribronchiolar cuffing or infiltration**: thickening of the bronchiolar wall and space around it. End on, such bronchi look like "donuts". In sagittal section they looks like "tram lines" (train or tram tracts). The normal arborization pattern to the normal bronchi appears like a tree with branches that taper. In a bronchiolar pattern the limbs may appear to be pruned.

• **Vascular pattern**: the fourth pattern; the vessels are either normal, increased or decreased. In a hypervascular pattern the vessels are larger than normal. They may become tortuous. Think of heartworm disease when large tortuous arteries are seen. When the veins are larger than the arteries, think of the left heart failing to deal with its preload.

Pulmonary edema: fluid in the lungs resulting in increased radiographic opacity of alveolar pattern.

SUMMARY - LUNG PATTERNS
Interstitial pattern: - slightly denser lung field (variable) - Air evident in lung - Vessels fuzzy, but evident 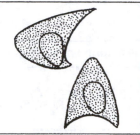
Anatomy: pg. 325
Alveolar pattern: - Opaque lung field - No air in the lung - No vasculature - Air bronchogram (black worm holes in white apple) Air bronchiogram 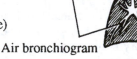

Bronchiolar pattern:
 - Peribronchiolar cuffing
   Donuts
   Tram lines
   "Donuts"
   "Tram lines" 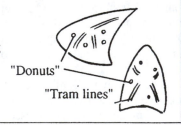

Vascular pattern - Enlarged vessels (hypervascularity) - Smaller vessels (hypovascular) - Normal vessels   - Loss of symmetry in size of arteries versus veins 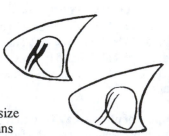

HEART

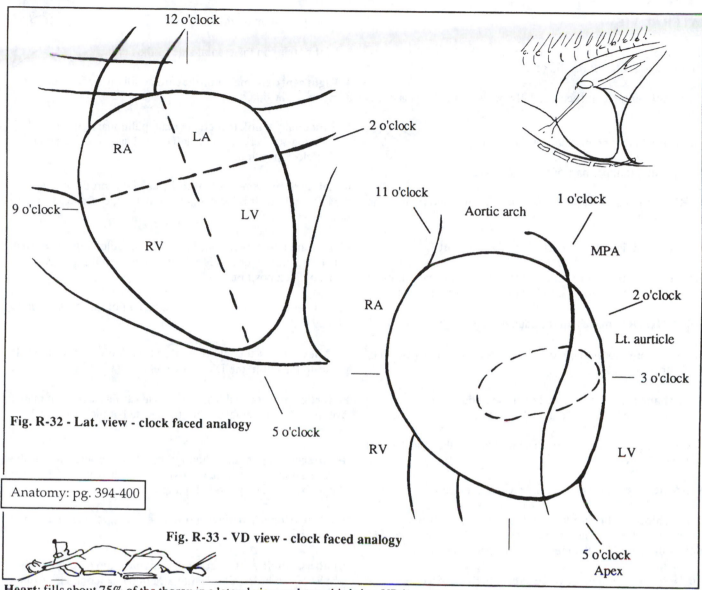

Fig. R-32 - Lat. view - clock faced analogy

Anatomy: pg. 394-400

Fig. R-33 - VD view - clock faced analogy

Heart: fills about 75% of the thorax in a lateral view and two thirds in a VD/DV view. Minimal heart enlargement will be hard to determine. The heart appears as a solid disk because it is muscle filled with blood (both water densities). Therefore, you will evaluate the borders or silhouette of the heart, not its cavities. (The heart should be less than 1/2 the width of the VD thorax at the level of the 9th rib.)

CHAMBERS OF THE HEART

Chambers of the heart: can be imagined on a lateral view by drawing two crossing perpendicular lines. The first one follows the axis of the heart and passes through the apex. This gives a rough estimate of the location of the chambers. Another learning aid is the clock-faced analogy. "Be very careful of this approach", it is not good when trying to figure out the chambers in heart enlargement. This is because the right ventricle wraps almost completely around the left ventricle, except for the caudal side. In right heart enlargement it can even project caudal to the left ventricle. In spite of this, the analogy can still aid the student in a three dimensional interpretation of the radiographs of a normal heart. Of special value is the location of the pulmonary trunk, aortic arch, apex and left auricle.

Heart - clock face analogy:

VD view:

11-1: Aortic arch
1-2 o'clock: pulmonary trunk (MPA)
2-3 o'clock: left atria appendage (auricle)
2-6 o'clock: left ventricle
5 o'clock: apex
6-9 o'clock: right ventricle
9-11 o'clock: right atria

Lateral view:

1-2 and 9 o'clock: waist of heart
11-12 o'clock: aortic arch
1-2 o'clock: left atrium
2-6 o'clock: left ventricle
5 o'clock: apex
6-9 o'clock: Right ventricle
9-11 o'clock: right atrium

621

HEART

LATERAL VIEW

1. Cranial vena cava: located cranial to the heart, usually its ventral edge is all that can be seen.

2. Caudal vena cava: seen caudally between the heart and the diaphragm.

Right side heart: cranial part of the heart.

3. Right atria: upper part of the cranial heart.

3'. Right auricular appendage: wraps around the front of the outflow tract.

4. Right ventricle: lower part of the cranial heart.

5. Pulmonary trunk or main pulmonary artery (MPA): can't be seen on a lateral projection because it is superimposed.

LEFT HEART: makes up the caudal aspect of the heart.

6. Left atrium: located on the upper part of the caudal aspect of the heart.

6'. Left auricle: superimposed over the middle of the heart so it is not visualized in the lateral or VD views.

7. Left ventricle: makes up the ventral part of the caudal aspect of the heart and the apex.

8. Aortic arch: comes out of the base of the heart.

9. Brachiocephalic trunk and left subclavian artery: come off the arch of the aorta and travel cranially. These can't be seen, unless there is air in the mediastinum (pneumomediastinum).

10. Descending aorta: travels caudally high in the thorax against the vertebral bodies to the abdomen. It is easily seen.

11. Cranial waist: located at the junction between the cranial vena cava and the right atrium. In this area there is the arch of the aorta, right auricular appendage and pulmonary trunk. Enlargement of any of these structures could cause a bulge and loss of the cranial cardiac waist.

12. Caudal waist: the coronary (atrioventricular) groove between the left atrium and left ventricle.

13. Sternopericardiac ligament: connects the ventral pericardium to the sternal floor of the thorax.

DV/VD VIEW:

1. Cranial vena cava: doesn't show up because of all the other structures in the cranial mediastinum.

2. Caudal vena cava: extends between the right side of the heart and the diaphragm on the right side.

3. Right atria: on the cranial side of the heart.

4. Right ventricle: makes up the cardiac silhouette from the apex along the right side.

5. Pulmonary trunk (called the main pulmonary artery [MPA] by radiologists): arises on the left cranial side of the heart at the 1 - 2 o'clock position.

6. Left atrium: summated over the caudal heart directly above the left ventricle. It is located just caudal to the tracheal bifurcation.

6'. Left auricle: superimposed over the middle of the heart so it is not visualized unless it is enlarged, and then it projects out at 2 to 3 o'clock position.

7. Left ventricle: makes up the caudal half of the left silhouette of the heart.

7'. Apex: part of the left ventricle at the 5 o'clock position. It points to the left in the DV/VD view.

8. Aortic arch: not visible in the DV view because it is summated over the cranial mediastinum. It is located at the 11 - 1 o'clock position.

10. Descending aorta: a line representing the left edge of the aorta is all that is seen due to overlapping densities. This edge should be seen in a good radiograph.

11. Phrenicopericardiac ligament: makes up the left margin of the mediastinum.

Contrast studies of the heart (angiocardiography): radiographs of the heart taken while a radiopaque contrast medium circulates through it. Insert a canula into the external jugular vein and into the right atrium with the aid of a fluoroscope. Inject the contrast medium quickly as a bolus and take a film. This lights up the right side of the heart. The right ventricle covers the cranial part of the cardiac silhouette. It actually covers most of the silhouette, except the caudal part. The pulmonic valve shows up as little black indentations in the beginning of the pulmonary trunk (MPA). The pulmonary arteries are seen extending away into the lung fields.

Left side of the heart: cannulate the common carotid in the dog. Thread the catheter into the aorta and into the left ventricle.

6. Aortic sinus: (Sinus of Val Salva) the pockets in the base of the aorta behind the aortic semilunar valve leaflets. The coronary arteries arise form the aortic sinuses as the first branches of the ascending aorta. The brachiocephalic trunk is the first branch of the aortic arch. The left subclavian artery is the second branch of the aortic arch.

HEART

Anatomy: pg. 394-400

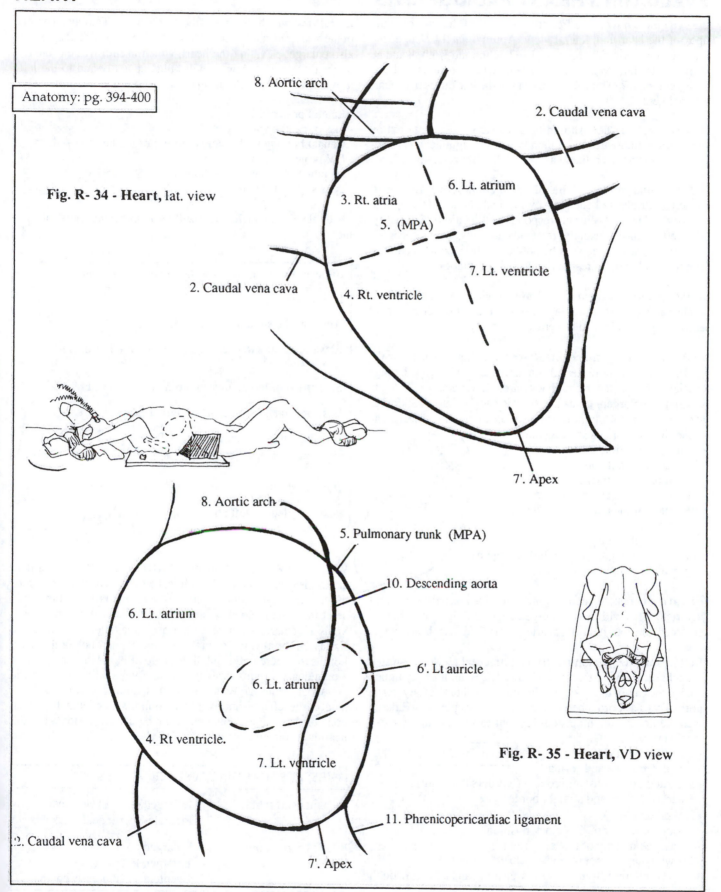

Fig. R- 34 - Heart, lat. view

8. Aortic arch

2. Caudal vena cava

6. Lt. atrium

3. Rt. atria

5. (MPA)

2. Caudal vena cava

7. Lt. ventricle

4. Rt. ventricle

7'. Apex

8. Aortic arch

5. Pulmonary trunk (MPA)

10. Descending aorta

6. Lt. atrium

6. Lt. atrium

6'. Lt auricle

4. Rt ventricle.

7. Lt. ventricle

Fig. R- 35 - Heart, VD view

11. Phrenicopericardiac ligament

2. Caudal vena cava

7'. Apex

623

EVALUATING HEART RADIOGRAPHS

2/5-3/5 rule: Draw a line from the "carina" of the trachea to the apex of the heart in a lateral view. Approximately 2/5th of the bulk of the heart should be in back of the line and 3/5th should be in front of the line. More than 2/5th behind the line infers left heart enlargement. More than 3/5th in front of the line infers right heart enlargement.

Sternal contact: there should be three sternebrae contacted by the cardiac silhouette. More than this infers right heart enlargement. This is not as reliable as the 2/5th-3/5th rule.

Signs of enlargement of the different chambers of the heart: the left ventricle is likened to a cylindrical pump and the right to a bellows. The right ventricle responds by dilatation quite readily. The left ventricle usually responds initially with concentric hypertrophy which may not be noticed without contrast studies. The thin-walled atria respond readily by dilatation.

Right atrial enlargement - Lateral view: elevation of the trachea and loss of the cranial waist. DV projection: enlargement of the 9 to 11 o'clock silhouette of the heart.

Right ventricular enlargement: seen as a cranial bulging on the lateral view with more sternal contact. In a VD view, it will bulge cranially and to the right (backwards or reverse "D"). Right ventricular enlargement causes fluid to back up into the abdomen and extremities. Pulmonic stenosis or heartworm disease can cause right ventricular enlargement.
- Lateral projection
- increased sternal contact
- elevation of the trachea
- elevation of the caudal vena cava
- elevation of the apex off the sternum
- DV projection:
- rounded right cardiac border
- inverted "D" sign with marked enlargement
- apex more to the left

• **Heart worms**: located in the pulmonary arteries and right ventricle. This will cause enlargement of the right ventricle and enlarged, tortuous pulmonary arteries in reactions to heart worms.

Left atrial enlargement: will cause tracheal and left mainstem bronchi elevation in the lateral view. These are not very noticeable in the cat. In the DV view the auricle will project beyond the normal cardiac border between the 2-3 o'clock position. Enlargement can cause the mainstem bronchi to spread out ("cowboy legs") (VD).
- Lateral projection:
- elevated trachea and carina
- separation of mainstem bronchi (left dorsal to right)
- enlarged atrium and straight border
- DV projection:
- auricle projects at 2-3 o'clock position
- increased density of the left atrium
- "cowboy legs" (mainstem bronchi)

Anatomy: pgs. 394-400

Left ventricular enlargement: seen as a caudal bulging on the lateral view which eliminates the caudal waist. The caudal border of the heart is normally straighter and more vertical. The apex will also enlarge, elevating the heart, which in turn will elevate the trachea. On a VD view, it will bulge caudally and to the left, moving the apex to the right. This is common in mitral valve insufficiency.
- Lateral projection:
- loss of caudal waist
- Caudal bulging to the caudal border of the heart
- DV projection:
- rounding of left ventricle border (3 - 5 o'clock)
- apex shifted to right

• **Mitral valve insufficiency**: will result in left ventricle enlargement.

Signs of heart chamber enlargement - indicate:
Lateral view
Apex off the sternum: right ventricle
Elevation of the trachea: right or left atria, left or right ventricle
Separation of the main stem bronchi: left atrial
Loss of caudal cardiac waist: left atria
Bowing out of caudal border - left ventricle
DV view
Backwards "D" - right ventricle
"Cowboy legs" - left atria

VESSEL EVALUATION of CARDIAC DISEASE: Cardiac disease is basically a pump failure. To avoid overinterpretation of the cardiac bulges, look for signs of hydrolic failure. If the right heart fails, the preload (systemic venous return) will overload. Signs are enlarged caudal vena (post) cava (should be the same size as the aorta), effusion in the peritoneal and/or pleural spaces. Left heart failure will result in back up of blood into the preload - pulmonary venous drainage. Therefore, you should see the pulmonary veins larger than the corresponding arteries, enlargement of the left atria and eventually pulmonary edema. If you see none of these signs, then there may be cardiac lesions, but the heart is still in compensation.

VESSELS - CARDIAC DISEASE	
Right heart faliure -	Enlarged caudal vena cava
	Pleural or peritoneal effusions
Left heart failure -	Enlarged pulmonary veins
	Enlarged left atria
	Eventually pulmonary edema

ABDOMENAL RADIOGRAPHS

Abdominal radiographs: taken during the pause after expiration. Positioning is very important and there should be no motion. Use the right or left lateral projection consistently to eliminate this as a variable. High latitude films are taken to see subtle shades of gray for the different water densities. This also burns through the distracting ribs in the cranial abdomen. Standard views of the abdomen are the lateral and VD/DV views. Standing lateral views use a horizontal beam direction through a standing animal to detect fluid levels in bowel or abdomen. Special lateral recumbency views direct the beam horizontally through a laterally recumbent animal in the VD direction. These are used to detect small amounts of air in the abdomen. Oblique views are shot through the animal placed in DV or VD position and rotated 15 to 30°. These are used to get a more complete examination of the esophagus, stomach, colon and urinary bladder by moving them away from the spinal column.

Peritoneal detail: depends on serosal fat surrounding the surface of the organs. Fat is radiographically less dense than water (appears darker), thus, contrasts the water densities. Fat is deposited in the omentum, the falciform ligament and in the retroperitoneal space.

• **Loss of serosal detail**: happens when fat is absent from the abdomen in neonatal or emaciated animals and when there is fluid in the abdomen. This causes the abdomen to have an overall gray appearance like "ground glass". The difference between absence of fat and extra fluid is assessed by the shape of the abdomen. A thin dog will be gaunt or "tucked up". A dog with a lot of peritoneal fluid will have a full, rotund or pendulous abdomen. Young dogs have poor serosal detail because they don't have the right type of fat. This is normal in dogs under 4 months of age.

- **Ground glass appearance**: classical description of an overall gray abdomen due to loss of serosal detail. This can be overcome by adding contrast material in the abdomen.

• **Focal loss of detail**: small areas where serosal detail is poor while the rest of the abdomen has good detail. An example would be pancreatitis with focal peritonitis. This causes loss of detail in the right cranial quadrant of the abdomen where the pancreas resides.

Gas: within the organs allows differentiation between the inside of the organs and helps to identify them (e.g., stomach).

Hydroabdomen(ascites): fluid in the abdomen due to hypoproteinemia, liver failure, heart failure, renal failure, portal hypertension.

Kidneys can become invisible if there is surrounding fluid in the retroperitoneal space (ruptured ureter, abscesses).

Air in the abdomen: will go to the independent site. Air first appears against the diaphragm. Usually only the lung side of the diaphragm is seen because the abdominal side is summated with the liver tissue. If both sides can be seen there is air in the abdomen. Horizontal views are used to detect a small amount of air in the abdomen. The animal is placed in left lateral recumbency (right side up). A small amount of gas present will be detected between the right lobes of the liver and the diaphragm.

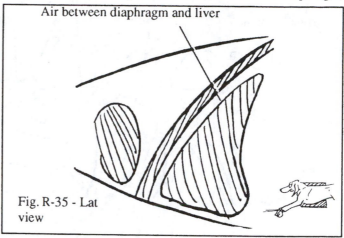

Air between diaphragm and liver

Fig. R-35 - Lat view

POSITIONING: The right lateral view (left lateral recumbency) is preferred to the left lateral view (right side up) to avoid gas in the fundus, which confuses what is seen. This view puts the fundus down so that gas will collect in the smaller pylorus (located on the right, thus, independent in this view).

Positioning of film:
• Center the umbilicus in the center of the film
• Include the entire abdomen from the pelvic inlet to the diaphragm
• Put the thickest end towards the cathode because of the heel effect

CONTRAST STUDIES: use of opaque media (positive contrast agents) or gas (negative contrast agent) to delineate portions of the GI tract. Survey radiographs must always precede any contrast studies.

Negative contrast agents: usually CO_2 or air, are used to see where organs are, such as the stomach. Blow air into the stomach or give the animal a carbonated beverage.

Positive contrast agents: mineral densities that appear very white on radiographs. They are used to detect or confirm gastric or small bowel disease and to outline size, shape, and position of segments of the GI tract. Barium Sulfate is a positive contrast agent. It is inert in the lungs but causes granulomatous responses in the peritoneal cavity. Avoid it if there is a possibility of perforation of the GI tract. Use barium in the stomach in case of aspiration into the lungs. Iodine is also a second positive contrast substance that is extremely hyperosmotic and can cause pulmonary edema but has little effect on the peritoneum. Because of its hyperosmolarity it dilutes itself decreasing its radio-opacity. It gives poor mucosal detail compared to barium. It is indicated if there is suspected perforation of the stomach.

COMPRESSION STUDIES: squeeze the contents of the abdomen with a wooden spoon or piece of Plexiglass to separate different structures, while taking radiographs.

625

ABDOMENAL RADIOGRAPHS

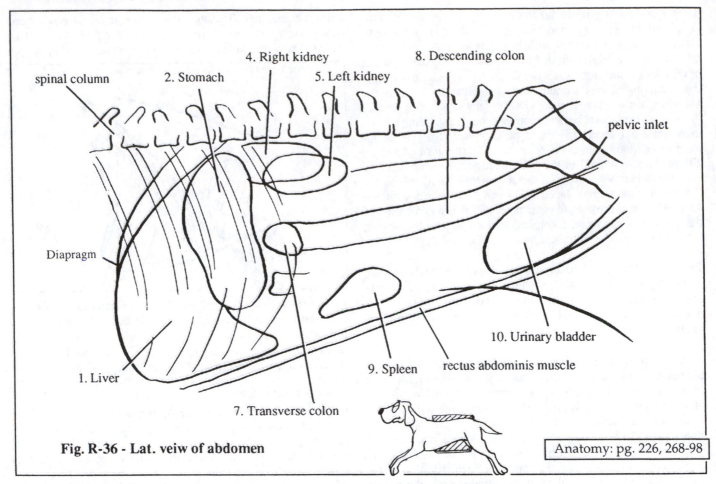

Fig. R-36 - Lat. veiw of abdomen

Anatomy: pg. 226, 268-98

Viewing abdominal films: just as in the thorax, viewing needs to be systematic and consistent (done the same way ever time). Frame of the picture first, look at the diaphragm, spine, musculature of sublumbar soft tissue, part of the pelvis in film, ventral body wall, falciform fat area and the caudal thorax. Look at the location of organs normally not seen on radiographs. If seen, something is amiss. Therefore, it is important to know anatomically where organs are located. Mobile structures of the abdomen, such as the small and large intestines, can be displaced. A displaced organ may be normal with an invisible, abnormal structure displacing it (indirect evidence).

BOUNDARIES OF ABDOMEN:

• Cranial - diaphragm
• Caudal- pelvic inlet
• Dorsal - spinal column
• Lateral and ventral- abdominal muscles
• Ventral - rectus abdominis muscle

QUADRANTS: draw two imaginary lines on the DV abdominal view. The first, down the midline and one perpendicular to it through the umbilicus. This divides the abdomen into four quadrants. Knowing what is in each quadrant helps viewing radiographs.The greatest number of individual structures are located in the cranial quadrants.

Lateral view of abdomen:

1. Liver abuts the diaphragm cranially.
2. Stomach is caudal to the liver.
3. Spleen: its distal part is seen on end as a triangle in the ventral abdominal wall just caudal to the liver.
4. Right kidney: seen high in the abdominal cavity. Its cranial pole is embedded in the caudate process of the liver, thus, not visualized.
5. Left kidney: 1/2 kidney length caudal to the right kidney and usually can be completely visualized. It is also usually somewhat ventral to the right kidney.
7. Transverse colon: crosses the abdomen caudal to the stomach and is seen end on if it contains any gas.
8. Descending colon: continues from the transverse colon caudally to the pelvis where it becomes the rectum.
9. Spleen: in ventral abdomen caudal to the liver.
10. Urinary bladder: caudoventral abdomen.

Abnormal mass: may be caused by enlargement of any structure present in the area.

ABDOMENAL RADIOGRAPHS

Anatomy: pg. 226, 268-98

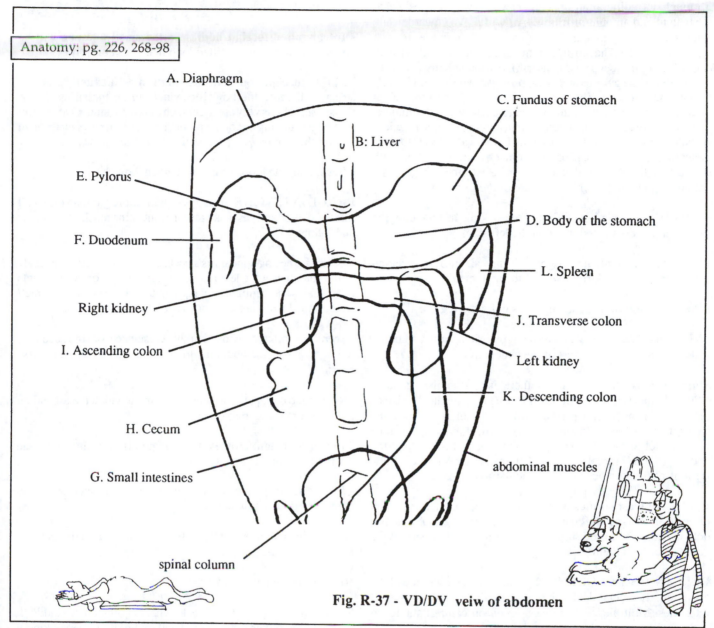

A. Diaphragm

C. Fundus of stomach

B: Liver

E. Pylorus

F. Duodenum

D. Body of the stomach

L. Spleen

Right kidney

J. Transverse colon

I. Ascending colon

Left kidney

K. Descending colon

H. Cecum

G. Small intestines

abdominal muscles

spinal column

Fig. R-37 - VD/DV veiw of abdomen

DV/VD view:

A. Diaphragm
B. Liver: between stomach and diaphragm
C. Fundus of stomach: located on the left side of the abdomen.
D. Body of the stomach: crosses the midline.
E. Pylorus: located on right side of the abdomen in dogs; on midline in cats.
F. Duodenum: passes down the right side of the abdomen.
G. Small intestines: hard to follow.
H. Cecum: located on the right side.
I. Ascending colon: located on the right side.
J. Transverse colon: crosses midline from right to left.
K. Descending colon: travels down the left side.
L. Spleen: located caudal to the stomach on the left side.

Quadrants - organs	
Right cranial quadrant	**Left cranial quadrant**
Pylorus	Fundus of stomach
Pancreas	Spleen
Duodenum	Left kidney
Right lobes of liver	
Gall bladder	
Ascending colon	
Right kidney	
Right caudal quadrant	**Left caudal quadrant**
Cecum	Descending colon
Small intestine	Left ovary
Right ovary	Left uterine horn
Right uterine horn	

627

ABDOMEN - RADIOGRAPH

Stomach: its radiographic appearance varies with the position of the patient and amount of filling. Air will move upward, while fluid is gravity dependent. Do not confuse fluid in the stomach with a mass (ball). The unfilled stomach is normally within the rib cage (doesn't project past the last rib). A foreign body can act as a ball valve in the pylorus and cause projectile vomiting. The cat's stomach is J-shaped. The cat's pyloric antrum is to the left of midline. The peristaltic rate of the stomach is 2 to 4 a minute. During fluoroscopy, look for emptying, contraction and function. A thumb print pattern is depressions in the wall of the stomach indicating an infiltrative process. Stomach rugae are visible with contrast studies. Gastric distention can be extremely large, causing great pain and possibly a rupture of the stomach.

• Right lateral recumbency (left side up) - air in fundic region located in the dorsal abdomen on the left side.

• Left lateral recumbency (right side up): air in pyloric region located in the ventral, right side of the abdomen.

• DV projection (dorsal side up): gas in fundic region.

• VD (ventral side up): gas will be in pyloric antrum and body, which are in the ventral part of the abdomen.

Stomach axis: can be seen if there is gas in the stomach. Clinically the axis of the stomach is used to evaluate the size of the liver. In the lateral projection the normal position of the stomach axis is between a line drawn vertical to the spine and a line parallel to the ribs. The pylorus is superimposed over the body or slightly cranial to it (10-11th ribs). In the VD or DV view the axis of the stomach is perpendicular to the spine.

Double contrast studies: use of air and contrast material in an organ. Barium is a good coating material providing good mucosal detail. The rugae of the stomach should be about the size of the valleys between them.

DESCENDING DUODENUM: located on the right side of the abdomen. It is classically larger than the rest of the small intestines. Multiple views must be seen on contrast studies to make a diagnosis of duodenal problems.

• **Lymphatic craters**: normal depressions in the wall of the duodenum that are seen in contrast studies. They are often mistaken for ulcers, and have been called pseudo-ulcers

SMALL INTESTINE: train yourself to routinely look for individual loops. The serosal surface of small intestines is smooth. The thickness of the bowel wall is 1/9 to 1/8th the width of the distended lumen. Mucosal detail can only be evaluated with contrast material or in air-filled segments.

• **Rule of thumb for intestinal size**: equals the height of a lumbar vertebral body or two rib widths. Small intestines wider than 2 1/2 rib widths may be abnormal.

• **Sentinel loops**: large distended loops of bowel named because

they indicate trouble.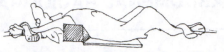

• **Intraluminal foreign bodies**: in the small intestine will be noticed by finding a gas filled loop that ends abruptly.

• **Linear foreign bodies in the small intestine**: items, such as string, will cause the bowel to bunch up on the string due to peristalsis. This is very apparent with a contrast study. Do not pull on a string sticking out of the mouth or anus or it can saw through the bunched up bowel (peritonitis). Remove surgically.

• **Ileus**: multiple loops of gas-distended bowel.

LARGE INTESTINE: usually contains more gas than the small intestine. Food and gas make the large intestine much easier to see and follow.

Cecum: in the dog appears as a corkscrew shape on the right side of the abdomen at the level of L_3. It can be seen on survey films if it contains some intraluminal gas. In the cat the cecum is a small cone-shaped structure. It is not visible on survey films.

Ascending colon: extends for a short distance from the cecum up the right side of the abdomen to be continued as the transverse colon.

• **Right colic or hepatic flexure**: the point at which the ascending colon becomes the transverse colon.

Transverse colon: crosses the abdomen from right to left and continues as the descending colon.

• **Left colic or splenic flexure**: where the transverse colon becomes the descending colon.

Descending colon: on the left side. Fecal material can usually be seen in it.

Rectum: in the pelvic cavity.

The colon often provides clues to what is going on around it. It is filled with either radiopaque fecal material or gas, making it generally quite visible. The colon is relatively mobile because of its relatively long mesentery. If it is focally displaced, look for what is displacing it. An enlarged left kidney may displace the left colic flexure. The pancreas and right kidney may displace the right colic flexure.

Medial iliac lymph nodes: located at the termination of the abdominal aorta and usually not seen radiographically.

LIVER: The largest organ in the abdomen, it is located in the cranial quadrants behind the diaphragm and in front of the stomach. Normally the edges are sharp. In adult dogs the liver doesn't extend past the last rib. It is relatively larger in the young animal. The liver is contrasted cranially by air filled lungs and caudally by gas in the stomach.

ABDOMEN - RADIOGRAPH

Gall bladder: a pear-shaped structure lying between the quadrate lobe and the right medial lobe. It is normally not visible unless it contains stones or gas.

Renal impression: cups the cranial pole of the right kidney. It is part of the caudate process of the caudate lobe.

Clinically the axis of the stomach is used to evaluate the size of the liver. Assess stomach fullness. A full stomach can fool you.

• Enlarged liver: indicated if the stomach extends back and exceeds the angle parallel to the ribs.

• Small liver: indicated if the axis of the stomach inclines cranially in front of the line perpendicular to the spine. Small liver size can be due to chronic liver disease or a portal-caval shunt.

• Try to 3-dimensionally visualize the size of the liver from the lateral and the VD view, using the stomach axis.

A crisp, triangular caudal margin of the liver in a left projection indicates normal liver. A blunt and rounded caudal liver margin infers liver enlargement.

Paradoxical liver: when the stomach slants cranially, indicating a small liver, but the caudal end of the liver extends past the costal arch indicating a large liver. It has a crisp triangular caudal margin inferring a normal liver. This is a normal occurrence in older dogs due to gravity causing slumping of the liver (splanchnoptosis). The liver is of normal size.

Liver enlargement: can be diffuse or focal. Enlargement of the right liver lobe will extend past the costal arch in the lateral projection. It will appear as a large area opacification in the right cranial quadrant. This can be confused with splenic enlargement. Masses in the center of the liver can distort the shape of the stomach.

PANCREAS: a soft tissue density normally not visible radiographically because of its small size and its similar density to the surrounding structures. Cranial displacement of the duodenum or pylorus may indicate pancreatitis. Pancreatic masses of the body and right limb of the pancreas will be in the right cranial quadrant. The mass may not be seen due to focal loss of serosal detail because of surrounding inflammation and a small amount of fluid. Contrast studies may show displacement of the pylorus and the descending duodenum by a pancreatic mass. Left limb pancreatic disease is also possible and is located in the left side of the abdomen.

SPLEEN: a tongue-shaped organ loosely attached to the greater curvature of the stomach in the left cranial abdomen. The tail of the spleen extends caudally; ventral and medial to the stomach. The head of the normal spleen is attached loosely to the stomach by the gastrosplenic ligament. The head is normally tucked over in the left cranial quadrant of the abdomen with the kidney right behind it in the DV view. Splenic enlargement assessment is completely subjective, and depends on experience. The spleen's

size is variable depending on the amount of engorgement. Barbiturates cause normal physiological enlargement of the spleen. Disease processes can cause the spleen to be enlarged normal-shaped spleen. Splenic tumors can be found in many places in the abdomen because the spleen is very mobile.

• Lateral projection of the spleen: appears as a soft tissue triangle in the middle of the ventral abdomen just behind the liver.

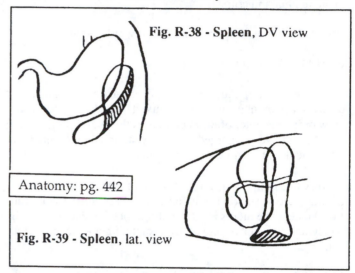

Fig. R-38 - Spleen, DV view

Anatomy: pg. 442

Fig. R-39 - Spleen, lat. view

• VD projection: the head of the spleen appears as a triangular shape adjacent and caudal to the stomach. Occasionally it may be seen superimposed over the caudal portion of the right kidney.

MESENTERIC LYMPH NODES: enlarged lymph nodes located in the root of the mesentery. Enlarged mesenteric lymph nodes can give a radiographic enlargement in the middle of the abdomen.

• Root of the mesentery is at about the level of L_2.

KIDNEYS: located in the dorsal cranial part of the abdomen. Normally both are smooth and of equal size and shape. Visualization of the renal borders is dependent on the amount of perirenal fat present. Cat's and obese dog's kidneys are easier to see than young and emaciated dogs. Compare the kidneys for size. Check that there are two, especially if you are removing one.

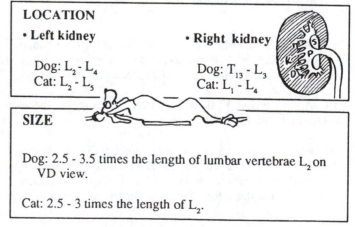

LOCATION

• **Left kidney**

Dog: $L_2 - L_4$
Cat: $L_2 - L_5$

• **Right kidney**

Dog: $T_{13} - L_3$
Cat: $L_1 - L_4$

SIZE

Dog: 2.5 - 3.5 times the length of lumbar vertebrae L_2 on VD view.

Cat: 2.5 - 3 times the length of L_2.

GENITALIA - RADIOGRAPH

URETERS: not visible on survey films because of their density and small size.

ADRENAL GLANDS: not visible on survey films.

URINARY BLADDER: has a vertex, body and neck. Normally it is an oval shape in the dog and elliptical in the cat. It is located in the caudal ventral abdomen, just cranial to the pubis and ventral to the rectum and colon.

URETHRA: not seen on normal survey radiographs.

FEMAL GENITAL TRACT:

• **Ovaries:** small, thus, not usually seen on radiographs. If enlarged a mass may be apparent caudal to the kidney on the DV view or in the center of the abdomen on the lateral projection. If they become very enlarged, they may stretch their ligamentous attachment and migrate more ventrally.

• **Uterus:** if nongravid, can't be seen on survey films. In obese dogs and cats the uterine body can be seen between the rectum and the bladder. The uterus is often radiographed to determine pregnancy and number of fetuses by visualizing and counting fetal skulls.

MALE GENITAL TRACT: the internal genitalia are not seen on survey films. The penis and testicles can be seen on the abdominal wall, but they are best assessed by physical examination.

• **Os penis:** in close association with the penile urethra.

• **Scrotum:** contains the testicles, the epididymis, and ductus deferens.

• **Prostate gland:** normally located in the pelvic cavity, around the neck of the bladder, ventral to the rectum and dorsal to the pubis. It is spherical to oval. Its position is influenced by age. It should not extend past the pelvic inlet. A prostate can be mistaken for a bladder. It is hard to see prostatic enlargement on a VD view because it is summated with the rectum, which is often filled with feces. The lateral view is better. Dorsal displacement of the colon can indicate prostatic enlargement. The bladder will not displace the colon.

SUBLUMBAR LYMPH NODE: located at the termination of the aorta in the caudodorsal abdomen. Enlargement of these lymph nodes will result in ventral displacement of the colon.

ORGANOMEGALY: there are three organs in the abdomen that normally enlarge.

• **Stomach:** can distend a tremendous amount due to the amount of food in it. It can take up 1/3 to 1/2 of the abdomen making it hard to interpret the other structures. This causes displacement of the GI tract and the spleen caudally. Gastric dilatation due to a disease process will also look like this. Prior to radiography the patient should have nothing per os from 12 to 24 hours and be given cleansing enemas to remove material from the descending colon. Food, relatively radiopaque, will mask anything that is in the same plane.

• **Urinary bladder:** can fill up to one third of the abdomen pushing everything cranially. Walk the dog and allow it to urinate before radiography.

• **Uterus:** A gravid uterus can occupy up to half the abdomen.

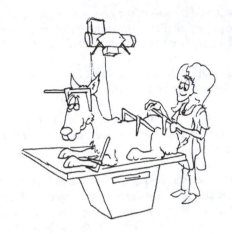

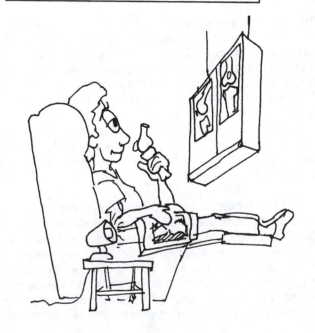

Anatomy: Ovaries: pg. 340
Uterus: pg 342
Testes: pg. 356
Accessory sex glands: pg. 364
Penis: pg 366

EQUINE - RADIOGRAPHS - RULES & VIEWS

Rules for reading and taking equine limb radiographs:

1. Distance: view radiographs first from a distance to get the overall picture; then move closer.

2. Most radiographic films of horse limbs should include four or more views. A minimum of two views is required to make three dimensional sense of a two dimensional image (radiograph) and equine limbs, which are so large, require more to be complete.

3. Highlight: try to highlight the lesion (place it on an edge) where there is greater contrast between the lesion (of bone) and the surrounding structures (soft tissue). The word silhouette would be a better word than highlighted, but is not proper*.

4. Shoot enough films when you travel in the field to avoid a second trip.

5. Bone preps: when reading films, use articulated bone preparations to line up the different views correctly.

Bone preps: radiologists use articulated bone preparations to exactly line up different views. This allows checking the exact part of each bone in question and yo determine if it is normal. Especially true of the hock and the carpus, the many confusing, overlapping lines are caused by the bones not being level, and thus, the same joint may have different representative lines on the radiograph. Such complicated configurations and possible subtle lesions make referring to bone preps essential.

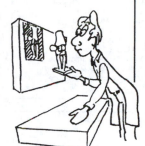

Views: named by listing the entrance and exit points of the radiographic beam.

- **DP** (**Dorsopalmar**/dorsoplantar view) or **AP** (anterior/posterior) or **CrCa** (craniocaudal): the beam passes through the dorsal/cranial side and out the palmar/plantar/caudal side.

- **Lateral** or **LM** (lateral-medial view): the beam passes through the lateral side and out the medial side of the bone or joint (or through the medial and then lateral sides).

- **Oblique views**: are taken to highlight different parts of a joint or bone. Standard for the carpus and tarsus due to the complexity and size of these joints, obliques views are also used for other areas such as the metacarpus, fetlock, digits, etc. Naming the oblique views is a major stumbling block for students. The official system of the Nomenclature Committee of the American College of Veterinary Radiology name the oblique views for the entrance and exit points of the beam. The entrance point is considered to always be on the dorsal surface (even if it isn't) to eliminate extra names. The degrees off the midsagittal plane may be placed between the dorsal and medial/lateral designations of the entrance point of the beam (e.g., D70°LPMO, D300°MPLO).

- **DMPLO** (**DorsoMedial-PalmaroLateral Oblique**): enters the dorsomedial (or palmarolateral) surface and exits the palmarolateral (or dorsomedial) surface. This is often called a **Lateral Oblique (LO)** that indicates the dorsal side highlighted (see box).

- **DLPMO** (**DorsoLateral-PalmaroMedial Oblique**: enters the dorsolateral (palmaromedial) surface and exits the palmaromedial (dorsolateral) surface. This is often called a **Medial Oblique (MO)** that indicates the dorsal side highlighted (dorsomedial)(see box).

- **Supplemental views**: are often added to the standard carpal or tarsal series.

- **Flexed lateral view**: flexes the joint(s) to open it (them) up.

- **Skyline** or **tangential view**: dorsoproximal-dorsodistal views, of which there might be at least three for the carpus.

It is common to deal with at least ten films of the carpus or tarsus.

Other oblique naming systems: due to the length of the standard names, it is common for clinicians to shorten them when working in the clinics. There are many different systems depending on the clinic (use the one your clinic uses).

- **LO and MO** (lateral and medial oblique): name the oblique view for the dorsal surface highlighted. These are shorthand for DMPLO and DLPMO, respectively. Note that they are the last two letters of the respective standard terms. This can be used to derive one from the other easily mentally. Placing a small "d" in front (dLO and dMO) will be reminder that they are named for the dorsal surface highlighted, differentiating it from the following MO and LO system. We will use this LO/MO system in this text.

- **LO**: highlights the dorsolateral. Thus, it translates into another name for the **DMPLO**, where the accessory carpal or calcanean tuberosity is overlapped.

- **MO**: another name for the **DLPMO**, where the accessory carpal or the calcanean tuberosity is completely highlighted.

- **MO and LO** (pMO and pLO): another system that names the oblique view for the palmar surface highlighted instead of the dorsal. These are shorthand for DMPLO and DLPMO, respectively. A small "p" may be used to indicate that the palmar surface is highlighted.
- **MO** (pMO): another name for the DMPLO, and thus, the accessory carpal or calcanean tuberosity is overlapped.
- **LO** (pLO): another name for the DLPMO, and thus, the accessory carpal or the calcanean tuberosity is completely highlighted.

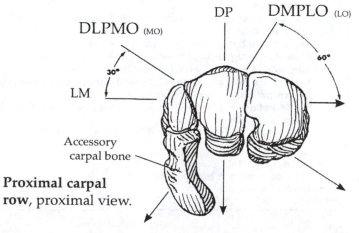

DLPMO (MO)   DP   DMPLO (LO)

30°   60°

LM

Accessory carpal bone

Proximal carpal row, proximal view.

---

*Silhouette: used in radiology of the abdomen or the thorax when a situation in which two organs of similar density are in contact and the contacting borders/margins are NOT visualized - the term is, thus, contrary to what we think of as silhouetting in which something is more visible or more easily seen. This was due to a respected radiologist's typist misusing the term in a paper that the journal's editor allowed to stand out of respect for radiologist.

Carpal Views

Lateral view, LM (lateral-medial view):

- 90° - 270°; the beam passes in through the lateral side & out the medial side
- Clue to naming: Accessory carpal bone (on the palmar side) - round & not very dense appearing. It has very little overlap with the other bones.
- **Surfaces silhouetted:** dorsal & palmar sides

Carpal anatomy: pgs. 82, 112

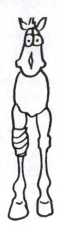

Clinical check list
- Chip fxs
  - Radius/radial carpal
  - Radial carpal/3rd carpal
  - Intermediate carpal/radius
- Slab fxs - 3rd carpal
- Joint diz
  - Fuzzy edges (exostosis)
  - "Lipping" (build up of exostosis)

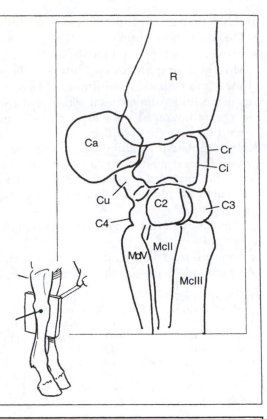

Cr. Radial carpal
Ci. Intermediate carpal bone
Cu. Ulnar carpal bone
Ca. Accessory carpal bone
C1. 1st carpal bone
C2. 2nd carpal bone
C3. 3rd carpal bone
C4. 4th carpal bone
R. Radius
McIII. 3rd metacarpal bone
McII. 2nd metacarpal bone
McIV. 4th metacarpal bone

DP view (dorsal palmar) or AP (anterior/posterior)

- 0° - 180°; the beam passes through the dorsal side & out the palmar side of the carpus
- **Silhouettes:** lateral & medial sides of the carpus
- **Clue to naming:** accessory carpal bone flat, very opaque & completely overlapped

Cr. Radial carpal
Ci. Intermediate carpal bone
Cu. Ulnar carpal bone
Ca. Accessory carpal bone
C1. 1st carpal bone
C2. 2nd carpal bone
C3. 3rd carpal bone
C4. 4th carpal bone
R. Radius
McIII. 3rd metacarpal bone
McII. 2nd metacarpal bone
McIV. 4th metacarpal bone

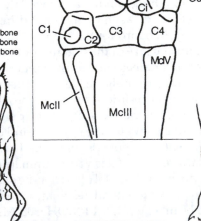

Identifying carpal bones in DP view: use the laterally-located accessory carpal bone to identify the other carpal bones. Carpal bones on the same side as the accessory carpal bone are on the lateral side; those on the opposite side are medial.

- **Proximal row**
  - Ulnar carpal bone: articulates w/ the accessory carpal bone on the lateral side of the carpus
  - Radial carpal bone: medial - on opposite side of accessory carpal
  - Intermediate carpal bone: between ulnar & radial carpal bones
- **Distal row** (bones numbered from **medial to lateral**)
  - 1st carpal bone: may or may not appear as a small bone on the medial side of the carpus
  - **2nd carpal bone**: med. side of carpus
  - **3rd carpal bone**: centered in the distal row overlapping both the 2nd & 4th carpal bones
    . It has a palmar projection that can appear like a different bone in the DP view
  - **4th carpal bone**: lateral
  - 5th is rarely (never say never) seen
- **Radial & 2nd** (1st if present) - medial side
- **Ulnar, accessory & fourth** - lateral side
- **Intermediate & 3rd** - center

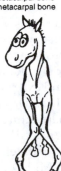

Clinical check list
- Closure of distal radius & physitis
- Angular deformities: bone alignment of forearm & cannon region
- DJD: evaluate joint spaces for narrowing
- Usually doesn't show fxs
- Complete list on a preceding page

OBLIQUE VIEWS - CARPUS
DLPMO (MO)
(Dorsolateral-palmaromedial oblique)(medial oblique, dMO)

- Enters the dorsolateral (or palmaromedial) surface and exits the palmaromedial (or dorsolateral) surface.
- MO (Medial oblique)(or dMO): used as a shorthand (note it is the last two letters of the long name), it indicates the dorsal side highlighted.
- **Highlights** DM (dorsomedial) and PL (palmarolateral) surfaces of the carpus.

Clinical problem highlighted in MO:
Chip fractures are on the **dorsomedial** surface of the carpus; (most common site in order of occurrence), are in the areas where the following bones come together:
- Radial carpal bone
- Distomedial radius
- Third carpal bone

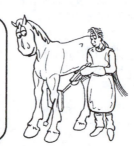

Chip fractures are seen when the beam passes through the fracture line, thus, the need for multiple views. Usually not seen on a DP view, the lateral view may show them, and the flexed lateral view shows them even better. The oblique views show them best if the beam passes through the fracture. Skyline views may also show them to advantage.

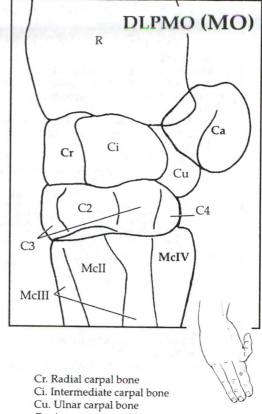

Cr. Radial carpal bone
Ci. Intermediate carpal bone
Cu. Ulnar carpal bone
Ca. Accessory carpal bone
C1. 1st carpal bone
C2. 2nd carpal bone
C3. 3rd carpal bone
C4. 4th carpal bone
R. Radius
McIII. 3rd metacarpal bone
McII. 2nd metacarpal bone'
McIV. 4th metacarpal bone

DMPLO (LO)
(Dorsomedial-palmarolateral oblique)(lateral oblique dMO)

- Enters the dorsomedial (or palmarolateral) surface and exits the palmarolateral (or dorsomedial) surface.
- LO (lateral oblique)(or dLO): used as a shorthand (note it is the last two letters of the long name), it indicates the dorsal side highlighted.
- **Highlights** DL (dorsolateral) and PM (palmaromedial) surfaces of the carpus.

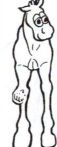

"Pinky-naming" obliques
- **Clue: accessory carpal bone and flexed pinky: palmar and lateral.**
- Check radiograph: film not a DP or Lateral, so oblique.
- Check Accessory carpal bone: completely seen (highlighted) or not (overlapped).
- Flex your little finger and hold your hand down
- Point your opposite index finger (1° beam) at the dorsal side of your hand so the amount of the pinky seen is like the accessory in the film.
- Name the entrance and exit point of your pointing finger through your hand and add oblique at the end.
.. DMPLO (if pinky and accessory carpal bone overlapped) or
.. DLPMO (if pinky and accessory carpal completely seen)

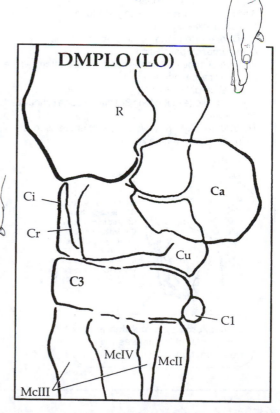

Flexed Lat. & Skyline - Carpus

Flexed lateral view:
- Usually added to the 4 standard views of the carpus
- Separates radial & intermediate carpal bones. The intermediate bone is more proximal in this view (help pinpoint a chip fx seen in a lateral view)
- Opens up the carpal joints & removes contacts betw. rows of carpal bones - silhouettes
   - Antebrachial ("radial") carpal joint opens wide
   - Middle carpal joint opens about 50% as much
   - Carpometacarpal joint opens very little
- "Kissing lesion" of the bone on the other side of the joint from the chip fracture, often not seen on radiographs, but are seen with arthroscopy

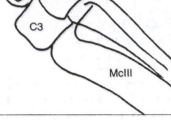

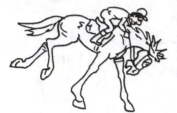

Cr. Radial carpal
Ci. Intermediate carpal bone
Cu. Ulnar carpal bone
Ca. Accessory carpal bone
C1. 1st carpal bone
C2. 2nd carpal bone
C3. 3rd carpal bone
C4. 4th carpal bone
R. Radius
McIII. 3rd metacarpal bone
McII. 2nd metacarpal bone
McIV. 4th metacarpal bone

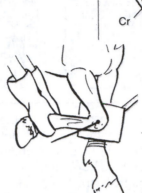

Clinical problems highlighted:
- Chip fxs
- Differentiating chip fx on radial carpal from intermediate carpal bone
- Kissing lesions possibly seen

Anatomy: pgs. 82, 112

Skyline or tangential view
- Dorsoproximal-dorsodistal views of which there may be at least three
- Carpus flexed maximally & beam directed across the dorsal surface of the distal radius, proximal row & distal row of carpal bones
- Skyline views & how to recognize them
   1. Distal radial skyline
      - Dorsal side of radius silhouetted - 1 line
   2. Proximal carpal skyline
      - Dorsal edge of 3 bones seen - radial, intermediate & ulnar carpal bones
   3. Distal carpal skyline
      - Dorsal edge of the long 3rd carpal bone silhouetted in the middle
- To interpret skyline views the exact angle used when taking the film must be known.

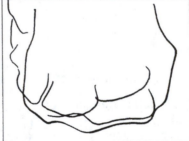

Distal radial skyline

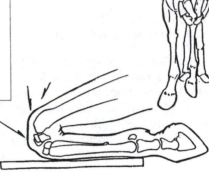

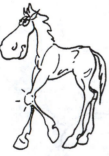

Cr. Radial carpal
Ci. Intermediate carpal bone
Cu. Ulnar carpal bone
Ca. Accessory carpal bone
C1. 1st carpal bone
C2. 2nd carpal bone
C3. 3rd carpal bone
C4. 4th carpal bone
R. Radius
McIII. 3rd metacarpal bone
McII. 2nd metacarpal bone
McIV. 4th metacarpal bone

Clinical problems highlighted
- Very small chip fractures
- Slab fractures

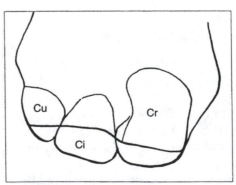

Proximal carpal skyline

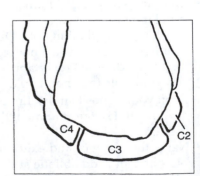

Distal carpal skyline

Radiographs - Tarsus

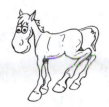

Tarsus

To understand radiographs of the tarsus 1st understand its anatomy. To get a handle on this complicated joint draw a schematic DPI view. Label the bones & the joint spaces.
- **Calcaneus**: lateral
- **Talus**: medial
- **4th tarsal bone**: 2 story bone on lateral side
- **Central tarsal bone**: medial side
- **Distal intertarsal joint** doesn't span the tarsus because of the 4th tarsal bone

- **Tarsal series**
  - 4 standard views: DP, Lat., DMO, DLO
    . Usually the Lat., DP & DMO are minimum views because bone spavin seen on DM (dorsomedial) aspect of tarsus
  - Supplemental views: Flexed lat., Plantar skyline
- **Procedure for 4 standard views:**
  - Bearing weight
  - Positioning: shot through dist. intertarsal & tarsometatarsal joints
    . Difficult to not get rotation while shooting so joints will be represented by multiple lines. Don't shoot too high!

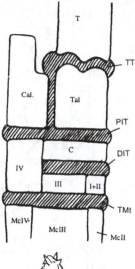

"Eyeball" naming Tarsal views

- **Calcaneus**: like the accessory carpal bone of the carpus is located on the lateral & "posterior" (plantar) side of the joint. It is your key to figuring out the radiographic view by its configuration & the amount it overlaps the other tarsal bones in each view.

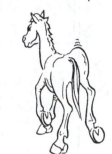

Lateral, LM (lateromedial) view:

- The beam passes from lat. to med. - 90° to 270°
- Landmarks for naming view
  - Calcaneus as large as possible & slightly overlapped
  - Sustentaculum seen as a distinct line
  - Front of the 3rd tarsal bone is flat
  - Confusing: Mt IV larger & more plantar than Mt II (not superimposed so view appears like an oblique, check sustentaculum tali)
- **Silhouettes**: dorsal & plantar sides of the tarsus

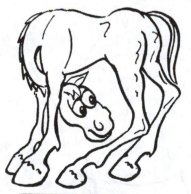

Clinical uses:
- Bone spavin
- Slab fxs of 3rd & central
- Calcanean fxs
- Fractures

C. Calcaneus: lateral
S. Sustentaculum tali
T. Talus: medial
Cen. Central
T1+2. Fused first & second tarsal bone
T3. 3rd tarsal bone
T4. 4th tarsal bone
TTj. Tarsocrural joint
PITj. Proximal intertarsal joint
DITj. Distal intertarsal joint
TMtj. Tarsal metatarsal joint
MtIII. Metatarsal III
MtII. Metatarsal II
Mt IV. Metatarsal IV

DP (Dorsoplantar) view:

- Shot 90° off the lateral view, from 0° to 180°
- Silhouettes the medial & lateral surfaces of the tarsus
- Landmarks for naming
  - Calcaneus completely overlapped by the rest of the hock
  - Ridges of the talus are as far apart as possible

Clinical uses
- DJD
  - Width of intertarsal joints

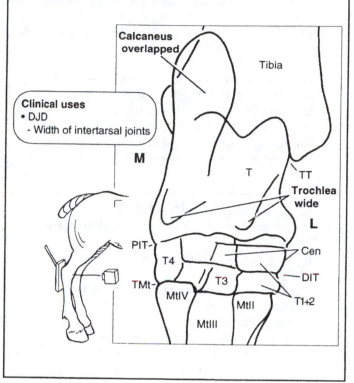

Anatomy: pgs. 123, 126, 100

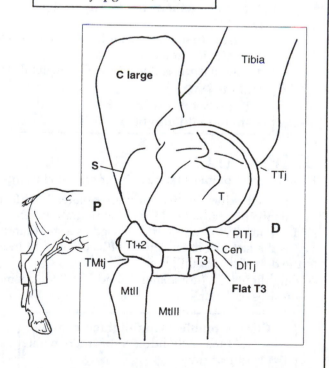

OBLIQUE VIEWS - TARSUS

DLPMO (MO)

(Dorsolateral-plantaromedial oblique)(medial oblique [dMO]).

- Enters the dorsolateral (or plantaromedial) surface and exits the plantaromedial (or dorsolateral) surface.
- MO (Medial oblique / dMO): used as a shorthand in some clinics (note it is the last two letters of the official name), it indicates the **dorsal** side is highlighted.
- Highlights the DM (dorsomedial) and PL (plantarolateral) surfaces of the tarsus.

> **Clinical problem highlighted in MO:**
> - Bone spavin (dorsomedial surface).
> - OC (osteochondrosis) on medial trochlear ridge.
> - Slab fractures of third and central tarsal bones.

Pinky naming obliques

- **Clue: calcaneus and flexed pinky: plantar and lateral.**
- Check radiograph: film not a DP or lateral, so oblique.
- Check calcaneus: completely seen (highlighted) or not (overlapped).
- Flex your little finger.
- Point opposite index finger at dorsal side of hand, look down it so the amount of the pinky seen is like the amount of the calcaneus seen in the film.
- Name the entrance and exit point of your pointing finger through your hand and add oblique at the end.

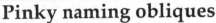

> **Alternate methods to identify obliques:**
> **DMPLO/LO**
> - **Fused first and second tarsal bones seen (medioplantar side).**
> - Lateral trochlear notch (on dorsolateral side).
>
> **DLPMO/MO:**
> - **Tarsal canal is seen.**
> - **4th tarsal highlighted**

DMPLO (LO)

(Dorsomedial-palmarolateral oblique)(lateral oblique dMO)

- Enters the dorsomedial (or plantarolateral) surface and exits the plantarolateral (or dorsomedial) surface.
- LO (lateral oblique)(or dLO): used as a shorthand (note it is the last two letters of the official name), it indicates the dorsal side highlighted.
- Highlights DL (dorsolateral) and PM (plantaromedial) surfaces of the tarsus.

> **Clinical problems highlighted in MO:**
> - OCD (osteochondrosis) of intermediate trochlear ridge.
> - OC of lateral trochlear ridge.

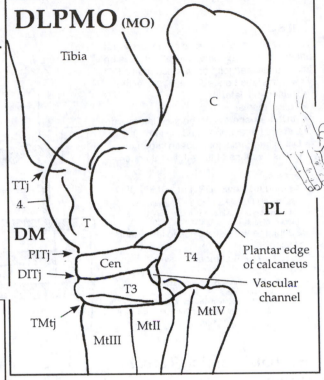

DLPMO (MO)

Tibia

C

TTj

4.

T

DM

PL

PITj →

Cen

T4

Plantar edge of calcaneus

DITj →

T3

Vascular channel

TMtj

MtIV

MtII

MtIII

C. Calcaneus: lateral.
S. Sustentaculum tali
T. Talus: medial.
Cen. Central tarsal bone.
T1+2. Fused first and second tarsal bones.
T3. 3rd tarsal bone.
T4. 4th tarsal bone.
TTj. Tarsocrural joint.
PITj. Proximal intertarsal joint.

DITj. Distal intertarsal joint.
MtII. Second metatarsal bone (medial splint).
MtIII. Third metatarsal (cannon).
MtIV. Fourth metatarsal bone (lateral splint).
1. Intermediate ridge
2. Lateral trochlear ridge
4. Medial trochlear ridge

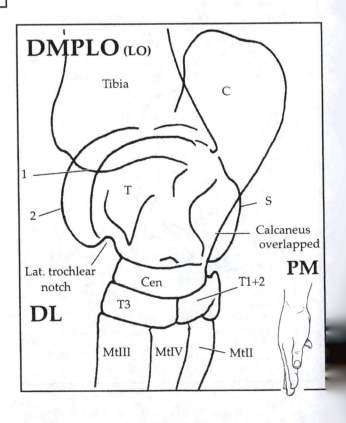

DMPLO (LO)

Tibia

C

1

T

2

S

Lat. trochlear notch

Cen

T1+2

PM

DL

T3

Calcaneus overlapped

MtIII

MtIV

MtII

636

Skyline - Flexed Lat. - Tarsus

Skyline, Flexed DP (dorsoplantar) view
(plantaroproximal-plantarodistal view)
- Procedure:
  - Flex tarsus as far behind the horse as possible (tranquilization often necessary)
  - Hold cassette parallel to plantar aspect of hock
  - Beam perpendicular to cassette

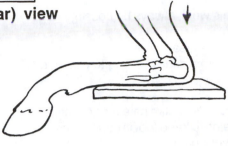

> **Clinical problems**
> - Evaluate calcaneus & sustentaculum tali

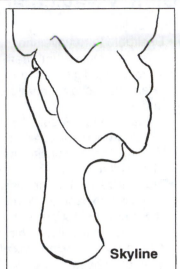

Skyline

Flexed lateral view
- Procedure:
  - Flex limb to 90°
  - Hold limb close to body to avoid rotation) avoid
  - Center beam through talus

Anatomy: pgs. 123, 126, 100

> **Clinical - areas silhouetted**
> - Proximal aspect of trochlear ridges of talus
> - Plantar aspect of tibia
> - Coracoid process of calcaneus

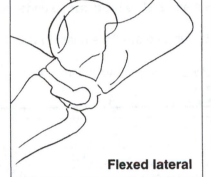

Flexed lateral

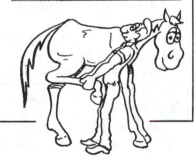

Clinical check list - Tarsus

- **Bone spavin - DJD #1** - poor correlation between radiographs & lameness 50% have radiographic signs & no lameness & 50% lame w/ no radiographic signs (occult spavin)
  - Dorsomedial surface of distal intertarsal & tarsometatarsal joints for bone spavin
  - No radiographic changes early - occult spavin or cunean bursitis
  - Cyst formation early (subchondral bone lysis)
  - Narrowing or loss of joint space, usually accompanied by subchondral sclerosis of involved bones
  - Check edges of 3rd, central & cannon bones
    . Fuzzy edges
    . Osteophytes (periarticular spurs)
  - Obliteration of tarsal canal w/ bone
  - Complete ankylosis of joints (eliminates pain, thus lameness)
- **Osteochondrosis** (DLO) (some OCD findings of little clinical significance)
  - Fragment of intermediate ridge of distal tibia - #1 (DLO)
  - Lat. trochlear ridge (DLO)
    . Irregularities
    . Radiolucent subchondral bone
  - Fragment or irregularities of dist. med. trochlear ridge (DMO)
  - Fragment of medial malleolus (DMO)
  - Fragments of lat. malleolus (less frequent than med.) (DLO)
  - Associated distention of tibiotarsal joint ("Bog spavin")
- **Slab fxs of 3rd & central tarsal bones**
- **Calcanean fxs (Skyline)**
- **Sustentaculum fxs (Skyline)**
- **Tarsal valgus (DP)**
  - Lines drawn down tibia & Mc3 cross each other
- **Incomplete ossification of tarsal bones (very young)**
  - Small tarsal bones, rounder than normal

- Compression of 3rd &/or central tarsal
  . Wedge shaped w/ or w/o fragment separation
- Luxation of tarsal joints (stressed radiographs)
- Sprains - capsule & ligaments
  - Extensive periosteal proliferation at attachment sites
  - Avulsion of lat. or med. malleolus
- Septic arthritis/epiphysitis - joint ill
  - Radiolucent lesions of tibial malleoli
  - Radiolucent lesions of metaphyseal region
  - Soft tissue swelling
  - Irregular widening of dist. tibial physis
  - Periosteal new bone growth
  - ± Subchondral bone cysts (lysis)
- General checks
  - "Joint space" width
    . Increases - lysis (septic arthritis)
    . Decreases (DJD)
  - Marginal joint changes
    . Osteophyte formation (DJD - advanced)
    . Lysis (septic arthritis)
  - Subchondral bone
    . Sclerosis (DJD)
    . Lysis (septic arthritis or OC)
  - Periarticular calcification (usually from steroid injection)

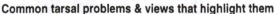

Common tarsal problems & views that highlight them
Problem	Views
Bone spavin - DJD #1	DMO, L
Osteochondrosis	
- Intermediate ridge	**DLO**
- Lateral trochlear ridge	**DLO**
- Medial trochlear ridge	**DMO**
Slab fxs of 3rd & central tarsals	DMO, L
Calcanean fxs	Skyline, L, DMO, DLO
Sustentaculum tali	Skyline
Fractures	All

COMMENTS on anatomy of tarsus
- In foals 1st & 2nd tarsal may be unfused, also in some adults
- Physis of calcaneus closes at 16-24 months
- Physis of lat. malleolus closes at 3 months
- Prox. physis of McIII closed at birth
- Apparent joint space larger in foals due to more cartilage
- Synovial fossa: normal irregular depression in intertrochlear groove of talus in adults (DMO view)
- Lat. trochlear ridge has a long notch on its dist. end (DLO)

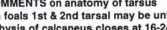

Digit & Navicular Films

Procedure:
- Desirable to remove shoes. This won't always be possible (e.g., horse is jumping that afternoon).
- #1 for good digit films: trim, pare & clean hoof
  - Remove rocks & gravel from commissures & frog to eliminate artifacts
  - Clean the foot & sole
  - Pack ground surface w/ PlayDoh® to eliminate air artifacts
- Holding up the opposite limb helps to keep foot in correct position
  - This will not be possible if severe pain
- Tranquilization m/b necessary
- All views, except the flexed fetlock, are shot in weight-bearing
  - **DP view**: do not place the foot directly on the cassette
    - Mount 2 sides of a 1" thick piece of plexiglass on 2 wood blocks
    - Stand horse on the plexiglass stand & slide the cassette under the plexiglass
  - **Lateral view**: elevate foot off the ground so all the phalanges & the hoof are included
    - Placing foot on a 2 by 6 block of wood w/ a groove that holds the cassette works nicely

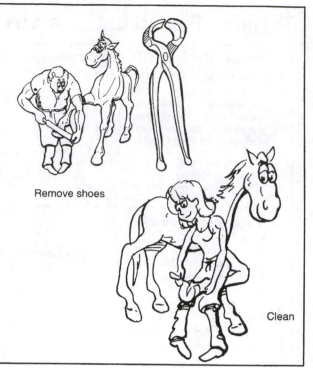

Remove shoes

Clean

45° DP

- Dorsopalmar/dorsoplantar view, Dorsoproximal-palmarodistal oblique view (D45Pr-PaDiO)
- Procedure:
  - Wooden block w/ a 45° angled slot used
  - Center beam 1" above coronet on midline, perpendicular to cassette
  - Anatomy seen
    - Phalangeal joint spaces
    - Navicular bone (dist. sesamoid) & its extremities
- To check if a fracture or cyst is in the navicular bone take a 65° DP view
  - Fracture line or cyst will move with bone

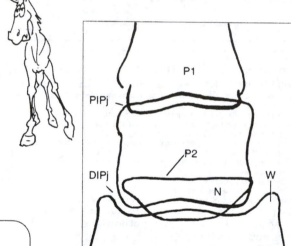

P1. Proximal phalanx
P2. Middle phalanx
P3. Distal phalanx
E. Extensor process of P3
W. Wings (palmar processes of P3)
N. Navicular bone
PIPj. Prox. interphalangeal joint
DIPj. Dist. interphalangeal joint

Clinical check list - 45° DP
- **Indications of navicular diz**
  - Synovial fossae - normally 1-7 along dist. border, should be pointed proximally in shape
    - Increased number & widening ("lollipops", "mushrooms")
  - "Spurs" on wings of navicular commonly (often normal w/ older horses)
  - Cysts in navicular bone
  - Generalized decrease in flexor bone compact capacity
  - "Shuttle shape" (change in contour of bone)
  - Significant percentage of horses with or without radiographic navicular signs may or may not have clinical navicular diz
    - Therefore positive radiographic signs only help to substantiate diagnosis
- Navicular fractures
- Low ringbone

Anatomy: pgs. 88, 114, 116

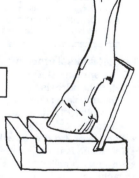

65° DP - Digit/Navicular

65° DP (Dorsopalmar/dorsoplantar)
(Dorsoproximalpalmarodistal oblique view (D65Pr-PaDiO)

- **Procedure:**
  - Position foot on protected cassette, or in angled block
  - Center beam on midline perpendicular to hoof wall (assess from side)
    - . P3 films: center on coronet
    - . Navicular film - center 1/2" above coronet
    - . 65° angle to ground
- **Technique:**
  - P3 film: use less technique bec. hoof & P3 are not dense
  - Navicular film: slightly increased technique for articular portion of P3 or navicular bone (grid will improve film)

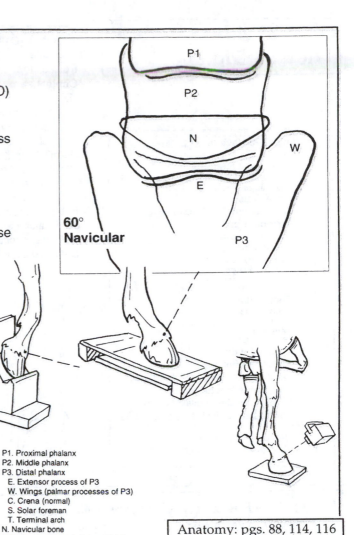

60° Navicular

P1. Proximal phalanx
P2. Middle phalanx
P3. Distal phalanx
 E. Extensor process of P3
 W. Wings (palmar processes of P3)
 C. Crena (normal)
 S. Solar foreman
 T. Terminal arch
N. Navicular bone
PIPj. Proximal interphalangeal joint
DIPj. Distal interphalangeal joint

Anatomy: pgs. 88, 114, 116

Navicular - Clinical same as in 45° DP
- **Indications of navicular diz**
  - Synovial fossae - normally 1-7 along dist. border, should be pointed proximally in shape
    - . Increased number & widening ("lollipops", "mush rooms") - abnormal
  - "Spurs" on wings of navicular commonly (often normal w/ older horses)
  - Cysts in navicular bone
  - Generalized decrease in flexor compact opacity
  - "Shuttle shape" (change in contour of bone)
  - Significant percentage of navicular horses will have no radiographic signs & percentage of sound horse will have radiographic signs
    - . Positive radiographic signs only help to substantiate diagnosis
- Navicular fractures
- Low ringbone

65° DP - Clinical check list - pedal bone
- **Pedal bone, coffin, P3**
  - **Pedal osteitis** (bone resorption [lysis] around the edges of P3)
    - . Vascular channels: all should normally be symmetrical; enlargement may indicate problem
  - Bone cysts
  - Penetrating wounds, abscesses - pedal bone lysis
  - Keratoma (hoof wall tumor) - circular erosion of pedal bone
  - Fragment proximal to extensor process - m/ or m/ not be significant
- Ossification of lateral cartilages (usually incidental finding)

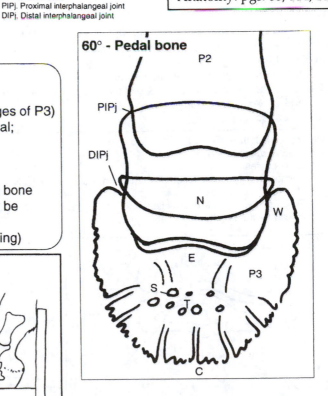

60° - Pedal bone

P3 - DP - Parallel ground
- Supplemental view
- Beam parallel to ground

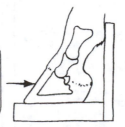

Clinical use:
- Evaluate conformation & relationship of coffin joint to ground
- Eliminate confusing frog sulcus air shadows when evaluating fractures

Lat. - Skyline - Oblique Views - Digit

Lateral View (LateroMedial) - Digit

Anatomy: pgs. 88, 114, 116

- Procedure:
  - Position foot on a wooden block to include whole foot
  - Center beam
    - Digit film: beam parallel to ground through midcoronet
      - Check film for superimposition of wings for proper placement
    - Navicular: parallel to ground slightly below coronary band towards palmar side of foot
    - Laminitis: put a metal strip or paint a stripe of barium sulfate on dorsal surface (toe) of hoof to make it easier to see rotation of P3
- Anatomy seen
  - Normally dors. wall of hoof should line up with dorsal surface of P3
  - Extensor process (may have a fragment which could be a normal 2° ossification center [round, smooth], or an avulsion fracture)
  - Palmar processes
  - Navicular bone

Clinical P3/Navicular - Lateral

- **P3**
  - **Rotational laminitis**
    - Alignment of dorsal P3 to dorsal hoof
    - Gas between P3 & dors. hoof wall
  - Bone cysts
  - **Chip & avulsion fractures (extensor process)**
  - **Articular lesions**
  - Low ring bone (coffin) DJD
    - Narrowed "joint space"
    - Marginal osteophytes
    - Subchondral bone sclerosis
    - Subchondral bone cysts (lysis)
  - Septic arthritis
    - Periarticular swelling
    - Joint capsule distention
    - Marginal bone lysis
    - Subchondral bone lysis
  - **Pyramidal disease**
  - **Pedal osteitis**
  - **Radiolucent nail lines** (shod horses)
  - **Sidebones/fractures**
  - **Foreign bodies** (nails & wires)
  - **Contrast medium into gravel tracts**
- **Navicular bone** - flexor surface
  - Cartilage erosion in later stages of navicular diz

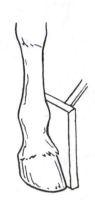

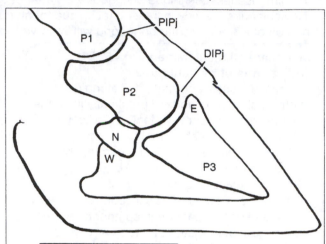

```
P1. Proximal phalanx
P2. Middle phalanx
P3. Distal phalanx
  E. Extensor process of P3
  W. Wings (palmar processes of P3)
N. Navicular bone
PIPj. Prox. interphalangeal joint
DIPj. Dist. interphalangeal joint
```

Navicular - Flexor (Skyline) view (Palmaroproximal-palmaro-distal oblique/Plantaroproximal - plantarodistal oblique)

- Procedure
  - Position foot on protected cassette with foot as far caudally as possible
  - Center beam between bulbs of heel, parallel to palmar/plantar aspect of digit (45-50° angle to ground)
- Navicular bone seen w/ minimal overlap
  - Flexor surface w/ sagittal ridge & distinct margin between medullary cavity & cortex seen clearly
- Palmar aspect of P3

Clinical check list:
- **Navicular disease signs**
  - Osteophytes
  - Palmar (flexor) cortex: loose differentiation of cortex & medullary cavity
  - Medullary cavity: sclerotic & lucent areas - cystic areas
  - Flexor surface lysis & destruction of sagittal ridge
- Navicular fractures (check if on 45° & 65° DP)

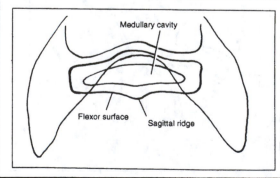

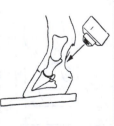

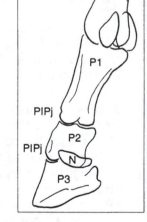

DLO/DMO (Dorsolateral/medial obliques), DMPLO/DLPMO

- Procedure:
  - Position foot on protected cassette, slightly to side of cassette (machine side)
- Beam center
  - Centered below coronary band
  - Through dorsomed./lat. hoof, 45° off midsagittal plane
  - 65° to the ground

Clinical area highlighted:
- Silhouettes wings of navicular bone

Pastern - Fetlock

Pastern studies

- Commonly done to evaluate acute or chronic trauma or joint disease
- Survey films often obtained in radiographic evaluation of fetlock or foot
- Procedure for specific pastern study: DP, Lat., DMO & DLO
  - Center beam midway between coronet & fetlock
  - Cassette held in contact w/ digit & rests on the floor
  - Beam: 30-45° angle to ground
    . DP m/b obtained with beam either parallel to ground or perpendicular to dorsal surface of pastern
  - Oblique views (DMO or DLO) shot at 35° off midline & 30-45° to ground

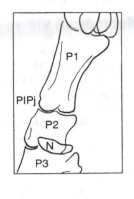

DP

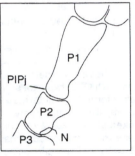

P1
PIPj
P2
N
P3

Oblique

Clinical check list - Pastern

- **Chip fxs** (distal P1 or prox. P2) best visualized in DMO & DLO
- **High ring bone** (DJD) (DP best) - advanced DJD
  - Articular high ringbone (Narrowed "joint space", Marginal osteophytes, Subchondral bone sclerosis, Subchondral bone cysts
  - Periarticular high ringbone - osteophytes but no joint involvement - mild DJD
- **Fracture lines** (DP, Lat., DMO & DLO)
- **Periosteal new bone** (DP, Lat., DMO & DLO)
- **Septic osteoarthritis** (DP, Lat., DMO & DLO), Periarticular swelling, Joint capsule distention, Marginal bone lysis, Subchondral bone lysis
- **OCD** (osteochondritis dissecans)
- **Distal sesamoidean ligament damage**
  - Usually middle (oblique) sesamoidean lig
  - Calcification where tears from palmar aspect of P1

P1. Proximal phalanx
P2. Middle phalanx
P3. Distal phalanx
N. Navicular bone
PIPj. Prox. interphalangeal joint

Anatomy: pgs. 88, 114, 116

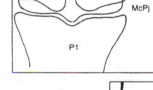

P1
PIPj
P2
P3
N

Fetlock studies

Anatomy: pgs. 88, 114, 116

- Fetlock series: DP, Lat., 35° DMO & DLO
  - Beam 20-25°° to ground & through the fetlock, except for lateral view (beam parrallel to ground)
- Supplemental views
  - Flexed lat.: separates prox. sesamoids from rest
- **125° DP - Distal cannon skyline** - supplemental view
  - Shot w/ foot on ground as far forward as possible
  - Beam almost parallel to ground
  - Silhouettes the condyles of distal cannon
    . Best for OC (osteochondritis), "gullwing arthrosis"
- Angle beam across abaxial surface of sesamoids to try to shoot through fracture line
- **Sagittal ridge of cannon bone**: divides head into a larger med. part & a smaller lat. part, see in DP view

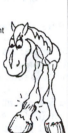

McIII
S
E
P1
P2

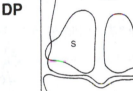

DP

McIII
S
McPj
P1

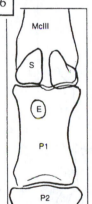

P1. Proximal phalanx
P2. Middle phalanx
McIII. Metacarpal III
S. Proximal sesamoid
E. Ergot
McPj. Metacarpophalangeal joint

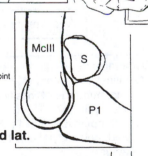

McIII
S
P1

Flexed lat.

Clinical check list - Fetlock:

- **Fractures of proximal sesamoids**
  - DP view: apical, mid-body & basilar fxs
  - Obliques: abaxial fxs involving articular surface
- **Sesamoiditis**
  - Lucent areas on abaxial border
- **Distal cannon fxs** - DP & obliques
- **Fxs of palmar eminences of P1**
- **Chip fxs** of P1 (DMO, DLO)
- **Osselets** (DJD) all views
  - Width of joint
  - Subchondral sclerosis
  - Remodelling of dist. articular surface of cannon
- **Septic arthritis**: Periarticular swelling, Joint capsule distention, Marginal bone lysis, Subchondral bone lysis
- **Capsulitis** - all views: Soft tissue shadows (joint capsule thickening & joint effusion)
- **Villonodular hypertrophic synovitis**: irregular periosteal new bone production on dorsomed. aspect of dist. cannon, Patchy reduction in opacity of underlying bone

- **OCD** (osteochondrosis)- Flattening of subchondral bone, Localized subchondral bone lysis, Subchondral bone fragments, 2° DJD m/b present
  - Sagittal ridge of Mc3
  - Palmar condyle of Mc3
- **Bone cysts**: close to articular surface & m/ communicate w/ joint, P1, sesamoids & dist. cannon
- **Physitis**: widened, irregular thickness to physis, lipping, angular limb deformity
- **Angular deformity** (usually varus [medial]) Dist. articular surface of cannon not perpendicular to long axis, Widening of metaphysis, Cortical thickening & wedging of epiphysis, Compensatory wedging of prox. epiphysis of P1
- **Calcification in suspensory lig.**
- **Distal sesamoidean lig. damage**
  - Calcification where tears from palmar aspect of P1
  - Complete disruption - prox. sesamoids displaced proximally

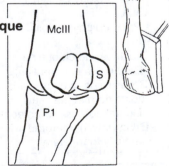

Oblique

McIII
S
P1

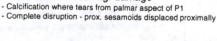

Metacarpus - Elbow

Metacarpal views

- Metacarpal series DP, Lat., DMO, DLO
  - Shot in weight bearing
  - Use long cassette to get whole metacarpus or number of films & jigsaw together
- Supplemental view:
  - DPr-PDiO (Dorsoproximal-palmarodistal oblique) shot 10° proximodistally to separate the sesamoid bones from the distal end of the cannon for incomplete condylar fxs

ID oblique

- DLO: 2nd carpal bone completely on top of McII (palmaromed. so dorsolat. opposite side silhouetted
  - Looks into interosseous space betw. McII & McIII, site of medial "splints", different than other situations because lesion not on the edge, but inside the radiographic edge
- DMO: 4th silhouetted on palmarolat side so opposite side dorsomed.
  - Bucked shin view because silhouettes dorsomed. surface

> **Clinical check list - metacarpus/metatarsus:**
> - **Splints** (DLO) betw. med. splint & cannon
>   - Callus formation **obliterates interosseous space**
> - **Osteomyelitis** (multiple views)
> - **Bucked shins** (stress fxs of dorsomed. cannon) (Lat., DMO)
> - **Stress fractures**: dorsolat. cannon (DLO, Lat.)
> - Dist. condylar fxs of cannon bone that spiral proximally

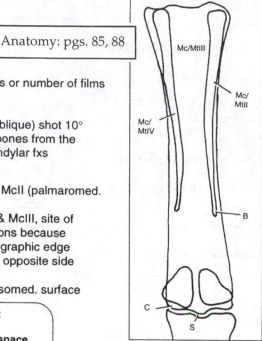

Anatomy: pgs. 85, 88

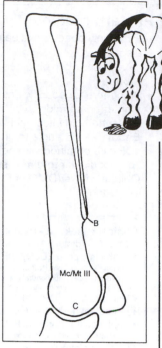

Dorsopalmar/ plantar view

McII. Metacarpal/metatarsal II
McIII. Mertacarpal/metatarsal III
McIV. Metacarpal/metatarsal IV
B. Button of splint
C. Condlyle
S. Sagittal ridge

Lat. view

Anatomy: pgs. 85, 89

Elbow films

- Procedure:
  - Horse standing, portable machine, grid not essential
- **Views:**
  - **Lateral** (pull limb foreward)
  - Craniocaudal
  - Obliques
    - CrLO (craniomedial-caudolat. oblique) easier to obtain than CrMO

Anatomy: pgs. 111, 78, 80

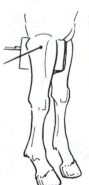

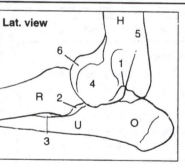

Lat. view

Craniocaud. view

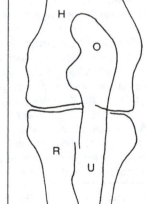

H. Humerus
R. Radius
U. Ulnar
O. Olecranon process
1. Anconeal process
2. Coronoid processes
3. Interosseous space
4. Epicondyles
5. Epicondylar crest
6. Condylar processes of femur
6. Radial tuberosity

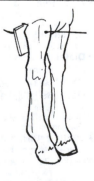

Comments

- Ossification centers
  - Distal humerus - 3 ossification centers
    - Diaphysis
    - Dist. epiphysis: join 11-24 mo
    - Med. epicondyle: join 11-24 mo
  - Radius
    - Prox. epiphysis: join 11-24 mo
  - Ulna
    - Prox. epiphysis: join 24-36 mo
- Adult
  - Trochlear notch of ulna
    - Dist. notch is nonarticular
  - Several lips to cran. margin of articular radius normal (lat. view)
    - Do not confuse w/ osteophytes
  - CrCa view: humeroradial joint space wider medially than laterally

> **Clinical check list - elbow:** (infrequent)
> - Demonstrate a fracture w/ displaced fragments
> - Fractures of olecranon
>   - Single or comminuted
>   - Access fx through trochlear notch if articular or nonarticular dist. trochlea
> - Salter Harris Type I fxs (physeal) of olecranon
>   - Compare to other limb
> - Infection - young foals
>   - Osteomyelitis & sequestrum in adults
>   - Contrast medium into puncture wound to see if communication w/ joint
> - 2° DJD (osteophytes - don't confuse normal "lips" w/ osteophytes)
> - Osteochondrosis (rare) med. condyle of humerus & med. prox radius, ununited anconeal process reported in 1 horse (young horse m/b secondary ossification center)
>   - Cyst - med. prox. radius
> - Ligament strains/tears: periosteal proliferation at insertions of biceps brachii m. & collateral ligaments

Shoulder - Stifle

Shoulder

- **Procedure:**
  - High output machine required, grid recommended
  - General anesthesia in lat. recumbency better than standing
- **Views:**
  - Lateral view
  - CrLO view (craniomed.-caudolat. oblique) best in standing horse

Comments

- Shoulder joint - young horse - ossification centers
  - Scapula - 4 ossification centers
    - . Scapular cartilage (not seen in shoulder films)
    - . Body of scapula
    - . Supraglenoid tubercle (fuses betw. 12-24 months)
    - . Cran. part of glenoid cavity (fuses by 5 months)
  - Prox. humerus - 3 ossification centers (close 24-36 months)
    - . Body
    - . Humeral head
    - . Greater tubercle

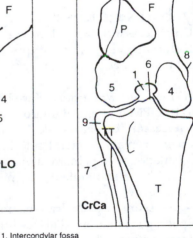

S. Scapula
H. Humerus
1. Supraglenoid tuberosity
2. Coracoid process
3. Neck
4. Glenoid cavity
5. Head
6. Greater tubercle
 6'. Cranial eminence
 6". Intermediate
7. Lesser tubercle

Lat.

CrLO

Anatomy: pgs. 110, 76, 78

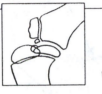

Clinical check list - Shoulder

- **Osteochondritis dissecans**
  - Humerus
    - . Flattening of caud. head
    - . Radiolucent areas surrounded by sclerosis in subchondral bone
    - . Discrete circular radiolucent areas
  - Sclerosis of subchondral bone - head &/or glenoid cavity
  - Glenoid cavity
    - . Irregularities in contour
    - . Decr. concavity - fuzzy
    - . Radiolucent areas in subchondral bone surrounded by sclerosis
  - Contrast arthrography for dissecting cartilage flaps
- **Subchondral bone cysts of scapula**
  - Distinct, large radiolucent areas in scapula
  - Single or multiple
  - Usually sclerotic rim
  - Initially close to articulation them move proximally
- Small radiolucent areas m/ or m/not cause lameness
- **DJD** Rare
  - Narrowed "joint space", marginal osteophytes, subchondral bone sclerosis, subchondral bone cysts
- **Septic arthritis**, most common in foal, subchondral radiolucent areas w/ or w/o sclerosis, new bone formation, involves dist. scapula, humeral epiphysis or prox. humeral physis, widening of joint space (excess synovial fluid)
- **Fractures**
  - **Supraglenoid tubercle**, cran. displacement: non-union fx, M/b calcification of bicipital tendon
  - **Fxs of body of scapula**, Horizontal & vertical fxs, Re-shot in 10-14 days if suspect & can't find
- **Calcification of bicipital tendon**, Sequela to supraglenoid tubercle fxs or DJD
- **Luxation of shoulder joint:** prox. & cran. displacement m/b or prox. & caudally, Oblique view tells if displacement also med. or lat.

Stifle

- **Views:**
  - CrLO - Craniolateral oblique (Plantarolateral (45°)-craniomedial oblique): easier to obtain than a true lateral
  - Skyline (cranioprox.-craniodist oblique): for patella & trochlear ridge studies
  - Lateral: difficult to obtain true lateral
  - Cr/Ca - Craniocaudal (Caudocranial): shot from caudally

Anatomy: pgs. 120, 122

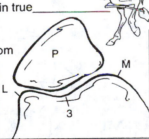

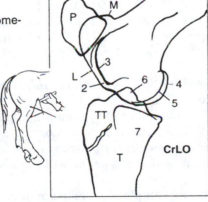

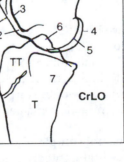

CrLO

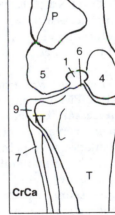

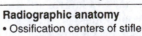

CrCa

Clinical check list - Stifle:

- **OCD**
  - **Lat. trochlea of femur (#1 site)**
    - . Marked irregularity of articular outline
    - . Radiolucencies & local sclerosis
    - . Flattening of ridge
    - . Joint mouse still attached or floating free
  - Med. trochlea
  - Articular apex of patella
  - Check other joints if OC findings in stifle
  - Subchondral bone cysts
    - . Medial condyle of femur
    - . Prox. tibia beneath Intercondylar spines
- **Patellar fxs**, ridge fxs
- **Roughening of patella & med. trochlear ridge**
- **DJD** (less common than in distal joints)
  - Periarticular osteophytes
  - Narrowing of joint space
  - Flattening of articular surfaces
- Sclerosis/lucencies of subchondral bone
- **Joint ill** (suppurative arthritis in foals) takes time to see changes
  - Radiolucent sequestration
  - Collapse & fragmentation of weakened bone
- **Collateral lig. damage:** new bone at attachments, stress radiographs
- **Meniscal damage**
  - Narrowing of joint space (med. usually) - need standing study
  - Med. lig. damage - marginal lipping of femorotibial joint
- **Cruciate damage**
  - Bony fragments in intercondyloid fossa
  - Periosteal new bone at cran. insertion (tibia)
  - 2° DJD
- **Middle patellar ligament injury**
  - Thickening & radiopacity to ligament
  - Periosteal reaction of attachment to patella
- **Calcinosis circumscripta** - rare
  - Large circumscribed radiodense mass close to but not involving the stifle

F. Femur
T. Tibia
P. Patella
M. Med. trochlea
L. Lat. troclea
TT. Tibial tuberosity

1. Intercondylar fossa
2. Extensor fossa
3. Intertrochlear groove
4. Med. femoral condyle
5. Lat. femoral condyle
6. Intercondylar eminence
7. Fibula
8. Med. epicondyle
9. Extensor groove

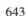

Radiographic anatomy

- **Ossification centers of stifle**
  - Dist. physis of femur (closes 24-30 months)
  - Prox. physis of tibia (closes 24-30 months)
  - Apophysis of tibial tuberosity (closes 30-36 months)
  - Patella
- **Med. & lat. trochlear ridges are same size at birth**
- **Fibula:** shows ossification at 1-2 months
  - Ossification often incomplete, don't confuse w/ fractures
- **Fabellae** occasionally occur prox. to caudal part of femoral condyles

NAMING OBLIQUES

Pinky naming oblique: figuring out the oblique view in radiographs without using a pen and paper.

- **Clue: accessory carpal bone is located palmar and lateral** like your **flexed little finger.**
- Check radiograph: decide if the film is NOT a DP or lateral film, and thus, is an oblique. Look at enough lateral and DP views (40 or 50) so that you can identify them readily.
  - Straight lateral (LM): the accessory carpal bone is as large as possible.
  - DP (dorsal palmar view): the accessory carpal bone is completely overlapped and as small as possible. Any view showing the accessory carpal bone in between these sizes is an oblique view.
  - . Accessory carpal bone: check if this landmark is completely highlighted or overlapped.
- **Flex your little finger** and hold that hand down.
  - . **Opposite hand's index finger**: represents the primary beam.
  - . Point your index finger on either the medial or lateral side of your dorsal hand, looking down the finger to match the amount of the pinky seen with the accessory carpal bone in the film, either highlighted or overlapped.
  - . Name view by saying the point you are touching on you hand, either as:
    - .. **Dorsomedial** (if pinky and accessory carpal bone overlapped), or
    - .. **Dorsolateral** (if pinky and accessory carpal bone are highlighted).
  - . Then, add the next part of its name by saying where the beam would exit your hand if it continued through it, either:
    - .. **DMPalmaroLateral**, or
    - .. **DLPalmaroMedial**
  - . Add O for oblique at the end to finish naming it
    - .. DMPL **Oblique (DMPLO)**, or
    - .. DLPM **Oblique (DLPMO)**.

Eyeball surfaces highlighted in obliques.

- **Clue: accessory carpal bone/calcaneus** located **palmar** and **lateral.**
- **Determine view is an oblique,** any that is **NOT** a DP or **Lateral.**
- **ID the Palmar surface** easily by the accessory carpal bone/calcaneus located on the palmar side.
- **ID the palmar/plantar surface highlighted: PL (palmaro/plantarolateral) or PM (palmar/plantaromedial).**
  - **Accessory carpal bone/calcaneus completely seen (highlighted)** = palmar/plantarolateral side highlighted: the accessory carpal's articulation with palmarolateral side of the carpus can be seen and the bone has a knob line on it. The whole plantar side of the calcaneus can be seen.
  - **Accessory carpal/calcaneus not completely seen (superimposed)** = palmar/plantaromedial side highlighted: the accessory carpal bones' articulation/whole calcaneus' plantar side can't be seen as they are almost completely overlapped.
- **ID opposite dorsal surface: DM or DL,** dorsomedial is opposite palmar/plantarolateral, dorsolateral is opposite palmar/plantaromedial. Knowing the surface highlighted allows you to identify structures on these sides(e.g., medial and lateral splints, medial and lateral trochlea, radial and ulnar carpal bones).

Dorsal surface highlighted can be used as an alternate method to name the oblique views.

- Add oblique to the dorsal surface highlighted.
  MO (dMO): dorsomedial surface highlighted (accessory carpal seen)
  LO (dLO): dorsolateral surface (accessory not seen completely seen).
- Add missing letters starting with D to come up with official name:
  DLPMO = MO + DLP
  DMPLO = LO + DMP

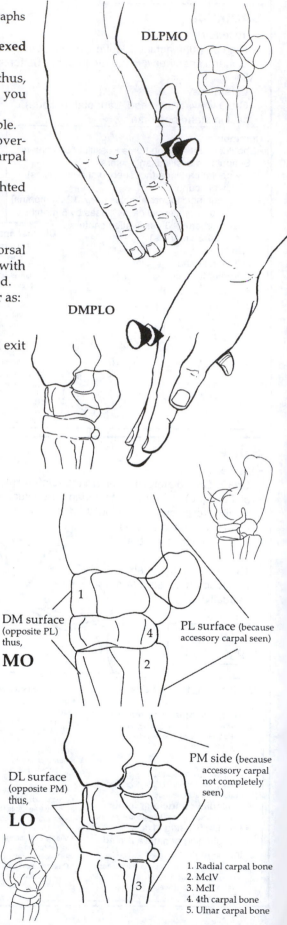

DLPMO

DMPLO

DM surface
(opposite PL)
thus,

MO

1

4

2

PL surface (because
accessory carpal seen)

DL surface
(opposite PM)
thus,

LO

PM side (because
accessory carpal
not completely
seen)

3

1. Radial carpal bone
2. McIV
3. McII
4. 4th carpal bone
5. Ulnar carpal bone

PAPER & PEN - ID CARPAL VIEWS

Pen and paper method using the accessory carpal bone to learn and name the different carpal views.

- Draw a schematic of the carpus as two ellipses.
- The smaller ellipse represents the accessory carpal bone (located lateral and palmar).
- Label the sides of the joint using the accessory carpal bone and the degree they correspond to as follows:
  Dorsal surface: D-0°
  Palmar: P-180°
  Lateral: L-90°
  Medial: M-270°
- Beam: draw the direction of the beam through your schematic, depending on the view.
- ID the highlighted edges (edge of the carpal bones in the radiograph next to soft tissue).
- Box the edges of the drawings parallel to the beam direction.
- Read the sides of the carpus on either end of the box for the obliques and the side the box it is on for the DP and lateral views. These will be the sides highlighted for each view.

DP (AP) and L (LM) views: identification is easy with a little practice.

- **DP (DorsoPalmar) view** (AP, anterior posterior): the accessory carpal is completely overlapped, small and dense.
- Highlights: medial and lateral surfaces.
- **Lateral (LateroMedial) view**: the accessory carpal bone is large, slightly overlapped and faint.
- Sides highlighted: dorsal and palmar.

Naming obliques:
- First note whether the film is not a DP or a Lateral view, thus, an oblique view.
- Look at the accessory carpal bone in the radiograph.
  . From its configuration and the amount of overlap, draw the direction of the beam through your schematic.
- **Box** the **highlighted sides** parallel to the beam.
- Then read your schematic for the different naming schemes.
- **DMPLO/ DLPMO system**: named for entrance and exit points. Read the labeled surface on either side of the entrance and exit points to name. You may put the degree the beam enters after the D (e.g., D70°LPMO, D300°MPLO)
- **DMPLO**: (accessory carpal bone not completely seen).
  . Dorsolateral and palmaromedial surfaces highlighted.
- **DLPMO**: (accessory carpal bone is seen)
  .Dorsomedial and palmarolateral surfaces highlighted.
- **LO, MO system** (dLO, dMO): named for the dorsal surface highlighted.
- LO: (accessory carpal is not completely seen).
  . Dorsolateral and palmaromedial surfaces highlighted.
- DMO: (accessory carpal seen).
  . Dorsomedial and palmarolateral surfaces highlighted.

Short cuts to translate last two system in your head:
  DMPLO/DLPMO: use last two letters = LO/MO
  LO/MO: put the missing letters in front starting with D = DMPLO/DLPMO

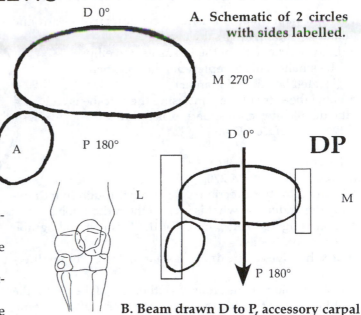

A. Schematic of 2 circles with sides labelled.

D 0°
L 90°
M 270°
A P 180°

DP

D 0°
L
M
P 180°

B. Beam drawn D to P, accessory carpal bone overlapped.

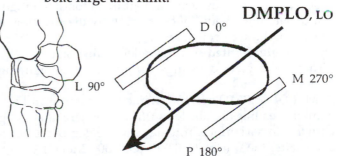

LM

D
L - 90°
M 270°
P

C. Beam drawn L to M, accessory carpal bone large and faint.

DMPLO, LO

D 0°
L 90°
M 270°
P 180°

D. Beam drawn DM to PL, accessory carpal bone not completely seen.

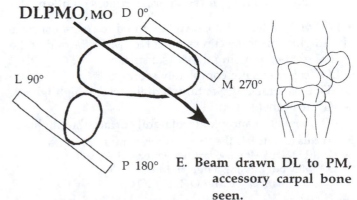

DLPMO, MO

D 0°
L 90°
M 270°
P 180°

E. Beam drawn DL to PM, accessory carpal bone seen.

*The P for palmar can be followed by a small a (Pa) to differentiate it from plantar (Pl) but hopefully you should be able to differentiate a tarsus from a carpus without this help.

645a

PAPER & PEN - ID TARSAL VIEWS

Pen and paper method using the calcaneus to learn and name the different tarsal views.

- Draw a schematic of the tarsus as two ellipses.
  - The smaller ellipse represents the calcaneus (located lateral and plantar)
- Label the sides of the joint using the calcaneus and the degree they correspond to as follows:

  Dorsal surface **D 0°**
  Plantar **P 180°**
  Lateral **L 90°**
  Medial **M 270°**

- Beam: draw the direction of the beam through your drawing, depending on what is seen in the radiograph.
- ID highlighted edges (edge of the tarsus in radiograph next to soft tissue).
  - Box the edges of the drawings parallel to the beam direction.
  - Read the sides of the tarsus on either end of the box for the obliques and the side the box is on for the DP and lateral views. These will be the sides highlighted for each view.

DP (AP) and L (LM) views: identification is easy with a little practice.

- **DP (DorsoPlantar) view** (AP, anterior-posterior): the calcaneus is completely overlapped.
  - Highlights: the medial and lateral surfaces.
- **Lateral (LateroMedial) view**: the calcaneus is large and the sustentaculum tali has a distinct appearance.
  - Sides highlighted: the dorsal and plantar.

Oblique views: naming by first noting the view is not a DP or Lateral, thus, it is an oblique view.

- Look at the calcaneus in the radiograph. From its configuration and the amount of overlap, draw the direction of the beam through your drawing.
- **Box the highlighted sides** parallel to the beam.
- Then read your drawings for the different naming schemes.
- **DMPLO/ DLPMO system***: name the entrance and exit points by reading the labelled surface on either side starting with the dorsal surface. You may put the degree the beam enters after the D (e.g., D70°LPMO, D300°MPLO)
  - **DMPLO**: (calcaneus partially overlapped).
    Dorsolateral and plantaromedial surfaces highlighted.
  - **DLPMO**: (calcaneus is seen).
    Dorsomedial and plantarolateral surfaces highlighted.

- **LO, MO system** (dLO, dMO): named for dorsal surface highlighted in some clinics, read L or M on the end of the highlight box crossing the dorsal surface.
  - LO: (calcaneus not completely seen).
    Dorsolateral and plantaromedial surfaces highlighted.
  - MO: (calcaneus seen).
    Dorsomedial and plantarolateral surfaces highlighted.

Short cuts to translate the above two systems in your head:
  DMPLO/DLPMO: use last two letters = LO/MO
  LO/MO: put missing letters in front starting
    with D = DMPLO/DLPMO

*The P for plantar can be followed by a small "l" (Pl) to differentiate it from palmar (Pa) but hopefully you should be able to differentiate a tarsus from a carpus without this help.

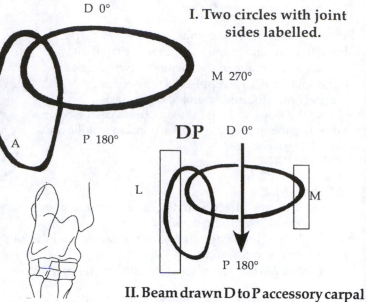

I. Two circles with joint sides labelled.

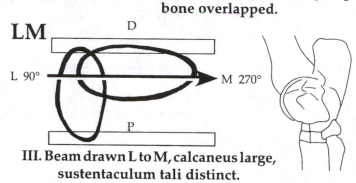

II. Beam drawn D to P accessory carpal bone overlapped.

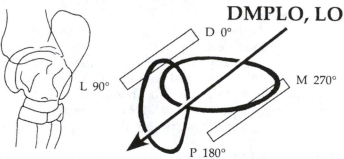

III. Beam drawn L to M, calcaneus large, sustentaculum tali distinct.

DMPLO, LO

IV. Beam drawn DM to PL, calcaneus not completely seen.

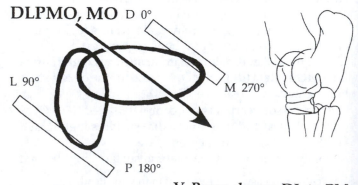

V. Beam drawn DL to PM, calcaneus seen.

DIAGNOSTIC ULTRASOUND (US) - HORSE

- Ultrasound: frequency of sound waves beyond range of human hearing
- Ultrasonic imaging of internal structures
  - Safe, noninvasive method
  - Standard diagnostic tool
- Follows History, Gait observation, Palpation of limb, Serial nerve blocks m/b

- **Procedure:**
  - Adequate skin contact (soak limb with water for a few minutes, then liberal amounts of aqueous gel (Aquasonic®) on skin. Clipping hair usually indicated, shaving improves, but not always necessary
  - Angle of beam important
    - . Transverse plane
    - . Sagittal plane

- **How ultrasound works**
  - Mechanical or lectronic sector scanner w/ a mutifrequency scan head
  - Produces a high frequency sound wave directed toward target tissue
  - Difference in acoustic impedance caused portions of sound beam to be reflected (echo)
  - Returning echoes interpreted by transducer onto the videoscreen (sonogram or scan)
  - High frequency transducers necessary (at least 7.5 MHz)
  - Serial photographs or videotapes of the monitor may be made

Anatomy: pgs. 116, 166, 167, 192

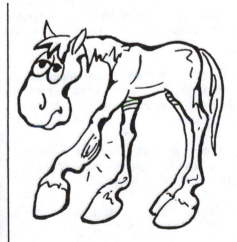

Normal tissues appearance on the sonogram
- **Echogenic** (echo-producing) appearance
  - Indicates relative echodensity
  - **Hyperechoic** (echo producing) - appear white i.e., bone, metal
  - **Anechoic** (without echoes) appear dark (i.e., blood, extracellular fluid)
  - **Hypoechoic** - appear as shade of gray, i.e., tendons & ligaments
- Size & shape
  - Increase with damage (edema)
  - Even small nonpalpable lesions m/b seen w/ US

Grading injuries rated on scale from 1-4
- **Grade 1** - slightly hypoechoic, darker than normal, minimum disruption of fiber pattern, infiltration & inflammatory fluid
- **Type 2 lesions**
  - . Half echogenic & half anechoic
  - . Disruption of fiber pattern & local inflammation
- **Type 3 lesions** - mostly anechoic
  - . Significant fiber tearing
- **Type 4 lesion** - totally anechoic
  - . Homogenous black areas - almost total tearing of structure w/ hematoma formation

Complete fibrosis - m/ appear hyperechoic

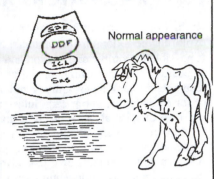

Normal appearance

Sagittal section: characteristic axial alignment of fibers (include in all studies)

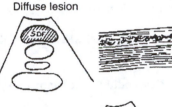

Diffuse lesion

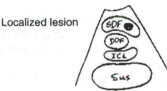

Localized lesion

SDF. Supf. digital flexor tendon
DDF. Deep digital flexor tendon
ICF. Check lig. of DDF
SUS. Suspensory lig.

Zones
- **Metacarpus** for specific location of scans
  - 1A, 1B, 2A. 2B, 3A, 3B all roughly 2" (4 cm)
- Metatarsus divided into 4 zones because of greater length (4A & 4B

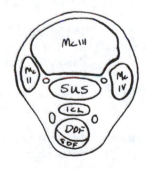

SDF.   Superficial digital flexor tendon
DDF.   Deep digital flexor tendon
SUS.   Suspensory ligament
SUS-Br. Branch of suspensory lig.
ICL.   Inferior check lig. (DDF)
Mc3.   Metacarpal 3
Mc2.   Metacarpal 2
Mc4.   Metacarpal 4
V.   Vessel
I.   Integument

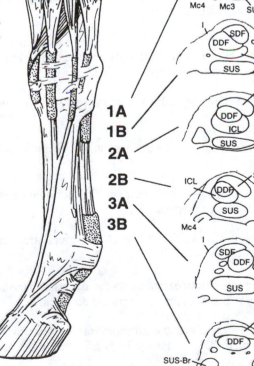

1A
1B
2A
2B
3A
3B

Clinical uses in lameness
- **Tendon injuries** - most common in SDF, also in suspensory lig. & deep digital flexor tendon
  - Precisely quantify size, location & severity of tendon & ligament damage
  - Monitoring healing to tell when training can start again
  - Photographic record of damage & healing process (photograph causes client to accept presence of lesion & follow treatment)
  - Differential diagnosis of bowed tendons below:
- **Edema**
- **Abscessation**
- **Cellulitis**
- **Distention of carpal sheath**

OX - EXPLORATORY RIGHT PARALUMBAR LAPAROTOMY

Right flank (paralumbar) laparotomy: a good approach for exploring the abdomen of ruminants. Standing flank laparotomy is possible for simple exploration and many surgical procedures (repositioning, untwisting, or deflating a structure). A lateral recumbency flank laparotomy is indicated if the animal may fall or for extended surgeries (e.g. intestinal resection). Calves, because of their small size, are best done in lateral recumbency. Exploratory surgery should be systematic. Try to develop a mental picture of how the viscera are positioned in the abdomen. A right paralumbar incision is placed in different positions within the paralumbar fossa depending on what structure you want to reach: small intestines, in the center of the paralumbar fossa; the cecum and proximal colon – in the cranial part of the fossa caudal and parallel to the last rib. The following is a systematic palpation of the abdomen:

STRUCTURES SEEN through a RIGHT PARALUMBAR INCISION:

1. Descending duodenum: crosses the dorsal end of the incision.

2, 3. "Omental curtain": the superficial and deep leaves of the greater omentum attached to the duodenum and extending ventrally along the abdominal wall to reach the rumen.

4. Mesoduodenum: attaches the duodenum to the dorsal abdominal wall.

The bulk of the viscera is behind the curtain formed by the greater omentum, duodenum, and mesoduodenum.

STRUCTURES PALPATED BETWEEN the OMENTAL CURTAIN and the RIGHT ABDOMINAL WALL: Run your hand cranially between the wall and the greater omentum. Identify the following structures:

5. Liver: located on the right side due to the rumen. Its edges should be sharp. Feel for abscesses, enlargement or irregularities. The right lobe is dorsal and the left lobe is ventral.

6. Gall bladder: hangs down from the center of the caudoventral edge of the liver.

Diaphragm: palpate it lateral to the liver and cranial to the reticulum.

Reticulum: against the diaphragm. Feel for adhesions, internal foreign bodies or magnet.

7. Omasum: felt as a firm (but not hard), round structure through the lesser omentum.

8. Lesser omentum: extends between the lesser curvature of the abomasum and the liver. It covers the omasum.

9. Abomasum: felt ventral to the omasum as it lies on the floor of the abdomen. The fundus and body are filled with fluid digesta.

10. Pylorus: can be found by following the descending duodenum cranially. It normally contains dry firm digesta. Exteriorize the pylorus for examination if the abomasum is not too full.

Cranial duodenum: feel the direct continuation of the pylorus as an S-shaped loop next to the liver.

1. Descending duodenum: travels down the right side of body attached to the mesoduodenum and the greater omentum.

11. Right kidney: located dorsal to the descending duodenum, between the mesoduodenum and the abdominal wall.

Right ureters: extend caudally from the kidney, retroperitoneally.

STRUCTURES BEHIND the OMENTAL CURTAIN (in the supraomental recess): Grasp the caudal edge of the omental curtain and move it cranially like a shower curtain. This exposes the supraomental recess and the viscera within it.

12. Left kidney: located high in the supraomental recess on the left side of the root of the mesentery and to the right of the rumen. Palpate its ureter.

13. Cecum: the blind-ended viscus located in the supraomental recess. It may extend out the caudal end of the recess. To identify the other intestinal structures, first find the easily identified cecum.

14. Ileum: located by following the cecum cranially to where the smaller ilium enters the junction between the cecum and the ascending colon.

15. "Flange": the section of the intestine with the longest mesentery. It consists of the distal part of the jejunum and the proximal part of the ileum. It is found by exteriorizing the intestine and following the ileum proximally.

16. Jejunum: located running proximally (orad) from the end of the "flange". Replace the flange and palpate the jejunum to the duodenojejunal flexure.

17. Great mesentery: suspends the ilium and jejunum from the dorsal abdominal wall.

18. Root of the mesentery: follow the great mesentery to the dorsal abdomen.

Return to the cecum and follow it cranially to the ileocecocolic junction:

19. Ileocecocolic junction: where the ileum joins the cecum and proximal loop of the ascending colon. Move the omental curtain as far cranially as possible to see this junction.

20. Proximal loop of ascending colon: located as the continuation of the cecum cranial to the ileocecocolic junction. Exteriorize

OX - EXPLORATORY RIGHT PARALUMBAR LAPAROTOMY

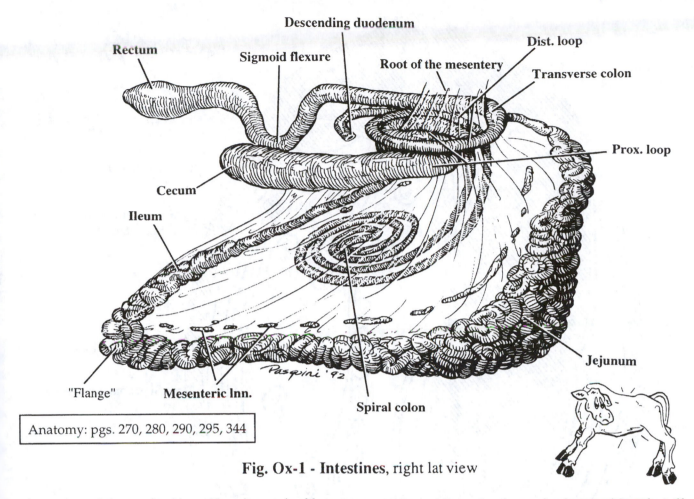

Descending duodenum
Rectum
Sigmoid flexure
Root of the mesentery
Dist. loop
Transverse colon
Prox. loop
Cecum
Ileum
Jejunum
"Flange"
Mesenteric lnn.
Spiral colon

Anatomy: pgs. 270, 280, 290, 295, 344

Fig. Ox-1 - Intestines, right lat view

the cecum and the proximal loop. Note the proximal loop turns caudally on itself on the right side of the mesentery. Follow it until it again turns, this time cranially, on the other side (left) of the root of the mesentery.

21. "Conjoined mesenteries": the short, fused mesenteries of the third part of the proximal loop, transverse colon, ascending duodenum, distal loop and first part of the descending colon. This makes a mass of the structures in the dorsal abdomen. It is impossible to distinguish each of these by palpation.

22. Spiral loop: reflect the "flange" of the intestine cranially to locate the disc-like spiral loop attached to its mesentery's left side. Note the inward spiraling centripetal coils, the outward spiraling centrifugal coils and the central flexure between the two. In the sheep and goat, follow the last centrifugal coil as it swings wide to pass just inside the jejunum. In the ox, the last coil does not stray.

23. Distal loop: can't be readily found because of the "conjoined mesenteries". It has a descending part on the left of the mesentery and an ascending part on the right side.

24. Transverse colon: can't be located because of the "conjoined mesenteries". It is situated cranial to the root of the mesentery.

25. Descending colon: its proximal part can't be palpated because of the "conjoined mesenteries". Its distal part runs in the dorsal abdomen on the left side of the mesentery and to the right of the rumen and can be palpated.

STRUCTURES LOCATED in the CAUDAL ABDOMEN:

Uterus and **ovaries:** note that the ovaries are located near the pelvic inlet. In the pregnant state the uterus will usually expand into the supraomental recess and make exploration difficult.

Urinary bladder: located over the brim of the pelvis below the uterus.

STRUCTURES LOCATED in the LEFT SIDE of the ABDOMEN

26. Rumen: fills the left half of the abdomen. Palpate it. Pass your hand caudally and dorsally around the caudal end of the rumen to palpate the left side of the rumen.

Spleen: palpated cranially on the left side of the rumen.

Left displaced abomasum: would be located between the rumen and the left body wall.

OX - EXPLORATORY RIGHT PARALUMBAR LAPAROTOMY

26

12

25

23'

1

1. Descending duodenum

Space between omental curtain & rt. abdominal wall

23"

20'''

20"

20'

17. Great mesentery

Supraomental recess

2, 3. Omental curtain

Fig. Ox-2 - Cross section of abdomen, caud. view

2. Supf. leaf of greater omentum

3. Deep leaf of greater omentum

Structures seen through a rt. paralumbar incision:
- 1. Descending duodenum
- 1". Ascending duodenum
- 2, 3. "Omental curtain"
  2. Superficial leaf of the greater omentum
  3. Deep leaf of the greater omentum
- 4. Mesoduodenum

Structures between omental curtain & rt. abdominal wall:
- 5. Liver
- 6. Gall bladder

- Diaphragm
- Reticulum
- 7. Omasum (under lesser omentum)
- 8. Lesser omentum
- 9. Abomasum
- 10. Pylorus
- Cranial duodenum
- 1. Descending duodenum
- 11. Right kidney
- Right ureters

Structures in supraomental recess:
- 12. Left kidney
- 13. Cecum
- 14. Ileum (Fig. Ox-1)

- 15. "Flange" (Fig. Ox-1)
- 16. Jejunum
- 17. Great mesentery
- 18. Root of the mesentery
- 19. Ileocecocolic junction (Fig. Ox-1)
- 20. Prox. loop of ascending colon
  20'. First part
  20". Second part
  20'''. Third part
- 21. "Conjoined mesenteries"
- 22. Spiral loop
- 23. Distal loop
  23' Descending part
  23". Ascending part

- 24. Transverse colon (Fig. Ox-1)
- 25. Descending colon
  25'. Sigmoid loop (Fig. Ox-1)

Structures in caud. abdomen:
- Uterus and ovaries
- Urinary bladder

Structures located in lt. side of abdomen:
- 26. Rumen
- Spleen
- Left displaced abomasum

OX - EXPLORATORY RIGHT PARALUMBAR LAPAROTOMY

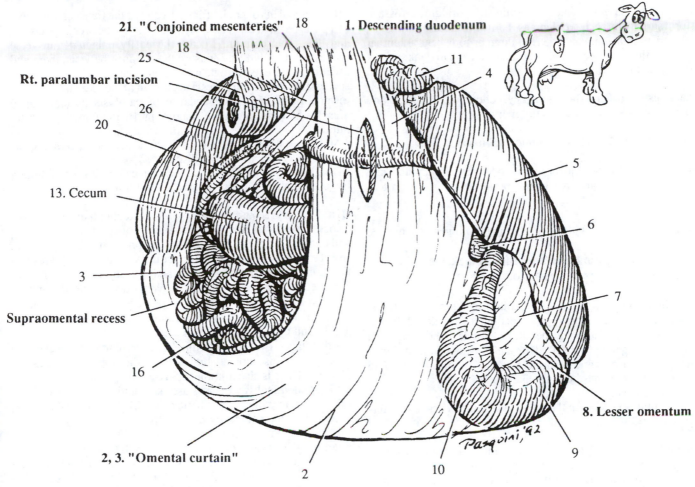

21. "Conjoined mesenteries" 18   **1. Descending duodenum**

18

25

Rt. paralumbar incision

26

20

13. Cecum

3

Supraomental recess

16

11

4

5

6

7

8. Lesser omentum

2, 3. "Omental curtain"

2

10

9

Pasquini, '92

Fig. Ox-3 - Abdomenal contents, right caudolateral
view   Drawn for Dr. Geraint Wyn-Jones

STRUCTURES - EXTERIORIZED - PALPABLE or IM-PALPABLE:

Exteriorization of structures is limited by the length of their mesenteries and their attachments. Many of those that can't be exteriorized can still be palpated.

Rumen, reticulum, omasum, and fundus and body of the abomasum: can't be exteriorized because of their attachment to each other and their position. They can be palpated.

PYLORUS: usually can be exteriorized if the abomasum is not to full of digesta.

S-loop of cranial duodenum, liver, gall bladder, and pancreas: can't be exteriorized, but can be palpated.

DESCENDING DUODENUM: easily exteriorized with attached mesoduodenum and greater omentum.

Ascending duodenum: can't be exteriorized or palpated because of its close association with the descending colon and the "conjoined mesenteries" in the dorsal abdomen.

JEJUNUM, ILEUM and **"FLANGE":** can be easily exteriorized, except the proximal 3-4 m of the jejunum.

CECUM: easily exteriorized.

Proximal loop of the ascending colon: easily exteriorized.

Distal loop: can't be exteriorized or palpated because of the "conjoined mesentery" of the structures in the dorsal abdomen.

Transverse colon and proximal part of the descending colon: can't be palpated or exteriorized because of the "conjoined mesenteries" in the dorsal abdomen.

SIGMOID LOOP of the DESCENDING COLON: Just caudal to the duodenocolic ligament, it has a long mesentery and may be pulled to the incision site.

Remaining caudal part of the descending colon and intraperitoneal part of the rectum: can be palpated, but not exteriorized.

Adapted from *Bovine Intestinal Surgery*, D. F. Smith, DVM, Food Animal, Nov. 1984

FLANK ANESTHESIA

Standing flank surgery in the ox: opening the paralumbar fossa to perform surgery on such problems as "hardware disease", dystocia, displaced abomasum, etc. The first three or four ventral lumbar nerves and the last thoracic nerve are anesthetized in flank surgery of the ox and horse.

Local anesthesia for a flank surgery: concerned with T_{13}, L_1 and L_2 nerves and can be done in a number of ways.

• **Line block:** infiltration of the intended incision line.

• **Inverted "L" block:** injections are done in the abdominal wall, from the subcutaneous area to the peritoneum, in the pattern shown.

• **Paravertebral block:** blocks all branches of the spinal nerves.

• **Distal paralumbar analgesia** or **Magda block:** blocks only the ventral and lateral dorsal branches of the spinal nerves.

Line block: infiltration of the intended incision line. This is probably the most commonly used technique. Multiple subcutaneous injections (1" 20-gauge needle) are made in the skin. Then a needle (3" 18 gauge) is inserted through the desensitized skin to infiltrate the muscles and peritoneum (10 - 100 ml). Allow 10 to 15 minutes for the anesthetic to take effect.
• Advantages: easy.
• Disadvantages: edema in the incision site and possible interference with healing.

Inverted "L" or "7" block: the line infiltration of anesthetic cranial and dorsal to the intended incision site, taking advantage of the caudoventral course of the nerves of the region. Two lines are laid down, one caudal to the last rib and one ventral to the transverse processes of the lumbar vertebrae. Up to 100 ml of anesthetic is injected. Allow 10 to 15 minutes for analgesic to take effect.
• Advantages: easy and is away from incision site.
• Disadvantages: amount of anesthetic required.

Proximal paravertebral analgesia, Farquharson technique: desensitizing the dorsal and ventral nerve branches T_{13}, L_1 and L_2 spinal nerves as they emerge from the intervertebral foramina. The injection sites are from 1 to 2 inches lateral to the dorsal midline over the cranial edge of transverse process of L_1 and the caudal edge of the transverse processes of L_1 and L_2. Prep and desensitize the skin over these areas with 3 ml of anesthetic subcutaneously. Push a 1/2 inch 14-gauge needle through the skin as a cannula. Pass a 2 to 6", 18-gauge spinal needle through the 14 gauge needle. To desensitize T_{13}, pass the needle ventrally to contact the transverse process of L_1. Walk the needle off the cranial edge of the transverse process and through the intertransverse fascia 1/2 inch (1 cm) below the transverse process. Inject 5 to 10 ml of anesthetic to desensitize the ventral branch of T_{13}. Withdraw the needle 1/2 to 1 inch above the transverse process and inject 5 ml of anesthetic to block the dorsal branch of T_{13}. Desensitization of L_1 and L_2 are done at similar levels with the same amounts of anesthetic as for T_{13}. The only difference is the transverse process and direction you walk off it. Walk the needle off the caudal border of the transverse process of L_1, for L_1;

off the caudal border of L_2 for L_2. Locating the transverse process of T_{13} can be difficult because it is in the angle between the last rib and the spinal column. Locate the easily palpated transverse processes of L_2 and L_3. Measure the distance between them and use this distance to estimate how far in front of L_2, T_{13} is. Signs of successful block are analgesia to the skin of the area and scoliosis toward the blocked side because of paralysis of the epaxial muscles. Analgesia usually begins in 10 minutes and last 90 minutes.
• Advantages: small amount of anesthetic needed, good analgesia and no anesthetic near wound site.
• Disadvantages: difficulty of technique, possibility of hitting large abdominal vessels, paresis of hind limb.

Distal paravertebral analgesia, Magda technique: desensitizes (blocks) the dorsal and ventral branches of spinal nerves T_{13}, L_1 and L_2 at the distal end of the transverse processes (L_1, L_2 and L_4). Insert a needle (3" 18-gauge) under the ventral tip of the respective transverse processes (L_1, L_2 and L_4). Inject 10 to 20 ml of anesthetic in a fan-shaped pattern. Withdraw the needle and reinsert it dorsal to the transverse process in a slightly caudal direction. Inject 5 ml of anesthetic around the dorsal branches of T_{13}, L_1 and L_2.
• Advantages over the proximal paravertebral analgesia: no scoliosis because not all branches of the dorsal branches are blocked. There is also minimum pelvic limb paresis, no danger of hitting abdominal vessels and uses standard needle sizes.
• Disadvantages: more anesthetic needed, effectiveness can vary, especially if the nerves vary.

Segmental dorsolumbar epidural analgesia, Arthur block: desensitization of the nerve roots as they leave the spinal cord by injecting into the epidural space through the dorsal space, between first and second lumbar vertebrae. Thorough restraint is necessary. Locate the space between the spinous process of L_1 and L_2 by palpating the transverse processes of L_2. Inject 2 to 4 ml subcutaneous at this site. Insert a 1/2" 14 gauge needle through the skin as a canula. Insert a 4 1/2" 18-gauge needle through the canula. The needle is directed ventrally at an angle of 10 to 15° to the vertical for 3 to 4 inches. Direct the needle through the interarcuate ligament into the epidural space. Inject anesthetic into the epidural space. The amount of anesthetic depends on the size of the animal and the nerves that you want to block. To block T_{13}, L_1 and L_2 of a 1100 pound cow, 8 ml of anesthetic is injected. Resistance will be felt as the needle passes through the interspinous ligament and the interarcuate ligament. If the needle hits the arch of a vertebrae then withdraw it and redirect it. Once the interarcuate ligament is penetrated you are in the epidural space. Do not go any further and remove the needle immediately after injection. Aspiration of CSF indicates the needle has crossed the epidural space, through the dura mater and arachnoid and into the subarachnoid space.

• Advantages over proximal and distal paravertebral analgesia: only one injection, small amount of anesthetic, and uniform analgesia.
• Disadvantages: difficult technique, motor loss to hind limbs, possibility of damage to spinal cord and venous sinuses.

FLANK ANESTHESIA

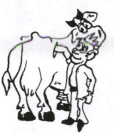

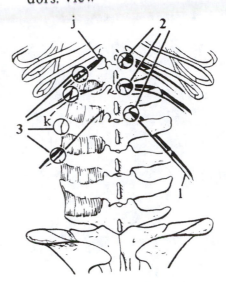

Ox - Lumbar vertebrae
dors. view

Ox - lat. view

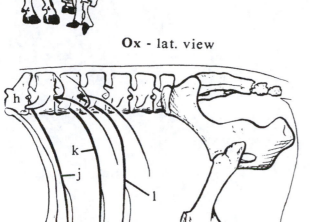

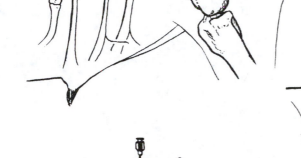

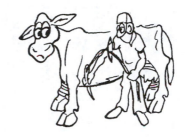

Fig. X-74 - Ox - Flank
- lat. view

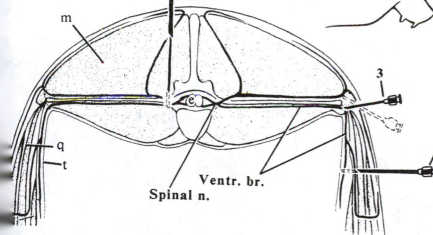

m

q

t

e

Ventr. br.

Spinal n.

Ox - 1st lumbar
vertebra - cross section

Anatomy: pg. 498

1. Inverted "L" block
2. Paravertebral block
3. Magda block

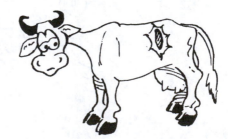

651

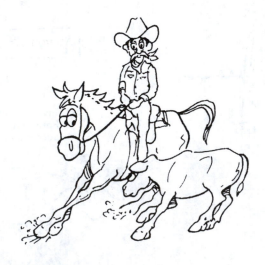

Index

Arteries

Bones

Bones

667

Muscles

673

Notes

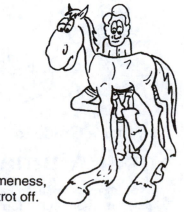

Flexion test to exacerbate lameness,
flex for time and immediately trot off.

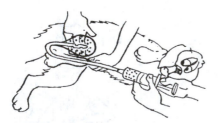
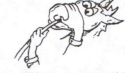
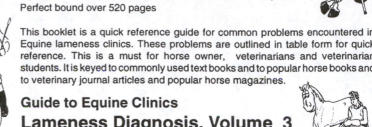
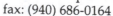

Student's Guide to Equine Clinics (1993) by Chris Pasquini and Susan Pasquini; published by Sudz Publishing Co., 1222 Hwy 377, P.O. Box 1199, Pilot Point, TX 76258; 388 pages; delightfully illustrated; $24.95.

The first thing you notice about this book is that it is really different. It breaks with tradition, opening up new, and interesting, ways to communicate a complicated subject. Everyone will enjoy this book because it is fun. The practitioner may find a point or two on which to disagree, but will certainly enjoy browsing, even absorbing, many parts of it.

The book is designed to be a quick reference guide to conditions found in horses. It is constructed in easy to read charts dealing with facts, causes, clinical signs, diagnosis and treatment of the most common conditions found in equine clinics— yes, every page in the book is a chart like the one below. It is packed with useful information for the student, but helpful to anyone interested in veterinary care of the horse. It provides an easy to use differential diagnosis list for most conditions. One chapter is dedicated to differential diagnosis lists. Key words are used to jog the student's memory. Its many levels allow different approaches to assimilating the information, either by skimming to get a handle on each condition, or delving deeper. Keyed to other veterinary texts for easy reference, it is an excellent starting point for studying for the national board exam.

The way in which this guide has been organized shows the teaching abilities of Chris Pasquini. He has received six teaching awards from his students. His other books include *The Atlas of Equine Anatomy, The Atlas of Bovine Anatomy, Anatomy of Domestic Species, Guide to Bovine Clinics*. Two of the books he worked on received the "Award of Excellence" by the Association of American Medical Illustrators, including *The Anatomy of Domestic Species*. They are all teaching texts clarifying learning anatomy. *The Student's Guide to Equine Clinics* creates a framework of reference on which students can build throughout their education.

This handbook has a unique sense of humor. It contains many cartoon-like illustrations which emphasize important points. It has an ingenious means of reference. Twenty major veterinary reference texts are listed in the front, each with a reference code which is used throughout the manual, with a page reference for that text. In this manner the Guide becomes an extensive index to these 20 classic texts. **WEJ**

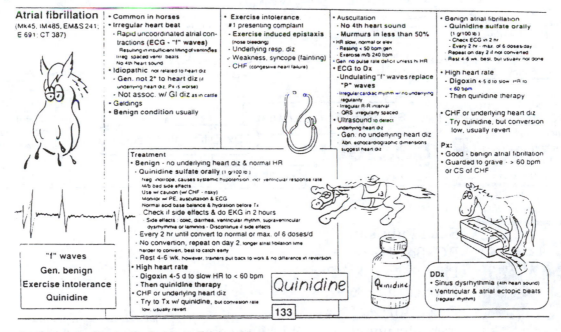

Above: a sample page from Student's Guide to Equine Clinics

Tshauner's Guide to

Small Animal Clinics

By Chris Pasquini & Susan Pasquini

799 pages in a soft bound format (8.5" X 5.5")
This booklet is a quick reference guide for the veterinary student and clinician alike, allowing easy accessibility to the diagnosis and treatment of specific conditions while giving references for later more in-depth investigation. We feel it will be of great value to any person interested in small animal medicine. Common problems encountered in small animal clinics are outlined in table form, as shown below. This is a must for veterinary students in small animal medicine and during small animal clinics.

Condition

References: See page ii

Facts/Cause: important information (cause, pathophysiology, Hx (history), transmission, etc.)

Presentation/CS: clinical signs that can be visualized from a distance, or that an owner might report

Diagnosis: CS, palpation, auscultation, lab tests, radiographs, postmortem, etc.

Treatment

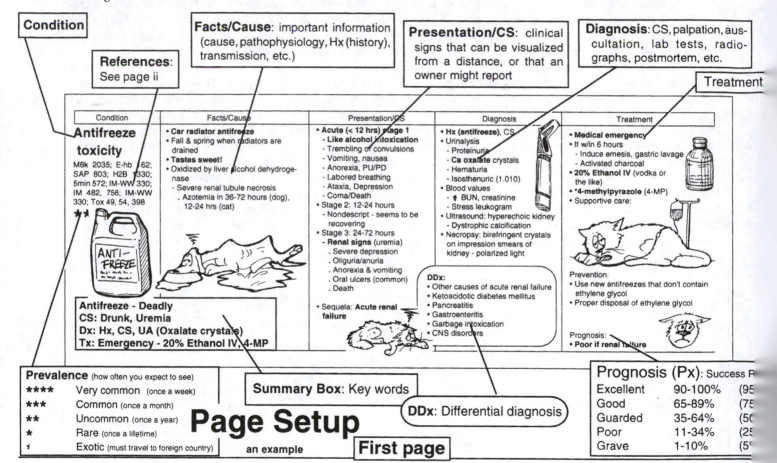

Condition	Facts/Cause	Presentation/CS	Diagnosis	Treatment
Antifreeze toxicity M8k 2035; E-hb 162; SAP 803; H2B 330; 5min 572; IM-WW 330; IM 482, 756; IM-WW 330; Tox 49, 54, 398 ✱ᴶ	• Car radiator antifreeze • Fall & spring when radiators are drained • **Tastes sweet!** • Oxidized by liver alcohol dehydrogenase - Severe renal tubule necrosis . Azotemia in 36-72 hours (dog), 12-24 hrs (cat)	• **Acute (< 12 hrs) stage 1** - **Like alcohol intoxication** - Trembling of convulsions - Vomiting, nausea - Anorexia, PU/PD - Labored breathing - Ataxia, Depression - Coma/Death • Stage 2: 12-24 hours - Nondescript - seems to be recovering • Stage 3: 24-72 hours - **Renal signs** (uremia) . Severe depression . Oliguria/anuria . Anorexia & vomiting . Oral ulcers (common) . Death • Sequela: **Acute renal failure**	• **Hx (antifreeze)**, CS • Urinalysis - Proteinuria - **Ca oxalate** crystals - Hematuria - Isosthenuric (1.010) • Blood values - ⬆ BUN, creatinine - Stress leukogram • Ultrasound: hyperechoic kidney - Dystrophic calcification • Necropsy: birefringent crystals on impression smears of kidney - polarized light **DDx:** • Other causes of acute renal failure • Ketoacidotic diabetes mellitus • Pancreatitis • Gastroenteritis • Garbage intoxication • CNS disorders	• **Medical emergency** • If w/in 6 hours - Induce emesis, gastric lavage - Activated charcoal • **20% Ethanol IV** (vodka or the like) • **4-methylpyrazole** (4-MP) • Supportive care: Prevention: • Use new antifreezes that don't contain ethylene glycol • Proper disposal of ethylene glycol Prognosis: • **Poor if renal failure**

Antifreeze - Deadly
CS: Drunk, Uremia
Dx: Hx, CS, UA (Oxalate crystals)
Tx: Emergency - 20% Ethanol IV, 4-MP

Prevalence (how often you expect to see)
✱✱✱✱	Very common	(once a week)
✱✱✱	Common	(once a month)
✱✱	Uncommon	(once a year)
✱	Rare	(once a lifetime)
ᴶ	Exotic	(must travel to foreign country)

Summary Box: Key words

Page Setup

First page

an example

DDx: Differential diagnosis

Prognosis (Px): Success R
Excellent	90-100%	(95
Good	65-89%	(75
Guarded	35-64%	(50
Poor	11-34%	(25
Grave	1-10%	(5⁹

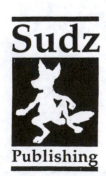

Sudz Publishing
P.O. Box 1199
Pilot Point, TX 76258
Phone(940) 686-9208
Fax: (940) 686-0164
web site: www.sudzpublishing.com
e-mail: sudzpub@mac.com
       sudzpub@hotmail.com

Call, fax or e-mail for information & orders